Let's Code It!

2026–2027 CODE EDITION

2026 Release

Shelley C. Safian, PhD, RHIA
MAOM/HSM/HI, CCS-P, COC, CPC-I, HCISPP, AHIMA-Approved ICD-10-CM/PCS Trainer

Mary A. Johnson, MBA-HM-HI, CPC
Central Carolina Technical College

Mc Graw Hill

LET'S CODE IT!, 2026 RELEASE

Published by McGraw Hill LLC, 1325 Avenue of the Americas, New York, NY 10019.

This book is printed on acid-free paper.

1 2 3 4 5 LBC 29 28 27 26 25

ISBN 978-1-266-72852-5 (bound)
MHID 1-266-72852-X (bound)
ISBN 978-1-26549018-8 (loose-leaf)
MHID 1-265-49018-X (loose-leaf)

Portfolio Manager: *Marah Bellegarde*
Product Developer: *Theresa Collins*
Content Project Manager: *Sherry Kane*
Manufacturing Project Manager: *Sandy Ludovissy*
Content Licensing Specialist: *Prineeth Priyan*
Cover Image: *Shutterstock/Juliy Koval*
Compositor: *Straive*

All credits appearing on page or at the end of the book are considered to be an extension of the copyright page.

Library of Congress Cataloging-in-Publication Data

Cataloging-in-Publication Data has been requested from the Library of Congress

mheducation.com/highered

ABOUT THE AUTHORS

Shelley C. Safian

Shelley C. Safian has been teaching medical coding and health information management for 25 years, at both on-ground and online campuses. In addition to her regular teaching responsibilities at Central Carolina Technical College and Colorado State University-Global, she regularly presents webinars/seminars and writes about coding for the *Just Coding* newsletters (in-patient and outpatient). Safian is the course author for multiple distance education courses on various coding topics, including ICD-10-CM, ICD-10-PCS, CPT, and HCPCS Level II coding.

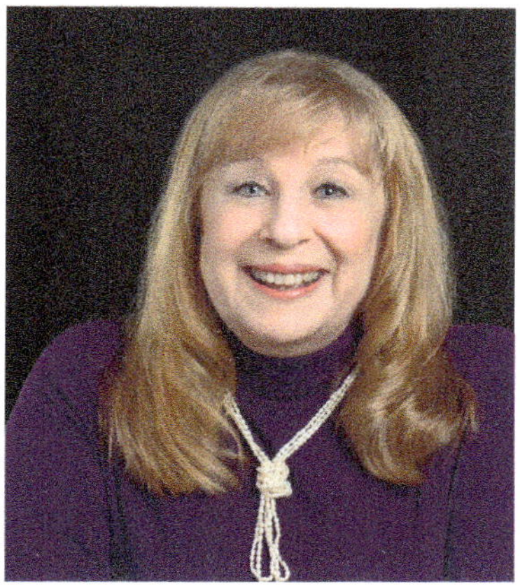

Shelley C. Safian

Safian is a Registered Health Information Administrator (RHIA) and a Certified Coding Specialist-Physician-based (CCS-P) from the American Health Information Management Association and a Certified Outpatient Coder (COC) and a Certified Professional Coding Instructor (CPC-I) from the American Academy of Professional Coders. She is also a Health Care Information Security and Privacy Practitioner (HCISPP) and a Certified HIPAA Administrator (CHA) and has earned the designation of AHIMA-Approved ICD-10-CM/PCS Trainer.

Safian completed her Graduate Certificate in Health Care Management at Keller Graduate School of Management. The University of Phoenix awarded her the Master of Arts/Organizational Management degree and a Graduate Certificate in Health Informatics. She earned her Ph.D. in Health Care Administration with a focus in Health Information Management.

Mary A. Johnson

Mary Johnson is the Health Information Management Director at Central Carolina Technical College in Sumter, South Carolina. She is also an adjunct faculty member for Southern New Hampshire University and Bryan University. Her background includes corporate training using both on-campus and online platforms. Johnson has over a decade of teaching experience in medical coding and Health Information Management and specializes in the design and implementation of customized coding curricula. Johnson received her Bachelor of Arts dual degree in Business Administration and Marketing from Columbia College and earned a Masters of Business Administration with a dual focus in Healthcare Management and Health Informatics from New England College. Johnson is a Certified Professional Coder (CPC) credentialed through the American Academy of Professional Coders (AAPC).

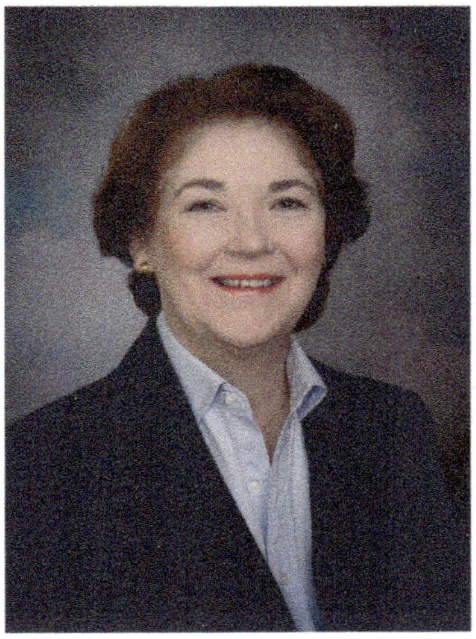

Jimmy Wood Photography

Dedications

–This book is dedicated to all of those who have come into my life sharing encouragement and opportunity to pursue work that I love; for the benefit of all of my students: past, present, and future.

–Shelley

–This book is dedicated to the loving memory of my parents, *Dr. and Mrs. Clarence J. Johnson Sr.,* for their love and support. Also, to those students with whom I have had the privilege to work and to those students who are beginning their journey into the world of medical coding.

–Mary

BRIEF CONTENTS

CONTENTS

GUIDED TOUR

Let's Code It! was developed with student success in mind: success in college, success taking the certification exam, and success in their future health care career.

Chapter Openers

Each chapter begins by clearly identifying the **Learning Outcomes** students need to master along with the **Key Terms** that they need to learn.

1

Introduction to the Languages of Coding

Key Terms

Classification Systems
Condition
Diagnosis
Eponym
External Cause
Inpatient
Medical Necessity
Nonessential Modifiers
Outpatient
Procedure
Reimbursement
Services
Treatments

Learning Outcomes

After completing this chapter, the student should be able to:

LO 1.1 Explain the four purposes of medical coding.
LO 1.2 Identify the structure of the ICD-10-CM diagnosis coding manual.
LO 1.3 Differentiate between the types of procedures and the various procedure coding manuals.
LO 1.4 Examine the HCPCS Level II coding manual used to report the provision of equipment and supplies.

CODING BITES

We use the concept of "*languages*" to help you relate medical coding—and its code sets—to an idea you already understand. In the health care

1.1 The Purpose of Coding

Around the world, languages exist to enable clear and accurate communication between individuals in similar groups or working together in similar functions. The purpose of using health care coding languages is to enable the sharing of information, in a specific and efficient way, between all those involved in health care.

Coding languages are constructed of individual codes that are more precise than words. (You will discover this as you venture through this textbook.) By communicating using codes rather than words, you can successfully convey to others involved (1) exactly what happened during a provider-patient encounter and (2) why it occurred. You, as the professional coding specialist, have the responsibility to accurately interpret health care terms and definitions

Coding Bites

These appear throughout the text to highlight key concepts and tips to further support understanding and learning.

CODING BITES

This is just an overview to help you orient yourself to the structure of the code book. You will learn, in depth, how to use the ICD-10-CM code set to report any and all of the reasons *why* a patient needs the care of a health care professional in ***Part II: Reporting Diagnoses***.

Examples, Let's Code It! Scenarios, and You Code It! Case Studies

EXAMPLES

B95.2 Enterococcus as the cause of diseases classified elsewhere
B96.3 *Haemophilus influenzae* [H. influenzae] as the cause of diseases classified elsewhere
B97.11 Coxsackievirus as the cause of diseases classified elsewhere

These code descriptions identify the specific pathogen to be reported along with the code describing the condition caused.

LET'S CODE IT! SCENARIO

Francie Holland, a 23-year-old female, came to see Dr. Kensington due to severe abdominal pain. She had a fever and stated that she has had bloody diarrhea for the past 2 days. Dr. Kensington's examination revealed that she was dehydrated as well. Francie stated she ate at a new restaurant at the beach where she had a salad and a vegetable plate. After taking some tests, he diagnosed Francie with Shigella dysenteriae *(bacillary dysentery).*

Let's Code It!

Dr. Kensington found Francie to be suffering from *Shigella dysenteriae*. Turn to the Alphabetic Index and find

Shigella (dysentery) (see Dysentery, bacillary)

Dysentery, bacillary A03.9

Turn to the Tabular List, and check the code's complete description:

✓4 **A03 Shigellosis**

There are no notations or directives, so read down the column to review all of the choices for the required fourth character. The code suggested by the Alphabetic Index:

A03.9 Shigellosis, unspecified

Is this the most accurate code? You will note that the other fourth-character code choices want specifics on which group

YOU INTERPRET IT!

What is the mode of transmission for each condition?

1. Hepatitis B ________
2. Measles ________
3. Cholera ________
4. Insect bites ________
5. Influenza ________

Examples are included throughout each chapter to help students make the connection between theoretical and practical coding. **Let's Code It! Scenarios** walk students through abstracting and the coding process, step-by-step, to determine the correct code. And **You Code It! Case Studies** provide students with hands-on practice coding scenarios and case studies throughout each chapter. In addition, **You Interpret It!** questions present opportunities for students to use critical-thinking skills to identify details needed for accurate coding.

Guidance Connections

GUIDANCE CONNECTION

Read the ICD-10-CM Official Guidelines for Coding and Reporting, section **III. Reporting Additional Diagnoses.**

Each of these boxes connects the concepts students are learning in the chapter to the related, specific Official Guidelines in order to further students' knowledge and understanding of coding resources.

End-of-Chapter Reviews

Most chapters end with the following assessment types to reinforce the chapter learning outcomes: Let's Check It! Terminology; Let's Check It! Concepts; Let's Check It! Guidelines; Let's Check It! Rules and Regulations; and You Code It! Basics.

CHAPTER 40 REVIEW
Reimbursement

connect
Enhance your learning by completing these exercises and more at mcgrawhillconnect.com!

Let's Check It! Terminology

Match each term to the appropriate definition.

Part I

1. **LO 40.2** A physician, typically a family practitioner or an internist, who serves as the primary care physician for an individual. This physician is responsible for evaluating and determining the course of treatment or services, as well as for deciding whether or not a specialist should be involved in care.
2. **LO 40.1** A type of health insurance coverage that controls the care of each subscriber (or insured person) by using a primary care provider as a central health care supervisor.
3. **LO 40.2** A type of health insurance that uses a primary care physician, also known as a gatekeeper, to manage all health care services for an individual.
4. **LO 40.2** A policy that covers loss or injury to a third party caused by the insured or something belonging to the insured.
5. **LO 40.1** The total management of an individual's well-being by a health care professional.
6. **LO 40.3** An insurance company pays a provider one flat fee to cover the entire course of treatment for an individual's condition.
7. **LO 40.2** The agency under the Department of Health and Human Services (DHHS) in charge of regulation and control over services for those covered by Medicare and Medicaid.
8. **LO 40.3** Payment agreements that outline, in a written fee schedule, exactly how much money the insurance carrier will pay the physician for each treatment and/or service provided.
9. **LO 40.3** An extra reduction in the rate charged to an insurer for services provided by the physician to the plan's members.
10. **LO 40.1** The amount of money, often paid monthly, by a policyholder or insured, to an insurance company to obtain coverage.
11. **LO 40.2** Auto accident liability coverage will pay for medical bills, lost wages, and compensation for pain and suffering for any person injured by the insured in an auto accident.
12. **LO 40.3** Agreements between a physician and a managed care organization that pay the physician a predetermined amount of money each month for each member of the plan who identifies that provider as his or her primary care physician.
13. **LO 40.2** A plan that reimburses a covered individual a portion of his or her income that is lost as a result of being unable to work due to illness or injury.
14. **LO 40.2** Individuals who are supported, either financially or with regard to insurance coverage, by others.

A. Automobile Insurance
B. Capitation Plans
C. Centers for Medicare & Medicaid Services (CMS)
D. Dependents
E. Disability Compensation
F. Discounted FFS
G. Episodic Care
H. Fee-for-Service (FFS) Plans
I. Gatekeeper
J. Health Care
K. Health Maintenance Organization (HMO)
L. Insurance Premium
M. Liability Insurance
N. Managed Care

Real Abstracting Practice with You Code It! Practice, You Code It! Application, and Capstone Case Studies Chapters

Gain real-world experience by using actual patient records (with names and other identifying information changed) to practice ICD-10-CM, ICD-10-PCS, CPT, and HCPCS Level II coding for both inpatients and outpatients. *You Code It! Practice* exercises give students the chance to practice coding with short coding scenarios. *You Code It! Application* exercises give students the chance to review and abstract physicians' notes documenting real patient encounters in order to code those scenarios. Both of these types of exercises can be found at the end of most chapters. *Capstone Chapters* come at the end of Parts II–V and include 15 additional real-life outpatient and inpatient case studies to help students synthesize and apply what they have learned through hands-on coding practice with each code set.

YOU CODE IT! Practice

Using the techniques described in this chapter, carefully read through the case studies and determine the most accurate ICD-10-CM code(s) and external cause code(s), if appropriate, for each case.

1. Ben Kenton, a 49-year-old male, presents today with a high fever, chills, nausea, and diarrhea. After an examination and reviewing the results of the blood tests, Dr. Daniels diagnoses Ben with West Nile fever.
2. Robin Pullen, a 36-year-old female, comes to see Dr. Ditolla because she is running a fever and has a sore throat and overall body aches. Test results are positive for H1N1. Robin is diagnosed with swine influenza.
3. Joan Kenney, a 27-year-old female, is having difficulty breathing. Dr. Aung documents a fever of 101 F and facial edema. Joan recently returned home from a trip to Asia. Joan said they were contending with some sort of larval infestation in Asia. Joan is diagnosed with nasopharyngeal myiasis.
4. Babbs Fisher, a 48-year-old female, just returned from an African vacation. Babbs is brought in by her husband, George, who noticed she was acting confused. Dr. Carla notes a low fever. Babbs states she feels tired and has a sore throat. She started vomiting this morning and admits to abdominal pain. Dr. Carla examines Babbs and orders an enzyme-linked immunosorbent assay (ELISA) test, which confirms the diagnosis of Ebola virus. Babbs is admitted to Weston Hospital for treatment.
5. Steven Jordan, a 51-year-old male, comes to see Dr. Kolb because he is experiencing nausea and vomiting and his stool is unusually light in color. Steven is accompanied by his wife, Sally. Sally says her husband seems confused and less alert lately. Upon examination, Dr. Kolb notes hepatosplenomegaly, jaundice, and RUQ tenderness. Steven is admitted to the hospital, where blood test results confirm the presence of IgG anti-HAV antibodies. Steven is diagnosed with acute hepatitis A.
6. Johnny Brennen, a 7-year-old male, is brought in by his parents. Johnny has developed a hard cough and says his sides hurt. Dr. Travis, Johnny's pediatrician, completes blood work and takes a CXR and nasopharyngeal specimen. A subconjunctival hemorrhage is noted in the left eye. Test results confirm a diagnosis of whooping cough due to *Bordetella pertussis* with pneumonia. Johnny is admitted to Weston Hospital.
7. Frances Lowder is having difficulty breathing. She also admits to a bad headache, sore throat, and no appetite. She is 28-weeks pregnant and was diagnosed with HIV 3 years ago. Dr. Mabry notes a temperature of 102 F and papules over her upper body. Blood tests confirm the diagnosis of varicella with pneumonia. Frances is admitted to Weston Hospital.
8. Jenny Cassidy, a 4-year-old female, is brought in by her parents to see her pediatrician, Dr. Harmon. Jenny has a fever and a rash on her back. Dr. Harmon notes a "strawberry tongue." The completed CBC test confirms a diagnosis of scarlet fever.

YOU CODE IT! Application

The following exercises provide practice in the application of abstracting the physicians' notes and learning to work with documentation from our health care facility, Anytown Anesthesiology Associates. These case studies are modeled on real patient encounters. Using the techniques described in this chapter, carefully read through the case studies and determine the most accurate anesthesia code(s) and modifier(s), if appropriate, for each case study:

ANYTOWN ANESTHESIOLOGY ASSOCIATES

241 MAIN STREET • ANYTOWN, FL 32711 • 407-555-1234

PATIENT: PERSILE, LORRAINE

ACCOUNT/EHR #: PERSLO001

Preoperative DX: Locked right knee, rule out medial meniscus tear

Postoperative DX: 1. Grade 2 tear, anterior, cruciate ligament

2. Medial meniscus tear, anterior, horn

3. Grade 2 chondrosis, medial femoral condyle

Procedure: 1. Arthroscopy

2. Partial anterior cruciate ligament debridement

3. Partial medial meniscectomy

Attending Physician: Renee O. Bracker, MD

Anesthesia: General

Anesthesiologist: Lawrence Miller, MD

INDICATIONS: The patient is a 33-year-old female who was in her usual state of good health until about 10 days ago when she sustained a twisting injury to the right knee with inability to fully extend the knee, with pain and swelling.

PROCEDURE: Estimated blood loss: None. Complications: None. Tourniquet time: See anesthesia notes. Specimens: None. Drains: None. Disposition: To the recovery room in stable condition.

Pt was taken to surgery and placed on the OR table in the supine position. After adequate general anesthesia was administered, she received a gram of intravenous Kefzol preoperatively. A proximal thigh tourniquet was applied. Examination revealed no significant Lachman or drawer and a moderate effusion. No varus or valgus instability. Distal pulses intact. The right lower extremity was placed in the arthroscopic leg holder; shaved, prepped, and draped in the usual meticulously sterile fashion for lower extremity surgery. Esmarch exsanguinations of the limb were performed, and the tourniquet was inflated. Proximal medial, anteromedial, and anterolateral portals were fashioned. A systematic evaluation of the knee was performed. The undersurface of the patella demonstrated normal tracking with no chondrosis.

The suprapatellar pouch, medial, and lateral gutters were well within normal limits, and in the notch a grade 2 tear of the anterior cruciate ligament was identified. There were some bloody fragments of the ACL that seemed to be impinging in the medial compartment. This was meticulously debrided. Approximately 50% of the ACL appeared to be intact. Attention was turned to the lateral compartment. The articular surface of the meniscus was normal. On the medial side, a grade 2 lesion in medial femoral condyle, lateral side, was noted. This was not debrided. Also, an anterior tear of the medial meniscus, which was frayed and torn, was another potential source of impingement. This was meticulously debrided to a smooth, stable mechanical limb, and the wound was irrigated and closed with 4-0 nylon simple interrupted sutures. Xeroform, 4 × 4s, Webril and Ace bandage from the tips of the toes to the groin completed the sterile dressing. There were no intraoperative or immediate postoperative complications. The prognosis is good, although it may be limited by potential for arthritis and instability in the future.

Determine the most accurate anesthesia code(s) and modifier(s), if appropriate.

In addition, all of the exercises in the Chapter Review can be assigned through Connect. Of particular note are the ***You Code It! Practice*** exercises, which offer our unique **CodePath** option. In Connect, students are presented with a series of questions to guide them through the critical thinking process to determine the correct code.

PREFACE

Welcome to *Let's Code It!* This product has been created to instruct students on how to become proficient in medical coding—a health care field that continues to be in high demand. The Bureau of Labor Statistics notes the demand for health information management professionals (which includes coders) will continue to increase much faster than average through 2033 and beyond.

Let's Code It! offers a 360-degree learning experience for anyone interested in the field of medical coding, with strong guidance down the path to coding certification. Theory is presented in easy-to-understand language and accompanied by lots of examples. Hands-on practice is included with real-life physician documentation, from both outpatient and inpatient facilities, to promote critical thinking analysis and evaluation. This is in addition to determination of accurate codes to report diagnoses, procedures, and ancillary services. All of this is assembled to support the reader's development of a solid foundation upon which to build a successful career after graduation.

Let's Code It! is designed to give your students the medical coding experience they need in order to pass their first medical coding certification exams, such as the CCS/CCS-P or CPC/COC. This product offers students a variety of practice opportunities by reinforcing the learning outcomes set forth in every chapter. The chapter materials are organized in short bursts of text followed by practice—keeping students active and coding!

What's new for the 2026 Code Edition: Our updated content includes key advancements from the last year and new items for 2026. For example, additional information on working with documentation from multiple healthcare practitioners and more emphasis on establishing medical necessity have been added to this edition. A section on Auditing Claims has been added to the Reimbursement chapter. All codes within the text and the Instructor Manual answer keys have been updated complying with the 2026 code sets: ICD-10-CM, CPT, HCPCS Level II, and ICD-10-PCS.

Here's What You Can Expect from *Let's Code It!*

- Each of the six parts of this product includes an Introduction to provide students with an overview of the information within that part and how they can use this knowledge.
    - Part I: Medical Coding Fundamentals
    - Part II: Reporting Diagnoses
    - Part III: Reporting Physicians Services and Outpatient Procedures
    - Part IV: DMEPOS & Transportation
    - Part V: Inpatient (Hospital) Reporting
    - Part VI: Legal, Ethical, and Reimbursement Issues
- **Part I: Medical Coding Fundamentals** helps students build a strong theoretical foundation regarding the various code sets. The chapters teach students how and when each code set is used and how to abstract documentation. These chapters also teach them how to use a solid coding process, including the importance of queries, how to write a legal query, exposure to the Official Guidelines, and confirmation of medical necessity.
- **Part II: Reporting Diagnoses** provides students with an incremental walkthrough of the ICD-10-CM code set.
- **Part III: Reporting Physicians Services and Outpatient Procedures** provides students with a progressive learning experience for using CPT® procedure codes.
- **Part IV: DMEPOS & Transportation** gives students insight into, and hands-on practice using, the HCPCS Level II code set to report the provision of durable medical equipment, prosthetics, orthotics, and other medical supplies.
- **Part V: Inpatient (Hospital) Reporting** shows students how to build an accurate ICD-10-PCS code to report inpatient procedures, services, and treatments.
- The coding chapters in Parts II–V all include real-life scenarios, as well as physician documentation mainly in the form of procedure notes and operative reports (both inpatient and outpatient) for students to practice abstracting and coding.
    - *Let's Code It! Scenarios* provide step-by-step instruction so students can learn to use their critical-thinking skills throughout the coding process to determine the correct code.
    - *You Code It! Case Studies* provide students with hands-on practice coding scenarios and case studies throughout each chapter.

    - *You Interpret It!* questions present additional opportunities for students to use critical-thinking skills to identify details required for accurate coding.
    - *Chapter Reviews* include assessments of chapter concepts:
        - Let's Check It! Terminology
        - Let's Check It! Concepts
        - Let's Check It! Guidelines
        - Let's Check It! Rules and Regulations
        - You Code It! Basics
        - You Code It! Practice Case Studies
        - You Code It! Application Case Studies

- *Examples* are included throughout each chapter to help students make the connection between theoretical and practical coding.
- *Coding Bites* highlight key concepts and tips to further support understanding and learning.
- *Guidance Connection* features point to the specific Official Guideline applicable for the concept being discussed.
- *Capstone Chapters* come at the end of Parts II–V with 15 additional real-life outpatient and inpatient case studies to help students synthesize and apply what they have learned through hands-on coding practice with each code set.
- **Part VI: Legal, Ethical, and Reimbursement Issues** provides a concise overview connecting these broad topics to a professional coding specialist's job requirements.
- *Examples* again take students through real-life scenarios to help them understand how they will use this information.
- *Coding Bites* provide tips and highlight key concepts.
- This part also includes material to teach students how to access credible resources on the Internet.
- *Codes of Ethics* from both AHIMA and AAPC are discussed as well as information on compliance plans.
- *You Interpret It!* questions present students with opportunities to use critical-thinking skills to identify details required for accurate job performance.
- *Chapter Reviews* include assessments of chapter concepts:
    - Let's Check It! Terminology
    - Let's Check It! Concepts
    - Let's Check It! Which Type of Insurance?
    - Let's Check It! Rules and Regulations
    - You Code It! Application Case Studies

CONNECT FOR LET'S CODE IT!

McGraw Hill Connect for *Let's Code It!* includes:

- All end-of-chapter questions.
- CodePath versions of You Code It! practice questions, in which students are presented with a series of questions to guide them through the critical thinking process to determine the correct code.
- Interactive Exercises, such as Matching, Sequencing, and Labeling activities.
- Testbank questions.
- Lecture-style videos, which provide additional guidance on challenging coding questions. With the 2026–2027 Code Edition, the videos are now assignable through the Question Bank with new assessment questions for students to complete after each video. The videos are also available in the Connect Media Bank.

INSTRUCTORS' RESOURCES

You can rely on the following materials to help you and your students work through the material in the book; Instructor's manual, PowerPoint presentations, testbank, and additional tools to plan your course. These materials are available in the Instructor Resources under the Library tab in *Connect* (available only to instructors who are logged in to *Connect*).

Want to learn more about this product? Attend one of our online webinars. To learn more about them, please contact your McGraw Hill learning technology representative. To find your McGraw Hill representative, go to www.mheducation.com and click "Get Support," select "Higher Ed" and then click the "Get Started" button under the "Find Your Sales Rep" section.

Need help? Contact the McGraw Hill Education Customer Experience Group (CXG). Visit the CXG website at www.mhhe.com/support. Browse our frequently asked questions (FAQs) and product documentation and/or contact a CXG representative.

McGraw Hill **connect**®

Your complete course platform

Connect enables you to build deeper connections with your students through cohesive digital content and tools, creating engaging learning experiences. We are committed to providing you with the right resources and tools to support all your students along their personal learning journeys.

90%
student satisfaction

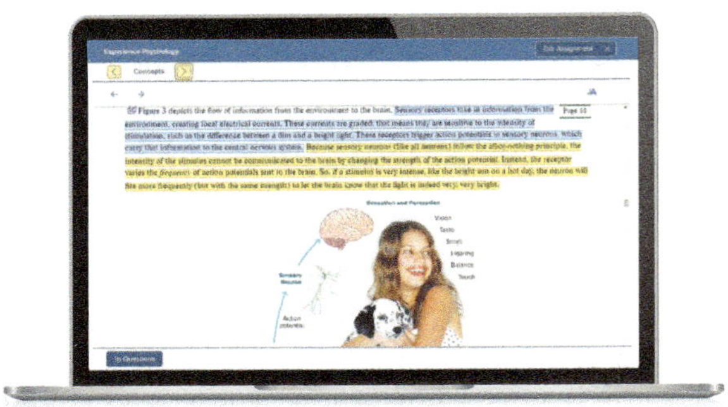

Laptop: Getty Images; Woman/dog: George Doyle/Getty Images

Every learner is unique

In Connect, instructors can assign an adaptive reading experience with SmartBook®. Rooted in advanced learning science principles, SmartBook delivers a personalized experience, focusing students on their learning gaps and ensuring the time they spend studying is time well spent.
mheducation.com/highered/connect/smartbook

Study anytime, anywhere

Encourage your students to download the free ReadAnywhere® app so they can access their online eBook, SmartBook, or Adaptive Learning Assignments when it's convenient, even when they're offline. Because the app automatically syncs with students' Connect accounts, all their work is available every time it is opened.
mheducation.com/readanywhere

"I really liked this app—it made it easy to study when you don't have your textbook in front of you."

Jordan Cunningham, a student at *Eastern Washington University*

Effective tools for efficient studying

Connect is designed to help students be more productive with simple, flexible, intuitive tools that maximize study time and meet students' individual learning needs and prepare them with real-world application. Get learning that works for everyone with Connect.

SUPPORT AT every step

Education for all

McGraw Hill works directly with Accessibility Services departments and faculty to meet the learning needs of all students. Please contact your Accessibility Services Office, and ask them to email **accessibility@mheducation.com**, or visit **mheducation.com/about/accessibility** for more information.

Affordable solutions, added value

Make technology work for you with LMS integration for single sign-on access, mobile access to the digital textbook, and reports to quickly show you how each of your students is doing. And with Affordable Access programs, you can provide all these tools at the lowest available market price to your students. Ask your McGraw Hill representative for more information.

Solutions for your challenges

A product isn't a solution. Real solutions are affordable, reliable, and come with training and ongoing support when you need it and how you want it. Visit **supportateverystep.com** for videos and resources both you and your students can use throughout the term.

Updated and relevant content

Our Evergreen™ Delivery Model provides you with the most relevant and updated content, tools, and accessibility. Engage students and freshen up assignments with up-to-date coverage of select topics and new questions, all without having to switch editions or build a new course.

ACKNOWLEDGMENTS

Reviewers

We would like to acknowledge the valuable contributions of the following reviewers. Their detailed feedback provides an additional dimension and perspective that we consider during our revision process.

Bev Bartholomew, *Wake Tech Community College*

Tanya Becker, *Bryan University Springfield*

Sandra Bhatnagar, *Arlington Career Institute*

Emma Brice, *Walla Walla Community College*

Barbara A. Jackson-Bryant, *St. Louis College of Health Careers*

Nicole Cobb, *Miller Motte College*

Teresa Diana, *Cape Fear Community College*

Eva Hearn, *Central Texas College*

Brandi Lippincott, *Merit Training Institute*

Julia Monk, *Blue Cliff College*

Heather E Morris, *Trident Technical College*

Joshua Pearson, *North Central Missouri College (Trenton, MO)*

Darcel Robinson, *Dorsey College*

Deborah Ryan, *Purdue Global University*

Shannon E Sharpe, *Green River College*

Shamva Wright-Shingler, *The College of Westchester*

Stephanie Slade, *South Piedmont Community College*

Slavica Tumminelli, *ACI Medical & Dental School*

Devonica Vaught, *Indian River State College*

Jennifer Washington, *Paris Junior College*

Kelly Williams, *Delgado Community College*

PART I

MEDICAL CODING FUNDAMENTALS

INTRODUCTION

Coding is not like anything you have ever studied before. No courses that you experienced in elementary, middle, or high school have prepared you for learning this skill. Biology and your science classes began your education that your anatomy and physiology class continued. Other courses you are taking as part of this program also typically connect to something, in some way, you have previously learned.

As you begin this educational journey, you will use your critical thinking skills as well as some experiences you may have had as a patient yourself (or as the loved one of a patient). For the most part, though, this will be different, so prepare yourself for a new learning experience.

In Part I, the chapters Introduction to the Languages of Coding, Abstracting Clinical Documentation, and The Coding Process share an overview of the concepts and skills you will apply in the chapters that follow. You will be introduced to the tools you have and will need to use as a professional coding specialist. Together, these three chapters create the foundation, the first layer, of a multilayered approach to learning coding. Then, the remaining parts will share with you, one by one, the best practices for how to use each of these tools correctly. You will then be given many opportunities for hands-on practice so that you can build your skills and reinforce the knowledge you have obtained.

1

Introduction to the Languages of Coding

Key Terms

Classification Systems
Condition
Diagnosis
Eponym
External Cause
Inpatient
Medical Necessity
Nonessential Modifiers
Outpatient
Procedure
Reimbursement
Services
Treatments

Learning Outcomes

After completing this chapter, the student should be able to:

LO 1.1 Explain the four purposes of medical coding.
LO 1.2 Identify the structure of the ICD-10-CM diagnosis coding manual.
LO 1.3 Differentiate between the types of procedures and the various procedure coding manuals.
LO 1.4 Examine the HCPCS Level II coding manual used to report the provision of equipment and supplies.

1.1 The Purpose of Coding

Around the world, languages exist to enable clear and accurate communication between individuals in similar groups or working together in similar functions. The purpose of using health care coding languages is to enable the sharing of information, in a specific and efficient way, between all those involved in health care.

Coding languages are constructed of individual codes that are more precise than words. (You will discover this as you venture through this textbook.) By communicating using codes rather than words, you can successfully convey to others involved (1) exactly what happened during a provider-patient encounter and (2) why it occurred. You, as the professional coding specialist, have the responsibility to accurately interpret health care terms and definitions (medical terminology) into numbers or number-letter combinations (alphanumeric codes) that specifically convey **diagnoses** and **procedures**.

Why is it so critical to code diagnoses and procedures accurately? The coding languages, known as **classification systems**, communicate information that is key to various aspects of the health care system, including

- Medical necessity
- Statistical analyses
- Reimbursement
- Resource allocation

CODING BITES

We use the concept of "*languages*" to help you relate medical coding–and its code sets–to an idea you already understand. In the health care industry, however, the various code sets, such as ICD-10-CM or HCPCS Level II, are referred to as **Classification Systems**.

Classification Systems
The term used in health care to identify ICD-10-CM, CPT, ICD-10-PCS, and HCPCS Level II code sets.

Diagnosis
A physician's determination of a patient's condition, illness, or injury.

Procedure
Action taken, in accordance with the standards of care, by the physician to accomplish a predetermined objective (result); a surgical operation.

Medical Necessity
The assessment that the provider was acting according to standard practices in providing a procedure or service for an individual with a specific diagnosis.

Medical Necessity

The diagnosis codes that you report explain the justification for the procedure, service, or treatment provided to a patient during their encounter. Every time a health care professional provides care to a patient, there must be a valid medical reason. Patients certainly want to know that health care professionals performed procedures or provided care for a specific, justified purpose, and so do third-party payers! This is referred to as **medical necessity**. Requiring medical necessity ensures that health care providers are not performing tests or giving injections without a good medical reason. Diagnosis codes explain *why* the individual came to see the physician and support the physician's decision about *what* procedures to provide.

Medical necessity is one of the reasons why it is so very important to code the diagnosis accurately and with all the detail possible. If you are one number off in your code selection, you could accidentally cause a claim to be denied because the diagnosis, identified by your incorrect code, does not justify the procedure.

Let's analyze an example:

EXAMPLE

Dr. Justini performs a colonoscopy on Shoshanna because a lab test identified that she had blood in her feces (melena).

CODING BITES

A **diagnosis** explains WHY the patient requires the attention of a health care provider and a **procedure** explains WHAT the physician or health care provider did for the patient.

CODING BITES

The WHY justifies the WHAT.

A colonoscopy involves the insertion of a camera, with surgical tools, into the patient's anus, rectum, and up through the large intestine. If you are Shoshanna, or if you are the one paying for this procedure, you want to make certain that this colonoscopy was done to support Shoshanna's good health and not any other reason. This is clearly communicated when you report the code K92.1 Melena (the presence of blood in feces). Now, whether for resource allocation or reimbursement, it is understood that Dr. Justini was caring properly for Shoshanna and her good health.

Statistical Analyses

Research organizations and government agencies statistically analyze the data provided by codes to develop programs, identify research areas, allocate funds, and write public health policies that will best address areas of concern for the health of our nation. For example, we can only know that a disease such as Alzheimer's needs diagnostic tests, treatments, and possibly a vaccine or a cure by studying statistics to see what individual signs and symptoms are being identified and treated around the country and around the world.

Reimbursement

In most cases, there are three parties involved in virtually every encounter: the health care provider, the patient, and the person or organization paying for the care provided (frequently, a health care insurance company). However, the insurance company is not always an actual insurance company, so the broader term "third-party payer" is used. Third-party payers use our coding data to determine how much they should pay health care professionals for the attention and services they provide patients. This is the role that coding plays in the **reimbursement** process. The codes make it easier for the organizations involved to evaluate and manage all their data.

Reimbursement
The process of paying for health care services after they have been provided.

CODING BITES

In most cases, there are three parties involved in reimbursement:

- The health care provider = First party
- The patient = Second party
- The insurance company or other organization financially responsible = Third-party payer

Resource Allocations

Whether a health care facility is a one-physician office or a large hospital, there are not unlimited resources available. Administrators and managers must ensure that all resources are employed in the most efficient and effective manner. Computer programs can easily and quickly organize data (the codes) to identify the largest patient population's diagnoses and the most frequently provided treatments and services. With these details, staff members, equipment, and money can be directed to those patients and locations that need them the most.

Can't AI Just Do This?

As you work your way through this textbook and your coding courses, you may find yourself wondering, "*Can't AI just do this?*" While artificial intelligence (AI) is advancing, research shows that well-trained *human* medical coding professionals outperform AI in accuracy by a three-to-one margin. More importantly, human coders consistently adhere to complex federal and state regulations, helping to avoid costly legal consequences such as fines, penalties, and even jail time. With continued strong job growth predicted by the Bureau of Labor Statistics, it's clear that the expertise, judgment, and compliance skills of *human* coders remain not only relevant but essential in today's health care landscape.

1.2 Diagnosis Coding

When a person goes to see a health care provider, there must have a reason–a health-related reason. After all, as much as you might like your physician, you probably wouldn't make an appointment, sit in the waiting room, and go through all the paperwork just to say, "hello." Whether the reason is a checkup, a flu shot, or something more serious, there is always a reason *why*. The physician will create notes, either written or dictated, recounting the events of the visit. The diagnosis, or diagnostic statement, in these notes will explain the reason *why* the patient was seen and treated.

The physician's notes explain, in writing, the reasons *why* the encounter occurred. The notes may document a specific condition or illness, the signs or symptoms of a yet-unnamed problem, or another reason for the encounter, such as a preventive service. As a coding specialist, it is your job to translate this explanation into a diagnosis code (or codes) so that everyone involved will clearly understand the issues of a particular patient at a particular time.

The International Classification of Diseases - 10th Revision - Clinical Modification (ICD-10-CM) code book contains all of the codes from which you will choose to report the reason *why* the health care professional cared for the patient during a specific encounter.

> **CODING BITES**
>
> This is just an overview to help you orient yourself to the structure of the code book. You will learn, in depth, how to use the ICD-10-CM code set to report any and all of the reasons *why* a patient needs the care of a health care professional in ***Part II: Reporting Diagnoses***.

> **Condition**
> The state of abnormality or dysfunction.

> **Eponym**
> A disease or condition named for a person.

Overview of the International Classification of Diseases – 10th Revision – Clinical Modification (ICD-10-CM) Code Book Sections

The ICD-10-CM code book (whether paper or electronic) is made up of several sections. Here is an overview of its parts and how you will utilize the information in these sections to determine the most accurate code or codes to report the reasons *why* an encounter occurred.

Index to Diseases and Injuries [aka Alphabetic Index]

The Alphabetic Index [Index to Diseases and Injuries] lists, in alphabetic order, the terms used by the physician to describe the reasons why the patient required attention from a health care professional.

The Alphabetic Index lists all diagnoses and other reasons to provide health care by their basic description alphabetically from A to Z (see **Figure 1-1**). Diagnostic descriptions are listed by

- **Condition** (e.g., infection, fracture, and wound)
- **Eponym** (e.g., Epstein-Barr syndrome and Cushing's disease)
- Other descriptors (e.g., personal history, family history)

Abnormal, abnormality, abnormalities (*see also* Anomaly)
acid–base balance (mixed) E87.4
albumin R77.0
alphafetoprotein R77.2
alveolar ridge K08.9
anatomical relationship Q89.9
apertures, congenital, diaphragm Q79.1
auditory perception H93.29-
  diplacusis—*see* Diplacusis
  hyperacusis—*see* Hyperacusis
  recruitment—*see* Recruitment, auditory
  threshold shift—*see* Shift, auditory threshold
autosomes Q99.9

FIGURE 1-1 ICD-10-CM Alphabetic Index, partial listing under main term Abnormal

Therefore, whichever type of words you read in the documentation, you should be able to find them in the Alphabetic Index in one form or another.

The Alphabetic Index can only suggest a possible code to report the patient's diagnosis, and you will use this suggestion to guide you to the correct page or subsection in the Tabular List (see the next subsection of this text, *Tabular List of Diseases and Injuries*). The Official Guidelines require you to always find a suggested code in the Tabular List to confirm it is accurate, or to find another code that might be better.

Tabular List of Diseases and Injuries

The Tabular List provides you with each and every available code in the ICD-10-CM code book, in order of the code characters—alphanumeric order. You need to carefully read the descriptions, beginning at the top of the three-character code category. When you begin reading at this point, you can make certain that you find the best code, to the highest level of specificity, according to the physician's documentation.

You will find that the Tabular List section shows all ICD-10-CM codes, first in alphabetic order and then in numeric order: A00 through Z99.89 (see **Figure 1-2**), along with additional details (notations and symbols) that guide you to the accurate code.

B67 Echinococcosis

INCLUDES *hydatidosis*

B67.0 Echinococcus granulosus infection of liver

B67.1 Echinococcus granulosus infection of lung

B67.2 Echinococcus granulosus infection of bone

B67.3 Echinococcus granulosus infection, other and multiple sites

B67.31 Echinococcus granulosus infection, thyroid gland

B67.32 Echinococcus granulosus infection, multiple sites

B67.39 Echinococcus granulosus infection, other sites

B67.4 Echinococcus granulosus infection, unspecified

Dog tapeworm (infection)

FIGURE 1-2 ICD-10-CM Tabular List, partial list of codes included in code category B67 Echinococcosis

CODING BITES

Notations in the Tabular List help make your coding process more accurate and a bit easier. For example, as you can see in **Figure 1-2**, the condition represented by code category B67 is Echinococcosis. Now, read the INCLUDES note directly below B67; it reads . . . INCLUDES hydatidosis. This notation lets you know that, if the physician wrote "echinococcosis" or "hydatidosis" in the documentation, this is the correct code category.

In ICD-10-CM, the INCLUDES note provides you with alternative words or phrases that the physician might use that mean the same condition. In English, they are known as synonyms. In ICD-10-CM, they are known as **nonessential modifiers**.

You will learn more about notations in the ***Introduction to ICD-10-CM*** chapter.

Ancillary Sections of ICD-10-CM

Neoplasm Table

The Neoplasm Table (**Figure 1-3**) itemizes all of the anatomical sites in the human body that may develop a tumor (neoplasm). Columns in this table further describe the type of neoplasm and suggest a code that may be accurate. As with other codes suggested by the Alphabetic Index, you will need to go to the Tabular List to look up any code found on the Neoplasm Table to confirm accuracy, additional characters required, and other details before you can determine the accurate code to report.

Nonessential Modifiers
Descriptors whose inclusion in the physician's notes are not absolutely necessary and that are provided simply to further clarify a code description; optional terms.

You will learn how to use the Neoplasm Table to report diagnoses of benign, malignant, and other types of neoplasms in the ***Coding Neoplasms*** chapter.

Table of Drugs and Chemicals

The Table of Drugs and Chemicals (**Figure 1-4**) lists pharmaceuticals and chemicals that may cause poisoning or adverse effects in the human body. The multiple columns in this table categorize the intent of how or why the patient became ill from the drug or chemical to suggest a possible code. As with all of these, this suggested code must be reviewed in the Tabular List to ensure completeness and accuracy before you can report it.

You will learn how to use the Table of Drugs and Chemicals in the chapter ***Coding Injury, Poisoning, and External Causes***.

	Malignant Primary	Malignant Secondary	Ca in situ	Benign	Uncertain Behavior	Unspecified Behavior
Neoplasm, neoplastic	C80.1	C79.9	D09.9	D36.9	D48.9	D49.9
abdomen, abdominal	C76.2	C79.8-	D09.8	D36.7	D48.7	D49.89
cavity	C76.2	C79.8-	D09.8	D36.7	D48.7	D49.89
organ	C76.2	C79.8-	D09.8	D36.7	D48.7	D49.89
viscera	C76.2	C79.8-	D09.8	D36.7	D48.7	D49.89
wall (*see also* Neoplasm, abdomen, wall, skin)	C44.509	C79.2-	D04.5	D23.5	D48.5	D49.2
connective tissue	C49.4	C79.8-	—	D21.4	D48.1	D49.2
skin	C44.509	—	—	—	—	—
basal cell carcinoma	C44.519	—	—	—	—	—
specified type NEC	C44.599	—	—	—	—	—
squamous cell carcinoma	C44.529	—	—	—	—	—

FIGURE 1-3 The Neoplasm Table from ICD-10-CM, listings for abdominal neoplasms

Substance	Poisoning, Accidental (Unintentional)	Poisoning, Intentional Self-harm	Poisoning, Assault	Poisoning, Undetermined	Adverse Effect	Underdosing
Acefylline piperazine	T48.6X1	T48.6X2	T48.6X3	T48.6X4	T48.6X5	T48.6X6
Acemorphan	T40.2X1	T40.2X2	T40.2X3	T40.2X4	T40.2X5	T40.2X6
Acenocoumarin	T45.511	T45.512	T45.513	T45.514	T45.515	T45.516
Acenocoumarol	T45.511	T45.512	T45.513	T45.514	T45.515	T45.516
Acepifylline	T48.6X1	T48.6X2	T48.6X3	T48.6X4	T48.6X5	T48.6X6
Acepromazine	T43.3X1	T43.3X2	T43.3X3	T43.3X4	T43.3X5	T43.3X6
Acesulfamethoxypyridazine	T37.0X1	T37.0X2	T37.0X3	T37.0X4	T37.0X5	T37.0X6
Acetal	T52.8X1	T52.8X2	T52.8X3	T52.8X4	—	—
Acetaldehyde (vapor)	T52.8X1	T52.8X2	T52.8X3	T52.8X4	—	—
liquid	T65.891	T65.892	T65.893	T65.894	—	—
P-Acetamidophenol	T39.1X1	T39.1X2	T39.1X3	T39.1X4	T39.1X5	T39.1X6
Acetaminophen	T39.1X1	T39.1X2	T39.1X3	T39.1X4	T39.1X5	T39.1X6

FIGURE 1-4 The Table of Drugs and Chemicals from ICD-10-CM, listings from Acefylline piperazine to Acetaminophen

Source: *ICD-10-CM Official Guidelines for Coding and Reporting*, The Centers for Medicare and Medicaid Services (CMS) and the National Center for Health Statistics (NCHS)

External Cause
An event, outside the body, that causes injury, poisoning, or an adverse reaction.

Index to External Causes

The Index to **External Causes** (**Figure 1-5**) lists the causes of injury and poisoning. These codes are used to explain *how* a patient got injured and *where* (place of occurrence) they were when the injury happened.

Abandonment (causing exposure to weather conditions) (with intent to injure or kill) NEC X58

Abuse (adult) (child) (mental) (physical) (sexual) X58

Accident (to) X58

aircraft (in transit) (powered) (*see also* Accident, transport, aircraft)

due to, caused by cataclysm—*see* Forces of nature, by type

animal-rider—*see* Accident, transport, animal-rider

animal-drawn vehicle—*see* Accident, transport, animal-drawn vehicle occupant

automobile—*see* Accident, transport, car occupant

bare foot water skier V94.4

boat, boating (*see also* Accident, watercraft)

striking swimmer

powered V94.11

unpowered V94.12

bus—*see* Accident, transport, bus occupant

cable car, not on rails V98.0

FIGURE 1-5 The Index to External Causes, first listings including main terms Abandonment, Abuse, and Accident

As with the other content in the Alphabetic Index, the code or codes shown here are only suggestions and must be confirmed in the Tabular List before you are permitted to report them. You will learn about the importance of reporting these codes as you progress through your learning experience, particularly in the chapter ***Coding Injury, Poisoning, and External Causes***.

The Format of ICD-10-CM Codes

A complete, valid ICD-10-CM code will always begin with a three (3)-character code category: a letter of the alphabet followed by a minimum of two (2) characters (either letters or numbers).

E54 Ascorbic acid deficiency (scurvy)

L26 Exfoliative dermatitis

A majority of the codes will require additional characters to communicate more specific information about the patient's condition. When an additional character is needed to complete the code, a symbol to the left of the code in the Tabular List will identify that additional characters are necessary. The symbol may be a bullet ● or it may be a box with a check mark ✓4, depending upon the publisher of your code book. You will find a legend to explain the meaning of each symbol at the bottom of the page in your code book. As you evaluate the options available for the additional character, make certain to place a dot (period) between the third and fourth characters.

Let's take a look at an example together:

✓4 **M17 Osteoarthritis of knee**

M17.0 Bilateral primary osteoarthritis of knee

The symbol to the left of code M17 alerts you that this code requires a fourth (4th) character. In looking at the second line of this example (M17.0), you can see that this fourth character shares additional, important information about the patient's condition. It is not enough to communicate that the patient has been diagnosed with osteoarthritis of the knee. You must explain the specific location (from our example, bilateral = both knees) and specific type of condition (from our example, primary osteoarthritis).

CODING BITES

When additional characters are required, those codes with fewer characters are invalid. The need for additional characters is mandatory, not a suggestion.

ICD-10-CM codes can be as short as three (3) characters and can add additional characters containing more specificity about the patient's condition . . . up to a total of seven (7) characters. These additional characters ensure that as much detail as possible about the patient's condition is communicated accurately and completely.

EXAMPLE

The Tabular List shows you which details to abstract from the documentation. All you have to do is keep reading. The portion of the ICD-10-CM Tabular List below shows options for additional characters and the information these characters convey.

S43.3 **Subluxation and dislocation of other and unspecified parts of shoulder girdle**

S43.30 **Subluxation and dislocation of unspecified parts of shoulder girdle**

Dislocation of shoulder girdle NOS

Subluxation of shoulder girdle NOS

S43.301 **Subluxation of unspecified parts of right shoulder girdle**

S43.302 **Subluxation of unspecified parts of left shoulder girdle**

S43.303 **Subluxation of unspecified parts of unspecified shoulder girdle**

S43.304 **Dislocation of unspecified parts of right shoulder girdle**

S43.305 **Dislocation of unspecified parts of left shoulder girdle**

S43.306 **Dislocation of unspecified parts of unspecified shoulder girdle**

MCGRAW GENERAL HOSPITAL

PATIENT: YOUNG, MATTHEW JAMES

HISTORY: Neonate is male, delivered yesterday at 1915 hours by C-section due to previous C-section. Mother is:

- gravida 2, para 2, AB 1
- blood type B positive
- GBS negative
- hepatitis B surface antigen negative
- rubella immune
- VDRL nonreactive

VITAL SIGNS:

Weight: 6 pounds 9 ounces

Height: 19-1/2 inches

Head circumference: 14 inches

GENERAL:

APGAR = 10 @1 min, 10 @ 5 min

SKIN: Portwine nevus on right ankle

NEUROLOGIC: Alert, vigorous cry, good tone, nonfocal

DISPOSITION:

The neonate was discharged to his mother. I instructed the mother to phone me PRN. I told her that I want to see both in my office in 10 days for a follow-up.

Let's Code It!

Dr. Michaels delivered Matthew James Young and examined him. Being born is the confirmed reason why the baby needed Dr. Michael's time and expertise. You need to translate the reason *why* into an ICD-10-CM diagnosis code. Therefore, begin in the Alphabetic Index of your ICD-10-CM manual. What should you look up? Matthew needed to be examined right after being born, so let's look up:

Birth . . . nothing here that matches.

Next, try: Newborn. We have a match!

(continued)

Newborn (infant) (liveborn) (singleton) Z38.2

Turn in the Tabular List to this code and begin by reading at the three-character code category:

✓4 Z38 Liveborn infants according to place of birth and type of delivery

NOTE: This category is for use as the principal code on the initial record of a newborn baby. It is to be used for the initial birth record only. It is not to be used on the mother's record.

You know that Matthew was just born, so this note confirms you are in the right place in the code book. Notes, notations, symbols, and other marks in the code book are there to help point you in the right direction and to support your determination of the correct code.

Our next step is to look at the mark to the left of the code . . . it may be a box with a check mark ✓4 , it may be a dot ●, or the following lines may just be indented. However your copy of the code book alerts you, it is clear . . . this code needs an additional character. And this is not a suggestion; it is mandatory.

There are three options for a fourth character:

✓5	Z38.0	Single liveborn infant, born in hospital
	Z38.1	Single liveborn infant, born outside hospital
	Z38.2	Single liveborn infant, unspecified as to place of birth

You can see in the record above that Matthew was born in McGraw General Hospital and, therefore, Z38.0 is the most accurate.

But we aren't done yet. There is a symbol to the left of code Z38.0. It is telling you that an additional character is required. Let's look at the two options:

Z38.00	Single liveborn infant, delivered vaginally
Z38.01	Single liveborn infant, delivered by cesarean

Go back to the documentation and read the information provided by the doctor. He noted that Matthew was born via a C-section (the C stands for cesarean).

There are no more symbols or notations here in the Tabular List. Next, double-check the **Official Guidelines, Section 1C. Chapter 21, subsection 12) Newborns and Infants** as well as **Chapter 16, subsection 6) Code all clinically significant conditions**. It appears that there are no further details or codes needed . . . so this is the code.

Good job! You were able to determine that code Z38.01 most accurately reports Matthew's birth. You did it!

1.3 Procedure Coding

Once the physician has determined the patient's condition or problem, he or she can then establish a treatment plan. Generally, there are three terms used to describe actions that the physician can take to support a patient's good health or to improve a current condition:

Procedures are actions, or a series of actions, taken to accomplish an objective (result). For example, surgically removing a mole or resectioning the small intestine.

Services are actions that will most often involve counseling, educating, and advising the patient, such as discussing test results or sharing recommendations for risk reduction.

Treatments are typically an application of a health care service, such as radiation treatments for tumor reduction or acupuncture.

These actions provided by the physician, or other health care professional, are done for one of three reasons:

Diagnostic tests or procedures are performed to provide the physician with additional information required to determine a confirmed diagnosis.

Preventive procedures and services are provided to keep a healthy patient healthy. In other words . . . to avoid illness or injury. These also include early detection testing, known as screenings.

CODING BITES

You will learn many more details about reporting diagnoses in ***Part II: Reporting Diagnoses***, with more in-depth introduction to ICD-10-CM as well as details by body system.

Services
Spending time with a patient and/or family about health care situations.

Treatment
The provision of medical care for a disorder or disease.

Therapeutic procedures, treatments, and services are performed with the intention of removing, correcting, or repairing an abnormality or condition.

There are three different code sets available for you to use to translate health care procedures, services, and treatments into codes. These three code sets are

Current Procedural Terminology (CPT)

International Classification of Diseases - 10th Revision - Procedure Coding System (ICD-10-PCS)

Healthcare Common Procedure Coding System (HCPCS) Level II

Current Procedural Terminology (CPT)

Outpatient
A patient who receives services for a short amount of time (less than 24 hours) in a physician's office or clinic, without being kept overnight.

CPT codes are used to describe procedures performed by a physician in any location. These services range from speaking with a patient about test results to performing surgery or determining a treatment plan. In addition, CPT codes are used to report the contribution made by **outpatient** facilities (a physician's office, a clinic, an ambulatory surgical center, or the emergency department of a hospital), such as a sterile procedure room, trained nursing and support staff, etc.

CODING BITES

CPT codes and sections run, generally, in numeric order; however, there are exceptions throughout. Bottom line . . . *read carefully and completely.*

The Organization of the CPT Code Book

The CPT book has two parts, which in turn have many sections.

The CPT book (see **Figure 1-6**) has six sections, which are generally presented in numeric order by code number:

- Evaluation and Management: 99202–99499
- Anesthesia: 00100–01999 and 99100–99140
- Surgery: 10004–69990
- Radiology: 70010–79999
- Pathology and Laboratory: 80047–89398, 0001U-0222U
- Medicine: 90281–99199, 99500–99607

pancreas, 49180 for abdominal or retroperitoneal mass, 50200 for kidney, 54500 for testis, 54800 for epididymis, 60100 for thyroid, 62267 for nucleus pulposus, intervertebral disc, or paravertebral tissue, 62269 for spinal cord)

(For evaluation of fine needle aspirate, see 88172, 88173)

Integumentary System

Skin, Subcutaneous, and Accessory Structures

Introduction and Removal

⊙ **10030** Image-guided fluid collection drainage by catheter (e.g., abscess, hematoma, seroma, lymphocele, cyst), soft tissue (e.g., extremity, abdominal wall, neck), percutaneous
➲ *CPT Changes: An Insider's View* 2014
➲ *CPT Assistant* Fall 13:6, May 14:3, 9
➲ *Clinical Examples in Radiology* Summer 14:9

(Report 10030 for each individual collection drained with a separate catheter)

(Do not report 10030 in conjunction with 75989, 76942, 77002, 77003, 77012, 77021)

Incision and Drainage

(For excision, see 11400, et seq)

10040 Acne surgery (e.g., marsupialization, opening or removal of multiple milia, comedones, cysts, pustules)
➲ *CPT Assistant* Fall 92:10, Feb 08:8

10060 Incision and drainage of abscess (e.g., carbuncle, suppurative hidradenitis, cutaneous or subcutaneous abscess, cyst, furuncle, or paronychia); simple or single
➲ CPT *Assistant* Sep 12:10

10061 complicated or multiple
➲ *CPT Assistant* Sep 12:10

10080 Incision and drainage of pilonidal cyst; simple
➲ *CPT Assistant* Fall 92:13, Dec 06:15, May 07:5

10081 complicated
➲ *CPT Assistant* Fall 92:13, Dec 06:15, May 07:5

(For excision of pilonidal cyst, see 11770-11772)

10120 Incision and removal of foreign body, subcutaneous tissues: simple
➲ *CPT Assistant* Sep 12:10, Apr 13:10, Dec 13:16

10121 complicated
➲ *CPT Assistant* Spring 91:7, Dec 06:15, Sep 12:10, Dec 13:16

(To report wound exploration due to penetrating trauma without laparotomy or thoracotomy, one 20100-20103, as appropriate)

FIGURE 1-6 CPT main section, showing codes 10030–10121

Source: American Medical Association, *CPT Professional Manual*

The second part of the CPT book also contains several sections, including

- *Category II codes:* used for supplemental tracking of performance measurements. These codes are not reimbursable but support research on specific physician actions taken on behalf of a patient's health.
- *Category III codes:* temporary codes used to report emerging technological procedures. Technology and health care are innovating and improving every day. These codes enable tracking physician adoption and the frequency of use to identify what should stay and what will be deleted.
- *Appendixes A–P:* modifiers and other relevant additional information.
- *Alphabetic Index:* all the CPT codes in alphabetical order by code description, presented in four types of entries (see **Figure 1-7**):
    - **a.** Procedures or services, such as bypass, decompression, insertion.
    - **b.** Anatomical site or organ, such as brain stem, spinal cord, lymph nodes.
    - **c.** Condition, such as pregnancy, fracture, abscess.
    - **d.** Eponyms, synonyms, or abbreviations, such as Potts-Smith Procedure or EEG.

> **CODING BITES**
>
> More information about Category II and Category III codes will be covered in the chapter ***Introduction to CPT.***

Activity, Glomerular Procoagulant — **Alanine Transaminase**

Activity, Glomerular Procoagulant
See Thromboplastin

Acupuncture
with Electrical Stimulation 97813, 97814
without Electrical Stimulation 97810, 97811

Acute Poliomyelitis
See Polio

Acylcarnitines 82016, 82017

Adamantinoma, Pituitary
See Craniopharyngioma

Adaptive Behavior Treatment Assessment

Adductor Tenotomy of Hip
See Tenotomy, Hip, Adductor

Adenoidectomy
See Adenoids, Excision

Adenoids
Excision 42830, 42836
with Tonsils 42820, 42821
Unlisted Services and Procedures 42999

Adenoma
Pancreas
Excision 48120
Parathyroid
Localization
Injection Procedure 78808
Thyroid Gland Excision 60200

Labial
Lysis 56441
Liver
Lysis 58660
Lungs
Pneumonolysis 32174, 32940
Nose
Lysis 30560
Pelvic
Lysis 58660, 58740
Penile
Lysis
Post-circumcision 54162
Preputial
Lysis 54450
Urethral
Lysis 53500

Adipectomy
See Lipectomy

ADL
See Activities of Daily Living

Administration
Immunization
Each Additional Vaccine/Toxoid 90472, 90474
with Counseling 90461
One vaccine/Toxoid 90471, 90473
with Counseling 90460
Occlusive Substance 31634
Pharmacologic Agent 93463

ADP
See Adenosine Diphosphate

Adult T Cell Leukemia Lymphoma Virus I
See HTLV-I

Advanced Life Support
Physician/Health Care Professional Direction 99288

Advancement
Genioglossus 21199
Tendon
Tibia 28238

Advancement Flap
See Skin, Adjacent Tissue Transfer

Aerosol Inhalation
See Pulmonology, Therapeutic
Pentamidine 94642

AFB
See Acid-Fast Bacilli (AFB)

Afferent Nerve
See Sensory Nerve

AFP
See Alpha-Fetoprotein (AFP)

After Hours Medical Services .. 99050

Agents, Anticoagulant
See Clotting Inhibitors

Agglutinin
Cold 86156, 86157
Febrile 86000

Index

FIGURE 1-7 CPT Alphabetic Index, partial listings from Activity, Glomerular Procoagulant to Agglutinin

Source: American Medical Association, *CPT Professional Manual*

The Formats of CPT Codes

Each code listed in the various CPT sections has a different structure:

CPT codes (Category I codes) are five-digit codes. They have all numbers (no letters, no punctuation). Example: 51100 Aspiration of bladder; by needle.

Category II codes are five-character codes, with four numbers followed by the letter "F." Example: 2001F Weight recorded (PAG).

Category III codes are five-character codes. These codes also have four numbers; however, Category III codes are followed by the letter "T." Example: 0208T Pure tone audiometry (threshold), automated; air only.

> **CODING BITES**
>
> You will learn many more details about reporting procedures in ***Part III: Reporting Physician Services and Outpatient Procedures.***

Modifiers (listed in **Appendix A** of your CPT code book) are two characters: two numbers, two letters, or one letter and one number. Modifiers are appended to CPT codes under special circumstances, such as the use of unusual anesthesia, two surgeons working on the same patient at the same time, or a multipart procedure performed over time. When required, a modifier is added after the main CPT code with a hyphen. Example: 47600-54 Cholecystectomy, surgical care only.

ICD-10-CM

LET'S CODE IT! SCENARIO

Corey Carter, a 55-year-old male, came to the McGraw Ambulatory Surgery Center, an outpatient facility, so Dr. Lucano could perform a percutaneous core needle biopsy on his thyroid. Corey's primary care physician referred him to Dr. Lucano after noting a lump on his thyroid during an annual physical.

Let's Code It!

Open your CPT book to the Alphabetic Index. Which term should you look up? Let's dissect the scenario:

Biopsy = the procedure

Percutaneous core needle = the type of biopsy

Thyroid = the anatomical site

Let's begin by finding Biopsy in the Alphabetic Index:

Biopsy

See Brush Biopsy; Needle Biopsy

Abdomen 49000, 49321

Notice that Abdomen is the beginning of a long list of anatomical sites on which a biopsy can be done. Read down the list to find:

Thyroid 60100

Now, turn into the Main Section of CPT to find code 60100. You can see:

60100 Biopsy thyroid, percutaneous core needle

This matches Dr. Lucano's documentation perfectly—you can report this procedure code with confidence!

International Classification of Diseases – 10th Revision – Procedure Coding System (ICD-10-PCS)

Inpatient
An individual admitted for an overnight or longer stay in a hospital.

The International Classification of Diseases - 10th Revision - Procedure Coding System (ICD-10-PCS) codes are used to describe the contribution made by the hospital to a procedure provided to an **inpatient** (a patient admitted into an acute care facility). These are known as "facility charges" because they report what the hospital provided during a specific procedure, service, or treatment, such as the skilled nursing staff, the operating room, the equipment, and whatever else is required.

ICD-10-PCS contains an Alphabetic Index and a Tables section (**Figure 1-8**). The Alphabetic Index is used in the same way you use this part of the other code books–to get an idea of where in the Tables section to find codes. However, the Tables section of this code set is very different. Rather than a listing of the codes in numeric or alphanumeric order, you will find Tables listing various characters and their meanings. Then, you will actually build the code, according to the physician's documentation.

Section **0** Medical and Surgical *Body System* **2** Heart and Greater Vessels *Operation* **5** Destruction: Physical eradication of all or a portion of a body part by the direct use of energy, force, or a destructive agent			
Body Part Character 4	*Approach* Character 5	*Device* Character 6	*Qualifier* Character 7
4 Coronary Vein **5** Atrial Septum **6** Atrium, Right **8** Conduction Mechanism **9** Chordae Tendineae **D** Papillary Muscle **F** Aortic Valve **G** Mitral Valve **H** Pulmonary Valve **J** Tricuspid Valve **K** Ventricle, Right **L** Ventricle, Left **M** Ventricular Septum **N** Pericardium **P** Pulmonary Trunk **Q** Pulmonary Artery, Right **R** Pulmonary Artery, Left **S** Pulmonary Vein, Right **T** Pulmonary Vein, Left **V** Superior Vena Cava **W** Thoracic Aorta, Descending **X** Thoracic Aorta, Ascending/Arch	**0** Open **3** Percutaneous **4** Percutaneous Endoscopic	**Z** No Device	**Z** No Qualifier
7 Atrium, Left	**0** Open **3** Percutaneous **4** Percutaneous Endoscopic	**Z** No Device	**K** Left Atrial Appendage **Z** No Qualifier

FIGURE 1-8 Table 025, one of the tables from the ICD-10-PCS Tables section

The Format of ICD-10-PCS Codes

ICD-10-PCS codes have seven (7) characters and are alphanumeric (both letters and numbers). Each of the seven positions in the code represents a specific piece of information relating to a procedure, service, or treatment provided. These meanings change for each section of the codebook. But don't worry. No memorization is required . . . the code book provides you with what you need to know. All you have to do is read carefully.

For example, in the Medical and Surgical Section, each character reports the:

1. *Section* of the ICD-10-PCS code set.
2. *Body system* upon which the procedure or service was performed.
3. *Root operation*, which explains the category or type of procedure.
4. *Body part*, which identifies the specific anatomical site involved in the procedure.
5. *Approach*, which reports which method was used to perform the service or treatment.
6. *Device*, which reports, when applicable, what type of device was involved in the service or procedure.
7. *Qualifier*, which adds any additional detail.

EXAMPLES

0DQ48ZZ	Repair of the esophagogastric junction, via natural opening endoscopic
0RRJ0J6	Replacement of shoulder joint humeral surface with synthetic substitute, right side, open approach

Whereas in the Imaging Section, each character reports the:

1. *Section* of the ICD-10-PCS code set.
2. *Body system* upon which the procedure or service was performed.
3. *Root type*, which explains the type of imaging, such as MRI or CT scan.
4. *Body part*, which identifies the specific anatomical site imaged and recorded.
5. *Contrast*, which reports if contrast materials were used in the imaging process.
6. *Qualifier*, which adds any additional detail.
7. *Qualifier*, which adds any additional detail.

EXAMPLES

B31M110	Intraoperative fluoroscopy of the spinal arteries, low osmolar contrast, laser
BB24ZZZ	Bilateral CT scan of lungs, no contrast

ICD-10-CM

LET'S CODE IT! SCENARIO

Marlena Takamoto, a 37-year-old female, contracted hepatitis seven years ago. The disease severely damaged her liver. She was admitted to Carolina Brookdale Hospital today so Dr. Lewis and his team can perform a liver transplantation, open approach. The liver donor was killed in a car accident early this morning.

Let's Code It!

The physicians will transplant a liver, using an open approach, from the donor to Marlena. The coder who works for Dr. Lewis will use CPT codes to report his services provided to Marlena. You work as the coder for Carolina Brookdale Hospital, so you need to use ICD-10-PCS to report the hospital's contribution in this surgery (the operating room, the support staff [surgical nurses, technicians], and other equipment).

The procedure is a transplant, so let's start by looking in the Alphabetic Index in ICD-10-PCS for transplant. In the index, we find

Transplantation
Liver 0FY00Z-

In this particular case, the Alphabetic Index provides you with the first six of the required seven characters. In other cases, you may find the Alphabetic Index will only provide you with three or four characters. Regardless, you must find this Table in the Tables section to complete the seven (7) characters. Using the first three characters provided by the Alphabetic Index, turn in the Tables section to the Table that begins with **0FY** (see below):

Section	**0**	Medical and Surgical
Body System	**F**	Hepatobiliary System and Pancreas
Operation	**Y**	Transplantation: Putting in or on all or a portion of a living body part taken from another individual or animal to physically take the place and/or function of all or a portion of a similar body part

(continued)

Body Part	*Approach*	*Device*	*Qualifier*
0 Liver **G** Pancreas	**0** Open	**Z** No Device	**0** Allogeneic **1** Syngeneic **2** Zooplastic

Now, with all of this information, let's build the correct code:

1. *Section* of the ICD-10-PCS code set = *Medical and Surgical 0*
2. *Body system* upon which the procedure was performed = *Hepatobiliary F*

Remember, the liver is an organ that is part of the Hepatobiliary System.

3. *Root operation*: the type of procedure = *Transplantation Y*
4. *Body part*: the specific anatomical site involved in the procedure = *Liver 0*
5. *Approach:* method used to perform the transplant = *Open 0*
6. *Device*, when applicable = *No Device Z*
7. *Qualifier*: any additional detail = *Allogeneic 0*

Before reporting this code . . . check the **Official Guidelines**, specifically **B3.16 Transplantation vs. Administration**. This confirms that you used the correct root operation term of Transplantation.

Good job! Now you have built the ICD-10-PCS code for this procedure: **0FY00Z0**.

It would not be unusual for one patient encounter, for a patient admitted into the hospital, to ultimately require interpretation into all three coding languages: ICD-10-CM, CPT, and ICD-10-PCS.

EXAMPLE

Injured in an accident, Terence McCarthy was admitted into McGraw General Hospital with a major contusion of the spleen. Terence was brought into the operating room, he was placed in the supine position, and general anesthesia was administered by Dr. London. Dr. Berring performed a total splenectomy.

Together, let's review all of the codes that will be reported for this surgical procedure:

- The professional coding specialist for Dr. Berring, the surgeon, will report:

    S36.021A **Major contusion of spleen, initial encounter**

    38100 **Splenectomy; total**

- The professional coding specialist for Dr. London, the anesthesiologist, will report:

    S36.021A **Major contusion of spleen, initial encounter**

    00790-P1 **Anesthesia for intraperitoneal procedures in upper abdomen including laparoscopy; not otherwise specified, a normal healthy patient**

- The professional coding specialist for McGraw General Hospital, the facility, will report:

    S36.021A **Major contusion of spleen, initial encounter**

    07TP0ZZ **Splenectomy, open approach**

CODING BITES

Use a medical dictionary whenever you do not know the meaning of a term:

Allogeneic means coming from a different individual of the same species.

Syngeneic means coming from a genetic identical, such as from an identical twin.

Zooplastic means the tissue or organ is coming from a donor of another species into a human.

CODING BITES

You will learn many more details about reporting inpatient procedures in ***Part V: Inpatient (Hospital) Reporting***.

HCPCS Level II Procedure Codes

In some cases, you might determine that the CPT code set does not contain a code that accurately and completely reports a procedure or service. It is possible that a HCPCS Level II code may do the job.

HCPCS (pronounced "hick-picks") is the abstraction for Healthcare Common Procedure Coding System.

- HCPCS Level I codes are actually called CPT codes. While CPT codes are maintained by the American Medical Association (AMA), this code set was adopted by our industry as the first level of HCPCS.
- HCPCS Level II codes are referred to as HCPCS Level II codes.

For the most part, health care services are listed in the HCPCS Level II section titled Procedures/Professional Services (Temporary) G0008–G9999 [but not exclusively, so be certain to check the Alphabetic Index first]. As always, reading carefully and completely is required. However, as you scan the codes and their descriptions in this section of HCPCS Level II, you may find some are very close to CPT code descriptions. But . . . not exactly. Let's look at the simple repair of a 2.1 cm superficial laceration on the patient's left hand being repaired with tissue adhesive.

In CPT, under REPAIR (CLOSURE), the in-section guidelines state: "*Use the codes in this section to designate wound closure utilizing sutures, staples, or tissue adhesives, either singly or in combination with each other or in combination with adhesive strips.*"

The definition in CPT of a simple repair includes "*. . . requires simple one layer closure.*" With this scenario, this would lead to code

12001 **Simple repair of superficial wounds of scalp, neck, axillae, external genitalia, trunk and/or extremities (including hands and feet); 2.5 cm or less**

Compare this with the most appropriate HCPCS Level II code:

G0168 **Wound closure utilizing tissue adhesive(s) only**

Which code reports the repair more accurately? You must go back to the documentation and read carefully, looking for the additional details included in the definition of Simple Repair in CPT. Was a one-layer closure performed? Was local anesthesia used? Was anything else done by the physician in addition to the application of the tissue adhesive?

If the answer to any of these questions is Yes, then you need to report the CPT code 12001. If the answers to all of these questions are No, then report G0168.

Let's look at an example that is perhaps a bit less complex. Compare and contrast these two codes, both of which are used for reporting speech therapy services:

92507 **Treatment of speech, language, voice, communication, and/or auditory processing disorder; individual**

S9128 **Speech therapy, in the home, per diem**

> **CODING BITES**
>
> Learn about the other types of HCPCS Level II codes in the section ***Equipment and Supplies*** in this chapter.
>
> And learn more about the HCPCS Level II code set in the chapter ***HCPCS Level II.***

These two codes report similar services: speech therapy provided to an individual. However, they differ with regard to location, length of the session, and possibly the professional providing the therapy. Be certain to read the CPT in-section guidelines related to the reporting of 92507 (and other codes in this subsection) before you decide. And, of course, you need to carefully abstract the details within the documentation from which you are coding and compare the specifics to each of the code descriptions, and perhaps to any others available. Then, and only then, can you determine which code to report.

Don't worry . . . one item, one detail, one concept at a time. It will take time, but we are confident you will be able to understand, learn, and master coding for health care services.

1.4 Equipment and Supplies

A large number of components of health care extend beyond what are usually referred to as procedures, services, and treatments you learned about earlier in **Section 1.3** of this chapter. This includes equipment that is provided for a patient's use at home, supplies that are not already included in other codes, and transportation services not described in the CPT book at all. HCPCS Level II also contains codes you can use to report them.

HCPCS Level II codes cover specific aspects of health care services, including

- Durable medical equipment (e.g., a wheelchair or a humidifier).
- Pharmaceuticals administered by a health care provider (e.g., a saline solution or a chemotherapy drug).
- Medical supplies provided for the patient's home use (e.g., an eye patch or gradient compression stockings).
- Dental services (e.g., all services provided by a dental professional).

- Transportation services (e.g., ambulance services).
- Vision and hearing services (e.g., trifocal spectacles or a hearing aid).
- Orthotic and prosthetic procedures (e.g., scoliosis brace or prosthetic arm).

HCPCS Level II codes are listed in sections, grouped by the type of service, the type of supply item, or the type of equipment they represent. However, you should not assume that a particular item or service is located in a specific section. Use the Alphabetic Index (**Figure 1-9**) to direct you to the correct section or subsection in the Alphanumeric Listing of the code book. One type of service or procedure might be located under several different categories depending upon the details.

Cyclosporine, J7502, J7515, J7516

Cytarabine, J9100

Cytarabine liposome, J9098

Cytomegalovirus immune globulin (human), J0850

D

Dacarbazine, J9130

Daclizumab, J7513

Dactinomycin, J9120

FIGURE 1-9 HCPCS Level II Alphabetic Index, partial listing from Cyclosporine to Dactinomycin

Medicare and Medicaid want you to use HCPCS Level II codes; however, not all insurance carriers accept these codes. It is your responsibility, as a coding specialist, to find out whether each third-party payer with which your facility works will permit the reporting of HCPCS Level II codes on a claim form. If not, you should ask for the payer's policies on reporting the services and supplies covered by HCPCS Level II so you don't have a claim delayed or denied.

The Format of HCPCS Level II Codes

The codes listed in the HCPCS Level II code book are all structured the same way: one letter followed by four numbers. No dots, no dashes (**Figure 1-10**).

A0225 **Ambulance service, neonatal transport, base rate, emergency transport, one way**

E0130 **Walker, rigid (pickup), adjustable or fixed height**

J3480 **Injection, potassium chloride, per 2 mEq**

L0130 **Cervical, flexible, thermoplastic collar, molded to patient**

V5050 **Hearing aid, monaural, in the ear**

ICD-10-CM

LET'S CODE IT! SCENARIO

Rita Widden, a 92-year-old female, was being transferred from Hampton Medical Center to the Sunflower Nursing Home across town. Cosentti Ambulance Service provided nonemergency transportation prepared with basic life support (BLS) services.

Let's Code It!

Cosentti Ambulance Service provided nonemergency BLS (basic life support) transportation for Rita. After looking carefully in your CPT and ICD-10-PCS code books, you find that this type of service is not represented. Therefore, you need to look in the HCPCS Level II code set.

(continued)

Begin in the Alphabetic Index, and find:

Transportation

Ambulance, A0021–A0999

This code set often will require some patience as you read through all of the code options, which were suggested by the Alphabetic Index, until you find the one that matches the services for which you are reporting:

A0428 Ambulance service, basic life-support, nonemergency transport, (BLS)

Good work! You got it!

HCPCS Level II **J7628**

J7512 Prednisone, Immediate release or delayed release, oral, 1 mg

J7513 Daclizumab, parenteral, 25 mg
Use this code for Zenapax.
CMS: 100-2,15,50.5; 100-4, 17, 80.3
AHA: 20, '05, 11

J7515 Cyclosporine, oral, 25 mg
Use this code for Neoral, Sandimmune, Gengraf, Sangcya.
CMS: 100-4, 17, 80.3

J7516 Cyclosporine, parenteral, 250 mg
Use this code for Neoral, Sandimmune, Gengraf, Sangcya.
CMS: 100-4, 17, 80.3

J7517 Mycophenolate mofetil, oral, 250 mg
Use this code for CeliCept.
CMS: 100-4, 17, 80.3

J7518 Mycophenolic acid, oral, 180 mg
Use this code for Myfortic Delayed Release.
CMS: 100-4, 17, 80, 3.1
AHA: 20, '05, 11

J7520 Sirolimus, oral, 1 mg
Use this code for Rapamune.
CMS: 100-2, 15, 50.5; 100-4, 17, 80.3

J7525 Tacrolimus, parenteral, 5 mg
Use this code for Prograt.
CMS: 100-2, 15, 50.5; 100-4, 17, 80.3

J7527 Everolimus, oral, 0.25 mg
Use this code for Zortress, Afinitor.

J7599 Immunosuppressive drug, not otherwise classified
Determine if an alternative HCPCS Level II or a CPT code Better describes the service being reported. This code should be used only if a more specific code is unavailable.
CMS: 100-2, 15, 50.5; 100-4, 17, 80.3
AHA: 2Q, '13, 3

Inhalation Solutions

J7604 Acetylcysteine, Inhalation solution, compounded product, administered through DME, unit dose form, per g

J7605 Arformoterol, inhalation solution, FDA approved final product, noncompounded, administered through DME, unit dose form, 15 mcg

J7611 Albuterol, inhalation solution, FDA-approved final product, noncompounded, administered through DME, unit dose, 1 mg
Use this code for Accuneb, Proventil, Respirol, Ventolin.
AHA: 20, '08, 10; 20, '07, 10

J7612 Levalbuterol, inhalation solution, FDA-approved final product, noncompounded, administered through DME, unit dose, 0.5 mg
Use this code for Xopenex.
CMS: 100-3, 200.2
AHA: 20, '08, 10; 20, '07, 10

J7615 Levalbuterol, inhalation solution, compounded product, administered through DME, unit dose, 0.5 mg
CMS: 100-3, 200.2

J7620 Albuterol, up to 2.5 mg and ipratropium bromide, up to 0.5 mg, FDA-approved final product, noncompounded, administered through DME

J7622 Betclomethasone, inhalation solution, compounded product, administered through DME, unit dose form, per mg
Use this code for Beclovent, Beconase.
AHA: IQ, '02, 5

J7624 Betamethasone, inhalation solution, compounded product, administered through DME, unit dose form, per mg
AHA: IQ, '02, 5

J7626 Budesonide, inhalation solution. FDA-approved final product, noncompounded, administered through DME, unit dose form, up to 0.5 mg
Use this code for Pulmicort, Pulmicort Flexhaler, Pulmicort Respules, Vanceril.
AHA: IQ, '02, 5

J7627 Budesonide, Inhalation solution, compounded product, administered through DME, unit dose form, up to 0.5 mg

J7628 Bitolterol mesylate, inhalation solution, compounded product, administered through DME, concentrated form, per mg

Drugs Administered Other Than Oral method

J7512 – J7628

FIGURE 1-10 One page from the HCPCS Level II Alphanumeric Listing, showing codes J7512–J7628

Source: Center for Medicare and Medicaid Services (CMS)

Chapter Summary

Essentially, the process of coding begins with the physician's documentation stating why the patient needed care and what was done for this patient during this visit. As a professional coding specialist, you will interpret the documentation in the patient's record from medical terminology into codes: diagnosis codes to explain *why*, along with *how* and *where* if the patient is injured; and procedure codes to report *what* the physician or facility did for the patient during this encounter. You will need to confirm that the diagnosis code or codes support medical necessity for the procedures, services, and treatments provided. As you proceed through this textbook, read carefully and completely. Coding is like nothing you have experienced before, and you want to learn how to be proficient.

CODING BITES

You will learn many more details about using the HCPCS Level II code set in ***Part IV: DMEPOS & Transportation***.

CODING BITES

ICD-10-CM . . . Diagnosis Codes

- Used by all health care providers and facilities
- Report WHY the patient needed care [medical necessity]
- ICD-10-CM diagnosis codes = A12.3K5A (up to seven (7) alphanumeric)

CPT . . . Procedure Codes

- Used by physicians to report services provided at any/all facilities
- Also used by outpatient care facilities [i.e., ambulatory surgery centers, hospital emergency rooms, hospital outpatient surgery centers]
- Report WHAT was done for the patient
- CPT procedure codes = 12345 (five numbers always)

ICD-10-PCS . . . Procedure Codes

- Used only by hospitals for reporting facility services to inpatients
- ICD-10-PCS procedure codes = 012B4LZ (seven characters always)

HCPCS Level II . . . Services and Supplies Codes

- Used to report services and supplies not already represented by a code in CPT [i.e., transportation, drugs administered by a health care professional, durable medical equipment]
- Used by any facility or provider
- Not all third-party payers accept the use of HCPCS Level II codes
- HCPCS Level II codes = A1234 (one letter, four numbers always)

CHAPTER 1 REVIEW
Introduction to the Languages of Coding

Mc Graw Hill connect

Enhance your learning by completing these exercises and more at mcgrawhillconnect.com!

Let's Check It! Terminology

Match each key term to the appropriate definition.

1. **LO 1.3** The provision of medical care for a disorder or disease.
2. **LO 1.2** The state of abnormality or dysfunction.
3. **LO 1.1** The determination that the health care professional was acting according to standard practices in providing a particular procedure for an individual with a particular diagnosis.
4. **LO 1.1** The process of paying for health care services after they have been provided.

A. Classification System
B. Condition
C. Diagnosis
D. Eponym
E. External Causes
F. Inpatient

5. **LO 1.2** The explanation of how a patient became injured or poisoned, as well as other necessary details about the event; a health concern caused by something outside of the body.
6. **LO 1.1** A physician's determination of a patient's condition, illness, or injury.
7. **LO 1.1** Action taken, in accordance with the standards of care, by the physician to accomplish a predetermined objective (result); a surgical operation.
8. **LO 1.1** The category term used in health care to identify ICD-10-CM, CPT, ICD-10-PCS, and HCPCS Level II code sets.
9. **LO 1.3** A patient admitted into a hospital for an overnight stay or longer.
10. **LO 1.3** Spending time with a patient and/or family about health care situations.
11. **LO 1.3** Health care services provided to individuals without an overnight stay in the facility.
12. **LO 1.2** A disease or condition named for a person.

G. Medical Necessity
H. Outpatient
I. Procedure
J. Reimbursement
K. Services
L. Treatment

Let's Check It! Concepts

Choose the most appropriate answer for each of the following questions.

1. **LO 1.1** Coding languages communicate information that is key to which of the following aspect(s) of the health care system?
   a. medical necessity **b.** reimbursement **c.** resources allocation **d.** all of these
2. **LO 1.1** Coding is accurately interpreting health care terms and definitions into _____ that specifically convey diagnoses and procedures.
   a. letter combinations **b.** number combinations
   c. number-letter combinations **d.** numbers or number-letter combinations
3. **LO 1.1** A diagnosis explains
   a. what the provider did for the patient. **b.** who the policyholder is.
   c. why the patient requires attention of the provider. **d.** where the patient was seen by the provider.
4. **LO 1.1** A procedure explains
   a. where the patient was seen by the provider. **b.** what the provider did for the patient.
   c. why the patient requires attention of the provider. **d.** who the policyholder is.
5. **LO 1.2** Which code book contains all of the codes to report the reason why the health care provider cared for the patient during a specific encounter?
   a. ICD-10-CM code book **b.** ICD-10-PCS code book
   c. CPT code book **d.** HCPCS Level II code book
6. **LO 1.2** What part of the ICD-10-CM code book do you use to confirm that a diagnostic code is accurate?
   a. the Alphabetic Index **b.** the Index to External Causes
   c. the Tabular List **d.** the Neoplasm Table
7. **LO 1.2** Diagnostic descriptions are listed by
   a. conditions such as fractures. **b.** eponyms such as Epstein–Barr syndrome.
   c. other descriptors such as family history. **d.** all of these.
8. **LO 1.2** Which of the following would be an example of an eponym?
   a. infections **b.** wounds **c.** Arnold-Chiari disease **d.** family history
9. **LO 1.2** The Index to External Causes lists the causes of
   a. injuries and poisoning **b.** diseases and syndromes **c.** injuries **d.** poisoning
10. **LO 1.2** An example of an ICD-10-CM code is
    a. H2031 **b.** 85460 **c.** H61.022 **d.** 08NTXZZ

11. **LO 1.1** When ICD-10-CM codes support medical necessity, this means that
    - **a.** there was a valid medical reason to provide care.
    - **b.** a preexisting condition was treated.
    - **c.** the patient was seen in a hospital.
    - **d.** a licensed health care professional was involved.
12. **LO 1.1** The why justifies the
    - **a.** who
    - **b.** where
    - **c.** what
    - **d.** when
13. **LO 1.3** Surgical removal of a skin tag is an example of a
    - **a.** treatment
    - **b.** procedure
    - **c.** service
    - **d.** diagnosis
14. **LO 1.3** _____ tests or procedures are performed to provide the physician with additional information to support the determination of a confirmed diagnosis.
    - **a.** Diagnostic
    - **b.** Preventive
    - **c.** Therapeutic
    - **d.** Conditional
15. **LO 1.3** The code set(s) available for the coding specialist to use to translate health care procedures, services, and treatments into codes is/are
    - **a.** CPT code book.
    - **b.** ICD-10-PCS code book.
    - **c.** HCPCS Level II code book.
    - **d.** all of these.
16. **LO 1.3** The main body of the CPT book has _____ sections.
    - **a.** 5
    - **b.** 6
    - **c.** 7
    - **d.** 8
17. **LO 1.3** An example of a Category II code is
    - **a.** 89398
    - **b.** 1134F
    - **c.** V95.9
    - **d.** 0241T
18. **LO 1.3** The code set used for hospital facility reporting of procedures, services, and treatments provided to a patient who has been admitted as an inpatient is
    - **a.** ICD-10-CM code book.
    - **b.** CPT code book.
    - **c.** ICD-10-PCS code book.
    - **d.** HCPCS Level II code book.
19. **LO 1.4** HCPCS Level II codes are presented as
    - **a.** five numbers.
    - **b.** one letter followed by four numbers.
    - **c.** four numbers followed by two letters.
    - **d.** one letter, a dash, and four numbers.
20. **LO 1.4** An example of a HCPCS Level II code is
    - **a.** J3285
    - **b.** D7056ZZ
    - **c.** 58940
    - **d.** T84.010D

Let's Check It! Rules and Regulations

Please answer the following questions from the knowledge you have gained after reading this chapter.

1. **LO 1.1** Explain what is meant by a third-party payer.
2. **LO 1.2** Describe the Tabular List of Diseases and Injuries, including its format and why it is important.
3. **LO 1.3** Explain the difference between diagnostic testing, preventive procedures, and therapeutic procedures.
4. **LO 1.1** Discuss medical necessity and its importance.
5. **LO 1.4** Do all insurance carriers accept HCPCS Level II codes, and what is the responsibility of the coding specialist in regard to billing third-party payers?

2

Abstracting Clinical Documentation

Key Terms

Abstracting
Assume
Co-morbidity
Demographic
Interpret
Manifestation
Query
Sequela
Signs
Symptoms

Learning Outcomes

After completing this chapter, the student should be able to:

LO 2.1 Identify which health care professional for whom you are coding.
LO 2.2 Describe the process of abstracting physician documentation and operative notes.
LO 2.3 Recognize the terms used to describe diagnoses in documentation.
LO 2.4 Distinguish between co-morbidities, manifestations, and sequelae.
LO 2.5 Determine those conditions that require external cause codes to be reported.
LO 2.6 Recognize the terms used to describe procedures, services, and treatments provided.
LO 2.7 Create a legal query to obtain documentation about a missing, ambiguous, or contradictory component in the existing documentation.

2.1 For Whom You Are Reporting

Most people do not realize how many coders are involved in reporting one patient's surgical procedure or other type of encounter. Let's look at a scenario and dissect it:

Carly Camden, a 27-year-old female, was admitted into the hospital to have surgery on her broken leg.

- The surgeon will have a coder to report what he does for Carly.
- The anesthesiologist will have a coder to report administration of anesthesia.
- The facility will have a coder to report what the hospital did for Carly (providing the nursing and other support staff, equipment, and room). In this case, the facility is an acute care hospital. In other cases, the facility may be a same day surgery center, a skilled nursing facility, an imaging center, or another health care organization.
- The radiologist will have a coder to report for any imaging (e.g., x-rays, MRI, CT scan).
- The pathologist will have a coder to report for any blood work or lab tests provided.

Therefore, the first question you, as the professional coder, will need to ask is . . . for whom are you reporting? Only then will you know which key terms to look for as you abstract the operative notes, the physician's notes, and the reports.

CODING BITES

Patient = *Who* is provided with care

Physician = *Who* is the health care provider you are representing

Diagnosis = *Why* the provider is caring for this individual during this encounter

External Cause = *How* and *Where* the patient became injured

Procedure = *What* the provider did for the individual

Facility = *Where* the services were provided

There may also be many professionals providing different types of care for one patient for different reasons. For example:

Allen Davidson, a 59-year-old male, was admitted to the hospital due to a myocardial infarction (heart attack). Allen has type 2 diabetes mellitus.

- A cardiologist (heart specialist) will diagnose and treat Allen's heart problem.
- An endocrinologist will diagnose and treat Allen's diabetes mellitus.
- The facility, such as a hospital, will provide care for Allen and all of his health concerns.

GUIDANCE CONNECTION

Read the **ICD-10-CM Official Guidelines for Coding and Reporting , Section B, 14.** ***Documentation by Clinicians Other than the Patient's Provider*** which informs medical coders when it is acceptable to determine which code to report based on the documentation of providers, other than the primary or attending physician, who are involved in the patient's care.

For all professionals involved in the care of a patient, the reason or reasons *why (diagnosis code or codes)* care was required are critical to establishing medical necessity for the *what (specific procedures, services, and treatments)* were provided. In a location, such as an acute care facility (hospital), there may be issues for you to evaluate and connect involving the input from multiple types of health care practitioners.

2.2 The Process of Abstracting

You are learning that documentation about the encounter between physician and patient will be your primary source for details that you will use to determine the most accurate codes to report. Physicians, though, do not write their documentation solely for coding; therefore, there will be pieces of information included that you will not use in your coding process. Reading the entire patient record and pulling out the details necessary for determining the correct codes is known as **abstracting**.

Abstracting
The process of identifying the relevant words or phrases in health care documentation in order to determine the best, most appropriate code(s).

Establishing Medical Necessity

You, as a professional medical coder, determine which codes you report to tell the whole story... the connection between what was provided and why it was necessary, in accordance with the standards of care. This detail is fundamental to reimbursement because the lack of medical necessity is a valid reason for a third-party payer to deny a claim. Think about it ... who would pay for a procedure to be performed that the patient doesn't need?

Whether an office visit or open-heart surgery, every claim must have at least one diagnosis code and at least one procedure code. Every patient must have a reason for needing the care from this health professional, as explained by ICD-10-CM code(s). Further, it is expected that the health professional will do something for this patient, related to that reason, during this encounter, as reported with CPT or ICD-10-PCS code(s).

Assume or Interpret

Always keep in mind the professional coding specialists' motto: "*If it isn't documented, it didn't happen. If it didn't happen, you can't code it!*"

If it *is* documented appropriately, there is no reason for you to **assume** any details; you only need to **interpret** what is documented.

Assume
Suppose to be the case, without proof; guess the intended details.

Interpret
Explain the meaning of; convert a meaning from one language to another.

One of the most challenging aspects of coding is the very fine line between assuming and interpreting. Yes, professional coding specialists must interpret the physician's documentation. This does not include assuming in any way. Assuming is making up details, filling in the blanks with your own specifics, guessing, or substituting your own knowledge for missing facts. Interpreting is an exact science; it involves changing information from one language to another. Just like *casa* = house (Spanish-to-English), fine needle aspiration = 10021 (medical terminology-to-CPT). This is why coding can be so challenging. We are responsible for not only translating from one language (medical terminology) to another (medical codes) but also for accurately figuring out into *which* language (CPT or ICD-10-CM or ICD-10-PCS or HCPCS Level II) medical terminology must be translated. Another major factor is that no one is a natural-born speaker of medical terminology, so you are required to learn a new language to understand the languages of medical coding. Imagine if you were born speaking English, but you had to learn to speak French before achieving your ultimate goal of interpreting French words into Spanish.

CODING BITES

Keep a medical dictionary by your side so that the minute you come upon a word you don't understand for an absolute fact, you can look it up right away. If you don't understand what you are reading, you will not be able to interpret it accurately.

EXCELLENT RESOURCE: ***MedlinePlus***, an online medical dictionary and encyclopedia, is an excellent and reliable source created and maintained by the U.S. National Library of Medicine.

Source Documents

The patient's health care record is at the center of health information management in general as well as the primary focus for you, as the professional coding specialist. Within this record, whether it is written on paper or typed into an electronic health record (EHR), are several important components that you will use to gather details necessary to determine the correct code or codes.

> **Demographic**
> Demographic details include the patient's name, address, date of birth, and other personal details, not specifically related to health.

Virtually every patient record should include all, or most, of these pages or sections:

- *Patient's Registration Form:* This document or section includes the patient's **demographic** information, as well as health insurance policy numbers and the name of the individual who will be financially responsible for the patient's care.
- *Referral Authorization Form:* If another physician or health care provider referred this patient for a consultation, you will need to know this to determine the correct evaluation and management code.
- *Physician's Notes/Operative Reports:* Written documentation of what occurred during the encounter between physician and patient is also known as clinical documentation. The physician's notes or operative reports are your most important source for details required to determine the most accurate code or codes. Your job is to interpret the words–medical terminology–into codes. Your ability to interpret accurately is dependent upon your knowledge of anatomy and physiology, as well as medical terminology.
- *Pathology and Laboratory Reports:* Results of testing performed on blood, tissue, and other specimens hold important keys to the patient's condition. The results can provide you with important details necessary for you to determine a specific, accurate code.
- *Imaging Reports:* Similar to pathology reports, these are reports written by a radiologist containing his or her interpretations of images taken of the patient [e.g., x-ray, CT scan, MRI].
- *Medication Logs:* If the facility is residential, such as an acute care hospital, skilled nursing facility, long-term care facility, the nursing staff must record every time they administer a medication to a patient, including the drug name, dosage, time administered, and route used for administration. All data must be reported.
- *Allergy List:* This list is included for the patient's safety so health care professionals can avoid giving the patient any substance to which he or she may be allergic.
- *History and Physical (H&P):* Essentially, this document, written by the admitting physician, explains the background and current issues used to make the decision to admit the patient into the hospital.
- *Consultation Reports:* When a specialist is asked by an attending physician to evaluate a patient's condition, a report is written and sent over to be included in the patient's medical record in the requesting physician's files, as well as those belonging to the consulting physician.
- *Discharge Summary:* At the time a patient is released from a facility, such as a hospital, the Discharge Summary provides the conclusions and results of the patient's stay in the facility in addition to follow-up advice.

CODING BITES

Principles of Documentation for Medical Records

Adapted from the Centers for Medicare and Medicaid Services

1. The documentation of each patient encounter should include:
   - the date;
   - the reason for the encounter;
   - appropriate history and physical exam in relationship to the patient's chief complaint;
   - review of lab, x-ray data, and other ancillary services, where appropriate;
   - assessment; and
   - a plan for care (including discharge plan, if appropriate).
2. Past and present diagnoses should be accessible.
3. The reasons for–and results of–x-rays, lab tests, and other ancillary services should be documented or included in the medical record.
4. Relevant health risk factors should be identified.
5. The patient's progress, including response to treatment, change in treatment, change in diagnosis, and patient noncompliance, should be documented.
6. The written plan for care should include, when appropriate:
   - treatments and medications, specifying frequency and dosage;
   - any referrals and consultations;
   - patient/family education; and
   - specific instructions for follow-up.

(continued)

7. The documentation should support the intensity of the patient evaluation and/or the treatment, including thought processes and the complexity of medical decision making as it relates to the patient's chief complaint for the encounter.
8. All entries to the medical record should be dated and authenticated.
9. The CPT/ICD-10-CM/ICD-10-PCS/HCPCS Level II codes reported on the claim form should be supported by the documentation in the medical record.

Abstracting the Documentation

Abstracting is the first step in the coding process. You must read all clinical documentation related to the specific encounter all the way through, slowly and carefully. Whether the encounter was a short visit in a physician's office, an hours-long surgical procedure documented in operative reports, or a five-day stay in a hospital, you cannot expect that one sentence will give you a clear and complete picture of *what* occurred (the procedures or services) and *why* they were provided (the diagnosis or diagnoses). You learned about understanding the *why* and *what* in the ***Introduction to the Languages of Coding*** chapter. You are required to code all conditions documented to be relevant during this encounter or hospital stay, not just those in the official diagnostic statement. The same stands for the procedures.

CODING BITES

One suggestion is to use scrap paper so you can jot down details as you read them, which may point toward *why* the patient required the attention of the physician (e.g., signs, symptoms, confirmed diagnoses), as well as *what* was provided (e.g., specific procedures, services, and treatments).

Reasons That Are Not Illness; Procedures That Are Not Actions

There are times when an individual comes to see a health care provider without having a particular illness or injury. In such cases, you might assign a diagnosis code that explains *why* the patient was seen that is not a current health condition or injury. A healthy person might go to see a physician for preventive care, for routine and administrative exams, or for monitoring care and screenings for someone with a personal history or family history of a condition. As you read through the documentation, you may discover that the reason *why* the encounter was necessary may be wellness, rather than illness or injury.

In the same fashion, the description of *what* the physician provided may not be a procedure, service, or treatment. It may be advice or a second opinion. The physician and patient may meet to discuss previously done test results, a recommendation for a specific treatment plan, suggestions for risk-factor reduction (e.g., stop smoking), or a referral to another physician or facility.

CODING BITES

Every health care professional/patient encounter must have at least one reportable [codeable] reason *why* and at least one reportable [codeable] explanation of *what*.

2.3 Deconstructing Diagnostic Statements

Diagnosis codes, for either reimbursement or statistical purposes, will report only those conditions addressed by the provider during a specific encounter and not the patient's entire health history. When there is no confirmed diagnosis to provide medical necessity for a procedure, service, or treatment performed, determining the diagnosis code to report will vary slightly, depending on whether you are coding for an inpatient or outpatient encounter.

- In an outpatient encounter, if there is no confirmed diagnostic statement, you will code the patient's **signs** and/or **symptoms** that led to the physician's decision for the next step in care.
- When an inpatient (admitted into the hospital) is being discharged without a confirmed diagnosis, you will code the suspected conditions listed on the discharge summary as if they were confirmed. You will not code the signs and symptoms.

Signs
Measurable indicators of a patient's health status.

Symptom
A subjective sensation or departure from the norm as related by the patient.

Dissect the Diagnostic Statement

Now that you have identified all of the statements in the documentation that explain *why* the patient was cared for, take each statement apart to determine which word identifies the disease, illness, condition, or primary reason for the visit (also known as the "main term"). Separate this term from any words that may simply describe the type of condition or the location of the condition (anatomical site/body site). Keep a medical dictionary close by so you can look up any terms you don't clearly understand. Remember, if you do not completely understand the terms, how can you possibly interpret them?

Why is the physician caring for the patient? Many diagnostic statements are made up of multiple words, with each providing additional information. As you analyze the examples below, dissect the condition for which the physician is seeing the patient and separate out those terms used to provide more detail about that condition.

- *Herpes zoster* . . . The disease is "herpes" and "zoster" is the type of herpes.
- *Acute bronchospasm* . . . The condition is a "spasm" (muscle contraction) of the bronchus (a part of the lungs) and the term "acute" (which means severe) describes what type of bronchospasm the patient has.
- *Personal history of lung cancer* . . . The issue of concern is "history"—why the patient is being seen. The type of history is "personal" and the secondary descriptor is "malignant neoplasm of the lung (lung cancer)" to explain "a history of what?"
- *Myocardial infarction* . . . The condition is "infarction" (area of dead tissue) and "myocardial" (heart muscle) is the anatomical site of the infarction.
- *Congenital pneumothorax* . . . The condition is "pneumothorax" (air in the chest cavity) and the term "congenital" (present at birth) describes the cause of the condition.
- *Family history of renal failure* . . . The issue of concern is "history"—why the patient is being seen. The type of history is "family" and the secondary descriptor is "renal failure" (loss of function of the kidneys) to explain "a history of what?"

CODING BITES

A diagnostic term might have a suffix like:

Dermatitis *derma* = skin + *-itis* = inflammation (a condition)

Acrophobia *acro* = heights + *-phobia* = fear (a condition)

A procedural term might have a suffix like:

Pancreatectomy *pancreat* = pancreas + *-ectomy* = to surgically remove (an action)

Conjunctivoplasty *conjunctivo* = conjunctiva (part of the eye) + *-plasty* = to repair (an action)

LET'S CODE IT! SCENARIO

Dr. Olivera diagnosed Kathleen Belsara with ulcerative blepharitis of the right upper eyelid. He treated her with an injection of gentamicin 80 mg, IM, and gave her a prescription for gentamicin ointment 0.3% q.i.d. for 7 to 10 days.

Let's Code It!

Why did Dr. Olivera care for Kathleen? *ulcerative blepharitis of the right upper eyelid.*

The condition is: *blepharitis*

The type of blepharitis: *ulcerative*

Anatomical site affected: *right upper eyelid*

NOTE: These first three steps will get you started when it comes to determining the correct diagnosis code in ICD-10-CM. You will learn more about this beginning in the chapter ***Introduction to ICD-10-CM***.

Also . . .

What did Dr. Olivera do for Kathleen? *an injection of gentamicin 80 mg, IM*

The drug: *gentamicin*

The dosage: *80 mg*

The route of administration: *IM (intramuscular) injection*

NOTE: These first three steps will get you started when it comes to determining the correct drug code in HCPCS Level II. You will learn more about this beginning in the chapter ***HCPCS Level II***.

Recognize Inclusive Signs and Symptoms

As you abstract the documentation, you will need to identify any signs and symptoms that are already part of the description of a confirmed diagnosis. Physicians are trained in medical school to add all of the data (history, signs, symptoms, test results) together, almost like a math equation, to arrive at a diagnosis. This sign + that symptom = this diagnosis. These equations are based on the standards of care accepted by the health care industry around the world.

Think about it: *John comes to see Dr. Finch complaining of chest congestion, runny nose, sneezing, headaches, being achy all over. Dr. Finch examines John, does a quick lab test, and tells John he has the flu.*

It is a fact that "chest congestion, runny nose, sneezing, headaches, being achy all over" are signs and symptoms of the flu. Therefore, when you report the code for the flu, there is no reason to also code the signs and symptoms of the flu . . . it is redundant.

GUIDANCE CONNECTION

Read the ICD-10-CM Official Guidelines for Coding and Reporting, section **I. Conventions, General Coding Guidelines and Chapter- Specific Guidelines**; subsections

- **B.4** ***Signs and Symptoms***
- **B.5** ***Conditions that are an integral part of a disease process***
- **B.6** ***Conditions that are not an integral part of a disease process***

LET'S CODE IT! SCENARIO

Ralph Carbonna, a 61-year-old male, came into the Emergency Department of McGraw General Hospital. Earlier in the day, Ralph felt lightheaded and a little dizzy. In addition, he complained that his heart was beating so wildly that he thought he may have had a heart attack. When interviewed by the nurse, Ralph revealed his previous diagnosis of type 1 diabetes mellitus, prompting Dr. Geller to order a blood glucose test. Dr. Geller also ordered an EKG (ECG) to check Ralph's heart. After getting the results of the tests, Dr. Geller determined that Ralph's lightheadedness and dizziness were a result of his abnormal glucose level. He spoke with Ralph about how to bring his diabetes mellitus under control and informed Ralph that the EKG was negative [normal], meaning there were no signs of a heart attack.

Let's Code It!

Dr. Geller confirmed that Ralph's *type 1 diabetes mellitus*, specifically his abnormal glucose level, caused his feelings of dizziness. Diabetes seems to be the only confirmed diagnosis in Dr. Geller's notes. You can report this with confidence, and this condition justifies performing the blood glucose test.

Dr. Geller also ordered an EKG (ECG). A diagnosis for diabetes does not provide any medical rationale for doing an EKG. In addition, the test was negative and, therefore, provided no diagnosis.

You still need a diagnosis code to report that there was a medical necessity to run the EKG. Why did Dr. Geller order the EKG? Because Ralph complained of a *rapid heartbeat*. A rapid heartbeat provides the medical necessity for performing the EKG.

Before you confirm any codes, be certain to read all notations and symbols and check the Official Guidelines. Now, you can continue with confidence.

For the encounter, you have one confirmed diagnosis (the diabetes) and one symptom unrelated to the confirmed diagnosis (rapid heartbeat).

GUIDANCE CONNECTION

Read the ICD-10-CM Official Guidelines for Coding and Reporting, section **I. Conventions, General Coding Guidelines and Chapter-Specific Guidelines**; subsection **B.18. Use of Sign/Symptom/Unspecified Codes**. "*If a definitive diagnosis has not been established by the end of the encounter, it is appropriate to report codes for sign(s) and/or symptoms in lieu of a definitive diagnosis.*"

Section **II. Selection of Principal Diagnosis**, subsection **H. Uncertain Diagnosis**. "*If the diagnosis documented at the time of discharge is qualified as 'probable', 'suspected', 'likely', 'questionable', 'possible', or 'still to be ruled out', or other similar terms indicating uncertainty, code the condition as if it existed or was established.*" NOTE: This guideline is applicable only to inpatient admissions to short-term, acute, long-term care, and psychiatric hospitals.

2.4 Identifying Manifestations, Co-morbidities, and Sequelae

Manifestations

Manifestation
A condition that develops as the result of another, underlying condition.

CODING BITES

The underlying condition is known as the etiology–the original source or cause for the development of a disease or condition.

There are some diseases (also known as *underlying conditions*) that actually cause patients to develop other conditions. This second condition, directly the result of the first condition, is known as a **manifestation**. In these cases, scientific evidence proves that the patient would not have the manifested disease or problem if the first condition had not already been present. The cause-and-effect relationship between the two conditions must be documented by the physician and supported by medical research to be coded as a manifestation.

A manifestation is a second condition CAUSED by a first condition. Let's use diabetes mellitus as an example. Diabetes is known to cause problems with patients' eyes. The physician determined that the patient has diabetic retinopathy with macular edema. This documentation confirms that diabetes CAUSED the retinopathy to develop. You often will find combination codes in ICD-10-CM. These codes report both the underlying condition and the manifestation. In our example, the combination code is

E11.3513 Type 2 diabetes mellitus with proliferative diabetic retinopathy with macular edema, bilateral

This one code, E11.3513, tells the whole story about this patient's condition. However, not all conditions and their manifestations have combination codes from which to choose. When an appropriate combination code is not available, you will need to select two codes (or more) to clearly communicate the complete story of a patient's diagnosis. One example is a patient who is admitted to the hospital with pulmonary histoplasmosis, a documented manifestation of the patient's HIV-positive status. In this case, there is no combination code, so two codes are needed to tell the whole story of this patient's condition.

B20 Human immunodeficiency virus [HIV] disease

B39.0 Acute pulmonary histoplasmosis capsulati

Co-Morbidities

Co-morbidity
A separate diagnosis existing in the same patient at the same time as an unrelated diagnosis.

A **co-morbidity** is a condition that is present in the same body at the same time as another problem or disease, but the two conditions are unrelated–there is no documented cause-and-effect relationship. These "other diagnoses" may be referred to in the physician's documentation. However, only those conditions that the physician has specifically evaluated, treated, or ordered additional testing for or those requiring additional monitoring, nursing care, or more time in the hospital should be reported with a code.

EXAMPLE

Lindsey, 28-weeks pregnant, fell and broke her leg. Therefore, the pregnancy and the fracture are co-morbidities—they are two conditions present in the same patient at the same time. You know that being pregnant does not cause a fracture and a fracture does not cause pregnancy.

Which code will you report first? The code that is the reason for the encounter with the physician. You are coding for Dr. Kessler, an orthopedist, and Lindsey comes in because her leg hurts. Dr. Kessler confirms her leg is fractured, so the fracture will be reported first because this is Dr. Kessler's primary concern–caring for the fracture. However, Dr. Kessler MUST take the pregnancy into consideration because pregnancy is a systemic condition and will impact the treatment plan for the fracture. The pregnancy code also will be reported (after the fracture code).

EXAMPLE

Mary-Ellen's history includes asthma. She is here to see the dermatologist to have a benign mole removed from her arm. Dr. Callen does not ask about Mary-Ellen's asthma. The asthma does not have any relationship at all to the benign mole or the care/treatment of the mole. You will only determine the correct diagnosis code for the benign mole. The asthma will NOT be reported at all.

EXAMPLE

Paul's history includes asthma. He is here to see Dr. Hannah, his family physician, for his annual checkup. Dr. Hannah asks Paul about his asthma and writes a prescription for a refill for his inhaler. In addition to the annual exam code, you also will need to report the code for the asthma because the physician paid attention to it during this encounter.

Sequelae

A **sequela** is the residual impact of a previous condition or injury that may need the attention of a physician. When the patient has come to see the health care professional for the treatment of a sequela (also known as a late effect), you must code the particular problem as a sequela only in the following situations:

- Scarring.
- Nonunion of a fracture.
- Malunion of a fracture.
- When the connection is specifically documented by the physician or health care professional confirming the new condition as a sequela (a late effect) of a previous condition.

Coding a sequela requires at least two codes, in the following order:

1. The sequela condition, which is the condition that resulted and is being treated, such as a scar or paralysis.
2. The sequela (late effect) or original-condition code with the seventh character "S."

GUIDANCE CONNECTION

Read the ICD-10-CM Official Guidelines for Coding and Reporting, section **III. Reporting Additional Diagnoses**.

Sequela
A cause-and-effect relationship between an original condition that has been resolved with a current condition; also known as a late effect.

EXAMPLE

Jenna Malaletto, an 18-year-old female, was using a hydrofluoric acid mixture to etch glass for an art class last spring and got some on her left forearm, causing a corrosion burn of the third degree. She came in today to see Dr. Rosen to discuss treatment options for the adherent scarring.

Dr. Rosen is discussing treatment options of the scars that were left behind after the third-degree corrosion burn had healed. This is known as a sequela, and it is the reason for this encounter. However, as you learned, you also will need to report what caused the scar—the corrosion burn.

L90.5	**Scar conditions and fibrosis of skin (adherent scar)**
T22.712S	**Corrosion of third degree of left forearm, sequela**

2.5 Reporting External Causes

You learned in the *Introduction to the Languages of Coding* chapter that in addition to the *why* and the *what*, if a patient is injured, you will need to abstract details about *how* and *where* the patient became injured. As you learn more about determining external cause codes, you will discover that a simple statement such as "the patient was hurt in a car accident" does not contain enough information to determine the accurate external cause code. The details of the accident are very important. For example:

CODING BITES

You will learn a lot more about reporting co-morbidities, manifestations, and sequelae in ***Part II: Reporting Diagnoses***.

- Was the patient the driver, a passenger, or outside of the vehicle?
- Was the vehicle a car, a pick-up truck, a van, or a heavy transport vehicle?
- Did the vehicle collide with another vehicle, a nonmotor vehicle, or a stationary object?
- Was this a traffic accident or a nontraffic accident?

ICD-10-CM

LET'S CODE IT! SCENARIO

Victor Lamza, a 13-year-old male, was brought into the Emergency Department complaining of pain after he banged his head. Dr. Farxia diagnosed him with a contusion of the scalp. When asked by Dr. Farxia what he was doing immediately before he got hurt, he reluctantly admitted that he had made a bet with his friends at Space Camp. They wanted to see who could stay the longest in the weightlessness simulator; Victor was in there for 6 hours.

Let's Code It!

Dr. Farxia documented that Victor's staying too long in the weightlessness simulator caused the contusion of his scalp. You will need to code why Dr. Farxia cared for Victor (his injury), how he became injured, and where he was when the injury occurred.

S00.03XA	**Contusion of scalp, initial encounter**
X52.XXXA	**Prolonged stay in weightless environment, initial encounter**
Y92.838	**Other recreation area as the place of occurrence of the external cause**
Y93.89	**Activity, other specified**
Y99.8	**Other external cause status (recreation or sport not for income or while a student)**

There are thousands of different ways a patient can become injured, and there is a different code for almost every incident: the typical, the silly, the unusual, and the surprising.

ICD-10-CM provides a separate *Index to External Causes*, usually found between the Index to Diseases and Injuries (Alphabetic Index) and the beginning of the Tabular List. This index will point you to the correct subsection in the Tabular List, within the code range of V00–Y99.

You will learn more details about how to code external causes later in this textbook in the chapter ***Coding Injury, Poisoning, and External Causes.***

2.6 Deconstructing Procedural Statements

In addition to abstracting the terms from the documentation related to the diagnosis code or codes, you also will need to identify those terms that relate to what was done for the patient.

Due to the structure of medical terminology, you might find that the word or term mentioned in the documentation describing what was done for the patient is a combination term identifying both the action taken and the anatomical site on which the action was performed.

EXAMPLES

i. Neuroplasty: *neuro* = nerves + *-plasty* = repair
ii. Thrombolysis: *thrombo* = blood clot + *-lysis* = dissolving
iii. Gastrectomy: *gastr* = stomach + *-ectomy* = surgical removal

Other times, the procedure will be identified by its name. This name may be

- a description of the action, such as ablation, debridement, or injection.
- an eponym (named after the individual who invented it), such as Abbe-Estlander procedure, Swan-Ganz catheter, or Dupuy-Dutemps operation.
- an abbreviation or acronym, such as ECG = electrocardiography; GTT = glucose tolerance test; PET = positron emission tomography; TAVR = transcatheter aortic valve replacement.

CODING BITES

Only the procedures, services, and treatments actually provided during a specific encounter, by a specific physician, health care professional, or facility, will be coded.

Review and practice your medical terminology and keep a medical dictionary close at hand. As you gain more experience, the process of deconstructing the statements in the various types of documentation will become easier (not really easy, but easier). You learned about the part of this career that involves interpreting and you cannot interpret the words if you don't know what they mean.

Interpreting for Each Code Set

You will find that you not only need to understand medical terminology overall to interpret the physician's documentation into codes; each code set may require you to interpret them differently.

LET'S CODE IT! SCENARIO

McGRAW GENERAL HOSPITAL

PATIENT: Christine Gordon
PREOPERATIVE DIAGNOSIS: Acute right lower abdominal pain.
POSTOPERATIVE DIAGNOSIS: Acute appendicitis.
OPERATION PERFORMED: Laparoscopic appendectomy.
SURGEON: Charles E. Manchester, MD
SEDATION: General endotracheal anesthetic.

PROCEDURE:

This 47-year-old female presented with signs and symptoms consistent with acute appendicitis. Preoperative CT scan indicates an inflamed appendix, rupture not probable. Patient signed written consent for a laparoscopic appendectomy.

Let's Code It!

The documentation created by Dr. Manchester clearly provides us with the details of what occurred during this encounter with this patient, Christine Gordon. She was having lower right side abdominal pain, which was determined to be appendicitis (*why* reported with ICD-10-CM code K35.80 Acute Appendicitis Not Otherwise Specified) and the doctor performed a surgical laparoscopic appendectomy (*what*). Seems very straightforward, doesn't it?

A good place to begin is the CPT Alphabetic Index; look up:

Appendectomy
Appendix Excision 44950, 44955, 44960
Laparoscopic 44970

Turn to the Main Section of CPT to find code 44970 because Dr. Manchester specifically documented that the appendectomy was done laparoscopically. Therefore, now you have found the correct code to report for Dr. Manchester's work:

44970 Laparoscopy, surgical, appendectomy

--*

Now, if you were the coder for the hospital at which the surgery occurred, you would need to report this same procedure using the ICD-10-PCS code set.

(continued)

Dr. Manchester performed this surgical procedure on Christine Gordon in the hospital. The hospital provided the support staff (nurses, technicians), as well as the equipment, the room, etc. You learned earlier that the hospital's coder would use ICD-10-PCS codes to report their participation and care for this patient. Let's look at the documentation again . . .

"the doctor performed a surgical laparoscopic appendectomy"

In the ICD-10-PCS code book's Alphabetic Index, you will see:

Appendectomy

see Excision, Appendix 0DBJ

see Resection, Appendix 0DTJ

Which is correct? The ICD-10-PCS code book includes the definitions right in the front of the code book:

Excision: Cutting out or off, without replacement, a portion of a body part

Resection: Cutting out or off, without replacement, all of a body part

You learned in medical terminology class that appendectomy = surgical removal of the appendix. Therefore, you have documentation that the entire appendix was surgically removed, and this is called "*Resection*" by ICD-10-PCS. Terrific! Now we will turn to the 0DT Table in ICD-10-PCS.

First character: Section: **Medical and Surgical 0**

This is correct because this was a surgical procedure.

Second character: System: **Gastrointestinal System D**

You know this is correct because you learned in anatomy class that the appendix is part of the gastrointestinal system.

Third character: Root Operation: **Resection T**

You confirmed this by reading the root operation term definition for "resection" and comparing it with the physician's documentation.

Fourth character: Body Part: **Appendix J**

The documentation clearly states the appendix is the body part that was removed.

Fifth character: Approach: **Percutaneous Endoscopic 4**

The documentation states that this procedure was performed laparoscopically. A laparoscope is an endoscope passed through the skin of the abdomen using small slits (percutaneously). Therefore, you know that this procedure was done using a percutaneous endoscopic approach.

Sixth character: Device: **None Z**

Seventh character: Qualifier: **None Z**

Great! Therefore, if you were the coder for the hospital where Dr. Manchester performed surgery, you would report ICD-10-PCS code

0DTJ4ZZ Resection of the appendix, via percutaneous endoscope

Good work!

You can see how the two procedure code sets, CPT and ICD-10-PCS, use different terms to describe and report the same procedure. Use your resources, like a medical dictionary, and you will be able to interpret all of the terms correctly.

2.7 How to Query

Query
To ask.

Once you have completed abstracting the documentation, you may find that details needed to determine a specific code are not included. Should this happen, you should **query** the physician who wrote the documentation to ask him or her to provide clarification or additional specifics. Every day, coders and health information management specialists find documentation with information that is

- Missing or incomplete
  - for example, *What specific type of fracture?*
- Ambiguous or inconsistent
  - for example, *Procedure notes state a single lead pacemaker was inserted; however, the equipment list states the pacemaker was dual lead.*
- Contradictory
  - for example, *In first paragraph, notes state, "Patient denies any cough or chest congestion."; however, last paragraph states patient was prescribed Tessalon (a cough suppressant).*

In **Section 2.2**, *The Process of Abstracting*, you learned the difference between assuming and interpreting. Therefore, you will need to ask the physician to add the details you need to the patient's record so you can move forward and determine the correct code. This process is known as creating a query, and it must be done in a very specific manner so as not to break the law.

Writing the Query

Remember that one important use of codes is to determine reimbursement. Different codes are paid at different amounts. [You will learn more about this in the ***Reimbursement*** chapter.] When writing a query, the law does not permit you to prompt or promote a specific response so you don't inadvertently influence the physician to opt for the higher-paying detail rather than the truth. This means you must ask for the details in a nonleading manner. Asking open-ended questions and providing multiple options for the answer are the best approaches.

EXAMPLES

Dr. Osage saw Jose Ramirez and documented him to have a displaced fracture of the metatarsal bone of the right foot.

After rereading the operative notes again, and reviewing the entire patient record, you discover that the detail of which specific bone was fractured is missing. Therefore, you need to query Dr. Osage.

Open-ended query:

Which metatarsal bone was fractured?

Multiple-choice query:

Which metatarsal bone was fractured?

A. First
B. Second
C. Third
D. Fourth
E. Fifth

--*

Dr. Stabler performed a total hysterectomy on Melinda Blaudon.

After rereading the operative notes again, and reviewing the entire patient record, you discover that the detail of which approach was used to perform the hysterectomy is missing. Therefore, you need to query Dr. Stabler.

Open-ended query:

What approach was used in the surgery?

Multiple-choice query:

What approach was used in the surgery?

A. Open
B. Percutaneous endoscopic [Laparoscopic]
C. Via natural orifice

> **CODING BITES**
>
> Before using an unspecified diagnosis code, query the physician to gain the details needed to use a more specific code. Unspecified or NOS (not otherwise specified) codes should only be used as a last resort when the physician cannot be contacted.

The query you write to request the specific details needed should be accompanied by the pertinent clinical information from the patient's chart. You want to make it clear to the physician what you need clarified or supported with more details. There are many query templates available and often larger organizations have their own versions, already approved by attorneys.

Query Pathways

The specific details will need to be added to the chart in a time-efficient manner; therefore, the way you deliver the query to the physician is important. Most facilities have an existing process for delivering a query to the attending physician. Certainly, in a physician's office or small clinic, it may be easier than in a hospital to connect with the physician to ask a question or questions and obtain a response or responses.

Some electronic health records (EHR) software programs include a query feature. Alternatively, using a secure, encrypted e-mail system can provide a swift route for asking for the details required as well as a written response. Remember our creed: "*If it's not documented, it didn't happen. If it didn't happen, you cannot code it!*" This reinforces the importance of obtaining those additional specifics in writing from the physician.

For those facilities still using paper patient records, query notes should be attached to the front of charts, so all relevant information about that patient, for that encounter, is at hand and easy for the physician to reference and annotate.

Chapter Summary

In preparation for you to learn the process of determining the specific code or codes, you must be able to gather the required information from the clinical documentation. You must read through the clinical documentation in the patient's record and understand everything you read so you can collect the specifics you need. If details are missing, ambiguous, or conflicting, you will need to query the physician to have the documentation amended. This is your responsibility and a critical part of the coding process.

CHAPTER 2 REVIEW
Abstracting Clinical Documentation

Let's Check It! Terminology

Match each key term to the appropriate definition.

1. **LO 2.2** Suppose to be the case, without proof; guess the intended details.
2. **LO 2.3** A patient's subjective description of feeling.
3. **LO 2.7** To ask; an official request to the attending physician for more specific information related to a patient's condition or treatment.
4. **LO 2.3** Measurable indicators of a patient's health status.
5. **LO 2.2** The patient's name, address, date of birth, and other personal details, not specifically related to health.
6. **LO 2.2** Explain the meaning of; convert a meaning from one language to another.
7. **LO 2.4** A cause-and-effect relationship between an original condition that has been resolved with a current condition; also known as a late effect.
8. **LO 2.4** A condition that develops as the result of another, underlying condition.
9. **LO 2.2** Identifying the key words or terms needed to determine the accurate code.
10. **LO 2.4** A separate condition or illness present in the same patient at the same time as another, unrelated condition or illness.

A. Abstracting
B. Assume
C. Co-morbidity
D. Demographic
E. Interpret
F. Manifestation
G. Query
H. Sequela
I. Signs
J. Symptoms

Let's Check It! Concepts

Choose the most appropriate answer for each of the following questions.

1. **LO 2.1** The first question you, as the professional coder, will need to ask is
   a. does the patient have health insurance? **b.** is there a preexisting condition?
   c. for whom are you reporting? **d.** is this encounter to treat a sequela?
2. **LO 2.1** The_______will have a coder to report for any imaging procedures.
   a. anesthesiologist **b.** radiologist **c.** cardiologist **d.** pathologist
3. **LO 2.1** Which of the following is an acute care facility?
   a. The physician's office **b.** A nursing facility
   c. A hospital **d.** An assisted-living facility
4. **LO 2.2** Converting a meaning from one language to another is called
   a. assuming. **b.** interpreting. **c.** querying. **d.** supposing.
5. **LO 2.2** The most important source for details required for the coding specialist to determine the most accurate code or codes is found in which part of the patient's record?
   a. Patient's Registration Form **b.** Referral Authorization Form
   c. Physician's Notes/Operative Reports **d.** Imaging Reports
6. **LO 2.2** What is the best way to begin abstracting clinical documentation?
   a. Listen to the nurse explain the encounter.
   b. Read all the way through the clinical documentation for the specific encounter.
   c. Talk to the technician.
   d. Read the patient's registration form.
7. **LO 2.2** Every patient encounter must have at least____reportable [codeable] reason(s) *why* and at least____reportable [codeable] explanation(s) of *what*.
   a. 1, 1 **b.** 2, 1 **c.** 1, 2 **d.** 3, 1
8. **LO 2.3** All of the following would be considered a diagnostic "main term" except
   a. herpes. **b.** acute. **c.** spasm. **d.** infarction.
9. **LO 2.3** The patient has been diagnosed with hypersecretion of thyroid stimulating hormone. Identify the condition.
   a. hormone **b.** thyroid **c.** stimulating **d.** hypersecretion
10. **LO 2.3** Which official guideline is concerned with conditions that are an integral part of a disease process?
    a. Section I.B.4 **b.** Section I.B.5 **c.** Section I.B.6 **d.** Section I.B.7
11. **LO 2.4** A manifestation is a_____ condition caused by the_____condition.
    a. first, second **b.** third, fourth **c.** second, first **d.** second, third
12. **LO 2.4** Coding a sequela requires at least ____ code(s).
    a. 1 **b.** 2 **c.** 3 **d.** 4
13. **LO 2.5** External causes explain ____ and ____ the patient became injured.
    a. why, what **b.** what, where **c.** how, where **d.** why, how
14. **LO 2.5** Which of the following would be an example of an external cause code?
    a. H26.053 **b.** M62.831 **c.** S00.03A **d.** Y92.838
15. **LO 2.6** The suffix *-plasty* means
    a. to dissolve. **b.** to repair. **c.** to crush. **d.** to remove.
16. **LO 2.6** The abbreviation *ECG* stands for
    a. electrocardiography. **b.** electroencephalography.
    c. electroconvulsive therapy. **d.** electrocautery.

17. **LO 2.7** When you find missing or incomplete information in the physician's notes, you should
   a. place the file at the bottom of the pile.
   b. figure out the information yourself; you should know what the doctor is thinking.
   c. ask a coworker.
   d. query the physician.
18. **LO 2.7** Before using an unspecified or NOS (not otherwise specified) code(s), you should
   a. code the case as unspecified and move to the next file.
   b. assume what the missing information is.
   c. query the physician to gain the details needed to use a more specific code.
   d. leave it for your coworker to do.
19. **LO 2.3** Tom is diagnosed with herpes zoster, conjunctivitis. Which ICD-10-CM diagnosis code would you assign?
   a. B02.9 **b.** B02.31 **c.** B02.0 **d.** B02.1
20. **LO 2.6** Terry presents for a unilateral mammography. Which procedural (CPT) code would you assign?
   a. 77053 **b.** 77054 **c.** 77065 **d.** 77066

Let's Check It! A Diagnosis or Procedure

First, identify the following statements as a diagnosis or a procedure, and then identify the main term.

Example: Factitial dermatosis:

a. *diagnosis or procedure: diagnosis* ***b.*** *main term: dermatosis*

1. **LO 2.3** Sprained wrist, left, initial encounter:
   a. diagnosis or procedure: ___________ **b.** main term: ___________
2. **LO 2.6** Tympanic neurectomy:
   a. diagnosis or procedure: ___________ **b.** main term: ___________
3. **LO 2.3** Acute bronchitis:
   a. diagnosis or procedure: ___________ **b.** main term: ___________
4. **LO 2.6** Cerebral thrombolysis:
   a. diagnosis or procedure: ___________ **b.** main term: ___________
5. **LO 2.3** Newborn circulatory failure:
   a. diagnosis or procedure: ___________ **b.** main term: ___________
6. **LO 2.6** Laryngeal web laryngoplasty:
   a. diagnosis or procedure: ___________ **b.** main term: ___________
7. **LO 2.3** Cutaneous abscess of chest wall, initial encounter:
   a. diagnosis or procedure: ___________ **b.** main term: ___________
8. **LO 2.6** Planned tracheostomy:
   a. diagnosis or procedure: ___________ **b.** main term: ___________
9. **LO 2.3** Stenosis of the esophagus:
   a. diagnosis or procedure: ___________ **b.** main term: ___________
10. **LO 2.6** Ulna osteomyelitis:
   a. diagnosis or procedure: ___________ **b.** main term: ___________

Let's Check It! Rules and Regulations

Please answer the following questions from the knowledge you have gained after reading this chapter.

1. **LO 2.2** What is the professional coding specialists' motto?
2. **LO 2.2** Explain the difference between assuming and interpreting.
3. **LO 2.3** Explain the ICD-10-CM Official Guidelines concerning Signs and Symptoms–Section I.B.4; include where the guideline directs you.
4. **LO 2.4** Discuss the ICD-10-CM Official Guidelines concerning Sequela–Section I.B.10; include where the guideline directs you.
5. **LO 2.4** Discuss co-morbidity and the correct coding sequence for the encounter.

3

The Coding Process

Key Terms

Alphabetic Index
Alphanumeric
Alphanumeric Section
Coding Process
Linking
Main Section
Notations
Official Guidelines
Symbols
Tables
Tabular List

Learning Outcomes

After completing this chapter, the student should be able to:

LO 3.1 Implement the six actions of the coding process.
LO 3.2 Locate main terms in the Alphabetic Index.
LO 3.3 Confirm the accurate code in the Tabular List, Main Section, or Tables.
LO 3.4 Apply the Official Guidelines to ensure accurate code determination.
LO 3.5 Analyze documentation and code selection to confirm medical necessity.

3.1 The Coding Process Overview

There are six specific actions that you should take as part of the **coding process**. As you gain experience, it will take you less time to go through these tasks. However, remember that time is not the number one consideration when coding—no matter what anyone says, accuracy is the most important factor. Following all of these actions every time you code will support your development of habits that will maintain accuracy throughout your career.

Coding Process
The sequence of actions required to interpret physician documentation into the codes that accurately report what occurred during a specific encounter between health care professional and patient.

Action 1. Abstract the Documentation

- Read completely through the documentation for the encounter, from beginning to end.
- Then, reread the documentation and identify the main words regarding the diagnoses (*why*) and procedures (*what*) of the encounter.
- Remember, if the patient was injured, you will need to identify the external causes (*how* and *where*) as well.

Action 2. Query, If Necessary

- Make a list of any questions you have regarding unclear or missing information necessary to code the encounter. Query the health care provider who cared for the patient. Never assume or guess. You are only allowed to code what you know from actual documentation. *If it is not documented, it did not happen. If it didn't happen, you cannot code it!*
- Create a query using nonleading questions, with open-ended or multiple-option formatting, to have the physician amend the documentation, so you can use those added details to determine the accurate code or codes. *NOTE:* In school, your queries should go to your instructor.

Action 3. Code the Diagnosis or Diagnoses

- Code each diagnosis and/or appropriate signs or symptoms describing *why* the health care provider treated this patient during this encounter, as documented in the notes, to tell the whole story. Use the best, most accurate code or codes available based on that documentation.
- Read the symbols and notations around the code in the Tabular List.
- Go to the Official Guidelines to review any coding rules with which you must comply.

NOTE: ***Part II: Reporting Diagnoses*** *of this textbook will share with you everything you need to know to determine the accurate diagnosis code or codes.*

Action 4. Code the Procedure or Procedures

- Determine for whom you are reporting: physician, outpatient facility, or inpatient facility. This way, you will know which code set to use: CPT or ICD-10-PCS.
- Code each procedure, service, or treatment, as stated in the notes, describing what the provider did for the patient during this encounter. You should not code any procedures that are simply recommended, suggested, or ordered; you can only code those that have already been provided to the patient during the encounter for which you are reporting. Use the best, most accurate codes available based on the documentation.
- Read the symbols and notations around the code in the Main Section. Check for guidelines (in front of this section as well as in the subsection) to review any coding rules with which you must comply.
- In some cases, you will also need to report a code or codes using the HCPCS Level II code set. You will learn more about this code set in ***Part IV: DMEPOS & Transportation***.

NOTE: ***Part III: Reporting Physician Services and Outpatient Procedures*** *of this textbook will share with you everything you need to know to determine the accurate procedure code or codes. This chapter is just an introduction.*

Action 5. Confirm Medical Necessity

- Ensure that each and every procedure code is supported by at least one diagnosis code to verify medical necessity.

Action 6. Double-Check Your Codes

You, as the professional coding specialist, have a responsibility to ensure that you are submitting only accurate, truthful information, supported by the physician's documentation. Yet, we are all human and anyone can make a mistake. *Now* is the time to build the habit of double-checking your work before you hit that submit button.

- Go back into the code books you have used and reread the full descriptions, all notations, and symbols for the codes you have assigned. Compare these details, once more, with the original documentation–just to be certain you did not misread anything.
- Read carefully, one letter at a time, one number at a time, so you can catch and correct any typos before your work becomes official.

Taking action to code precisely will result in a greater number of your claims getting paid quickly, and your reports will represent accurate data. You owe this to your facility, your patients, and yourself.

> **CODING BITES**
>
> One diagnosis code can provide the explanation of medical necessity for more than one procedure code. One procedure code may be provided to treat more than one diagnosis, but there must be at least one diagnosis code to explain why each procedure was medically necessary.
>
> For inpatient settings, the admission into the facility must also be justified–explained by a diagnosis code or codes. You will learn more about this later in this chapter, **Section 3.5**, *Confirming Medical Necessity*.

> **CODING BITES**
>
> Begin to build the habit, right now, of reading slowly, carefully, and completely. There are so many times, when reviewing a coding error, we have heard, "*Oh, I can't believe I didn't read that!*" It is better for you to find and correct your own mistakes than have anyone else find your mistakes and suffer the consequences.

3.2 The Alphabetic Indexes

Once you have abstracted the main terms that describe the diagnosis (*why*) and the procedure (*what*) from within the physician documentation or operative reports, the next action is to determine the codes that accurately report these details. You will begin by matching those main terms to an entry in the appropriate code book's **Alphabetic Index**.

> **Alphabetic Index**
> The section of a code book showing all codes, from A to Z, by the short code descriptions.

In the ***Introduction to the Languages of Coding*** chapter, you learned to connect the details you abstracted from the medical documentation to the correct code set:

Diagnoses (*why*) = ICD-10-CM code set
Physician services (*what*) = CPT code set
Outpatient facility services (*what*) = CPT code set
Inpatient (hospital) facility services (*what*) = ICD-10-PCS code set
Transportation, equipment, drugs (*what*) = HCPCS Level II code set

Each of these codes set books includes a section, or part, that is called the Alphabetic Index. Each Alphabetic Index lists all of the main terms that are represented by codes within its set, in alphabetic order (A to Z). Therefore:

In ICD-10-CM's Alphabetic Index, you will see terms such as:

Abscess
Carcinoma
Hyperemia
Pneumonia
Shock
Ulcer

In CPT's Alphabetic Index, you will see terms such as:

Angioplasty
Bypass
Discography
Insertion
Psychotherapy
Reconstruction

In ICD-10-PCS's Alphabetic Index, you will see terms such as:

Cannulation
Detachment
Extraction
Laryngoplasty
Repair
Supplement

In HCPCS Level II's Alphabetic Index, you will see terms such as:

Commode
IPPB machine
Nebulizer
Wheelchair

Once you find the main term that matches the word or words that you abstracted from the medical documentation, you may find an indented list containing adjectives providing more detail about that specific main term. It may be an additional description, such as chronic or laparoscopic, or it may be the anatomical site that was involved.

EXAMPLES

ICD-10-CM: ABDOMINAL ABSCESS

Condition: Abscess

Anatomical Site: Abdominal

CPT: INSERTION OF A GASTROSTOMY TUBE

Procedure: Insertion

Device: Gastrostomy Tube

ICD-10-PCS: REPAIR OF MANDIBLE

Procedure: Repair

Anatomical Site: Mandible

HCPCS LEVEL II: NEBULIZER FILTER

Medical Equipment: Nebulizer

Supply: Filter

Often, you will find that further details will be necessary, and options will be provided in another list, indented from the previous indented list.

EXAMPLES

ICD-10-CM: ABSCESS IN THE WALL OF THE ABDOMINAL CAVITY

Condition: Abscess
- Anatomical Site: Abdominal
  - Specific Anatomical Site: Cavity
  - Additional Anatomical Site Detail: Wall

CPT: PERCUTANEOUS INSERTION OF GASTROSTOMY TUBE

Procedure: Insertion
- Device: Gastrostomy Tube
  - Approach: Percutaneous

ICD-10-PCS: REPAIR OF THE RIGHT MANDIBLE

Procedure: Repair
- Anatomical Site: Mandible
  - Laterality: Right

HCPCS LEVEL II: NON-DISPOSABLE NEBULIZER FILTER

Equipment: Nebulizer
- Accessory: Filter
  - Type of Accessory: Non-disposable

You are required to keep making choices, matching the documentation, all the way to the most specific detail. Once at the most specific level, you will see that the Alphabetic Index will suggest a code or codes.

EXAMPLES

ICD-10-CM: ABSCESS IN THE WALL OF THE ABDOMINAL CAVITY

Condition: Abscess
- Anatomical Site: Abdominal
  - Cavity K65.1
  - Wall L02.211

CPT: PERCUTANEOUS INSERTION OF GASTROSTOMY TUBE

Procedure: Insertion
- Device: Gastrostomy Tube
  - Laparoscopic 43653
  - Percutaneous 43246

ICD-10-PCS: REPAIR OF THE RIGHT MANDIBLE

Procedure: Repair
- Anatomical Site: Mandible
  - Left 0NQV
  - Right 0NQT

(continued)

HCPCS LEVEL II: NON-DISPOSABLE NEBULIZER FILTER

Equipment: Nebulizer
Accessory: Filter
Disposable A7013
Non-disposable A7014

You are not done with the coding process yet. These codes will guide you to find the suggested code in the Main Section, Tabular List, or Tables of that code book. You are not permitted, by law, to report a code from the Alphabetic Index without first confirming that it is the best possible option in the Tabular List, Main Section, or Tables.

Symbols
Marks, similar to emojis, that provide additional direction to use codes correctly and accurately.

Notations
Alerts and warnings that support more accurate use of codes in a specific code set.

CODING BITES

The Main Section and Tabular List of the code books all contain additional **symbols** and **notations** to help you determine the most accurate code. The book actually can help you determine the accurate code or codes!

More about these in chapters later in this book.

Tabular List
The section of the ICD-10-CM code book listing all of the codes in alphanumeric order.

Main Section
The section of the CPT code book listing all of the codes in numeric order.

Tables
The section of the ICD-10-PCS code book listing all of the codes in alphanumeric order, based on the first three characters of the code.

Alphanumeric Section
The section of the HCPCS Level II code book listing all of the codes in alphanumeric order.

Alphanumeric
Containing both letters and numbers.

3.3 The Tabular List, Main Section, Tables, and Alphanumeric Section

Think of the Alphabetic Index as a very cheap GPS mapping app. You cannot count on it to give you accurate information because it is not designed to get you to your precise destination. Sometimes, yes, it will get you to the correct front door. Sometimes, however, it will mistakenly take you to the house down the block, and you will have to look at all of the houses and all of the addresses in the area to see which one is correct. You begin with a suggested code from the Alphabetic Index to get you to the correct neighborhood. However, you cannot report this code until you have confirmed it is correct and complete, using the ICD-10-CM's **Tabular List**, CPT's **Main Section**, ICD-10-PCS's **Tables** section, or HCPCS Level II's **Alphanumeric Section** of the appropriate code book.

These sections list all of the codes available in that code set, only this time, they are listed in numeric or **alphanumeric** order by the code first, followed by the words describing exactly what that code represents. Here, you will find several things to help you get to absolute accuracy.

Full Code Descriptions

In these sections, you will be able to read the full code description, not the shortened version used in the Alphabetic Index. Let's continue with our examples from the previous section, **Section 3.2**, *The Alphabetic Indexes:*

EXAMPLES

ICD-10-CM

The Alphabetic Index gave you:

-- Abscess, Abdominal, Cavity K65.1

-- Abscess, Abdominal, Wall L02.211

(continued)

The Tabular List gives you:

-- K65.1 Peritoneal abscess (mesenteric abscess)

-- L02.211 Cutaneous abscess of abdominal wall

CPT

The Alphabetic Index gave you:

-- Insertion, Gastrostomy Tube, Laparoscopic 43653

-- Insertion, Gastrostomy Tube, Percutaneous 43246

In the Main Section, you will read:

-- 43653 Laparoscopy, surgical; gastrostomy, without construction of gastric tube (e.g., Stamm procedure)

-- 43246 Esophagogastroduodenoscopy, flexible, transoral; with directed placement of percutaneous gastrostomy tube

ICD-10-PCS

The Alphabetic Index gave you:

-- Repair, Mandible, Left 0NQV

-- Repair, Mandible, Right 0NQT

In the Tables Section, you must build the code out to seven (7) characters based on the additional details in the operative notes:

-- 0NQV0ZZ Repair of mandible, left side, open approach

-- 0NQTXZZ Repair of mandible, right, external approach

HCPCS LEVEL II

The Alphabetic Index gave you:

-- Nebulizer, Filter, Disposable A7013

-- Nebulizer, Filter, Non-disposable A7014

In the Alphanumeric List, you will read:

-- A7013 Filter, disposable, used with aerosol compressor or ultrasonic generator

-- A7014 Filter, non-disposable, used with aerosol compressor or ultrasonic generator

Look at all the additional details provided in the complete code descriptions. As you can see with just our few examples, there are specifics that may require you to go back to the documentation to confirm these additional details are still accurate. While you are here, you also need to read the complete code descriptions for all of the other codes in this code category. It is not uncommon that you may find another code that is a better match for the documentation.

Conventions (Notations and Symbols)

In addition to full code descriptions, you also will find conventions (notations and symbols) in the Tabular List (ICD-10-CM) and Main Section (CPT) that include tips and hints pointing you toward the correct code. This section is a preview of more in-depth discussions about symbols that will come in future chapters. Therefore, for now, just a little glance.

ICD-10-CM

In the Tabular List above K65.1 is a notation that states:

Use additional code **to identify infectious agent**

K65.1 Peritoneal abscess (mesenteric abscess)

A "*Use additional code*" notation reminds you that you will need to include a second code reporting the detail identified in the notation. This notation helps you ensure you are reporting complete information about a patient's diagnosis that will support medical necessity for the appropriate treatment.

CODING BITES

You will learn more about ICD-10-CM conventions, notations, and symbols in the chapter titled ***Introduction to ICD-10-CM***.

> **CODING BITES**
>
> You will learn more about CPT conventions, notations, and symbols in the chapter titled ***Introduction to CPT.***

CPT

In the Main Section to the left of code 97803 is a star symbol:

★ 97803 Medical nutrition therapy; re-assessment and intervention, individual, face-to-face with the patient, each 15 minutes

Both at the bottom of the page in CPT and in the "Introduction" in the front of the CPT code book, you can see that this symbol ★ informs you, the coder, that if this service was provided using audio/video synchronous equipment (i.e., Skype, FaceTime), you will need to append modifier 95 to this code. This small symbol helps you avoid committing fraud.

> **CODING BITES**
>
> You will learn more about ICD-10-PCS conventions in the chapter titled ***Introduction to ICD-10-PCS.***

ICD-10-PCS

The majority of the codes suggested in the Alphabetic Index of ICD-10-PCS are not complete codes. This fact will not let you forget that you have to go into the Tables section to build the code out to seven (7) characters (based on the additional details in the operative notes). To report a complete, valid code, you must go into the Tables section.

0NQV0ZZ Repair of mandible, left side, open approach

0NQRXZZ Repair of maxilla, external approach

NOTE: Even in those occasions when the Alphabetic Index provides you with all seven characters for the code, you still should go to the appropriate Table to confirm. It will only take a few seconds, and you can be certain you are reporting the complete and accurate code.

> **CODING BITES**
>
> You will learn more about HCPCS Level II conventions, notations, and symbols in the chapter titled ***HCPCS Level II.***

HCPCS LEVEL II

In the Alphanumeric Section, to the left of code J8705 is a symbol:

☑ J8705 Topotecan, oral, 0.25 mg

The symbol ☑, in some versions of the HCPCS Level II book, alerts you that this code description includes a specific quantity. When seeing this, you should confirm the quantity documented with the quantity in the code description. The code may need to be reported multiple times.

3.4 The Official Guidelines

> **Official Guidelines**
> A listing of rules and regulations instructing how to use a specific code set accurately.

With all these code sets and all these codes, you can see that the process to get from documentation to code is more complicated than simply finding a word here and a code there. Coding is important work, so you want to get it accurate every time. To accomplish this, it is essential to have help and support exactly when you need it. Moreover, you have that help right at your fingertips within each code set's book. Always there, just the turn of a few pages, is the guidance from those who created these code sets and who oversee their legal and correct use. These are the published **Official Guidelines** with which you must comply. You don't need to memorize them; you just need to remember they are there and refer to them every time you are working to determine a code.

ICD-10-CM

Usually in the front of this code book, you will find the section titled "***ICD-10-CM Official Guidelines for Coding and Reporting.***"

CPT

In the front of each individual main section, you will find the guidelines applicable to that part of the CPT codes. Therefore, in front of the *Evaluation and Management (E/M) Services* codes are the pages containing the ***E/M Services Guidelines***; in front of the *Anesthesia* code section are the ***Anesthesia Guidelines***; etc.

In addition, it is important to note that the CPT book also includes official guidelines within the sections, at some subsections, with advice and direction for accurate coding of just those procedures, services, and treatments. This means you must get in the habit of reading from the beginning of each section *and* the beginning of the subsection before determining a code. It only takes a few seconds, and it can make the difference between accuracy and fraudulent reporting.

ICD-10-PCS

Usually in the front of this code book, you will find the section titled "*ICD-10-PCS Official Guidelines for Coding and Reporting.*"

Guidance Connection

Throughout this book, you will see special boxes titled GUIDANCE CONNECTION that will point you to a specific guideline in that particular code set directly related to whatever concept or aspect is being discussed. Take a minute and turn to that guideline in your personal code book and read it, think about it, and identify how you would apply this guideline to your work as a professional coding specialist. There is no need to memorize these details because they will always be there for you, right inside your code book, at your fingertips.

LET'S CODE IT! SCENARIO

PATIENT: GENE FERGUSON

PREOPERATIVE DIAGNOSIS: Acute upper abdominal pain

POSTOPERATIVE DIAGNOSIS: Liver tumor

OPERATION PERFORMED: Diagnostic laparoscopy; Laparoscopic ablation, using radiofrequency

SURGEON: Harrison Brusk, MD

SEDATION: General endotracheal anesthetic

ESTIMATED BLOOD LOSS: Minimal.

COMPLICATIONS: None.

INDICATIONS FOR PROCEDURE:

This 57-year-old male presented with signs and symptoms consistent with liver malfunction. Laparoscopic investigation to confirm suspected liver tumor, and if so, ablation. The informed consent form was signed.

DESCRIPTION OF OPERATION:

The patient was brought to the operating room and placed in a supine position on the operating table. After administration of general anesthetic, I prepped and draped the upper abdomen in the usual sterile fashion.

A small incision was made into the umbilicus through which a bladeless 11 mm trocar was inserted without difficulty. After the pneumo-peritoneum was established, the patient was moved into the Trendelenburg position. Two additional 5 mm trocar insertions were made. The liver was visualized and two tumors were identified, one on the distal portion of the liver and one on the proximal surface. The diagnostic laparoscopy was then converted to a surgical procedure so we could remove the tumors. Using radiofrequency techniques, both tumors were successfully ablated.

Let's Code It!

The documentation created by Dr. Brusk clearly provides us with the details of what occurred during this encounter with this patient, Arthur Ferguson. He was having upper abdominal pain that was determined to be two liver tumors (*why* reported with ICD-10-CM code *D13.4 Benign neoplasm of liver*) and the doctor performed a diagnostic laparoscopy, followed by a surgical laparoscopic ablation of liver tumors (*what*). Seems very straightforward, doesn't it?

(continued)

A good place to begin: in the CPT Alphabetic Index, look up:

Ablation

Liver (Tumor)
Cryosurgical 47381, 47383
Laparoscopic. 47370, 47371
Radiofrequency. 47380-47382

Turn to the Main Section of CPT to find code 47370 because Dr. Brusk specifically documented that the ablation was done laparoscopically. Directly above code 47370 are some official guidelines that provide important direction:

"Surgical laparoscopy always includes diagnostic laparoscopy. To report a diagnostic laparoscopy (peritoneoscopy) (separate procedure), use 49320."

Without this direction, you might have gone to the trouble to report both 49320 and 47370. Therefore, now you saved yourself some time and found the correct code to report for Dr. Brusk's work:

47370 Laparoscopy, surgical, ablation of 1 or more liver tumor(s); radiofrequency

If you had reported both codes, this could constitute overcoding—which would be fraud.

See . . . the guidelines help you code accurately, and legally.

Good work!

3.5 Confirming Medical Necessity

No one believes physicians or other health care professionals should be permitted to do whatever they want to a patient without a valid reason. In our industry, this valid reason is known as medical necessity, and you learned about it in the ***Introduction to the Languages of Coding*** chapter. The code or codes that you report to identify the reasons *why* the patient required the attention of a health care professional justify *what* the physician or health care professional did to the patient or for the patient . . . but only when they are in accordance with the standards of care.

Outpatient Settings

Linking
Confirming medical necessity by pairing at least one diagnosis code to at least one procedure code.

In an outpatient setting, once you have determined the accurate diagnosis codes and procedure codes, you must confirm that you are reporting at least one diagnosis code to identify medical necessity by **linking** it to at least one procedure code. Multiple procedure codes can link to one diagnosis code, and multiple diagnosis codes can link to one procedure code. But there must be at least one of each to support the encounter.

You must take this action to ensure that the diagnosis codes you are reporting accurately represent the documented reasons *why* the physician made the decisions he or she made and provided care to this patient, based on those reasons. You must make certain you did not miss anything in the documentation. You must make certain you did not jot down, or enter, the code incorrectly [a typo?].

LET'S CODE IT! SCENARIO

Ahmed Obodeh, a 23-year-old male, came in to see Dr. Starkey because he hit his head on a cabinet and has had a headache for 2 days nonstop. Dr. Starkey examined Ahmed and ordered an MRI of his brain to be taken. Just before the nurse took him down to imaging, Ahmed told Dr. Starkey that he also banged his left knee and was having pain when walking. So Dr. Starkey told the nurse to have radiology take an x-ray of his left knee while he was there. Afterwards, Dr. Starkey gave Ahmed instructions for care of a mild concussion, and suggested an ace bandage for his knee and over-the-counter pain relievers for 1 week.

(continued)

Let's Code It!

Dr. Starkey diagnosed Ahmed with a mild concussion and provided an MRI of the brain and an x-ray of the left knee. Let's analyze this. The concussion is a traumatic impact of the brain and skull. This matches with the MRI of the brain. Perfect.

But there is no diagnosis to justify the x-ray of the knee. Did Dr. Starkey order an unnecessary test? Was he trying to cheat the insurance company and take advantage of Ahmed? No. He is a good doctor, and he was doing a good job by ordering the x-ray of Ahmed's knee. How will you communicate that he was properly caring for his patient?

Go back to the documentation. What was written about Ahmed's knee? "*was having pain when walking*" The report of pain by a patient is a symptom and a valid reason for the provision of an x-ray. Therefore, you will determine the diagnosis code to explain that pain in the knee was the medical necessity.

Diagnosis		*Procedure*
Brain concussion [S06.0X0A]	*–Links to–*	MRI brain [70551]
Pain in left knee [M25.562]	*–Links to–*	X-ray of knee, left [73560-LT]

You are really learning!

Inpatient Setting

In an inpatient setting, the diagnosis code or codes reported must support the medical necessity for the patient to require acute care in a hospital setting–24-hour care from trained health care professionals.

For example, *uncomplicated mild intermittent asthma* [J45.20], occasional narrowing of the bronchi causing diminished breathing, relieved with a prescription inhaler, is not a reason to admit a patient into the hospital to receive round-the-clock care; however, *mild intermittent asthma with status asthmaticus* [J45.22], a life-threatening asthma attack that is not responding to normal treatments such as an inhaler or nebulizer, certainly might be.

ICD-10-CM

LET'S CODE IT! SCENARIO

ADMITTING DIAGNOSIS: Suspected bowel obstruction

CHIEF COMPLAINT: Severe abdominal pain, vomiting, bloating

HISTORY OF PRESENT ILLNESS: Patient is a 29-year-old male with a history of Crohn's disease of the large intestine. The patient came to the ER for an episode of vomiting, continuous, 36 hours. Patient states crampy abdominal pain and bloating. Abdominal ultrasound shows thickening of the bowel wall resulting in acute stricture of the descending colon. Patient is admitted with suspected Crohn's disease with bowel obstruction. Consult with gastroenterology is requested.

Let's Code It!

The admitting diagnosis appears to be clear:

K50.112 Crohn's disease of large intestine with intestinal obstruction

You could see the problem getting reimbursed for this hospital stay if, by mistake, this code was reported:

K50.10 Crohn's disease of large intestine without complications

The little details are important!

CODING BITES

Action 1. Abstract the documentation

Action 2. Query, if necessary

Action 3. Code the diagnosis or diagnoses

Action 4. Code the procedure or procedures

Action 5. Confirm medical necessity

Action 6. Double-check your codes

Chapter Summary

In this chapter, you learned how to take the data culled from the physician's documentation and interpret the data into another language, a medical code (ICD-10-CM, CPT, HCPCS Level II, or ICD-10-PCS). Following each and every one of the six actions required will help you ensure that you are accurately interpreting what occurred between physician and patient during a specific encounter or during a patient's stay in a hospital. In the next part of this book, you will delve more deeply into diagnosis coding using the language of ICD-10-CM.

CHAPTER 3 REVIEW
The Coding Process

Let's Check It! Terminology

Match each key term to the appropriate definition.

1. **LO 3.2** The section of a code book showing codes, from A to Z, by the short code descriptions.
2. **LO 3.3** The section of the ICD-10-PCS code book listing all of the codes in alphanumeric order, based on the first three characters of the code.
3. **LO 3.1** The sequence of actions required to interpret physician documentation into the codes that accurately report what occurred during a specific encounter between health care professional and patient.
4. **LO 3.3** A code consisting of both numbers and letters.
5. **LO 3.5** Confirming medical necessity by pairing at least one diagnosis code to at least one procedure code.
6. **LO 3.3** The section of the CPT code book listing all of the codes in numeric order.
7. **LO 3.4** A listing of rules and regulations instructing how to use a specific code set accurately.
8. **LO 3.2** Alerts and warnings that support more accurate use of codes in a specific code set.
9. **LO 3.2** Marks, similar to emojis, that provide additional direction to use codes correctly and accurately.
10. **LO 3.3** The section of the ICD-10-CM code book listing all of the codes in alphanumeric order.

A. Alphabetic Index
B. Alphanumeric
C. Coding Process
D. Official Guidelines
E. Linking
F. Main Section
G. Notations
H. Symbols
I. Tables
J. Tabular List

Let's Check It! Concepts

Choose the most appropriate answer for each of the following questions.

1. **LO 3.1** There are ____ specific actions that you should take to construct your proper coding process.

   a. 3   **b.** 4   **c.** 5   **d.** 6

2. **LO 3.1** The most important factor in coding is
   a. speed of the coding process.
   b. accuracy of codes.
   c. level of codes
   d. quantity of codes.
3. **LO 3.1** *Abstract the documentation* is Action ___ in the coding process.
   a. 1
   b. 2
   c. 3
   d. 4
4. **LO 3.1** Action 5 in the coding process is to
   a. code the diagnosis or diagnoses.
   b. code the procedure or procedures.
   c. confirm medical necessity.
   d. double-check your codes.
5. **LO 3.1** Every encounter between a patient and health care professional must have at least ___ diagnosis code(s) and at least ___ procedure code(s).
   a. 2, 2
   b. 1, 2
   c. 1, 1
   d. 2, 1
6. **LO 3.2** After abstracting the main terms, a coder will go next to the
   a. external cause codes.
   b. Tabular listings.
   c. Alphabetic Index.
   d. Appendix C.
7. **LO 3.2** Pneumonia would be an example of a term found in which Alphabetic Index?
   a. ICD-10-CM
   b. CPT
   c. ICD-10-PCS
   d. HCPCS Level II
8. **LO 3.2** IPPB machine would be an example of a term found in which Alphabetic Index?
   a. ICD-10-CM
   b. CPT
   c. ICD-10-PCS
   d. HCPCS Level II
9. **LO 3.2** The Main Section and Tabular List of the code books all contain additional ___ and ___ to help you determine the most accurate code.
   a. notations, modifiers
   b. symbols, notations
   c. figures, icons
   d. transformers, symbols
10. **LO 3.3** Which of the following code books lists the codes in numeric order?
    a. ICD-10-CM
    b. HCPCS Level II
    c. CPT
    d. ICD-10-PCS
11. **LO 3.3** Which of the following is a full code description?
    a. Carbuncle of trunk L02.23
    b. Furuncle of trunk L02.22
    c. Cutaneous abscess of chest wall L02.213
    d. Impetigo L01.0
12. **LO 3.3** In the ICD-10-CM Tabular List above code K70.31 there is a notation. What is the notation?
    a. Use additional code to identify alcohol abuse and dependence
    b. Code first underlying diseases
    c. Code also, if applicable, viral hepatitis
    d. Code first poisoning due to drug or toxin, if applicable
13. **LO 3.3** If you see this symbol + (plus sign) in the CPT code book's main section beside a code, it tells you that
    a. the code is a revised code.
    b. moderate sedation is included in this code.
    c. the code is an add-on code.
    d. the code is a new code.
14. **LO 3.3** Which code set requires you, the coder, to build the code out to seven characters?
    a. ICD-10-CM
    b. HCPCS Level II
    c. CPT
    d. ICD-10-PCS
15. **LO 3.3** What is the correct ICD-10-PCS code for the repair of mandible, left side, open approach?
    a. 0NQT0ZZ
    b. 0NQRXZZ
    c. 0NQR0ZZ
    d. 0NQV0ZZ
16. **LO 3.3** What is the correct CPT code for a Laparoscopy, surgical; gastrostomy, without construction of gastric tube?
    a. 43246
    b. 43653
    c. 48001
    d. 43830
17. **LO 3.4** Official____ is(are) a listing of rules and regulations instructing you how to use a specific code set accurately.
    a. Guidelines
    b. linking
    c. tables
    d. appendix
18. **LO 3.4** The Official Guidelines for ICD-10-CM can usually be found in the
    a. back of the code book.
    b. Alphabetic Index.
    c. Tabular List.
    d. front of the code book.

19. **LO 3.5** The why justifies the
   a. where. b. who. c. what. d. when.

20. **LO 3.5** ____ confirm(s) medical necessity by pairing at least one diagnosis code to at least one procedure code.
   a. Tables b. Linking c. Guidelines d. Appendix

Let's Check It! Guidelines

Part I

Refer to the ICD-10-CM Official Guidelines and match each section number to the corresponding guideline.

1. Diagnostic Coding and Reporting Guidelines for Outpatient Services.
2. Selection of Principal Diagnosis.
3. Conventions, general coding guidelines and chapter-specific guidelines.
4. Reporting Additional Diagnoses.

A. Section I
B. Section II
C. Section III
D. Section IV

Part II

Refer to the ICD-10-CM Official Guidelines and match each section number to the corresponding guideline.

1. **LO 3.4** Sequela (Late Effects)
2. **LO 3.4** Format and Structure
3. **LO 3.4** Abbreviations - Tabular List abbreviations
4. **LO 3.4** Etiology/manifestation convention ("code first", "use additional code" and "in diseases classified elsewhere" notes)
5. **LO 3.4** "Code Also" note
6. **LO 3.4** Conditions that are an integral part of a disease process
7. **LO 3.4** Placeholder character
8. **LO 3.4** Conditions that are not an integral part of a disease process
9. **LO 3.4** Signs and symptoms
10. **LO 3.4** Laterality

A. Section I.A.2
B. Section I.A.4
C. Section I.A.6.b
D. Section I.A.13
E. Section I.A.17
F. Section I.B.4
G. Section I.B.5
H. Section I.B.6
I. Section I.B.10
J. Section I.B.13

Let's Check It! Rules and Regulations

Please answer the following questions from the knowledge you have gained after reading this chapter.

1. **LO 3.1** List the six actions of the coding process and explain each action in your own words.
2. **LO 3.2** Discuss the Alphabetic Index and the role it plays in the coding process.
3. **LO 3.3** Explain the ICD-10-CM Tabular List, how the codes are listed, and why it is important.
4. **LO 3.4** Describe what the Official Guidelines are, why they are important, where they are located, and if you are required to comply with these guidelines.
5. **LO 3.5** Discuss the importance of linking a diagnosis code to a procedure code.

4

Medical Coding Fundamentals Capstone

Learning Outcomes

After completing this chapter, the student should be able to:

LO 4 Apply the concepts learned, and correctly identify the most accurate practice to employ when faced with a professional coding process.

INTRODUCTION

In Part I, the chapters Introduction to the Languages of Coding, Abstracting Clinical Documentation, and The Coding Process share an overview of the concepts and skills you will need as a successful medical coding specialist. Together, these three chapters helped you create the foundation, the first layer of a multilayered approach to learning coding.

Select the most accurate answer to each of the following questions:

1. Equipment and supplies provided to a patient are most often reported with codes from the ______
   a. ICD-10-CM code set.
   b. HCPCS Level II code set.
   c. CPT code set.
   d. ICD-10-PCS code set.
2. The first letter of every ICD-10-PCS code identifies the
   a. body system being treated.
   b. root operation term.
   c. approach used by the physician to reach the anatomical site.
   d. section of ICD-10-PCS from which the procedure is reported.
3. ICD-10-CM codes explain _____ health care services were provided.
   a. to whom
   b. which
   c. why
   d. when
4. A confirmed diagnosis explains the patient's
   a. illness, injury, or other reason for services.
   b. insurance coverage.
   c. surgical history.
   d. amount of co-payment required.
5. When a medical coding specialist must report what services a physician provided to a patient, code from _____ must be reported, regardless of the location.
   a. ICD-10-CM
   b. ICD-10-PCS
   c. CPT
   d. HCPCS Level II

6. A CPT code always has ____
   a. 7 alphanumeric characters.
   b. 5 numbers.
   c. 3–7 alphanumeric characters.
   d. 1 letter followed by 4 numbers.
7. An ICD-10-PCS code always has ____
   a. 7 alphanumeric characters.
   b. 5 numbers.
   c. 3–7 alphanumeric characters.
   d. 1 letter followed by 4 numbers.
8. A HCPCS Level II code always has ____
   a. 7 alphanumeric characters.
   b. 5 numbers.
   c. 3–7 alphanumeric characters.
   d. 1 letter followed by 4 numbers.
9. An ICD-10-CM code always has ____
   a. 7 alphanumeric characters.
   b. 5 numbers.
   c. 3–7 alphanumeric characters.
   d. 1 letter followed by 4 numbers.
10. Dr. Marin just completed an annual physical for Mrs. Roddenberry, in his office, as he does every year. This is considered a(n) ____
    a. inpatient encounter.
    b. same day surgical center visit.
    c. consultation.
    d. outpatient care.
11. All of these are source documents, located with the patient chart from which the coder can use to support coding, EXCEPT
    a. note from school nurse.
    b. medication logs.
    c. operative reports.
    d. history and physical.
12. Medical coding specialists must understand medical terminology so the details in the ____ can be accurately interpreted.
    a. operative report.
    b. procedure notes.
    c. consultation reports.
    d. all documents written by clinicians.
13. Eileen tells her physician that she has had a fever and coughing for several days. Dr. Benjamin diagnoses her with the flu. The fever and cough are ____
    a. not as severe, so they are not coded.
    b. also coded, along with the flu.
    c. inclusive signs and symptoms not separately coded.
    d. identified before the flu, so they are reported first.

14. When a patient is found to have two different conditions at the same time, which are not related to each other [such as a pregnant woman who has a broken ankle], these two conditions are known as _____
    a. manifestations.
    b. co-morbidities.
    c. sequela.
    d. inclusive.

15. Sally had burned her hand while cooking. The burn has healed, but a scar remains. The scar is medically known as _____ to the burn.
    a. inclusive sign.
    b. manifestation.
    c. co-morbidity.
    d. sequela.

16. When a patient has been injured, it is important to also report how and where the injury occurred along with other details. The codes used to explain these factors are known as _____
    a. accident location codes.
    b. external cause codes.
    c. action report codes.
    d. accessory codes.

17. When a physician provides care to a patient, it is reported with CPT codes, and may be a procedure, service, treatment, or _____
    a. a recommendation.
    b. a test.
    c. an injection.
    d. an x-ray.

18. When a medical coding specialist explains the meaning of a medical diagnosis or a procedure using a code, this process is known as _____
    a. assuming.
    b. exchanging.
    c. interpreting.
    d. translating.

19. The last time Kevin saw Dr. Freida, a year ago, he had a blister on his foot. Today, he is here for his annual flu shot. The medical coder should _____
    a. code both the blister and the flu shot.
    b. code only the flu shot because the blister is resolved.
    c. code only the flu shot because the blister was last year.
    d. code only the blister because the flu shot is preventative.

20. Every health care professional/patient encounter must have at least _____
    a. one codable reason why [diagnosis].
    b. one codable reason what [procedure or service].
    c. one codable reason why [diagnosis] and one codable reason what [procedure or service].
    d. one codable reason why [diagnosis] or one codable reason what [procedure or service].

21. The sequence of actions required to interpret physician documentation into the codes that accurately report what occurred during a specific encounter between health care professional and patient, is known as the _____
    a. clinical documentation.
    b. coding process.
    c. standard of care.
    d. indexes.

22. Confirming medical necessity by pairing at least one diagnosis code to at least one procedure code is known as ______
    a. pinning.
    b. abstracting.
    c. connection.
    d. linking.

23. A code that is constructed with both letters and numbers is known as a(n) ______ code.
    a. alphanumeric
    b. numerator
    c. dual-constructed
    d. categorized

24. The _____ report the medical necessity for the _____.
    a. procedure codes ...; diagnosis codes
    b. policy number ...; procedure codes
    c. diagnosis codes ...; procedure codes
    d. conventions and guidelines ...; diagnosis codes

25. A listing of rules and regulations instructing how to use a specific code set accurately is known as the ______
    a. notations and symbols.
    b. official guidelines.
    c. conventions.
    d. tabular list.

26. If the documentation contains contradictory, ambiguous, or is missing details necessary for the determination of a specific code, the medical coding specialist is required to ______
    a. assume the details to report.
    b. conduct research and reflect what the literature states.
    c. code the closest details available.
    d. query the provider who wrote the documentation for the required details.

27. To report why the patient needed care from a health care professional, the medical coding specialist must use ______
    a. CPT codes.
    b. HCPCS Level II codes.
    c. ICD-10-CM codes.
    d. ICD-10-PCS codes.

28. To report what a physician did to or for a patient, the medical coding specialist must use ______
    a. CPT codes.
    b. HCPCS Level II codes.
    c. ICD-10-CM codes.
    d. ICD-10-PCS codes.

29. After the cast on the patient's leg was applied, the patient was provided with a pair of crutches. To report the provision of the crutches, the medical coding specialist must use ______
    a. CPT codes.
    b. HCPCS Level II codes.
    c. ICD-10-CM codes.
    d. ICD-10-PCS codes.

30. The last step in your personal coding process should always be ______
    a. determine the most accurate procedure code or codes.
    b. use a medical dictionary.
    c. query the provider who wrote the documentation.
    d. double-check your codes carefully.

PART II

REPORTING DIAGNOSES

INTRODUCTION

For the second layer of your learning, you will focus on interpreting and reporting the key terms and details about the diagnoses, signs, and symptoms–the reasons why the physician provided care to the patient during a specific encounter. As you learned in Part I of this book, this is known as medical necessity.

The concept of medical necessity is as simple as it sounds–the determination that a medical procedure, service, or treatment needed to be provided to a patient because of an identified health care issue or concern. Overall, the industry uses the accepted standards of care by which to measure the rationale–the justification–for every action taken on behalf of an individual patient.

For example, atrial fibrillation [irregular heartbeats in the upper chambers of the heart] may be a diagnosis that supports the insertion of a pacemaker; however, ventricular fibrillation [irregular heartbeats in the lower chambers of the heart] does not. A diagnosis of dysphasia [problems with speech] justifies the provision of a speech evaluation; however, a diagnosis of dysphagia [problems with swallowing] does not. The physician's confirmation of a hydrocele [collection of fluid in tunica vaginalis, spermatic cord, or testis] can only be diagnosed in a male patient and the determination of a hematometra [accumulated blood in the uterus] can only be diagnosed in a female.

When you think about it–why would anyone pay for, or accept, the provision of medical treatment to patients who do not need treatment? The way you will explain that the physician's actions were reasonable and correct is by reporting the accurate diagnosis code or codes.

5

Introduction to ICD-10-CM

Key Terms

Acute
Adverse Effect
Alphabetic Index
Anatomical Site
Chronic
Condition
Confirmed
Differential Diagnosis
Eponym
External Cause
First-Listed
Index to External Causes
Inpatient Facility
Manifestation
Neoplasm Table
Nonessential Modifiers
Not Elsewhere Classifiable (NEC)
Not Otherwise Specified (NOS)
Other Specified
Outpatient Services
Principal Diagnosis
Sequela (Late Effects)
Systemic Condition
Table of Drugs and Chemicals
Tabular List of Diseases and Injuries
Underlying Condition
Unspecified

Learning Outcomes

After completing this chapter, the student should be able to:

LO 5.1 Explain the official conventions used in ICD-10-CM.
LO 5.2 Translate the Official Guidelines and how they impact the way codes are reported.
LO 5.3 Use the Alphabetic Index in ICD-10-CM properly.
LO 5.4 Employ the information within the Tabular List to determine the accurate code to report.
LO 5.5 Distinguish which conditions mentioned in the documentation to report.
LO 5.6 Utilize what you learned in this chapter to determine the correct diagnosis code to report.

STOP! Remember, you need to follow along in your ICD-10-CM code book for an optimal learning experience.

5.1 Introduction and Official Conventions

In the chapters ***Introduction to the Languages of Coding*** and ***The Coding Process***, you were provided with a brief overview of the various code sets. Now, let's begin to dig deeper into the specifics of the ICD-10-CM code set and how to implement it as part of the coding process.

Introduction

In the very front of the ICD-10-CM code book is the *Introduction*. Here you can learn about the history of ICD-10-CM and how we got to this tenth revision. The use of codes to describe the reasons *why* a patient would need the care of a health care professional is an ever-evolving process. These codes, and coding overall, will continue to change throughout your career as a professional coder, so you will need to learn to adapt and change as the needs of health care progress.

ICD-10-CM Official Conventions

The Official Conventions are a very important part of the ICD-10-CM code set. You need to learn the specifics of how codes are presented, and what symbols and notations mean, so you can use them accurately.

Throughout the ICD-10-CM code book, directions, tips, symbols, and helpful notations are available to guide you to the accurate code for a patient encounter. Let's go through common notations and abbreviations, with examples, so you can develop a clear understanding of their meanings.

CODING BITES

NOTE: This code set is maintained by the U.S. federal government; however, there are many different publishers. Each publisher may present the symbols and notations in its own way. Don't worry. The conventions section in the very front of your code book, in Section I.A of the Official Guidelines, as well as the legend along the bottom of every page, will always explain what means what. All you have to do is read.

Punctuation

Punctuation in ICD-10-CM adds information and helps you further your quest for the best, most appropriate code.

Brackets [ ]

Found in the Tabular List, *brackets* will show you alternate terms, alternate phrases, and/or synonyms to provide additional detail or explanation to the description. In the following example, the provider may have diagnosed the patient with foodborne intoxication due to either *Clostridium perfringens* or *C. welchii.* In either case, A05.2 would be the correct code. The same for our other examples: If the documentation reads either "benign recurrent meningitis" or "Mollaret's," code G03.2 can be reported, and if either "third nerve palsy" or "palsy of the oculomotor nerve" is documented, code H49.02 is valid.

EXAMPLES

A05.2 Foodborne *Clostridium perfringens* [*Clostridium welchii*] intoxication

G03.2 Benign recurrent meningitis [Mollaret]

H49.02 Third [oculomotor] nerve palsy, left eye

Italicized or Slanted Brackets *[ ]*

Italicized, or *slanted brackets*, used in the Alphabetic Index, will surround an additional code or codes (i.e., secondary codes) that *must* be included with the initial code. It is the Alphabetic Index's way of telling you that you may need to report more than one code, as well as in what order to sequence these codes.

The italic brackets tell you that if the patient has been diagnosed with schistosomiasis due to granuloma, you have to use two codes: first, B65.9 for the underlying condition (the schistosomiasis) and, second, G07 for the granuloma itself.

EXAMPLE

Granuloma L92.9

  brain (any site) G06.0

    schistosomiasis B65.9 *[G07]*

Parentheses ( )

Throughout the code set, *parentheses* show you additional terms or phrases that are also included in the description of a particular code. The additional terms are called **nonessential modifiers**. The modifiers can be used to provide additional definition but do not change the description of the condition. The additional terms are not required in the documentation, so if the provider did not use the additional term, the code description is still valid.

Nonessential Modifiers
Descriptors whose inclusion in the physician's notes are not absolutely necessary and that are provided simply to further clarify a code description; optional terms.

Take a look at the first example below. Whether the physician wrote the diagnosis as "malaria," "malarial," or "malarial fever," code B54 would still be a valid suggestion.

In the Tabular List example, code H18.52 would be valid for a diagnosis written by the physician as "epithelial corneal dystrophy" or "juvenile corneal dystrophy."

EXAMPLES

In the Alphabetic Index:

Malaria, malarial (fever) B54

Injury, thyroid (gland) NEC S19.84

(continued)

In the Tabular List:

H18.521	Epithelial (juvenile) corneal dystrophy, right eye
H44.631	Retained (old) magnetic foreign body in lens, right eye

Colon :

A *colon* (two dots, one on top of the other), used in the Tabular List, emphasizes that one or more of the following descriptors are *required* to make the code valid for the diagnosis.

EXAMPLE

venous embolism and thrombosis (of):

cerebral (I63.6, I67.6)

coronary (I21–I25)

You would read these as:

venous embolism and thrombosis (of), cerebral (I63.6, I67.6)

venous embolism and thrombosis (of), coronary (I21–I25)

CODING BITES

Health care is an industry that uses many, many abbreviations and acronyms. Keep a medical dictionary close at hand so you can look up any with which you are not familiar.

Not Elsewhere Classifiable (NEC)
Specifics that are not described in any other code in the ICD-10-CM book; also known as *not elsewhere classified.*

Abbreviations

NEC

Not elsewhere classifiable (NEC), or *not elsewhere classified*, indicates that the physician provided additional details of a condition but that the ICD-10-CM book did not include those extra details in any of the other codes in the book. NEC may appear in either the Alphabetic Index or the Tabular List, as you can see in our examples here.

Before reporting a code with NEC in its description, you want to check and double-check that there is not another code with a more complete description that matches the details documented in the physician's notes.

EXAMPLES

K73.0 Chronic persistent hepatitis, not elsewhere classified

Infection, coronavirus NEC B34.2

NOS

Not Otherwise Specified (NOS)
The absence of additional details documented in the notes.

Not otherwise specified (NOS) means that the physician did not document any additional details that are identified in any of the other available code descriptions. On occasion, you may find an NOS in the Alphabetic Index, but most often, you will see these notations in the Tabular List. Or you might see a code description include "unspecified," a shorter way to state the same thing.

Before reporting a code with NOS in the description, you need to reread the physician's documentation and complete patient chart to make certain the specifics you need to report a more complete code are not there. And, even then, you should query the physician to obtain the details, as you learned in the chapter ***Abstracting Clinical Documentation***. An NOS code should be a very last resort to report.

EXAMPLES

R10.811	Right upper quadrant abdominal tenderness NOS
Z30.09	Encounter for other general counseling and advice on contraception (Encounter for family planning advice NOS)

GUIDANCE CONNECTION

Read the ICD-10-CM Official Guidelines for Coding and Reporting, section **I. Conventions, General Coding Guidelines and Chapter-Specific Guidelines**, subsection **A. Conventions for the ICD-10-CM**, paragraph **6. Abbreviations**.

General Notes

Includes, Excludes1, and Excludes2

Let's begin the explanations of INCLUDES, EXCLUDES1, and EXCLUDES2 notations with an example. Turn, in the ICD-10-CM Tabular List, to code F31:

F31 BIPOLAR DISORDER

INCLUDES	**manic-depressive illness**
	manic-depressive psychosis
	manic-depressive reaction
EXCLUDES1	**bipolar disorder, single manic episode (F30.-)**
	major depressive disorder, single episode (F32.-)
	major depressive disorder, recurrent (F33.-)
EXCLUDES2	**cyclothymia (F34.0)**

These notations are in the Tabular List to help you determine the correct code. They provide you with additional terms as well as alternate codes that you might find better match what the physician wrote. Notations are all designed to make the coding process easier and more accurate.

INCLUDES

The INCLUDES notation provides you with additional terms and diagnoses that are included in the above code (this code's description). These notations provide you with additional terms, and variations of descriptors, that expand the meaning of this code's description, making it easier to match what the physician wrote in the documentation. Take a look at our example: The INCLUDES notation explains to you that diagnoses of *bipolar disorder, manic-depressive illness, manic-depressive psychosis*, and *manic-depressive reaction* are all reported from code category F31.

EXCLUDES1

There are times when two diagnostic statements may be close to each other, yet actually conflict with each other. The EXCLUDES1 notation identifies codes that cannot be used together on the same health claim form with the originally listed code. The notation explains that the two codes

- Are contradictory to each other.
- Cannot coexist in the same person at the same time.
- Are redundant.

Using our example above, this notation tells you that F32 Major-depressive disorder, single episode is mutually exclusive to (cannot be reported with) F31 Bipolar disorder.

EXAMPLE

Turn in your ICD-10-CM code book, Tabular List, and find code:

J99 Respiratory disorders in diseases classified elsewhere

EXCLUDES1 *respiratory disorders in:*

amebiasis (A06.5)

blastomycosis (B40.0–B40.2)

You would read the excluded diagnoses as . . .

EXCLUDES1 respiratory disorders in amebiasis (A06.5)

EXCLUDES1 respiratory disorders in blastomycosis (B40.0–B40.2)

EXCLUDES 2

An EXCLUDES2 notation is a warning to *Stop and Double-Check the Documentation* so you don't report the code above the notation when a code shown in the notation may be more accurate. You will see specific conditions listed in the notation that are *not* a part of the code above and a suggestion for an alternate code that may be a more accurate match to the physician's notes. In some cases, the EXCLUDES2 notation may be alerting you that an additional code may be needed to complete telling the story about the patient's condition. Using our example, you can see that the EXCLUDES2 notation tells you that F34.0 Cyclothymia is not the same as F31 Bipolar disorder. Now you can go back to the physician's notes, double-check the information, and determine which is the more accurate code to report, or if you need to report both codes.

EXAMPLE

Turn in your ICD-10-CM Tabular List to:

✓4 **M66.1** Rupture of synovium

EXCLUDES2 rupture of popliteal cyst (M66.0)

The EXCLUDES2 notation alerts you to *Stop and Double-Check the Documentation* to confirm which type of cyst the physician documented. If the documentation states a synovial cyst, then continue determining the correct additional characters for **M66.1**. If the documentation states that the cyst was a popliteal cyst, then you need to report **M66.0** to be more accurate.

GUIDANCE CONNECTION

Read the ICD-10-CM Official Guidelines for Coding and Reporting, section **I. Conventions, General Coding Guidelines and Chapter-Specific Guidelines**, subsection **A. Conventions for the ICD-10-CM**, paragraphs **10. Includes notes**; **11. Inclusion terms**; and **12. Excludes notes**.

Underlying Condition
One disease that affects or encourages another condition.

Manifestation
A condition that develops as the result of another, underlying condition.

Code First

Certain conditions and diseases can cause other problems in the body. Individuals with diabetes, for example, are known to have problems with their eyes or circulation, just to name a few, as a direct result of having diabetes. Patients found to be HIV-positive are prone to conditions such as pneumonia, again as a direct result of the fact that they have human immunodeficiency virus infection. In these examples, diabetes and HIV are what are known as **underlying conditions**. The resulting conditions (e.g., circulation problems, pneumonia) are called **manifestations**.

The *Code first* notation is a reminder that you are going to need another code to identify the underlying disease that caused the diagnosed condition. This notation also tells you the sequence in which to report the two codes: the underlying condition first, followed by the manifestation (see **Figure 5-1**). Often, the notation will reference the most common underlying diseases for a manifestation (along with their codes)! Cool!

13. Etiology/manifestation convention ("code first," "use additional code," and "in diseases classified elsewhere" notes)

Certain conditions have both an underlying etiology and multiple body system manifestations due to the underlying etiology. For such conditions, ICD-10-CM has a coding convention that requires the underlying condition to be sequenced first, if applicable, followed by the manifestation. Wherever such a combination exists, there is a "use additional code" note at the etiology code, and a "code first" note at the manifestation code. These instructional notes indicate the proper sequencing order of the codes, etiology followed by manifestation.

In most cases the manifestation codes will have the code title, "in diseases classified elsewhere." Codes with this title are a component of the etiology/manifestation convention. The code title indicates that it is a manifestation code. "In diseases classified elsewhere" codes are never permitted to be used as first-listed or principal diagnosis codes. They must be used in conjunction with an underlying condition code and they must be listed following the underlying condition. See category F02, Dementia in other diseases classified elsewhere, for an example of this convention.

There are manifestation codes that do not have "in diseases classified elsewhere" in the title. For such codes, there is a "use additional code" note at the etiology code and a "code first" note at the manifestation code and the rules for sequencing apply.

In addition to the notes in the Tabular List, these conditions also have a specific Alphabetic Index entry structure. In the Alphabetic Index both conditions are listed together with the etiology code first followed by the manifestation codes in brackets. The code in brackets is always to be sequenced second.

An example of the etiology/manifestation convention is dementia in Parkinson's disease. In the Alphabetic Index, code G20 is listed first, followed by code F02.80 or F02.81 in brackets. Code G20 represents the underlying etiology, Parkinson's disease, and must be sequenced first, whereas codes F02.80 and F02.81 represent the manifestation of dementia in diseases classified elsewhere, with or without behavioral disturbance.

"Code first" and "Use additional code" notes are also used as sequencing rules in the classification for certain codes that are not part of an etiology/manifestation combination.

See Section I.B.7. Multiple coding for a single condition.

FIGURE 5-1 ICD-10-CM Convention I.A.13. Etiology/manifestation convention

Source: CDEC.gov

The *Code first* notation is ICD-10-CM's way of informing you that

1. You may need to report another code in addition to the code above to accurately tell the whole story of a diagnosis.
2. This other code should be reported first, before the code above the *Code first* notation.

EXAMPLE

I26.01 Septic pulmonary embolism with acute cor pulmonale

Code first **underlying infection**

This notation tells you that

1. You need to report both code I26.01 and a code for an infection (see the physician's notes to determine the exact infection).
2. You need to report the code for the infection first, followed by I26.01.

CODING BITES

An underlying condition must come first and then a manifestation develops from it. Think of an underlying condition as the trunk of a tree and a manifestation as a branch that grows out from that trunk. If the tree trunk didn't exist, there would be no branch.

Use Additional Code

Similar to the *Code first* notation, the *Use additional code* notation is ICD-10-CM's way of informing you that

1. You may need to report another code *in addition* to the code above to accurately tell the whole story of a diagnosis.
2. This extra (additional) code should be reported *after* the code above the *Use additional code* notation.

EXAMPLE

G00.2 Streptococcal meningitis

Use additional code **to further identify the organism (B95.0–B95.5)**

(continued)

This notation tells you that

1. You need to report both code G00.2 and a code from the range B95.0–B95.5 (as per the physician's notes).
2. You need to report G00.2 first, followed by the code from B95.0 to B95.5.

CODING BITES

Sometimes notations appear under the three-character code at the top of a category but are not repeated after each additional code in its section. This is another reason why it is important to start reading at the three-character code, even when the Alphabetic Index directs you to a code with more characters. You don't want to miss any important directives, such as INCLUDES, EXCLUDES, *Code first*, or *Use additional code* notations.

GUIDANCE CONNECTION

Read the ICD-10-CM Official Guidelines for Coding and Reporting, section **I. Conventions, General Coding Guidelines and Chapter-Specific Guidelines**, subsection **A. Conventions for the ICD-10-CM**, paragraph **17. "Code also note."**

Code Also

The *Code also* notation is similar to the *Code first* and *Use additional code* notations, just without the predetermination of sequencing. ICD-10-CM is alerting you that the physician's notes may contain some additional condition or issue that should be reported with a separate code, in addition to the code above this notation. This notation leaves it up to you to decide whether or not the additional code is needed to tell the whole story. If it is needed, you will need to use the Official Guidelines, Sections II and III, to determine the reporting order.

EXAMPLE

H18.041 Kayser-Fleischer ring, right eye

***Code also* any associated Wilson's disease (E83.01)**

This ***Code also*** notation alerts you to check the documentation to see if there is a diagnosis of Wilson's disease mentioned in connection with the Kayser-Fleischer ring of the patient's right eye.

If so, then . . .

1. You need to report both code H18.041 and code E83.01 (as per the physician's notes).
2. You need to determine from the physician's documentation, and using the **Official Guidelines, Section II. Selection of Principal Diagnosis, and Section III. Reporting Additional Diagnoses**, which code to report first.

Category Notes

Occasionally, you may see informational notes under the description of a three-character code or at the top of a subsection in the Tabular List. These notes share important information and clarifications that you need to know before you determine the code or codes to report.

EXAMPLES

I69 Sequelae of cerebrovascular disease

Note: Category I69 is to be used to indicate conditions in I60–I67 as the cause of sequelae. The "**sequelae**" include conditions specified as such or as residuals that may occur at any time after the onset of the causal condition.

--*

Chapter 15. Pregnancy, Childbirth and the Puerperium (O00–O9A)

Note: Codes from this chapter are for use only on maternal records, never on newborn records. Codes from this chapter are for use for conditions related to or aggravated by the pregnancy, childbirth, or by the puerperium (maternal causes or obstetric causes).

Sequela
A cause-and-effect relationship between an original condition that has been resolved with a current condition; also known as a late effect.

And

The guidelines for the accurate use of ICD-10-CM instruct you to interpret the use of the word *and* in a code description as "and/or." Therefore, if the physician's notes include only one part of a code description but not the other, the code may still be correct.

EXAMPLE

J38.01 Paralysis of vocal cords and larynx, unilateral

You would be correct to report code J38.01 on the basis of physician's notes that confirm a diagnosis of paralysis of the vocal cords only, paralysis of the larynx only, or paralysis of both the vocal cords and larynx.

GUIDANCE CONNECTION

Read the ICD-10-CM Official Guidelines for Coding and Reporting, section **I. Conventions, General Coding Guidelines and Chapter-Specific Guidelines**, subsection **A. Conventions for the ICD-10-CM**, paragraph **14. "And."**

With

The term "with" can be seen in both the Alphabetic Index and the Tabular List, and you should read this as a connection **confirmed** by the physician. A phrase you may see in the physician's documentation is "associated with." To use a combination code containing "with," you do not need the physician to document the connection between the two diagnoses. The **Official Guidelines** direct us to avoid using a combination code when the physician's documentation specifies that the conditions are *not* related or associated with each other.

Confirmed
Found to be true or definite.

GUIDANCE CONNECTION

Read the ICD-10-CM Official Guidelines for Coding and Reporting, section **I. Conventions, General Coding Guidelines and Chapter-Specific Guidelines**, subsection **A. Conventions for the ICD-10-CM**, paragraph **15. "With."**

EXAMPLE

Lorrie Demming, a 31-year-old female, G1, P0, came to see Dr. Southland because of bleeding. She is in her third trimester and very worried about the baby. Dr. Southland confirmed the hemorrhage was associated with her placenta previa.

O44.13 Placenta previa with hemorrhage, third trimester

Other Specified

The phrase **other specified** means the same thing as NEC: The physician specified additional information that the ICD-10-CM book doesn't have in any of the other codes in the category.

Other Specified
Additional information the physician specified that isn't included in any other code description.

EXAMPLE

Dr. Josephs diagnosed Allen Halverson with portal cirrhosis of the liver. Turn to the ICD-10-CM Tabular List code category:

✓4 K74 Fibrosis and cirrhosis of liver

K74.3 Primary biliary cirrhosis

K74.4 Secondary biliary cirrhosis

✓5 K74.6 Other and unspecified cirrhosis of liver

K74.60 Unspecified cirrhosis of liver

K74.69 Other cirrhosis of liver

You can see that *Portal cirrhosis of the liver* is not specified in codes K74.3 or K74.4. You cannot honestly report K74.60 because the physician DID specify the type of cirrhosis. Therefore, to be accurate, you must report **K74.69 Other cirrhosis of liver**.

Unspecified
The absence of additional specifics in the physician's documentation.

Unspecified

Unspecified has the same meaning as NOS, explaining that the physician did not provide more details in his or her notes. Query the physician for specifics so you can avoid using an unspecified code. Using these codes should always be a last resort.

CODING BITES

Before choosing any code with NOS or *unspecified* in the description, double-check the notes and patient record to be certain you cannot find specific details to support a specific code. If not, then query the provider and ask for the additional details you need to determine a more accurate code. An unspecified or NOS code should always be a last resort.

EXAMPLES

K64.9 Unspecified hemorrhoids

Tumor, yolk sac, unspecified site, male C62.90

See

GUIDANCE CONNECTION

Read the ICD-10-CM Official Guidelines for Coding and Reporting, section **I. Conventions, General Coding Guidelines and Chapter-Specific Guidelines**, subsection **A. Conventions for the ICD-10-CM**, paragraph **16. "See" and "See Also."**

In the Alphabetic Index of ICD-10-CM, you may look up a term and notice that the book instructs you to *see* another term. This is an instruction in the index that the information you are looking for is listed under a different term.

EXAMPLES

Entamoeba, entamebic, entamebiasis —*see* Amebiasis

Amebiasis A06.9

with abscess – *see* Abscess, amebic

acute A06.00

chronic (intestine) A06.1

with abscess—*see* Abscess, amebic

--*

Glue

sniffing (airplane)—*see* Abuse, drug, inhalant

Abuse

drug

inhalant F18.10

See Also

In other places in the Alphabetic Index, you may see that the instruction *see also* is next to the term you are investigating. *See also* explains that additional details may be found under a different term. The index is providing you with an alternate main term that may show descriptions more accurate to the physician's documentation.

EXAMPLE

Angiofibroma (*see also* Neoplasm, benign, by site)

juvenile

specified site—*see* Neoplasm, benign, by site

unspecified site D10.6

You can see that the *See Also* notation provides you with an additional path to get to the correct code.

See Condition

The Alphabetic Index also may point you in a less concrete way, such as when you look up a term and the notation tells you to *see condition*. This can be confusing. The index is not telling you to look up the term *condition*. What it is instructing you to do is to find the term that describes the health-related situation involved with this diagnosis and look up that term. You will see this most often next to the listing for an **anatomical site**.

Anatomical Site
A specific location within the anatomy (body).

EXAMPLES

Heart—*see* condition

Leg—*see* condition

Patellar—*see* condition

This instruction comes back to the reason you are looking for a code in the first place. Remember, you are looking for a code to explain *why* the physician cared for the patient during the encounter. Using our example, having a heart is not a reason for a physician to meet with a patient. Everyone has a heart. Therefore, the index is telling you to look, instead, for the term that describes the condition of this patient's heart–the problem or concern about his or her heart that brought the patient together with the physician at this time. Therefore, as an example, instead of *heart*, *cervix*, or *lung*, you need to look up *atrophy*, *fracture*, or *deformity* . . . whatever the reason *why* the patient would need the care of a health care professional.

Additional Characters Required

Box with a Checkmark and Number ✓4

A *box with a checkmark and number* located to the left of a code in the Tabular List is a symbol that notifies you that an additional character is required. The number tells you which character–fourth, fifth, sixth, or seventh–is needed. Some publishers of ICD-10-CM code books use a bullet ● rather than a box. In addition, some versions of the ICD-10-CM book will use a ✓xx7, alerting you to the need for a placeholder–the letter **X**–to be used prior to the 7th character.

CODING BITES

If you ever forget what one of these symbols, abbreviations, or notations means, look for the pages in your ICD-10-CM book titled ***ICD-10-CM Official Guidelines for Coding and Reporting, Section I.A. Conventions for the ICD-10-CM***. On these pages, you will find the explanation for all of the footnotes, symbols, instructional notes, and conventions used.

In addition, most versions of ICD-10-CM include a legend across the bottom of the pages throughout the Tabular List with the symbols used and a brief description.

EXAMPLE

✓4 H20 Iridocyclitis

✓5 H20.0 Acute and subacute iridocyclitis

✓6 H20.01 Primary iridocyclitis

H20.013 Primary iridocyclitis, bilateral

You can see that, as each additional character is added to the code, more specific details are included in the code description. As a professional coding specialist, it is your obligation to always report the most detail possible. This is referred to as the "*highest level of specificity*." Therefore, when the ICD-10-CM code book directs you to keep reading to find an additional character, you are required to do this.

Hyphen -

A *hyphen* is used in the Alphabetic Index to indicate that additional characters are required. This alerts you to an incomplete code.

> **EXAMPLES**
>
> Cogan's syndrome H16.32-
> Discontinuity, ossicles, ear H74.2-
> Fahr Volhard disease (of kidney) I12.-

5.2 ICD-10-CM Official Guidelines for Coding and Reporting

As you work your way through this content, you may be thinking, "How can I possibly remember all of this information?" Here is the good news . . . you don't have to memorize because your code book contains the important information you need to code accurately. All you have to do is read carefully and completely.

In the front of your code book are the rules and directions for accurate reporting of diagnosis codes. You don't have to memorize them. All you have to do is remember that they are available, right at your fingertips, so you can make certain that the codes you report (1) are presented in the legal manner and (2) support clear communications with all parties involved in the care and reimbursement of patients (See **Figure 5-2**).

> **a. Diabetes mellitus**
>
> The diabetes mellitus codes are combination codes that include the type of diabetes mellitus, the body system affected, and the complications affecting that body system. As many codes within a particular category as are necessary to describe all of the complications of the disease may be used. They should be sequenced based on the reason for a particular encounter. Assign as many codes from categories E08 to E13 as needed to identify all the associated conditions that the patient has.
>
> **(1) Type of diabetes**
>
> The age of a patient is not the sole determining factor, though most type 1 diabetics develop the condition before reaching puberty. For this reason type 1 diabetes is also referred to as juvenile diabetes.
>
> **(2) Type of diabetes mellitus not documented**
>
> If the type of diabetes mellitus is not documented in the medical record the default is E11.-, Type 2 diabetes mellitus.
>
> **(3) Diabetes mellitus and the use of insulin**
>
> If the documentation in a medical record does not indicate the type of diabetes but does indicate that the patient uses insulin, code E11, Type 2 diabetes mellitus, should be assigned. Code Z79.4, Long-term (current) use of insulin, or Z79.84, Long-term (current) use of oral hypoglycemic drugs, should also be assigned to indicate that the patient uses insulin or oral hypoglycemic drugs. Code Z79.4 should not be assigned if insulin is given temporarily to bring a type 2 patient's blood sugar under control during an encounter.

FIGURE 5-2 An excerpt from the Official Guidelines for Coding and Reporting, section I.C. Chapter-Specific Coding Guidelines, chapter 4: Endocrine, Nutritional, and Metabolic Diseases (E00-E89), subsection a. Diabetes mellitus, parts 1 through 3

Source: *ICD-10-CM Official Guidelines for Coding and Reporting*, The Centers for Medicare and Medicaid Services (CMS) and the National Center for Health Statistics (NCHS).

Section I. Conventions, General Coding Guidelines and Chapter-Specific Guidelines

As you can tell from this header, Section I has three parts:

A. Conventions for the ICD-10-CM
B. General Coding Guidelines
C. Chapter-Specific Coding Guidelines

This section contains the rules and guidelines for determining and reporting accurate, valid diagnosis codes. Take a moment and review the information in A and B. You will discover that most of these reiterate what you read in the ***Introduction and Official Conventions*** section. These may describe each of the items differently, so be certain to read both to ensure that you understand the guidelines.

There are a few additional elements that are important and, therefore, emphasized here.

Section I.A. Conventions for the ICD-10-CM and Section I.B. General Coding Guidelines

Multiple and Additional Codes

If the patient has several conditions or concerns, the physician might possibly indicate more than one diagnosis. Sometimes, the doctor will list the diagnoses, making it easier for you to know which additional codes are needed.

> **GUIDANCE CONNECTION**
>
> Read the ICD-10-CM Official Guidelines for Coding and Reporting, section **I. Conventions, General Coding Guidelines and Chapter-Specific Guidelines**, subsection **B. General coding guidelines**, paragraph **7. Multiple coding for a single condition.**

HOW MANY CODES DO YOU NEED?

A professional coding specialist's job is to tell the *whole story* about the encounter between the health care provider and the patient. With diagnosis codes, you relate the whole story about *why* the physician provided the services, treatments, and procedures to the patient at this time. You must support *medical necessity* for all of these procedures.

Let's use a scenario as an example:

> *Jenna Wilson, a 29-year-old female, came to a walk-in clinic complaining of a terrible headache in her forehead and pain in her cheeks. She stated that this is the third time over the last few months she has had this pain. Dr. Jackson evaluated her, did a physical exam, and took a culture from her nasal cavity. The in-house lab identified the cause of her sinusitis as Streptococcus pneumoniae. Dr. Jackson diagnosed Jenna with acute recurrent frontal sinusitis due to Streptococcus pneumoniae and gave her a prescription for Amoxicillin.*

Therefore, how many codes do you need?

You need as many codes as necessary to tell the *whole story* about *why* Jenna required Dr. Jackson's care at this visit. Why did Dr. Jackson examine Jenna, take the culture, perform the lab test, and then write a prescription? Because Jenna has acute frontal sinusitis caused by *Streptococcus pneumoniae*. When you look for **Sinusitis, Acute**, in the Alphabetic Index, it leads you to the Tabular List at code category

✓4	**J01**	**Acute Sinusitis**
	J01.10	**Acute frontal sinusitis, unspecified**
	J01.11	**Acute recurrent frontal sinusitis**

Dr. Jackson noted that Jenna's sinusitis was recurrent, leading you to J01.11 as the correct code. However, this does not tell the WHOLE story, does it? You need to also explain the cause of the sinusitis.

Take a look at the notations beneath J01:

Use additional code ***(B95-B97) to identify infectious agent***

This tells you that the second code to report will explain the cause of the sinusitis. You are already using what you have learned in just this short amount of time. You can find the correct second code by turning in your Tabular List to B95 and read all of the code descriptions in these code categories carefully. Did you find:

B95.3 Streptococcus pneumoniae as the cause of diseases classified elsewhere

> **CODING BITES**
>
> The sinusitis is considered a *"disease classified elsewhere"* because it is a condition that is reported with a code from elsewhere in this code set. The word "classified" is used to mean assigned a code in this code set.

Therefore, you will report:

J01.11 Acute recurrent frontal sinusitis

B95.3 Streptococcus pneumoniae as the cause of diseases classified elsewhere

Now you can see that, with these two codes, you and anyone reading these codes clearly can understand that Dr. Jackson cared for Jenna because she had a recurring acute frontal sinus infection caused by *Streptococcus pneumoniae*. Without BOTH codes, you don't have the *whole story*. Therefore, for every case, every encounter, every scenario, you are responsible for telling *the WHOLE STORY about the encounter.*

CODE SEQUENCING

> **Principal Diagnosis**
> The condition, after study, that is the primary, or main, reason for the admission of a patient to the hospital for care; the condition that requires the largest amount of hospital resources for care.

When more than one diagnosis code is required to tell the whole story of the encounter accurately, you then must determine in which order the codes should be listed. [Yes, it does matter!] The code reporting the most important reason for the encounter is called the **principal diagnosis.**

Sometimes the ICD-10-CM book will tell you which code should come first and which should come second with the *Code first* and *Use additional code* notations. Section II and Section III of the Official Guidelines will help you with those instances when there are no notations to guide you with sequencing.

> **EXAMPLE**
>
> Carl Rossen was diagnosed with myocarditis due to *E. coli*. You will find notations directing you on how to sequence these two codes.
>
> I40.0 Infective myocarditis
>
> *Use additional code* **(B95-B97) to identify infectious agent**
>
> I41 Myocarditis in diseases classified elsewhere
>
> *Code first* **underlying disease, such as: typhus (A75.0–A75.9)**

> **CODING BITES**
>
> If two (or more) diagnoses are of equal severity, then report them in order of anatomical site–head to toe.

In cases when there are multiple confirmed diagnoses identified, the guidelines instruct you to list the codes in order of severity from the most severe to the least severe. Take a look at the encounter Dr. Jackson documented with Jenna Wilson. You knew to report B95.3 AFTER J01.11 because the notation beneath J01 directed you to *Use additional code,* providing you with the detail

1. that you needed a second code to complete your explanation of why Jenna required treatment and
2. that clarified the order in which to place the codes.

Acute and Chronic Conditions

If a patient has a health concern diagnosed by a physician as being both acute (severe) and chronic (ongoing) and the condition offers you separate codes for the two descriptors, you should report the code for the acute condition first, as directed by the guidelines. Remember, from your medical terminology lessons–acute is more serious than chronic.

> ICD-10-CM
>
> **YOU CODE IT! CASE STUDY**
>
> *Lorraine Pankow has acute lymphoblastic leukemia and chronic lymphocytic leukemia of B-cell type, now in remission. She is seeing Dr. Huang today for a checkup of this condition.*
>
> *(continued)*

You Code It!

Can you determine the correct codes for Lorraine's visit with Dr. Huang?

Step #1: Read the case carefully and completely.

Step #2: Abstract the scenario. Which main words or terms describe why the physician cared for the patient during this encounter?

Step #3: Are there any details missing or incomplete for which you would need to query the physician? [If so, ask your instructor.]

Step #4: Check for any relevant guidance, including reading all of the symbols and notations in the Tabular List and the appropriate sections of the Official Guidelines.

Step #5: Determine the correct diagnosis code or codes to explain why this encounter was medically necessary.

Step #6: Double-check your work.

Answer:

Did you determine the correct codes?

C91.01 Acute lymphoblastic leukemia, in remission

C91.11 Chronic lymphocytic leukemia of B-cell type in remission

Great job!

Combination Codes

If one code exists with a description that includes two or more diagnoses identified in one patient at the same time, you must choose the code that includes as many conditions as available. You may not code each separately.

When the physician's notes indicate that the patient suffered with both **acute** respiratory failure and **chronic** respiratory failure, you must use the code J96.2-. You are not allowed to use J96.0- and J96.1-, even though, technically, you are reporting the patient's conditions accurately. It is required that you use the combination code, as discussed in the Official Guidelines.

Acute
Severe; serious.

Chronic
Long duration; continuing over an extended period of time.

EXAMPLES

J96.0- Acute respiratory failure

J96.1- Chronic respiratory failure

J96.2- Acute and chronic respiratory failure

GUIDANCE CONNECTION

Read the ICD-10-CM Official Guidelines for Coding and Reporting, section **I. Conventions, General Coding Guidelines and Chapter-Specific Guidelines**, subsection **B. General Coding Guidelines**, paragraphs **8. Acute and Chronic Conditions** and **9. Combination Code.**

In addition, there are combination codes throughout ICD-10-CM that enable you to report an underlying condition along with a manifestation.

EXAMPLES

E10.21 Type 1 diabetes mellitus with diabetic nephropathy

. . . This one code reports two diagnoses: type 1 DM + diabetic nephropathy.

I73.01 Raynaud's syndrome with gangrene

. . . This one code reports two diagnoses: Reynaud's syndrome + gangrene.

K55.21 Angiodysplasia of colon with hemorrhage

. . . This one code reports two diagnoses: Angiodysplasia of colon + hemorrhage.

Two or More Conditions—Only One Confirmed Diagnosis

There may be cases where the physician documents treatment of two (or more) complaints and only one is identified by a confirmed diagnosis.

ICD-10-CM

LET'S CODE IT! SCENARIO

Cahlen Achmed, a 61-year-old male, came to see Dr. Miller. Earlier in the day, he was lightheaded and a little dizzy. In addition, he complained that his heart was beating so wildly that he thought he was having a heart attack. Due to his previous diagnosis of type 1 diabetes, Dr. Miller ordered a blood glucose test. He also performed an EKG to check Cahlen's heart. After getting the results of the tests, Dr. Miller determined that Cahlen's lightheadedness and dizziness were a result of his glucose being too high and administered a shot of insulin subq, 5U. He spoke with Cahlen about how to bring his diabetes under control. He also told him that the EKG was negative and that there were no signs of a heart attack.

Let's Code It!

Dr. Miller confirmed that Cahlen's *type 1 diabetes mellitus* was the cause of his lightheadedness and dizziness. Turn to the Alphabetic Index and find:

Diabetes

Turn to the Tabular List and see:

✓4 **E10 Type 1 diabetes mellitus**

E10.9 Type 1 diabetes mellitus without complications

CODING BITES

Cahlen Achmed's case illustrates that sometimes asking yourself, "*Why* did the physician provide a specific test, treatment, or service?" can help you find the necessary diagnostic key words for an encounter.

Type 1 diabetes mellitus seems to be the only confirmed diagnosis in Dr. Miller's notes. However, the doctor performed an EKG. A diagnosis for diabetes does not provide any medical necessity for doing an EKG. In addition, the test was negative and, therefore, provided no diagnosis. Therefore, you still need a diagnosis code to report the medical necessity for running the EKG. Why did Dr. Miller perform the EKG? Because Cahlen complained of a *rapid heartbeat.* The Alphabetic Index suggests:

Rapid, heart(beat) R00.0

The Tabular List confirms

✓4 **R00 Abnormalities of heartbeat**

R00.0 Tachycardia, unspecified

For the encounter, you have one confirmed diagnosis (the diabetes) and one symptom (rapid heartbeat).

Check the top of this subsection and the head of this chapter in ICD-10-CM. There is a NOTE, an EXCLUDES1 notation, and an EXCLUDES2 notation. Read carefully. Do any relate to Dr. Miller's diagnosis of Cahlen? No. Turn to the Official Guidelines and read Section I.C.4, particularly a. Diabetes mellitus. There is nothing specifically applicable here either.

The guidelines state that a confirmed diagnosis should precede a sign or symptom, so you will list the diabetes code first and then the tachycardia.

E10.9 **Type 1 diabetes mellitus without complications**

R00.0 **Tachycardia, unspecified**

CODING BITES

An electrocardiogram may be referred to as either an ECG or an EKG. *Tachycardia* is the medical term for rapid heart-beat.

Differential Diagnosis

In the case where a provider indicates a **differential diagnosis** by using the word *versus* or *or* between two diagnostic statements, you need to code both as if they were confirmed, and either may be listed first. This means that the physician has determined that the patient's signs and symptoms lead equally to two different diagnoses.

Differential Diagnosis
When the physician indicates that the patient's signs and symptoms may closely lead to two different diagnoses; usually written as "diagnosis A versus diagnosis B."

YOU CODE IT! CASE STUDY

Gilbert Albun, a 57-year-old male complaining of chest pain and shortness of breath, was seen by his family physician. Dr. Pressman admitted him into the hospital with a differential diagnosis of congestive heart failure versus pleural effusion with respiratory distress.

You Code It!

Review the notes of the encounter between Dr. Pressman and Gilbert Albun, and determine the applicable diagnosis code(s).

Step #1: Read the case carefully and completely.
Step #2: Abstract the scenario. Which main words or terms describe why the physician cared for the patient during this encounter?
Step #3: Are there any details missing or incomplete for which you would need to query the physician? [If so, ask your instructor.]
Step #4: Check for any relevant guidance, including reading all of the symbols and notations in the Tabular List and the appropriate sections of the Official Guidelines.
Step #5: Determine the correct diagnosis code or codes to explain why this encounter was medically necessary.
Step #6: Double-check your work.

Answer:

Did you determine the correct codes?

I50.9 **Congestive heart failure, unspecified**

J90 **Pleural effusion, not elsewhere classified**

R06.00 **Dyspnea, unspecified**

Other Current Conditions

Another important issue that needs to be coded is a current condition that might be subtly addressed by the physician. It might be the writing of a prescription refill or a short discussion on the state of the patient's well-being as the result of ongoing therapy for a matter other than that which brought the patient to see the physician today.

YOU CODE IT! CASE STUDY

Deanna Franklin, a 45-year-old female, came to see Dr. Carter for a follow-up on a previous diagnosis of paroxysmal atrial fibrillation. Dr. Carter examined Deanna and did a blood test to monitor the effectiveness of the prescription medication Coumadin, a blood thinner. Dr. Carter told Deanna he was very pleased with her progress and that she was doing well. Before leaving, Deanna asked Dr. Carter for a refill of trinalin, her allergy medication. This time of year typically provoked her allergy to pollen, which caused a lot of inflammation and irritation in her nose (rhinitis). Dr. Carter wrote the refill prescription.

You Code It!

Read Dr. Carter's notes regarding this encounter with Deanna, and determine the correct diagnostic code or codes.

Step #1: Read the case carefully and completely.
Step #2: Abstract the scenario. Which main words or terms describe why the physician cared for the patient during this encounter?
Step #3: Are there any details missing or incomplete for which you would need to query the physician? [If so, ask your instructor.]
Step #4: Check for any relevant guidance, including reading all of the symbols and notations in the Tabular List and the appropriate sections of the Official Guidelines.
Step #5: Determine the correct diagnosis code or codes to explain why this encounter was medically necessary.
Step #6: Double-check your work.

Answer:

Did you determine the correct codes?

I48.0 Paroxysmal atrial fibrillation

J30.1 Allergic rhinitis, due to pollen (hayfever)

Z79.01 Long-term (current) use of anticoagulants

The code for the atrial fibrillation supports the office visit and exam, the code for long-term use of the Coumadin (an anticoagulant) justifies the blood test, and the code for the allergic rhinitis supports the medical necessity for the trinalin prescription.

Placeholder Character

There are times when a fifth, sixth, or seventh character is required, yet there are no fourth, fifth, or sixth characters. In these cases, ICD-10-CM uses a placeholder character, the letter "X," so the following characters will fall into their correct locations. The symbols in the Tabular List will lead you to filling out your code accurately. Just pay attention to each character as well as in what position each character belongs. Let's look at ✓xx7 as an example. This symbol tells you that you will need to add a placeholder X in the fifth position and a placeholder X in the sixth position before determining which of the seventh character options to place at the end of the code.

EXAMPLES

O32.1XX2	Maternal care for breach presentation, fetus 2
T47.2X2D	Poisoning by stimulant laxatives, intentional self-harm, subsequent encounter
W89.1XXS	Exposure to tanning bed, sequela
W85.XXXA	Exposure to electric transmission lines, initial encounter

As you can see, all of these codes require a seventh character, yet the initial codes were shorter. These codes are examples of how the placeholder character "**X**" is used so that all of the characters fall into their proper placement.

GUIDANCE CONNECTION

Read the ICD-10-CM Official Guidelines for Coding and Reporting, section **I. Conventions, General Coding Guidelines and Chapter-Specific Guidelines**, subsection **A. Conventions for the ICD-10-CM**, paragraph **4. Placeholder character**.

Seventh Character

Some ICD-10-CM codes require a seventh character. Different subsections of the code book use this position–the seventh character–to add varying types of information. Most often, the character choices are listed at the top of the code category to be used for all codes within that category. With this in mind, you must always begin reading at the top of the code category or subsection for this information.

GUIDANCE CONNECTION

Read the ICD-10-CM Official Guidelines for Coding and Reporting, section **I. Conventions, General Coding Guidelines and Chapter-Specific Guidelines**, subsection **A. Conventions for the ICD-10-CM**, paragraph **5. 7th Characters**.

The Tabular List contains all the details you need. All you have to do is read the options and determine which is the most accurate, as per the physician's documentation.

Section I.C. Chapter-Specific Coding Guidelines

This subsection of the Official Guidelines is further divided and sorted by the chapters in the Tabular List. The process of determining the code or codes for a specific encounter will lead you to various places throughout the ICD-10-CM code set. It is important to always reference these chapter-specific Official Guidelines to ensure you are considering all of the facets of this complex job before you report a code on an assessment in class or on a claim form or report when you are on the job.

CODING BITES

Inpatient coding calls the most serious diagnosis code, the code that is reported first, the **principal diagnosis** code.

Outpatient coding calls the most serious diagnosis code the **first-listed** diagnosis code.

Principal Diagnosis
The condition, after study, that is the primary, or main, reason for the admission of a patient to the hospital for care; the condition that requires the largest amount of hospital resources for care.

First-Listed
"First-listed diagnosis" is used, when reporting outpatient encounters, instead of the term "principal diagnosis."

Section II. Selection of Principal Diagnosis and Section III. Reporting Additional Diagnoses

Earlier in this chapter, you learned about reporting multiple diagnosis codes and about the basics of sequencing codes. It might seem straightforward right now, but there are times when sequencing and reporting multiple codes become more complicated. Determining the sequencing of the diagnosis codes reported is very important, so you want to get it right every time. With the Official Guidelines readily available for you to reference while you are coding, you can report codes with confidence.

Section IV. Diagnostic Coding and Reporting Guidelines for Outpatient Services

Outpatient Services
Health care services provided to individuals without an overnight stay in the facility.

This section of the Official Guidelines covers specific differences when reporting for an **outpatient service**, including a hospital emergency department, same-day surgical center, walk-in clinic, or physician's office.

Essentially, the guidelines for inpatient and outpatient coding are the same or similar when it comes to reporting the reasons *why* a patient needs care except for one main difference—unconfirmed diagnoses.

GUIDANCE CONNECTION

Read the ICD-10-CM Official Guidelines for Coding and Reporting, section **IV. Diagnostic Coding and Reporting Guidelines for Outpatient Services,** subsection **H. Uncertain Diagnosis.**

Unconfirmed Diagnoses

The Official Guidelines are different for reporting unconfirmed diagnoses for patients who are treated as outpatient versus inpatient.

Outpatient Services

The guideline Section IV. H, Uncertain diagnosis states that you are to use the code or codes that identify the condition to its highest level of certainty. This means that you code only what you know for a fact. You are *not permitted* to assign an ICD-10-CM diagnosis code for a condition that is described by the provider as *probable*, *suspected*, *possible*, *questionable*, or *to be ruled out*. If the health care professional has not been able to confirm a diagnosis, then you must code the signs, symptoms, abnormal test results, or other element stated as the reason for the visit or service.

EXAMPLE

Ellyn Cragen, a 27-year-old female, came to see Dr. Jenisha in his office because of nausea and absence of her period for 2 months. After doing a thorough examination, Dr. Jenisha suspects that Ellyn may be pregnant, so he orders a blood test. If the blood test comes back *positive* to confirm her pregnancy (after the physician documents it in the file), you would use the following code:

Z32.01 Encounter for pregnancy test, result positive

If the blood test comes back *negative*, this confirms that Ellyn is not pregnant. Therefore, you would need to report what you know to be true:

N91.2 Amenorrhea, unspecified

R11.0 Nausea

Z32.02 Encounter for pregnancy test, results negative

Inpatient Services

Inpatient Facility
An establishment that provides health care services to individuals who stay overnight on the premises.

The rules for coding uncertain diagnoses for patients of an **inpatient facility** are different from those for outpatients. As directed by the guideline Section II. H, Uncertain Diagnosis, if the diagnosis is described as probable, possible, suspected, likely, or still to be ruled out at the time of discharge, you must code that condition as if it existed. This directive applies only when you are coding services provided in a short-term, acute, long-term care, or psychiatric hospital or facility. It is one of the few circumstances in which you will find the guidelines differ between coding for outpatient and inpatient services.

GUIDANCE CONNECTION

Read the ICD-10-CM Official Guidelines for Coding and Reporting, section **II. Selection of Principal Diagnosis**, subsection **H. Uncertain Diagnosis**.

YOU CODE IT! CASE STUDY

Howard Tamar, a 61-year-old male, was admitted to the hospital for observation after he complained of having severe chest pain radiating to his left shoulder and down his left arm. After 24 hours in the telemetry unit, Dr. Norwalk discharged him with a diagnosis of suspected variant angina pectoris.

You Code It!

As the hospital's coder, go through the steps of coding and determine the diagnosis code or codes that should be reported for this encounter between Dr. Norwalk and Howard Tamar.

Step #1: Read the case carefully and completely.
Step #2: Abstract the scenario. Which main words or terms describe why the physician cared for the patient during this encounter?
Step #3: Are there any details missing or incomplete for which you would need to query the physician? [If so, ask your instructor.]
Step #4: Check for any relevant guidance, including reading all of the symbols and notations in the Tabular List and the appropriate sections of the Official Guidelines.
Step #5: Determine the correct diagnosis code or codes to explain why this encounter was medically necessary.
Step #6: Double-check your work.

Answer:

Did you determine this to be the code?

I20.1 Angina pectoris with documented spasm (variant angina)

Good job!

Appendix I. Present-On-Admission Reporting Guidelines

You will learn more about Present-On-Admission (POA) indicators in the chapter ***Inpatient (Hospital) Diagnosis Coding***. These indicators are only used for reporting diagnoses for patients treated in a hospital as an inpatient. The Appendix I rules about how to use POA indicators will come in very handy later in your learning.

5.3 The Alphabetic Index and Ancillaries

In the ***Abstracting Clinical Documentation*** chapter, you learned how to identify the diagnosis-related main words abstracted from the physician's notes (the terms that explain *why* the physician needed to care for the patient during the encounter). Let's practice looking for the main term or terms in the Alphabetic Index of your ICD-10-CM code book [also titled *ICD-10-CM Index to Diseases and Injuries*] (see **Figure 5-3**), as well as the ancillary sections of the code set.

Index to Diseases and Injuries (aka Alphabetic Index)

Index to Diseases and Injuries, most often referred to as the **Alphabetic Index**, is the part of the code book that lists all of the diagnoses and other reasons to provide health care by their main word or term, alphabetically from A to Z.

Alphabetic Index
The section of a code book showing all codes, from A to Z, by the short code descriptions.

You will use the Alphabetic Index to guide you to the correct page or area in the Tabular List. Codes in the Alphabetic Index are only suggested codes. Often, the code shown in the Index will require additional characters, will need to be coupled with another code, or will be the wrong interpretation altogether.

A

Aarskog's syndrome Q87.1

Abandonment—*see* Maltreatment

Abasia (-astasia) (hysterical) F44.4

Abderhalden-Kaufmann-Lignac syndrome (cystinosis) E72.04

Abdomen, abdominal—*see also* condition

acute R10.0

angina K55.1

muscle deficiency syndrome Q79.4

Abdominalgia—*see* Pain, abdominal

Abduction contracture, hip or other joint—*see* Contraction, joint

FIGURE 5-3 Example from ICD-10-CM Alphabetic Index: Main terms Aarskog's syndrome through Abduction contracture, hip. or other joint

Source: *ICD-10-CM Official Guidelines for Coding and Reporting*, The Centers for Medicare and Medicaid Services (CMS) and the National Center for Health Statistics (NCHS).

Condition
The state of abnormality or dysfunction.

Eponym
A disease or condition named for a person.

Conditions are shown in the Alphabetic Index by:

- **Condition** (e.g., infections, fractures, and wounds).
- **Eponyms** (e.g., Epstein-Barr syndrome and Cushing's disease).
- Other descriptors (e.g., history, family history).

CODING BITES

Find the condition or issue ("main term") in the ICD-10-CM Alphabetic Index.

If you cannot identify a "main term" from all the words in the diagnostic statement, just look up all the words, one at a time, in the ICD-10-CM Alphabetic Index. You will get to the correct "main term" and find the suggested code. Write the suggested code down on a piece of scratch paper and move to the next step.

After you abstract the documentation and open the Alphabetic Index, you will realize that looking for a main word of a diagnosis in the Alphabetic Index may, sometimes, be easy and direct, and you will be able to determine the code right away!

For example, suppose you read that "*Dr. Gaseor diagnosed Belinda Alfonzo with Tourette's disorder.*"

Turn in the Alphabetic Index in your codebook to the section shown in **Figure 5-4**. The Alphabetic Index's suggestion is clear:

Tourette's syndrome F95.2

There are times, however, when finding the suggested code requires a bit more work. Consider this diagnostic statement, "*Dr. Mulford noted that Charlie has suffered an abrasion on his chin.*" Did you determine the main term to be "abrasion"? Good job! Let's find this term in the Alphabetic Index (**Figure 5-5**).

This is not as straightforward, is it? Notice that the long list indented below the main term **Abrasion** (and you can see in your ICD-10-CM book that it is much longer than what is shown here) is a list, in alphabetic order, of anatomical sites: abdomen, alveolar, ankle, etc. Go back to the diagnostic statement: "*Dr. Mulford noted that Charlie has suffered an abrasion on his chin.*" On what anatomical site was Charlie's abrasion? His chin. Now read down the long list and find the suggested code:

Abrasion, chin S00.81

Good work! You are really learning.

It is important for you to remember that the ICD-10-CM code book has information that can really help you do your job well. Consider Dr. Johnson, a pediatrician, caring for Melinda, who has a problem with her right eye. Dr. Johnson documents that Melinda has "*pink eye.*" Pink eye is not actually a medical term. It is a common term. But this is all you have to go on, so let's take a chance with this in the Alphabetic Index. Eye is an anatomical site, so you know that having an eye is not a reason to see the physician. Look for the term "**pink**" and find, not a suggested code, but a reference (see **Figure 5-6**).

Torture, victim of Z65.4
Torula, torular (histolytica) (infection)—*see* Cryptococcosis
Torulosis—*see* Cryptococcosis
Torus—*see* (mandibularis) (palatinus) M27.0
  fracture—*see* Fracture, by site, torus
Touraine's syndrome Q79.8
Tourette's syndrome F95.2
Tourniquet syndrome—*see* Constriction, external, by site
Tower skull Q75.0
  with exophthalmos Q87.0
Toxemia R68.89
  bacterial—*see* Sepsis
  burn—*see* Burn

FIGURE 5-4 ICD-10-CM, Alphabetic Index, partial, from Torture to Toxemia

Source: *ICD-10-CM Official Guidelines for Coding and Reporting*, The Centers for Medicare and Medicaid Services (CMS) and the National Center for Health Statistics (NCHS).

Abrasion T14.8
  abdomen, abdominal (wall) S30.811
  alveolar process S00.512
  ankle S90.51-
  antecubital space—*see* Abrasion, elbow
  anus S30.817
  arm (upper) S40.81-
  auditory canal—*see* Abrasion, ear
  auricle—*see* Abrasion, ear
  axilla—*see* Abrasion, arm
  back, lower S30.810
  breast S20.11-
  brow S00.81
  buttock S30.810
  calf—*see* Abrasion, leg
  canthus—*see* Abrasion, eyelid
  cheek S00.81
    internal S00.512
  chest wall—*see* Abrasion, thorax
  chin S00.81
  clitoris S30.814
  cornea S05.0-
  costal region—*see* Abrasion, thorax
  dental K03.1
  digit(s)
    foot—*see* Abrasion, toe
    hand—*see* Abrasion, finger

(continued)

ear S00.41-
elbow S50.31-
epididymis S30.813
epigastric region S30.811
epiglottis S10.11
esophagus (thoracic) S27.818
  cervical S10.11
eyebrow—*see* Abrasion, eyelid
eyelid S00.21-
face S00.81
finger(s) S60.41-
  index S60.41-
  little S60.41-
  middle S60.41-
  ring S60.41-
flank S30.811
foot (except toe(s) alone) S90.81-
  toe—*see* Abrasion, toe
forearm S50.81-
  elbow only—*see* Abrasion, elbow
forehead S00.81

FIGURE 5-5 ICD-10-CM Alphabetic Index, partial, from Abrasion to Abrasion, forehead

Source: *ICD-10-CM Official Guidelines for Coding and Reporting*, The Centers for Medicare and Medicaid Services (CMS) and the National Center for Health Statistics (NCHS).

Pinhole meatus (*see also* Stricture, urethra) N35.9
Pink
  disease—see subcategory T56.1
  eye—*see* Conjunctivitis, acute, mucopurulent
Pinkus' disease (lichen nitidus) L44.1

FIGURE 5-6 ICD-10-CM Alphabetic Index, partial, from Pinhole meatus through Pinkus' disease

Source: *ICD-10-CM Official Guidelines for Coding and Reporting*, The Centers for Medicare and Medicaid Services (CMS) and the National Center for Health Statistics (NCHS).

CODING BITES

Never, never, never code *only* from the Alphabetic Index. *You are required to check* every code in the Tabular List. Only then can you read the entire code description and all notations to determine the most accurate code.

The ICD-10-CM Alphabetic Index actually tells you the medical term for "pink eye" and that you need to look this up using this term. Turn in the Alphabetic Index to find the main term, **Conjunctivitis** (see **Figure 5-7**).

Similar to the situation with Abrasion, you see a long list indented beneath this main term, meaning you need more details from the documentation, or, in this case, the previous Alphabetic Index notation. Check back to what you read when you looked at **Pink**, eye—*see* Conjunctivitis, acute, mucopurulent. Now, read the indented list beneath **Conjunctivitis** carefully and find acute. Then, indented beneath that, find:

Conjunctivitis, acute, mucopurulent H10.02-

You may find that a medical dictionary also can help you find synonyms for terms used in the physician documentation that does not match an item in the Alphabetic Index. Build the habit to use all of your resources to help you determine the accurate code.

Conjunctiva—*see* condition

Conjunctivitis (staphylococcal) (streptococcal) **NOS** H10.9

  Acanthamoeba B60.12

  acute H10.3-

    atopic H10.1-

    chemical (see also Corrosion, cornea) H10.21-

    mucopurulent H10.02-

      follicular H10.01-

    pseudomembranous H10.22-

    serous except viral H10.23-

      viral—*see* Conjunctivitis, viral

    toxic H10.21-

  adenoviral (acute) (follicular) B30.1

  allergic (acute)—*see* Conjunctivitis, acute, atopic

    chronic H10.45

      vernal H10.44

  anaphylactic—*see* Conjunctivitis, acute, atopic

  Apollo B30.3

  atopic (acute)—*see* Conjunctivitis, acute, atopic

  Béal's B30.2

  blennorrhagic (gonococcal) (neonatorum) A54.31

  chemical (acute) (*see also* Corrosion, cornea) H10.21-

FIGURE 5-7 ICD-10-CM Alphabetic Index, partial, Conjunctiva to Conjunctivitis, chemical

Source: *ICD-10-CM Official Guidelines for Coding and Reporting*, The Centers for Medicare and Medicaid Services (CMS) and the National Center for Health Statistics (NCHS).

Neoplasm Table

The **Neoplasm Table** is a breakout section of the Alphabetic Index, listing the suggested codes for benign and malignant neoplasms. These pages are set up as a seven (7) column table (**Figure 5-8**) organized by the information in column 1—the anatomical location of the tumor, in alphabetic order. Moving to the right, the following six columns show the suggested code in the following order:

- Malignant Primary
- Malignant Secondary
- Ca in situ
- Benign
- Uncertain Behavior
- Unspecified Behavior

As you have learned, there are many different variations of diseases, especially neoplasms. When the documentation uses one of these alternate terms, you can still look up the main term used by the physician, and, again, the ICD-10-CM Alphabetic Index will help you find your way in the code book.

Adenosarcoma—*see* Neoplasm, malignant, by site

You will learn more about this Table in the chapter on ***Coding Neoplasms***.

Neoplasm Table
The Neoplasm Table lists all possible codes for benign and malignant neoplasms, in alphabetic order by anatomical location of the tumor.

CODING BITES

Neoplasm Table: A table that lists the suggested codes for benign and malignant neoplasms (tumors). The list is organized in alphabetic order by the anatomical location of the neoplasm.

	Malignant Primary	Malignant Secondary	Ca in situ	Benign	Uncertain Behavior	Unspecified Behavior
Neoplasm, neoplastic	C80.1	C79.9	D09.9	D36.9	D48.9	D49.9
abdomen, abdominal	C76.2	C79.8-	D09.8	D36.7	D48.7	D49.89
cavity	C76.2	C79.8-	D09.8	D36.7	D48.7	D49.89
organ	C76.2	C79.8-	D09.8	D36.7	D48.7	D49.89
viscera	C76.2	C79.8-	D09.8	D36.7	D48.7	D49.89
wall—*see also Neoplasm, abdomen, wall, skin*	C44.509	C79.2-	D04.5	D23.5	D48.5	D49.2

FIGURE 5-8 Excerpt from the Neoplasm Table, partial listing for Abdominal neoplasm

Source: *ICD-10-CM Official Guidelines for Coding and Reporting*, The Centers for Medicare and Medicaid Services (CMS) and the National Center for Health Statistics (NCHS).

Table of Drugs and Chemicals

Table of Drugs and Chemicals
The section of the ICD-10-CM code book listing drugs, chemicals, and other biologicals that may poison a patient or result in an adverse reaction.

Similar to the Neoplasm Table, the seven (7) columns in the **Table of Drugs and Chemicals** section (see **Figure 5-9**) provide suggested codes related to the cause of a patient being poisoned or of having an adverse reaction to a medication. This table's first column shows a list of most drugs and chemicals with which a patient might interact, listed in alphabetic order. The six columns that follow, to the right, are:

Substance	Poisoning, Accidental (unintentional)	Poisoning, Intentional Self-Harm	Poisoning, Assault	Poisoning, Undetermined	Adverse Effect	Underdosing
Acetomorphine	T40.1X1	T40.1X2	T40.1X3	T40.1X4	—	—
Acetone (oils)	T52.4X1	T52.4X2	T52.4X3	T52.4X4	—	—
chlorinated	T52.4X1	T52.4X2	T52.4X3	T52.4X4	—	—
vapor	T52.4X1	T52.4X2	T52.4X3	T52.4X4	—	—
Acetonitrile	T52.8X1	T52.8X2	T52.8X3	T52.8X4	—	—
Acetophenazine	T43.3X1	T43.3X2	T43.3X3	T43.3X4	T43.3X5	T43.3X6
Acetophenetedin	T39.1X1	T39.1X2	T39.1X3	T39.1X4	T39.1X5	T39.1X6
Acetophenone	T52.4X1	T52.4X2	T52.4X3	T52.4X4	—	—
Acetorphine	T40.2X1	T40.2X2	T40.2X3	T40.2X4	—	—
Acetosulfone (sodium)	T37.1X1	T37.1X2	T37.1X3	T37.1X4	T37.1X5	T37.1X6

FIGURE 5-9 Excerpt from Table of Drugs and Chemicals, Acetomorphine through Acetosulfone (sodium)

Source: *ICD-10-CM Official Guidelines for Coding and Reporting*, The Centers for Medicare and Medicaid Services (CMS) and the National Center for Health Statistics (NCHS).

Poisoning, Accidental (unintentional)
Poisoning, Intentional Self-Harm
Poisoning, Assault
Poisoning, Undetermined
Adverse Effect
Underdosing

Later in this book, the chapter titled ***Coding Injury, Poisoning, and External Causes*** will provide you with full explanations for using this table.

> **CODING BITES**
>
> **Table of Drugs and Chemicals:** A table that lists pharmaceuticals and chemicals that may cause poisoning or **adverse effects** in the human body.

Adverse Effect
An unexpected bad reaction to a drug or other treatment.

Index to External Causes

To make it easier to determine the correct code or codes to report *how* the patient became injured or poisoned, and *where* the patient was (Place of Occurrence) when the injury or poisoning occurred, you can use the **Index to External Causes** (see **Figure 5-10**) to find a suggested code for the main terms you abstract from the physician's documentation.

Index to External Causes
The alphabetic listing of the external causes that might cause a patient's injury, poisoning, or adverse reaction.

Fall, falling (accidental) W19
- building W20.1
  - burning (uncontrolled fire) X00.3
- down
  - embankment W17.81
  - escalator W10.0
  - hill W17.81
  - ladder W11
  - ramp W10.2
  - stairs, steps W10.9
- due to
  - bumping against
    - object W18.00
      - sharp glass W18.02
      - specified NEC W18.09
      - sports equipment W18.01

FIGURE 5-10 An excerpt from the Index to External Causes, main term Fall

Source: *ICD-10-CM Official Guidelines for Coding and Reporting*, The Centers for Medicare and Medicaid Services (CMS) and the National Center for Health Statistics (NCHS).

Later in this book, the chapter titled ***Coding Injury, Poisoning, and External Causes*** will provide you with full explanations for using this index.

> **CODING BITES**
>
> **Index to External Causes:** The alphabetic list with short descriptions of the **external causes** of injury and poisoning.

External Cause
An event, outside the body, that causes injury, poisoning, or an adverse reaction.

5.4 The Tabular List

Once you have a suggested code from the *Alphabetic Index*, *Neoplasm Table*, *Table of Drugs and Chemicals*, and/or the *Index to External Cause Codes*, you will need to find that code in the **Tabular List of Diseases and Injuries**. Remember, you may never report a code directly from the Alphabetic Index without checking it in the *Tabular List*.

This suggested code will point you to a section or subsection inside a chapter of the Tabular List (see **Table 5-1** for a list of the Tabular List chapters).

Beginning at the top of each chapter and subchapter, you will need to carefully read *all* associated code descriptions. This part of the process helps you ensure that you determine the most accurate code to the highest level of specificity:

- Matching the details in the physician's documentation.
- Regarding only one particular encounter .
- In compliance with the rules and guidelines.

Tabular List
The section of the ICD-10-CM code book listing all of the codes in alphanumeric order.

The **Tabular List** section of the ICD-10-CM book lists every code and its complete description in alphanumeric order by code. Starting at A00, the codes go all the way through to Z99.89 (see **Figure 5-11**). Let's investigate the various components of this section.

TABLE 5-1 Chapters in ICD-10-CM Tabular List

Chapter	Code Range	Title
1	A00–B99	Certain Infectious and Parasitic Diseases
2	C00–D49	Neoplasms
3	D50–D89	Diseases of the Blood and Blood-Forming Organs and Certain Disorders Involving the Immune Mechanism
4	E00–E89	Endocrine, Nutritional, and Metabolic Diseases
5	F01–F99	Mental, Behavioral, and Neurodevelopmental Disorders
6	G00–G99	Diseases of the Nervous System
7	H00–H59	Diseases of the Eye and Adnexa
8	H60–H95	Diseases of the Ear and Mastoid Process
9	I00–I99	Diseases of the Circulatory System
10	J00–J99	Diseases of the Respiratory System
11	K00–K95	Diseases of the Digestive System
12	L00–L99	Diseases of the Skin and Subcutaneous Tissue
13	M00–M99	Diseases of the Musculoskeletal System and Connective Tissue
14	N00–N99	Diseases of the Genitourinary System
15	O00–O9A	Pregnancy, Childbirth, and the Puerperium
16	P00–P96	Certain Conditions Originating in the Perinatal Period
17	Q00–Q99	Congenital Malformations, Deformations, and Chromosomal Abnormalities
18	R00–R99	Symptoms, Signs, and Abnormal Clinical and Laboratory Findings, Not Elsewhere Classified
19	S00–T88	Injury, Poisoning, and Certain Other Consequences of External Causes
20	V00–Y99	External Causes of Morbidity
21	Z00–Z99	Factors Influencing Health Status and Contact with Health Services
22	U00–U85	Codes for Special Purposes

Source: *ICD-10-CM Official Guidelines for Coding and Reporting*, The Centers for Medicare and Medicaid Services (CMS) and the National Center for Health Statistics (NCHS).

Tabular List Chapter Heads

Many of the 21 chapters within the Tabular List start out with valuable information that will support your determination of the accurate code to report. For example, the ICD-10-CM code book's ***Chapter 1: Certain Infectious and Parasitic Diseases (A00–B99)*** (**Figure 5-12**) begins with several instructions that will affect your code decisions. As you practice your coding process, be certain to include checking the very beginning of the chapter so you can benefit from these important notations.

B68 Taeniasis

EXCLUDES1 cysticercosis (B69.-)

B68.0 Taenia solium taeniasis

Pork tapeworm (infection)

B68.1 Taenia saginata taeniasis

Beef tapeworm (infection)

Infection due to adult tapeworm *Taenia saginata*

B68.9 Taeniasis, unspecified

B69 Cysticercosis

INCLUDES cysticerciasis infection due to larval form of *Taenia solium*

B69.0 Cysticercosis of central nervous system

B69.1 Cysticercosis of eye

B69.8 Cysticercosis of other sites

B69.81 Myositis in cysticercosis

B69.89 Cysticercosis of other sites

B69.9 Cysticercosis, unspecified

B70 Diphyllobothriasis and sparganosis

B70.0 Diphyllobothriasis

Diphyllobothrium (adult) (latum) (pacificum) infection

Fish tapeworm (infection)

EXCLUDES2 larval diphyllobothriasis (B70.1)

B70.1 Sparganosis

FIGURE 5-11 Example of a page from ICD-10-CM Tabular List: code categories B68 through B70

Source: *ICD-10-CM Official Guidelines for Coding and Reporting*, The Centers for Medicare and Medicaid Services (CMS) and the National Center for Health Statistics (NCHS).

Chapter 1

Certain infectious and parasitic diseases (A00–B99)

INCLUDES diseases generally recognized as communicable or transmissible

Use additional code to identify resistance to antimicrobial drugs (Z16.-)

EXCLUDES1 certain localized infections—*see* body system-related chapters

EXCLUDES2 carrier or suspected carrier of infectious disease (Z22.-)

infectious and parasitic diseases complicating pregnancy, childbirth, and the puerperium (O98.-)

infectious and parasitic diseases specific to the perinatal period (P35–P39)

influenza and other acute respiratory infections (J00–J22)

FIGURE 5-12 ICD-10-CM Tabular List, chapter 1 opening notations

Source: *ICD-10-CM Official Guidelines for Coding and Reporting*, The Centers for Medicare and Medicaid Services (CMS) and the National Center for Health Statistics (NCHS).

CODING BITES

The Alphabetic Index will suggest a possible diagnosis code. Then you must find the code suggested by the Alphabetic Index in the Tabular List. This step is not a suggestion–it is mandatory. The Tabular List provides more detail in the code description as well as additional notations such as *includes* and *excludes* notes and directives for the requirement of additional characters and codes. *NEVER, NEVER, NEVER code from the Alphabetic Index.*

CODING BITES

Different publishers do things differently. Therefore, your specific version of the ICD-10-CM code book may provide you with the meanings of the symbols in other ways, and other places. Be certain to spend a few minutes becoming familiar with YOUR code book and where things are placed. Inserting tabs on specific pages may help you find quick access to the details you need when you need them.

The Legends

Across the bottom of every page throughout the Tabular List you will find short explanations for many of the symbols you will see among the codes and their descriptions. These legends are an abbreviation of the more complete explanations of each symbol in the front of your code book, found on the pages titled ***Overview of ICD-10-CM Official Conventions*** and ***Additional Conventions***. Once you become familiar with each symbol and notation, the legends will provide you with a quick reference to confirm you are making the correct interpretation.

Using the Tabular List

Earlier in this chapter, in **Section 5.3**, *The Alphabetic Index and Ancillaries*, you learned to use the Alphabetic Index to find suggested codes that matched diagnostic statements. Let's take each of these to the next step . . . confirming the code in the Tabular List.

Case #1 Tourette's Disorder

The first scenario you worked with in the previous section, ***The Alphabetic Index and Ancillaries***, was "*Dr. Gaseor diagnosed Belinda Alfonzo with Tourette's disorder.*" And you found code F95.2 suggested by the Alphabetic Index. In your ICD-10-CM code book, turn to code category F95 in the Tabular List.

✓4 F95 Tic disorder

F95.0 Transient tic disorder Provisional tic disorder

F95.1 Chronic motor or vocal tic disorder

F95.2 Tourette's disorder Combined vocal and multiple motor tic disorder [de la Tourette] Tourette's syndrome

F95.8 Other tic disorders

F95.9 Tic disorder, unspecified Tic NOS

It appears that, at this point, F95.2 is the correct code to report this diagnosis. You are not done yet. Now, backtrack to the subchapter header to see if there are any notations that may apply to this case. [*HINT:* It is directly above code F90. See **Figure 5-13**.]

Behavioral and emotional disorders with onset usually occurring in childhood and adolescence (F90–F98)

Note: Codes within categories F90–F98 may be used regardless of the age of a patient. These disorders generally have onset within the childhood and adolescent years, but may continue throughout life or not be diagnosed until adulthood.

FIGURE 5-13 Example of a subchapter section note, from above code F90

Source: *ICD-10-CM Official Guidelines for Coding and Reporting*, The Centers for Medicare and Medicaid Services (CMS) and the National Center for Health Statistics (NCHS).

This is good information but has no impact to this specific encounter. Next, backtrack to the very beginning of this ICD-10-CM **chapter 6** (see **Figure 5-14**) to check for any notations that you need to apply in reporting Belinda's diagnosis.

Chapter 5. Mental, Behavioral, and Neurodevelopmental Disorders (F01–F99)

INCLUDES disorders of psychological development

EXCLUDES2 symptoms, signs, and abnormal clinical laboratory findings, not classified elsewhere (R00–R99)

FIGURE 5-14 Chapter opening notations, example from chapter 5

Source: *ICD-10-CM Official Guidelines for Coding and Reporting*, The Centers for Medicare and Medicaid Services (CMS) and the National Center for Health Statistics (NCHS).

Again, good information, but none of these notations related to reporting Belinda's diagnosis. One more step to take–check the ***ICD-10-CM Official Guidelines for Coding and Reporting, Section I.C.5. Mental, Behavioral, and Neurodevelopmental Disorders (F01–F99)***. Read all of the guidelines in this section to see if there is any guidance you need to properly report code F95.2. No? Great.

Now . . . you can report code F95.2 with confidence that it is accurate and correct to report *why* Dr. Gaseor cared for Belinda during this encounter. Good work!

Case #2 Abrasion

Let's look at the second case we covered in the section ***The Alphabetic Index and Ancillaries***, "*Dr. Mulford noted that Charlie has suffered an abrasion on his chin.*" And you found code Abrasion, chin S00.81. Turn in your ICD-10-CM Tabular List to the code category:

✓4 **S00 Superficial injury of head**

EXCLUDES1 diffuse cerebral contusion (S06.2-)

focal cerebral contusion (S06.3-)

injury of eye and orbit (S05.-)

open wound of head (S01.-)

The appropriate 7th is to be added to each code from category S00.

A Initial encounter

D Subsequent encounter

S Sequela

None of these diagnoses in the EXCLUDES1 notation relate to Charlie's case; however, it is a good thing you started reading here because there is a box containing the available seventh characters for you to use in this code category.

Read down through all of the available fourth characters in this code category to ensure you don't find something more accurate than that suggested by the Alphabetic Index:

✓5 S00.0 Superficial injury of scalp

✓5 S00.1 Contusion of eyelid and periocular area

✓5 S00.2 Other and unspecified superficial injuries of eyelid and periocular area

✓5 S00.3 Superficial injury of nose

✓5 S00.4 Superficial injury of ear

✓5 S00.5 Superficial injury of lip and oral cavity

✓5 S00.8 Superficial injury of other parts of the head

✓5 S00.9 Superficial injury of unspecified part of head

It looks like the Alphabetic Index was sending us in the right direction. S00.8 is the best option. A fifth character is needed. Read all of the options carefully. Did you determine this?

✓7 **S00.81 Abrasion of other part of head**

You see how different this code description is from what you read in the Alphabetic Index? This is one reason why it is important to use both the Alphabetic Index and the Tabular List. Each has its own details to share. Good. However, one thing the Alphabetic Index didn't let you know is that this code must have a seventh character. Turn back to that box at the beginning of this subsection. Which is the correct character to report for Charlie's encounter with Dr. Mulford for care related to his abrasion?

The appropriate 7th is to be added to each code from category S00.
A Initial encounter
D Subsequent encounter
S Sequela

Did you abstract from the scenario that this was the first encounter? And you noticed that you will need to insert a placeholder letter **X** after the fifth character, so that the seventh character **A** lands in the correct spot.

S00.81XA Abrasion of other part of head, initial encounter

Look back to the beginning of this ICD-10-CM chapter to check for any notations that you might need to consider before you report this code (see **Figure 5-15**).

Chapter 19. Injury, Poisoning and Certain Other Consequences of External Causes (S00–T88)

Note: Use secondary code(s) from **Chapter 21**, External causes of morbidity, to indicate cause of injury. Codes within the T section that include the external cause do not require an additional external cause code.

Use additional code to identify any retained foreign body, if applicable (Z18.-)

EXCLUDES1 birth trauma (P10–P15)

obstetric trauma (O70–O71)

Note: The chapter uses the S section for coding different types of injuries related to single body regions and the T section to cover injuries to unspecified body regions as well as poisoning and certain other consequences of external causes.

FIGURE 5-15 ICD-10-Tabular List, chapter 19 opening notations

Source: *ICD-10-CM Official Guidelines for Coding and Reporting*, The Centers for Medicare and Medicaid Services (CMS) and the National Center for Health Statistics (NCHS).

This is important information, but none of it relates to Charlie's abrasion.

One more step, check the *ICD-10-CM Official Guidelines for Coding and Reporting, Section I.C.19. Injury, Poisoning, and Certain Other Consequences of External Causes (S00–T88)*. Read all of the guidelines in this section to see if there is any guidance you need to properly report code S00.81XA. No? Great. Good work!

Case #3 Pink Eye (Conjunctivitis)

Our third scenario in the section ***The Alphabetic Index and Ancillaries*** was from Dr. Johnson's care for Melinda's pink eye. You used the Alphabetic Index properly to lead you to the suggested code:

Conjunctivitis, acute, mucopurulent H10.02-

In this case, the Alphabetic Index did notify you that an additional character is required by including the hyphen after the first five characters. In your ICD-10-CM's Tabular List, find the code category

✓4 **H10 Conjunctivitis**

EXCLUDES1 **keratoconjunctivitis (H16.2-)**

This is a match for the alternate term provided by the Alphabetic Index, and the EXCLUDES1 notation is not related to Melinda's case, so continue reading down to investigate the fourth-character options. Did you determine which one matches best?

✓5 **H10.0 Mucopurulent conjunctivitis**

You are making good progress! A fifth character is required, so read carefully and determine which you should use:

✓6 **H10.02 Other mucopurulent conjunctivitis**

This is the best because there was nothing about the pink eye diagnosis that stated it could be acute follicular conjunctivitis.

As you read the options for the sixth character, you should notice that you need a new piece of information . . . which eye was diagnosed? Right? Left? Or both (bilateral)? Go back to the documentation and read: "*Dr. Johnson . . . caring for Melinda, who has a problem with her right eye.*"

H10.021 Other mucopurulent conjunctivitis, right eye

Good work! Check the beginning of the subsection. There are no notations at all. Now, check the very beginning of this ICD-10-CM chapter (see **Figure 5-16**).

A lot of good information here, yet it is not related to Melinda's diagnosis, so you have only one more place to check: the *ICD-10-CM Official Guidelines for Coding and Reporting, Section I.C.7. Diseases of the Eye and Adnexa (H00–H59)*. Read all of the guidelines in this section to see if there is any guidance you need to properly report code H10.021. No? Great. You can now report H10.021 Other mucopurulent conjunctivitis, right eye with confidence.

Chapter 7. Diseases of the Eye and Adnexa (H00–H59)

Note: Use an external cause code following the code for the eye condition, if applicable, to identify the cause of the eye condition

EXCLUDES2 certain conditions originating in the perinatal period (P04–P96)
certain infectious and parasitic diseases (A00–B99)
complications of pregnancy, childbirth, and puerperium (O00–O9A)
congenital malformations, deformations, and chromosomal abnormalities (Q00–Q99)
diabetes mellitus related eye conditions (E09.3-, E10.3-, E11.3-, E13.3-)
endocrine, nutritional and metabolic diseases (E00–E88)
injury (trauma) of eye and orbit (S05.-)
injury, poisoning, and certain consequences of external causes (S00–T88)
neoplasms (C00–D49)
symptoms, signs and abnormal clinical and laboratory findings, not elsewhere classified (R00–R94)
syphilis related eye disorders (A50.01, A50.3-, A51.43, A53.71)

FIGURE 5-16 Tabular List, chapter 7, Diseases of the Eye and Adnexa, opening notations

Source: *ICD-10-CM Official Guidelines for Coding and Reporting*, The Centers for Medicare and Medicaid Services (CMS) and the National Center for Health Statistics (NCHS).

5.5 Which Conditions to Code

As you abstract the provider's notes, you are looking for the information that will direct you to those codes that explain or describe the answer to the question, "*Why* did this health care provider care for and treat this individual during *this* encounter?" That is it. The codes do not report the individual's complete medical history.

GUIDANCE CONNECTION

Read the ICD-10-CM Official Guidelines for Coding and Reporting, section **I. Conventions, General Coding Guidelines and Chapter-Specific Guidelines**, subsection **B. General coding guidelines**, specifically paragraphs **4. Signs and symptoms**, **5. Conditions that are an integral part of a disease process**, and **6. Conditions that are not an integral part of a disease process**.

Unrelated Conditions

The attending physician may include information in his or her documentation that reports a condition or diagnosis that is unrelated to this encounter. Remember that the physician does not write the notes just for you to code from. The notes have other, important purposes, such as documenting past history. You must learn to distinguish among notations. You will code only those diagnoses, signs, and/or symptoms related to procedures, services, treatments, and/or medical decision-making occurring during this visit. ICD-10-CM guidelines specifically direct you to omit (do not code) any diagnoses or conditions from a patient's history that have no impact on the current treatment or service. Therefore, you will have to read carefully.

Keep in mind, in some situations, the attention to a condition may be subtle. For example, the physician may renew a previous prescription for a chronic condition. You will need to report that condition to support the writing of the prescription, even if it is not the principal reason the patient is being cared for at this encounter.

Systemic Conditions

If a patient has a **systemic condition**, this means that this condition affects the entire body, for example, diabetes mellitus, hypertension, or pregnancy. The physician, therefore, must take this into consideration in the medical decision-making for virtually any other condition.

Systemic Condition
A condition that affects the entire body and virtually all body systems, therefore requiring the physician to consider this in his or her medical decision-making for any other condition.

LET'S CODE IT! SCENARIO

MaeBelle Abernathy, a 29-year-old female, came to see Dr. Cypher complaining of severe pain in her shoulder. She stated that she was working in the garden and a loose branch fell out of her magnolia tree onto her left shoulder. MaeBelle is 15-weeks pregnant. Normally, Dr. Cypher would have sent MaeBelle for an x-ray. However, because she is pregnant, he decided to examine her, diagnosed her with a sprained coracohumeral shoulder, and strapped her shoulder and arm. He also double-checked the pain medication he prescribed to ensure that it was safe for pregnant women.

Let's Code It!

Dr. Cypher diagnosed MaeBelle with a *sprained shoulder.* Turn to the Alphabetic Index and look up *sprain, shoulder.*

Sprain, shoulder joint S43.40-

In the Tabular List, begin reading at code category S43 and read the INCLUDES and EXCLUDES2 notes carefully. There is nothing here that relates to this patient, so continue reading.

✓4 **S43 Dislocation and sprain of joints and ligaments of shoulder girdle**

You can see that you need additional characters, so continue reading down the column. Match the terms to the physician's notes. The fact is that Dr. Cypher did not provide any further specifics, so the most accurate code is:

S43.412A Sprain of left coracohumeral (ligament), initial encounter

This is the only diagnosis confirmed by Dr. Cypher at this encounter. However, the notes clearly indicate that MaeBelle's pregnancy influenced the way the doctor treated her. Therefore, the codes need to tell that part of the story. The code for the pregnancy must be included to accurately report this visit. The Alphabetic Index suggests

Pregnancy incidental finding Z33.1

In the Tabular List, you will find:

✓4 **Z33 Pregnant state**

Keep reading to review the fourth-character choices. The most accurate is

Z33.1 Pregnant state, incidental

This code explains the situation perfectly. MaeBelle is pregnant and that pregnancy was involved in the treatment of her shoulder injury, but it was not the principal reason she came to see Dr. Cypher. This code means that her pregnancy was a factor included in the patient's treatment plan but not a part of the principal diagnosis. Perfect!

Do you remember when you read the chapter ***Abstracting Clinical Documentation*** that you will need external cause codes for this encounter between MaeBelle and Dr. Cypher because she was injured? Therefore, you also would include three other codes:

W20.8XXA Other cause of strike by thrown, projected, or falling object

Y93.H2 Activity, gardening and landscaping

Y99.8 Other external cause status (leisure activity)

[Don't worry . . . more details about determining external cause codes are in the upcoming chapter titled ***Coding Injury, Poisoning, and External Causes***.]

Check the top of each subsection and the head of each chapter in ICD-10-CM. There are notations at the beginning of this chapter: an INCLUDES notation, a ***Use Additional Code*** note, an EXCLUDES1 notation, and an EXCLUDES2 notation. Read carefully. Do any relate to Dr. Cypher's diagnosis of MaeBelle? No. Turn to the **Official Guidelines** and read **Sections I.C.19, I.C.20, and I.C.21**. There is nothing here that will change what you have already determined, this time.

(continued)

The bottom line . . . there will be five codes to report the reasons why Dr. Cypher needed to care for MaeBelle at this encounter:

S43.412A	**Sprain of left coracohumeral (ligament), initial encounter**
Z33.1	**Pregnant state, incidental**
W20.8XXA	**Other cause of strike by thrown, projected, or falling object**
Y93.H2	**Activity, gardening and landscaping**
Y99.8	**Other external cause status (leisure activity)**

In some encounters you, will not report a condition, just because there was a mention of it in the documentation.

ICD-10-CM

LET'S CODE IT! SCENARIO

Arthur Fleurs, a 47-year-old male, came to Dr. Davenport at the clinic because he was having a nosebleed that wouldn't stop. Arthur was in a single-car accident and his airbag expanded, hitting him in the nose, causing it to bleed. He is otherwise healthy with a history of allergic asthma. Dr. Davenport examined Arthur's nasal passages and packed the nostrils. The doctor then told Arthur to go home and rest and return the next day for a follow-up.

Let's Code It!

Arthur came to see Dr. Davenport because he had a *nosebleed*. Turn to the Alphabetic Index and look up the diagnosis.

Nosebleed R04.0

Surprised it was that easy? Well, sometimes it is. Check the code in the Tabular List, and you will see

✓4 **R04** **Hemorrhage from respiratory passages**

The nose is on the head, so you are in the correct category. Continue reading down the column to review your choices for the fourth-digit:

R04.0 Epistaxis

Hemorrhage from nose; nosebleed

Yes. I guess it was easy. Is that all you need to code? The notes state that Arthur has a history of asthma. However, it has nothing to do with the reason he came to the doctor, and it did not affect the way Dr. Davenport treated Arthur. Therefore, you will not code it for this encounter because it had nothing to do with this visit.

Check the top of this subsection and the head of this chapter in ICD-10-CM. There is a **NOTE** and an EXCLUDES2 notation. Read carefully. Do any relate to Dr. Davenport's diagnosis of Arthur? No. Turn to the **Official Guidelines** and read **Section I.C.18**. There is nothing specifically applicable here either.

Now you can report **R04.0** with confidence.

Screenings and Other Preventive Services

When a screening test is performed (patient has no signs, symptoms, or diagnosis of a condition), you still will need to report a code to explain the reason why Fiona had her annual mammogram or Roger, after his 50th birthday, had a colonoscopy. Many times, you can identify such instances because they are usually determined not by the patient's feelings, signs, symptoms, or other active health issue, but by the calendar.

EXAMPLES

Z00.00 Encounter for general adult medical examination without abnormal findings

. . . this code reports what is commonly known as an annual physical, which is an encounter prompted by the calendar to ensure preventive measures and early detection testing are employed to support good health.

Z02.1 Encounter for preemployment examination

. . . some employers require a candidate to have a physical prior to being officially hired. This code is used to report this reason *why* the individual would see the physician.

Z12.31 Encounter for screening mammogram for malignant neoplasm of breast

. . . every woman over the age of 40 should be doing this annually, or every other year, to identify the presence of a malignancy at the earliest possible time, when treatment is less invasive, less intensive, and less costly. This code explains that this woman has no signs or symptoms; she and her physician just want to be smart about her health.

Test Results

Even though you didn't go to medical school, you still need to know the difference between a positive test result and a negative test result. However, you are not permitted to affirm a diagnosis from a test result without the physician's documentation. This rule applies to laboratory tests, x-rays and other imaging, pathology, and any other screening or diagnostic testing done for a patient. In such cases, especially when the health care professional has ordered additional tests based on an abnormal finding, you should query, or ask, the physician whether or not you should document the results. Be certain to get your answer in writing in the patient's record. *If it's not in writing, you can't code it!*

EXAMPLE

Laboratory report in patient's file shows:

Glucose 155 Norm Range: 65–105 mg/dL

You can see that the patient's glucose is abnormally high. However, you cannot code *hyperglycemia* without a physician's written interpretation and diagnostic statement.

If a physician or other health care professional has already interpreted the test results and the final report has been placed in the patient's file with a diagnostic statement, you should include the code.

EXAMPLE

Report from radiology states: "X-ray shows an open fracture of the anatomical neck of the humerus, right arm. Signed: Flor Rodriquez, MD, Chief of Radiology."

The report, signed by a physician, includes a specific diagnostic statement that should be coded. However, you should always check with the attending physician and permit him or her the opportunity to update the patient's chart with the confirmed diagnosis. You should do this as a sign of respect.

Preoperative Evaluations

Whenever a patient is scheduled for a surgical procedure (on a nonemergency basis), there are typical tests that must be done to ensure that the patient is healthy enough to have the operation. Cardiovascular, respiratory, and other examinations often are done a couple of days prior to the date of surgery. Often these tests do not necessarily relate directly to the diagnostic reason the surgery will be performed. Therefore, they will need a different diagnosis code to report medical necessity.

Coding those encounters carries a specific guideline. In such cases, the principal, or first-listed, diagnosis code will be from the following category:

Z01.8 Encounter for other specified special examinations

Follow that code with the code or codes that identify the condition(s) documented as the reason for the upcoming surgical procedure.

EXAMPLE

Kenzie Hannon was diagnosed with carpal tunnel syndrome in her right wrist. Dr. Isaacs recommended a surgical solution. Because of her history of atrial fibrillation, Kenzie was required to get approval from her cardiologist before she could have the procedure.

G56.01, Carpal tunnel syndrome, right upper limb, is the code that will be used to report the medical necessity for the surgery on Kenzie's wrist. However, it will not support the examination performed by her cardiologist. Think about it . . . who would agree to pay for a cardiologist to examine a patient with a diagnosis of carpal tunnel syndrome? The cardiologist is not qualified to do the job; that is better suited for an orthopedist.

Z01.810, Encounter for preprocedural cardiovascular examination, will support the cardiologist's time and expertise to clear Kenzie for the procedure on her wrist.

GUIDANCE CONNECTION

Read the ICD-10-CM Official Guidelines for Coding and Reporting, sections **II. Selection of Principal Diagnosis** and **III. Reporting Additional Diagnoses.**

Preoperative/Postoperative Diagnoses

You may have already noticed that procedure and operative reporting usually include both a preoperative diagnosis and a postoperative diagnosis. For cases where the two statements differ, the guidelines state that you should code the postoperative diagnosis because it is expected that it is the more accurate of the two.

5.6 Putting It All Together: ICD-10-CM Basics

Now that you have learned about how to use all of the parts of the ICD-10-CM code book, let's put all your new knowledge to the test.

LET'S CODE IT! SCENARIO

Michael Smithstone, a 45-year-old male, came in to see Dr. Opell, his internist. He complains of a fever, sweating, headaches, and pain in his muscles, joints, and back. He stated that he also has felt fatigued. Dr. Opell documents that Michael has just returned from working for a week at a goat farm in an impoverished area. He said that he was supposed to stay longer but came home early because of his illness, "whatever it is."

Dr. Opell ordered a CBC and other blood tests, which revealed that Michael was suffering from Cypress Fever, a bacterial infection caused by Brucella abortus. Dr. Opell gave Michael a prescription for Doxycycline, 100 mg PO q 12 hr on the first day, then once daily for 6 weeks; and another for Rifampin, 600 mg BID for 6 weeks.

Let's Code It!

First, let's identify the confirmed diagnosis of the bacterial infection:

Cypress Fever, caused by Brucella abortus

(continued)

Next, which word is the main term . . . the reason why Michael needed Dr. Opell's care. You can always look up all of the words; however, as you gain more experience in identifying the main term, it will save you time. For this case, the main term is *Fever*.

Open your ICD-10-CM code book to the Index to Diseases and Injuries—more commonly referred to as the Alphabetic Index—and find the main term in bold: FEVER.

Fever (inanition) (of unknown origin) (persistent) (with chills) (with rigor) R50.9
- abortus A23.1
- Aden (dengue) A90
- African tick-borne A68.1
- American
  - mountain (tick) A93.2
  - spotted A77.0
- aphthous B08.8
- arbovirus, arboviral A94
  - hemorrhagic A94
  - specified NEC A93.8
- Argentinian hemorrhagic A96.0
- Assam B55.0
- Australian Q A78
- Bangkok hemorrhagic A91
- Barmah forest A92.8
- Bartonella A44.0
- bilious, hemoglobinuric B50.8
- blackwater B50.8
- blister B00.1
- Bolivian hemorrhagic A96.1
- Bonvale dam T73.3
- boutonneuse A77.1
- brain—*see* Encephalitis
- Brazilian purpuric A48.4
- breakbone A90
- Bullis A77.0
- Bunyamwera A92.8
- Burdwan B55.0
- Bwamba A92.8
- Cameroon—*see* Malaria
- Canton A75.9
- catarrhal (acute) J00
  - chronic J31.0
- cat-scratch A28.1
- Central Asian hemorrhagic A98.0

(continued)

cerebral—*see* Encephalitis
cerebrospinal meningococcal A39.0
Chagres B50.9
Chandipura A92.8
Changuinola A93.1
Charcot's (biliary) (hepatic) (intermittent)—*see* Calculus, bile duct
Chikungunya (viral) (hemorrhagic) A92.0
Chitral A93.1
Colombo—*see* Fever, paratyphoid
Colorado tick (virus) A93.2
congestive (remittent)—*see* Malaria
Congo virus A98.0
continued malarial B50.9
Corsican—*see* Malaria
Crimean-Congo hemorrhagic A98.0
Cyprus—*see* Brucellosis
dandy A90
deer fly—*see* Tularemia
dengue (virus) A90
    hemorrhagic A91

You can see the long, long list of types of fevers that a person can have. Notice these additional terms are shown in alphabetic order, so . . . what kind of fever did Michael have? Cypress Fever. Read carefully down the long list and see if you can find Cypress.

Fever
    Cyprus—*see* Brucellosis

Still in the Alphabetic Index, turn to find the main term, Brucellosis.

Bruce sepsis A23.0
Brucellosis (infection) A23.9
abortus A23.1
canis A23.3
dermatitis A23.9
melitensis A23.0
mixed A23.8
sepsis A23.9
    melitensis A23.0
    specified NEC A23.8
suis A23.2
Bruck-de Lange disease Q87.1

(continued)

There are several choices here as well. Go back to Dr. Opell's notes. Are there any terms that will help with this decision?

. . . *a bacterial infection caused by* Brucella abortus

Therefore, *Brucellosis abortus* leads you to a suggested code **A23.1**—good. Now you have a suggested code to work with.

Turn in the Tabular List of your ICD-10-CM code book and find the code category **A23**. Remember, you must always begin reading in the Tabular List at the three-character code category.

A23 Brucellosis

INCLUDES Malta fever

Mediterranean fever

undulant fever

A23.0 **Brucellosis due to Brucella melitensis**

A23.1 **Brucellosis due to Brucella abortus**

A23.2 **Brucellosis due to Brucella suis**

A23.3 **Brucellosis due to Brucella canis**

A23.8 **Other brucellosis**

A23.9 **Brucellosis, unspecified**

Check the INCLUDES notation. This does not relate to this case. Check for any other notations. There are none. Do you need a second code to identify the specific bacteria that caused Michael's infection? No, because this is a combination code and it already includes that detail.

One final step . . . turn to the **ICD-10-CM Official Guidelines for Coding and Reporting, Section I.C.1. Certain Infectious and Parasitic Diseases (A00–B99).** Read through the subsections. Are there any related to Cypress Fever or Brucellosis? No.

Terrific! Now you can feel confident that reporting **A23.1 Brucellosis due to Brucella abortus** will justify Dr. Opell's care for Michael.

Good job! You are really learning.

Chapter Summary

As you look back over this chapter, you should notice one very important thing: The ICD-10-CM book will almost always guide you to the correct code. The Alphabetic Index will guide you to the correct chapter and subsection in the Tabular List, so you can read all of the notations and symbols, evaluate all the options, and determine the best, most accurate code. If no codes seem to match the attending physician's notes, just go back and keep looking.

Two principles important to becoming a good ICD-10-CM coder:

1. Abstract the main term(s) from the physician's documentation so that you can determine the best, most accurate code or codes.
2. In case of an injury, poisoning, or adverse effect, you will need to add an external cause code.

The Official Coding Guidelines are always there at your fingertips in the book for you to reference–no memorization! All the information can point you in the right direction toward the best, most accurate code. Just look and read. And when the time comes, you will have no problem transitioning from student to professional coding specialist.

The ICD-10-CM code book will lead you, step-by-step, to the correct, complete code to report medical necessity–*why* the health care provider cared for the patient–for this encounter with the highest level of specificity. However, not all diagnostic statements follow a straight line. Sometimes, you have to really read carefully and use your critical thinking skills to interpret accurately. Other times, you may have to use alternate terms from those used in the notes to determine the correct code description. A medical dictionary will help you, so it is recommended that you keep one by your side (especially now, while you are early in your learning). Familiarize yourself with the terms used as well as the critical thinking and interpretation skills that are part of the coding process.

CODING BITES

ICD-10-CM CODE BOOK CONTENTS

- Introduction
- Official Conventions
- Official Guidelines for Coding and Reporting
- The Alphabetic Index
- The Neoplasm Table
- The Table of Drugs and Chemicals
- The Index to External Causes
- The Tabular List

CHAPTER 5 REVIEW
Introduction to ICD-10-CM

connect

Enhance your learning by completing these exercises and more at mcgrawhillconnect.com!

Let's Check It! Terminology

Match each key term to the appropriate definition.

Part I

1. **LO 5.4** The section of the ICD-10-CM code book listing all of the codes in alphanumeric order.
2. **LO 5.3** The section of a code book showing all codes, from A to Z, by the short code descriptions.
3. **LO 5.3** The section of the ICD-10-CM code book listing drugs, chemicals, and other biologicals that may poison a patient or result in an adverse reaction.
4. **LO 5.3** A list of all possible codes for benign and malignant neoplasms, in alphabetic order by anatomical location of the tumor.
5. **LO 5.3** The alphabetic listing of the multitude of external causes that might result in a patient's injury.

A. Alphabetic Index
B. Index to External Causes
C. Neoplasm Table
D. Table of Drugs and Chemicals
E. Tabular List of Diseases and Injuries

Part II

1. **LO 5.1** A specific location or part of the human body.
2. **LO 5.1** Found to be true or definite.
3. **LO 5.3** A condition named after a person.
4. **LO 5.5** A condition that affects the entire body and virtually all body systems, therefore requiring the physician to consider this in his or her medical decision-making for any other condition.
5. **LO 5.2** An establishment that provides acute care services to individuals who stay overnight on the premises.
6. **LO 5.1** Cause-and-effect relationship between an original condition, illness, or injury and an additional problem caused by the existence of that original condition.
7. **LO 5.2** Health care services provided to individuals without an overnight stay in the facility.
8. **LO 5.3** The state of abnormality or dysfunction.

A. Adverse Effect
B. Anatomical Site
C. Condition
D. Confirmed
E. Eponym
F. External Cause
G. Inpatient Facility
H. Outpatient Services
I. Sequela (Late Effect)

9. **LO 5.3** An unexpected, bad result.
10. **LO 5.3** An event, outside the body, that causes injury, poisoning, or an adverse reaction.

J. Systemic Condition

Part III

1. **LO 5.1** Descriptors that are not absolutely necessary to have been included in the physician's notes and are provided simply to further clarify a code description; optional terms.
2. **LO 5.1** Specifics that are not described in any other code in the ICD-10-CM book.
3. **LO 5.2** Long duration; continuing over a long period of time.
4. **LO 5.1** A condition caused or developed from the existence of another condition.
5. **LO 5.1** One disease that affects or encourages another condition.
6. **LO 5.1** The absence of additional specifics in the physician's documentation.
7. **LO 5.1** Additional information that the physician specified and isn't included in any other code description.
8. **LO 5.2** The condition that is the primary, or main, reason for the encounter.
9. **LO 5.1** An indication that more detailed information is not available from the physician's notes.
10. **LO 5.2** Severe; serious.
11. **LO 5.2** When the physician indicates that the patient's signs and symptoms may closely lead to two different diagnoses.

A. Acute
B. Chronic
C. Differential Diagnosis
D. Manifestation
E. Nonessential Modifier
F. Not Elsewhere Classifiable (NEC)
G. Not Otherwise Specified (NOS)
H. Other Specified
I. Principal Diagnosis
J. Underlying Condition
K. Unspecified

Let's Check It! Concepts

Choose the most appropriate answer for each of the following questions.

1. **LO 5.4** Which code range identifies the diseases of the digestive system?
   a. E00–E89 **b.** G00–G99 **c.** K00–K95 **d.** R00–R99
2. **LO 5.1** Turn to Hypertension in the ICD-10-CM Alphabetic Index. All of the following are listed as nonessential modifiers *except*
   a. accelerated. **b.** benign. **c.** idiopathic. **d.** organic.
3. **LO 5.2** Refer to the ICD-10-CM Official Guidelines Section II. What is section II's title?
   a. Conventions, General Coding Guidelines, and Chapter-Specific Guidelines
   b. Selection of Principal Diagnosis
   c. Reporting Additional Diagnoses
   d. Diagnostic Coding and Reporting Guidelines for Outpatient Services
4. **LO 5.2** The ICD-10-CM Official Guidelines I.A.16 are guidelines with instructions concerning which word(s)?
   a. "And" **b.** "With" **c.** "See" and "See Also" **d.** "Code Also" note
5. **LO 5.1** A code surrounded within *italicized*, or *slanted brackets*
   a. is optional. **b.** must be included.
   c. is a previously deleted code. **d.** is a manifestation.
6. **LO 5.1** NEC means
   a. the hospital didn't provide more details.
   b. the physician didn't provide more details.
   c. the ICD-10-CM book didn't provide a code with more details.
   d. the patient didn't provide more details.

7. **LO 5.3** An example of a condition is
   a. Cushing's disease. **b.** Danlos syndrome. **c.** Beck's. **d.** a wound.
8. **LO 5.6** The correct code for acute and chronic respiratory failure with hypoxia is
   a. J96.01 **b.** J96.12 **c.** J96.21 **d.** J96.92
9. **LO 5.5** Which of the following would not be considered a systemic condition?
   a. diabetes mellitus **b.** sprain of left coracohumeral
   c. pregnancy **d.** hypertension
10. **LO 5.6** Morgan is starting a new job and is required to complete a preemployment examination. Dr. Rogers completed the exam and signs the paperwork. How is this encounter coded?
   a. Z02.1 **b.** Z00.00 **c.** Z12.31 **d.** Z02.2

Let's Check It! Guidelines

Refer to the Official Guidelines and fill in the blanks according to the Conventions and General Coding Guidelines Section I, subsections A and B.

Tabular	3	Neoplasms	separate
reported	Diseases	Excludes2	right
first	highest	placeholder	Drugs
acute	discharge	Alphabetic	same
related	External Causes	both	not
verify	once	expansion	confirmed
left	invalid	Excludes1	established
unspecified	insufficient		

1. The ICD-10-CM is divided into the ____ Index, an alphabetic list of terms and their corresponding code, and the ______ List, a structured list of codes divided into chapters based on body system or condition.
2. The Alphabetic Index consists of the following parts: the Index of ____ and Injury, the Index of ______ of Injury, the Table of ___, and the Table of ____ and Chemicals.
3. All categories are ____ characters.
4. A code that has an applicable seventh character is considered ____ without the seventh character.
5. The "X" is used as a ____ at certain codes to allow for future ____ .
6. Codes titled ____ are for use when the information in the medical record is ____ to assign a more specific code.
7. A type ____ note is a pure excludes note. It means "NOT CODED HERE!"
8. A type ____ note represents "Not included here."
9. To select a code in the classification that corresponds to a diagnosis or reason for a visit documented in a medical record, ____ locate the term in the Alphabetic Index, and then ____ the code in the Tabular List.
10. Diagnosis codes are to be used and _____ at their ____ number of characters available.
11. Codes that describe symptoms and signs, as opposed to diagnoses, are acceptable for reporting purposes when a ____ definitive diagnosis has ____ been ____ (confirmed) by the provider.
12. If the same condition is described as both acute (subacute) and chronic, and ____ subentries exist in the Alphabetic Index at the ____ indentation level, code ____ and sequence the ____ code first.
13. Each unique ICD-10-CM diagnosis code may be reported only ____ for an encounter.
14. If no bilateral code is provided and the condition is bilateral, assign separate codes for both the ____ and ____ side.
15. If the provider documents a "borderline" diagnosis at the time of _____, the diagnosis is coded as ____, unless the classification provides a specific entry (e.g., borderline diabetes).

Let's Check It! Rules and Regulations

Please answer the following questions from the knowledge you have gained after reading this chapter.

1. **LO 5.2** Explain the difference in the guidelines between coding for outpatient services and coding for inpatient services.
2. **LO 5.3** When is it appropriate to code from the Alphabetic Index?
3. **LO 5.1** Explain a *code first* notation.
4. **LO 5.4** Explain the importance of the Tabular List.
5. **LO 5.5** When the preoperative and the postoperative diagnoses differ, which diagnosis is coded and why?

YOU CODE IT! Basics

First, identify the main term in the following diagnoses; then code the diagnosis.

Example: Factitial dermatosis:

a. main term: dermatosis **b.** diagnosis: *L98.1*

1. Acute cystitis without hematuria:
   a. main term: _____ **b.** diagnosis: _____
2. Pulmonary necrosis:
   a. main term: _____ **b.** diagnosis: _____
3. Fibrocystic disease of the pancreas:
   a. main term: _____ **b.** diagnosis: _____
4. Chronic daily headache:
   a. main term: _____ **b.** diagnosis: _____
5. Inflammation of the jaw:
   a. main term: _____ **b.** diagnosis: _____
6. Mobile kidney:
   a. main term: _____ **b.** diagnosis: _____
7. Lymphoid interstitial pneumonia:
   a. main term: _____ **b.** diagnosis: _____
8. Adrenal fibrosis:
   a. main term: _____ **b.** diagnosis: _____
9. Upper respiratory infection, chronic:
   a. main term: _____ **b.** diagnosis: _____
10. Acute conjunctivitis, right:
    a. main term: _____ **b.** diagnosis: _____
11. Ulcer of lower limb, left calf with muscle necrosis:
    a. main term: _____ **b.** diagnosis: _____
12. Aortic endocarditis:
    a. main term: _____ **b.** diagnosis: _____
13. Tuberculous cystitis:
    a. main term: _____ **b.** diagnosis: _____
14. Acute appendicitis:
    a. main term: _____ **b.** diagnosis: _____
15. Systemic lupus erythematosus with lung involvement:
    a. main term: _____ **b.** diagnosis: _____

YOU CODE IT! Practice

Using the techniques described in this chapter, carefully read through the case studies and determine the most accurate ICD-10-CM code(s) and external cause code(s), if appropriate, for each case.

1. Ralph Flower, a 27-year-old male, presents today for his annual flu vaccination.
2. Erina Castles, a 43-year-old female, presents today with a few pimples on her chest. Dr. Moss noted some slight redness and swelling in the area and orders blood tests. The results of the blood tests confirm the diagnosis that Erina is a carrier of staphylococcal, methicillin resistant (MRSA).

(continued)

3. Herman Carson, a 32-year-old male, presents with a severe headache and occasional nosebleeds. Dr. Wells completed an examination recording a blood pressure reading of 180/110. Herman is hospitalized, where an ECG and echocardiogram confirm the diagnosis of malignant hypertension.
4. Anna Blanks, a 68-year-old female, presents with a cyst on the anterior wall of her vagina. After an examination, Dr. Hervey takes a tissue biopsy and orders a CT scan. Anna is diagnosed with a primary malignant neoplasm of the Skene's gland.
5. Jan McKenzie, a 68-year-old female, presents today to see Dr. McLeod due to restlessness and being anxious. Jan retired 3 months ago. Dr. McLeod diagnosis Jan with problems adjusting to retirement.
6. Margaret Carll, a 28-year-old female, presents today with the complaint of feeling dizzy and has some headaches. Dr. Dithomas notes a fever and completes an ECG, which shows an ST depression. PMH and PFH are noncontributory. Margaret is admitted to the hospital, where further blood tests, a chest CT scan, and a ventilation scan confirm the diagnosis of hyperventilation (tetany).
7. Elizabeth Hagun, a 35-year-old female, spent yesterday afternoon outside in the full sun; now she is experiencing severe itching. She comes to see Dr. Jerod, who completes an examination and notes skin redness and blistering. Elizabeth is diagnosed with acute dermatitis due to solar radiation. Code the dermatitis.
8. Audrey Harkey, a 33-year-old female, comes to see Dr. Blankenship. Audrey is accompanied by her husband, Henry. Audrey complaints of fever, a stiff neck, and headaches. Henry states he is concerned because he has noticed some confusion. Audrey is admitted to the hospital, where a lumbar puncture is performed; 5 ml of cerebrospinal fluid is drawn. Test results confirm Dr. Blankenship's diagnosis of tuberculous meningitis.
9. Gloria Leugers, a 37-year-old female, comes to see Dr. Lewis with a fever, weakness, and abdominal pain. Blood tests reveal a hemoglobin of 8.6 and UA is positive for blood. Gloria is admitted to Weston Hospital and diagnosed with schistosomiasis disorder in the kidney.
10. Lauren Wheatle, a 68-year-old female, presents today with chest discomfort when resting. Dr. Billings completes an examination with ECG. The ECG reveals an elevated ST segment. Lauren is admitted to the hospital, where blood tests show elevated cardiac enzymes and a cardiac echo confirms the diagnosis of variant angina.
11. Carolyn Mann, a 34-year-old female, presents today with intense itching and a burning sensation of her anus. Dr. Neal completes an examination and diagnoses her with pruritus ani, stage 2.
12. Sylvia McCray, a 17-year-old female, presents today with a headache and dull facial pain between and behind her eyes. Dr. Clayton orders a CT scan, which confirms the diagnosis of acute ethmoidal sinusitis, infection due to staphylococcus.
13. Shawn Phillips, a 6-year-old male, is brought in by his parents to see Dr. Smoak, his pediatrician. Shawn was eating his lunch and swallowed a piece of chicken bone, which is stuck in his esophagus. Shawn is having difficulty breathing. Dr. Smoak notes that the bone is causing tracheal compression. Dr. Smoak was able to remove the bone and Shawn's breathing returned to normal.
14. Christopher Crawford, a 47-year-old male, presents today with swollen, red gums that are painful to touch, but are not bleeding. Dr. Hubert diagnosed Christopher with acute gingivitis, non-plaque induced.
15. Paul Plum, an 8-month-old male, is brought in by his mother to see Dr. Wallace, Paul's pediatrician. Paul's stomach feels hard and he is also having some diarrhea and vomiting. Dr. Wallace notes Paul is failing to thrive and hospitalizes him. After blood tests and a hydrogen breath test are completed, Paul is diagnosed with congenital lactase deficiency.

YOU CODE IT! Application

The following exercises provide practice in abstracting physician documentation from our health care facility, Prader, Bracker, & Associates. These case studies are modeled on real patient encounters. Using the techniques described in this chapter, carefully read through the case studies and determine the most accurate ICD-10-CM code(s) for each case study. Remember to include external cause codes, if appropriate.

(continued)

PRADER, BRACKER, & ASSOCIATES

A Complete Health Care Facility

159 Healthcare Way • SOMEWHERE, FL 32811 • 407-555-6789

PATIENT: Kassandra, Kelly

ACCOUNT/EHR #: KASSKE001

Attending Physician: Oscar R. Prader, MD

S: Pt is a 19-year-old female who has had a sore throat and cough for the past week. She states that she had a temperature of 101.5 F last night. She also admits that it is painful to swallow. No OTC medication has provided any significant relief.

O: Ht 5′5″ Wt. 148 lb. R 20. T 101 F. BP 125/82. Pharynx is inspected, tonsils enlarged. There is pus noted in the posterior pharynx. Neck: supple, no nodes. Chest: clear. Heart: regular rate and rhythm without murmur.

A: Acute pharyngitis

P: 1. Send pt for Strep test

2. Recommend patient gargle with warm salt water and use OTC lozenges to keep throat moist

3. Rx if needed once results of Strep test come back

4. Return in 2 weeks for follow-up

Determine the most accurate ICD-10-CM code(s).

WESTON HOSPITAL

629 Healthcare Way • SOMEWHERE, FL 32811 • 407-555-6541

PATIENT: DAVIS, HELEN

ACCOUNT/EHR #: DAVIHE001

Attending Physician: Renee O. Bracker, MD

Patient, an 82-year-old that presents today to see Dr. Newson. Dr. Newson saw this patient 10 days ago in office, where she was diagnosed with a UTI and prescribed nitrofurantoin po. Today she presents with the complaints of dysuria, low back pain, abdominal pain, nausea, and diarrhea. After a positive UA she was admitted to Weston Hospital.

PE: Ht: 5′3″, Wt: 112 lb., T: 97.3, P: 70, R: 19, BP: 133/62, O_2 sat 97%. Dr. Newson notes LLQ tenderness and poor nutritional intake. Blood work results: WBC-16.5, RBC-5.70, HCT-50.5 indicating infection. Urine culture showed Staphylococcus. CT scan of abdomen and pelvis reveals mild diverticulitis. Chest clear, lungs clear—sounds bilaterally S1 & S2 heard. Active bowel sound. Strong muscle strength in all extremities. Pulse is regular. Skin is intact, noted redness in coccyx area. Mucous membrane is moist and pink. Functioning independently.

Laboratory results:

Sodium—133 (L); Potassium—4.7

Chloride—95 (L); CO_2—23

Glucose-Serum—122 (H); BUN—16

Creatinine—0.8; Protein—8.2

Albumin—4.7; Total Bilirubin—1.3

WBC—15.5 (H); RBC—5.70 (H)

HGB—15.9; HCT—50.5 (H)

Platelet—326; Neutrophils—65.4

(continued)

Lymphocytes—27.0; Monocytes—6.3

Eosinophils—0.4; Basophils—0.9

ALT—13; AST—31; Alkaline Phosphatase—106

Patient was started on Vancomycin 200 mg/IV q 6 hr, Docusate sodium 100 mg/hr, and Zofran 24 mg po. Patient responded to treatment and is alert & oriented x 3. If she continues to improve, she will be discharged home tomorrow.

Dx: Staphylococcal UTI, Large intestine diverticulitis

Determine the most accurate ICD-10-CM code(s).

PRADER, BRACKER, & ASSOCIATES

A Complete Health Care Facility

159 Healthcare Way • SOMEWHERE, FL 32811 • 407-555-6789

PATIENT: HOBARTH, CHANTEL

ACCOUNT/EHR #: HOBACH001

Attending Physician: Oscar R. Prader, MD

S: Pt is a 45-year-old female diagnosed with bladder cancer 4 years ago. She underwent chemotherapy and radiation treatments and is now malignant-free for 18 months. Since being malignant-free she comes in for an abdominal scan every 6 months. Pt has no signs or symptoms indicating a return of the malignancy.

O: Ht 5′5″. Wt. 137 lb. R 18. T 99. BP 128/81. Abdomen appears to be normal upon manual examination. Results of CT scan indicated no abnormalities.

A: Personal history of bladder cancer

P: Pt to return PRN

Determine the most accurate ICD-10-CM code(s).

PRADER, BRACKER, & ASSOCIATES

A Complete Health Care Facility

159 Healthcare Way • SOMEWHERE, FL 32811 • 407-555-6789

PATIENT: ROMANO, JOSEPH

ACCOUNT/EHR #: ROMAJO001

Attending Physician: Renee O. Bracker, MD

S: Pt is a 32-year-old male who works at a local restaurant. While at work he was preparing a chicken and cut the back of his right index finger. He states he stopped the bleed with pressure, but now he can't extend his finger. Pt. had last tetanus toxoid administered last year. He has no past history of serious illnesses, operations, or allergies. Social history and family history are noncontributory.

O: Examination reveals a 3.6-cm laceration, dorsum of right index finger, with laceration of extensor tendon, proximal to the interphalangeal joint. The patient cannot extend the finger. Pt was prepped, and a digital nerve block using 1% Carbocaine was administered. When the block was totally effective, the wound was irrigated with normal saline. The joint capsule was repaired with two sutures of 5-0 Dexon. The tendon repair was then carried out using 4-0 nylon. Dressings were applied, and a splint was applied holding the interphalangeal joint in neutral position, in full extension. The Pt tolerated the procedure well.

A: 3.6-cm laceration, dorsum of right index finger

(continued)

P: 1. Rx Percocet, q4h prn for pain

2. Rx Augmentin, 250 mg tid

3. Follow-up in 3 days

Determine the most accurate ICD-10-CM code(s) for the laceration.

WESTON HOSPITAL

629 Healthcare Way • SOMEWHERE, FL 32811 • 407-555-6541

PATIENT: FLORA, VINCENT

ACCOUNT/EHR #: FLORVI001

Attending Physician: Oscar R. Prader, MD

S: Pt is a 37-year-old female who was on vacation with friends. On a wager she parachuted from a plane and landed in a tree. She hit her head against a rock when she fell from the tree and lost consciousness for approximately 5 minutes. She says she has a headache and is a bit nauseated.

O: Ht 5′6″ Wt. 130 lb. R 18. T 98.1. BP 122/83. HEENT unremarkable. PERRLA. Dr. Prader notes slight slurred speech. EEG shows indication of a head trauma. CT scan confirmed the brain concussion. Patient was admitted to the hospital for observation.

A: Concussion with brief loss of consciousness

P: 1. Watch for 24 hours

2. Discharge home if no further complications.

Determine the most accurate ICD-10-CM code(s) for the concussion.

6

Coding Infectious Diseases

Key Terms

Acute
Asymptomatic
Bacteria
Chronic
Fungi
Human Immunodeficiency Virus (HIV)
Infection
Infectious
Inflammation
Nosocomial
Parasites
Pathogen
Sepsis
Septic Shock
Septicemia
Severe Sepsis
Systemic
Systemic Inflammatory Response Syndrome (SIRS)
Tuberculosis
Viruses

Learning Outcomes

After completing this chapter, the student should be able to:

LO 6.1 Interpret the details required to report an accurate code for an infection.
LO 6.2 Clarify the details about bacterial infections.
LO 6.3 Determine the specifics needed to report viral infections.
LO 6.4 Translate information about parasitic and fungal infections into diagnosis codes.
LO 6.5 Abstract documentation to identify important details about the specific pathogen causing a diagnosis.
LO 6.6 Ascertain the correct code or codes to report immunodeficiency conditions.
LO 6.7 Apply the guidelines for reporting blood infections.
LO 6.8 Analyze the documentation to identify the code or codes required to report antimicrobial resistance.

STOP! Remember, you need to follow along in your ICD-10-CM code book for an optimal learning experience.

6.1 Infectious and Communicable Diseases

Many conditions and illnesses can be disseminated from one individual to another. **Infectious** diseases are spread by personal contact, such as a handshake or the exchange of bodily fluids, while other diseases can be spread by the touch of a doorknob that has been handled by someone else. Some of these conditions, such as meningitis, hepatitis, **tuberculosis**, and **human immunodeficiency virus (HIV)**, have been in the media, and others you may never have heard of before. This chapter will help you understand how to report all of these diseases using ICD-10-CM codes.

Infectious
A condition that can be transmitted from one person to another.

Tuberculosis
An infectious condition that causes small rounded swellings on mucous membranes throughout the body.

Human Immunodeficiency Virus (HIV)
A condition affecting the immune system.

CODING BITES

Keep references close at hand. Bookmark or mark as a favorite reliable sources such as the MedlinePlus online medical encyclopedia. This will help you increase your understanding of any infectious disease, and its inclusive signs and symptoms, that you encounter in physician documentation.

Infections and Inflammation

There are wars going on constantly throughout your body as **pathogens** (vehicles of disease) insert themselves into your cells and multiply. There are many types of pathogens, and each carries its own threat to your health. **Infection** happens once a pathogen successfully invades the body and begins to replicate. This multiplication of the organism, known as *colonization*, causes damage to cell structures and can remain localized in one area (such as an infected

Pathogen
Any agent that causes disease; a microorganism such as a bacterium or virus.

Infection
The invasion of pathogens into tissue cells.

toe), spread to a larger area (such as infection of the foot and leg), or become **systemic** (spreading throughout the entire body). The human body is designed to alert the individual and the doctor to the existence of infection by exhibiting specific signs and symptoms:

Systemic
Spread throughout the entire body.

- Increased body temperature (commonly known as a *fever*).
- Increased white blood cell count.
- Increase (tachycardia) or decrease (bradycardia) in heart rate.
- Increase (hyperventilation) or decrease (dyspnea) in respiratory rate.

CODING BITES

Remember, inclusive signs and symptoms are not coded separately. This is why you need to learn what they are for each illness or disease so you know what should not and what should be coded.

In some cases, a patient might not be aware that there is an infection in his or her body. This is known as a *subclinical* or **asymptomatic** infection. In other cases, the condition can become **acute** (severe), and a specific area may show signs of **inflammation**. When located in the epidermis, inflammation can be visible; it causes signs and symptoms, such as erythema (reddening), swelling, warmth to the touch, and often pain. When located internally, the inflammation can cause lack of function, especially when found within a joint. When inflammation is left untreated, or if treatment is ineffective, the condition can become **chronic** (ongoing). Any of these details may be required to determine an accurate code. You will know by reading the complete code descriptions in the Tabular List.

Asymptomatic
No symptoms or manifestations.

Acute
Severe; serious.

Inflammation
The reaction of tissues to infection or injury; characterized by pain, swelling, and erythema.

Chronic
Long duration; continuing over an extended period of time.

Nosocomial
A hospital-acquired condition; a condition that develops as a result of being in a health care facility.

EXAMPLE

A39.2	Acute meningococcemia
B39.1	Chronic pulmonary histoplasmosis capsulati
Z21	Asymptomatic human immunodeficiency virus [HIV] infection status

Communicable Diseases

People interact in society, and, therefore, the transmission of pathogens cannot be avoided. The level of interaction and the severity of the pathogen (how aggressive it may be) will impact how many individuals are infected. There are many ways that patients can be exposed to an infection and become ill.

Health care–acquired infections (HAIs), also known as **nosocomial** infections, are those conditions that are contracted solely due to interactions with a health care facility, during which exposure to various types of pathogens occurs. Take note that HAIs are infections that occur in hospitals, nursing homes, and other health care provider locations. HAIs are not just the concern of inpatient acute care facilities.

A cough or a sneeze may send pathogens into the air, and a doorknob or a telephone receiver easily transfers pathogens to the skin that touches it next–these are methods of transportation for bacteria or viruses to travel from an infected person to another soon-to-be-infected person. Some diseases require more intimate contact, such as the exchange of bodily fluids (during sex, exposure to blood, or contact with mucus).

- *Touch exposure:* Physical interaction with blood, bodily fluids, nonintact skin, and mucous membranes can enable a long list of bloodborne pathogens to make their way from one person to another.
- *Airborne exposure:* Some pathogens travel in small particles that remain contagious in the air, such as chickenpox. Measles can live in the air of a room for 2 hours after the infected person leaves. Breathing in contaminated air by merely entering an examination room or patient area can expose someone to the disease.
- *Droplet exposure*: Some diseases, such as influenza, can be dispersed in large droplets, such as those transmitted by coughing, spitting, talking, and sneezing.
- *Contact exposure*: As with touch exposure, some infections, such as herpes simplex virus, are communicated by skin-to-skin contact or skin to other surfaces (e.g., countertops, paper).
- *Needlestick/sharps injury exposure*: Bloodborne pathogens, including HIV, hepatitis B, and hepatitis C, can be highly contagious when contaminated needles or other sharp objects (e.g., scalpels, dental wire) penetrate the protective outer layer of the skin.
- *Insect bites*: Mosquitoes, deer ticks, fleas, and other insects/parasites spread disease as well. Zika is transmitted by mosquitoes, deer ticks transmit Lyme disease, and fleas spread the plague.
- *Food and water:* There are many diseases, such as *E. coli* or cholera, that are spread by ingestion of substances.

Reporting the Infectious Agent

In some cases, the code you determine to report an infection may be complete with the specific type of pathogen, such as tuberculosis, which is only caused by *Mycobacterium tuberculosis* or *Mycobacterium bovis*. This means that the specific pathogen is included in the diagnostic statement and therefore the code.

CODING BITES

Later on, in the chapter titled ***Inpatient (Hospital) Diagnosis Coding***, you will learn how to use Present-On-Admission indicators to report nosocomial conditions.

EXAMPLE

Tuberculosis (A15-A19)

INCLUDES infections due to *Mycobacterium tuberculosis* and *Mycobacterium bovis*

Sometimes, you will find a combination code that includes the name of the pathogen in the code description.

EXAMPLES

J02.0 Streptococcal pharyngitis

J09.X3 Influenza due to identified novel influenza A virus with gastrointestinal manifestations

These code descriptions are known as combination codes because they include both the condition and the specific pathogen.

Other times, an infection might be caused by any one of several different pathogens. In these cases, you will need to report a second code to specify the bacterial or viral infectious agent.

EXAMPLES

B95.2 Enterococcus as the cause of diseases classified elsewhere

B96.3 *Haemophilus influenzae* [H. influenzae] as the cause of diseases classified elsewhere

B97.11 Coxsackievirus as the cause of diseases classified elsewhere

These code descriptions identify the specific pathogen to be reported along with the code describing the condition caused.

The part of the code description that states "*diseases classified elsewhere*" means that the condition has its own code within this code set. This underscores the fact that this is not a combination code and you will need two codes to report the condition.

EXAMPLE

✓4 N30 Cystitis

Use additional code **to identify infectious agent (B95–B97)**

Very often, the ICD-10-CM will tell you that you will need this second code to identify the specific pathogen.

YOU INTERPRET IT!

What is the mode of transmission for each condition?

1. Hepatitis B __________
2. Measles __________
3. Cholera __________
4. Insect bites __________
5. Influenza __________

6.2 Bacterial Infections

Types of Bacteria

> **Bacteria**
> Single-celled microorganisms that cause disease.

Bacteria are single-celled organisms named by their shape (see **Figure 6-1**). Rod-shaped bacteria, called *bacilli*, are responsible for the development of diphtheria, tetanus, and tuberculosis, among others. *Spirilla*, bacterial organisms shaped like a spiral, may cause cholera or syphilis, while dot-shaped bacteria known as *cocci* cause gonorrhea, tonsillitis, scarlet fever, and bacterial meningitis.

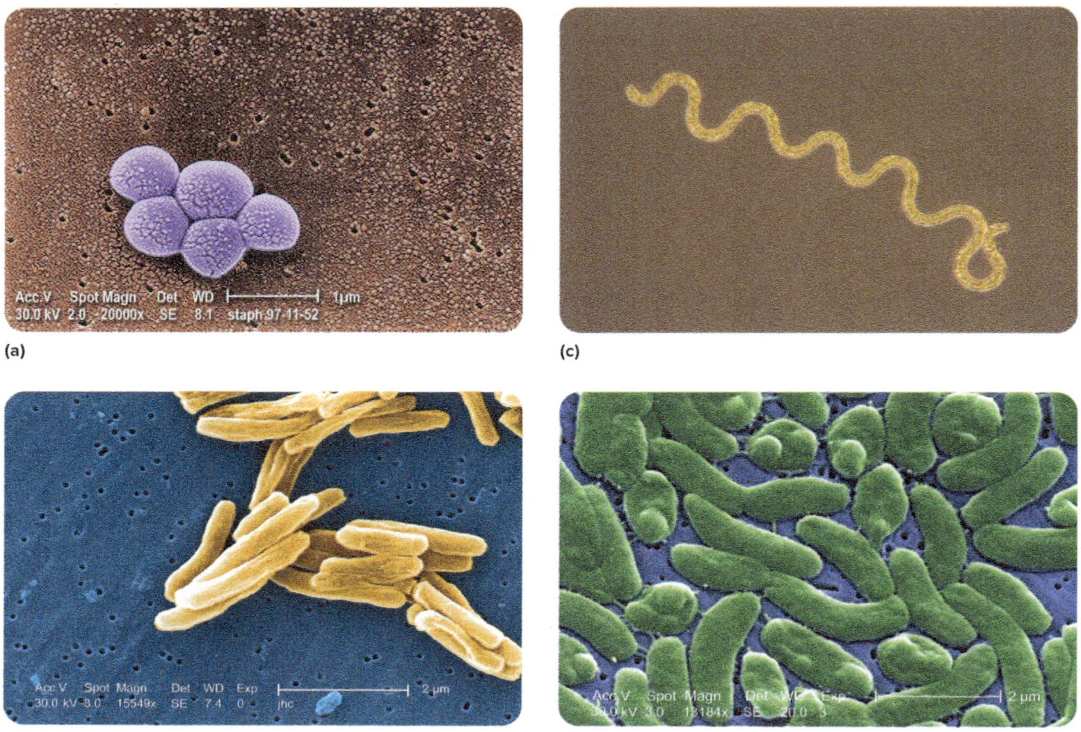

(a) (c) (b) (d)

FIGURE 6-1 Types of bacteria: (a) coccus, (b) bacillus, (c) spirillum, and (d) vibrio

(a) Janice Carr/CDC; (b) Janice Carr/CDC; (c) MELBA PHOTO AGENCY/Alamy Stock Photo; (d) Janice Carr/CDC

EXAMPLES

A05.4 Foodborne *Bacillus cereus* intoxication

A27.9 Leptospirosis, unspecified

A49.1 Streptococcal infection, unspecified site

This is a great example of why professional coders-to-be need to know these details . . . so you can recognize the name of a bacterium in diagnostic terms and phrases. Until you learn them, use your medical dictionary to confirm.

Conditions Caused by Bacteria

Impetigo

Impetigo is a common illness affecting children, caused by either a streptococcal or a staphylococcal pathogen. This means that MRSA (methicillin-resistant *Staphylococcus aureus*) is a real concern. This disease spreads through contact with fluid oozing from a bullous–or blister. Visually, impetigo is evidenced by the appearance of rings that can range from pea-size to large rings.

They may itch. These blisters may ooze yellow or honey-colored fluid and then crust. Of course, the itching may result in the patient scratching, which then spreads the rash. The physician may also document swollen lymph nodes, particularly in the body areas close to the infection site. Impetigo is often reported with a code from code category L01 with additional required characters to provide additional specificity.

EXAMPLE

A specific, complete diagnostic statement is required to determine an accurate code for a case of impetigo:

L01.01 Non-bullous impetigo

L01.02 Brockhart's impetigo

L01.03 Bullous impetigo

L01.09 Other impetigo [ulcerative impetigo]

Yet, notice . . . not all impetigo diagnoses are reported from this one code category . . .

L40.1 Generalized pustular psoriasis [impetigo herpetiformis]

Foodborne Illness

Some bacterial infections that you will encounter in a typical health care facility are those that are foodborne, commonly called *food poisoning*. Do not let the word "poisoning" fool you. These diagnoses are not poisonings; they are actually infections. Some of the most frequently seen bacterial infections, and their sources, are shown in **Table 6-1**.

TABLE 6-1 Common Bacterial Infections, Their Sources, and Their Codes

Name	Source	Code
Campylobacter	From foods including raw poultry, raw meat, untreated milk	A04.5
Listeria	Untreated milk, dairy products, raw salads and vegetables	A32.-
Salmonella	Raw poultry, eggs, raw meat, untreated milk and dairy products	A02.9
Shigella	Untreated water, milk and dairy products, raw vegetables and salads, shellfish, turkey, apple cider	A03.-
Vibrio	Raw and lightly cooked shellfish	A00.-
Clostridium perfringens	Animal and human excreta, soil, dust, insects, raw meat	B96.7
Escherichia coli (E. coli O157)	Human and animal gut, sewage, water, raw meat	A49.8

EXAMPLES

Clostridium botulinum is the bacterium that causes A05.1 Botulism food poisoning.

Foodborne *Clostridium perfringens*, the bacterium that causes enteritis necroticans, is reported with code A05.2.

Foodborne staphylococcal intoxication is reported with A05.0.

Salmonella foodborne intoxication and infection are reported from code category A02, which requires additional information related to the infection resulting from this bacterium.

Listeriosis [listerial foodborne infection] is reported from code category A32 and requires additional detail about the patient's condition.

Almost all infections shown in **Table 6-1** induce symptoms of diarrhea, abdominal pain, nausea, fever, and vomiting. Other serious effects include dehydration, headache, and kidney damage or failure. Therefore, you must be careful not to report unnecessary codes for signs and symptoms that are actually included in a definitive diagnosis that has been made.

LET'S CODE IT! SCENARIO

Francie Holland, a 23-year-old female, came to see Dr. Kensington due to severe abdominal pain. She had a fever and stated that she has had bloody diarrhea for the past 2 days. Dr. Kensington's examination revealed that she was dehydrated as well. Francie stated she ate at a new restaurant at the beach where she had a salad and a vegetable plate. After taking some tests, he diagnosed Francie with Shigella dysenteriae *(bacillary dysentery).*

Let's Code It!

Dr. Kensington found Francie to be suffering from *Shigella dysenteriae*. Turn to the Alphabetic Index and find

Shigella (dysentery) (see Dysentery, bacillary)

Dysentery, bacillary A03.9

Turn to the Tabular List, and check the code's complete description:

✓4 **A03 Shigellosis**

There are no notations or directives, so read down the column to review all of the choices for the required fourth character. The code suggested by the Alphabetic Index:

A03.9 Shigellosis, unspecified

Is this the most accurate code? You will note that the other fourth-character code choices want specifics on which group (A, B, C, or D) of the *Shigella* infection is present. Do you know? Dr. Kensington did specify in the notes—*Shigella dysenteriae*, which matches the description for

A03.0 Shigellosis due to Shigella dysenteriae

Check the top of this subsection and the head of this chapter in ICD-10-CM. There are notations at the beginning of this chapter: an INCLUDES notation, a ***Use Additional Code*** note, an EXCLUDES1 notation, and an EXCLUDES2 notation. Read carefully. Do any relate to Dr. Kensington's diagnosis of Francie? No. Turn to the Official Guidelines and read Section I.C.1. There is nothing specifically applicable here either.

Therefore, A03.0 is the most accurate code available. Excellent!!

Cellulitis

CODING BITES

When the documentation states that an external cause, such as an animal bite, provided entry for the pathogen, external cause codes may be required. More about these in the chapter ***Coding Injury, Poisoning, and External Causes.***

Cellulitis is a serious infection of the skin that may be either a staph infection (the staphylococcal bacteria) or a strep infection (the streptococcal bacteria). These pathogens typically enter the body through an abnormal opening in the epidermal layer of the skin—for example, a burn, puncture wound, abrasion (also known as a scrape), or even a bite—either animal or human.

Cellulitis begins with the typical signs of inflammation: erythema (redness), heat arising from the area of infection, pain, and edema (swelling). Vesicles or bullae may appear in the infected area. In addition, the patient may develop a fever with chills, experience tachycardia (a rapid heartbeat), suffer a headache, have hypotension (low blood pressure), and, at times, become mentally confused.

Report a diagnosis of cellulitis with a code—in many cases—from code category L03. You will need specific information on the precise anatomical site affected by the condition.

EXAMPLES

L03.012	Cellulitis of left finger
L03.113	Cellulitis of right upper limb
L03.314	Cellulitis of groin

These are examples of the need to identify the specific anatomical site of the cellulitis to determine an accurate code.

There is an EXCLUDES2 notation beneath L03.211, the code used to report cellulitis of the face. This long list of specific anatomical sites that might normally be included within the face are actually reported with different codes from different areas of the ICD-10-CM code book . . . such as cellulitis of the ear, reported with code H60.1, or cellulitis of the mouth, which is reported with code K12.2. As always, you must read all of the notations, carefully and completely.

L03.31–the code used to report cellulitis of the trunk–also has a list of specific anatomical sites located on the torso that are reported with codes from other chapters, such as cellulitis of anal and rectal regions, which is reported with a code from the K61 Abscess of anal and rectal regions code category, or cellulitis of the breast, which is reported from code category N61 Inflammatory disorders of the breast.

Tetanus (Lockjaw)

You are probably more familiar with the tetanus vaccine than you are with the disease. Tetanus is an infection of the nervous system and is caused by the entry of bacteria into the body through a break in the skin. It causes death in about 11% of all cases. The illness can be prevented by the administration of the tetanus toxoid, included in the DTaP, DT, and Td vaccines.

When a patient has come for inoculation with the tetanus toxoid only, you will use Z23. However, read the notes carefully. If the development of tetanus is a complication arising from the vaccination, use code T88.1. If tetanus is a result of an incident, such as stepping on a rusty nail, report it with code A35 plus an external cause code. Should this disease occur with or following an abortion or ectopic pregnancy, then you will report it as a complication of pregnancy, using A34 or O08.89. And in cases where the tetanus is affecting a neonate, it will be reported with code A33.

Tuberculosis

Mycobacterium tuberculosis, the causative agent of tuberculosis (TB), is a bacterial infection that is transmitted through the air. One version of TB is called *latent tuberculosis infection (LTBI)* because it is dormant and may not show symptoms right away. Not everyone who has been infected is symptomatic, so a test is required to confirm the diagnosis. Most types of TB and LTBI are successfully treated with medication.

There is a specific cultural group of people who will get a positive result to the skin test but not actually have the disease. A simple chest x-ray confirms that situation. Should you have a patient in such a circumstance, you will use this code:

R76.11 Nonspecific reaction to tuberculin skin test without active tuberculosis

When the documentation confirms a diagnosis of TB, you will choose the best, most appropriate code from the range A15–A19 Tuberculosis based on the specific anatomical site affected.

EXAMPLES

A15.0	Tuberculosis of lung
A17.1	Meningeal tuberculoma
A18.81	Tuberculosis of thyroid gland
A19.1	Acute miliary tuberculosis of multiple sites

The codes in these four code categories illustrate the extensive list of anatomical sites that may be affected with TB. Read the documentation and diagnosis carefully (as always).

As you look through the section, you will notice that TB is a disseminated disease. While most people think of TB as a pulmonary infection, infiltrating only the lungs, it can actually leach throughout the body and be identified in many different anatomical sites. You have to abstract which anatomical site is infected with the TB bacterium so that you can find the most accurate code.

YOU CODE IT! CASE STUDY

Audra Swenson was brought into the emergency department (ED) by ambulance because she was having suprapubic pain, pain in her lower back, and nocturia. Dr. Balthazar diagnosed Audra with renal tuberculosis, also known as urogential TB, confirmed histologically, with pyelonephritis.

You Code It!

Go through the steps of coding, and determine the diagnosis code or codes that should be reported for this encounter between Dr. Balthazar and Audra Swenson.

Step #1: Read the case carefully and completely.
Step #2: Abstract the scenario. Which main words or terms describe why the physician cared for the patient during this encounter?
Step #3: Are there any details missing or incomplete for which you would need to query the physician? [If so, ask your instructor.]
Step #4: Check for any relevant guidance, including reading all of the symbols and notations in the Tabular List and the appropriate sections of the Official Guidelines.
Step #5: Determine the correct diagnosis code or codes to explain why this encounter was medically necessary.
Step #6: Double-check your work.

Answer:

Did you determine the correct code?

A18.11 Tuberculosis of kidney and ureter

Terrific!

Infectious
A condition that can be transmitted from one person to another.

Viruses
Microscopic particles that initiate disease, mimicking the characteristics of a particular cell; viruses can reproduce only within the body of the cell that they have invaded.

6.3 Viral Infections

Types of Viruses

There are a large number of viral **infectious** diseases that you may have to code, depending upon the type of facility that employs you, combined with geographic and other factors.

Viruses are tiny microorganisms that are not easily treated with medication because they embed themselves within their host's cells and are, therefore, difficult to isolate (see **Figure 6-2**). These invaders can remain dormant (latent) for long periods of time.

EXAMPLES

A85.0 Enteroviral encephalitis
B18.0 Chronic viral hepatitis B with delta-agent
B33.21 Viral endocarditis

Sometimes, the code description identifies the viral pathogen involved in a diagnosis. When a combination code is available, you will need to report it, as long as it matches the physician's documentation.

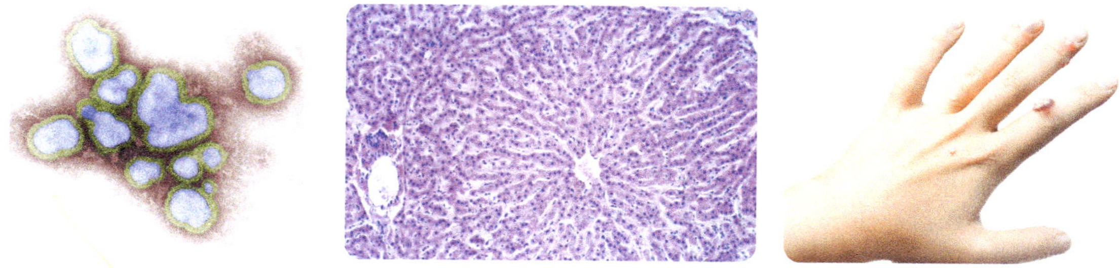

(a) (b) (c)

FIGURE 6-2 Types of viruses: (a) influenza, (b) hepatitis, and (c) warts

(a) F.A. Murphy/CDC; (b) Victor P. Eroschenko; (c) Zoonar GmbH/Alamy Stock Photo

Conditions Caused by Viruses

Viral Warts

Viral warts are most common in children and are rarely seen in the elderly. This virus can be spread from person to person during sexual contact or an individual with a viral wart can see it spread from one anatomical site to another.

There are several different types of warts, as you can see in **Figure 6-3**, so it is important that the specifics are documented. Take a look at the suggested codes, here in the Alphabetic Index: A63.0, B07.9, H18.49, L82.0 . . . located in several different chapters throughout the Tabular List. You must read the documentation carefully, including the pathology report, to point you toward the correct codes from which to choose.

Wart (due to HPV) (filiform) (infectious) (viral) B07.9
- anogenital region (venereal) A63.0
- common B07.8
- external genital organs (venereal) A63.0
- flat B07.8
- Hassal-Henle's (of cornea) H18.49
- Peruvian A44.1
- plantar B07.0
- prosector (tuberculosis) A18.4
- seborrheic L82.1
- inflamed L82.0
- senile (seborrheic) L82.1
- inflamed L82.0
- tuberculosis A18.4
- venereal A63.0

FIGURE 6-3 ICD-10-CM Alphabetic Index, partial listing under the main term Wart

Source: *ICD-10-CM Official Guidelines for Coding and Reporting*, The Centers for Medicare and Medicaid Services (CMS) and the National Center for Health Statistics (NCHS).

Viral Hepatitis

Hepatitis (*hepat* = liver; *-itis* = inflammation) actually refers to several different viral infections. According to the Centers for Disease Control and Prevention (CDC), viral hepatitis is the most prevalent cause of malignant neoplasms of the liver. As you know, prevention is a much better path than treatment. For those coming to your facility to get a hepatitis vaccine, you will report one of these codes:

Z20.5	**Contact with or (suspected) exposure to other viral hepatitis**
Z22.330	**Carrier of Group B Streptococcus**
Z23	**Encounter for immunization**

For those who are already infected with one of the strains of hepatitis, it's critical to understand the different types in order to code the encounter(s) correctly.

Viral Hepatitis, Type A

The CDC estimates that an additional 25,000 people each year become infected with viral hepatitis, type A, a viral infection of the liver caused by the hepatitis A virus (HAV). The virus can travel from person to person by personal contact, as with other infections. However, in addition, one can become infected through exposure to contaminated water or ice. Shellfish harvested from sewage-contaminated water as well as fruits, vegetables, and other foods that have been contaminated and eaten uncooked may also carry the HAV.

In some cases, a patient may develop hepatic encephalopathy (hepatic coma). This occurs when, because of the infection, the liver is unable to remove toxins from the blood, resulting in a loss of brain function.

Viral hepatitis A is reported with either:

B15.0 **Hepatitis A with hepatic coma**

or

B15.9 **Hepatitis A without hepatic coma**

Viral Hepatitis, Type B

Caused by the hepatitis B virus (HBV), viral hepatitis, type B is transmitted through contact with infected bodily fluids, such as blood or semen. The infection also can be spread by the use of equipment that has been contaminated with the virus, which is why when getting a tattoo, body piercing, or even a fingernail application one must be careful that the needles and files have been sterilized properly. The CDC estimates 43,000 new cases of hepatitis B are diagnosed each year.

To determine the most accurate code, you have to abstract these details from the documentation:

- Is the patient documented as in a hepatic coma?
- Is the condition identified as acute (code category B16) or chronic (code category B18)?
- Is hepatitis D (also known as hepatitis delta, or delta-agent) involved?

B16.0 **Acute hepatitis B with delta-agent with hepatic coma**
B16.1 **Acute hepatitis B with delta-agent without hepatic coma**
B16.2 **Acute hepatitis B without delta-agent with hepatic coma**
B16.9 **Acute hepatitis B without delta-agent and without hepatic coma**

Viral Hepatitis, Type C

The hepatitis C virus (HCV) infection is estimated by the CDC to chronically affect 3.2 million people in the United States. It is considered to be the most widespread chronic bloodborne infection. Those individuals at the highest risk for infection are those using injected drugs. Each year, it is believed that an additional 17,000 individuals become hepatitis C positive. Report this diagnosis with one of these codes:

B17.10 **Acute hepatitis C without hepatic coma**
B17.11 **Acute hepatitis C with hepatic coma**
B18.2 **Chronic hepatitis C**
B19.20 **Unspecified viral hepatitis C without hepatic coma**

Viral Hepatitis, Type D

Also known as *hepatitis delta*, this is a serious liver disease that requires the HBV to replicate itself. This condition is not seen often in the United States. Hepatitis D is transmitted through direct contact with infected blood, similar to how hepatitis B is passed from one person to another. Currently, there is no vaccine for hepatitis D. Hepatitis D is referred to as *hepatitis delta* in the code descriptions, and reported with this code:

B17.0 **Acute delta-(super) infection of hepatitis B carrier**

Viral Hepatitis, Type E

Occurrences of hepatitis E in the United States are rare; it is known to be common in countries with poor sanitation and contaminated water supplies. This liver disease, caused by the hepatitis E virus (HEV), does not lead to chronic infection. There is no vaccine currently approved by the FDA for hepatitis E. Report this diagnosis with

B17.2 Acute hepatitis E

LET'S CODE IT! SCENARIO

David Tranccione, a 55-year-old white male, came into our office. He complains that he feels tired all the time, no matter how much he sleeps. His muscles are sore, his stomach is upset, and he has experienced frequent bouts of diarrhea. He made an appointment with his regular physician, Dr. Cameron, when he noticed his urine was dark.

Dr. Cameron ordered blood tests, and the pathology report confirmed the diagnosis of acute hepatitis B virus.

Let's Code It!

Dr. Cameron confirmed that David has acute hepatitis B virus. Open your ICD-10-CM code book to the Alphabetic Index to:

Hepatitis K75.9

Before you turn to this code category in the Tabular List, read down the long list indented beneath, just to see if you can find a listing that is more specific and in agreement with Dr. Cameron's documentation.

Hepatitis K75.9

B B19.10

with hepatic coma B19.11

acute B16.9

Four different listings and three very different codes. It is a good thing you keep reading. Turn to code category B16 in the Tabular List:

✓4 **B16 Acute hepatitis B**

Read the four options for the required fourth character. What details do you need from the documentation to choose: with or without delta-agent and with or without hepatic coma? Go back to the scenario. There is no mention of either delta-agent or hepatic coma, so you can report:

B16.9 Acute hepatitis B without delta-agent and without hepatic coma

Check the top of this subsection, which has an EXCLUDES1 and an EXCLUDES2 notation. Neither relates to David's case this time, so next, check the head of this chapter in ICD-10-CM. Above code A00, you will find an INCLUDES notation, a ***Use additional code*** note, an EXCLUDES1 notation, and an EXCLUDES2 notation. Read carefully. Do any relate to Dr. Cameron's diagnosis of David? No. Turn to the Official Guidelines and read Section I.C.1. There is nothing specifically applicable here either.

Now you can report B16.9 for David's diagnosis with confidence.

Good coding!

Influenza

There is a reason why so much commotion is made annually about individuals getting their flu shots. A seemingly ordinary infection, influenza (commonly called the *flu*) can be deadly. It is caused by the influenza A or B virus and can be transmitted by casual contact, such as a handshake or touching a contaminated doorknob. It is estimated that as many as 36,000 people die in the United States each year from influenza.

The most common symptoms of the flu are

- Body or muscle aches
- Chills
- Cough
- Fever
- Headache
- Sore throat

The diagnosis of influenza will be reported with a code from these categories:

✓4 **J09** **Influenza due to certain identified influenza viruses**

✓4 **J10** **Influenza due to other identified influenza viruses**

✓4 **J11** **Influenza due to unidentified influenza viruses**

The required additional characters will enable you to report the specific virus, such as novel influenza A, as well as manifestations of this virus.

EXAMPLES

J09.X1	Influenza due to identified novel influenza A virus with pneumonia
J10.2	Influenza due to other identified influenza virus with gastrointestinal manifestations
J11.1	Influenza due to unidentified influenza virus with other respiratory manifestations

The physician's documentation, along with the pathology report, should provide you with the details you need.

COVID-19

In 2020, the world experienced something not seen in 100 years. . . a global pandemic. We all got to become familiar with an infection due to SARS-CoV-2 virus, the 2019 novel coronavirus disease, known more commonly as COVID-19. This event has initiated the creation of new codes, and a new Chapter in the ICD-10-CM coding manual, ***Chapter 23****. Codes for Special Purposes (U00-U85).*

GUIDANCE CONNECTION

Read the ICD-10-CM Official Guidelines for Coding and Reporting, section **I. Conventions, General Coding Guidelines and Chapter-Specific Guidelines**, subsection **C. Chapter- Specific Coding Guidelines**, chapter **1. Certain Infectious and Parasitic Diseases**, subsection **g. Coronavirus infections.**

EXPOSURE

If a patient has been exposed to COVID-19, and is showing no signs or symptoms (asymptomatic), you will report the reason for this encounter with code:

Z20.828 **Contact with and (suspected) exposure to other viral communicable diseases**

EXHIBITING SIGNS AND SYMPTOMS

If the patient is reporting signs and symptoms, and, there is no confirmed diagnosis yet, you need to report the codes for those specific signs and symptoms, for example:

R06.02 **Shortness of breath**

R50.9 **Fever, unspecified**

When the documentation also states that the patient was exposed to COVID-19, report Z20.828, as well.

CONFIRMED DIAGNOSIS

Should the test come back positive, you will see a confirmed diagnosis of COVID-19 in the physician's documentation. Then, you need to report this with:

U07.1 COVID-19

There are cases when some patients, confirmed to have COVID-19 positive, also exhibit manifestations–other conditions caused by this infection. When these are documented, report the COVID-19 code U07.1 first, followed by the codes reporting the specific manifestation(s).

LET'S CODE IT! SCENARIO

Lillie Karnowski, a 25-year-old female, was admitted with acute bronchitis. She tested positive for COVID-19 last week after spending the weekend at the beach with her friends. Dr. Mancuso admits her with COVID-19-related acute bronchitis

Let's Code It!

Lillie has been confirmed for COVID-19 and has now developed acute bronchitis as a result. The Official Coding Guidelines direct us to report the COVID-19 diagnosis first. Let's turn in the Alphabetic Index to:

Coronavirus (infection)

Coronavirus-19 U07.1

COVID-19 U07.1

SARS-associated B97.21

This is straightforward. The thing to remember here is that the Chapter in the coding manual for the new U codes is not in alphabetic order like the rest, it is after the Z code chapter at the very end of the coding manual.

U07.1 COVID-19

Read carefully. There is a ***Use additional code*** note, which confirm what the Official Guideline states. . . this code must be reported first, followed by the code for Lillie's acute bronchitis. Also, there is an EXCLUDES1 notation with three conditions shown. Do any of these apply to this one case? No. Good, so you can report this code with confidence.

Next, you need to report Lillie's diagnosis of acute bronchitis. Let's go back to the Alphabetic Index and find bronchitis. Read the list below this main term and find acute.

Acute or subacute (with bronchospasm or obstruction) J20.9

There was no mention in the scenario about bronchospasms or obstruction, so let's keep reading. A little further down the column, see

Acute or subacute

Viral NEC J20.8

Well, this fits! The documentation states the bronchitis was caused by the coronavirus. Turn to the Tabular list and find

J20 Acute bronchitis

Followed by a long list of INCLUDES, EXCLUDES1, and EXCLUDES2 notations. Read them all, carefully. None apply to this specific scenario. Now examine the code descriptions for all of the codes in this code category. The only one that fits accurately is

J20.8 Acute bronchitis due to other specified organisms

The organism is specified—COVID-19—but there is no specific code description that matches more accurately. So, you now have the two codes to report the reasons for Lillie's hospital admission: U07.1, J20.8. Good coding!

FOLLOW-UP ENCOUNTERS

The longer the world deals with this pandemic, the greater the opportunity you may have to report a reason for a follow-up visit, after the patient has cleared the virus. For these visits, and for those where the patient has now tested negative, report one of two codes, determined by the specifics in the documentation:

Z09 **Encounter for follow-up examination after completed treatment for conditions other than malignant neoplasm**

Z86.19 **Personal history of other infectious and parasitic diseases**

At an encounter where the patient is coming back in for a COVID-19 antibody test, you need to report

Z01.84 **Encounter for antibody response examination**

Varicella

> **CODING BITES**
>
> Varicella is commonly called *chickenpox*.

Varicella, commonly known as *chickenpox*, is generally not perceived to be serious, most particularly for children. Complications from varicella, however, may include pneumonia in adults and bacterial infections of the skin and soft tissue in affected children. The infections can be severe and can lead to septicemia, toxic shock syndrome, necrotizing fasciitis, osteomyelitis, bacterial pneumonia, and septic arthritis. There may also be a connection between varicella and development of herpes zoster, also known as *shingles*, later in life. The availability of the varicella vaccine has made the risk of contracting the infection almost nil.

Code varicella from B01.- if the patient has been diagnosed. If the patient has come to receive a varicella vaccine, then use code Z23. However, if the patient has been exposed to varicella, the code will change to Z20.820.

Rubeola

The risk of catching the childhood illness of rubeola, commonly referred to as *measles*, is very low because of the success of the measles vaccine. Your coding experience relating to measles should be limited to office visits for administering the vaccine.

When an individual has come to get vaccinated against rubeola only, code the encounter using Z23. However, a patient who is seeing a health care professional because of having been exposed to rubeola will be reported with Z20.828. A diagnosis of rubeola (measles) should be reported with code B05.-.

YOU CODE IT! CASE STUDY

Gregg Espinoza brought his 3-year-old son, Raymond, to his pediatrician, Dr. Nunez, with complaints of a 102 degree F fever for 3 days' duration. The boy was coughing, had signs of a runny nose, and had conjunctivitis in both eyes. Upon examination, Dr. Nunez notes Koplik's spots inside his cheeks and lips. Also noted are small, generalized, maculopapular erythematous rashes on his scalp. When asked, the father agreed that the boy had been scratching his head and he had been tugging at his ears.

Dr. Nunez confirmed that Raymond had measles keratoconjunctivitis.

You Code It!

Read the scenario carefully and determine the diagnosis code or codes to report for this encounter with Dr. Nunez.

Step #1: Read the case carefully and completely.

Step #2: Abstract the scenario. Which main words or terms describe why the physician cared for the patient during this encounter?

(continued)

Step #3: Are there any details missing or incomplete for which you would need to query the physician? [If so, ask your instructor.]

Step #4: Check for any relevant guidance, including reading all of the symbols and notations in the Tabular List and the appropriate sections of the Official Guidelines.

Step #5: Determine the correct diagnosis code or codes to explain why this encounter was medically necessary.

Step #6: Double-check your work.

Answer:

Did you determine this to be the code?

B05.81 Measles keratitis and keratoconjunctivitis

Good job!

Rubella

Rubella, an acute viral disease that can affect anyone of any age, is thought of by many to be a children's disease known as the *German measles*. While the symptoms are most often not more than a mild rash, the health danger of rubella can be serious to a pregnant woman in her first trimester. When contracted during the early months of pregnancy, rubella can be associated with a condition known as *congenital rubella syndrome (CRS)*. CRS may cause any of a large number of birth defects, including deafness and possibly fetal death. The rubella vaccine has almost eliminated CRS.

Rubella is coded with B06.- when it has been diagnosed. For those cases in which a patient is being vaccinated against rubella alone, you will use Z23, and if the patient has been exposed to rubella, report this with code Z20.4.

Herpes Simplex Virus

The *herpes simplex virus*, often referred to by the abbreviation HSV, is transmitted by direct contact between individuals. Small vesicles (fluid-filled lesions) appear on reddened skin in clusters or groups, particularly in the mucous membranes. HSV type 1 may be associated with orofacial disease and type 2 is associated with infections in the genitalia.

B00 is the code category dedicated to reporting herpes simplex infections–with the exception of congenital herpesviral infection, reported with code P35.2.

EXAMPLE

✓4 B00 Herpesviral [herpes simplex] infections

EXCLUDES1 congenital herpesviral infections (P35.2)

EXCLUDES2 anogenital herpesviral infection (A60.-)

gammaherpesviral mononucleosis (B27.0-)

herpangina (B08.5)

Specific documentation is critical to determine an accurate code. You want to avoid reporting B00.9 Herpesviral infection NOS, so be certain to query your physician if you need more details to determine which of these codes to report.

Herpes Zoster

Herpes zoster or *postherpetic neuralgia* is commonly known as *shingles*. Herpes zoster is an infection of the varicella zoster virus–the same pathogen that causes chickenpox. Those patients who actually had chickenpox previously are at the greatest risk for developing this painful disease. Patients will feel a burning sensation or shooting pain, accompanied often by tingling or itching on only one side of the body.

Finding shingles in the ICD-10-CM Alphabetic Index will require you to search for *Herpes, zoster* . . . reported with a code from code category B02. The required additional characters will identify specific details about the anatomical location and activity of the virus.

EXAMPLE

✓4 B02 Zoster [herpes zoster]

INCLUDES shingles
zona

B02.0 Zoster encephalitis

B02.24 Postherpetic myelitis

You may be aware of the shingles vaccine, made recently available. For those patients coming to your health care facility to take advantage of this preventive medicine, the likely ICD-10-CM diagnosis code to provide medical necessity will be Z86.19 Personal history of other infectious and parasitic diseases.

Of course, the specific disease would be varicella–commonly known as chickenpox. The documentation will need to specify this personal history to support the provision of this vaccine. Also, make note of any other qualifiers set forth by third-party payers. Some require the patient to be aged 65 or over.

Zika Virus Infections

When a physician documents a confirmed diagnosis of the Zika virus, you are going to report code A92.5 Zika virus disease. However, if the physician includes any terms of doubt, such as describing this diagnosis as "suspected" or "possible," do not report the A92.5 code. Instead, you must report either:

- the codes for the specific symptoms that are included in the documentation, such as joint pain, fever.

or

- Z20.021 Contact with and (suspected) exposure to Zika virus

GUIDANCE CONNECTION

Read the ICD-10-CM Official Guidelines for Coding and Reporting, section **I. Conventions, General Coding Guidelines and Chapter-Specific Guidelines**, subsection **C. Chapter-Specific Coding Guidelines**, chapter **1. Certain Infectious and Parasitic Diseases**, subsection **f. Zika virus infections**.

YOU INTERPRET IT!

Is the infection bacterial or viral?

6. Strep throat (a) Bacteria (b) Virus

7. The flu (a) Bacteria (b) Virus

8. Plantar wart (a) Bacteria (b) Virus

9. Measles (a) Bacteria (b) Virus

10. Staph infection (a) Bacteria (b) Virus

6.4 Parasitic and Fungal Infections

Parasitic Infestations

Parasites are tiny living things that can invade and feed off other living things–like humans. They are one-celled organisms (protozoa), insects (lice and mites), and worms (helminths) among others (see **Figure 6-4**) that can interfere with a healthy body. Tapeworms, hookworms, and pinworms are internal parasites. Parasites can be transmitted in food (e.g., protozoa like *Giardia intestinalis* and *Cyclospora cayetanensis*); spread by mosquitoes and other insects through the bloodstream (as in malaria and leishmaniasis); or ingested in contaminated water (as in amebiasis and schistosomiasis).

Parasites
Tiny living things that can invade and feed off other living things.

EXAMPLES

B86	Scabies
B71.9	Cestode infection, unspecified
B87.2	Ocular myiasis

Diagnoses with a pathogen that is parasitic may not always be clearly defined. Keep that medical dictionary close at hand.

CODING BITES

These terms from Greek and Latin can be complex. However, physicians are more likely to use these terms in documentation. Therefore, keep that medical dictionary close at hand. You will need the support and accuracy of the definitions to help you determine the correct code.

Protozoal diseases are caused by a single-celled, microscopic organism. There are several types of diagnoses that fall into this category:

✓4	**B50-B54**	**Malaria**
✓4	**B57**	**Chagas' disease (infection due to Trypanosoma cruzi)**
✓4	**B58**	**Toxoplasmosis (infection due to Toxoplasma gondii)**

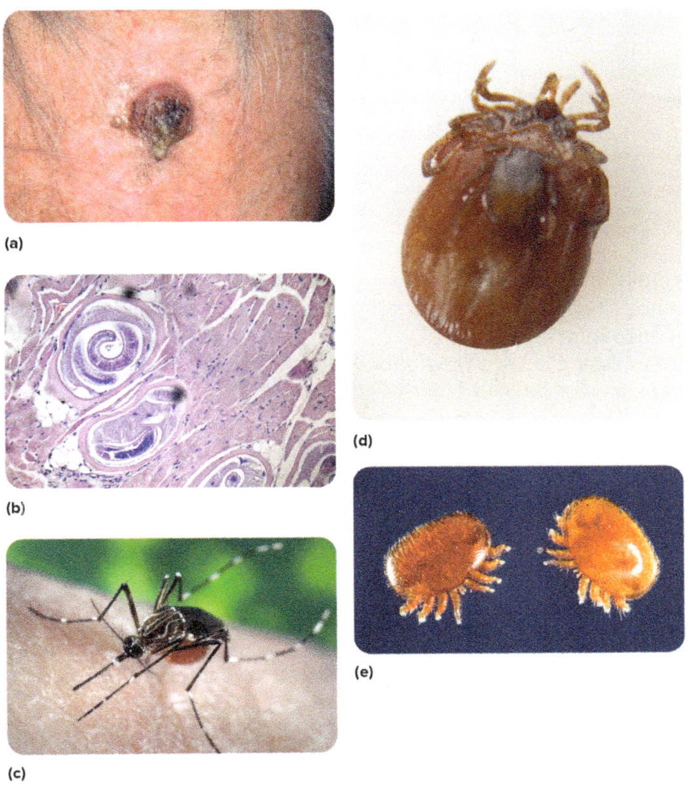

FIGURE 6-4 Parasitic worms: (a) tapeworms and (b) *Trichinella*. Parasitic insects: (c) mosquitoes, (d) deer ticks, and (e) mites

(a) DR P. Marazzi/Science Photo Library/Alamy Stock Photo; (b) D. Kucharski K. Kucharska/Shutterstock; (c) James Gathany/CDC; (d) Svetoslav Radkov/Shutterstock; (e) Scott Bauer/USDA

Helminths (from the Greek word for worms) are large organisms that grow to be visible with the naked eye (see **Figure 6-5**). Platyhelminths (flatworms) are commonly called tapeworms, like acanthocephalins, which seek out the gastrointestinal tract. Ascariasis is the medical term used to describe a case of roundworm infection.

	B68.1	**Taenia saginata taeniasis (infection due to adult tapeworm Taenia saginata)**
✓4	**B76**	**Hookworm diseases**
✓4	**B77**	**Ascariasis (roundworm infection)**
	B85.3	**Phthiriasis (infestation by crab-louse)**

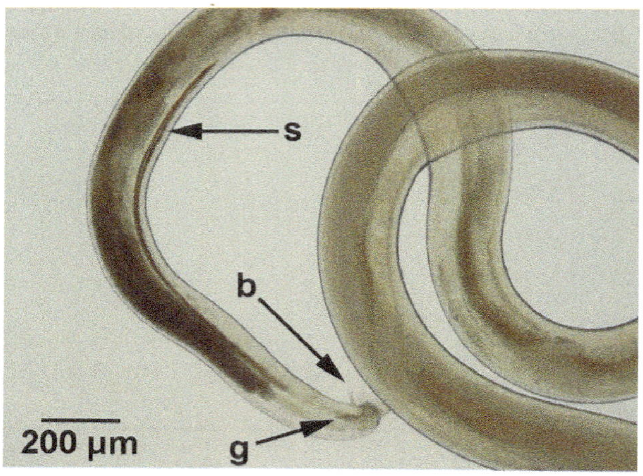

FIGURE 6-5 Angiostrongyliasis due to *Parastrongylus cantonensis*, reported with code B83.2

Michael S. Duffy

YOU CODE IT! CASE STUDY

Michael McCarthey brought his 6-year-old daughter, Johannah, to see Dr. Benzzoni, complaining that his daughter keeps scratching her head. After a thorough exam, Dr. Benzzoni explains that Johannah has a case of head lice. He instructs Michael to buy Nix, an over-the-counter permethrin, and provides an instruction sheet on how to rid his child and their household of the parasites.

You Code It!

Step #1: Read the case carefully and completely.

Step #2: Abstract the scenario. Which main words or terms describe why the physician cared for the patient during this encounter?

Step #3: Are there any details missing or incomplete for which you would need to query the physician? [If so, ask your instructor.]

Step #4: Check for any relevant guidance, including reading all of the symbols and notations in the Tabular List and the appropriate sections of the Official Guidelines.

Step #5: Determine the correct diagnosis code or codes to explain why this encounter was medically necessary.

Step #6: Double-check your work.

Answer:

Did you determine the correct code?

B85.0 **Pediculosis due to Pediculus humanus capitis [head louse infestation]**

Great work!

Fungal Infections

There are many versions of **fungi** (the plural form of *fungus*) in our lives. Mushrooms on your pizza or in your salad and yeast in your bread or beer are tasty. Mold, a form of fungus, can be delicious when it is called blue cheese or feta cheese, and it can be helpful when developed in a pill containing penicillin. Then there are fungi that cause illness, such as *Aspergillus*, which may cause lower respiratory tract dysfunction, or *Candida albicans*, which causes infection in the oral mucosa and the walls of the vagina. *Onychomycosis* is the most common nail fungal infection.

Fungi
Group of organisms, including mold, yeast, and mildew, that cause infection [singular: fungus].

EXAMPLES

P37.5	Neonatal candidiasis
B44.81	Allergic bronchopulmonary aspergillosis
B40.3	Cutaneous blastomycosis

With fungal infections, it may not be easy or straightforward from reading the diagnostic statement. You may need to do some research, or check in your medical dictionary.

Except in patients with compromised immune systems, fungal infections are not life-threatening.

✓4 **B35 Dermatophytosis**

Ectoparasites are organisms that attach, or burrow, into the epidermis and dermis and remain there, such as ticks, fleas, lice, and mites. Often, the medical term "tinea" is used in the diagnostic statement, such as tinea pedis (commonly known as athlete's foot) or tinea cruris (also known as jock itch).

✓4 **B44 Aspergillosis**

There can be serious concerns with a fungal infection when it affects the pulmonary organs, skin, or adrenal glands, known as histoplasmosis.

✓4 **B38.0 Acute pulmonary coccidioidomycosis** *(also known as Valley Fever; this is an infection of the lungs)*

✓4 **B39.3 Disseminate histoplasmosis capsulati**

YOU INTERPRET IT!

How are these diseases transmitted?

11. Lyme disease (a) Parasite (b) Fungus
12. *Candida albicans* (a) Parasite (b) Fungus
13. Zika (a) Parasite (b) Fungus
14. *Aspergillus* (a) Parasite (b) Fungus
15. Blastomycosis (a) Parasite (b) Fungus
16. Ring worm (a) Parasite (b) Fungus

6.5 Infections Caused by Several Pathogens

Up to this point, you have been reading about infectious and communicable diseases that are known to be caused by either a bacterium, virus, or other specific pathogen. However, there are some diagnoses that can be caused by a virus, a bacterium, or even a fungus. This means that you must abstract not only the name of the condition but also the specific type of underlying pathogen to determine an accurate code. Lab tests are required to confirm a diagnosis. Therefore, reading the pathology reports in the patient's chart can provide these details.

Pneumonia

Pneumonia is not an uncommon infection of the lungs. Actually, it is estimated that more than 3 million diagnoses of pneumonia are made each year in the United States. Yet, as a professional coder, you need to know the specific type of pathogen that caused this infection before you can accurately determine the code.

Types of Pneumonia

Several different types of pathogens can result in fluid and pus filling the air sacs (alveoli)–the underlying cause of pneumonia. Integral signs and symptoms include cough with phlegm or pus, fever, chills, and difficulty breathing. When you look under the main term **PNEUMONIA** in the ICD-10-CM Alphabetic Index, you can see the very long list of additional descriptors needed to get to a specific code recommendation.

Bacterial Pneumonia

The *Streptococcus pneumoniae* bacterium, also known as pneumococcus, causes the most common type of pneumonia. Atypical pneumonia, commonly referred to as walking pneumonia, also is caused by bacteria, but different bacteria, including *Legionella pneumophila*, *Mycoplasma pneumoniae (M. pneumoniae)*, and *Chlamydophila pneumoniae*.

Aspiration pneumonia is a bacterial infection that develops after the patient has inhaled food, a liquid, or vomit. The particles deteriorate and bacteria grow, causing the infection and inflammation.

ICD-10-CM

LET'S CODE IT! SCENARIO

Anna Carland, an 81-year-old female, was admitted to the hospital with pneumonia. She was placed on oxygen to help her breathe while labs were done to determine the type of pneumonia. Dr. Premin diagnosed her with streptococcal pneumonia. The pathology report specifies Streptococcus pneumoniae *group B.*

Let's Code It!

Anna was diagnosed with streptococcal pneumonia by Dr. Premin. Turn to the Alphabetic Index in your ICD-10-CM code book and find the main term:

Pneumonia (acute) (double) (migratory) (purulent) (septic) (unresolved) J18.9

Read carefully down the long, indented list beneath and find

Pneumonia

in (due to)

all the way down this list to . . .

Streptococcus J15.4

group B J15.3

pneumoniae J13

specified NEC J15.4

Knowing that Anna has "*Streptococcus pneumoniae*" is not enough. Remember that we are required to always code to the greatest specificity, and the code book is reminding you that you need additional details. Go back to the documentation, not only the physician's notes but the pathology report, too. Aha! The pathology report specifies "*Streptococcus* group B." Now, turn to the Tabular List to the code category J15.

✓4 **J15 Bacterial pneumonia, not elsewhere classified**

Code First **associated influenza, if applicable (J09.X1, J10.0-, J11.0-)**

Code Also **associated lung abscess, if applicable (J85.1)**

(continued)

EXCLUDES1 chlamydial pneumonia (J16.0)
congenital pneumonia (P23.-)
Legionnaires' disease (A48.1)
spirochetal pneumonia (A69.8)

Read these notations carefully and determine if any of them relate to Anna's case. Not this time. Good! So, read down all of the fourth-character options and determine which matches Dr. Premin's documentation.

J15.3 Pneumonia due to streptococcus, group B

Check the head of this chapter in ICD-10-CM. There are notations at the beginning of this chapter: a **NOTE**, a *Use Additional Code* notation, and an EXCLUDES2 notation. Read carefully. Do any relate to Dr. Premin's diagnosis of Anna? No. Turn to the Official Guidelines and read Section I.C.1. There is nothing specifically applicable here either.

Now you can report J15.3 for Anna's diagnosis with confidence.

Good coding!

Viral Pneumonia

There are some viruses that are known to cause inflammation and swelling in the lungs. The influenza A and B viruses, as well as *Hemophilus influenzae (H. influenzae)*, can develop into viral pneumonia if not treated quickly. *Cytomegalovirus* (CMV) is most often seen in patients with a suppressed immune system, such as one going through chemotherapy or one suffering with an immunodeficiency condition.

EXAMPLES

✓5 J11.0 Influenza due to unidentified influenza virus with pneumonia

✓4 J12 Viral pneumonia not elsewhere classified

J14 Pneumonia due to Hemophilus influenzae

Fungal Pneumonia

The fungus *Pneumocystis jirovecii* is the cause of a fungal pneumonia, previously known as *Pneumocystis carini* or PCP pneumonia, in patients whose immune system is diminished. This is a known manifestation in those diagnosed with advanced HIV infection.

Pneumonia due to *Aspergillus* is the result of inhaling this form of mold.

Secondary Pneumonia

There are some diseases that can manifest a case of pneumonia. These conditions include rheumatic fever, schistosomiasis, and Q fever. There is a difference between this type of pneumonia and those we have just been discussing, so read carefully and possibly query the physician. This diagnosis is reported with the following code:

J17 Pneumonia in diseases classified elsewhere

CODING BITES

The incidence of pneumonia is also categorized by the environment in which the patient may have contracted this condition.

Community-acquired pneumonia (CAP) identifies that pneumonia has developed in a patient who has not recently been in the hospital or another health care facility such as a nursing home or rehab facility.

Hospital-acquired pneumonia identifies those patients who contract pneumonia while in a residential health care facility.

Meningitis

Meningitis is the inflammation of the meningeal membranes of the brain and/or the spinal cord. Meningitis can be caused by a bacterial pathogen, such as *Meningococcus*; however, it is more often the result of a viral infection. When meningitis is caught early, the prognosis is good and complications are rare.

In order to code a diagnosis of meningitis, you have to know the specific virus or bacterium at the core of the inflammation. This will typically be found in the pathologist's report as well as the physician's documentation.

EXAMPLES

Some bacterial causes of meningitis would be reported with

A39.0 Meningococcal meningitis

A54.81 Gonococcal meningitis

G00.2 Streptococcal meningitis ***Use additional code*** **to further identify organism (B95.0–B95.5)**

EXAMPLES

Some viral causes of meningitis would be reported with

A87.1 Adenoviral meningitis

A87.0 Echoviral meningitis

B26.1 Mumps (virus) meningitis

In some cases, ICD-10-CM will identify the requirement of a second code.

EXAMPLES

Meningitis due to poliovirus A80.9 *[G02]*

A80.9 Acute poliomyelitis, unspecified

G02 Meningitis in other infectious and parasitic diseases classified elsewhere

G00.2 Streptococcal meningitis ***Use additional code*** **to further identify organism (B95.0–B95.5)**

6.6 Immunodeficiency Conditions

Some conditions cause the body's immune system to stop working, meaning that infection and pathogens cannot be fought off effectively. You may remember learning about T cells, B cells, and lymphoid tissues from your physiology class. A defect involving any of these is known as a *primary (congenital) immunodeficiency* condition. A *secondary (acquired) immunodeficiency* is a manifestation caused by something that is blocking the proper immune response or depressing the response to an ineffective level. There are some viruses that trigger secondary immunodeficiency, such as with acquired immunodeficiency syndrome (AIDS). However, there are a number of potential external causes of secondary immunodeficiency, ranging from exposure to an infection, a toxic chemical, or radiation to suffering severe burns.

Primary immunodeficiency disorders include

- X-linked agammaglobulinemia (XLA).
- Common variable immunodeficiency (CVID).
- Severe combined immunodeficiency (SCID), also known as "boy in a bubble" disease.
- Alymphocytosis (deficiency of lymphocytes in the blood).

Secondary immunodeficiency conditions include

- AIDS.
- Leukemia and other cancers of the immune system.
- Viral hepatitis and other immune-complex diseases.
- Multiple myeloma (a cancer of the plasma cells).

Human Immunodeficiency Virus

Human immunodeficiency virus (HIV) infection is a serious illness. Sadly, as if this illness were not enough for a patient to deal with, it also carries a huge societal stigma. Therefore, whether you are coding for an inpatient facility (an exception to the guideline discussed earlier) or an outpatient facility, you will code this illness *only* when it has been *clearly specified in the physician's notes* that the patient is HIV-positive.

GUIDANCE CONNECTION

Read the ICD-10-CM Official Guidelines for Coding and Reporting, section **I. Conventions, General Coding Guidelines and Chapter-Specific Guidelines**, subsection **C. Chapter-Specific Coding Guidelines**, chapter **1. Certain Infectious and Parasitic Diseases**, subsections **a. Human immunodeficiency virus (HIV) infections** and **a.2)(h) Encounters for testing for HIV**.

Anyone possibly exposed to HIV should be tested. Similar to so many other conditions, like malignancies, the earlier a diagnosis is made, the sooner treatment can begin. Early treatment translates into a longer, better-quality life for the patient.

CODING BITES

In some states, information in the patient's record relating to HIV testing (positive or negative result), HIV AIDS status, sexually transmitted diseases, genetic information (such as the results of any genetic testing), mental health conditions, and substance abuse is categorized as *superconfidential* information. This information has additional legal protection, above the requirements of HIPAA, with regard to disclosure and use. Be certain to find out if your state has this additional protection for patients as well as the requirements for compliance.

Coding HIV Testing, Test Results, and Symptoms

Documenting Medical Necessity of HIV Testing

When an individual with no symptoms comes to a health care facility to be tested for a condition, you will need a diagnosis code to provide medical necessity for the test. As with other preventive health care encounters, you will use a Z code to document the need for HIV testing. For a first office visit to discuss possible exposure to HIV, you will use this code:

Z20.6 Contact with and (suspected) exposure to human immunodeficiency virus [HIV]

For the diagnosis code used to support the actual test, generally, you will use this code:

Z11.4 Encounter for screening for human immunodeficiency virus [HIV]

However, if the patient is documented by the physician as a member of a known high-risk group, you may use one of these codes:

Z72.5- High-risk sexual behavior

Z72.8- Other problems related to lifestyle

Remember, until there is a specific diagnostic statement in the physician's notes, you are not to report anything connected to HIV. If the patient is tested because of specific signs and/or symptoms, you will code those signs and symptoms, rather than any of the above.

LET'S CODE IT! SCENARIO

Michael Callahan got drunk and had unprotected intercourse last night. He comes to Dr. Ansara's office to discuss his concerns about possible exposure to HIV.

Let's Code It!

Michael went to see Dr. Ansara because he was concerned that he had been *exposed to HIV*. Let's turn to the Alphabetic Index and look up *exposure*:

Exposure (to)

human immunodeficiency virus (HIV) Z20.6

(continued)

Confirm the complete code description in the Tabular List; start reading at the top of the chapter subsection titled

Persons with potential health hazards related to communicable diseases (Z20–Z29)

Be certain to read the EXCLUDES1 and EXCLUDES2 notes. While these excluded diagnoses do not relate to our current case of Michael's visit to Dr. Ansara, always reading up and down and around the code that was suggested by the Alphabetic Index is a critical habit that you need to build. This time, the notes do not apply, but next time, they might. Continue reading down the column.

✓4 **Z20 Contact with or (suspected) exposure to communicable diseases**

This fits the documentation, which notes that Michael is concerned that he has been "exposed." Keep reading down the column to find that required fourth digit. You will see this code:

Z20.6 Contact with and (suspected) exposure to human immunodeficiency virus [HIV]

Directly beneath this code is another EXCLUDES1 notation:

Asymptomatic human immunodeficiency virus [HIV] infection status (Z21)

This reminds you that contact or exposure is not the same as a positive status asymptomatic HIV diagnosis.

Check the top of this subsection and the head of this chapter in ICD-10-CM. There is a **NOTE** at the beginning of this chapter. Read carefully. Does it relate to Dr. Ansara's diagnosis of Michael? No. Turn to the Official Guidelines and read Section I.C.1. There is nothing specifically applicable here, either.

Now you can report code Z20.6 with confidence!

CODING BITES

Positive status means that laboratory tests have confirmed that the patient does have the virus in his or her system (positive status).

Asymptomatic means that the patient is currently not exhibiting any signs or symptoms of the disease.

Test Negative

There are rapid HIV tests using oral swabs or finger sticks that can provide results in minutes. Other HIV tests may take several days to provide an answer. Therefore, a return visit to the health care provider will sometimes be required.

The entire experience of being tested and then having to wait for the results can be psychologically difficult, even when the news is good and the test is negative. It is the health care professional's responsibility to counsel the patient on how to prevent future risk. Therefore, when an individual returns to get the results of an HIV test, even when the results are negative, counseling should be provided. For that reason, when documented, report:

Z71.7 Human immunodeficiency virus [HIV] counseling

Test Inconclusive

It can happen that the serology (pathology testing) comes back inconclusive for HIV. There can be no specific diagnosis for HIV or any direct manifestations of the illness because there is nothing to confirm or deny HIV-positive status. In such cases, you have to use this code:

R75 Inconclusive laboratory evidence of human immunodeficiency virus [HIV]

Test Positive but Asymptomatic

Thanks to research and the development of new drug therapies, patients who have HIV are living longer and with a better quality of life. Therefore, testing positive for HIV is not quite as devastating as it was years ago. When a patient comes to receive the HIV test results that are positive, but the patient has no signs, symptoms, or manifestations, the patient is **asymptomatic**. You will assign this code:

Z21 Asymptomatic human immunodeficiency virus [HIV] infection status

When the physician provides counseling for the patient, discusses therapeutic treatments, and/or any other elements of dealing with the disease, you should report the counseling code as well.

Test Positive with Symptoms or Manifestations

Once the individual has been diagnosed and exhibits any manifestations associated with HIV, the code to report the condition will change from Z21 to

B20 Human immunodeficiency virus [HIV] disease

Code B20 includes a diagnosis of acquired immune deficiency syndrome (AIDS), which is essentially HIV with manifestations. When you use code B20, you have to follow it with a code or codes to identify the specific manifestations, such as pneumonia or HIV-2 infection. There is a notation in the ICD-10-CM book, below code B20's description in the Tabular List, reminding you to do this. If the patient is seen for a condition or illness directly related to his or her HIV-positive status, list code B20 first, followed by the code or codes for the conditions.

GUIDANCE CONNECTION

Read the ICD-10-CM Official Guidelines for Coding and Reporting, section **I. Conventions, General Coding Guidelines and Chapter-Specific Guidelines**, subsection **C. Chapter-Specific Coding Guidelines**, chapter **1. Certain Infectious and Parasitic Diseases**, subsection **a.2)(f) Previously diagnosed HIV-related illness**.

CODING BITES

Once a patient has been diagnosed with manifestations of HIV-positive status, you are no longer permitted to use code Z21, even when the manifestations are no longer present.

CODING BITES

NEVER report a code for HIV infection or illness without a specific physician diagnostic statement–a confirmed diagnosis.

LET'S CODE IT! SCENARIO

Alfredo Zimoso has been HIV-positive for 10 years. He comes to see Dr. Chang because of severe headaches and vision problems. After a complete physical examination (PE) and appropriate tests, Dr. Chang diagnoses Alfredo with noninfectious acute disseminated encephalomyelitis, secondary to HIV.

Let's Code It!

Alfredo has been diagnosed with *noninfectious acute disseminated encephalomyelitis, secondary to HIV.* Do you know whether the noninfectious acute disseminated encephalomyelitis is an HIV-related manifestation? There are two ways to tell. First, the physician's notes state that the condition is *secondary to HIV.* This means that not only are the two conditions related to each other but that the HIV is also the underlying condition (it came first). The second way to tell is shown in the Tabular List. Let's first go to the Alphabetic Index to find encephalomyelitis. The indented descriptions of encephalomyelitis include terms used by the physician in her notes.

Encephalomyelitis

acute disseminated (ADEM) (postinfectious) G04.01

Notice that this description also includes the term *postinfectious.* Alfredo was diagnosed with noninfectious encephalomyelitis. Keep reading down and find:

Encephalomyelitis, acute disseminated, noninfectious G04.81

That seems to match the doctor's notes, so now, let's turn to the Tabular List and read the complete descriptions. Start reading at

✓4 **G04 Encephalitis, myelitis, and encephalomyelitis**

This code category contains INCLUDES, EXCLUDES1, and EXCLUDES2 notes, which you need to read carefully. Is there anything that leads you away from this code category? No, there isn't, so you need to read down the column to find the most accurate, required fourth digit:

✓5 **G04.8 Other causes of encephalitis, myelitis, and encephalomyelitis**

(continued)

None of the other descriptions match Dr. Chang's notes, so this looks like the best option. Take a look at your choices for the required fifth digit:

G04.81 Other encephalitis and encephalomyelitis

G04.89 Other myelitis

Check the notes and you will see that Alfredo was diagnosed with encephalomyelitis, leading you directly to code:

G04.81 Other encephalitis and encephalomyelitis; noninfectious acute disseminated encephalomyelitis (noninfectious ADEM)

That matches Dr. Chang's notes exactly.

Now you need the code for Michael's HIV-positive status. You know that the encephalomyelitis is a manifestation of that status and you should be clear as to what the code should be. In the Alphabetic Index, find:

Human immunodeficiency virus (disease) (infection) B20

asymptomatic status Z21

Which one should you follow? You know from the notes that Alfredo does have symptoms and has manifested a secondary illness. Therefore, turn to the Tabular List to confirm:

B20 Human immunodeficiency virus [HIV] disease

You now have two codes to report the reasons Dr. Chang cared for Alfredo at this encounter. Which gets listed first? The notation below the description reminds you to "***use additional code(s)*** to identify all manifestations of HIV." This tells you that B20 is listed first.

Check the top of this subsection and the head of this chapter in ICD-10-CM. There are notations at the beginning of this chapter: an INCLUDES notation, a ***Use additional code*** note, an EXCLUDES1 notation, and an EXCLUDES2 notation. Read carefully. Do any relate to Dr. Chang's diagnosis of Alfredo? No. Turn to the Official Guidelines and read Section I.C.1. Read subparagraph a. Human immunodeficiency virus (HIV) infections, particularly 2) Selection and sequencing of HIV codes, (a) Patient admitted for HIV-related condition.

So your report for Dr. Chang's encounter with Alfredo will show:

B20 Human immunodeficiency virus [HIV] disease

G04.81 Other causes of encephalitis, noninfectious acute disseminated encephalomyelitis

Good job!

HIV Status with Unrelated Conditions

An individual who is HIV-positive can still be affected by conditions, illnesses, or injuries that have nothing to do with his or her HIV status. As you have learned, the first-listed code should answer the question, "Why did the health care provider care for the patient at this encounter?" Therefore, the code for the condition that caused the patient to visit the physician should come first. Because HIV is a systemic disease, affecting the entire body, you have to include a code for that condition as well. Even if it has nothing to do with the services or treatment provided by the physician, it will have an impact on the physician's decision-making and therefore must be included.

GUIDANCE CONNECTION

Read the ICD-10-CM Official Guidelines for Coding and Reporting, section **I. Conventions, General Coding Guidelines and Chapter-Specific Guidelines**, subsection **C. Chapter-Specific Coding Guidelines**, chapter **1. Certain Infectious and Parasitic Diseases,** subsection **a.2)(b)**: *"If a patient with HIV disease is admitted for an unrelated condition (such as a traumatic injury), the code for the unrelated condition (e.g., the nature of injury code) should be the principal diagnosis. Other diagnoses would be B20 followed by additional diagnosis codes for all reported HIV-related conditions."*

GUIDANCE CONNECTION

Read the ICD-10-CM Official Guidelines for Coding and Reporting, section **I. Conventions, General Coding Guidelines and Chapter-Specific Guidelines**, subsection **C. Chapter-Specific Coding Guidelines,** chapter **1. Certain Infectious and Parasitic Diseases,** subsection **a.2)(f) Previously diagnosed HIV-related illness.**

GUIDANCE CONNECTION

Read the ICD-10-CM Official Guidelines for Coding and Reporting, section **I. Conventions, General Coding Guidelines and Chapter-Specific Guidelines**, subsection **C. Chapter-Specific Coding Guidelines** , chapter **1. Certain Infectious and Parasitic Diseases,** subsection **a.2)(i) History of HIV managed by medication.**

EXAMPLE

Gayle Robbins came to see Dr. Tigliano because she slipped on the ice this morning and hurt her ankle. Dr. Tigliano examined her and took x-rays that confirmed a sprain of the deltoid ligament of the left ankle. Gayle was diagnosed with HIV 2 years ago and is asymptomatic.

S93.422A	Sprain, of deltoid ligament of left ankle, initial encounter
Z21	Asymptomatic human immunodeficiency virus [HIV]

EXAMPLE

Yuri Kastachen fell off a ladder and hurt his lower back. Dr. Lang determined that Yuri had a fractured coccyx. Last year, Yuri was hospitalized with HIV-related pneumonia.

S32.2XXA	Fracture of coccyx, initial encounter
B20	Human immunodeficiency virus [HIV] disease

HIV Status in Obstetrics

When a woman with HIV-positive status is pregnant, giving birth, or in the postpartum period, the systemic disease must be a consideration in determining her care. Therefore, whether or not she has symptoms or manifestations of the HIV condition, the first-listed code must be

O98.7- Human immunodeficiency virus [HIV] disease complicating pregnancy, childbirth, or the puerperium

This should be followed by the appropriate HIV-positive status code: Z21 or B20.

YOU CODE IT! CASE STUDY

Maureen Dunbar, a 27-year-old female, 23-weeks pregnant, was playing tennis when she felt a pain in her right knee. She went to see her physician, Dr. Rummur, who diagnosed her problem as a derangement of the anterior horn of the lateral cystic meniscus. Maureen has been HIV-positive and asymptomatic for 5 years.

(continued)

You Code It!

Go through the steps of coding, and determine the diagnosis code(s) to be reported for this encounter between Dr. Rummur and Maureen Dunbar.

Step #1: Read the case carefully and completely.
Step #2: Abstract the scenario. Which main words or terms describe why the physician cared for the patient during this encounter?
Step #3: Are there any details missing or incomplete for which you would need to query the physician? [If so, ask your instructor.]
Step #4: Check for any relevant guidance, including reading all of the symbols and notations in the Tabular List and the appropriate sections of the Official Guidelines.
Step #5: Determine the correct diagnosis code or codes to explain why this encounter was medically necessary.
Step #6: Double-check your work.

Answer:

Did you determine the correct codes?

M23.041 **Cystic meniscus, anterior horn of lateral meniscus, right knee**

O98.712 **Human immunodeficiency virus [HIV] disease complicating pregnancy, childbirth, or the puerperium, antepartum condition, second trimester**

Z21 **Asymptomatic human immunodeficiency virus [HIV] infection status**

Good job!

Are you wondering why the knee condition is listed first when the guideline for HIV infection in pregnancy states the O98.7- code category should be listed first? In this case, you have two guidelines that need to be followed:

Section I.C.1.a.2)(b) Patient with HIV disease admitted for unrelated condition

Section I.C.1.a.2)(g) HIV infection in pregnancy, childbirth, and the puerperium

To break the tie, let's look at one more guideline, either

Section II. Selection of Principal Diagnosis (for inpatient encounters)

or

Section IV. Diagnostic Coding and Reporting Guidelines for Outpatient Services, Subsection H (for outpatient encounters)

Whether you are coding for outpatient or inpatient services, the guidelines agree that the principal, or first-listed, diagnosis code should be the condition "chiefly responsible" for the encounter. In Maureen's case, the reason she went to the doctor for care was the pain in her knee–not the pregnancy and not the HIV. Then why code them at all? Because Dr. Rummur must take Maureen's pregnant status and her HIV status into consideration in his medical decision-making process to determine the best way to treat her knee.

YOU INTERPRET IT!

Which condition code is sequenced first [principal diagnosis]?

17. HIV-positive patient admitted with fractured leg ____________

18. Patient admitted with pneumocystis carinii, HIV-positive since 2015 ____________

19. Patient, 38-weeks pregnant, HIV-positive, delivers ____________

20. Patient seen for type 1 diabetes, HIV-positive ____________

6.7 Septicemia and Other Blood Infections

Blood infections are very dangerous, as you might imagine, because of their potential effect on the entire body. Blood circulates through the body and touches all the cells and organs in some fashion. So you can understand that if the blood circulating through the body is carrying a disease, it can have the potential to cause serious problems. There are several types of blood infections, and each needs to be coded differently.

Septicemia

Essentially, **septicemia** is identified as the presence of a microorganism or toxin in the bloodstream. The organism might be a virus, a fungus, a bacterium, or another pathologic substance. Septicemia is very serious. A physician may refer to this condition as *bacteremia*; however, they are really not the same. Bacteremia may not be clinically significant, but septicemia is always significant.

> **Septicemia**
> Generalized infection spread through the body via the bloodstream; blood infection.

The code used for a diagnosis of septicemia may be taken from category

A41.9 Sepsis, unspecified sepsis (Septicemia NOS)

GUIDANCE CONNECTION

Read the ICD-10-CM Official Guidelines for Coding and Reporting, section **I. Conventions, General Coding Guidelines and Chapter-Specific Guidelines**, subsection **C. Chapter-Specific Coding Guidelines**, chapter **1. Certain Infectious and Parasitic Diseases**, subchapter **d. Sepsis, severe sepsis, and septic shock**.

You will need to determine a more accurate code by the pathogen or toxin found in the blood, such as streptococcus or staphylococcus.

A diagnosis of **systemic inflammatory response syndrome** (SIRS) is used when the basic cause, or *pathogen*, is unknown. The human body is amazing and is designed to fight any and all intruders (disease or infection). The system's response to infection may be

> **Systemic Inflammatory Response Syndrome (SIRS)**
> A definite physical reaction, such as fever, chills, etc., to an unspecified pathogen.

- Increased body temperature.
- Change in heart rate.
- Change in respiratory rate.
- Increased white blood cell count.

Systemic inflammatory response syndrome (SIRS) of non-infectious origin R65.10

Systemic inflammatory response syndrome (SIRS) of non-infectious origin with acute organ dysfunction R65.11

YOU CODE IT! CASE STUDY

Priscilla Christopher, a 17-year-old female, was brought by her mother to see Dr. Fasold. Priscilla claimed that her muscles ache, she has been sweating, and she has chills at the same time. She stated that she has been coughing and short of breath for several days. After running some tests, Dr. Fasold diagnosed Priscilla with sepsis due to Hemophilus influenzae.

You Code It!

Go through the steps of coding, and determine the diagnosis code or codes that should be reported for this encounter between Dr. Fasold and Priscilla.

(continued)

Step #1: Read the case carefully and completely.
Step #2: Abstract the scenario. Which main words or terms describe why the physician cared for the patient during this encounter?
Step #3: Are there any details missing or incomplete for which you would need to query the physician? [If so, ask your instructor.]
Step #4: Check for any relevant guidance, including reading all of the symbols and notations in the Tabular List and the appropriate sections of the Official Guidelines.
Step #5: Determine the correct diagnosis code or codes to explain why this encounter was medically necessary.
Step #6: Double-check your work.

Answer:

Did you determine the correct code?

A41.3 Sepsis due to Hemophilus influenzae

Terrific!

Sepsis

Sepsis
Condition typified by two or more systemic responses to infection; a specified pathogen.

When an individual exhibits two or more systemic responses or when the presence of a specific pathogen has been identified in the bloodstream, the diagnosis is typically **sepsis.**

Reporting a diagnosis of sepsis will begin with the identification of the underlying systemic infection–the pathogen that initiated the septic condition. This code will come from category A40.- or A41.-. You may find this detail in the physician's documentation or the pathology report.

On occasion, a physician might diagnose a patient with *urosepsis*. This is not a synonym for sepsis and cannot be coded as sepsis. Should you find this term used in the documentation, you will need to query the physician for clarification.

A patient may be diagnosed with sepsis and acute organ failure during the same encounter, without a relationship (or cause and effect) between the two. In these situations, the organ failure is a co-morbidity and is reported separately from the sepsis.

EXAMPLE

Bernard Madison was in the hospital and diagnosed with group A streptococcus sepsis.

A40.0 Sepsis due to streptococcus, group A

Severe Sepsis

Severe Sepsis
Sepsis with signs of acute organ dysfunction.

When left untreated, sepsis may become severe and cause an organ to fail–a life-threatening condition. In some cases, this can occur when treatment is provided but is ineffective. A diagnosis of sepsis in combination with acute organ failure due to the septic condition is reported as **severe sepsis.** The physician's notes that contain a diagnosis of severe sepsis will be reported with

- *First:* the code for the underlying systemic infection, such as streptococcus or other bacteria (e.g., a code from A40.- or A41.-). If the organism is not known, you may report A41.9 Sepsis, unspecified organism.
- *Followed by:* a code from subcategory R65.2 Severe sepsis. An additional character is required to report whether or not the physician has documented that the patient is in "septic shock."
- *Followed by:* a code to report the specific organ failure caused by the septic condition. To remind you, code subcategory R65 has a ***Use additional code*** notation.

GUIDANCE CONNECTION

Read the ICD-10-CM Official Guidelines for Coding and Reporting, section **I. Conventions, General Coding Guidelines and Chapter-Specific Guidelines**, subsection **C. Chapter-Specific Coding Guidelines**, chapter **1. Certain Infections and Parasitic Diseases**, subsection **d.3) Sequencing of severe sepsis**, which warns you that a code from subcategory **R65.2 Severe sepsis** is *never* permitted to be the first-listed or principal diagnosis code reported.

LET'S CODE IT! SCENARIO

Dr. Kahanni admitted Burton Chapel with acute renal failure due to severe sepsis resulting from Streptococcal pneumonia.

Let's Code It!

Dr. Kahanni diagnosed Burton with "acute renal failure due to severe sepsis resulting from Streptococcal pneumonia." Remember the Official Guideline at Section I.C.1.d.1(b): The coding of severe sepsis requires first a code for the underlying systemic infection, followed by a code from R65.2-, and then the code for the acute organ dysfunction. Turn to the Alphabetic Index and find

Sepsis

Pneumococcal A40.3

Turn to the Tabular List to confirm this code:

✓4 **A40 Streptococcal sepsis**

Read the fourth-character choices and find

A40.3 Sepsis due to Streptococcus pneumoniae (Pneumococcal sepsis)

Next, let's turn to R65.2- and see what will accurately report Dr. Kahanni's diagnosis for Burton.

✓5 **R65.2 Severe sepsis**

Read the fifth-character descriptions, and determine which one matches:

R65.20 Severe sepsis without septic shock

The notations above this code help you further. They remind you to "***Code first underlying infection***," which you have done already with the pneumococcal sepsis code. The second notation directs you to

Use additional code **to specify acute organ dysfunction, such as: acute kidney failure (N17.-)**

Next, confirm the code for the acute renal (kidney) failure:

✓4 **N17 Acute kidney failure**

Carefully read the ***Code also*** and EXCLUDES1 notes. There is no relevance here to Burton's diagnosis at this encounter, so read down the column to review all of your choices for the required fourth character. With no documentation of any lesions on Burton's kidneys, the best choice is

N17.9 Acute renal failure, unspecified

Check the top of this subsection and the head of this chapter in ICD-10-CM. There are notations at the beginning of this chapter: an INCLUDES notation, a ***Use additional code*** note, an EXCLUDES1 notation, and an EXCLUDES2 notation. Read carefully. Do any relate to Dr. Kahanni's diagnosis of Burton? No. Turn to the Official Guidelines and read Section I.C.1, particularly d. Sepsis, Severe Sepsis, and Septic Shock.

Now you can report, with confidence, these codes in the order specified by the guidelines: A40.3, R65.20, N17.9 . . .

Good job!

Septic Shock

Septic Shock
Severe sepsis with hypotension; unresponsive to fluid resuscitation.

CODING BITES

The code for septic shock may not be the principal or first-listed diagnosis.

Should a patient also develop hypotension (low blood pressure) in addition to having severe sepsis, the diagnosis becomes **septic shock**. Septic shock cannot be present without the existence of severe sepsis–and it all must be documented. When coding septic shock, report the codes in the following order:

1. The code for the systemic infection (e.g., A40.-).
2. The code for the severe sepsis with septic shock (e.g., R65.21).
3. The code for the organ dysfunction.

GUIDANCE CONNECTION

Read the ICD-10-CM Official Guidelines for Coding and Reporting, section **I. Conventions, General Coding Guidelines and Chapter-Specific Guidelines**, subsection **C. Chapter-Specific Coding Guidelines**, chapter **1. Certain Infectious and Parasitic Diseases**, subsection **d.2) Septic shock**.

Post-Procedural Infection and Post-Procedural Septic Shock

If the physician documents a diagnosis of post-procedural septic shock, the codes required to accurately report this condition are:

The codes required to report sepsis due to a post-procedural infection, followed by:

T81.12X- Post-procedural septic shock

Code first **underlying infection**

Use additional code **to identify any associated acute organ dysfunction, if applicable**

Code R65.21 Severe sepsis with septic shock should not be reported for this diagnosis.

Sepsis and Septic Shock Relating to Pregnancy or Newborns

Sepsis during Labor

During the process of giving birth, a woman might develop a septic infection. In this case, code O75.3 Other infection during labor (Sepsis during labor) is reported. A code from B95–B97 Bacterial and viral infectious agents should follow to specify the pathogen causing the infection.

Puerperal Sepsis

Puerperal sepsis, also known as *postpartum sepsis*, *puerperal peritonitis*, or *puerperal pyemia*, results from an infection that develops in a woman's reproductive organs and that was initiated during or following miscarriage or childbirth. This diagnosis is reported with code O85 Puerperal sepsis.

In addition, a code from B95–B97 Bacterial and viral infectious agents is required to specify the pathogen causing the infection. If severe sepsis is documented, a code from R65.2- also should be reported.

Neonatal Sepsis

A fetus may contract an infection in utero, during the birth process (delivery), or during the first 28 days after birth. In these cases, when a neonate is diagnosed with sepsis, the code will be reported from category P36 Bacterial sepsis of newborn. An additional character is required to identify the pathogen that caused the infection. If severe sepsis is documented, a code from R65.2- also should be reported.

GUIDANCE CONNECTION

Read the ICD-10-CM Official Guidelines for Coding and Reporting, section **I. Conventions, General Coding Guidelines and Chapter-Specific Guidelines,** subsection **C. Chapter-Specific Coding Guidelines,** chapter **1. Certain Infectious and Parasitic Diseases,** subsection **d. 5) Sepsis due to a postprocedural infection.**

Septic Condition Resulting from Surgery

Should a patient develop sepsis from an infection as a complication of a surgical procedure, and the relationship between the infection and the procedure is specifically documented by the physician, you will list a code for that situation first. In the Alphabetic Index, find

Sepsis, postprocedural T81.44X-

In the Tabular List, find

T81.4XX- Infection following a procedure

You can see, included with other nonessential modifiers, *Sepsis following a procedure* is listed. When you read the additional characters' definitions, you will see that this code category includes other infections, not only sepsis.

Carefully read the six diagnoses listed in the EXCLUDES2 note.

bleb associated endophthalmitis (H59.4-)

infection due to infusion, transfusion and therapeutic injection (T80.2-)

infection due to prosthetic devices, implants and grafts (T82.6–T82.7, T83.5–T83.6, T84.5–T84.7, T85.7)

obstetric surgical wound infection (O86.0-)

post-procedural fever NOS (R50.82)

post-procedural retroperitoneal abscess (K68.11)

Don't forget the *Use Additional Code* notations also:

Use additional code **to identify infection**

Use additional code **(R65.2-) to identify severe sepsis, if applicable**

Then, continue with the usual coding sequence for sepsis, as reviewed earlier in this section. Remember to refer to the physician's documentation and the pathology report to gather all of the details you need to code accurately. *NOTE:* All of these codes require a 7th character.

T81.41X- Infection following a procedure, superficial incisional surgical site

T81.42X- Infection following a procedure, deep incisional surgical site

T81.43X- Infection following a procedure, organ and space surgical site

T81.44X- Sepsis following a procedure

Use additional code **to identify the sepsis**

YOU CODE IT! CASE STUDY

Gregory Parrale, a 31-year-old male, had his appendix taken out last week. He comes to Dr. Gorman's office for his post-surgical follow-up visit. Dr. Gorman finds the surgical wound is erythematous, swollen, and painful to the touch. He takes a swab of the fluid oozing from the site. The lab confirms a postoperative staph infection.

(continued)

You Code It!

Go through the steps of coding, and determine the diagnosis code(s) to be reported for this encounter between Dr. Gorman and Gregory Parrale.

Step #1: Read the case carefully and completely.
Step #2: Abstract the scenario. Which main words or terms describe why the physician cared for the patient during this encounter?
Step #3: Are there any details missing or incomplete for which you would need to query the physician? [If so, ask your instructor.]
Step #4: Check for any relevant guidance, including reading all of the symbols and notations in the Tabular List and the appropriate sections of the Official Guidelines.
Step #5: Determine the correct diagnosis code or codes to explain why this encounter was medically necessary.
Step #6: Double-check your work.

Answer:

Did you determine the correct codes?

T81.4XXA **Infection following a procedure, initial encounter**

B95.8 **Unspecified staphylococcus as the cause of diseases classified elsewhere**

Good job!

Systemic Inflammatory Response Syndrome (SIRS) without Infection

Systemic inflammatory response syndrome (SIRS) can develop in patients who have not developed an infection. Instead the reaction may occur due to the presence of a burn or other trauma, a malignant neoplasm, or the presence of pancreatitis. In such cases, coding the condition will change slightly. You will code the following sequence:

1. The code for the underlying condition (e.g., T22.311- Third-degree burn of right forearm).
2. The code for SIRS from the subcategory R65.1- Systemic inflammatory response syndrome (SIRS) of non-infectious origin.
3. The code for the acute organ dysfunction, when applicable.

If the documentation indicates that the patient later developed an infection, you will code the diagnosis for the infection as shown earlier in this section, along with the additional code for the underlying trauma or condition.

GUIDANCE CONNECTION

Read the ICD-10-CM Official Guidelines for Coding and Reporting, section **I. Conventions, General Coding Guidelines and Chapter-Specific Guidelines**, subsection **C. Chapter-Specific Coding Guidelines**, chapter **18. Symptoms, signs, and abnormal clinical laboratory findings, not elsewhere classified**, subsection **g. SIRS due to Non-Infectious Process**.

6.8 Antimicrobial Resistance

There are individuals who go to the doctor or clinic demanding a prescription for an antibiotic for the slightest sniffle. Touch a cart at the supermarket? Wipe antimicrobial gel on your hands. Unfortunately, there is an ongoing war on germs and, it turns out, the pathogens are winning. A natural phenomenon of adaptation to survive is one of the reasons why antimicrobial drugs are no longer working. Biologists call this "adaptive immunity" . . . a concept similar to the process of vaccinations affording a patient ultimate resistance to the effects of a specific pathogen. Only, in this case, it is the pathogen building its own immunity.

In 1928, bacteriologist Alexander Fleming realized that a mold growing on a culture plate actually had antibacterial benefit. The mold became known as "penicillin," and it was found to be very effective against *staphylococci* bacteria–a serious and life-threatening human infection. This discovery saved millions of lives as penicillins and other antibiotics were able to kill infection and prevent patients from dying. More than eight decades later, antibiotics are no longer halting the spread of infectious disease. And, in one perspective, they actually may be contributing to the spread.

The World Health Organization (WHO) defines "antimicrobial resistance (AMR)" as the "*. . . resistance of a micro-organism to an antimicrobial medicine to which it was originally sensitive.*" In addition to adaptive immunity, AMR is caused by the overuse of antibiotics. In the United States, antibiotics are prescribed for patients who actually do not need them an estimated 50% of the time. The CDC recommends that physicians wait for the results of cultures and lab tests before writing that prescription to ensure the bacteria or virus proven to cause the patient's infection can be fought off with the most effective drug. And these tests also will identify when no prescription is in the patient's best interests, saving the money that would have been spent on medication that would not work anyway.

Both inpatient and outpatient facilities are guilty of having less than effective infection control and prevention–the third underlying cause of AMR. The invisibility of these tiny organisms makes it difficult for some individuals to believe and remember to wash up or, at least, access antibacterial gel/foam.

Several codes are available to you to report AMR.

Coding for AMR

The CDC identified three pathogens as urgent threats: *Clostridium difficile (C. diff)*, carbapenem-resistant *Enterobacteriaceae*, and drug-resistant *Neisseria gonorrhoeae*. Let's look at some details about these three concerns.

Primarily, one code category is used to report AMR. There is a note and a notation for you:

✓4 **Z16 Resistance to antimicrobial drugs**

NOTE: The codes in this category are provided as ***Use additional codes*** to identify the resistance and non-responsiveness of a condition to antimicrobial drugs.

Code first **the infection.**

Clostridium difficile (C. diff)

C. diff is a spore-forming, gram-positive anaerobic bacillus that causes life-threatening diarrhea and that has been documented as causing about 250,000 infections each year, which have resulted in about 14,000 deaths. Of those patients aged 65 and older infected with *C. diff*, more than 90% died. In total, *C. diff* costs us an estimated $1 billion in excess health care costs. At greatest risk for contracting *C. diff* are hospitalized patients, those who have been recently hospitalized, and those who have recently received medical care with a course of antibiotic therapy.

The CDC is calling for more data as it tracks these AMRs. ICD-10-CM gives us the tools to collect and submit these details. For example, these codes may be reported for a patient with *C. diff* who is not responding to antibiotics:

Z16.23 Resistance to quinolones and fluoroquinolones

Z16.24 Resistance to multiple antibiotics

Carbapenem-Resistant *Enterobacteriaceae* (CRE)

CRE refers to a collection of microorganisms that have developed resistance to antibiotics. This grouping, or family, includes *Klebsiella* species and *Escherichia coli (E. coli)*. Carbapenem antibiotics are beta-lactam antibiotics used as a last resort for many bacterial infections (brand names include Invanz®, Primaxin®, and Merrem®); however, increased resistance to these antibiotics has made them virtually ineffective.

Klebsiella pneumoniae carbapenemase (KPC) and *New Delhi Metallo-beta-lactamase* (NDM), both types of CRE, are the enzymes responsible for rendering carbapenems ineffective. CRE causes a variety of diseases, ranging from pneumonia to urinary tract infections to serious bloodstream or wound infections. Patients who are ill, exposed to hospital environments, and in long-term care facilities are most susceptible to CRE infection.

Z16.19 Resistance to other specified beta lactam antibiotics

CODING BITES

A *Physician's Desk Reference* (PDR) or a Drug Guide can help you connect the name of a specific drug to a family name of drugs. For example, the quinolones are a family of synthetic broad-spectrum antibiotics. Ciprofloxacin, also known as Cipro, and levofloxacin, also known as Levaquin, are part of the quinolones family of drugs.

Neisseria gonorrhoeae Bacterial Infection

Gonorrhea is caused by the *Neisseria gonorrhoeae* bacterium and is most often transmitted by sexual contact. This microorganism replicates easily in the warm, moist areas of the reproductive tract, as well as in the mouth, throat, eyes, and anus. Approximately 30% of gonorrhea infections are found to be drug resistant, and, often, patients infected with drug-resistant *Neisseria gonorrhoeae* do not exhibit any signs or symptoms. This disease can have long-lasting effects on the patient, including pelvic inflammatory disease that can result in infertility in women and epididymitis (an inflammation of the structure within the testis that stores sperm and transports the sperm to the vas deferens) in men. A patient who has contracted gonorrhea is more susceptible to contracting the HIV.

When the physician's documentation states the patient is resistant to one of these antibiotics, normally prescribed to combat a diagnosis of *Neisseria gonorrhoeae*, report one of these codes in addition to the code for the infection (based on the anatomical site). Code Z16.19 or Z16.29 explains why the physician prescribed a different antibiotic.

Z16.19 **Resistance to other specified beta lactam antibiotics (resistance to cephalosporins)**

Z16.29 **Resistance to other single specified antibiotic (resistance to macrolides) (resistance to tetracyclines)**

Methicillin-Resistant *Staphylococcus aureus* Infection

Methicillin-resistant *Staphylococcus aureus* (MRSA) is a bacterial (staph) infection that is essentially unaffected by certain antibiotics. MRSA is spread from one person to another by direct contact with the infection, such as touching a skin bump or infection that is draining pus. MRSA can be spread directly, for example, by touching an infected person's rash, or it can be spread indirectly, such as by touching a used bandage contaminated with MRSA or by sharing a towel or razor that has come in contact with infected skin. One of the most frequent anatomical sites of MRSA colonization is the nose; bacteria can be found in nasal secretions.

To properly report these diagnoses, code the current infection due to MRSA and the MRSA infection separately with codes:

A49.02 **Methicillin resistant Staphylococcus aureus infection, unspecific site**

B95.62 **Methicillin resistant Staphylococcus aureus infection as the cause of diseases classified elsewhere**

Combination Codes

There are some infections commonly known to be caused by the patient's current MRSA status. In these cases, ICD-10-CM provides a combination code that can be used–the one code instead of two different codes. Two examples of these combination codes are

A41.02 **Sepsis due to Methicillin resistant Staphylococcus aureus**

J15.212 **Pneumonia due to Methicillin resistant Staphylococcus aureus**

Notice that the code descriptions include both the MRSA and another infection: septicemia in the first code and pneumonia in the second.

GUIDANCE CONNECTION

Read the ICD-10-CM Official Guidelines for Coding and Reporting, section **I. Conventions, General Coding Guidelines and Chapter-Specific Guidelines**, subsection **C. Chapter-Specific Coding Guidelines**, chapter **1. Certain Infectious and Parasitic Diseases**, subsection **e. Methicillin Resistant Staphylococcus aureus (MRSA) Conditions**.

EXAMPLE

Sally Hayes-Meyer was diagnosed with acute cystitis due to MRSA.

N30.00 Acute cystitis without hematuria

B95.62 Methicillin resistant Staphylococcus aureus infections as the causes of diseases classified elsewhere

Methicillin-Resistant *Staphylococcus aureus* Colonization

When a patient is documented as having a MRSA screening or nasal swab test that is positive yet there is no current illness, this is called colonization. Colonization indicates that the patient is a carrier. When this is the case, report either

Z22.321 Carrier or suspected carrier, Methicillin susceptible Staphylococcus aureus (MSSA)

or

Z22.322 Carrier or suspected carrier, Methicillin resistant Staphylococcus aureus (MRSA)

The coding guidelines state that it is possible for one patient to be a MRSA carrier *and* have a current MRSA infection at the same encounter. When this is the case, you are permitted to report code Z22.322 and a code for the MRSA infection.

YOU CODE IT! CASE STUDY

REFERRING PHYSICIAN: Audra Starch, MD

REASON FOR CONSULTATION: MRSA pneumonia, fever.

HISTORY OF PRESENT ILLNESS: This 77-year-old male has a history of recent stroke. Garden Nursing Home, where he is a resident, requested a consultation due to his increased cough, along with some pulmonary congestion. Dr. Starch prescribed an extended spectrum penicillin (Zosyn, 4.5 g q6hr via IV bedside) for the patient's low-grade fever. Sputum cultures evidenced MRSA, leading to the request for this consultation.

Patient is post-CVA aphasic. Daughter is present and serves as primary relator. Nurse's notes document that the patient has been aspirating in conjunction with the increasing frequency of cough. Overall status has decreased due to these situations. At this time, the patient appears to be resting comfortably without any complaints.

ASSESSMENT AND PLAN:

1. Pathology report shows: positive sputum cultures with methicillin-resistant *Staphylococcus aureus*.

2. Fever, most likely secondary to pneumonia.

RX: Vancomycin, 500 mg q6hr IV x 10 days to treat MRSA
ceftriaxone, 2 g q12, IM x 7 days to treat UTI/*E. coli*

You Code It!

Read Dr. Starch's documentation about this patient's condition and determine the accurate diagnosis code or codes.

Step #1: Read the case carefully and completely.
Step #2: Abstract the scenario. Which main words or terms describe why the physician cared for the patient during this encounter?
Step #3: Are there any details missing or incomplete for which you would need to query the physician? [If so, ask your instructor.]
Step #4: Check for any relevant guidance, including reading all of the symbols and notations in the Tabular List and the appropriate sections of the Official Guidelines.
Step #5: Determine the correct diagnosis code or codes to explain why this encounter was medically necessary.
Step #6: Double-check your work.

Answer:

Did you determine this to be the correct code?

J15.212 Pneumonia due to methicillin resistant Staphylococcus aureus

Good job!

NOTE: The fever is not reported separately because it is an inclusive sign of the pneumonia.

> **CODING BITES**
>
> *Did you know . . .?*
>
> - Number of visits to physician offices for infectious and parasitic diseases: 23 million (2025)
> - Number of new tuberculosis cases: 10,347 (2024)
> - Number of new salmonella cases: 1.28 million (est per year)
> - Number of new Lyme disease cases: 89,375 (2023)
> - Number of new meningococcal disease cases: 438 (2023)

Chapter Summary

The contagious nature of infectious diseases makes them very serious. The coding of such conditions, and their treatments, has statistical significance, in addition to the importance of reimbursement.

Ordinary day-to-day activities, such as sneezing, coughing, having sex, or playing baseball, may pass an infectious disease from one person to another. Health care advancements have enabled the use of vaccines to prevent such conditions as measles, mumps, varicella, or human papillomavirus (HPV). Other conditions require behavioral or lifestyle changes to prevent their spread.

In any case, the health care industry is charged with helping patients, and it is, or will be, your job to code all of these infectious diseases correctly.

You Interpret It! Answers

1. Needlestick, **2.** Airborne, **3.** Drinking water, **4.** Insect bites, **5.** Droplets, **6.** Bacteria (streptococcus bacteria), **7.** Virus (influenza virus A or B), **8.** Virus (human papillomavirus [HPV]), **9.** Virus (measles virus), **10.** Bacteria (staphylococcus bacteria), **11.** Parasite (deer tick), **12.** Fungus (bodily fluid exchange), **13.** Parasite (mosquito), **14.** Fungus (airborne, contaminated water), **15.** Parasite (lice), **16.** Fungus (microsporum), **17.** Fracture, **18.** HIV, **19.** Complication of pregnancy, **20.** Type 1 diabetes.

CHAPTER 6 REVIEW
Coding Infectious Diseases

Let's Check It! Terminology

Match each key term to the appropriate definition.

Part I

1. **LO 6.1** A hospital-acquired condition.
2. **LO 6.2** A single-celled microorganism that causes disease.
3. **LO 6.1** A condition that can be transmitted from one person to another.
4. **LO 6.1** Long-lasting; ongoing.
5. **LO 6.1** A condition affecting the immune system.
6. **LO 6.4** Group of organisms, including mold, yeast, and mildew, that cause infection.
7. **LO 6.1** Severe.
8. **LO 6.1** The invasion of pathogens into tissue cells.
9. **LO 6.1** No symptoms or manifestations.
10. **LO 6.1** The reaction of tissues to infection or injury; characterized by pain, swelling, and erythema.

A. Acute
B. Asymptomatic
C. Bacteria
D. Chronic
E. Fungi
F. Human Immunodeficiency Virus (HIV)
G. Infection
H. Infectious
I. Inflammation
J. Nosocomial

Part II

1. **LO 6.3** Microscopic particles that initiate disease, mimicking the characteristics of a particular cell, and can reproduce only within the body of the cells that they have invaded.
2. **LO 6.4** Tiny living things that can invade and feed off of other living things.

A. Parasites
B. Pathogen
C. Sepsis

3. **LO 6.1** Any agent that causes disease; a microorganism such as a bacterium or virus.
4. **LO 6.7** Generalized infection spread through the body via the bloodstream; blood infection.
5. **LO 6.7** Sepsis with signs of acute organ dysfunction.
6. **LO 6.7** A definite physical reaction, such as fever, chills, etc., to an unspecified pathogen.
7. **LO 6.1** Spread throughout the entire body.
8. **LO 6.2** An infectious condition that causes small rounded swellings on mucous membranes throughout the body.
9. **LO 6.7** Condition typified by two or more systemic responses to infection; a specified pathogen.
10. **LO 6.7** Severe sepsis with hypotension; unresponsive to fluid resuscitation.

D. Septic Shock
E. Septicemia
F. Severe Sepsis
G. Systemic
H. Systemic Inflammatory Response Syndrome (SIRS)
I. Tuberculosis
J. Viruses

Let's Check It! Concepts

Choose the most appropriate answer for each of the following questions.

1. **LO 6.1** The body's response to an infection may include the sign or symptom of
   - **a.** rash.
   - **b.** blurred vision.
   - **c.** increased body temperature.
   - **d.** reduced body temperature.
2. **LO 6.2** ________is a serious infection of the skin that may be either a staph infection (staphylococcal bacteria) or a strep infection (streptococcal bacteria).
   - **a.** Impetigo
   - **b.** Cellulitis
   - **c.** Hepatitis
   - **d.** Meningitis
3. **LO 6.3** Grant Harris, a 19-year-old male, is diagnosed with herpes zoster keratoconjunctivitis. How is this coded?
   - **a.** B02.30
   - **b.** B02.31
   - **c.** B02.32
   - **d.** B02.33
4. **LO 6.4** All of the following are parasites *except*
   - **a.** lice.
   - **b.** mites.
   - **c.** warts.
   - **d.** worms.
5. **LO 6.5** Aspiration pneumonia is a
   - **a.** viral infection.
   - **b.** bacterial infection.
   - **c.** fungal infection.
   - **d.** parasitic infection.
6. **LO 6.6** A woman with HIV-positive status is pregnant and in her second trimester. What must be the first-listed code?
   - **a.** O98.7
   - **b.** O98.71
   - **c.** O98.711
   - **d.** O98.712
7. **LO 6.6** Exposure to HIV will be coded with which code?
   - **a.** Z20.4
   - **b.** Z20.5
   - **c.** Z20.6
   - **d.** Z20.7
8. **LO 6.7** When coding for SIRS in a patient who has *not* developed an infection, you would code in which sequence?
   - **a.** the code for the acute organ dysfunction, the code for SIRS, the code for the underlying condition
   - **b.** the code for SIRS, the code for the acute organ dysfunction, the code for the underlying condition
   - **c.** the code for the underlying condition, the code for SIRS, the code for the acute organ dysfunction
   - **d.** none of these
9. **LO 6.7** The code for septic shock may be all of the following *except*
   - **a.** the first-listed diagnosis code.
   - **b.** an additional code.
   - **c.** used to identify the inclusion of hypotension.
   - **d.** added to the codes required for severe sepsis.
10. **LO 6.8** Methicillin-resistant *Staphylococcus aureus* (MRSA) is spread from one person to another by
    - **a.** direct contact.
    - **b.** indirect contact.
    - **c.** both direct and indirect contact.
    - **d.** none of these.

Let's Check It! Guidelines

*Refer to the Official Guidelines and fill in the blanks according to **Chapter 1**, Certain Infectious and Parasitic Diseases, Chapter-Specific Coding Guidelines.*

I.C.16.f	R65.2	infection	synonymous
follow up	confirmed		underlying
Septic	B95.62	2	inconclusive
unrelated	documentation	sepsis	organ
R75	severe	urosepsis	Z71.7
postprocedural	queried	principal	

1. Code only _____ cases of HIV infection/illness. This is an exception to the hospital inpatient guideline _____.
2. If a patient with HIV disease is admitted for an _____ condition, the code for the unrelated condition should be the _____ diagnosis.
3. Patients with documentation of _____ HIV serology, may be assigned code _____.
4. When a patient presents for _____ regarding their HIV test results and the test result is negative, assign code _____, Human immunodeficiency virus [HIV] counseling.
5. The term _____ is a nonspecific term. It is not to be considered _____ with sepsis. Should a provider use this term, they must be _____ for clarification.
6. The coding of severe sepsis requires a minimum of _____ codes: first code for the _____ systemic infection, followed by a code from subcategory _____, Severe sepsis.
7. _____ shock generally refers to circulatory failure associated with_____sepsis, and therefore, it represents a type of acute _____ dysfunction.
8. As with all _____ complications, code assignment is based on the provider's _____ of the relationship between the _____ and the procedure.
9. Newborn _____ See Section _____. Bacterial sepsis of Newborn.
10. When there is documentation of a current infection due to MRSA, and that infection does not have a combination code that includes the causal organism, assign the appropriate code to identify the condition along with code _____.

Let's Check It! Rules and Regulations

Please answer the following questions from the knowledge you have gained after reading this chapter.

1. **LO 6.2/6.3** Explain the difference between a bacterial infection and a viral infection, and give examples of each.
2. **LO 6.4** What is the difference between a parasitic and a fungal infection? Include an example of each in your answer.
3. **LO 6.1** What is a nosocomial infection, and where do such infections occur?
4. **LO 6.7** Discuss the difference between septicemia and SIRS.
5. **LO 6.8** What is MRSA and how is it spread?

YOU CODE IT! Basics

First, identify the main term in the following diagnoses; then code the diagnosis.

Example: Neonatal candidiasis:

a. main term: *candidiasis* **b.** diagnosis: *P37.5*

1. Allergic bronchopulmonary aspergillosis:
   a. main term: _____ **b.** diagnosis: _____
2. Chronic active hepatitis:
   a. main term: _____ **b.** diagnosis: _____
3. Sepsis, streptococcal, group B:
   a. main term: _____ **b.** diagnosis: _____

(continued)

4. Pulmonary cryptococcosis:
   a. main term: _____ b. diagnosis: _____
5. Herpes zoster meningitis:
   a. main term: _____ b. diagnosis: _____
6. Chronic otitis media, right ear:
   a. main term: _____ b. diagnosis: _____
7. Jungle yellow fever:
   a. main term: _____ b. diagnosis: _____
8. Kaposi's sarcoma of the lymph nodes:
   a. main term: _____ b. diagnosis: _____
9. Cellulitis of upper right limb:
   a. main term: _____ b. diagnosis: _____
10. Generalized blastomycosis:
   a. main term: _____ b. diagnosis: _____
11. Acute disseminated, noninfectious, encephalomyelitis:
   a. main term: _____ b. diagnosis: _____
12. Laryngeal diphtheria:
   a. main term: _____ b. diagnosis: _____
13. Retroperitoneal tuberculosis:
   a. main term: _____ b. diagnosis: _____
14. Shigellosis, group C:
   a. main term: _____ b. diagnosis: _____
15. Ringworm honeycomb:
   a. main term: _____ b. diagnosis: _____

ICD-10-CM

YOU CODE IT! Practice

Using the techniques described in this chapter, carefully read through the case studies and determine the most accurate ICD-10-CM code(s) and external cause code(s), if appropriate, for each case.

1. Ben Kenton, a 49-year-old male, presents today with a high fever, chills, nausea, and diarrhea. After an examination and reviewing the results of the blood tests, Dr. Daniels diagnoses Ben with West Nile fever.
2. Robin Pullen, a 36-year-old female, comes to see Dr. Ditolla because she is running a fever and has a sore throat and overall body aches. Test results are positive for H1N1. Robin is diagnosed with swine influenza.
3. Joan Kenney, a 27-year-old female, is having difficulty breathing. Dr. Aung documents a fever of 101 F and facial edema. Joan recently returned home from a trip to Asia. Joan said they were contending with some sort of larval infestation in Asia. Joan is diagnosed with nasopharyngeal myiasis.
4. Babbs Fisher, a 48-year-old female, just returned from an African vacation. Babbs is brought in by her husband, George, who noticed she was acting confused. Dr. Carla notes a low fever. Babbs states she feels tired and has a sore throat. She started vomiting this morning and admits to abdominal pain. Dr. Carla examines Babbs and orders an enzyme-linked immunosorbent assay (ELISA) test, which confirms the diagnosis of Ebola virus. Babbs is admitted to Weston Hospital for treatment.
5. Steven Jordan, a 51-year-old male, comes to see Dr. Kolb because he is experiencing nausea and vomiting and his stool is unusually light in color. Steven is accompanied by his wife, Sally. Sally says her husband seems confused and less alert lately. Upon examination, Dr. Kolb notes hepatosplenomegaly, jaundice, and RUQ tenderness. Steven is admitted to the hospital, where blood test results confirm the presence of IgG anti-HAV antibodies. Steven is diagnosed with acute hepatitis A.
6. Johnny Brennen, a 7-year-old male, is brought in by his parents. Johnny has developed a hard cough and says his sides hurt. Dr. Travis, Johnny's pediatrician, completes blood work and takes a CXR and nasopharyngeal specimen. A subconjunctival hemorrhage is noted in the left eye. Test results confirm a diagnosis of whooping cough due to *Bordetella pertussis* with pneumonia. Johnny is admitted to Weston Hospital.
7. Frances Lowder is having difficulty breathing. She also admits to a bad headache, sore throat, and no appetite. She is 28-weeks pregnant and was diagnosed with HIV 3 years ago. Dr. Mabry notes a temperature of 102 F and papules over her upper body. Blood tests confirm the diagnosis of varicella with pneumonia. Frances is admitted to Weston Hospital.
8. Jenny Cassidy, a 4-year-old female, is brought in by her parents to see her pediatrician, Dr. Harmon. Jenny has a fever and a rash on her back. Dr. Harmon notes a "strawberry tongue." The completed CBC test confirms a diagnosis of scarlet fever.

(continued)

9. Lee Greenwalt, a 9-year-old male, is brought in by his parents. Lee is not feeling well and is losing weight. Mrs. Greenwalt states Lee seems to be sweating at night. Dr. Moon documents a bitonal cough, a temperature of 100 F, and a general weakening. Lee is admitted to Weston Hospital. Test results confirm a diagnosis of tuberculosis of tracheobronchial lymph nodes.
10. Donald Rampey, a 72-year-old male, was admitted to the hospital with severe sepsis due to streptococcus, group B. Donald developed acute hepatic failure.
11. Mendenhall Aguirre, a 37-year-old male, presents today with a burning sensation during urination. Dr. Boykin collects a penile swab specimen for a microscopic examination, which confirms trichomonal prostatitis.
12. Gayle Cassels, a 12-year-old female, is brought in by her mother to see Dr. Kellum. Gayle has had a fever for 3 days with a head cold. Dr. Kellum notes conjunctivitis, an erythematous rash on the head and neck, as well as Koplik's spots on the inside of Gayle's mouth. The salivary measles-specific IgA test confirmed the diagnosis of measles.
13. Steven Crooks, a 16-year-old male, presents today with a sore throat. Dr. Hoffman notes acute pharyngitis with a low-grade fever, as well as petechiae on the roof of the mouth. A serological test confirms the diagnosis of Epstein–Barr infectious mononucleosis.
14. Donna Burgess, a 33-year-old female, comes to see Dr. Freeman today with a headache, fever, and chest pain. The ELISA serological test confirms a diagnosis of Coxsackie B virus infection with pericarditis.
15. Victor Lockhart, a 29-year-old male, presents today with a fever of 100.6 F. He says one minute he is sweating and the next he is shivering and his stomach hurts. Dr. Osterlund documents paleness and tenderness in the right hypochondria region. Victor is admitted to Weston Hospital, where blood tests, a liver function test, and a CT scan confirm the diagnosis of amebic liver abscess due to *Entamoeba histolytica*.

ICD-10-CM YOU CODE IT! Application

The following exercises provide practice in abstracting physicians' documentation from our textbook's health care facility, Prader, Bracker, & Associates. These case studies are modeled on real patient encounters. Using the techniques described in this chapter, carefully read through the case studies and determine the most accurate ICD-10-CM code(s) for each case study.

WESTON HOSPITAL

629 Healthcare Way • SOMEWHERE, FL 32811 • 407-555-6541

PATIENT: GALEANA, ROBERT

ACCOUNT/EHR #: GALERO001

Attending Physician: Oscar R. Prader, MD

This 33-year-old male was admitted for a high fever, abdominal pain, and a noted moderate decrease in alertness. Robert has been on oral antibiotics for a left ear infection for approximately 7 days. I last saw the patient in the office 4 days ago when his left ear spontaneously drained.

PE: Ht: 5′11″, Wt: 194, T: 101.2, R: 19, BP: 134/86. Pt seems confused. Left ear drainage continues.

CSF analysis reveals normal pressure, a slightly thicker viscosity with a cloudy appearance. Results of CSF exam showed 6875 WBC, 35 g/L protein, and 23 mg/dL glucose.

Arbovirus is identified in two blood cultures. Pt responds positively to antimicrobial therapy.

DX: Meningitis due to arbovirus, urban yellow fever; acute suppurative otitis media

Determine the most accurate ICD-10-CM code(s).

(continued)

WESTON HOSPITAL

629 Healthcare Way • SOMEWHERE, FL 32811 • 407-555-6541

PATIENT: MURPHY, ADRIENNE

ACCOUNT/EHR #: MURPAD001

Attending Physician: Renee O. Bracker, MD

Pt is admitted with a chief complaint of shortness of breath of approximately 7- to 10-days duration and a feeling of uneasiness and discomfort. Pt was found to be HIV-positive in May 2018, and diagnosed with AIDS in February 2019. Patient also complains of vision loss. She states she can't see and it hurts when you touch her eyes and face.

PE: Ht: 5′4″, Wt: 126, T: 101.6. The physician notes pustules on forehead, right eye, and bridge of nose. A Tzanck smear with methylene blue stain was performed; results positive.

DX: Herpesviral keratoconjunctivitis (simplex), secondary to AIDS

Plan: Acyclovir, IV: 10 mg/kg q8hr

Determine the most accurate ICD-10-CM code(s).

PRADER, BRACKER, & ASSOCIATES

A Complete Health Care Facility

159 Healthcare Way • SOMEWHERE, FL 32811 • 407-555-6789

PATIENT: LUPO, THERESA

ACCOUNT/EHR #: LUPOTH001

Attending Physician: Renee O. Bracker, MD

Pt presented to office with a laceration to the left knee that occurred approximately 10 days ago. Theresa states that she fell as she was getting up from a chair in her backyard. She cleaned the area and put an OTC antibiotic ointment on the bandage before applying it to the wound. She has changed the bandage daily.

PE: Ht: 5′2″, Wt: 120, T: 99.6, R: 18, BP: 128/78. After removing the bandage, a widely infected wound was found with small pieces of gravel, with resulting cellulitis to the knee. Extensive irrigation and debridement using sterile water were performed, but closure was not attempted pending resolution of the infection. Culture of the wound revealed streptococcus D.

1,200 units of Bicillin CR IM was given.

Rx for oral antibiotics was given to Pt.

Pt to return in 3 days for follow-up.

Determine the most accurate ICD-10-CM code(s). Do not code external causes.

PRADER, BRACKER, & ASSOCIATES

A Complete Health Care Facility

159 Healthcare Way • SOMEWHERE, FL 32811 • 407-555-6789

PATIENT: PLATTENBAUM, BENJAMIN

ACCOUNT/EHR #: PLATBE001

Attending Physician: Oscar R. Prader, MD

(continued)

Pt, a 32-year-old male, presents with continued complaints of nasal drainage, pressure behind his eyes, and a sore throat. I last saw Ben 2 weeks ago when he was diagnosed with acute frontal sinusitis due to *Staphylococcus aureus*. Prescription for amoxicillin 250 mg q8hr was given.

PE: Ht: 6′2″, Wt: 210, T 100.1, R 20, BP: 134/86. Nasal endoscopy confirms the diagnosis that acute sinusitis is still present. MRSA, specifically to penicillins, is apparent. IV injection levofloxacin, 500 mg.

Rx: Levofloxacin, 250 mg q24hr x 10 days

Recommendation for bed rest, lots of fluids. Pt to return prn.

Determine the most accurate ICD-10-CM code(s). Do not code external causes.

WESTON HOSPITAL

629 Healthcare Way • SOMEWHERE, FL 32811 • 407-555-6541

PATIENT: SAMUELS, BERNARD

ACCOUNT/EHR #: SAMUBE001

Attending Physician: Oscar R. Prader, MD

This 82-year-old male was admitted to the hospital with high fever, myalgia, headache, rhinitis, and a nonproductive cough. He also shows signs of confusion.

PE: Ht: 5′9″, Wt: 173, T: 103.2, R: 22, BP: 90/59. Pt's condition deteriorated with definite signs of septic shock, pneumonia, and hypotension. He is now in acute renal failure.

DX: Influenza with pneumonia due to *E. coli*; septic shock, acute renal failure.

Determine the most accurate ICD-10-CM code(s).

7

Coding Neoplasms

Key Terms

Benign
Carcinoma
Ectopic
Functional Activity
Malignant
Mass
Metastasize
Morphology
Neoplasm
Overlapping Boundaries
Topography

Learning Outcomes

After completing this chapter, the student should be able to:

LO 7.1 Identify the medical necessity for screenings and diagnostic testing for malignancies.
LO 7.2 Discern the various types of neoplasms.
LO 7.3 Interpret the Table of Neoplasms accurately.
LO 7.4 Employ the directions provided in the Chapter Notes at the head of the Neoplasms section of the Tabular List.
LO 7.5 Apply the guidelines for sequencing admissions due to complications of neoplasms and/or their treatments.

STOP! **Remember, you need to follow along in your ICD-10-CM code book for an optimal learning experience.**

7.1 Screening and Diagnosis

Screenings

You may already know about screenings. Screenings are provided with the intention of identifying a disease or abnormality as early as possible. When a neoplasm is detected and treated early in its formation, the treatment is less intense, making the process easier on the patient and less costly. Also important is the proven fact that the earlier a malignancy is dealt with, the better the chances of recovery and survival. Patients with *no* signs or symptoms are typically scheduled for various screenings based on guidelines related to age, family history, or personal history.

When you are coding for a patient encounter for a screening for a possible malignant neoplasm, such as a mammogram or a colonoscopy, you will report a code from this category:

Z12 Encounter for screening for malignant neoplasms

> **GUIDANCE CONNECTION**
>
> Read the ICD-10-CM Official Guidelines for Coding and Reporting, section **I. Conventions, General Coding Guidelines and Chapter-Specific Guidelines**, subsection **C. Chapter-Specific Coding Guidelines**, chapter **21. Factors influencing health status and contact with health services (Z00–Z99)**, subsection **c.5) Screening**.

EXAMPLE

You would report code:

Z12.5 Encounter for screening for malignant neoplasm of prostate

for an encounter when a 59-year-old man goes in for a screening prostate exam, as per recommendations for men aged 55 to 69 years of age.

Read the notation directly below the Z12 code category:

> **Screening is the testing for disease or disease precursors in asymptomatic individuals so that early detection and treatment can be provided for those who test positive for the disease.**

Also, read the next notation carefully:

> *Use additional code* **to identify any family history of malignant neoplasm (Z80.-)**

ICD-10-CM reminds you that an additional code should be reported when the prompting factor for the screening is not age but family history. Family history means that someone in the patient's past bloodline had been diagnosed with the condition being screened for, and it is known that this places the patient at a higher risk for developing the condition.

EXAMPLE

You would report code:

Z80.42 Family history of malignant neoplasm of prostate

in addition to code Z12.5 for an encounter when a 44-year-old man goes in for a screening prostate exam because his father and brother were both diagnosed with prostate cancer, dramatically increasing his risk.

A personal history code (Z85.-) should be reported for those patients who may receive screening tests more frequently than others. For example, a woman with a history of breast cancer may get mammograms every 6 months rather than annually. The personal history of breast cancer code will support medical necessity for this increase in the frequency of testing.

EXAMPLE

You would report code:

Z85.3 Personal history of malignant neoplasm of breast

in addition to code **Z12.31 Encounter for screening mammogram for malignant neoplasm of breast** for an encounter when a 57-year-old female goes in for a screening mammogram every 6 months, instead of the usual (once a year), because the fact that she had a malignant neoplasm of her breast a few years ago dramatically increases her risk for a recurrence.

GUIDANCE CONNECTION

Read the ICD-10-CM Official Guidelines for Coding and Reporting, section **I. Conventions, General Coding Guidelines and Chapter-Specific Guidelines**, subsection **C. Chapter-Specific Coding Guidelines**, chapter **21. Factors influencing health status and contact with health services (Z00-Z99)**, subsection **c.4) History (of)**.

The Z12 code category also carries an EXCLUDES1 notation to remind you of the difference between a diagnostic test, which is performed when a patient *does* exhibit signs or symptoms, and a screening test, which is performed with the intention of early detection of disease without signs or symptoms.

> EXCLUDES1 **encounter for diagnostic examination—code to sign or symptom**

EXAMPLE

You would report code:

N63.- Unspecified lump in breast

for an encounter when a 62-year-old female goes in for a mammogram because she felt a lump in her breast during her monthly self-check and her gynecologist confirmed it was suspicious.

Confirming a Diagnosis

Once the patient exhibits signs, such as a lump found during a physical examination or an abnormality identified during a screening test, a pathologist must determine the essence of the neoplasm. This is the only way to factually distinguish between benign cells and malignant cells.

Generally, specimens may be provided to the laboratory in various forms: blood (capillary or vein), urine, semen, sputum, swabs (that carry tissue cells, pus, or other excretion), or tissue specimens (surgical samples taken during a biopsy). Most often with neoplasms, a biopsy is necessary. You will need to ensure that an accurate ICD-10-CM diagnosis code is presented with the specimen to confirm medical necessity for the diagnostic testing, such as signs and symptoms.

CODING BITES

The only way to confirm a diagnosis of a malignancy is for the physician to perform a biopsy (surgical removal of all or part of the tumor tissue) and submit that tissue for pathological examination. Therefore, you can understand why reporting a malignancy and not specifying the anatomical location of the tumor would be unlikely.

EXAMPLES

R91.8 Other nonspecific abnormal finding of lung field (mass on lung)

R93.1 Abnormal findings on diagnostic imaging of heart and coronary circulation

Abnormal findings of diagnostic tests justify the need for additional tests and procedures.

Blood tests can also provide important information with regard to malignancies in the body. For example, an increased white blood cell (WBC) count, also known as *leukocytosis*, may be a sign that neoplastic cells have been produced in the bone marrow and released into the bloodstream—common in conditions such as leukemic neoplasia and other myeloproliferative disorders. Many types of pathological and imaging tests can provide critical information to the physician seeking to confirm, or deny, a diagnosis of a malignancy. Tests available depend upon the anatomical site and the type of malignancy (see **Table 7-1**).

TABLE 7-1 Some Common Tests Performed When Various Types of Malignancies Are Suspected

Malignant Neoplasm of the Cervix
• Abdominal ultrasound • Cervical biopsy • Colposcopy • CT scan of the abdomen and pelvis
Malignant Neoplasm of the Colon and Rectum
• Barium enema • Carcinoembryonic antigen (CEA) • Colonoscopy • Stool for occult blood
Leukemia/Lymphoma
• Blood smear • Bone marrow biopsy • Cell surface immunophenotyping • Cryoglobulins
Malignant Neoplasm of the Lung
• Alpha-1 antitrypsin • Bone scan • Bronchoscopy • Chest x-ray • Lung biopsy

Malignant Neoplasm of the Ovary
• CA-125 • Laparoscopy • Paracentesis • Pyelography
Malignant Neoplasm of the Prostate
• Acid phosphatase • CT scan of the pelvis • Cystoscopy • MRI of the prostate • Prostate specific antigen (PSA)

Source: cancer.gov

Test Results

You will see pathology reports in the patient's chart, whether you work in a hospital or a physician's office. Some examples of reports include

- Histopathology: a punch biopsy of the overlying skin reveals an adenocarcinoma with diffuse involvement of the dermis and extensive invasion of the dermal lymphatics. The adenocarcinoma is composed of irregular nests with some areas forming tubercles. Mitotic figures, including atypical forms, are seen. The tumor was ER −, PR −, Her2 +, CK7 +, and CK 20 −.
- Tissue biopsy culture: negative for any growth.
- Lumbar puncture: negative for organisms.
- Blood culture: 2/2 positive for *Neisseria meningitidis*.
- Labs: WBC: 8.6, Hgb/Hct: 9.4/26.3, Platelets: 222, BUN: 71, Creatinine: 6.8, U/A: 2+ protein, 3+ blood, ANA: negative, Hepatitis B surface antigen: negative, Hepatitis C antibody: negative, Serum cryoglobulins: negative, HIV: negative, cANCA: positive (1:1280), Tissue culture: negative, Initial blood cultures: negative, CXR: bilateral opacities.

Pathology reports also may provide information on the grading and/or staging of the tumor. Grading a tumor is the microscopic analysis of the tumor cells and tissue to describe how abnormal they appear. Staging, however, evaluates the size and location of the tumor, as well as determination of any signs or evidence of metastasis. In some cases, you will need to know the grade of a patient's tumor so you can determine the correct code.

EXAMPLES

C82.07 Follicular lymphoma grade I, spleen

C82.16 Follicular lymphoma grade II, intrapelvic lymph nodes

These two codes are examples of those with code descriptions that require you to check the physician's documentation and pathology reports to identify the grade of the tumor.

The pathologist also will stage the tumor tissue specimen (see **Table 7-2** for more details on the stages of cancer).

TABLE 7-2 Cancer Stages

Tumor Stage	What the Stage Describes
Stage 0	Abnormal cells are present but have not spread to nearby tissue. Also known as carcinoma in situ, or CIS. CIS is not malignant, but it may evolve into malignancy.
Stage I, Stage II, Stage III	Malignant cells are present. The higher the number, the larger the malignant tumor and the more it has metastasized to nearby tissues.
Stage IV	Malignant cells have metastasized to distant parts of the body.

Physicians, most often oncologists, use tumor grading in addition to staging, a patient's age, and overall health to determine a prognosis and create a treatment plan. Cancer registries collect population-based cancer incidence data, as required under federal law, to support research and government funding to support the impact of cancer on a community.

CODING BITES

Find out more about Cancer Registries at https://www.cdc.gov/cancer/npcr/value/index.htm

YOU INTERPRET IT!

Is this order for a screening or a diagnostic test?

1. Susie's annual mammogram — **(a)** Screening **(b)** Diagnostic
2. Dr. McFadden felt a lump in Arthur's arm. Dr. McFadden did a biopsy. — **(a)** Screening **(b)** Diagnostic
3. Edith told her doctor she is coughing, is wheezing, and suffers from unexplained weight loss. Her doctor ordered a lung CT. — **(a)** Screening **(b)** Diagnostic
4. At Roger's annual checkup, Dr. Concord ordered a PSA test to be completed. — **(a)** Screening **(b)** Diagnostic

7.2 Abstracting the Details about Neoplasms

When normal cells mutate, they may create a **neoplasm**, also known as a *tumor*. A tumor is an overgrowth or abnormal mass of tissue, and it may be either benign or malignant (cancerous). In all cases, a physician should check the abnormality and determine a course of action.

Neoplasm
Abnormal tissue growth; tumor.

Once a diagnosis is confirmed, you will need to accurately report it with the specific code or codes. Begin by ensuring you understand the details.

In some cases, you will see the term **mass** used to describe a patient's condition. Mass is *not* the same as a neoplasm. More often, mass is used to identify a cyst or other thickening of tissue.

Mass
Abnormal collection of tissue.

While many people think that *neoplasm* and *cancer* are synonymous, they are not. Cancer is the common term for **carcinoma** (see **Figure 7-1**).

Carcinoma
A malignant neoplasm or cancerous tumor.

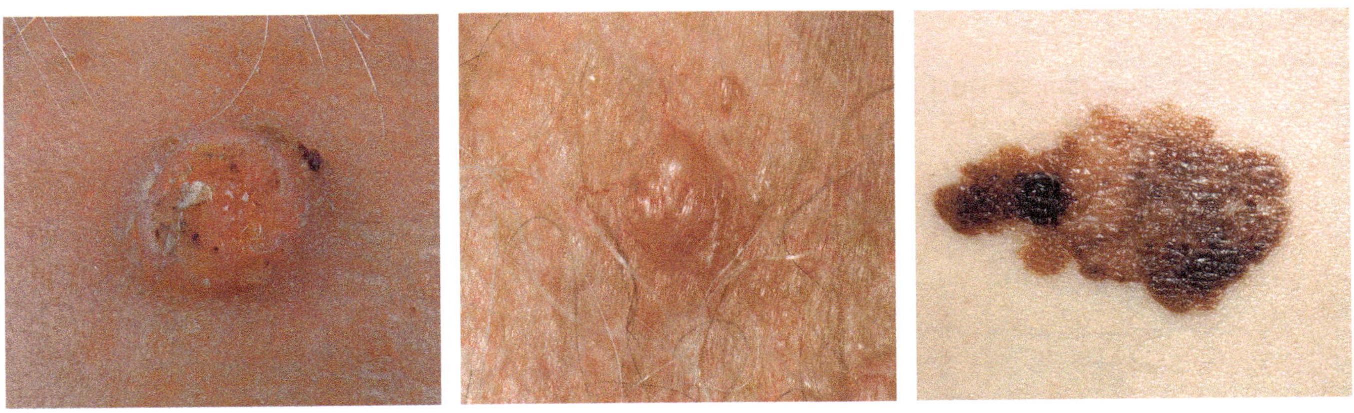

FIGURE 7-1 Types of skin cancer: (a) squamous cell carcinoma, (b) basal cell carcinoma, and (c) malignant melanoma

(a) BSIP SA/Alamy Stock Photo; (b) Dr. P. Marazzi/Science Source; (c) National Cancer Institute (NCI)

Terms Used to Identify Neoplasms

Malignant
Invasive and destructive characteristic of a neoplasm; possibly causing damage or death.

Benign
Nonmalignant characteristic of a neoplasm; not infectious or spreading.

CODING BITES

In medical terminology, the suffix *-oma* means tumor.

Neoplasms might be **malignant** or **benign** or have aspects of both characteristics. In diagnoses, neoplasms also may be defined by an individual name. The physician's notes may state a different term. Some examples of these terms are

- Adenoma
- Melanoma
- Leukemia
- Papilloma

When the physician uses a term such as adenoma, melanoma, or other specific name rather than the more generic term of *neoplasm*, it is more efficient for you to look for that specific term in the Alphabetic Index first, before looking under the term *neoplasm*. At the very least, the Alphabetic Index can tell you if that type of tumor is known to be malignant or benign.

Often, when you look up one of these specific neoplasm terms in the Alphabetic Index, it will provide you with some specific information about the tumor. Let's take a look in the ICD-10-CM Alphabetic Index under the term written by the physician . . .

Fibroxanthoma (see also Neoplasm, connective tissue, benign)

atypical — *see* Neoplasm, connective tissue, uncertain behavior

malignant — *see* Neoplasm, connective tissue, malignant

Fibroxanthosarcoma — *see* Neoplasm, connective tissue, malignant

You can see that while you might not know if a fibroxanthoma is malignant or benign, the Alphabetic Index will tell you.

LET'S CODE IT! SCENARIO

Abby Shantner, a 41-year-old female, comes to see Dr. Branson to get the results of her biopsy. Dr. Branson explains that Abby has an alpha cell adenoma of the pancreas. Dr. Branson spends 30 minutes discussing treatment options.

Let's Code It!

Dr. Branson has diagnosed Abby with an *alpha cell adenoma of the pancreas.* You have been working with Dr. Branson as his coder for a while, so you know that an adenoma is a neoplasm, but what kind of neoplasm is it—benign or malignant? To help you determine this, instead of going to *neoplasm*, let's see if there is a listing in the Alphabetic Index under *adenoma*. When you find *adenoma*, the book refers you to

Adenoma (*see also* Neoplasm, benign, by site)

This tells you an adenoma is a benign tumor. Or you can continue down this list to the indented term, and find

Adenoma

alpha-cell

pancreas D13.7

Turn to the Tabular List and read the complete description of code category D13:

(continued)

✓4 **D13 Benign neoplasm of other and ill-defined parts of digestive system**

The EXCLUDES1 note does not relate to this patient's diagnosis for this encounter, so continue reading down the column to review all of the choices for the required fourth character.

D13.7 Benign neoplasm of endocrine pancreas

That matches Dr. Branson's diagnosis.

Check the top of this subsection and the head of this chapter in ICD-10-CM. There are several **NOTES**. Read carefully. Do any relate to Dr. Branson's diagnosis of Abby? No. Turn to the Official Guidelines and read Section I.C.2. There is nothing specifically applicable here, either.

Good job!

Malignant Primary

The term *primary* indicates the anatomical site (the place in the body) where the malignant neoplasm was first seen and identified. If the physician's notes do not specify primary or secondary, then the site mentioned is primary.

Malignant Secondary

The term *secondary* identifies the anatomical site to which the malignancy **metastasized**. One very strange thing about cancerous cells is that they travel through the body and do not necessarily spread to adjoining body parts. Cancer can be identified in the breast as the primary site and metastasize to the liver without actually affecting anything in between. Notes will state that a site is "secondary to" *(primary site)*, "metastasized from" *(primary site)*, or *(primary site)* "metastasized to" *(secondary site)*.

The terms *disseminated cancer*, *generalized cancer*, or *widely metastatic* would indicate that the malignancy has infiltrated the body throughout and affects all or most of the patient's anatomy. This would be coded as a malignant neoplasm without specification of site (code C80.0). In such cases, it is not that the physician forgot to specify the site. It is that there are too many sites to list.

Ca in Situ

The term *Ca in situ* indicates that the tumor has undergone malignant changes but is still limited to the site where it originated (i.e., it has not spread). *Ca* is short for carcinoma, and you can remember *situ* as in the word *situated*. So think of it as a cancerous tumor that is staying in place.

Benign

The term *benign* means there is no indication of invasion of adjacent cells. Essentially, benign means not cancerous.

Uncertain

The classification *uncertain* indicates that the pathologist is not able to specifically determine whether a tumor is benign or malignant because indicators of both are present.

Unspecified Behavior

Choose codes that describe "*Unspecified Behavior*" when the physician's notes do not include any specific information regarding the nature of the tumor. Before choosing one of these codes, please query the physician and make certain that a laboratory report is not available or on its way with the information you need.

CODING BITES

Always begin with the terms the physician writes in his or her notes. Then, only when that does not bring you to a suggested code, you can look up alternate terms. This rule of thumb will save you a lot of time.

Metastasize
To proliferate, reproduce, or spread.

CODING BITES

To determine the code to report a neoplasm, you need to know

1. Where in the body (specifically, which anatomical site) is the neoplasm located?
2. Is the neoplasm benign, malignant, in situ, or uncertain? Uncertain is a pathologic determination and is *not* the same as unspecified.
3. If the neoplasm is malignant, is this the first diagnosis of malignancy for this patient? If so, this is the primary site. If not, this is a secondary malignancy because it metastasized from the primary.

YOU INTERPRET IT!

What type of neoplasm is this: benign or malignant; primary or secondary?

5. Metastatic lung cancer ____________

6. Melanoma ____________

7. Squamous cell carcinoma ____________

8. Pancreatic lymph gland neoplasm ____________

9. Adenoma ____________

CODING BITES

If you turn to the term ***Neoplasm*** in the Alphabetic Index in the regular alphabetic order, you will see the notation *(see also Table of Neoplasms).*

7.3 Reporting the Neoplastic Diagnosis

Once you have determined the anatomical location and type of tumor that has been documented, you will need to find a suggested code in the ICD-10-CM Neoplasm Table, found directly after the Alphabetic Index.

The Neoplasm Table is a seven-column table set in alphabetic order by the anatomical site (the part of the body where the tumor is located), shown in the first column. To the right of the first column, there are six columns across: Malignant Primary, Malignant Secondary, Ca in situ, Benign, Uncertain Behavior, and Unspecified Behavior (see **Figure 7-2**) . . . the types of neoplasms you read about previously in this chapter. It is here, in this table, that you can find the suggested code to report the specific type and location of the tumor documented by the physician.

	Malignant Primary	Malignant Secondary	Ca in situ	Benign	Uncertain Behavior	Unspecified Behavior
Neoplasm, neoplastic	C80.1	C79.9	D09.9	D36.9	D48.9	D49.9
- abdomen, abdominal	C76.2	C79.8-	D09.8	D36.7	D48.7	D49.89
-- cavity	C76.2	C79.8-	D09.8	D36.7	D48.7	D49.89
-- organ	C76.2	C79.8-	D09.8	D36.7	D48.7	D49.89
-- viscera	C76.2	C79.8-	D09.8	D36.7	D48.7	D49.89
-- wall — *see also Neoplasm, abdomen, wall, skin*	C44.509	C79.2-	D09.5	D23.5	D48.5	D49.2
--- connective tissue	C49.4	C79.8-	—	D21.4	D48.1-	D49.2
--- skin	C44.509	—	—	—	—	—
---- basal cell carcinoma	C44.519	—	—	—	—	—
---- specified type NEC	C44.599	—	—	—	—	—
---- squamous cell carcinoma	C44.529	—	—	—	—	—
- abdominopelvic	C76.8	C79.8-	—	D36.7	D48.7	D49.89

FIGURE 7-2 The Neoplasm Table, in part, showing codes for various abdominal neoplasms and abdominopelvic neoplasms

After abstracting the physician's documentation to identify the anatomical site of the tumor, turn to the Neoplasm Table and find that anatomical site in the first column in the table. Remember to carefully review indented lists below the main term of the anatomical site so you can determine the code for the greatest specificity.

EXAMPLE

Epiglottis

anterior aspect or surface

cartilage

free border (margin)

junctional region

posterior (laryngeal) surface

You can see in this one example that knowing the anatomical site of the tumor—the *epiglottis*—is not enough information. You need to identify, from the documentation, where the tumor is located on the epiglottis.

Once you have found the most specific match for the anatomical site identified as the location of the tumor in the documentation, go back to the physician's notes. This time, look for the type of neoplasm in the diagnosis: Malignant Primary, Malignant Secondary, Ca in situ, Benign, Uncertain Behavior, or Unspecified Behavior. Now, back in the Neoplasm Table, read straight across to the right of the anatomical site line. At the top of the page, each of these six columns has a title. Find which column has the title that matches the diagnosis, and then go down until you hit the conjunction of the anatomical site line and the type of neoplasm in question. This is your suggested code.

EXAMPLE

Dr. Tomlinsonn diagnosed Elsa with a malignant neoplasm of the abdominal viscera, noted as Ca in situ.

	Malignant Primary	Malignant Secondary	Ca in situ	Benign	Uncertain Behavior	Unspecified Behavior
Neoplasm, neoplastic	C80.1	C79.9	D09.9	D36.9	D48.9	D49.9
- abdomen, abdominal	C76.2	C79.8-	D09.8	D36.7	D48.7	D49.89
-- cavity	C76.2	C79.8-	D09.8	D36.7	D48.7	D49.89
-- organ	C76.2	C79.8-	D09.8	D36.7	D48.7	D49.89
-- viscera	C76.2	C79.8-	D09.8	D36.7	D48.7	D49.89
-- wall — *see also Neoplasm, abdomen, wall skin*	C44.509	C79.2-	D04.5	D23.5	D48.5	D49.2

In the Neoplasm Table, in the first column, find **Abdomen**, then indented below that the specific site **-- viscera**.

Then, across to the right you can see suggested codes for each type of tumor. For Elsa's diagnosis, code D09.8 is *suggested.*

Next, turn in the Tabular List to check this code, and all of the notations. Because the Neoplasm Table is a part of the Alphabetic Index, the rule still applies . . . never, never report a code directly from here. You must check the suggested code in the Tabular List, read the symbols and notations, read the complete code description and all of the options, and check the Official Guidelines before you can confirm and report a code.

LET'S CODE IT! SCENARIO

Aaron Docker, a 65-year-old male, returns to see Dr. Cabrera. The results of his colonoscopy and laboratory tests on the biopsy have come back. Dr. Cabrera confirms Aaron has a benign neoplasm of the ascending colon.

Let's Code It!

Dr. Cabrera confirmed Aaron has *a benign neoplasm of the ascending colon.* Turn to the Neoplasm Table in your ICD-10-CM code book. Go down the list of anatomical sites until you reach *colon.* There is a notation that directs you to *"see also* Neoplasm, intestine, large." The ascending colon is actually the portion of the large intestine that goes from the cecum to the transverse colon. Indented under *colon* are the words *and rectum.* Go back to Dr. Cabrera's notes. His diagnosis does not include the rectum, so follow the book's advice and turn to the listing for *intestine, large*, and read what is shown there.

Continue through the list until you get to *intestine, intestinal.* Beneath the term *intestine*, you will find the word *large* indented. Indented under *large* is *colon.* Indented under *colon*, you see *ascending.* This matches Dr. Cabrera's diagnosis of Aaron's neoplasm exactly! Now, read across the table to the right to the "Benign" column. Here, the code D12.2 is suggested. Remember the rule: Never, never code from the Alphabetic Index, and that includes the Neoplasm Table, so turn to the Tabular List to confirm this suggested code. Start reading at the three-character code category:

✓4 **D12 Benign neoplasm of colon, rectum, anus, and anal canal**

The EXCLUDES1 note does not relate to this patient's diagnosis for this encounter, so continue reading down the column to review all of the choices for the required fourth character.

D12.2 Benign neoplasm of ascending colon

Check the top of this subsection and the head of this chapter in ICD-10-CM. There are several **NOTES** at the beginning of this chapter. Read carefully. Do any relate to Dr. Cabrera's diagnosis of Aaron? No. Turn to the Official Guidelines and read Section I.C.2. There is nothing specifically applicable here, either.

Now you can report D12.2 for Aaron's diagnosis with confidence.

Good coding!

A Pregnant Patient with a Malignancy

Conditions that may complicate a pregnancy have their very own chapter in ICD-10-CM. You will learn about this in depth in the chapter ***Coding Genitourinary, Gynecology, Obstetrics, Congenital, and Pediatrics Conditions***. However, when a pregnant woman is diagnosed with a malignancy, a code from code subcategory O9A.1- Malignant neoplasm complicating pregnancy, childbirth, and the puerperium will be reported as the principal diagnosis, followed by the code for the primary malignancy. To reinforce this, you can see the notation beneath this code subcategory that reminds you to *Use additional code to identify neoplasm.*

EXAMPLE

Fran has been diagnosed with malignant melanoma on her right shoulder. She is 21-weeks pregnant.

O9A.112	Malignant neoplasm complicating pregnancy, second trimester
C43.61	Malignant melanoma of right upper limb, including shoulder
Z3A.21	21-weeks gestation of pregnancy

Malignancies in Remission or Relapse

There are certain types of malignancies, such as multiple myeloma (malignancy of the plasma cells in the bone marrow), lymphoma (malignancy of the white blood cells), or leukemia (malignancy of the bone marrow and bone-forming tissues), that may be described differently. For example:

C90.00	**Multiple myeloma not having achieved remission**
C90.01	**Multiple myeloma in remission**
C90.02	**Multiple myeloma in relapse**

These categorizations are not available for all malignancies; however, when they are, you already know to match the code description to the documentation. Remission is described as an absence of all signs and symptoms of the cancer previously diagnosed. In the 2025 code set, there are 47 new codes for malignancies in remission. This indicates good news for our fight against cancers.

CODING BITES

Professional coding specialists must be cautious when determining the difference between a patient *in remission* and a patient with a *personal history of a condition*. If the documentation is not absolutely clear on this, you must query the physician for clarification. There is a big difference between these two diagnostic identifications.

LET'S CODE IT! SCENARIO

PATIENT: Roberta Wolfe
CONSULTING PHYSICIAN: Oliver Cannon, MD
REQUESTING PHYSICIAN: Theresa Calabressi, MD

Thank you for referring the patient for medical oncology consultation.

HISTORY OF PRESENT ILLNESS: The patient is a 29-year-old female with noninvasive left breast cancer. The patient had a screening mammogram 4 months ago, which revealed a left upper-outer breast abnormality. Stereotactic biopsy previously confirmed ductal carcinoma in situ. The patient underwent needle localization excision with pathology confirming ductal carcinoma in situ grade 2, ER positive, PR positive. She received ipsilateral breast radiation. Her course has been complicated by apparent incision site infection, which has resulted in persistent low-grade oozing of blood and occasional extrusion of pus. She has been treated with several courses of antibiotics. However, the scant bloody discharge continued. Over the past 1 week, she has noted increasing tenderness at the site of bleeding and apparent infection. She otherwise offers no complaints.

PAST MEDICAL HISTORY: Remarkable for anemia attributed to iron deficiency for which she takes iron supplements. Unremarkable for hypertension, diabetes, hypercholesterolemia, or prior cardiac, pulmonary, or hepatic dysfunction. Normal monthly cycles; however, the last cycle has been particularly prolonged at 9 days.

MEDICATIONS: She takes no regular prescription medications.

ALLERGIES: No known allergies.

FAMILY HISTORY: Remarkable for sister with diagnosis of breast cancer at age 43, presently 51, in remission. No other known family history of breast or ovary cancer. Father died at age 82 of cardiac disease, mother aged 79 with history of heart disease; two brothers, three sons, and two daughters are healthy.

SOCIAL HISTORY: Married. Denies cigarettes, alcohol, drugs.

REVIEW OF SYSTEMS: Denies fever, chills, sweats, headaches, seizures, syncope, blurred vision, dysphagia, cough, chest pain, shortness of breath, abdominal pain, nausea, vomiting, diarrhea, constipation, melena, hematochezia, dysuria, hematuria, flank pain, back pain, abnormal bleeding, bruising, lymph node swelling, or focal paresthesias or weakness.

PHYSICAL EXAMINATION

GENERAL: The patient is well developed, well nourished, in no acute distress.
VITAL SIGNS: Temperature 98.8, heart rate 63, blood pressure 110/81, weight 135.4 pounds, and height 57 inches.
SKIN: Skin clear. No visible rash, ecchymosis, or petechia.
HEENT: Normocephalic. No scleral icterus. No mucosal lesions.
NECK: Supple without thyromegaly.

(continued)

LYMPH NODES: No secondary neck, axillary, or inguinal nodes.

BREASTS: Without dominant mass bilaterally. There is moderate induration of approximately 2.8 cm across, underlying the left upper outer quadrant incision. There is no fluctuance or erythema and patient denies significant tenderness to the area.

CHEST: Clear to auscultation and percussion.

CARDIAC: Regular rate and rhythm. No murmur, rub, or gallop.

ABDOMEN: Soft and nontender. No masses or hepatosplenomegaly.

RECTAL AND GENITAL: Deferred.

EXTREMITIES: No clubbing, cyanosis, or edema.

MUSCULOSKELETAL: No back tenderness. No bony or joint deformity.

NEUROLOGIC: Alert and oriented. Cranial nerves, sensory and motor system, and gait are normal.

IMPRESSION: Ductal carcinoma in situ, left breast, stage 0 (Tis N0 M0), ER positive, PR positive, status post lumpectomy to negative surgical margins and has set up breast radiation. Overall prognosis is excellent with estimated risk of local recurrence in the 5% range. Risk of systemic metastasis is negligible. Thus, adjuvant systemic therapy is not warranted. She is, of course, at increased risk for second malignancy; thus, tamoxifen chemoprevention would be a reasonable option.

RECOMMENDATIONS AND PLAN: Diagnosis, prognosis, and management options were discussed in detail with the patient and questions were answered. Tamoxifen chemoprevention was discussed in detail and she, at this time, appears agreeable to initiation of therapy. I provided a prescription for tamoxifen 20 mg daily. On the assumption that she desires continuing oncologic follow-up, any follow-up appointment will be made in 6 months. Alternatively, if she should decline tamoxifen chemoprevention or if her gynecologic physician, Dr. Calabressi, would be willing to prescribe tamoxifen and provide continuing oncologic follow-up, then medical oncology follow-up will be on an as-needed basis.

Let's Code It!

Dr. Cannon examined and evaluated Roberta Wolfe with regard to her post-procedural condition for breast cancer. Read the entire documentation. Can you find his conclusion or impression of her condition? In the section marked IMPRESSIONS, he documents, "*Ductal carcinoma in situ, left breast.*"

Turn in your ICD-10-CM Alphabetic Index, Table of Neoplasms. What is the anatomical site of this neoplasm? "breast, duct." Find this in the first column:

breast (connective tissue) (glandular tissue) (soft parts)

Read all of the specific components of the breast shown in the indented list below this. Can you find "duct"? Neither can I. However, you know that this is the location within the breast that has the neoplasm. Hmm. Read across to the third column to the right, titled Ca in situ. Notice that the majority of these have the same code category suggested: D05. Perhaps we can find a more specific description for the duct in the Tabular List. Turn to find D05 in the Tabular List.

✓4 **D05 Carcinoma in situ of breast**

Check the **EXCLUDES1** notation. None of these diagnoses relates to Roberta's diagnosis, so read down and review the four options you have for a fourth character. One seems to be what you are looking for:

✓5 **D05.1 Intraductal carcinoma in situ of breast**

Read the three options for the required fifth character. Which one matches Dr. Cannon's documentation?

D05.12 Intraductal carcinoma in situ of left breast

However, before you can report this code, you must check the top of this subsection and the **INCLUDES** note above code D00. Next, check the notations at the head of this chapter in ICD-10-CM. There are notations at the beginning of this chapter; you will learn more about these specific notations in the next part of this chapter. Read carefully. Do any relate to Dr. Cannon's diagnosis of Roberta? No. Turn to the Official Guidelines and read Section I.C.2. There is nothing specifically applicable here either.

Now you can report D05.12 for Roberta's diagnosis with confidence.

D05.12 Intraductal carcinoma in situ of left breast

Good work!

7.4 Neoplasm Chapter Notes

In the ICD-10-CM Tabular List, take a look at the beginning of ***Chapter 2: Neoplasms (C00–D49)*** (directly above code C00). There are four notes here to help you determine the most accurate neoplasm code.

Functional Activity

The functional activity of a neoplasm notes whether or not the tumor is causing the secretion of hormones. This would be documented in the pathology report and may need to be reported.

The first note in the ICD-10-CM code book's ***Chapter 2: Neoplasms (C00–D49)*** helps you when certain neoplasms require an additional code to report **functional activity**. This note states:

> **Functional Activity**
> Glandular secretion in abnormal quantity.

Note: All neoplasms are classified in this chapter, whether they are functionally active or not. An additional code from Chapter 5 may be used to identify such functional activity associated with any neoplasm.

The note in the ICD-10-CM code book's Tabular List beneath the heading for ***Chapter 4: Endocrine, Nutritional, and Metabolic Diseases (E00–E89)*** (directly above code E00) reminds you of this detail:

Note: All neoplasms, whether functionally active or not, are classified in Chapter 2. Appropriate codes in this chapter (i.e., E05.8, E07.0, E16–E31, E34.-) may be used as additional codes to indicate either functional activity by neoplasms and ectopic endocrine tissue or hyperfunction and hypofunction of endocrine glands associated with neoplasms and other conditions classified elsewhere.

What this note means is that if a patient has been diagnosed with a neoplasm affecting the individual's glandular function, you have to identify the functional activity (of the gland) with an additional code.

For example, take a look beneath code category C56 Malignant neoplasm of ovary. There is a notation that says:

Use additional code **to identify any functional activity**

This note regarding functional activity also appears under the following terms:

Benign neoplasm of ovary
Malignant neoplasm of endocrine glands
Benign neoplasm of endocrine glands
Malignant neoplasm of islets of Langerhans
Benign neoplasm of islets of Langerhans
Malignant neoplasm of the testis
Benign neoplasm of the testis
Malignant neoplasm of thyroid glands
Benign neoplasm of thyroid glands

EXAMPLES

Catecholamine-producing malignant pheochromocytoma of thyroid

C73	Malignant neoplasm of thyroid gland
E27.5	Adrenomedullary hyperfunction

Ovarian carcinoma, right side, with hyperestrogenism

C56.1	Malignant neoplasm of right ovary
E28.0	Estrogen excess

Basophil adenoma of pituitary with Cushing's disease

C75.1	Malignant neoplasm of pituitary gland
E24.0	Pituitary-dependent Cushing's disease

LET'S CODE IT! SCENARIO

Daniel Coleman, a 41-year-old male, came to see Dr. Lucano for a checkup. He was diagnosed with functioning thyroid carcinoma. Dr. Lucano reviews with Daniel the results of his latest thyroid scan, TSH and TRH stimulation tests, and an ultrasonogram. Dr. Lucano informs Daniel that he has developed hyperthyroidism.

Let's Code It!

Dr. Lucano has diagnosed Daniel with *functioning thyroid carcinoma* and *hyperthyroidism.* The hyperthyroidism is the functional activity of the thyroid carcinoma. Turn to the Alphabetic Index and look for

Carcinoma — *see also* Neoplasm, by site, malignant

Look down the list. Neither the term *functioning* nor the term *thyroid* is shown here, so you will need to turn to the Neoplasm Table and find

Neoplasm, thyroid, malignant, primary C73

Let's go to the Tabular List, to confirm:

C73 Malignant neoplasm of thyroid gland

Use additional code **to identify any functional activity**

This code is correct, and the ICD-10-CM book is telling you that you need an additional code to report the functional activity. The only other detail Dr. Lucano included in her diagnostic statement is hyperthyroidism. Turn back to the Alphabetic Index and look up hyperthyroidism:

Hyperthyroidism (latent) (preadult) (recurrent) E05.90

Turn to the Tabular List to confirm this suggested code.

✓4 **E05 Thyrotoxicosis [hyperthyroidism]**

The EXCLUDES1 note mentions nothing that relates to this encounter for our patient, so read down the column to review the choices for the required fourth character.

✓5 **E05.9 Thyrotoxicosis unspecified**

This matches the notes, so you are in the correct place. The symbol to the left of the code tells you that an additional character is required.

E05.90 Thyrotoxicosis unspecified without mention of thyrotoxic crisis or storm

Did you notice that this code is located in **Chapter 5** and is describing the functional activity of the neoplasm? Great!

Check the top of this subsection and the head of this chapter in ICD-10-CM. A **NOTE** and an EXCLUDES1 notation are shown at the beginning of this chapter. Read carefully. Do any relate to Dr. Lucano's diagnosis of Daniel? Yes. Both chapters have **NOTES** regarding the coding of neoplasms and functional activity. Double-check to make certain you are complying with these directions. Next, turn to the Official Guidelines and read both Sections I.C.2 and I.C.4. There is nothing specifically applicable here either.

Now, you can report C73 and E05.90 for this encounter with Daniel with confidence.

Good coding!

Morphology (Histology)

The second note at the top of the ICD-10-CM code book's *Chapter 2: Neoplasms (C00–D49)* relates to the classifications of neoplasms.

Note: Chapter 2 classifies neoplasms primarily by site (topography) with broad groupings for behavior, malignant, in situ, benign, etc. The Table of Neoplasms should be used to identify the correct topography code. In a few cases, such as for malignant melanoma and certain neuroendocrine tumors, the morphology (histologic type) is included in the category and codes.

In addition to the code for a neoplasm, you may be required to include a separate code with additional information about the tumor's morphology. "Morphology of Neoplasms" is available as a separate book, the ***International Classification of Diseases for Oncology*** (ICD-O). Morphology codes are not structured like the other diagnosis codes. The codes always begin with the letter "M," which is followed by four characters, a slash (/), and a single character. A neoplasm's histology is described by the first four characters of the M code.

Topography
The classification of neoplasms primarily by anatomical site.

Morphology
The study of the configuration or structure of living organisms.

M codes are used for providing specific data about the site (topography) and the histology (morphology) of the affected tissue to tumor and cancer registries. Pathologists also may use the codes to provide more detail about a particular tissue sample. Normally, M codes are not used for reimbursement and are not placed on insurance claim forms. Cancer registries use them in their cataloging of data.

CODING BITES

The phrase "**subcategory/ code .8**" refers to the fourth character of 8.

Primary Malignant Neoplasms Overlapping Site Boundaries

The third note here, at the head of the ICD-10-CM code book's *Chapter 2: Neoplasms (C00–D49)*, is concerned with primary malignant tumors that overlap anatomical sites.

Note: A primary malignant neoplasm that overlaps two or more contiguous (next to each other) sites should be classified to the subcategory/code .8 ("overlapping lesion"), unless the combination is specifically indexed elsewhere. For multiple neoplasms of the same site that are not contiguous, such as tumors in different quadrants of the same breast, codes for each site should be assigned.

The nature of a malignant neoplasm includes its potential to spread to adjoining tissue. As you learned earlier in this chapter, you code malignancies by their anatomical site in the order in which the malignancy developed: primary and secondary. However, there are cases where the condition of the patient involves more than one code subcategory. Neoplasms with **overlapping boundaries**, also known as *contiguous*, may blur anatomical descriptors.

Overlapping Boundaries
Multiple sites of carcinoma without identifiable borders.

EXAMPLES

C05.8	Malignant neoplasm of overlapping sites of palate
C17.8	Malignant neoplasm of overlapping sites of small intestine
C57.8	Malignant neoplasm of overlapping sites of female genital organs

For cases in which the physician cannot identify a specific site, usually because the malignancy has metastasized so dramatically, the code category C76 enables you to report the malignancy by identifying only the section of the patient's body, such as head, abdomen, or lower limb.

EXAMPLES

C76.0	Malignant neoplasm of head, face, and neck
C76.51	Malignant neoplasm of right lower limb

Malignant Neoplasms of Ectopic Tissue

Ectopic
Out of place, such as an organ or body part.

The last note at the head of the ICD-10-CM code book's ***Chapter 2: Neoplasms (C00–D49)*** in the Tabular List states:

Note: Malignant neoplasms of ectopic tissue are to be coded to the site mentioned, e.g., ectopic pancreatic malignant neoplasms are coded to pancreas, unspecified (C25.9).

This notation provides you with direction on how to determine the code for a case when the neoplasm is located in an unusual and hard-to-determine location in the body. The term *ectopic* means outside of an organ. Therefore, if the diagnostic statement describes the tumor as being ectopic, report the condition to the nearest, identified organ.

EXAMPLE

Dr. Laveign documented that Evan's biopsy confirmed that he has an ectopic malignant neoplasm of the prostate.

Report this with the following code:

C61 Malignant neoplasm of prostate

7.5 Admissions Related to Neoplastic Treatments

When you are coding encounters with a patient who has been diagnosed with a neoplasm, whether benign or malignant, the same rule for identifying the principal diagnosis still applies.

Why did the health care professional care for this patient today?

Admission for Treatment of Malignancy

If a patient's encounter is only for therapeutic treatment of a malignancy, such as the administration of chemotherapy, immunotherapy, or radiation therapy, then the principal (first-listed) code will report this fact, followed by a code or codes to report details about the malignancy being treated.

One of these codes would be reported as the principal diagnosis code:

Z51.0 **Encounter for antineoplastic radiation therapy**

Z51.11 **Encounter for antineoplastic chemotherapy**

Z51.12 **Encounter for antineoplastic immunotherapy**

Note that there is a notation for the Z51 code category that reminds you to

Code also **condition requiring care**

This would be the code or codes with the details about the malignancy, the reason *why* the patient would need this radiation, chemotherapy, or immunotherapy treatment.

EXAMPLE

Warren Spencer was admitted to McGraw General Hospital for his third chemotherapy infusion . . . treatment for the malignant neoplasm on the tail of his pancreas.

Z51.11 Encounter for antineoplastic chemotherapy

C25.2 Malignant neoplasm of tail of pancreas

Because Warren was admitted for the purpose of receiving his chemotherapy treatment, his chemotherapy is reported first (the principal diagnosis code), followed by the reason Warren needs this chemotherapy—pancreatic cancer.

Excised Malignancies/Personal History

Thanks to modern medical science and technology, health care professionals are more successful than ever at getting rid of certain neoplasms (tumors), often by excising them (surgically cutting them out). Postoperatively, the patient no longer has the anatomical site where the malignancy was located. Therefore, the patient can no longer have that condition. At that time, the code will change from a malignancy code (C00–C96) to a personal history of a malignancy code (category Z85).

Codes Z85.0- through Z85.7- are used to identify the previous site of a primary malignancy only. Reporting a former site of a secondary malignancy may be reported with Z85.8-.

EXAMPLE

Martha Peterson was diagnosed with a malignant neoplasm of the upper-inner quadrant of the right breast. The diagnosis code was

C50.211 Malignant neoplasm of upper-inner quadrant of right female breast

She underwent a mastectomy, a surgical procedure to remove her breast. Once the anatomical site (her breast) that contained the malignant neoplasm was removed, she no longer had the disease, and no additional treatment was needed. From this point on, the diagnosis code is

Z85.3 Personal history of malignant neoplasm, breast

GUIDANCE CONNECTION

Read the ICD-10-CM Official Guidelines for Coding and Reporting, section **I. Conventions, General Coding Guidelines and Chapter-Specific Guidelines**, subsection **C. Chapter-Specific Coding Guidelines**, chapter **2. Neoplasms**, subsection **d. Primary malignancy previously excised**.

Suppose a patient has a primary site of malignancy and the disease has already metastasized to a second location. If the primary site is removed, the secondary malignancy is still coded as secondary but listed first. Confusing? Let's look at an example.

EXAMPLE

Ronald Albertson was diagnosed with prostate cancer. It spread to his liver before he was able to have surgery. The diagnosis codes, in this sequence, are

C61 Malignant neoplasm of the prostate

C78.7 Secondary malignant neoplasm of liver, and intrahepatic bile duct

Dr. Isaacson removes Ronald's prostate successfully. He no longer required any treatment. The new codes are

C78.7 Secondary malignant neoplasm of liver, and intrahepatic bile duct

Z85.46 Personal history of malignant neoplasm, prostate

Once Ronald has the site of his primary malignancy removed, his prostate condition becomes "history." The code for his secondary malignancy in the liver moves up in order, but it will always be the *secondary* site at which Ronald developed a malignancy.

GUIDANCE CONNECTION

Read the ICD-10-CM Official Guidelines for Coding and Reporting, section **I. Conventions, General Coding Guidelines and Chapter-Specific Guidelines**, subsection **C. Chapter-Specific Coding Guidelines**, chapter **2. Neoplasms**, subsection **b. Treatment of secondary site**.

YOU CODE IT! CASE STUDY

Frederick Westchester, a 53-year-old male, came to see Dr. Henner, his dermatologist, for an annual checkup. Two years ago, Dr. Henner removed a malignant melanoma from Frederick's left forearm. The malignancy was totally removed, but he comes to see his physician for a checkup once a year.

You Code It!

Go through the steps of coding, and determine the diagnosis code or codes that should be reported for this encounter between Dr. Henner and Frederick.

Step #1: Read the case carefully and completely.
Step #2: Abstract the scenario. Which main words or terms describe why the physician cared for the patient during this encounter?
Step #3: Are there any details missing or incomplete for which you would need to query the physician? [If so, ask your instructor.]
Step #4: Check for any relevant guidance, including reading all of the symbols and notations in the Tabular List and the appropriate sections of the Official Guidelines.
Step #5: Determine the correct diagnosis code or codes to explain why this encounter was medically necessary.
Step #6: Double-check your work.

Answer:

Did you determine the following diagnosis code?

Z85.820 Personal history of malignant melanoma of skin

Good job!

Complications and Complications of Treatment

You probably are aware that some of the most frequently used treatments to eradicate malignant cells, such as chemotherapy and radiation, manifest other conditions.

In those cases where the patient is admitted for therapy (radiation, chemotherapy, or immunotherapy) and develops complications during the encounter, report Z51.0, Z51.11, or Z51.12 as the principal diagnosis code, *followed* by the code or codes to report the specific complications, such as uncontrolled nausea and vomiting or dehydration.

When the patient is admitted for treatment of anemia that is a manifestation of the malignancy, and only the anemia is treated during this stay, report the code for the neoplasm as the principal diagnosis *followed* by code D63.0 Anemia in neoplastic disease.

However, if the patient is admitted for treatment of anemia that is the result of the neoplastic treatment (chemotherapy or immunotherapy), you will report a code for the anemia first, *followed* by code T45.1X5- Adverse effect of antineoplastic and immunosuppressive drugs [seventh character is required to identify the encounter].

Anemia that is manifested as an effect from radiation treatments is reported a bit differently. For this patient, the code to report the anemia is reported as the principal diagnosis, *followed* by the code explaining the neoplasm for which the radiation was administered, *followed* by code Y84.2 Radiological procedure and radiotherapy as the cause of abnormal reaction of the patient, or of later complication, without mention of misadventure at the time of the procedure.

When the patient is admitted for treatment of dehydration, manifestation from the malignancy, and only the dehydration is treated during this stay, report the code for the dehydration as the principal diagnosis, *followed* by the code for the neoplasm that was the reason the treatment was needed.

GUIDANCE CONNECTION

Read the ICD-10-CM Official Guidelines for Coding and Reporting, section **I. Conventions, General Coding Guidelines and Chapter-Specific Guidelines**, subsection **C. Chapter-Specific Coding Guidelines**, chapter **2. Neoplasms**, subsection **c. Coding and sequencing of complications**.

Treatment of Secondary Site Only

There are instances where a physician may treat only the secondary site of malignancy for a patient in a given encounter. In this case, you would report the secondary site as the principal diagnosis and the primary site malignancy after this.

EXAMPLE

Marvin's prostate cancer has spread to his lungs. Today, he has come to see Dr. Dunbar, a pulmonologist specializing in lung cancer, for evaluation and treatment.

Report the codes in this order:

1. Secondary lung cancer
2. Primary prostate cancer

Note that the primary cancer site is still identified and coded as "primary" even though it is the second code reported.

GUIDANCE CONNECTION

Read the ICD-10-CM Official Guidelines for Coding and Reporting, section **I. Conventions, General Coding Guidelines and Chapter-Specific Guidelines**, subsection **C. Chapter-Specific Coding Guidelines**, chapter **2. Neoplasms,** subsection **l. Sequencing of neoplasm codes**.

YOU CODE IT! CASE STUDY

Eric Swanson is a 43-year-old male with a malignant neoplasm of the laryngeal cartilage. He has become dehydrated due to the course of radiation therapy treatments. Dr. Leistner admitted Eric today to receive rehydration therapy.

You Code It!

Abstract the details related to the reasons why Dr. Leistner met with Eric.

Step #1: Read the case carefully and completely.
Step #2: Abstract the scenario. Which key words or terms describe why the physician cared for the patient during this encounter?
Step #3: Are there any details missing or incomplete for which you would need to query the physician? [If so, ask your instructor.]
Step #4: Check for any relevant guidance, including reading all of the symbols and notations in the Tabular List and the appropriate sections of the Official Guidelines.
Step #5: Determine the correct diagnosis code or codes to explain why this encounter was medically necessary.
Step #6: Double-check your work.

(continued)

Answer:

Did you determine these to be the correct codes?

E86.0 **Dehydration**

C32.3 **Malignant neoplasm of laryngeal cartilage**

Prophylactic Organ Removal

Advances in science have given us genetic predisposition testing and other identification exams. The information these tests provide, along with personal and family histories, enables patients and health care professionals to predict an individual's risk for cancer and other diseases more accurately. Studies show, for example, that a woman who has inherited a mutation in the BRCA1 or BRCA2 gene faces a dramatically higher risk for developing breast cancer by age 65. A strong family history of colon cancer may lead an individual to be tested for a variant in the APC gene. There are many genes that can now be tested for various hereditary or familial conditions.

GUIDANCE CONNECTION

Read the ICD-10-CM Official Guidelines for Coding and Reporting, section **I. Conventions, General Coding Guidelines and Chapter-Specific Guidelines,** subsection **C. Chapter-Specific Coding Guidelines,** chapter **2. Neoplasms,** subsection **s. Breast implant associated anaplastic large cell lymphoma.**

Prophylactic, or preventive, surgery can reduce risk of cancer in these situations by as much as 90%. In the case of breast cancer, preventive action would mean having a double mastectomy (the surgical removal of both breasts) while a patient is still healthy and without any signs or symptoms of carcinoma.

As a coder, the question becomes: How do you code a diagnosis for a surgical procedure on a healthy anatomical site? You will use a code from this subcategory:

Z40.0- **Encounter for prophylactic surgery for risk factors related to malignant neoplasms (Admission for prophylactic organ removal)**

Use additional code **to identify risk factor**

For those patients who have had genetic testing with a confirmed abnormal gene, you will also use a second code from category Z15 Genetic susceptibility to disease.

If the reason for the preventive surgery is due to a family history of cancer, you will add another code from the Z80 Family history of primary malignant neoplasm category.

YOU CODE IT! CASE STUDY

Angelina Constantine, a 27-year-old female, was admitted today for the prophylactic removal of her breasts. Her grandmother, mother, and sister have all had breast cancer, so she had genetic testing performed. It indicated that she did have a genetic susceptibility to breast cancer. She elected to have the surgery instead of taking chances with her health.

You Code It!

Go through the steps of coding, and determine the diagnosis code or codes that should be reported for Angelina's surgery.

(continued)

Step #1: Read the case carefully and completely.
Step #2: Abstract the scenario. Which main words or terms describe why the physician cared for the patient during this encounter?
Step #3: Are there any details missing or incomplete for which you would need to query the physician? [If so, ask your instructor.]
Step #4: Check for any relevant guidance, including reading all of the symbols and notations in the Tabular List and the appropriate sections of the Official Guidelines.
Step #5: Determine the correct diagnosis code or codes to explain why this encounter was medically necessary.
Step #6: Double-check your work.

Answer:

Did you determine the following diagnosis codes?

Z40.01 Prophylactic removal of breast

Z15.01 Genetic susceptibility to malignant neoplasm of breast

Z80.3 Family history of malignant neoplasm, breast

Good job!

Chapter Summary

In this chapter, you learned how to identify the key words in physicians' documentation and test results reports that can guide you toward the most accurate code or codes. You learned the differences in the types of neoplasms and the proper sequencing of codes. In addition, you reviewed the correct way to sequence the codes when a patient has had a malignant site excised or been admitted for treatment or a complication.

There have been, and continue to be, incredible advancements made in the treatments of all types of neoplasms, as well as modifications to sociological behaviors to help prevent the development of those insidious health concerns. As a professional coding specialist, your ability to properly code the medical necessity for diagnostic tests and therapeutic procedures used in the care of individuals can open many job opportunities for you.

CODING BITES

Did you know that medical coders have foundational knowledge to become **Cancer Registrars**?

Run by the CDC, the National Program of Cancer Registries (NPCR) collates data amassed by local cancer registries. This important health information provides public health professionals with the ability to assess and make plans for ways to alleviate the cancer burden on patients, families, and the community more effectively.

According to the National Cancer Registrars Association (NCRA), *"cancer registrars capture a complete summary of the history, diagnosis, treatment, and disease status for every cancer patient. Registrars' work leads to better information that is used in the management of cancer, and ultimately, cures."*

Cancer registrars work in hospitals, state and regional cancer registries, federal government agencies, pharmaceutical companies, and other locations working with these data.

You Interpret It! Answers

1. (a) Screening, **2.** (b) Diagnostic, **3.** (b) Diagnostic, **4.** (a) Screening, **5.** Malignant, secondary, **6.** Malignant, primary, **7.** Malignant, primary, **8.** Malignant, secondary, **9.** Benign

CHAPTER 7 REVIEW
Coding Neoplasms

Mc Graw Hill connect

Enhance your learning by completing these exercises and more at mcgrawhillconnect.com!

Let's Check It! Terminology

Match each key term to the appropriate definition.

1. **LO 7.2** Invasive and destructive characteristic of a neoplasm; possibly causing damage or death.
2. **LO 7.4** Glandular secretion in abnormal quantity.
3. **LO 7.2** Nonmalignant characteristic of a neoplasm; not infectious or spreading.
4. **LO 7.2** A malignant neoplasm or cancerous tumor.
5. **LO 7.2** Abnormal tissue growth; tumor.
6. **LO 7.2** To proliferate, reproduce, or spread.
7. **LO 7.4** Out of place, such as an organ or body part.
8. **LO 7.4** The classification of neoplasms primarily by anatomical site.
9. **LO 7.4** Multiple sites of carcinoma without identifiable borders.
10. **LO 7.2** Abnormal collection of tissue.
11. **LO 7.4** The study of the configuration or structure of living organisms.

A. Benign
B. Carcinoma
C. Ectopic
D. Functional Activity
E. Malignant
F. Mass
G. Metastasize
H. Morphology
I. Neoplasm
J. Overlapping Boundaries
K. Topography

Let's Check It! Concepts

Choose the most appropriate answer for each of the following questions.

1. **LO 7.2** A neoplasm is the same as a
   a. tumor. **b.** cancer. **c.** malignancy. **d.** metastasis.
2. **LO 7.2** Different types of neoplasms include all of the following *except*
   a. adenoma. **b.** melanoma. **c.** papilloma. **d.** chemotherapy.
3. **LO 7.2** The term _____ indicates that the tumor has undergone malignant changes but is still limited to the site where it originated.
   a. uncertain **b.** Ca in situ **c.** benign **d.** secondary
4. **LO 7.4** Morphology codes are used
   a. for reimbursement.
   b. to describe treatment.
   c. to describe the topography and histology of the neoplasm.
   d. for identification of manifestations.
5. **LO 7.5** At subsequent encounters after the surgical removal of a neoplasm and no additional treatment, the diagnosis code changes to a
   a. personal history of malignancy code. **b.** malignancy code.
   c. late effects code. **d.** co-morbidity code.
6. **LO 7.5** When a patient is admitted for chemotherapy to treat a malignant neoplasm and that is the extent of treatment, the first code listed is the code for
   a. the primary malignancy. **b.** the secondary malignancy.
   c. the chemotherapy. **d.** observation in a hospital.

7. **LO 7.5** When a patient is admitted for treatment for a complication, such as anemia or dehydration, as the result of a neoplastic treatment, the code for this complication should be listed
   - **a.** after the primary malignancy.
   - **b.** first.
   - **c.** after the chemotherapy or radiation code.
   - **d.** as a Z code.
8. **LO 7.3** The correct code for a solitary plasmacytoma in remission is
   - **a.** C90.3
   - **b.** C90.30
   - **c.** C90.31
   - **d.** C90.32
9. **LO 7.1** All of the following are common diagnostic tests for a suspected malignancy of the lung *except*
   - **a.** alpha-1 antitrypsin.
   - **b.** CA-125.
   - **c.** bronchoscopy.
   - **d.** bone scan.
10. **LO 7.2** When coding a neoplasm, you must know
    - **a.** the anatomical site.
    - **b.** whether it is primary or secondary.
    - **c.** whether it is benign or malignant.
    - **d.** all of these.

Let's Check It! Guidelines

Refer to the Official Guidelines and fill in the blanks according to ***Chapter 2****, Neoplasms, Chapter-Specific Coding Guidelines.*

benign	Z85	anemia	primary
Z51.11	principal	extent	Z51.12
first-listed	malignancy	properly	M84.5
pathological	metastasis	dehydration	first
excised	principal/first-listed	Z51.0	

1. To ______ code a neoplasm it is necessary to determine from the record if the neoplasm is ______, in-situ, malignant, or of uncertain histologic behavior.
2. If the treatment is directed at the malignancy, designate the malignancy as the ______ diagnosis.
3. When a patient is admitted because of a ______ neoplasm with ______ and treatment is directed toward the secondary site only, the secondary neoplasm is designated as the principal diagnosis even though the primary malignancy is still present.
4. When admission/encounter is for management of an ______ associated with the malignancy, and the treatment is only for anemia, the appropriate code for the malignancy is sequenced as the principal or ______ diagnosis followed by the appropriate code for the anemia.
5. When the admission/encounter is for management of ______ due to the malignancy and only the dehydration is being treated (intravenous rehydration), the dehydration is sequenced first, followed by the code(s) for the ______.
6. When a primary malignancy has been previously ______ or eradicated from its site and there is no further treatment directed to that site and there is no evidence of any existing primary malignancy, a code from category ______, Personal history of malignant neoplasm, should be used to indicate the former site of the malignancy.
7. If a patient admission/encounter is chiefly for the administration of chemotherapy, immunotherapy or external beam radiation therapy for the treatment of a neoplasm, assign code ______, Encounter for antineoplastic radiation therapy, or ______, Encounter for antineoplastic chemotherapy, or ______, Encounter for antineoplastic immunotherapy as the first-listed or principal diagnosis.
8. When the reason for admission/encounter is to determine the ______ of the malignancy or for a procedure such as paracentesis or thoracentesis, the primary malignancy or appropriate metastatic site is designated as the principal or first-listed diagnosis, even though chemotherapy or radiotherapy is administered.
9. If the reason for the encounter is for treatment of a primary malignancy, assign the malignancy as the ______ diagnosis.
10. When an encounter is for a ______ fracture due to a neoplasm, and the focus of treatment is the fracture, a code from subcategory ______, Pathological fracture in neoplastic disease, should be sequenced ______, followed by the code for the neoplasm.

Let's Check It! Rules and Regulations

Please answer the following questions from the knowledge you have gained after reading this chapter.

1. **LO 7.2** Explain the difference between benign and malignant.
2. **LO 7.2** What is the difference between primary, secondary, Ca in situ, uncertain, and unspecified behavior?
3. **LO 7.4** Explain what overlapping boundaries are, and give another term for overlapping boundaries.
4. **LO 7.4** What is morphology, and why is it important?
5. **LO 7.5** Discuss prophylactic organ removal, its advantage, and how this should be coded.

YOU CODE IT! Basics

First, identify the main term in the following diagnoses; then code the diagnosis.

Example: Malignant primary neoplasm of lung, right upper lobe:

a. main term: ___*neoplasm*___ **b.** diagnosis _*C34.11*____

1. Acute megakaryocytic leukemia in relapse:
   a. main term: _______ **b.** diagnosis: _______
2. Benign neoplasm of uterine ligament, broad:
   a. main term: _______ **b.** diagnosis: _______
3. Papillary adenocarcinoma, intraductal, left breast:
   a. main term: _______ **b.** diagnosis: _______
4. Malignant carcinoid tumor of the colon:
   a. main term: _______ **b.** diagnosis: _______
5. Hemangioma of intra-abdominal structures:
   a. main term: _______ **b.** diagnosis: _______
6. Adenoma of the liver cell:
   a. main term: _______ **b.** diagnosis: _______
7. Follicular grade III lymphoma, lymph nodes of inguinal region and lower limbs:
   a. main term: _______ **b.** diagnosis: _______
8. Acral lentiginous, right heel melanoma:
   a. main term: _______ **b.** diagnosis: _______
9. Lipoma of the kidney:
   a. main term: _______ **b.** diagnosis: _______
10. Primary malignant neoplasm of right male breast, upper-outer quadrant:
    a. main term: _______ **b.** diagnosis: _______
11. Malignant odontogenic tumor, upper jaw bone:
    a. main term: _______ **b.** diagnosis: _______
12. Secondary malignant neoplasm of vallecula:
    a. main term: _______ **b.** diagnosis: _______
13. Carcinoma in situ neoplasm of left eyeball:
    a. main term: _______ **b.** diagnosis: _______
14. Benign neoplasm of cerebrum peduncle:
    a. main term: _______ **b.** diagnosis: _______
15. Myelofibrosis with myeloid metaplasia:
    a. main term: _______ **b.** diagnosis: _______

YOU CODE IT! Practice

Using the techniques described in this chapter, carefully read through the case studies and determine the most accurate ICD-10-CM code(s) and external cause code(s), if appropriate, for each case study.

1. George Donmoyer, a 58-year-old male, presents today with a sore throat, persistent cough, and earache. Dr. Selph completes an examination and appropriate tests. The blood-clotting parameters, the thyroid function studies, as well as the tissue biopsy confirm a diagnosis of malignant neoplasm of the extrinsic larynx.
2. Monica Pressley, a 37-year-old female, comes to see Dr. Wheaten today because she has been having diarrhea and abdominal cramping and states her heart feels like it's quivering. The MRI scan confirms a diagnosis of benign pancreatic islet cell adenoma.

(continued)

3. Suber Wilson, a 57-year-old male, was diagnosed with a malignant neoplasm of the liver metastasized from the prostate; both sites are being addressed in today's encounter.
4. William Amerson, a 41-year-old male, comes in for his annual eye examination. Dr. Leviner notes a benign right conjunctiva nevus.
5. Edward Bakersfield, a 43-year-old male, presents with shortness of breath, chest pain, and coughing up blood. After a thorough examination, Dr. Benson notes stridor and orders an MRI scan. The results of the MRI confirmed the diagnosis of bronchial adenoma.
6. Elizabeth Conyers, a 56-year-old female, presents with unexplained weakness, weight loss, and dizziness. Dr. Amos completes a thorough examination and does a workup. The protein electrophoresis (SPEP) and quantitative immunoglobulin results confirm the diagnosis of Waldenström's macroglobulinemia.
7. James Buckholtz, a 3-year-old male, is brought in by his parents. Jimmy has lost his appetite and is losing weight. Mrs. Buckholtz tells Dr. Ferguson that Jimmy's gums bleed and he seems short of breath. Dr. Ferguson notes splenomegaly and admits Jimmy to Weston Hospital. After reviewing the blood tests, MRI scan, and bone marrow aspiration results, Jimmy is diagnosed with acute lymphoblastic leukemia.
8. Kelley Young, a 39-year-old female, presents to Dr. Clerk with the complaints of sudden blurred vision, dizziness, and numbness in her face. Kelley states she feels very weak and has headaches. Dr. Clerk admits Kelley to the hospital. After reviewing the MRI scan, her hormone levels from the blood workup, and urine tests, Kelley is diagnosed with a primary malignant neoplasm of the pituitary gland.
9. Ralph Bradley, a 36-year-old male, comes to see Dr. Harper because he is weak, losing weight, and vomiting and has diarrhea with some blood showing. Ralph was diagnosed with HIV 3 years ago. Dr. Harper completes an examination noting paleness, tachycardia, and tachypnea. Ralph is admitted to the hospital. The biopsied tissue from an endoscopy confirms a diagnosis of Kaposi's sarcoma of gastrointestinal organ.
10. Ben Jameson, a 31-year-old male, was admitted today for the prophylactic removal of his prostate. Both Ben's father and brother have prostate cancer that has spread to the lungs and liver. Ben decides to have a laparoscopic radical prostatectomy while he is still healthy.
11. Phillip DeLorne, a 21-year-old male, presents with a sore on his left ear of approximately 5 weeks duration. Philip says it just won't get well. Dr. Duruy notes a pink lump on Philip's pinna and a biopsy is taken, which confirms a diagnosis of melanoma in situ of the left external ear.
12. Mitchell Lane, a 48-year-old male, presents with the complaints of night sweats and weight loss. Dr. Clark completes an examination noting hemoptysis and takes a chest x-ray, which reveals a mass. Mitchell is admitted to Weston Hospital where a CT-guided needle biopsy is then performed. Mitchell is diagnosed with a malignant primary neoplasm of the posterior mediastinum.
13. Raykeem McFadden, a 63-year-old female, was last seen in this office 6 months ago for her annual checkup; no concerns were noted at that time. She presents today because of excessive itching after a warm bath. She also complains of a burning sensation in her arms, especially her left arm. Dr. Dingle completes a physical exam and notes aphasia, hepatosplenomegaly, and some loss of physical coordination. Raykeem is admitted to the hospital. The laboratory tests and bone marrow aspiration confirm a diagnosis of polycythemia vera.
14. Terry Shelton, a 33-year-old female, had chemotherapy 3 days ago for gallbladder cancer. She presents today to see Dr. China due to extreme weakness and chest pain. Dr. China notes an irregular heartbeat and a CBC reveals a hemoglobin of 8.3 g/dL. Terry is diagnosed with anemia due to antineoplastic chemotherapy and admitted to Weston Hospital for treatment of her anemia.
15. Kewane Childs, a 44-year-old female, has a history of smoking cigarettes for 15 years; she quit last year. Kewane sees Dr. Cope for a dry cough, hoarse voice, and coughing up blood. Dr. Cope notes crepitation and dyspnea. Kewane is admitted to the hospital. The MRI scan and lung function tests confirm a diagnosis of neoplasm of the trachea, malignant primary.

YOU CODE IT! Application

The following exercises provide practice in abstracting physicians' documentation from our health care facility, Prader, Bracker, & Associates. These case studies are modeled on real patient encounters. Using the techniques described in this chapter, carefully read through the case studies and determine the most accurate ICD-10-CM code(s) and external cause code(s), if appropriate, for each case study.

(continued)

WESTON HOSPITAL

629 Healthcare Way • SOMEWHERE, FL 32811 • 407-555-6541

PATIENT: KAHN, SERENA

ACCOUNT/EHR #: KAHNSE001

Attending Physician: Oscar R. Prader, MD

HPI: This patient is being admitted to Weston Hospital for wide excision of a level 2 melanoma, right side of the face. She was referred from Dr. Robinson. Patient states she has had the lesion forever. Dr. Robinson found it disturbing and decided to take a biopsy; results, melanoma, level 2.

This lesion is located just anterior to the ear on the right zygomatic region; we should get a reasonably good margin.

PAST MEDICAL HISTORY: Hypothyroidism and takes thyroid replacement medication.

PAST SURGICAL HISTORY: The patient had carcinoma of the breast and underwent a left mastectomy in 2012. She had a hysterectomy for benign ovarian tumors in 2015.

ALLERGIES: NKA

SOCIAL HISTORY: Nonsmoker. Drinks alcohol socially.

FAMILY HISTORY: The patient's sister is diabetic.

ROS: Negative.

PHYSICAL EXAMINATION: Ht: 5′6″, Wt: 142, T: 98.6, R: 18, BP 170/70. HEENT: Head is atraumatic, normocephalic; there is a pigmented lesion just anterior to the right ear over the zygomatic region, which is slightly irregular in shape and different shades of brown. Biopsied site is noted and healing within normal limits.

NECK: Negative.

CHEST: Clear and symmetrical

HEART: Regular rhythm, no murmurs

ABDOMEN: Soft, nontender, no masses or organomegaly

EXTREMITIES: No cyanosis, clubbing, or edema

NEUROLOGIC: Grossly intact

IMPRESSION: Melanoma of the right cheek, level 2

PLAN: Wide excision with flap advancement closure

Determine the most accurate ICD-10-CM codes.

WESTON HOSPITAL

629 Healthcare Way • SOMEWHERE, FL 32811 • 407-555-6541

PATIENT: DAWSON, WILSON

ACCOUNT/EHR #: DAWSWI001

Attending Physician: Renee O. Bracker, MD

Pt is a 47-year-old male with left breast carcinoma, terminal stage, metastatic to the brain and liver. Wilson is undergoing chemotherapy and has become dehydrated, showing signs of confusion and disorientation. He is admitted to Weston Hospital for rehydration. Procalamine 3%, IV, 50 mL/hr was given for 12 hours. Patient stabilized and was discharged home with no other treatment.

Determine the most accurate ICD-10-CM codes.

(continued)

WESTON HOSPITAL

629 Healthcare Way • SOMEWHERE, FL 32811 • 407-555-6541

PATIENT: OAKWOOD, QUENTIN

ACCOUNT/EHR #: OAKWQU001

Attending Physician: Oscar R. Prader, MD

Pt is a 63-year-old male who was diagnosed with prostate cancer 3 years ago. 18 months ago he had a radical prostatectomy. 1 year ago he was diagnosed with bone and liver metastasis. Patient has a high level of pain associated with his liver cancer and is being admitted for an insertion of a tunneled centrally inserted port-a-cath VAD (venous access device) with a sub q port for delivery of pain control medication.

Determine the most accurate ICD-10-CM codes.

PRADER, BRACKER, & ASSOCIATES

A Complete Health Care Facility

159 Healthcare Way • SOMEWHERE, FL 32811 • 407-555-6789

PATIENT: CHARLES, KAREN

ACCOUNT/EHR #: CHARKA001

Attending Physician: Renee O. Bracker, MD

Patient, a 43-year-old female, presents today to discuss pathological findings of recent exploratory laparotomy. Patient is 4 days' status post lysis of adhesions; total abdominal hysterectomy; bilateral salpingo-oophorectomy; partial omentectomy; excision of small and large bowel implants; pelvic-abdominal peritoneal stripping; placement of intraperitoneal port-a-cath; and enterolyses.

The ovaries were found to be poorly differentiated; serous carcinoma extended to the left fallopian tube. The right fallopian tube was found to have serosal fibrosis consistent with tubo-ovarian adhesion. A broad-based endometrial polyp was found in the endometrium while the myometrium showed leiomyomata, adenomyosis, and multifocal serosal implants of poorly differentiated ovarian serous carcinoma.

The specimen from the omentum was found to be metastatic adenocarcinoma consistent with ovarian origin.

Lastly, the specimens from both the small and large bowel were positive for metastatic, poorly differentiated ovarian serous carcinoma.

The histomorphologic features of poorly differentiated ovarian serous carcinoma closely resemble that of a poorly differentiated fallopian tube primary adenocarcinoma. The bilateral ovarian involvement supports the primary ovarian origin of the neoplasm.

ASSESSMENT: Metastatic adenocarcinoma of the omentum; metastatic carcinoma of the small and large intestines.

Determine the most accurate ICD-10-CM codes.

WESTON HOSPITAL

629 Healthcare Way • SOMEWHERE, FL 32811 • 407-555-6541

PATIENT: BENTONN, VERNON

ACCOUNT/EHR #: BENTVE001

Attending Physician: Oscar R. Prader, MD

(continued)

PREOP DIAGNOSIS: Lower extremity ischemia with rest pain and gangrene of the right third toe, probable atheroembolic disease to the right lower extremity.

POSTOP DIAGNOSIS: Atheroembolic disease to the right lower extremity.

PROCEDURE: Right, axillary femoral-femoral bypass utilizing an 8.0-mm ringed Gore-Tex axillary-to-femoral graft and a 6.0-mm ringed Gore-Tex femoral cross-over graft, right third toe amputation.

OPERATIVE INDICATIONS: This is a 69-year-old male, presenting with local rectal carcinoma, recurrent, with miliary metastases to the liver.

PATHOLOGICAL FINDINGS: Specimen: Third right toe consistent with ischemic necrosis.

PLAN/RECOMMENDATIONS: At this time, given known early liver metastases and extensive local regional recurrence in the pelvis, I do not feel that further antineoplastic therapy will be of great benefit.

Specifically, patient has had chemotherapy up until September of this year and this disease has recurred. In addition, he has a history of full radiotherapy to the pelvis.

Secondly, evidence-based medicine for recurrent colorectal cancer has shown that secondline chemotherapy has been of little to no value.

Pain management: I would recommend continuing his Duragesic patch, advise the addition of a low dose of Elavil to help reduce neurogenic pain. Efforts will be made to improve mobility.

Determine the most accurate ICD-10-CM codes.

8

Coding Conditions of the Blood and Immunological Systems

Key Terms

Agglutination
Antibodies
Antigen
Blood
Blood Type
Coagulation
Hematopoiesis
Hemoglobin (hgb or Hgb)
Hemolysis
Hemostasis
Plasma
Platelets (PLTs)
Red Blood Cells (RBCs)
Rh (Rhesus) Factor
Transfusion
White Blood Cells (WBCs)

Learning Outcomes

After completing this chapter, the student should be able to:

LO 8.1 Differentiate between various blood conditions and how this affects the determination of the code.
LO 8.2 Determine the codes to report coagulation defects and hemorrhagic conditions accurately.
LO 8.3 Identify the different types of blood and the importance of Rh factoring involved in malfunction.
LO 8.4 Interpret the details of white blood cell disorders and diseases of the spleen.
LO 8.5 Evaluate the factors involved in immunodeficiency disorders.

STOP! Remember, you need to follow along in your ICD-10-CM code book for an optimal learning experience.

8.1 Reporting Blood Conditions

As with any other part of the body, malfunction of the blood-forming organs, the blood itself, or one of its components can result in problems affecting the entire body.

Blood is actually a type of connective tissue consisting of **red blood cells** (RBCs), **white blood cells** (WBCs), and **platelets** (PLTs)—all contained within liquid **plasma**. It is the transportation system used to deliver oxygen (nourishment) for cells throughout the body and to carry carbon dioxide (cell waste products) so it can be expelled from the body. The average adult has between 5 and 6 liters of blood constantly circulating throughout.

Blood
Fluid pumped throughout the body, carrying oxygen and nutrients to the cells and wastes away from the cells.

Red Blood Cells (RBCs)
Cells within the blood that contain hemoglobin responsible for carrying oxygen to tissues; also known as *erythrocytes.*

White Blood Cells (WBCs)
Cells within the blood that help to protect the body from pathogens; also known as *leukocytes.*

Platelets (PLTs)
Large cell fragments in the bone marrow that function in clotting; also known as *thrombocytes.*

Plasma
The fluid part of the blood.

Hematopoiesis
The formation of blood cells.

The Formation of Blood

Blood is created in the red bone marrow (see **Figure 8-1**) during a series of steps called **hematopoiesis**. During gestation, blood cells originate in the yolk sac from the mesenchyme (the section of the embryo in which blood, lymphatic vessels, bones, cartilage, and connective tissues form). As the fetus continues to develop, the liver, spleen, and thymus begin to produce blood cells. Then, at about the 20th week of gestation, the red bone marrow also begins to contribute to production. Once the baby is born, blood cell formation becomes the responsibility of the red bone marrow only, specifically in the sternum, ribs, and vertebrae. Red bone marrow produces red blood cells (erythrocytes) through a process called *erythropoiesis* and white blood cells (leukocytes) through a process called *leukopoiesis*.

How many blood cells does a healthy body need? Normal counts (per microliter of blood) are

- *Red blood cell count:* 4 to 6 million cells.
- *White blood cell count:* 4,000 to 11,000 cells.
- *Platelet count:* 150,000 to 400,000 platelets.

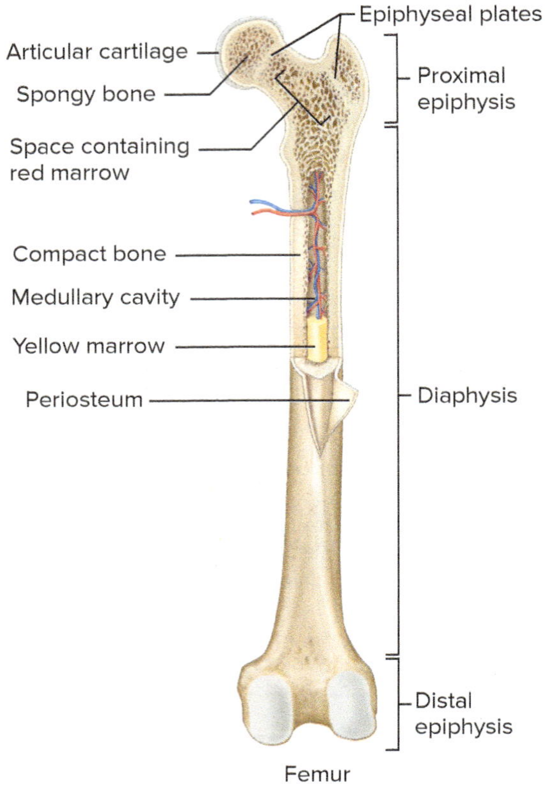

FIGURE 8-1 Bone marrow

> **CODING BITES**
>
> While professional coding specialists are not permitted to diagnose a patient, understanding these details from a pathology or lab report can support your understanding of the documentation or explain medical necessity–or it may alert you, as the coder, to query the physician about missing or ambiguous notes.

Too many cells or too few cells may indicate a problem. This is why one of the first diagnostic tests run when a physician is trying to figure out what is wrong with the patient is a complete blood count (CBC).

Blood Roles

Blood's primary job is transporting oxygen from the lungs and delivering it to tissue cells throughout the body. As the oxygen passes from the lungs to the blood, it binds to the RBCs and the **hemoglobin (hgb or Hgb)** inside those RBCs (see **Figure 8-2**), so it can travel through the heart and out through the body via the arteries. After delivering the oxygen (O_2) to the cells, the blood picks up carbon dioxide (CO_2) and carries it back to the lungs for expulsion from the body.

> **Hemoglobin (hgb or Hgb)**
> The part of the red blood cell that carries oxygen.

Anemias

While many believe anemia is the result of an iron deficiency, this is only one cause of an abnormally low count of hemoglobin, hematocrit, and/or RBCs. The low volume of RBCs reduces the amount of oxygen being transported, causing tissue hypoxia (low levels of oxygen). Blood loss, lack of red blood cell production, and high rates of red blood cell destruction are the three most common causes of anemia. Classic signs and symptoms include tachycardia, dyspnea, and sometimes fatigue.

Nutritional anemia, reported with a code from the D50-D53 range, is caused by an insufficient intake or absorption into the body of certain key nutrients. For example, pernicious anemia is a genetic condition that causes dysfunction of the ileum so it cannot properly absorb vitamin B_{12}; iron deficiency anemia may be caused by a diet lacking iron-rich foods.

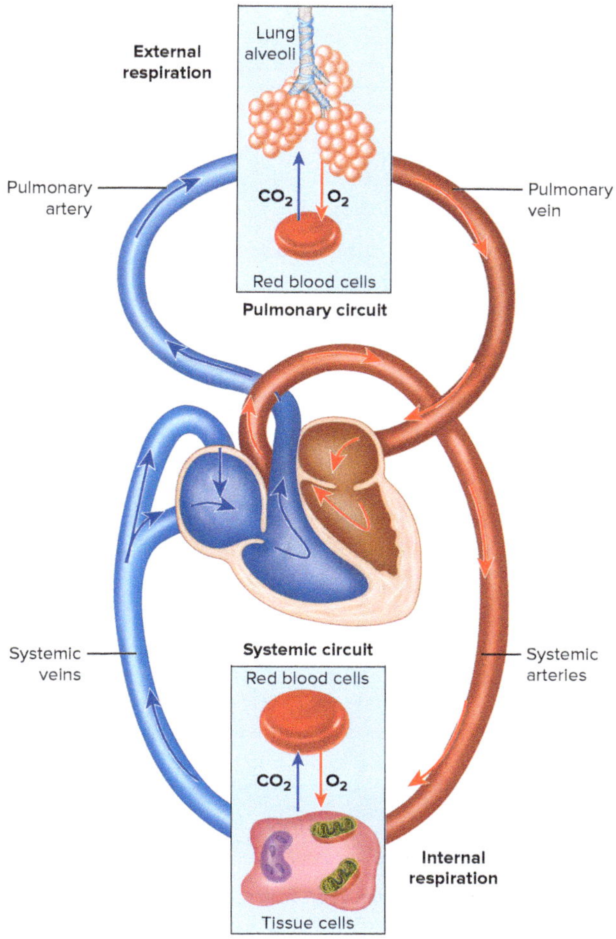

FIGURE 8-2 Oxygen and carbon dioxide exchanging in blood

EXAMPLES

D50.0	Iron deficiency anemia secondary to blood loss (chronic)
D51.0	Vitamin B_{12} deficiency anemia due to intrinsic factor deficiency (pernicious (congenital) anemia)
D52.0	Dietary folate deficiency anemia
D53.2	Scorbutic anemia

Specific details about the underlying cause of the anemia are required to report an accurate code.

Hemolytic anemia (codes D55-D59) results from an insufficient number of healthy RBCs due to abnormal or premature destruction, thereby retarding the delivery of oxygen to the tissues throughout the body. This premature destruction of the RBCs may be caused by a genetic defect, an infection, or exposure to certain toxins. Hemolytic anemia also can be caused by a mismatched blood transfusion.

EXAMPLES

D55.1	Anemia due to other disorders of glutathione metabolism
D56.4	Hereditary persistence of fetal hemoglobin

Sickle-cell disorders are included in this subsection. See upcoming section for more on these diagnoses.

Aplastic anemia (code category D61) is the inability of the bone marrow to manufacture enough new blood cells required by the body for proper function.

EXAMPLES

D61.01 Constitutional (pure) red blood cell aplasia

D61.2 Aplastic anemia due to other external agents ***Code first*****, if applicable, toxic effects of substances chiefly nonmedicinal as to source (T51–T65)**

Sickle-cell disorders are included in this subsection. See upcoming section for more on these diagnoses.

Hemorrhagic anemia, also called *blood loss anemia* or *posthemorrhagic anemia* (code D62 Acute posthemorrhagic anemia), can occur after the patient has lost a great deal of blood. This can be after a traumatic injury or internal bleeding, such as an untreated gastric ulcer.

LET'S CODE IT! SCENARIO

Carter McMannus, an 18-month-old male, was brought by his mother to Dr. Hampshire, a pediatrician specializing in hematologic (blood) disorders. Dr. Hampshire noted jaundice, an enlarged spleen on palpation, and other signs of failure to thrive. Dr. Hampshire recognized these signs and symptoms and confirmed with blood tests a diagnosis of Cooley's anemia.

Let's Code It!

Dr. Hampshire diagnosed Carter with *Cooley's anemia.* Turn to the Alphabetic Index and find

Anemia

Are you surprised by the long-indented list of different types of anemia? Read down the list and find

Anemia

Cooley's (erythroblastic) D56.1

Now let's go to the Tabular List to confirm this code. Remember, always begin reading at the three-character category.

✓4 **D56 Thalassemia**

Thalassemia is an inherited group of hemolytic anemias (*hemo* = blood + *-lytic* = involving lysis, the decomposition of a cell). Cooley's anemia, also known as *thalassemia major*, is one type of beta thalassemia, the most common form of this condition.

Read down the fourth-character choices and find

D56.1 Beta thalassemia (Cooley's anemia)

Check the top of this subsection and the head of this chapter in ICD-10-CM. There is an **EXCLUDES2** notation at the beginning of this chapter. Read carefully. Does this relate to Dr. Hampshire's diagnosis of Carter? No. Turn to the Official Guidelines and read Section I.C.3. Interesting, there are no guidelines for this chapter.

Now you can report D56.1 for Carter's diagnosis with confidence.

Good job!

Sickle Cell Disease and Sickle Cell Trait

Sickle cell disease (SCD) is not actually one diagnosis, but represents several genetically passed disorders of the RBCs. Normal RBCs are round, whereas an individual with SCD develops RBCs that are a C-shape and are unusually firm and sticky. The shape of these abnormal cells resembles a tool known as a sickle, leading to the name for this condition. In addition to the shape and nature of these cells, they have a shorter life span, resulting in a continuing shortage of RBCs. The sticky texture of these cells also increases the opportunity for the cells to stick to the walls of the blood vessels, manifesting obstructions and an ineffective delivery of oxygen via the hemoglobin.

SCD can be diagnosed in utero or in newborn blood screenings. The earlier the diagnosis, the sooner treatments can be implemented.

> **CODING BITES**
>
> Be certain to read the notation at the code category of ✓4 **D57 Sickle-cell disorders,** which directs you to
>
> *Use additional code* **for any associated fever (R50.81)**

As a professional coder, you will need to know more than a diagnosis of SCD; you will need to know specifics about the condition, as well as any manifestations.

Hb-SS

D57.00 Hb-SS disease with crisis, unspecified

D57.01 Hb-SS disease with acute chest syndrome

D57.02 Hb-SS disease with splenic sequestration

D57.03 Hb-SS disease with cerebral vascular involvement

D57.09 Hb-SS disease with crisis with other specified complications

Hb-SS disease is a condition in which the patient has inherited two sickle cell genes ("S"), one from each parent. Commonly referred to as *sickle cell anemia*, this is typically the most acute form of this condition.

Hb-C, Hb-S, or Hb-SC

D57.20 Sickle-cell/Hb-C disease without crisis

D57.211 Sickle-cell/Hb-C disease with acute chest syndrome

D57.212 Sickle-cell/Hb-C disease with splenic sequestration

D57.219 Sickle-cell/Hb-C disease with crisis, unspecified

D57.213 Sickle-cell/Hb-C disease with cerebral vascular involvement

D57.218 Sickle-cell/Hb-C disease with crisis with other specified complications

Sometimes known as Hb-SC or Hb-S disease, this patient has inherited a sickle cell gene ("S") from one parent and a gene for abnormal hemoglobin called "C" from the other parent.

Hb-S Beta Thalassemia

D57.40 Sickle-cell thalassemia without crisis

D57.411 Sickle-cell thalassemia, unspecified, with acute chest syndrome

D57.412 Sickle-cell thalassemia, unspecified, with splenic sequestration

D57.413 Sickle-cell thalassemia, unspecified, with cerebral vascular involvement

D57.418 Sickle-cell thalassemia, unspecified, with crisis with other specified complications

D57.419 Sickle-cell thalassemia, unspecified, with crisis, unspecified

This form of SCD manifests when the patient inherits one sickle cell gene ("S") from one parent and the gene for beta thalassemia from the other parent.

The sub-category D57.4- has codes to enable reporting: D57.42 Sickle-cell thalassemia beta zero without crisis, D57.43- Sickle-cell thalassemia beta zero with crisis [additional character required], D57.44 Sickle-cell thalassemia beta plus without crisis, D57.45- Sickle-cell thalassemia beta plus with crisis [additional character required].

Hb-SD and Hb-SE

D57.80	**Other sickle-cell disorders without crisis**
D57.811	**Other sickle-cell disorders with acute chest syndrome**
D57.812	**Other sickle-cell disorders with splenic sequestration**
D57.813	**Other sickle-cell disorders with cerebral vascular involvement**
D57.818	**Other sickle-cell disorders with other specified complications**
D57.819	**Other sickle-cell disorders with crisis, unspecified**

When a patient inherits one sickle cell gene ("S") and one gene with an abnormal type of hemoglobin ("D," "E," or "O"), it would be documented as Hb-SD, Hb-SE, or Hb-S.

Sickle Cell Trait

D57.3 **Sickle-cell trait**

Sickle cell trait (SCT) develops when the patient has inherited one sickle cell gene ("S") from one parent and a normal gene ("A") from the other parent. Individuals diagnosed with SCT do not typically exhibit any signs or symptoms of the disease. When this patient considers having children, this should be noted because this can be passed along to future children.

CODING BITE

New for the 2024 code set, ICD-10-CM has added codes related to Hb-SS and Sickle cell to specifically report the additional condition of dactylitis:

D57.04	**Hb-SS disease with dactylitis**
D57.214	**Sickle-cell/Hb-C disease with dactylitis**
D57.414	**Sickle-cell thalassemia, unspecified, with dactylitis**
D57.434	**Sickle-cell thalassemia beta zero with dactylitis**
D57.454	**Sickle-cell thalassemia beta plus with dactylitis**
D57.814	**Other sickle-cell disorders with dactylitis**

Hematologic Malignancies

Both lymphomas and leukemias are included in this category. Leukemia is the presence of malignant cells within the bone marrow that produces blood cells (hematopoietic tissues), causing a reduction in the production of RBCs, WBCs, and PLTs. This anemic state makes the patient very susceptible to infections and hemorrhaging.

There are several types of leukemia reported from several ICD-10-CM code categories:

code category C92	**Myeloid leukemia**
code category C93	**Monocytic leukemia**
code category C94	**Other leukemia of specified cell type**
code category C95	**Leukemia of unspecified cell type**

The aspiration of bone marrow (known as a bone marrow biopsy) is typically taken from the posterior superior iliac spine. This specimen is tested to quantify the WBCs. When a rapid reproduction of immature WBCs is evidenced, this confirms a diagnosis of acute leukemia. In addition, the results of a differential leukocyte count can specifically identify the type of cell, and a lumbar puncture (aka spinal tap) can reveal whether or not there is involvement of the meninges.

8.2 Coagulation Defects and Other Hemorrhagic Conditions

In addition to transporting oxygen, blood also controls **hemostasis** (stopping the bleeding process) via **coagulation** (clotting).

> **Hemostasis**
> The interruption of bleeding.

> **Coagulation**
> Clotting; the change from a liquid into a thickened substance.

Essentially, there are two types of clotting disorders: hemostatic and thrombotic. A *hemostatic disorder* is a failure in the system to repair a damaged blood vessel. Because there is no clot to stop it, the vessel continues to bleed. These coagulation deficiencies–where clotting does not occur as it should (see **Figure 8-3**)–may be seen with bleeding into the muscles, joints, and viscera or with the appearance of purpura (dysfunction of blood vessels). Hemophilia is a common hemostatic condition, reported with code D66 Hereditary factor VIII deficiency (Classical hemophilia).

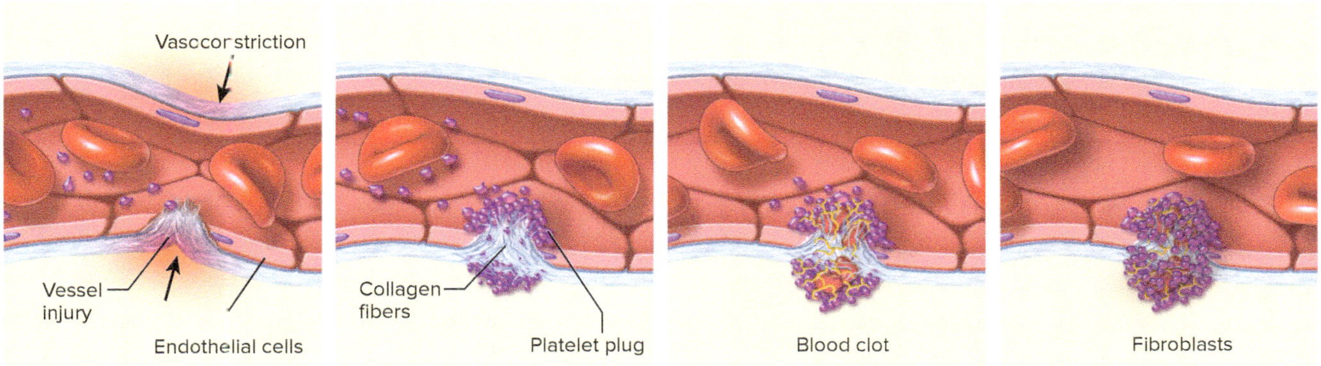

(a) Blood vessel spasm **(b)** Platelet plug formation **(c)** Blood clotting **(d)** Fibrinolysis

FIGURE 8-3 The four main events in hemostasis

Thrombotic disorders are the opposite: The blood clots without purpose, forming thrombi (blood clots) within the vessels, causing a blockage. Beyond the dangers from the thrombi themselves, should a clot dislodge (embolus) and travel through the blood vessels, it might get caught going through the lungs or heart, causing a blockage that could be deadly. Thrombophilia is an example of a thrombotic condition, reported with, for example, ICD-10-CM code D68.59 Other primary thrombophilia (Hypercoagulable state NOS).

Hemophilia

Hemophilia is a genetic mutation that establishes a deficiency lacking a protein (clotting factor) in the blood necessary in the clotting process. Therefore, the patient's blood will not clot when needed to prevent hemorrhaging. The lower the quantity of the clotting factor, the higher the probability that the patient might hemorrhage and have it become life-threatening.

The majority of patients diagnosed with hemophilia have a deficiency of either factor VIII or factor IX.

Types of Hemophilia

There are four types of hemophilia: A, B, C, and Acquired.

Hemophilia A (Classic Hemophilia) . . . deficiency of clotting factor VIII. This is reported with one of two codes:

D66 Hereditary factor VIII deficiency
(Hemophilia A)
(Deficiency factor VIII with functional defect)

D68.0 Von Willebrand's disease
(factor VIII deficiency with vascular defect)

Hemophilia B (Christmas Disease) . . . deficiency of clotting factor IX.

D67 Hereditary factor IX deficiency
(Hemophilia B)
(Deficiency factor IX with functional defect)
(Christmas disease)

Hemophilia C (Rosenthal's Disease) . . . deficiency of clotting factor XI.

D68.1 Hereditary factor XI deficiency
(Hemophilia C)
Plasma thromboplastin antecedent [PTA] deficiency
(Rosenthal's disease)

Acquired hemophilia (secondary hemophilia) . . . actually an autoimmune disease that occurs when antibodies are created that mistakenly attack healthy tissue, specifically clotting factor VIII. In these cases, the bleeding pattern is quite different from classical hemophilia. With acquired hemophilia, spontaneous hemorrhaging moves into the muscles, skin, soft tissue, and mucous membranes. Bleeding episodes are frequently acute and can become life-threatening.

D68.311 Acquired hemophilia
(Secondary hemophilia)

D68.4 Acquired coagulation factor deficiency
(Deficiency of coagulation factor due to liver disease)
(Deficiency of coagulation factor due to vitamin K deficiency)

LET'S CODE IT! SCENARIO

Dr. Victor ordered a coagulation profile, including a partial thromboplastin time (PTT) and prothrombin time (PT), to be done on Louis Langer prior to scheduling his surgery. The pathology report showed an abnormally prolonged PTT. The surgery will be delayed until Dr. Victor can confirm the cause.

Let's Code It!

The lab report identified an abnormal coagulation profile, and Dr. Victor did not provide any confirmed diagnosis. Therefore, this is all you know for a fact, and this is what must be reported. Turn to the Alphabetic Index and find

Abnormal

This is going to take some analysis. There is no listing under *Abnormal* for *Test* or *Coagulation.* Think about this. What is the body's reason for coagulation? To stop bleeding. Look for *Blood* or *Bleeding.* Did you find

Abnormal

Bleeding time R79.1

Now let's go into the Tabular List to check this out. Remember, always begin reading at the three-character category.

✓4 **R79 Other abnormal findings of blood chemistry**

Read down the fourth-character choices and find

R79.1 Abnormal coagulation profile (abnormal or prolonged partial thromboplastin time [PTT])

Read the **EXCLUDES1** and **EXCLUDES2** notations directly below this code.

Check the top of this subsection; there is an **EXCLUDES1** notation. Read it carefully to see if any of those conditions apply. At the head of this chapter in ICD-10-CM, you will find a long **NOTE** and an **EXCLUDES2** notation. Read carefully. Do any relate to Dr. Victor's diagnosis of Louis? Yes, so confirm that there is no more specific diagnosis that can be reported instead. There is not. Now, turn to the Official Guidelines and read Section I.C.18. There is nothing specifically applicable here either.

Now you can report R79.1 for Louis's diagnosis with confidence.

Good job!

Thrombocytopenia

This is a low platelet count most often due to increased platelet destruction, decreased platelet production, or malfunctioning PLTs. Underlying conditions might include splenomegaly (enlarged spleen); destruction of bone marrow by medication, chemotherapy, or radiation therapy; or aplastic anemia. The condition will be reported most often with a code from ICD-10-CM code category D69 Purpura and other hemorrhagic conditions, although not exclusively. For example, postpartum puerperal thrombocytopenia is reported with code O72.3 Postpartum coagulation defects and neonatal, transitory thrombocytopenia is reported with code P61.0 Transient neonatal thrombocytopenia.

ICD-10-CM

YOU CODE IT! CASE STUDY

Marissa Rubine, a 27-year-old female, came to see Dr. Post with complaints of bruising "suddenly appearing" on her arms and legs. She states she had two recent episodes of epistaxis but denies any other bleeding. She denied taking any drugs or smoking, and states she has no risk factors for HIV. Physical examination revealed the spleen was not palpable. Petechiae are noted scattered on her legs bilaterally.

Blood work results:

- *hemoglobin (138 g/L)—normal*
- *white cell count—normal*
- *platelet count of 10 × 10^9/L—low (normal >150 × 10^9/L)*
- *erythrocyte sedimentation rate was 6 mm/hr*
- *direct Coombs' test—negative*
- *antinuclear—absent*
- *DNA-binding antibodies—absent*
- *rheumatoid factor—absent*

Bone marrow aspiration: high number of normal megakaryocytes but otherwise normal

Dx: Immune thrombocytopenia purpura

She is placed on a short course of prednisolone.

You Code It!

Go through the steps of coding, and determine the code or codes that should be reported for this encounter between Dr. Post and Marissa.

Step #1: Read the case carefully and completely.
Step #2: Abstract the scenario. Which main words or terms describe why the physician cared for the patient during this encounter?
Step #3: Are there any details missing or incomplete for which you would need to query the physician? [If so, ask your instructor.]
Step #4: Check for any relevant guidance, including reading all of the symbols and notations in the Tabular List and the appropriate sections of the Official Guidelines.
Step #5: Determine the correct diagnosis code or codes to explain why this encounter was medically necessary.
Step #6: Double-check your work.

Answer:

Did you determine this to be the correct code?

D69.3 Immune thrombocytopenic purpura

Great work!

8.3 Conditions Related to Blood Types and the Rh Factor

Antigens on Red Blood Cells

> **Antigen**
> A substance that promotes the production of antibodies.

> **Antibodies**
> Immune responses to antigens.

Antigens sit on the surface of RBCs, while **antibodies** are located within the blood plasma. Antigens are proteins that cause antibodies to form, and each antibody can connect with only one specific type of antigen. Antigens that are located on RBCs are categorized in two ways: blood type and Rh factor.

> **Blood Type**
> A system of classifying blood based on the antigens present on the surface of the individual's red blood cells; also known as *blood group*.

Blood Type

You may know what **blood type** you have: type A, type B, type AB, or type O. This is something that is inherited from your parents.

- An individual with type A blood has only antigen A on their RBCs.
- An individual with type B blood has only antigen B on their RBCs.
- An individual with type AB blood has both antigens—A and B.
- An individual with type O blood has neither antigen—neither A nor B.

> **Rh (Rhesus) Factor**
> An antigen located on the red blood cell that produces immunogenic responses in those individuals without it.

Rh Factor

Another antigen that may or may not be present on the surface of a red blood cell is called **Rh (Rhesus) factor**. This is also an inherited situation.

- An individual identified as Rh-negative does *not* have the Rh antigen.
- An individual identified as Rh-positive *does* have the Rh antigen.

Because Rh factor is inherited, there is concern about additional complications if an Rh-negative woman becomes pregnant with a Rh-positive fetus (the father is Rh-positive). The good news is, often, the placenta will prevent the mother's blood from mixing with the baby's blood, keeping both mother and baby safe.

EXAMPLE

O36.012 Maternal care for anti-D (Rh) antibodies, second trimester

Z31.82 Encounter for Rh incompatibility status

When the mother is seen so Rh compatibility can be determined and, if necessary, dealt with, these codes are examples for reporting why the encounter was medically necessary.

When the mother is Rh-negative and her body makes antibodies to her fetus's Rh-positive blood cells, and the antibodies cross the placenta, it can result in Rh incompatibility, resulting in a large number of RBCs in the fetus's bloodstream that may be destroyed, known as hemolytic disease of the newborn.

EXAMPLES

P55.0 Rh isoimmunization of newborn [hemolytic disease (newborn)]

P55.1 ABO isoimmunization of newborn

A neonate affected by the Rh factor may be diagnosed with a hemolytic disease.

When proper precautions have not been taken while the baby is in utero, hydrops fetalis due to hemolytic disease, also known as immune hydrops fetalis, can develop. This is a known complication of Rh incompatibility and leads the neonate's entire body to swell, interfering with the proper function of body organs and systems.

P56.0 Hydrops fetalis due to isoimmunization

LET'S CODE IT! SCENARIO

Neonate Alvarez, male, was born vaginally yesterday, at 15:25 without incident. Apgar scores: 1 min.—10, 5 min.—10.

Four hours later, extensive purpura became visible on his abdomen, arms, and legs. No jaundice was observed. His 29-year-old mother was given a blood transfusion for a postpartum hemorrhage after her first pregnancy 3 years earlier. The mother's serum was found to contain IgG antibodies to the father's platelets and to some of a panel of platelets from normal, unrelated donors. These antibodies were typed as specific anti-HPA-1A antibodies and had been incited by the previous pregnancy and transfusion.

These antibodies crossed the placenta, manifesting as alloimmune thrombocytopenia in this neonate. Additionally, the neonate was found to have red cell incompatibility.

An exchange transfusion was performed to compensate for hemolysis. While it is unusual for an ABO incompatibility to require an exchange transfusion, it worked. The neonate's platelet count returned to normal quickly due to free reactant antibody to platelets having been removed by the exchange.

We kept the neonate for observation for another 48 hours and then discharged him to his mother. She was told to follow up in 1 week at the office or phone PRN.

Let's Code It!

The baby was born and diagnosed with *alloimmune thrombocytopenia*. In the Alphabetic Index, let's find our key term:

Thrombocytopenia

As you read down the indented list, there are two choices that may pop out at you:

Thrombocytopenia

Congenital D69.42

Neonatal, transitory P61.0

Due to

Exchange transfusion P61.0

Congenital means "present at birth," and this condition was. However, the patient is a neonate, and the documentation states that this condition is due to the exchange with his mother. One thing to always remember: You can always look up both terms in the Tabular List. So let's do just that—take a look at them both:

D69.42 Congenital and hereditary thrombocytopenia purpura

P61.0 Transient neonatal thrombocytopenia

Let's go back to the documentation. The physician notes that the baby contracted this condition as a result of the transfusion his mother received previously. So, this is not actually inherited because it is not the result of genetics; it is the result of circumstances. In addition, the treatment worked, so the baby no longer has the blood problem, meaning the thrombocytopenia was temporary (transient). This points us toward the accurate code of

P61.0 Transient neonatal thrombocytopenia

Check the top of this subsection as well as the head of this chapter in ICD-10-CM. You will find a **NOTE**, an INCLUDES notation, and an EXCLUDES2 notation at the beginning of this chapter. Read carefully. Do any relate to this neonate's diagnosis? No. Turn to the Official Guidelines and read Section I.C.16. There is nothing specifically applicable here either.

Now you can report P61.0 for baby boy Alvarez's diagnosis with confidence.

Good work!

Transfusion
The provision of one person's blood or plasma to another individual.

Transfusions

Due to the existence of antigens located on the surface of the patient's RBCs, any time a patient requires a **transfusion** of blood, it must be checked for compatibility with regard to type and Rh factor; otherwise, serious consequences could occur.

People with type O blood have neither antigen; anyone can accept this blood type. Individuals with type O blood are known as *universal donors*. So, a patient with type A blood can receive a transfusion of *only* type A or type O blood. An individual with type B blood can receive *only* type B or type O blood. Those with type AB blood have both types of antigens, so they can receive type A blood, type B blood, or type O blood. For this reason, they are known as *universal recipients*.

Agglutination
The process of red blood cells combining together in a mass or lump.

Hemolysis
The destruction of red blood cells, resulting in the release of hemoglobin into the bloodstream.

However, attention must still be paid to Rh factor compatibility. A patient with Rh-positive blood can receive either Rh-positive or Rh-negative blood. However, patients with Rh-negative blood should only receive Rh-negative blood. Because of these facts, in an emergency, when time cannot be taken to test the patient's blood, Rh-negative blood is used.

The concern about both blood type and Rh factor compatibility arises from the dangers that can happen when the correct antibodies and antigens are not in place. For example, if an Rh-negative patient receives Rh-positive blood, anti-Rh antibodies would be created, causing red blood cell **agglutination** and **hemolysis**. Agglutination occurs when antibodies merge with antigens, causing RBCs to clump together. Hemolysis is the process of cells rupturing–destroying RBCs and releasing hemoglobin into the bloodstream.

EXAMPLES

Complications of incompatibility can occur when a transfusion is administered without a valid match to the patient. Because this condition is a complication of the transfusion, this diagnosis is not reported from Chapter 15 in ICD-10-CM. As the result of an External Cause, this is reported from the following code category:

✓4	T80	Complications following infusion, transfusion, and therapeutic injection
	T80.411A	Rh incompatibility with delayed hemolytic transfusion reaction, initial encounter
	T80.310A	ABO incompatibility with acute hemolytic transfusion reaction
	T80.A10A	Non-ABO incompatibility with acute hemolytic transfusion reaction

8.4 Disorders of White Blood Cells and Blood-Forming Organs

White Blood Cell Disorders

Remember from when you took anatomy class, there are five major types of WBCs, each of which can malfunction and be unable to perform its job keeping the body working properly.

- *Neutrophils* contain enzymes that work to destroy parts of bacterial pathogens that have been consumed by phagocytes.
- *Lymphocytes* are critical in the immune response.
- *Monocytes* are large blood cells that travel throughout the body and destroy damaged RBCs.
- *Eosinophils* destroy some parasites in addition to controlling inflammation and allergic reactions.
- *Basophils* create heparin, a blood-thinning agent that prevents inappropriate blood clotting, and create histamines, involved in allergic reactions.

Neutropenia

Neutropenia is a condition when the patient's bone marrow produces an abnormally low number of WBCs. This may be an ineffective number of cells being created or a loss of neutrophils at a rate faster than they can be replaced by new cells. Remember that WBCs fight infection. Once created in the bone marrow, these cells are released into the bloodstream, so they can move about the body to wherever they are needed.

A diagnosis of neutropenia may be a congenital condition, an adverse reaction to chemotherapy or other medications, or a malfunction of the hematopoiesis process.

D70.0 **Congenital agranulocytosis**
(congenital neutropenia)
(Kostmann's disease)

D70.1 **Agranulocytosis secondary to cancer chemotherapy**
Code also **underlying neoplasm**
Use additional code **for adverse effect, if applicable, to identify drug (T45.1X5)**

D70.2 **Other drug-induced agranulocytosis**
Use additional code **for adverse effect, if applicable, to identify drug (T36–T50 with fifth or sixth character 5)**

D70.3 **Neutropenia due to infection**

D70.4 **Cyclic neutropenia**

Leukopenia and Leukocytosis

In leukopenia, the body is not producing the required number of leukocytes.

D72.810 **Lymphocytopenia**

D72.819 **Decreased white blood cell count, unspecified**

Of course, while an insufficient quantity of cells is not going to accomplish what is needed by the body, too many also can cause havoc. In leukocytosis, the body creates too many leukocytes. This may be a correct action because these cells are part of the immune response to certain pathogens. In that case, the elevated white blood cell count would be a sign that an infection is present, and not reported separately. Without a reason stated, this may be a malfunction, and its own condition.

D72.820 **Lymphocytosis (symptomatic)**

D72.829 **Elevated white blood cell count, unspecified**

> **CODING BITES**
>
> Leukemia is a malignancy of the white blood cells, resulting in the bone marrow producing abnormal white blood cells that do not function as needed. This is why it is reported from the Neoplasms section of ICD-10-CM, specifically the C91-C95 code categories.

Monocytic, Eosinophilic, and Basophilic Conditions

It is logical that the malfunctions causing too few, or too many, neutrophils and leukocytes might also occur to the other types of WBCs.

D72.818 **Other decreased white blood cell count**
(Basophilic leukopenia)
(Eosinophilic leukopenia)
(Monocytopenia)

D72.821 **Monocytosis (symptomatic)**

D72.823 **Leukemoid reaction**
(Basophilic leukemoid reaction)
(Monocytic leukemoid reaction)
(Neutrophilic leukemoid reaction)

Splenic Dysfunction

The spleen is part of the lymphatic system, but it contains WBCs that work to fight infection. Damage to this organ can be caused by disease or trauma. Problems with the spleen caused by pathogens are reported from this section of ICD-10-CM.

> **EXAMPLES**
>
> D73.0 Hyposplenism (Atrophy of spleen)
>
> D73.3 Abscess of spleen
>
> A pathogen or other disease that interferes with the proper function of the spleen is reported from this chapter of ICD-10-CM.

However, an injury to the spleen caused by a traumatic event would be reported from the ICD-10-CM code book's ***Chapter 20: Injury, Poisoning, and Certain Other Consequences of External Causes (S00–T88)***.

EXAMPLES

S36.021A Major contusion of spleen, initial encounter

S36.030A Superficial (capsular) laceration of spleen, initial encounter

Even though the spleen is part of the immune system, traumatic injuries are still reported from the appropriate chapter in ICD-10-CM.

When the problem with the spleen is a congenital anomaly, the appropriate codes will be found in the ICD-10-CM code book's ***Chapter 18: Congenital Malformations, Deformations, and Chromosomal Abnormalities (Q00–Q99)***.

EXAMPLES

Q89.01 Asplenia (congenital)

Q89.09 Congenital malformations of spleen

These codes explain that the malfunction of this organ (the spleen) occurred in utero.

Manifestations of Other Diseases

When a condition causes a malfunction in the blood system and/or the blood-forming organs, it might be a manifestation. If this is the case, the underlying condition will be reported first, followed by this code:

D77 Other disorders of blood and blood-forming organs in diseases classified elsewhere

YOU CODE IT! CASE STUDY

PATIENT: Frank Copeland

DISCHARGE SUMMARY

ADMISSION DIAGNOSIS: Neutropenic fever.

DISCHARGE DIAGNOSES:

1. Neutropenic fever.
2. Acute myelogenous leukemia, status post induction and three cycles of high-dose Ara-C.
3. Thrombocytopenia.

PROCEDURES PERFORMED:

1. Two-view chest x-ray.
2. One unit of PRBC transfusion.

HOSPITAL COURSE: The patient is a very pleasant 54-year-old male with acute myelogenous leukemia who has undergone three cycles of high-dose Ara-C. He was transferred here after he presented to an outside facility with a 1-day onset of fevers and chills. He had a measured temperature at the outside hospital at that time of 102 degrees. He was transferred to this facility and admitted to the oncology service.

He was initially placed on cefepime, and blood cultures were drawn. All cultures throughout the course of his hospitalization turned out to be negative. He, however, remained febrile for the majority of his hospitalization. Upon presentation, he did complain of 1-day onset of profuse watery diarrhea that was extremely foul smelling. Of note, he was on p.o. prophylactic Levaquin due to his neutropenia. He was also on prophylactic acyclovir. Due to his being on antibiotics and history of diarrhea, a stool PCR was collected but resulted negative. Before the stool PCR resulted, he was placed on Flagyl as empiric coverage for suspected *C. diff* colitis. After the stool PCR resulted negative, Flagyl was discontinued.

(continued)

During the short 24 hours when he was on Flagyl, he seemed to have defervesced, and his fever curve trended down. However, after the Flagyl was discontinued, he started having worsened diarrhea and the fevers went back up again. For this reason, a *C. diff* PCR was ordered and the Flagyl was resumed. The *C. diff* PCR was also negative. Until that point, he remained on cefepime and the Flagyl was also decided to be continued since the patient seemed to improve with it. The thinking was that he may have had some colitis that was not related to *C. diff.*

Six days into his hospitalization, he continued to have fever. At this juncture, vancomycin was added to see if this would help. Repeat blood cultures were negative. Cultures were even drawn from the port that he had. There was some discussion as to whether his fevers may have been caused by the cefepime. The cefepime was discontinued. At this time, however, his fever curve had already started slightly trending down. Over the next 48 hours, he remained afebrile.

The vancomycin and Flagyl were discontinued the day before discharge, and he remained afebrile that night. His diarrhea had resolved over the last 4 to 5 days of his hospitalization and he received Imodium for this. The remainder of his hospitalization was unremarkable and he felt well. Of note, he did complain of poor appetite. We advised him to try to eat as much as he can and at the very least remain hydrated with Gatorade, and he understood that it may take some time for his appetite to completely return to normal.

He did frequently have hypokalemia and hypomagnesemia. This was presumed to be secondary to the diarrhea. Both of these electrolytes were replaced appropriately. However, even after the diarrhea resolved, he continued to have hypokalemia despite replacement. He later notified us that this issue is not new and that he actually takes potassium supplementation at home. He reported that he had p.o. potassium chloride at home and that he did not need medication or a refill for this. He could not, however, recall the dosage. We do not know the etiology of his hypokalemia as this was not worked up while he was inpatient due to again thinking that his hypokalemia was a result of his diarrhea.

On the day of discharge, he was also instructed to resume his prophylactic Levaquin and acyclovir.

DISCHARGE MEDICATIONS:

1. Acyclovir 400 mg p.o. b.i.d.
2. HCTZ 25 mg p.o. daily.
3. Lopressor 25 mg p.o. b.i.d.
4. Pravastatin 10 mg p.o. at bedtime.
5. Norethindrone 5 mg p.o. daily.
6. Levaquin 500 mg p.o. daily.
7. Zofran 4 mg sublingually q8hr p.r.n. nausea.
8. Norco 5/325 one tablet p.o. q4hr p.r.n. pain.

FOLLOW-UP APPOINTMENT: Dr. Constantine Revorsky in 1 week for follow-up for chemotherapy.

FOLLOW-UP LABS AND STUDIES: CBC, CMP before appointment with Dr. Revorsky.

DISCHARGE DIET: Regular as tolerated.

DISCHARGE ACTIVITY: As tolerated.

You Code It!

Read this Discharge Summary for Frank Copeland and determine only the principal diagnosis code.

Step #1: Read the case carefully and completely.
Step #2: Abstract the scenario. Which main words or terms describe why the physician cared for the patient during this encounter?
Step #3: Are there any details missing or incomplete for which you would need to query the physician? [If so, ask your instructor.]
Step #4: Check for any relevant guidance, including reading all of the symbols and notations in the Tabular List and the appropriate sections of the Official Guidelines.
Step #5: Determine the correct diagnosis code to explain why this encounter was medically necessary.
Step #6: Double-check your work.

Answer:

Did you determine this to be the principal diagnosis code?

D70.9 Neutropenia, unspecified

8.5 Disorders Involving the Immune System

The immune system is the armed forces network that develops special forces, known as antibodies, produced by plasma cells in the blood to protect the body from pathogens and other invaders (antigens) that may disrupt proper function. In the previous section, you learned about the role that the different types of WBCs play in guarding the good health of the body . . . your immune system.

Researchers continue to study and learn more about the actual mechanisms in place, to employ in the development of more effective and efficient treatments when the body cannot fight alone. The integration of technology and the greater availability of genetic details support these efforts to eliminate past and current illness and disease, and to fight off or prevent new conditions from evolving.

Immunodeficiencies

Immunodeficiency disorders are conditions when the patient's immune response is diminished or totally ineffective. Typically, immunodeficiency disorders occur when T or B lymphocytes (special WBCs) do not work properly. Immunodeficiency disorders may be inherited (genetically passed from parent to child) or acquired, an adverse effect to another illness, such as HIV-positive status or some malignancies; long-term use of certain medications, such as corticosteroids; chemotherapy treatments; or a manifestation of a splenectomy (the surgical removal of the spleen).

- Hereditary hypogammaglobulinemia, also known as autosomal recessive agammaglobulinemia, is an inherited immunodeficiency disorder often causing pulmonary and digestive disorders—reported with code D80.0 Hereditary hypogammaglobulinemia.
- Agammaglobulinemia with immunoglobulin-bearing B-lymphocytes is a nonfamilial (acquired) defect in the body's antibodies—reported with code D80.1 Nonfamilial hypogammaglobulinemia.

CODING BITES

Generally, allergies are reported by either the substance or object to which the patient is allergic or by the response suffered by the patient.

K52.2-	Allergic and dietetic gastroenteritis and colitis
J30.1	Allergic rhinitis due to pollen
J30.81	Allergic rhinitis due to animal (cat) (dog) hair and dander

Allergies

An allergy is actually an immune system false alarm, responding to something as if it were a pathogen able to harm the body, when, in reality, it is not. In medical terminology, this is known as a hypersensitivity reaction. These reactions are divided into four classes. Classes I, II, and III are caused by antibodies, IgE or IgG, which are produced by B cells in response to an allergen. Class IV reactions are caused by T cells. In these cases, the T cells might turn traitor and cause damage to the body, or they may ignite macrophages and eosinophils, which, in turn, may damage host cells.

CODING BITES

- One-third (about 33%) of people with DVT/PE will have a recurrence within 10 years.
- Approximately 5 to 8% of the U.S. population has one of several genetic risk factors, also known as inherited thrombophilia, in which a genetic defect can be identified that increases the risk for thrombosis.

Source: http://www.cdc.gov/ncbddd/dvt/data.html

Sarcoidosis

The specific etiology of sarcoidosis is still unknown; however, most researchers believe it is a combination of a genetic susceptibility with a certain exposure to something that triggers the immune system to release chemicals that are ineffective at combating inflammation. Instead, the cells clump together and become granulomas (tumors that result from an ulcerated infection) situated within certain organs throughout the body, such as the lungs, liver, or skin. This diagnosis is reported with a code from category D86 Sarcoidosis.

EXAMPLES

D86.0	Sarcoidosis of lung
D86.3	Sarcoidosis of skin
D86.84	Sarcoidosis pyelonephritis

As you can see from these three examples, you will need to know the specific anatomical site of the sarcoidosis before you can determine an accurate code.

Wiskott–Aldrich Syndrome

When a patient suffers from Wiskott-Aldrich syndrome, this genetic mutation causes WBCs to malfunction, increasing the body's susceptibility to inflammatory diseases and other immunodeficiency disorders. Eczema, thrombocytopenia, and pyogenic infections often develop and put the patient at a higher-than-normal risk of autoimmune diseases. This condition is reported with code D82.0 Wiskott-Aldrich syndrome.

ICD-10-CM

YOU CODE IT! CASE STUDY

Carol-Anne Nieman, a 41-year-old female, came in complaining of discomfort and tenderness under her arms and in her neck. Dr. Rothenberg performed a physical exam, revealing swollen lymph nodes. Lab work showed she was suffering with sarcoidosis of her lymph nodes.

You Code It!

Go through the steps of coding, and determine the code or codes that should be reported for this encounter between Dr. Rothenberg and Carol-Anne.

Step #1: Read the case carefully and completely.
Step #2: Abstract the scenario. Which main words or terms describe why the physician cared for the patient during this encounter?
Step #3: Are there any details missing or incomplete for which you would need to query the physician? [If so, ask your instructor.]
Step #4: Check for any relevant guidance, including reading all of the symbols and notations in the Tabular List and the appropriate sections of the Official Guidelines.
Step #5: Determine the correct diagnosis code or codes to explain why this encounter was medically necessary.
Step #6: Double-check your work.

Answer:

Did you determine this to be the correct code?

D86.1 Sarcoidosis of lymph nodes

Great work!

Chapter Summary

Blood flows through your arteries and veins, transporting oxygen (O_2) to nourish tissues and carrying away the waste (CO_2) from those cells. Production of the components of the blood, including RBCs, WBCs, and PLTs, occurs within the red bone marrow, specifically, within the sternum, ribs, and vertebrae in the adult. Because blood is systemic (traveling throughout the entire body), blood tests are an excellent diagnostic tool because the minor invasiveness of venipuncture can yield massive amounts of information about the health of the body. When the blood system malfunctions, serious health consequences result.

CHAPTER 8 REVIEW
Coding Conditions of the Blood and Immunological System

Let's Check It! Terminology

Match each key term to the appropriate definition.

1. **LO 8.3** A system of classifying blood based on the antigens present on the surface of the individual's red blood cells.
2. **LO 8.1** Cells within the blood that help to protect the body from pathogens.
3. **LO 8.3** The process of red blood cells combining together in a mass or lump.
4. **LO 8.3** Immune responses to antigens.
5. **LO 8.2** Clotting; the change from a liquid into a thickened substance.
6. **LO 8.2** The interruption of bleeding.
7. **LO 8.3** An antigen located on the red blood cell that produces immunogenic responses in those individuals without it.
8. **LO 8.3** The provision of one person's blood or plasma to another individual.
9. **LO 8.1** Fluid pumped throughout the body, carrying oxygen and nutrients to the cells and wastes away from the cells.
10. **LO 8.1** The fluid part of the blood.
11. **LO 8.1** Cells within the blood that contain hemoglobin responsible for carrying oxygen to tissues.
12. **LO 8.1** The part of the red blood cell that carries oxygen.
13. **LO 8.3** The destruction of red blood cells resulting in the release of hemoglobin into the bloodstream.
14. **LO 8.1** Large cell fragments in the bone marrow that function in clotting.
15. **LO 8.1** The formation of blood.
16. **LO 8.3** A substance that promotes the production of antibodies.

A. Agglutination
B. Antibody
C. Antigen
D. Blood
E. Blood Type
F. Coagulation
G. Hematopoiesis
H. Hemoglobin
I. Hemolysis
J. Hemostasis
K. Plasma
L. Platelets (PLTs)
M. Red Blood Cells (RBCs)
N. Rh Factor
O. Transfusion
P. White Blood Cells (WBCs)

Let's Check It! Concepts

Choose the most appropriate answer for each of the following questions.

1. **LO 8.1** Blood is composed of all of the following *except*

   a. RBCs. **b.** WBCs. **c.** PLTs. **d.** HCT.

2. **LO 8.1** Red bone marrow produces white blood cells through which process?

   a. erythrocytes **b.** leukopoiesis **c.** lymphocytes **d.** erythropoiesis

3. **LO 8.3** An individual with blood type B− can receive only which type(s) of blood in a transfusion?

   a. type B− **b.** type B+ **c.** type O+ **d.** type B− or type O−

4. **LO 8.4** _____ create heparin, a blood-thinning agent that prevents inappropriate blood clotting, and create histamines, involved in allergic reactions.

   a. Neutrophils **b.** Lymphocytes **c.** Eosinophils **d.** Basophils

5. **LO 8.1** Which type of anemia results from an insufficient number of healthy red blood cells due to abnormal or premature destruction?

   a. aplastic anemia **b.** hemolytic anemia **c.** nutritional anemia **d.** hemorrhagic anemia

6. **LO 8.2** _____ is a low platelet count most often due to increased platelet destruction, decreased platelet production, or malfunctioning platelets.
   a. Pancytopenia
   b. Leukocytopenia
   c. Thrombocytopenia
   d. Erythrocytopenia
7. **LO 8.1** Donny Cobin, a 19-year-old male, has been diagnosed with sickle-cell thalassemia with acute chest syndrome. How would you code this?
   a. D57.40
   b. D57.411
   c. D57.811
   d. D57.812
8. **LO 8.3** Antigens are _____ that sit on the surface of red blood cells.
   a. proteins
   b. sugars
   c. markers
   d. chromosomes
9. **LO 8.5** Typically, immunodeficiency disorders occur when _____ do not work properly.
   a. T lymphocytes
   b. B lymphocytes
   c. T or B lymphocytes
   d. None of these
10. **LO 8.5** The genetic mutation causing white blood cells to malfunction, increasing the body's susceptibility to inflammatory diseases and other immunodeficiency disorders, is known as _____________.
    a. Clarke-Hadfield Syndrome
    b. Heubner-Herter Syndrome
    c. Wiskott-Aldrich Syndrome
    d. Lennox-Gastaut Syndrome

Let's Check It! Rules and Regulations

Please answer the following questions from the knowledge you have gained after reading this chapter.

1. **LO 8.1** Discuss what blood is, how it is created, and what it consists of; include how many blood cells are needed for a healthy body.
2. **LO 8.2** Explain the two types of clotting disorders.
3. **LO 8.3** When a patient requires a transfusion of blood, it must first be checked for compatibility. What does this mean?
4. **LO 8.4** Discuss the difference between neutropenia, leukopenia, and leukocytosis.
5. **LO 8.5** What are immunodeficiency disorders and are they inherited or acquired?

ICD-10-CM

YOU CODE IT! Basics

First, identify the main term in the following diagnoses; then code the diagnosis.

Example: Posthemorrhagic anemia, chronic

a. main term: *anemia* b. diagnosis: *D50.0*

1. Hemoglobin H disease:
   a. main term: _____ b. diagnosis: _____
2. Purpura fulminans:
   a. main term: _____ b. diagnosis: _____
3. Anemia due to vitamin B_{12} intrinsic factor deficiency:
   a. main term: _____ b. diagnosis: _____
4. Cyclic hematopoiesis:
   a. main term: _____ b. diagnosis: _____
5. Antineoplastic chemotherapy-induced pancytopenia:
   a. main term: _____ b. diagnosis: _____
6. Minor alpha thalassemia:
   a. main term: _____ b. diagnosis: _____
7. Medullary hypoplasia:
   a. main term: _____ b. diagnosis: _____
8. Infantile pseudoleukemia:
   a. main term: _____ b. diagnosis: _____
9. Deficiency factor VIII:
   a. main term: _____ b. diagnosis: _____
10. Congenital neutropenia:
    a. main term: _____ b. diagnosis: _____

(continued)

11. Sickle-cell Hb-C with crisis disease:
    a. main term: _____ b. diagnosis: _____
12. Agranulocytosis due to infection:
    a. main term: _____ b. diagnosis: _____
13. Hemolytic-uremic syndrome:
    a. main term: _____ b. diagnosis: _____
14. Polycythemia due to erythropoietin:
    a. main term: _____ b. diagnosis: _____
15. Non-Langerhans cell histiocytosis:
    a. main term: _____ b. diagnosis: _____

ICD-10-CM

YOU CODE IT! Practice

Using the techniques described in this chapter, carefully read through the case studies and determine the most accurate ICD-10-CM code(s) and external cause code(s), if appropriate, for each case study.

1. James Abney, a 7-month-old male, is brought in by his parents to see Dr. Fay, his pediatrician. Dr. Fay notes a temperature of 106 F, jaundice, and generalized weakness and admits James to Weston Hospital for a full work-up. The CBC and Coombs test results confirm the diagnosis of favism anemia.
2. Sam Goodman, a 9-year-old male, presents today for a sports physical in order to play on his school baseball team. Dr. Inabinet notes splenomegaly. The results from the CBC test and peripheral blood smear confirm a diagnosis of Hb-C disease.
3. Arthur Hylton, a 45-year-old male, presents today with the complaint of general weakness and overall tiredness. Arthur works for an industrial factory and has been exposed to a large quantity of benzene. Dr. Burger completes an examination, noting an irregular heartbeat and hand tremors. Arthur is admitted to the hospital. The results of the bone marrow biopsy confirm a diagnosis of aplastic anemia due to accidental poisoning by benzene.
4. Rosalyn Burkett, a 37-year-old female, presents today with the complaint of migraines and blurred vision. After an examination and a review of the laboratory tests, Dr. Flick diagnoses Rosalyn with Lupus anticoagulant syndrome.
5. Tilley Cabe, a 9-month-old female, is brought in to see Dr. Peterson, her pediatrician. Tilley has had a persistent low-grade fever for 4 days that has not diminished. Dr. Peterson notes a temperature of 100.2 and splenomegaly. Tilley is not thriving. Dr. Peterson admits her to the hospital. The laboratory results reveal Tilley has a low natural killer cell activity and cytopenia, which confirm the diagnosis of hemophagocytic lymphohistiocytosis (HLH).
6. Glenn Carballero, a 15-year-old male, presents today with the complaint of weakness and generalized muscular pains. Dr. Douglass notes an erythematous periorofacial macular rash. After a thorough examination and laboratory tests are completed, Glenn is diagnosed with biotinidase deficiency.
7. Sadie Thompson, an 18-month-old female, was born with TAR syndrome (thrombocytopenia with absent radius). Sadie is brought in today by her mother with the complaint of excessive bruising without significant trauma. After an examination and the laboratory tests are completed, Dr. Dotson diagnosis Sadie with congenital thrombocytopenia purpura.
8. Victor Motts, a 6-month-old male, is brought in by his mother to see his pediatrician, Dr. Stewart. Victor experienced a type of spasm. Dr. James notes skeletal abnormalities and cyanosis as well as some hearing difficulties and admits him to Weston Hospital. A fluorescence in situ hybridization (FISH) blood test confirms a diagnosis of Di George's syndrome.
9. Lindsey Williams, a 33-year-old female, has not been feeling well and is seen by Dr. Goldburg, who notes jaundice. Lindsey admits to feeling weak and being dizzy. Blood tests return a hemoglobin of 6.3 g/dL. Lindsey is admitted to the hospital for a blood transfusion; while there, a peripheral blood smear was performed that showed echinocytes, confirming a diagnosis of pyruvate kinase deficiency anemia.
10. Antonio Scott, a 47-year-old male, presents today with the complaint of a cough, runny nose, and a sore throat. Dr. Benton completes an examination and reviews the results of the CBC test and diagnoses Antonio with lymphocytopenia.

(continued)

11. Ivory Presnell, a 75-year-old female, comes in today complaining of fever, chills, and night sweats. She says she feels tired and has lost 5 lbs. within a week. Dr. Shirley notes nail clubbing and completes an in-house CBC test; results: hemoglobin of 7.9 g/dL. Ivory is admitted to Weston Hospital, where a tissue biopsy is taken, returning a positive reading for extra-pulmonary tuberculosis. Ivory is diagnosed with anemia due to tuberculosis.
12. Buddy Dent, a 59-year-old male with chronic kidney disease, stage 4, comes to see Dr. Wilberly complaining of extreme weakness. Dr. Wilberly completes a full blood workup and notes the following results: hemoglobin–8.2 g/dL, creatinine–52 mg/dL, and BUN–102 mg/dL. Buddy is diagnosed with anemia due to chronic kidney disease and is scheduled for a transfusion.
13. Juanita Ilderton, a 41-year-old female, received a blood transfusion 12 hours ago; now she is experiencing fever, chills, and dizziness. A direct Coombs test is performed, which confirms a diagnosis of acute hemolytic Rh blood transfusion incompatibility after a transfusion.
14. Richard Greene, a 33-year-old male, comes to see Dr. Walter with the complaints of tiredness and weakness. Dr. Walter completes bloodwork and a bone marrow biopsy. Richard is diagnosed with chronic lymphocytic, B-cell type leukemia.
15. Billy Stevenson, a 10-year-old-male, is brought in by his father to see Dr. Loveichelle. Billy has developed a cough and fever. Billy says he feels really tired. Mr. Stevenson also stated they can't get Billy to eat. Dr. Loveichelle completes an examination and an in-house CBC. Billy's hemoglobin is 7.4 g/dL. Billy is admitted to the hospital for a full workup. Once all the laboratory results have been reviewed, Billy is diagnosed with hookworm anemia.

ICD-10-CM

YOU CODE IT! Application

The following exercises provide practice in abstracting physicians' documentation from our health care facility, Prader, Bracker, & Associates. These case studies are modeled on real patient encounters. Using the techniques described in this chapter, carefully read through the case studies and determine the most accurate ICD-10-CM code(s) and external cause code(s), if appropriate, for each case study.

PRADER, BRACKER, & ASSOCIATES

A Complete Health Care Facility

159 Healthcare Way • SOMEWHERE, FL 32811 • 407-555-6789

PATIENT: KRIESEL, BROOKE

ACCOUNT/EHR #: KRIEBR001

Attending Physician: Oscar R. Prader, MD

Brooke Kriesel, a 41-year-old female, presents today with the complaint of fatigue—2-week duration. She admits to moderate shortness of breath with exertion; denies chest pain with exertion or at rest. No bright red blood per rectal exam or melena. She has had heavy menstrual periods—1-year duration.

PAST MEDICAL HISTORY: Noncontributory

FAMILY HISTORY: Noncontributory

OTC medication—aspirin, 81 mg daily—3-month duration.

PHYSICAL EXAM:

General appearance: Pale, no acute distress.

Vital signs: Ht: 5′7″, Wt: 146, T: 99.8, R: 15, HR: 81 and regular, BP: 128/81. Pale conjunctiva; mucous membranes, moist with no apparent lesions; chest, clear; heart, regular rate and rhythm, no murmurs, rubs, or gallops. The abdomen—soft, nontender, and nondistended; no hepatosplenomegaly; rectal examination—no masses and heme negative, brown stool is present.

Hemoglobin level—7.4 g/dL. There is evidence of marked microcytosis and hypochromia with a decreased hemoglobin level.

DIAGNOSIS: Anemia due to iron deficiency

Determine the most accurate ICD-10-CM code(s).

(continued)

PRADER, BRACKER, & ASSOCIATES

A Complete Health Care Facility

159 Healthcare Way • SOMEWHERE, FL 32811 • 407-555-6789

PATIENT: LAKEMONT, CALEB

ACCOUNT/EHR #: LAKECA001

Attending Physician: Oscar R. Prader, MD

Caleb Lakemont, a 29-year-old male, came to see me with complaints of bruising easily and prolonged nosebleeds. He also showed me a rash, nonpainful/nonitchy, on his ankles and shins. He denies making any recent changes in body soap or household detergents. Dr. Prader notes bruises on his arms and trunk; patient denies any type of trauma that would cause bruising.

PE: Ht: 5′11″, Wt: 185, T: 98.4, R: 13, HR: 57, BP: 115/79. No lymphadenopathy or hepatosplenomegaly. Stool sample testing is guaiac positive.

Laboratory results: CBC and peripheral smear confirm patient is thrombocytopenic. There is no evidence of a coagulation disorder.

DIAGNOSIS: Autoimmune thrombocytopenia (ITP)

Determine the most accurate ICD-10-CM code(s).

WESTON HOSPITAL

629 Healthcare Way • SOMEWHERE, FL 32811 • 407-555-6541

PATIENT: FUENTES, ERIN

ACCOUNT/EHR #: FUENER001

Attending Physician: Renee O. Bracker, MD

Pt is a 9-year-old female brought in by her parents to see Dr. Bracker. I last saw Erin 6 months ago, at which time she was thriving. Erin has experienced several nosebleeds over the last week. After questioning Erin, she admits she gets tired easily and doesn't feel much like eating.

PE: Ht: 52.5″, Wt: 60 lb., T: 101.2, R: 18, HR: 81, BP: 125/70. Dr. Bracker notes that Erin is having difficulty focusing and articulating. Weight loss of 3 lb. since last visit. A CBC is performed; results show a hemoglobin of 6.8 g/dL. Erin is admitted.

CV: Normal S1, S2, regular.

Pulm: Unlabored respiration, clear, bilaterally.

Abd: Soft, nontender, nondistended, without organomegaly or mass.

Extr: Warm, well perfused, no edema, notable for several 3 cm ecchymoses on the forearms and thighs bilaterally; in addition, there is a petechial rash over the ankles and feet bilaterally.

Neuro: Alert and oriented

Laboratory results:

Hemoglobin—6.7 g/dL

Platelet count—35 × 10/L

Leukocyte count–3.1 × 10/L

Neutrophil count—1.4 × 10/L

INR—1.5

PT—16.2

(continued)

Bone marrow aspirate was performed—20% promyelocytes.

Dx: Acute promyelocytic leukemia (APL)

P: Chemotherapy with ATRA

Determine the most accurate ICD-10-CM code(s).

WESTON HOSPITAL

629 Healthcare Way • SOMEWHERE, FL 32811 • 407-555-6541

PATIENT: FLOWERS, CATLYNNE

ACCOUNT/EHR #: FLOWCA001

Attending Physician: Renee O. Bracker, MD

S: Catlynne Flowers, a 22-year-old female, presents to the emergency room today with dyspnea and cough.

O: Ht: 5′3″, Wt: 131 lb., R: 30, T: 101.2, BP: 110/67. Catlynne was diagnosed with sickle cell disease 3 years ago. Patient appears to be in crisis. Chest x-ray confirms pulmonary infiltration. A broncho-alveolar lavage was performed; specimen was taken for culture, which confirmed the diagnosis.

A: Sickle cell/Hb-C crisis with acute chest syndrome ACS

P: Admit to inpatient

Determine the most accurate ICD-10-CM code(s).

WESTON HOSPITAL

629 Healthcare Way • SOMEWHERE, FL 32811 • 407-555-6541

PATIENT: ARNOLD, CAMERON

ACCOUNT/EHR #: ARNOCA001

Attending Physician: Oscar R. Prader, MD

Cameron Arnold, a 39-year-old female, comes in to see Dr. Prader with complaints of weakness and several spontaneous nosebleeds that last approximately 10 minutes—10-days duration. She states that she bruises easily without any injury—3 times in the last month alone—and her menstrual periods have been notably heavier. Dr. White, the referring physician, asks that we rule out coagulopathy. PMH: noncontributory. PFH: no history of family bleeding.

Preliminary laboratory results reveal a hemoglobin of 6.7 g/dL. The mean corpuscular volume (MCV) is 71 fl. PT and APTT are within normal range.

A von Willebrand factor antigen assay, a von Willebrand factor activity assay, and factor VIII measurement were ordered; results confirm the diagnosis of von Willebrand disease.

Determine the most accurate ICD-10-CM code(s).

9

Coding Endocrine Conditions

Key Terms

Cushing's Syndrome
Diabetes Mellitus (DM)
Dyslipidemia
Gestational Diabetes Mellitus (GDM)
Hyperglycemia
Hypoglycemia
Hypoglycemics
Hypothyroidism
Parathyroid Glands
Polydipsia
Polyuria
Secondary Diabetes Mellitus
Thyroid Gland
Type 1 Diabetes Mellitus
Type 2 Diabetes Mellitus

Learning Outcomes

After completing this chapter, the student should be able to:

LO 9.1 Identify the various disorders affecting the thyroid gland.
LO 9.2 Evaluate the details about a diabetes mellitus diagnosis to determine the correct code.
LO 9.3 Assess the relationship between diabetes mellitus and its manifestations.
LO 9.4 Interpret the documentation related to the reporting of other endocrinologic diseases.
LO 9.5 Identify the aspects of nutrition and weight required for accurate code determination.
LO 9.6 Analyze the details related to metabolic disorder diagnoses to determine the correct code.

STOP! Remember, you need to follow along in your ICD-10-CM code book for an optimal learning experience.

Thyroid Gland
A two-lobed gland located in the neck that reaches around the trachea laterally and connects anteriorly by an isthmus. The thyroid gland produces hormones used for metabolic function.

9.1 Disorders of the Thyroid Gland

Thyroid Gland

The **thyroid gland** is located in the neck. Each of its two lobes reaches around the trachea laterally; they connect anteriorly by an isthmus (see **Figure 9-1**).

The anterior pituitary gland transmits thyroid-stimulating hormone (TSH) to the thyroid, which then extracts iodine from the blood system to create two hormones. The two hormones secreted by this gland–triiodothyronine (T_3) and thyroxine (T_4)–are collectively known as *thyroid hormone (TH)*. TH is responsible for stimulating the production of proteins in virtually every tissue in the body, controlling the body's metabolic rate, and increasing the quantity of oxygen used by each cell. In addition, calcitonin is produced here from the C cells located in the follicles. This hormone, secreted in response to hypercalcemia (too much calcium in the blood), promotes the deposit of calcium and works in the formation of bone.

EXAMPLES

E03.1	Congenital hypothyroidism without goiter
E07.81	Sick-euthyroid syndrome

Parathyroid Glands
Four small glands situated on the back of the thyroid gland that secrete parathyroid hormone.

Parathyroid Glands

In the posterior aspect of the thyroid gland are four partially embedded **parathyroid glands**. When stimulated by hypocalcemia (too little calcium in the blood), they produce parathyroid hormone (PTH). PTH works in the opposite way of how calcitonin (produced by the thyroid) works.

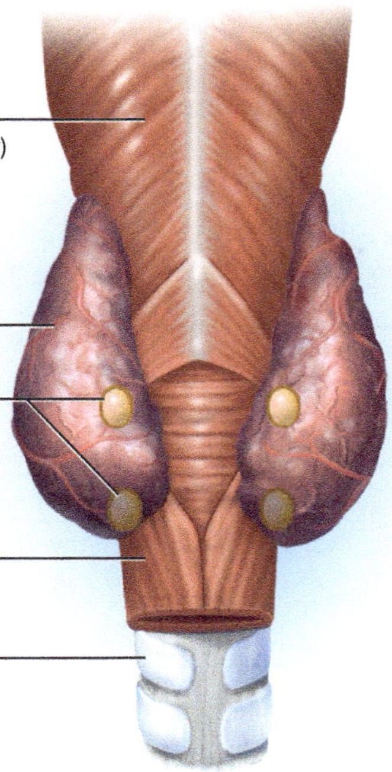

FIGURE 9-1 The thyroid gland, illustrated as part of the anatomical sites within the neck

EXAMPLES

E20.1 Pseudohypoparathyroidism

E21.0 Primary hyperparathyroidism

Hypothyroidism (Adults)

Hypothyroidism is caused by an insufficient production of TH. When a patient has hypothyroidism, the thyroid converts energy more slowly than normal, resulting in an otherwise unexplained weight gain and fatigue. In addition, hypercholesterolemia, unexplained increase in weight, forgetfulness, and even unusual sensitivity to colder temperatures may be evidence of early signs of this condition.

Hypothyroidism
A condition in which the thyroid converts energy more slowly than normal, resulting in an otherwise unexplained weight gain and fatigue.

This might be the result of irradiation therapy, infection, Hashimoto's disease (chronic autoimmune thyroiditis), or pituitary failure to produce the required amount of TSH.

To confirm this diagnosis, radioimmunoassay and/or lab tests are performed to look at the levels of TSH. Lab tests can identify the patient's TSH levels; however, reference ranges may fluctuate depending upon the patient's age and family history. Treatment for hypothyroidism includes medication, such as levothyroxine, to replace TH.

EXAMPLES

E03.1 Congenital hypothyroidism without goiter

E03.2 Hypothyroidism due to medicaments and other exogenous substances
Code first **poisoning due to drug or toxin, if applicable (T36–T65 with fifth or sixth character 1–4 or 6)**
Use additional code **for adverse effect, if applicable, to identify drug (T36–T50 with fifth or sixth character 5)**

E03.3 Postinfectious hypothyroidism

As you can see, the underlying cause of the hypothyroidism is key to determining an accurate code.

> **CODING BITES**
>
> If you recognize a patient's condition from a lab report, but the physician did not document a confirmed diagnosis, you must *query* the physician. You may *not* code from the lab report.

Hyperthyroidism

Hyperthyroidism, also known as *thyrotoxicosis*, is a condition in which the thyroid secretes too many hormones, more than the body needs to function properly. Interestingly, hyperthyroidism is most often a manifestation of another disease, including Graves' disease or thyroiditis.

Signs and symptoms include unexplained weight loss, rapid heart rate, and sensitivity to heat. Also, because the body systems are faster due to the excess of these hormones, irritability, trouble sleeping, hand tremors, and mood swings also may be exhibited.

> **EXAMPLES**
>
> E05.00 Thyrotoxicosis with diffuse goiter without thyrotoxic crisis or storm (Graves' disease)
> E05.11 Thyrotoxicosis with toxic single thyroid nodule with thyrotoxic crisis or storm
> E05.20 Thyrotoxicosis with toxic multinodular goiter without thyrotoxic crisis or storm
>
> As you can see from these few examples, the term *thyrotoxicosis* is used by the code descriptions, rather than the more common term *hyperthyroidism*.

Graves' Disease

Graves' disease (toxic diffuse goiter) is an autoimmune disorder. This malfunction of the immune system creates an antibody called *thyroid stimulating immunoglobulin (TSI)* that affixes itself to thyroid cells. TSI then accelerates the overproduction of the TH.

Thyroid Nodules

Thyroid nodules are adenomas, benign neoplasms that grow in the thyroid. These nodules may stimulate the thyroid to become overactive. A toxic multinodular goiter is an accumulation of several thyroid nodules multiplying the effects, and the quantity of TH that is overproduced.

Thyroiditis

Thyroiditis is an inflammation of the thyroid that causes TH stored within the thyroid gland to leak out. Initially, the leakage can be identified by increased hormone levels showing in the blood. If the leak continues, this can cause hyperthyroidism.

E06.0 Acute thyroiditis
(Abscess of thyroid)
(Pyogenic thyroiditis)
Use additional code **(B95–B97) to identify infectious agent**

E06.1 Subacute thyroiditis
(de Quervain thyroiditis)
(Giant cell thyroiditis)
EXCLUDES1 **autoimmune thyroiditis (E06.3)**

E06.2 Chronic thyroiditis with transient thyrotoxicosis
EXCLUDES1 **autoimmune thyroiditis (E06.3)**

E06.3 Autoimmune thyroiditis
(Hashimoto's thyroiditis)
(Lymphocytic thyroiditis)

E06.4 Drug-induced thyroiditis
Use additional code **for adverse effect, if applicable, to identify drug (T36–T50 with fifth or sixth character 5)**

E06.5 Other chronic thyroiditis
(Chronic fibrous thyroiditis)
(Ligneous thyroiditis)
(Riedel thyroiditis)

Postpartum thyroiditis develops during the postpartum period.

O90.5 Postpartum thyroiditis

Other Disorders of the Thyroid

Additional disorders of the thyroid include

- *Nontoxic goiter*, reported from code category E04
- *Hashimoto's thyroiditis*, reported with code E06.3
- *Myxedema*, a type of hypothyroidism, reported with code E03.9

LET'S CODE IT! SCENARIO

ICD-10-CM

PATIENT: Angela Tanner

Preprocedural Diagnosis: Right thyroid tumor

Postprocedural Diagnosis: Benign tumor of right thyroid

Procedure: Isthmectomy, Right thyroidectomy

Surgeon: Samuel Rodriguez, MD

DESCRIPTION OF OPERATION: The patient was intubated with a Xomed nerve monitor endotracheal tube. The neck was extended with a shoulder roll and a transverse cervical incision was made along the skin crease, leaning to the right side. The skin incision was made and the platysma was divided. A superior flap was developed to the thyroid notch and inferior flap to the sternal notch. Crossing jugular veins were ligated with 2-0 and 3-0 silk ties. The strap muscles were separated in the midline. The right strap muscles were then lifted off of a markedly enlarged right thyroid gland. The lateral border of the gland was identified. The middle thyroid vein and its branches were doubly ligated with 3-0 silk ties and divided. The recurrent laryngeal nerve was identified at the base of the neck and we traced this superiorly. The inferior thyroid vascular bundle was noted to be quite anterior to this. We doubly ligated this with 2-0 silk ties and divided it as it entered the thyroid gland. The inferior right parathyroid gland was identified. It was noted to be adherent to the thyroid gland. We separated the two glands and placed the right inferior parathyroid gland in the base of the neck. We then identified the superior pole of the right thyroid gland. The superior thyroid vascular bundle was doubly ligated with 2-0 silk ties and divided. The right upper parathyroid gland was separated from the thyroid gland. This was also adherent to the thyroid gland. We then mobilized the gland medially. A small amount of thyroid tissue was left behind in the upper pole. The stump was doubly ligated with 2-0 silk ties and divided. This allowed us to mobilize the thyroid gland medially, and we slowly separated the nerve from the posterior surface of the thyroid gland. This nerve was adherent to the thyroid gland. The gland was left intact as we separated the thyroid gland from it, and then we lifted the thyroid gland off of the trachea. Dissection was then carried beyond the isthmus, and with the right thyroid gland in the isthmus lifted off of the trachea, we then clamped the medial aspect of the right thyroid lobe and we then excised the specimen. The stump was then suture ligated with running 2-0 silk stitch. Specimen was sent for pathology, and on analysis, there was no evidence of a malignancy. The thyroid stump was inspected. No bleeding was noted. No bleeding was noted from the right upper or lower parathyroid glands. The recurrent laryngeal nerve was noted to be functional throughout its course, and the inferior and superior vascular bundles were noted to be hemostatic. With assurance of hemostasis, the strap muscles were closed with running 4-0 Vicryls, platysma was closed with interrupted 4-0 Vicryls, and 5-0 Monocryls were used for subcuticular skin closure. Local anesthesia was infiltrated. The patient tolerated the procedure well. Sponge and needle counts were correct. Blood loss was minimal. The patient was extubated and taken to the recovery room in stable condition.

Let's Code It!

Dr. Rodriguez operated on Angela to remove her right thyroid because there was a tumor on it. How do you know that the tumor was benign? The documentation states, "*Specimen was sent for pathology, and on analysis, there was no evidence of a malignancy.*"

Turn to the Neoplasm Table in your ICD-10-CM code book and find Thyroid in the first column . . .

Thyroid (gland)

Carefully read across, on that same row, to the fourth column to the right, the column titled, "Benign." Code D34 is suggested.

Now turn in the Tabular List to:

D34 Benign neoplasm of thyroid gland

(continued)

This matches. But wait, there is a notation beneath this code:

Use additional code **to identify any functional activity**

Hmm. There is nothing in the procedure note about functional activity, and there would not be. This would be noted in the diagnostic statement. In real life, you would need to look at the other parts of the patient's record, or query the physician about this detail. For now, consider that there is documentation in the patient's medical record that the functional activity with this tumor is corticoadrenal insufficiency.

Turn back to the Alphabetic Index and find

Insufficiency, insufficient

. . . read all the way down the list to find the indented . . .

corticoadrenal E27.40

primary E27.1

In the Tabular List, find

✓4 E27 Other disorders of adrenal gland

E27.1 Primary adrenocortical insufficiency

✓5 E27.4 Other and unspecified adrenocortical insufficiency

E27.40 Unspecified adrenocortical insufficiency

Before you report these codes, be certain to check the top of this subsection; there is an EXCLUDES1 notation above code E20. This has no relation to this case. At the beginning of the chapter, you will find a **NOTE** and an EXCLUDES1 notation. Read carefully. Do any relate to Dr. Rodriguez's diagnosis of Angela? No. Turn to the Official Guidelines and read Section I.C.4. There is nothing specifically applicable here either.

Now you can report these two codes for Angela's diagnosis, evidencing the medical necessity for this procedure, with confidence.

D34 **Benign neoplasm of thyroid gland**

E27.40 **Unspecified adrenocortical insufficiency**

Good work!

YOU CODE IT! CASE STUDY

Emily Benko, a 2-month-old female, was having dyspnea, and her cry sounded hoarse. In addition, Dr. Jenkins noticed her skin color was jaundiced. Her mother, Danielle, stated that she is a good baby and sleeps all the time. After running a TSH blood test and performing a thyroid scan, Dr. Jenkins diagnosed Emily with infantile cretinism, also known as congenital hypothyroidism. Dr. Jenkins also noted mild cognitive impairment, which is associated with the cretinism. He explained to Emily's mother that the mental impairment is likely to be progressive.

You Code It!

Go through the steps of coding, and determine the code or codes that should be reported for this encounter between Dr. Jenkins and Emily.

Step #1: Read the case carefully and completely.

Step #2: Abstract the scenario. Which main words or terms describe why the physician cared for the patient during this encounter?

Step #3: Are there any details missing or incomplete for which you would need to query the physician? [If so, ask your instructor.]

Step #4: Check for any relevant guidance, including reading all of the symbols and notations in the Tabular List and the appropriate sections of the Official Guidelines.

(continued)

Step #5: Determine the correct diagnosis code or codes to explain why this encounter was medically necessary.

Step #6: Double-check your work.

Answer:

Did you determine these to be the correct codes?

E03.1 Congenital hypothyroidism without goiter
G31.84 Mild cognitive impairment, so stated

Good for you!

9.2 Diabetes Mellitus

Diabetes Mellitus

Diabetes mellitus (DM) is a chronic disease and a result of insulin deficiency or resistance due to a malfunction of the pancreatic beta cells. The body has a difficult time metabolizing carbohydrates, proteins, and fats. It is estimated that 16 million people have DM; however, many (possibly as many as 50%) do not know it yet.

Diabetes Mellitus (DM)
A chronic systemic disease that results from insulin deficiency or resistance and causes the body to improperly metabolize carbohydrates, proteins, and fats.

A physician can diagnose diabetes with a glucose lab test and the presence of the following signs and symptoms:

- Excessive thirst **(polydipsia)**
- Excessive appetite
- Increased urination **(polyuria)**
- Unusual weight change (loss or gain)
- Fatigue
- Nausea, vomiting
- Blurred vision
- Frequent vaginal infections (females)
- Yeast infections (both males and females)
- Dry mouth
- Slow-healing sores or cuts
- Itchy skin, especially in the groin or vaginal area

Polydipsia
Excessive thirst.

Polyuria
Excessive urination.

Measures for detecting diabetes include a glucose tolerance test (GTT) and evaluation of the results. Diabetes may be indicated by

- A casual plasma glucose value greater than or equal to 200 mg/dL.
- A fasting plasma glucose level greater than or equal to 126 mg/dL.
- A plasma glucose value in the 2-hour sample of the oral GTT greater than or equal to 200 mg/dL.

(*Note:* Normal blood glucose levels are less than 110 mg/dL.)

There are four types of diabetes mellitus:

- **Type 1 DM**: The malfunction of the pancreatic beta cells, resulting in no production of insulin naturally, is the underlying cause of type 1 (juvenile) diabetes mellitus, although there is no documented known etiology for idiopathic DM. Therapeutically, type 1 DM patients must administer insulin every day in addition to following specific diet and exercise programs. Implanted insulin pumps may be used for those requiring multiple dose regimens. This diagnosis will be reported from ICD-10-CM code category E10 with additional characters required to identify specific information about complications (manifestations).

Type 1 Diabetes Mellitus
A sudden onset of insulin deficiency that may occur at any age but most often arises in childhood and adolescence; also known as *insulin-dependent diabetes mellitus (IDDM)*, *juvenile diabetes*, or *type I*.

Type 2 Diabetes Mellitus
A form of diabetes mellitus with a gradual onset that may develop at any age but most often occurs in adults over the age of 40; also known as *non-insulin-dependent diabetes mellitus (NIDDM)* or *type II*.

Dyslipidemia
Abnormal lipoprotein metabolism.

- **Type 2 DM**: In type 2 patients, the pancreatic beta cells do produce insulin; however, the glucose transport is ineffective, thereby failing to deliver the required amount to the rest of the body. Type 2 diabetics often suffer pathologic effects, including increased body fat (obesity), especially when the individual does not exercise regularly. Family history of DM, co-morbidities of hypertension or **dyslipidemia**, or a personal history of gestational DM will increase the likelihood of developing this condition. In addition, patients of African American, Latino, or Native American heritage are found to have a high risk. Diet and exercise are the first level of treatment and may resolve the condition. However, oral antidiabetic medications, such as sulfonylureas, may be prescribed to stimulate pancreatic beta cell function if diet and exercise fail to show sufficient improvement. Some type 2 DM patients require the administration of insulin. A type 2 diagnosis will be reported from ICD-10-CM code category E11 with additional characters required to identify specific information about complications (manifestations).

- **Type 2 DM in remission** is possible, thanks to the accomplishments of healthcare researchers. In these cases, the patient will have consistently maintained a fasting plasma glucose level below 126 mg/dL or a hemoglobin A1c (HbA1C) level below 6.5% for at least 3 months *without* the use of any glucose-lowering medication. This new 2026 ICD-10-CM code, E11.A *Type 2 diabetes mellitus without complications in remission* can only be reported with the physician documentation marking this status. Clear instructions for using this new code are included in a new 2026 Official Guideline 4.a.1)(b) Type 2 diabetes mellitus in remission: "*If the documentation is unclear as to whether the Type 2 diabetes mellitus has achieved remission, the provider should be queried.* For example, the term 'resolved' is not synonymous with remission." NOTE: For more information on querying the provider, see **Chapter 2, section 2.7 How to Query** in this text.

Secondary Diabetes Mellitus
Diabetes caused by medication or another condition or disease.

- **Secondary DM**: Certain drugs or chemicals can negatively affect the pancreatic beta cells and may prevent them from producing the required amount of insulin. Also, other diseases and conditions, such as Cushing's syndrome, can cause the patient to develop diabetes mellitus. This diagnosis is reported from code category E08 Diabetes mellitus due to underlying condition, E09 Drug or chemical induced diabetes mellitus, or E13 Other specified diabetes mellitus; additional characters are required to provide specific information about complications. The underlying condition, drug, or chemical causing the secondary DM will be reported first, and any codes required to identify specific manifestations will be reported following the E08, E09, or E13 code.

Gestational Diabetes Mellitus (GDM)
Usually a temporary diabetes mellitus occurring during pregnancy; however, such patients have an increased risk of later developing type 2 diabetes.

- **Gestational DM** (GDM): When a woman is pregnant, the weight gain, along with the higher levels of estrogen and the increase of placental hormones, may retard the production of insulin. This is considered a temporary type of DM due to the fact that, typically, the problem with the pancreatic beta cells resolves itself after the baby is delivered. Report this with a code from the ICD-10-CM code subcategory O24.4 Gestational diabetes mellitus, with an additional character to report additional details.

Diabetic Manifestations

Due to its involvement with the blood system as well as muscle and fat tissue, there can be serious manifestations–the development of other illnesses and conditions–caused by suffering with DM long term, especially when the condition goes untreated.

GUIDANCE CONNECTION

Read the ICD-10-CM Official Guidelines for Coding and Reporting, section **I. Conventions, General Coding Guidelines and Chapter-Specific Guidelines**, subsection **C. Chapter-Specific Coding Guidelines**, chapter **4. Endocrine, Nutritional, and Metabolic Diseases (E00-E89)**, subsection **a. Diabetes mellitus**, and chapter **15. Pregnancy, childbirth, and the puerperium**, subsections **g. Diabetes mellitus in pregnancy** and **i. Gestational (pregnancy-induced) diabetes.**

Ophthalmic Manifestations

The problems that diabetics frequently experience with their eyes are actually related to vascular concerns. *Diabetic retinopathy*, one of the leading causes of irreversible blindness, may be one of several types:

- *Background retinopathy:* blood vessel damage with no current vision problems.
- *Maculopathy:* damage to the macula part of the eye, resulting in a considerable loss of vision.
- *Proliferative retinopathy:* a microvascular complication of diabetes in which the small vessels of the eye become diseased as a result of diminishing oxygen.
- *Other eye problems often suffered by diabetics:* diabetic cataracts and macular edema.

Diabetic retinopathy is evidenced by microcirculatory changes in the eye that interfere with the blood supply and therefore the health of the eye. Nonproliferative diabetic retinopathy is seen in the blood vessels of the retina leaking plasma or fatty substances, resulting in diminished blood flow. Proliferative diabetic retinopathy encourages neovascularization (the growth of new blood vessels) in the vitreous of the eye; these vessels then rupture, causing a hemorrhage and sudden loss of vision. Without treatment, this can cause blindness. A diagnosis of type 1 diabetic retinopathy would be reported with a code from ICD-10-CM code subcategory E10.3 Type I diabetes mellitus with ophthalmic complications, with the required additional characters determined by the specifics (proliferative/nonproliferative, with/without macular edema, mild/moderate/severe).

Neurologic Manifestations

Uncontrolled diabetes can cause damage to the patient's nerves, causing diabetic neuropathy–in particular, sensory diabetic neuropathy, or a lack of feeling. Sensory diabetic neuropathy can be dangerous because the damaged nerves do not transmit feelings of heat, cold, or pain. Such a patient might be burned or cut and not know it. The injuries might become infected, causing additional health problems. In addition, the nerve damage can retard healing, making additional complications more viable.

Renal Manifestations

Diabetic nephropathy develops due to the reduced control of blood sugar. Almost 30% of diabetics develop diabetic nephropathy (kidney disease) or other kidney-related problems, such as bladder infections and nerve damage to the bladder. The nephrons within the kidneys thicken, and the scarring that forms results in leakage of albumin (protein) into the urine. Quantitative lab tests examine the levels of albumin in the patient's urine (microalbuminuria), as well as other levels such as blood urea nitrogen (BUN) and serum creatinine. Diabetic kidney disease can cause severe illness and possibly death. Therefore, early diagnosis and treatment to prevent the progression of the condition are important. Angiotensin-converting enzyme (ACE) inhibitors as well as angiotensin receptor blockers (ARB) are considered the best medications in these cases. A diagnosis of type 2 diabetic nephropathy is reported from ICD-10-CM subcategory E11.2 Type 2 diabetes mellitus with kidney complications, with an additional character to report a chronic or other condition.

You may need a second code to identify the exact nature of the renal complication, such as the stage of the chronic kidney failure. Type 2 diabetes-related chronic kidney disease may be reported with E11.22 Type 2 diabetes mellitus with diabetic chronic kidney disease; diabetic nephropathy may be reported with E10.21 Type 1 diabetes mellitus with diabetic nephropathy.

Circulatory Manifestations

Peripheral vascular disease is another likely complication because diabetes mellitus disturbs the blood flow, increasing the development of ulcers. It is estimated that as many as 10% of diabetics develop foot ulcers. Gangrene, a condition by which necrosis (tissue death) occurs as a result of lack of blood, is another relatively common manifestation. When gangrene is not caught early enough, the resulting treatment to stop the spread of the necrosis is often amputation. You might report one of these diagnoses with code E09.52 Drug or chemical induced diabetes mellitus with diabetic peripheral angiopathy with gangrene or E11.51 Type 2 diabetes mellitus with diabetic peripheral angiopathy without gangrene.

ICD-10-CM

LET'S CODE IT! SCENARIO

Brittany Hatthaway, a 53-year-old female, came to see Dr. DeRupo for her annual checkup. She is a type 1 insulin-dependent diabetic and has been feeling fine. There are no diabetic-related manifestations noted.

(continued)

Let's Code It!

Dr. DeRupo's notes state that Brittany has *type 1 diabetes mellitus* with *no complications.* When you turn to the Alphabetic Index, you see

Diabetes, diabetic (mellitus) (sugar) E11.9

When you turn to the Tabular List, you confirm:

✓4 **E11 Type 2 diabetes mellitus**

Oh, wait a minute. This code category is for type 2 diabetes. Dr. DeRupo's notes document that Brittany has type 1 diabetes. Turn the pages and review this whole section to see if you can find a more accurate code category. Did you find this code category?

✓4 **E10 Type 1 diabetes mellitus**

There is an INCLUDES note as well as an EXCLUDES1 notation listing several diagnoses. Take a minute to review them and determine if any apply to Brittany's condition. No, none of them do, so continue down and review all of the fourth-character choices. Which matches Dr. DeRupo's notes?

E10.9 Type 1 diabetes mellitus without complications

Perfect!

Diabetes-Related Drug Use

Non-Insulin Antidiabetic Drug Use

In the 2025 code set, there are new Use Additional Code notations for code categories: E08 Diabetes mellitus due to underlying condition; E11 Type 2 diabetes mellitus; and E13 Other specified diabetes mellitus.

***Use Additional** injectable non-insulin antidiabetic drugs (Z79.85)*

Z79.85 Long-term (current) use of injectable non-insulin antidiabetic drugs

Some of the drugs included in this category, known as injectable GLP-1 receptor agonists are:

- Dulaglutide (Trulicity)
- Exenatide (Byetta)
- Exenatide extended-release (Bydureon)
- Liraglutide (Victoza)
- Lixisenatide (Adlyxin)
- Injectable semaglutide (Ozempic)

Long-Term Drug Use

Long-Term Insulin Use

There are cases where a patient, who has been diagnosed with type 2 diabetes, gestational diabetes, or secondary diabetes, has been prescribed insulin on a regular basis. This is not a standard of care, so you will have to include a code stating this fact:

Z79.4 Long-term (current) use of insulin

You can see the notation at the beginning of the E11 Type 2 diabetes mellitus code category to remind you:

Use additional code **to identify control using: insulin (Z79.4) oral antidiabetic drugs (Z79.84) oral hypoglycemic drugs (Z79.84)**

Long-Term Hypoglycemic Use

There are now several new drugs, known as **hypoglycemics**. These medications are not insulin; however, they work to lower a patient's glycemic level. You may see names of drugs such as Orinase, Glucotrol, Avandia, or Glucophage in the physician's documentation. When a diabetic patient has been using one of these medications for a while, you will need to add a code:

Z79.84 Long-term (current) use of oral hypoglycemic drugs

Be careful not to confuse code Z79.84 with code Z79.4. Insulin and hypoglycemic drugs are different. And remember, both of these codes report that the use of the insulin or hypoglycemic drug is not a one-time or temporary treatment.

Hypoglycemics
Prescription, non-insulin medications designed to lower a patient's glycemic level.

CODING BITES

The code for long-term insulin use is not reported for patients with type 1 diabetes mellitus. Remember, type 1 DM is known as insulin-dependent diabetes, making Z79.4 unnecessary.

Long-Term Use of More Than One Type of Drug

For those patients who are prescribed both an insulin medication as well as an injectable antidiabetic (non-insulin) drug, report both Z79.4 and Z79.899 Other long-term (current) drug therapy.

When a patient is prescribed both an oral hypoglycemic (antidiabetic) drug and an injectable antidiabetic report both Z79.84 and Z79.899.

GUIDANCE CONNECTION

Read the ICD-10-CM Official Guidelines for Coding and Reporting, section **I. Conventions, General Coding Guidelines and Chapter-Specific Guidelines**, subsection **C. Chapter-Specific Coding Guidelines**, chapter **4. Endocrine, Nutritional, and Metabolic Diseases (E00–E89)**, subsections **a.3) Diabetes mellitus and the use of insulin and oral hypoglycemics** and **a.6)(a) Secondary diabetes mellitus and the use of insulin or hypoglycemic drugs**.

ICD-10-CM

YOU CODE IT! CASE STUDY

Alec Kustra, a 37-year-old male, was diagnosed with type 2 diabetes a year ago. Dr. Lockhart had prescribed tolbutamide to stimulate his pancreatic insulin release. However, 6 months ago, he became concerned that the medication was not working and started Alec on a regime of insulin injections. Alec is here today for Dr. Lockhart to check his insulin levels.

You Code It!

Go through the steps of coding, and determine the code or codes that should be reported for this encounter between Dr. Lockhart and Alec Kustra.

Step #1: Read the case carefully and completely.

Step #2: Abstract the scenario. Which main words or terms describe why the physician cared for the patient during this encounter?

Step #3: Are there any details missing or incomplete for which you would need to query the physician? [If so, ask your instructor.]

Step #4: Check for any relevant guidance, including reading all of the symbols and notations in the Tabular List and the appropriate sections of the Official Guidelines.

Step #5: Determine the correct diagnosis code or codes to explain why this encounter was medically necessary.

Step #6: Double-check your work.

(continued)

Answer:

Did you determine these to be the correct codes?

E11.9 **Type 2 diabetes mellitus without complications**
Z79.4 **Long-term (current) use of insulin**

9.3 Diabetes-Related Conditions

Hyperglycemia and Hypoglycemia

Hyperglycemia
Abnormally high levels of glucose.

Hypoglycemia
Abnormally low glucose levels.

A patient with **hyperglycemia** is *not* diagnosed with diabetes. Hyperglycemia, just like **hypoglycemia**, is a separate condition.

Chronic hyperglycemia may impair one's resistance to infection, resulting in diabetic skin problems and urinary tract infections. A diabetic patient that has hypoglycemia may have administered too much insulin or antidiabetic medication.

In the 2025 code set, there are three new codes to report hypoglycemia, specifically by the level of severity:

E16.A1	Hypoglycemia level 1
E16.A2	Hypoglycemia level 2
E16.A3	Hypoglycemia level 3

Of course, you need to read the documentation, but in addition to the physician's notes, it might be helpful to refer to the lab test results as well.

Hypoglycemia level 1 is identified as a glycemic level below 70 mg/dL in a diabetic patient. This is identified as an "alert" value to encourage behaviors that will help avoid more severe hypoglycemia. Hypoglycemia level 2 can be recognized by a glucose concentration of less than 54 mg/dL and the appearance of neuroglycopenic symptoms, such as nervousness, confusion, short temper, blurred vision, and difficulty walking. Hypoglycemia level 3 is evidenced by an altered mental state possibly accompanied by problems with physical function.

ICD-10-CM

LET'S CODE IT! SCENARIO

Jessica Gundersen, a 61-year-old female, has been feeling excessively tired and irritable. She tells Dr. Vickers that she has felt edgy and nervous while experiencing cold sweats and trembling. Dr. Vickers performs a glucose-screening test using a reagent strip, resulting in a reading of less than 45 mg/dL. He orders a lab test to confirm a diagnosis of reactive hypoglycemia and provides Jessica with a diet to follow and a referral to a nutritionist.

Let's Code It!

Jessica has been diagnosed with *reactive hypoglycemia*. Let's turn to the Alphabetic Index and look it up:

Hypoglycemia (spontaneous) E16.2

Read all the way down the indented list to find

Reactive (not drug-induced) E16.1

The Tabular List describes the code as

✓4 **E16** **Other disorders of pancreatic internal secretion**

(continued)

There are no notations or directives, so keep reading down the column.

E16.1 Other hypoglycemia

E16.2 Hypoglycemia, unspecified

How do you decide between these two codes? Let's think about this. Dr. Vickers *did* specify the type of hypoglycemia that Jessica has, so you cannot report that this detail was "unspecified." This eliminates E16.2 and confirms that E16.1 Other hypoglycemia is accurate.

Notice that the **EXCLUDES1** note under code E16.1 states that neither hypoglycemia in infant of diabetic mother (P70.1) nor neonatal hypoglycemia is to be reported with this code. Does it apply to Jessica's case? Dr. Vickers indicated that Jessica is an adult; therefore, it does not apply.

The correct diagnosis code for the encounter between Dr. Vickers and Jessica is this:

E16.1 Other hypoglycemia

Excellent!

Insulin Pumps

Technology has provided patients with an easier and more controlled manner by which to get their insulin: an insulin pump. However, nothing is perfect, so there may be a concern with the patient as a result of the insulin pump not working correctly.

Underdose of Insulin

It can be very dangerous for a patient to receive less than the proper amount of insulin, as prescribed by the physician, on schedule. If that occurs and is the reason the physician is caring for the patient at the encounter, your first-listed code should be this:

T85.614A Breakdown (mechanical) of insulin pump, initial encounter

Follow that code with the proper diabetes mellitus code and any other appropriate codes, including codes for any effects, or conditions, caused by the insulin underdose.

If the patient's ill health is caused by an underdose of insulin that the patient injects by hand (not using a pump), meaning that the patient is not taking the correct amount as often as it was prescribed, you might use the following code:

Z91.120 Patient's intentional underdosing of medication regimen due to financial hardship

Also note that beneath code Z91.12 and Z91.13 is a notation:

Code first **underdosing of medication (T36–T50) with fifth or sixth character 6**

This T code will enable you to report which specific medication was underdosed. So, in this example, you would also report this code:

T38.3X6D Underdosing of insulin and oral hypoglycemic (antidiabetic) drugs, subsequent encounter

GUIDANCE CONNECTION

Read the ICD-10-CM Official Guidelines for Coding and Reporting, section **I. Conventions, General Coding Guidelines and Chapter-Specific Guidelines**, subsection **C. Chapter-Specific Coding Guidelines**, chapter **4. Endocrine, Nutritional, and Metabolic Diseases (E00–E89)**, subsection **a.5) Complications due to insulin pump malfunction**.

YOU CODE IT! CASE STUDY

Tori Anderson, a 19-year-old female, was diagnosed with type 1 diabetes 2 years ago. Starting college, Tori kept forgetting to take her insulin as prescribed. She comes into the University Health Center because she feels dizzy, weak, and confused. Dr. Griffith, the on-call physician, finds her to have poor skin turgor and dry mucous membranes. He diagnoses her with dehydration caused by insulin deficiency and diabetes mellitus, type 1, uncontrolled.

(continued)

You Code It!

Go through the steps of coding, and determine the code or codes that should be reported for this encounter between Dr. Griffith and Tori Anderson.

Step #1: Read the case carefully and completely.

Step #2: Abstract the scenario. Which main words or terms describe why the physician cared for the patient during this encounter?

Step #3: Are there any details missing or incomplete for which you would need to query the physician? [If so, ask your instructor.]

Step #4: Check for any relevant guidance, including reading all of the symbols and notations in the Tabular List and the appropriate sections of the Official Guidelines.

Step #5: Determine the correct diagnosis code or codes to explain why this encounter was medically necessary.

Step #6: Double-check your work.

Answer:

Did you determine these to be the correct codes?

E86.0 **Dehydration**

E10.9 **Type 1 diabetes mellitus without complications**

T38.3X6A **Underdosing of insulin and oral hypoglycemic (antidiabetic) drugs, initial encounter**

Z91.138 **Patient's unintentional underdosing of medication regimen for other reason**

Overdose of Insulin

Patients with an insulin pump that malfunctions can dose with a higher quantity of insulin than prescribed by the attending physician. For such a case, you will use the following code (which is the same as the code for an underdose):

T85.614A **Breakdown (mechanical) of insulin pump, initial encounter**

Follow that code with a poisoning code, for example:

T38.3X1A **Poisoning by insulin and oral hypoglycemic (antidiabetic) drugs, accidental (unintentional), initial encounter**

Follow that code with the appropriate diabetes mellitus code and any other appropriate codes, including the codes identifying the reaction or conditions caused by the overdose.

If the patient delivers a dose of insulin manually and suffers an overdose, you will code it the same way you do any other poisoning, including the determination of the cause of the overdose (such as accident, attempted suicide, or assault). Unless the health concern with the patient is an adverse reaction to the insulin and not related to the actual dosage, you will not use the code reporting therapeutic usage.

9.4 Other Endocrine Gland Disorders

Diabetes Insipidus

Another type of diabetes that few people have heard of is *diabetes insipidus (DI)*. DI is a disorder of water metabolism that is the result of an antidiuretic hormone (ADH) deficiency. Intracranial neoplastic or metastatic lesions, hypophysectomy or other neurosurgery, or skull fractures or other head trauma that damages the neurohypophyseal structures can all incite DI. The condition also can result from infection. DI also is known as *pituitary diabetes insipidus* and is coded using E23.2 from the subsection for disorders of the pituitary gland.

Nephrogenic DI, another form of DI, is a very rare congenital disturbance of water metabolism resulting from a renal tubular resistance to vasopressin. Interestingly, it is not coded from the congenital anomalies but is reported using code N25.1 Nephrogenic diabetes insipidus.

YOU CODE IT! CASE STUDY

Roy Holvang, a 25-year-old male, comes to see Dr. Fletcher with complaints of extreme thirst and muscle weakness. During examination, Dr. Fletcher identifies that Roy has poor tissue turgor, dry mucous membranes, and hypotension. UA results show urine of low osmolality at 75 mOsm/kg. Dr. Fletcher diagnoses Roy with diabetes insipidus and prescribes vasopressin IM qid.

You Code It!

Go through the steps of coding, and determine the code or codes that should be reported for this encounter between Dr. Fletcher and Roy Holvang.

Step #1: Read the case carefully and completely.

Step #2: Abstract the scenario. Which main words or terms describe why the physician cared for the patient during this encounter?

Step #3: Are there any details missing or incomplete for which you would need to query the physician? [If so, ask your instructor.]

Step #4: Check for any relevant guidance, including reading all of the symbols and notations in the Tabular List and the appropriate sections of the Official Guidelines.

Step #5: Determine the correct diagnosis code or codes to explain why this encounter was medically necessary.

Step #6: Double-check your work.

Answer:

Did you determine this to be the correct code?

E23.2 Diabetes insipidus

Good job!

Cushing's Syndrome

Cushing's syndrome is caused by excessive production of corticotropin (ACTH) in the hypothalamus and too much secretion from the adenohypophysis (pituitary gland). This may be caused by a tumor in another organ affecting this process–possibly a bronchogenic tumor or a malignant neoplasm of the pancreas. Approximately 30% of such cases are the result of a benign neoplasm of the adrenal gland.

Cushing's Syndrome
A condition resulting from the hyperproduction of corticosteroids, most often caused by an adrenal cortex tumor or a tumor of the pituitary gland.

Cushing's syndrome may cause diabetes mellitus, hypokalemia (low potassium in the blood), pathologic fractures, slow wound healing, hypertension, irritability, and other conditions. Lab tests for plasma steroid levels measured by 24-hour urine samples can be used to confirm a diagnosis of Cushing's syndrome. An adrenal tumor can be seen on an ultrasound, CT scan, or angiography, while MRI and CT scans can illuminate the presence of a pituitary tumor.

Administration of radiation therapy, drug therapy with a medication such as aminoglutethimide, or surgery to remove the tumor can be successful to control or reverse the effects of Cushing's syndrome. ICD-10-CM code category E24 Cushing's syndrome requires an additional character to provide more specific information about the condition.

EXAMPLES

E24.0 Pituitary-dependent Cushing's disease

E24.2 Drug-induced Cushing's disease
Use additional code **for adverse effect, if applicable, to identify drug (T36–T50 with fifth or sixth character 5)**

E24.4 Alcohol-induced pseudo-Cushing's disease

As you can see, you will need to abstract additional details related to the diagnosis of Cushing's disease in order to determine a specific code.

Postprocedural Endocrine System Complications

Due to the incredible connections between all aspects of the human body, there are times when a procedure employed to treat one condition results in a malfunction elsewhere in the body.

Should a malfunction in the endocrine system be a documented postprocedural complication, you must report this using a designated code category: E89 Postprocedural endocrine and metabolic complications and disorders, not elsewhere classified.

CODING BITES

The postprocedural time frame is generally considered the time from the surgical procedure's conclusion until the physician releases the patient from care. This typically aligns with the global period standard for the specific procedure provided.

EXAMPLES

E89.0 Postprocedural hypothyroidism

E89.3 Postprocedural hypopituitarism

E89.5 Postprocedural testicular hypofunction

These complications may be predictable. For example, it would be expected, after the surgical removal of the patient's thyroid, that hypothyroidism would develop. However, this is not always the case.

9.5 Nutritional Deficiencies and Weight Factors

Nutritional Deficiencies

My mother said it a thousand times, as do physicians and the media . . . eat good food so you can get all your vitamins. Even with the large number of supplements available on the market, individuals still lack certain vitamins and other vital nutrients required for a healthy body.

Vitamin A deficiencies can manifest with diagnosed ophthalmological conditions. You will need to know this when reporting the vitamin A deficiency diagnosis. Two examples:

E50.0 Vitamin A deficiency with conjunctival xerosis
E50.4 Vitamin A deficiency with keratomalacia

Niacin, riboflavin, calcium, magnesium . . . and so many more deficiencies are reported from the Other Nutritional Deficiencies (E50–E64) subsection of the ICD-10-CM code book's *Chapter 4: Endocrine, Nutritional, and Metabolic Diseases (E00–E89).*

E52 Niacin deficiency [pellagra]
E56.0 Deficiency of vitamin E
E61.1 Iron deficiency

CODING BITES

Remember, in earlier chapters you learned the difference between a manifestation and a sequela. When a patient is diagnosed with a sequela of malnutrition or other nutritional deficiency, report the condition (the sequela) first, followed by a code from the E64 code category:

E64.0	Sequela of protein-calorie malnutrition
E64.1	Sequela of vitamin A deficiency
E64.2	Sequela of vitamin C deficiency
E64.3	Sequela of rickets
E64.8	Sequela of other nutritional deficiencies

ICD-10-CM

YOU CODE IT! CASE STUDY

Shakeia and Robert Malabwa just adopted Benjamin, a 3-year-old male, from an orphanage in Africa. They brought him in to see Dr. D'Onofrio, a pediatrician, for his first American checkup. After reviewing what was available about his history, and a complete physical examination, Dr. D'Onofrio diagnosed Ben with moderate protein-energy malnutrition. They sat together and discussed a treatment plan and diet to help him improve. Lactose intolerance can manifest, so he suggested that they avoid foods with lactose.

You Code It!

Go through the steps of coding, and determine the code or codes that should be reported for this encounter between Dr. D'Onofrio and Benjamin Malabwa.

Step #1:	Read the case carefully and completely.
Step #2:	Abstract the scenario. Which main words or terms describe why the physician cared for the patient during this encounter?
Step #3:	Are there any details missing or incomplete for which you would need to query the physician? [If so, ask your instructor.]
Step #4:	Check for any relevant guidance, including reading all of the symbols and notations in the Tabular List and the appropriate sections of the Official Guidelines.
Step #5:	Determine the correct diagnosis code or codes to explain why this encounter was medically necessary.
Step #6:	Double-check your work.

Answer:

Did you determine the correct diagnosis code?

E44.0 Moderate protein-calorie malnutrition

Obesity

The definitions of *overweight*, *obese*, and *morbidly obese* can get lost in societal norms and self-perception. Of course, the health care industry has its own official determinations of these conditions, further specified by reporting the patient's body mass index (BMI).

Overweight merely means weighing too much. This can be a reference to the individual's muscles, bones, fat, or fluid retention when calculated along with the person's height. This condition is calculated as a BMI of 25 to 29.9 in adults.

Obesity is a condition calculated as a BMI of 30 to 38.9 in adults. Typically, a person becomes obese when more calories are consumed than expended. While some critics believe extra pounds are caused only by eating too much and not exercising enough, the facts are that one's genetics and current medications (including herbal supplements) also can influence this condition. New codes for 2025 require more detail with specific classifications for the severity of obesity, identified as class 1, 2, or 3.

Obesity class 1 is low-risk, with no complications and a BMI measure of 30–34.9.

Obesity class 2 is considered moderate-risk, with a BMI of 35–39.9, and the patient exhibiting one or more obesity-related complications.

Obesity class 3 identifies a patient with a BMI of 40 or higher considered high-risk, experiencing one or more severe obesity-related complications.

Being diagnosed as obese is a true health condition that not only can result in self-esteem problems and social anxiety but also may increase the risk of developing complications such as hypertension, coronary heart disease, gallbladder disease, bone and joint problems, liver concerns, and kidney malfunction. As you may know, these complications can lead to chronic conditions including: diabetes, heart disease, arthritis, stroke, and even certain malignancies.

Morbid obesity is diagnosed when a patient's current overweight status increases to the extent that it actually interferes with normal, daily activities. This condition is calculated as a BMI over 39.

EXAMPLES

code category E66 Overweight and obesity

Use additional code **to identify Body Mass Index (BMI) if known, for adults (Z68.1–Z68.45) or pediatrics (Z65.-)**

E66.01	Morbid (severe) obesity due to excess calories
E66.09	Other obesity due to excess calories
E66.1	Drug-induced obesity
E66.2	Morbid (severe) obesity with alveolar hypoventilation
E66.3	Overweight
E66.8	Other obesity E66.811 Obesity, class 1 E66.812 Obesity, class 2 E66.813 Obesity, class 3
E66.9	Obesity, unspecified

CODING BITES

Several different types of health care professionals, such as a dietitian or a nutritionist, may be involved in the care of a patient determined to be overweight, obese, or morbidly obese. However, the first time this diagnosis code is reported, it may be coded only from physician documentation.

As you can see, ICD-10-CM reminds you to use an additional code to specify the patient's BMI.

Body Mass Index

It is important for health care professionals to determine specifically what is a healthy amount of body fat and what falls or rises to an unhealthy level. Body mass index (BMI) is a calculation using an individual's actual weight and current height to determine a workable measure of body fat. However, some people, such as athletes, may have a BMI that indicates they are overweight even though there is no excess body fat. This can occur because BMI does not actually measure body fat but instead determines a ratio with which to work. BMI is just an indicator of potential health risks related to an individual's being outside the normal weight range.

BMI ranges are listed differently for adults than they are for children and teens. The pediatric ranges, used for individuals aged 2 to 20 years, are based on the growth charts of the Centers for Disease Control and take into account the normal differences in body fat for various ages as well as differences between boys and girls.

Z68 Body Mass Index [BMI]

Adult BMI codes range from Z68.1–Z68.45. The pediatric BMI code is

Z68.5- Body Mass Index [BMI] pediatric

GUIDANCE CONNECTION

BMI codes should only be assigned when the associated diagnosis (such as overweight or obesity) meets the definition of a reportable diagnosis. Read the ICD-10-CM Official Guidelines for Coding and Reporting, section **III. Reporting Additional Diagnoses.**

Do not assign BMI codes during pregnancy. Read the ICD-10-CM Official Guidelines for Coding and Reporting, section **I. B.14 Documentation by clinicians other than the patient's provider.**

Underweight

With all the discussion regarding how many people in the United States are overweight or clinically obese, the opposite–being underweight–also can cause health concerns. Unlike the codes for overweight conditions, codes for reporting an abnormal weight loss or underweight condition are listed in the ICD-10-CM code book's *Chapter 19: Symptoms, Signs, and Abnormal Clinical and Laboratory Findings, Not Elsewhere Classified (R00–R99)*. In certain cases, the BMI also will need to be reported.

EXAMPLES

R63.4 Abnormal weight loss

R63.6 Underweight
Use additional code **to identify Body Mass Index (BMI) if known (Z68.-)**

When a patient is diagnosed with anorexia, you may need more information from the physician before determining the correct code.

R63.0 Anorexia

This is used when the cause of the anorexia has not been determined as organic [physiological] or nonorganic [psychological]. However, once a psychiatrist, or other qualified health-care professional, has confirmed this as a chronic condition, the documentation must reveal the type and severity of the patient's condition. Severity, reported with an additional character, will be measured as Mild, Moderate, Severe, Extreme, or in Remission.

CODING BITES

While you may see issues of overweight status accompanying diagnoses such as diabetes mellitus or hypertension, in cases of underweight patients, be alert to initial or additional diagnoses of malnutrition.

F50.0- Anorexia nervosa F50.01- Anorexia Nervosa, Restricting Type F50.02- Anorexia Nervosa, Binge Eating/ Purging Type

F50.2- Bulimia nervosa

F50.8- Other eating disorders

YOU CODE IT! CASE STUDY

PATIENT: Eric Micoh

REASON FOR CONSULTATION: Preoperative evaluation for bariatric surgery

HISTORY OF PRESENT ILLNESS: The patient is a 47-year-old morbidly obese male with a BMI of 46.3 and multiple medical problems including hypertension, diabetes, and dyslipidemia. He has been overweight most of his life. The patient was considering bariatric surgery and he is planning to go for a lap band procedure. He says that snoring is not a very common complaint of his wife. He snores mainly when he drinks; otherwise, it could be soft snoring or sometimes no snoring at all. There was no mention of witnessed apneas. He does not wake himself up choking or gasping for air. He is a very quiet sleeper with not much tossing and turning. He wakes up feeling refreshed for the most part, unless he sleeps for 5 hours or so. He goes on with his day with no difficulty as far as excessive daytime sleepiness or fatigue. He is only tired if he had a really busy long day. His Epworth sleepiness score today was between 5 and 6. He has never fallen asleep behind the wheel or got himself in an accident. His weight has been steady. He has been

(continued)

overweight since he was 15 years old. He never had any symptoms suggestive of cataplexy, sleep paralysis, or hypnagogic or hypnopompic hallucinations. He denies any symptoms of restless legs. No symptoms of parasomnia. No sleep onset or sleep maintenance insomnia.

ASSESSMENT AND PLAN:

1. Even though this patient does not have any of the cardinal symptoms of obstructive sleep apnea including snoring, witnessed apneas, or excessive daytime sleepiness, he does have physical features that increase the risk for sleep apnea including obesity, large neck circumference, crowded airway with a high Mallampati class, as well as his multiple associated cardiovascular and metabolic disorders including hypertension that is not very well controlled on different blood pressure medicines, diabetes, and dyslipidemia.
2. I had a long discussion with him today about the need for a sleep study to rule out obstructive sleep apnea, even though he does not have the classic symptoms. I also explained to him the risks in the perioperative period for patients with obstructive sleep apnea that has not been treated. At this point, he wants to wait and think about it as well as talk it over with the bariatric surgery team. He does not think he has sleep apnea. He does not think he would be able to perform the sleep study, as he will have a hard time sleeping outside his house.
3. I explained to him the risks involved with untreated moderate-to-severe obstructive sleep apnea, including worsening cardiovascular disease, arrhythmias, risk of stroke, and increased overall mortality.
4. I also mentioned to him that there is a possibility of doing a portable sleep study at home if that would be something he is willing to pursue.
5. In the meantime, he should continue to lose weight, avoid alcohol and sedatives, exercise routinely, and avoid driving if drowsy.
6. We will follow up with him as needed if he is willing to pursue this further.

You Code It!

Read this evaluation of Eric Micoh and determine the diagnosis code or codes to report.

Step #1: Read the case carefully and completely.

Step #2: Abstract the scenario. Which main words or terms describe why the physician cared for the patient during this encounter?

Step #3: Are there any details missing or incomplete for which you would need to query the physician? [If so, ask your instructor.]

Step #4: Check for any relevant guidance, including reading all of the symbols and notations in the Tabular List and the appropriate sections of the Official Guidelines.

Step #5: Determine the correct diagnosis code or codes to explain why this encounter was medically necessary.

Step #6: Double-check your work.

Answer:

Did you determine these to be the correct codes?

E66.01 **Morbid (severe) obesity due to excess calories**

E11.9 **Type 2 diabetes mellitus without complications**

I10 **Essential (primary) hypertension**

E78.5 **Hyperlipidemia, unspecified**

Z68.42 **Body mass index [BMI] 45.0–49.9, adult**

9.6 Metabolic Disorders

When you eat, it is your metabolism that processes nutrition into energy. The chemicals in the digestive system portion out glucose and acids from the carbohydrates, fats, and proteins in the food. This process is known as *metabolization*. The energy created by this process can be used right away—for example, when someone eats before taking a test or running a race. If the body doesn't need the energy at this time, the tissues in the liver and the muscular system, as well as the adipose (body fat), can store it for future use.

Dysfunction of the metabolic processes can interfere with the various systems of the body getting what they need to work properly. This may be realized as too little of a chemical needed, such as when the pancreas cannot create enough insulin (a condition known as *diabetes mellitus*). You have already learned about what havoc can be caused in the other organs and systems when this disorder continues. Metabolic disorders can also result in too much of a chemical being present in the body. For example, hyperchloremia is an excessive level of chloride anion in the blood and can cause tachycardia (rapid heartbeat), hypertension, dyspnea (shortness of breath), and agitation.

The long list of metabolic diagnoses includes:

- Acid lipase disease
- Amyloidosis
- Barth's syndrome
- Central pontine myelinolysis
- Farber's disease
- G6PD deficiency
- Gangliosidoses
- Hunter's syndrome
- Hyperoxaluria
- Lesch-Nyhan syndrome
- Lipid storage diseases
- Metabolic myopathies
- Mitochondrial myopathies
- Mucolipidoses
- Mucopolysaccharidoses (MPS)
- Oxalosis
- Pompe's disease
- Trimethylaminuria
- Type I glycogen storage disease
- Urea cycle disorder

Let's take a look at some of the more common metabolic conditions, and review the details required to accurately code them.

Cystic Fibrosis

Cystic fibrosis (CF) is a hereditary malfunction of the secretory glands. Many laypeople think of this as a malfunction of the pulmonary system. However, as you can see by the code descriptions, the effects of this genetic condition reach to other body systems as well.

A defect in the CFTR gene affects the glands that produce mucus and sweat, resulting in the creation of thick, sticky mucus and very salty sweat. There are manifestations that can develop in the respiratory, digestive, and reproductive systems, as well as other maladies.

E84.0 **Cystic fibrosis with pulmonary manifestations**
Use additional code **to identify any infectious organism present, such as Pseudomonas (B96.5)**

E84.11 **Meconium ileus in cystic fibrosis**

E84.19 **Cystic fibrosis with other intestinal manifestations**

E84.8 **Cystic fibrosis with other manifestations**

Other manifestations, reported with E84.8, include male neonates born without a vas deferens or females who may have an overproduction of mucus blocking the cervix.

Dehydration may result due to the large loss of salt in the CF patient's perspiration; clubbing and low bone density may both occur later in life.

YOU CODE IT! CASE STUDY

Rachel Ward brought her 3-year-old son Ethan to his pediatrician, Dr. Inger. She was very distressed because Ethan had eruptions on his arms, legs, and face that appeared after he had spent the day at the beach. She also had noticed that his urine appeared to be reddish in color. Dr. Inger examined Ethan and discovered that he had splenomegaly (enlargement of the spleen). The blood test came back positive for hemolytic anemia. Both of these conditions are signs of erythropoietic porphyria, also known as Gunther's disease. Dr. Inger diagnosed Ethan with this condition.

You Code It!

Go through the steps of coding, and determine the code or codes that should be reported for this encounter between Dr. Inger and Ethan Ward.

Step #1: Read the case carefully and completely.

Step #2: Abstract the scenario. Which main words or terms describe why the physician cared for the patient during this encounter?

Step #3: Are there any details missing or incomplete for which you would need to query the physician? [If so, ask your instructor.]

Step #4: Check for any relevant guidance, including reading all of the symbols and notations in the Tabular List and the appropriate sections of the Official Guidelines.

Step #5: Determine the correct diagnosis code or codes to explain why this encounter was medically necessary.

Step #6: Double-check your work.

Answer:

Did you determine this to be the correct code?

E80.0 Hereditary erythropoietic porphyria

Good job!

Lactose Intolerance

If you know anyone with a lactose intolerance, you understand how challenging this can be to quality of life. While the symptoms of this condition evidence in the digestive system, this is a metabolic disorder because a lactose intolerance develops after the small intestine is unable to digest lactose due to abnormally low production of lactase (also known as lactase deficiency).

As you have learned many times, while this sounds like a complete diagnostic statement, you will need to abstract the type of lactase deficiency before you will be able to determine the accurate code.

- *Congenital lactase deficiency* is an extremely rare, genetic disorder in which there is a failure of the small intestine to produce any, or enough, of the lactase enzyme. This diagnosis is reported with code E73.0 Congenital lactase deficiency.
- *Secondary lactase deficiency* manifests when an infection or disease causes the small intestine to malfunction in this way. These cases can be reversed with successful treatment of the underlying disease. This diagnosis is reported with code E73.1 Secondary lactase deficiency.
- *Other lactose intolerance* may be prompted by *developmental lactase deficiency*, a short-term condition seen in premature neonates, or *primary lactase deficiency (lactase nonpersistence)*, the most frequently seen type of lactase deficiency. Typically, in these patients, the small intestine's production of lactase begins to decline around 2 years of age. Any of these diagnoses are reported with code E73.8 Other lactose intolerance.

Chapter Summary

The glands of the endocrine system produce and release various types of hormones that are used by numerous organs throughout the body—all a part of the function of a healthy body. When a component of this system does not function properly, the harm can cascade and reveal itself as signs and symptoms evident with other body systems, such as the urinary system or reproductive system. Diabetes mellitus is probably the most common of the conditions and diseases affecting the endocrine system. From the hypothalamus of the brain to the genitals, every part of this system, like all of the others that make up the human body, can malfunction or become diseased.

Organs Included in the Endocrine System

Organs Included in the Endocrine System

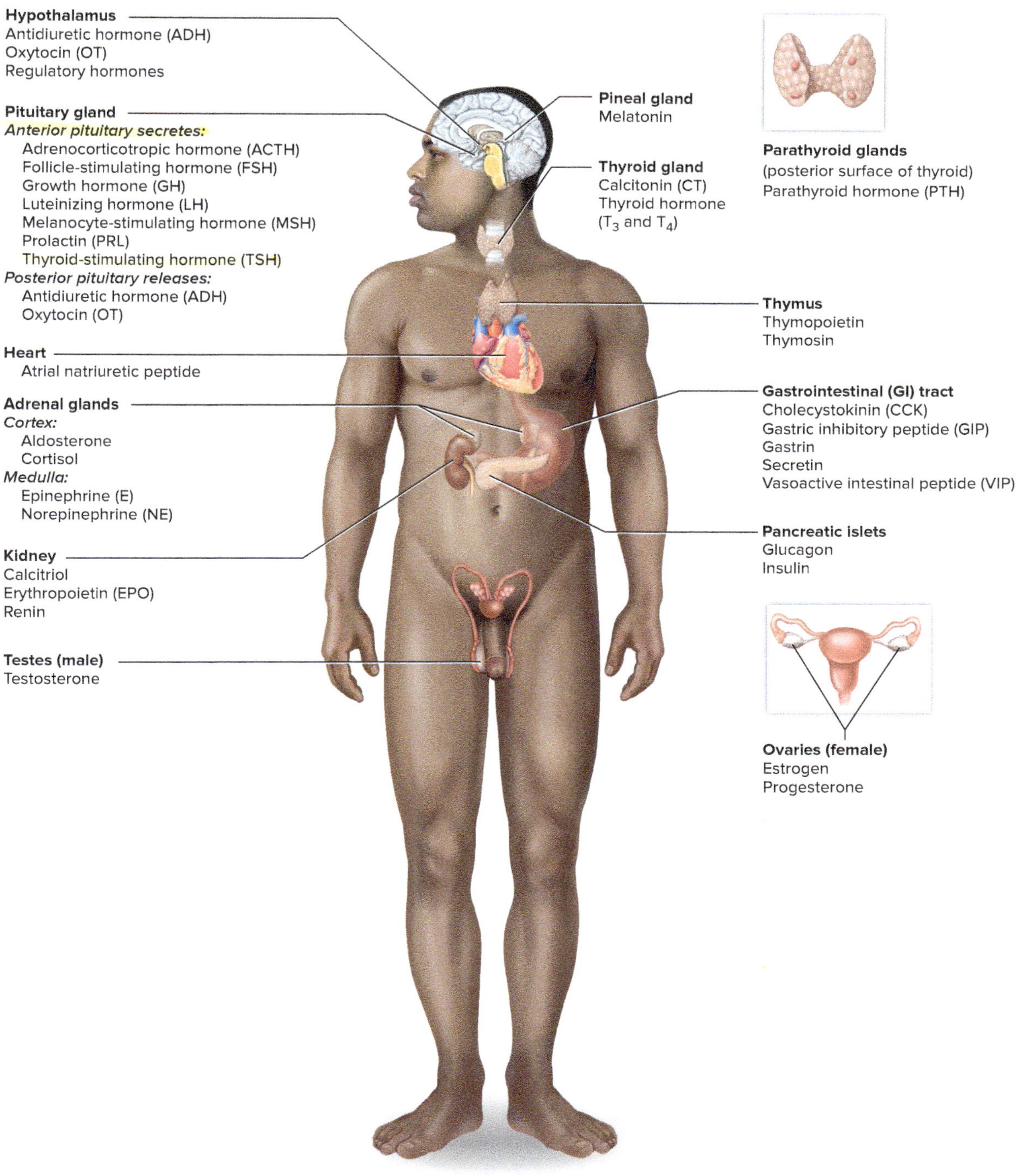

CHAPTER 9 REVIEW
Coding Endocrine Conditions

Let's Check It! Terminology

Match each key term to the appropriate definition.

1. **LO 9.2** A form of diabetes mellitus with a gradual onset.
2. **LO 9.2** A chronic systemic disease that results from insulin deficiency or resistance and causes the body to improperly metabolize carbohydrates, proteins, and fats.
3. **LO 9.2** A temporary diabetes mellitus occurring during pregnancy.
4. **LO 9.3** Abnormally high levels of glucose.
5. **LO 9.2** Excessive thirst.
6. **LO 9.2** Diabetes caused by medication or another condition or disease.
7. **LO 9.2** Excessive urination.
8. **LO 9.2** Abnormal lipoprotein metabolism.
9. **LO 9.3** Abnormally low glucose levels.
10. **LO 9.1** A condition in which the thyroid converts energy more slowly than normal, resulting in an otherwise unexplained weight gain and fatigue.
11. **LO 9.2** A sudden onset of insulin deficiency.
12. **LO 9.4** A condition resulting from the hyperproduction of corticosteroids, most often caused by an adrenal cortex tumor or a tumor of the pituitary gland.
13. **LO 9.1** Four small glands situated on the back of the thyroid gland that secrete parathyroid hormone.
14. **LO 9.1** Two lobes located in the neck that reach around the trachea laterally and connect anteriorly by an isthmus.
15. **LO 9.3** Prescription, non-insulin medications designed to lower a patient's glycemic level.

A. Cushing's Syndrome
B. Diabetes Mellitus
C. Dyslipidemia
D. Gestational Diabetes Mellitus (GDM)
E. Hyperglycemia
F. Hypoglycemia
G. Hypoglycemics
H. Hypothyroidism
I. Parathyroid Glands
J. Polydipsia
K. Polyuria
L. Secondary DM
M. Thyroid gland
N. Type 1 DM
O. Type 2 DM

Let's Check It! Concepts

Choose the most appropriate answer for each of the following questions.

1. **LO 9.3** Daniel Gupta is seen at his physician's office with a previous lab test result of positive for hyperglycemia. Dr. Ansewa writes in his chart that his diagnosis is suspected diabetes mellitus. The correct diagnosis code would report
   - **a.** diabetes mellitus with unspecified complication.
   - **b.** hyperglycemia.
   - **c.** hyperglycemia; diabetes mellitus uncomplicated.
   - **d.** diabetes mellitus with specified complication.
2. **LO 9.2** Karin is diagnosed with diabetes mellitus, type 2, with Kimmelstiel-Wilson disease. What is the correct code for this diagnosis?
   - **a.** E11.00
   - **b.** E11.01
   - **c.** E11.21
   - **d.** E11.29
3. **LO 9.2** Diabetic retinopathy may be manifested in all of the following *except*
   - **a.** background.
   - **b.** maculopathy.
   - **c.** proliferative.
   - **d.** neurologic.
4. **LO 9.2** Gestational diabetes is a condition that can affect only an individual
   - **a.** over the age of 65.
   - **b.** under the age of 4.
   - **c.** who is pregnant.
   - **d.** with hypertension.
5. **LO 9.5** What are the correct codes for a patient with type 1 DM who is overweight and has been diagnosed with Refsum's disease?
   - **a.** E10.51, E66.09, G60.8
   - **b.** E11.9, E66.3, G60.2
   - **c.** E11.49, E66.01, G60.0
   - **d.** E10.9, E66.3, G60.1

6. **LO 9.1** Amanda is being seen today for her hypothyroidism, which was induced when she took sulfonamide as prescribed by her physician, initial encounter. What is/are the correct code(s) for this condition?
   a. E03.2, T37.0X1A **b.** T37.0X5A, E03.2 **c.** E03.2, T37.0X5A **d.** T37.0X5A
7. **LO 9.1** When a patient has ________, the thyroid converts energy more slowly than normal, resulting in an otherwise unexplained weight gain and fatigue.
   a. hypothroidism **b.** myxedema **c.** hyperthyroidism **d.** thyroiditis
8. **LO 9.4** Which of the following conditions is a disorder of water metabolism that is the result of an ADH deficiency?
   a. type I DM **b.** diabetes insipidus **c.** secondary DM **d.** gestational DM
9. **LO 9.5** When the patient is diagnosed with obesity, their body mass will be between
   a. 20 and 24.9. **b.** 25 and 29.9. **c.** 30 and 38.9. **d.** 40 and 45.0.
10. **LO 9.6** Which of the following is a metabolic diagnosis?
   a. G6PD deficiency **b.** mucopolysaccharidoses **c.** hyperoxaluria **d.** all of these

Let's Check It! Guidelines

Refer to the Official Guidelines and fill in the blanks according to Chapter 4, Endocrine, Nutritional, and Metabolic Diseases, Chapter-Specific Coding Guidelines.

T85.6-	not	T85.6-	E08–E13
body system	E13	T38.3X6-	age
E09	T38.3X1-	combination	Z79
puberty	E89.1	temporarily	E11.-
	type	E08	

1. The diabetes mellitus codes are ________ codes that include the type of diabetes mellitus, the ________ affected, and the complications affecting that body system.
2. Assign as many codes from categories ________ as needed to identify all of the associated conditions that the patient has.
3. The ________ of a patient is not the sole determining factor, though most type 1 diabetics develop the condition before reaching ________.
4. If the ________ of diabetes mellitus is not documented in the medical record, the default is ________, type 2 diabetes mellitus.
5. An underdose of insulin due to an insulin pump failure should be assigned to a code from subcategory ________, Mechanical complication of other specified internal and external prosthetic devices, implants and grafts, that specifies the type of pump malfunction, as the principal or first-listed code, followed by code ________, Underdosing of insulin and oral hypoglycemic [antidiabetic] drugs.
6. The principal or first-listed code for an encounter due to an insulin pump malfunction resulting in an overdose of insulin should also be ________, Mechanical complication of other specified internal and external prosthetic devices, implants and grafts, followed by code ________, Poisoning by insulin and oral hypoglycemic [antidiabetic] drugs, accidental (unintentional).
7. Codes under categories ________, Diabetes mellitus due to underlying condition, ________, Drug or chemical induced diabetes mellitus, and ________, Other specified diabetes mellitus, identify complications/manifestations associated with secondary diabetes mellitus.
8. For patients with secondary diabetes mellitus who routinely use insulin or hypoglycemic drugs, or injectable non-insulin drugs, additional code(s) from category _____ should be assigned to identify long-term (current) use of insulin or oral hypoglycemic drugs.
9. Code Z79.4 should ________ be assigned if insulin is given ________ to bring a secondary diabetic patient's blood sugar under control during an encounter.
10. For postpancreatectomy diabetes mellitus (lack of insulin due to the surgical removal of all or part of the pancreas), assign code ________, Postprocedural hypoinsulinemia.

Let's Check It! Rules and Regulations

Please answer the following questions from the knowledge you have gained after reading this chapter.

1. **LO 9.1** Discuss Graves' disease. When you look up Graves' disease in the Alphabetic Index, where does it send you?
2. **LO 9.2** Explain the difference between diabetes mellitus type 1 and diabetes mellitus type 2; include the ICD-10-CM category code for each.
3. **LO 9.3** How would you code an overdose of insulin caused by a malfunction of an insulin pump?
4. **LO 9.4** Explain Cushing's syndrome, including the ICD-10-CM code category as well as an example of another diagnosis that may result from having Cushing's.
5. **LO 9.6** What is cystic fibrosis, and what gene is defective? Include an example of where manifestations can appear.

YOU CODE IT! Basics

First, identify the main term in the following diagnoses; then code the diagnosis.

Example: Diabetes mellitus, type 1, with dermatitis:

a. main term: *diabetes* **b.** diagnosis *E10.620*

1. Endemic hypothyroid cretinism:
   a. main term: ______ **b.** diagnosis: ______
2. Diabetes mellitus with hyperglycemia:
   a. main term: ______ **b.** diagnosis: ______
3. Abscess of the thyroid:
   a. main term: ______ **b.** diagnosis: ______
4. Type I glycogen storage disease:
   a. main term: ______ **b.** diagnosis: ______
5. Urea cycle metabolism disorder:
   a. main term: ______ **b.** diagnosis: ______
6. Thyroid nodules with thyrotoxicosis:
   a. main term: ______ **b.** diagnosis: ______
7. Hashimoto's disease:
   a. main term: ______ **b.** diagnosis: ______
8. 5-alpha-reductase deficiency:
   a. main term: ______ **b.** diagnosis: ______
9. Wernicke's encephalopathy:
   a. main term: ______ **b.** diagnosis: ______
10. Hartnup's disease:
    a. main term: ______ **b.** diagnosis: ______
11. Beta hyperlipoproteinemia:
    a. main term: ______ **b.** diagnosis: ______
12. Cystic fibrosis with intestinal manifestations:
    a. main term: ______ **b.** diagnosis: ______
13. Respiratory acidosis:
    a. main term: ______ **b.** diagnosis: ______
14. Postprocedural hypoparathyroidism:
    a. main term: ______ **b.** diagnosis: ______
15. Dysmetabolic syndrome X:
    a. main term: ______ **b.** diagnosis: ______

YOU CODE IT! Practice

Using the techniques described in this chapter, carefully read through the case studies and determine the most accurate ICD-10-CM code(s) and external cause code(s), if appropriate, for each case study.

1. Jason Peak, a 33-year-old male, comes to see Dr. James with the complaint that he is having difficulty sleeping, is sweating a lot, and has diarrhea. Dr. James completes an examination and notes muscle weakness and skin warmth with moistness. Dr. James also notes eyelid retraction with exophthalmos. Jason is diagnosed with Graves' disease.

(continued)

2. Pauline Allyson, a 2-week-old female, is brought in by her mother to see her pediatrician, Dr. Goldburg. Pauline is having feeding difficulties with vomiting. She also has diarrhea. Dr. Goldburg notes the child is failing to thrive, as well as having hepatosplenomegaly and abdominal distention. Pauline is admitted to the hospital, where lab tests confirm the absence of lysosomal lipase acid (LIPA). Pauline is diagnosed with Wolman's disease.
3. Joyce Meadows, a 42-year-old female, was found unconscious by her husband, George, who rushed his wife to the nearest ED. Dr. Herald asked about her medical history, and George said she was diagnosed with type 2 diabetes about 3 years ago. After lab work, Joyce is admitted in a diabetic hypoglycemic coma.
4. Richard Sullivan, a 12-year-old male, presents with the complaint of tiredness. Richard is accompanied by his mother. Mrs. Sullivan tells Dr. Gilbert that Richard has been clumsy lately and seems confused. After a thorough examination, Dr. Gilbert notes slight muscle stiffness and Kayser–Fleischer rings bilaterally. Richard is admitted to Weston Hospital, where a liver biopsy confirmed the diagnosis of Wilson's disease.
5. April Sundell, a 48-year-old female, presents today with the complaint of generally being "out of sorts" or a feeling of uneasiness. Dr. Loveichelle notes muscle weakness and mild hyperventilation. The laboratory results confirm the diagnosis of hyperkalemia.
6. Latoya Nexsen, a 61-year-old female with diabetes type 1, presents today with the complaint that her left lower leg is cold and she has a sore that won't heal. Dr. Benson notes gangrene in Latoya's left extremity and admits her to Weston Hospital. After a thorough physical exam, lab workup, and an angiography, Latoya is diagnosed with atherosclerosis and gangrene of the left lower extremity due to type 1 diabetes mellitus.
7. Lee Summers, a 3-year-old male, is brought in by his parents for a checkup. The parents have no specific concerns. Lee does have a history of ear infections and colds. Dr. Shirley, his pediatrician, notes a prominent forehead, a flattened nose bridge, and a slightly enlarged tongue. Dr. Shirley completes a urine test, which reveals the presence of mucopolysaccharides. Lee is admitted to the hospital, where further laboratory tests confirm the diagnosis of Hunter's syndrome.
8. Loretta Sims, a 14-year-old female, presents today with the complaint of abdominal bloating and cramps with vomiting. Mrs. Sims, her mother, says this usually occurs shortly after Loretta has drunk milk or eaten yogurt. Dr. Albany completes an examination and the hydrogen breath test confirms the diagnosis of primary lactose intolerance.
9. Billy Siau, an 8-month-old male with a congenital cataract, was referred to an ophthalmologist by his pediatrician, Dr. Wilberly. Billy and his mother present today to discuss the results of Billy's tests. Dr. Wilberly also notes that Billy has hypotonia and below-normal reflexes. The ophthalmologist's report confirms glaucoma. Dr. Wilberly diagnoses Billy with Lowe's syndrome.
10. Anita Kucherin, a 27-year-old female, is at 29-week gestation. This is Anita's first baby and she has not felt the baby move all day, so she presents to the ED. Anita was diagnosed with diabetes type 2 approximately 3 years ago. Anita states she has tried to keep her diabetes under control. Anita is admitted to the hospital for observation.
11. James Bucklew, a 38-year-old male, presents for the results of the blood tests taken last week. Dr. Walter documents central obesity, hypertension, decreased serum HDL cholesterol (fasting), elevated serum triglyceride level (fasting), and pre-diabetes. James's BMI is 35.4. Dr. Walter diagnoses James with dysmetabolic syndrome X.
12. Diana Gamble, a 56-year-old female, had her pancreas removed and is now experiencing headaches, blurred vision, and weight loss. Diana admits she has not been taking her medications as prescribed. Dr. Caldwell notes a blood sugar of 305 mg/dL postprandial and admits Diana. After a complete workup, Diana is diagnosed with postpancreatectomy hyperglycemia.
13. Mark Hennecy, a 32-year-old male, presents today with the complaints of feeling tired all the time, difficulty concentrating, and abdominal pain. Dr. Mather notes mild jaundice. After a thorough examination and review of the laboratory results, Mark is diagnosed with Gilbert's syndrome.
14. Erica Lamotte, a 63-year-old female, has been diagnosed with insulin-dependent (type 1) diabetic nephropathy and chronic renal failure, stage 4. She is now requiring regular dialysis treatments.
15. Sue Pittman, a 46-year-old female, presents today with the complaints of tiredness and numbness. Sue was diagnosed with hypertension 2 years ago. Dr. Charmers notes muscle weakness with slight paralysis. Sue is admitted to the hospital, where blood tests reveal a high level of calcium. After a complete workup, Sue is diagnosed with familial aldosteronism, type I.

(continued)

YOU CODE IT! Application

The following exercises provide practice in abstracting physicians' documentation from our health care facility, Prader, Bracker, & Associates. These case studies are modeled on real patient encounters. Using the techniques described in this chapter, carefully read through the case studies and determine the most accurate ICD-10-CM code(s) and external cause code(s), if appropriate, for each case study.

PRADER, BRACKER, & ASSOCIATES

A Complete Health Care Facility

159 Healthcare Way • SOMEWHERE, FL 32811 • 407-555-6789

PATIENT: FUENTES, GILES

ACCOUNT/EHR #: FUENGI001

Attending Physician: Renee O. Bracker, MD

This 61-year-old male returns today to review the results of his blood tests, ordered last week. Patient had come in with complaints of hyperactive deep tendon reflexes, muscle cramps, and carpopedal spasm.

Pathology report shows abnormally decreased blood calcium levels. I discussed the details of this condition and reviewed treatment options. He wants to discuss this with his wife, and he will call within the next few days.

DX: Hypocalcemia

Determine the most accurate ICD-10-CM code(s).

PRADER, BRACKER, & ASSOCIATES

A Complete Health Care Facility

159 Healthcare Way • SOMEWHERE, FL 32811 • 407-555-6789

PATIENT: MOLINAZZI, JAMES

ACCOUNT/EHR #: MOLIJA001

Attending Physician: Oscar R. Prader, MD

S: Pt is a 52-year-old male, comes in for a 6-week follow-up since his diagnosis of secondary diabetes mellitus due to hyperthyroidism. Patient states he has been taking his methimazole, as prescribed.

O: H: 6′0″, W: 168, T: 99.1, BP: 125/82; HEENT: unremarkable. Heart rhythm is regular and steady. Lung sounds are also normal. EKG unremarkable. I emphasized the importance of medication and diet. I reviewed the plan to control the secondary diabetes with diet and exercise as first treatment choice.

A: Hyperthyroidism with secondary diabetes mellitus

P: 1. Rx: Propranolol to manage tachycardia. Methimazole continued.

2. Rx: TSH blood test. Patient to go to lab for test within the week.

3. Patient to return in 10–14 days.

Determine the most accurate ICD-10-CM code(s).

(continued)

PRADER, BRACKER, & ASSOCIATES

A Complete Health Care Facility

159 Healthcare Way • SOMEWHERE, FL 32811 • 407-555-6789

PATIENT: CARTER, KIMBERLY

ACCOUNT/EHR #: CARTKI001

Attending Physician: Renee O. Bracker, MD

Pt, a 61-year-old female, comes in for her regular checkup. She has insulin-dependent diabetes mellitus, type 2, with bilateral, mild, nonproliferative retinal edema and chronic kidney disease, stage I. In addition, she suffers from hypertensive heart disease with episodes of congestive heart failure. After the exam, some time is spent talking about her day-to-day activities, her diet and overall eating habits, whether or not she is engaging in regular exercise, and her overall mental attitudes as well as physical well-being. The patient states it can be difficult to get around by herself due to the problems with her eyes, and she is finding it more and more difficult to give herself the insulin injections. Both pupils are dilated, a further eye exam revealed distortion of the vessels and tiny retinal hemorrhages. I provided her with some information about an insulin pump and she states she will go over it and discuss it with her son.

Determine the most accurate ICD-10-CM code(s).

PRADER, BRACKER, & ASSOCIATES

A Complete Health Care Facility

159 Healthcare Way • SOMEWHERE, FL 32811 • 407-555-6789

PATIENT: WILLRODT, VICTORIA

ACCOUNT/EHR #: WILLVI001

Attending Physician: Oscar R. Prader, MD

S: Pt is a 28-year-old female complaining of discoloration of her right lower eyelid. She states the discoloration is of 4-week duration with no evidence of healing despite multiple home remedies and over-the-counter treatments. Pt is a type 1 diabetic for 10 years.

O: Wt: 146 lb, Ht: 5′5″, T: 98.6, BP: 131/58; HEENT: unremarkable. Dr. Prader notes premature graying of the right eyelashes and eyebrows and discoloration of the right lower eyelid. Ultraviolet light treatment and micropigmentation are discussed as treatment options.

A: 1. Type 1 diabetes mellitus with diabetic dermatitis

2. Dermatitis of right lower eyelid secondary to diabetes

P: Discussed skin care and glycemic control. Prescribed 0.1% tacrolimus ointment, apply b.i.d. Follow up in 4 weeks.

Pt to return in 2 weeks for follow-up

Determine the most accurate ICD-10-CM code(s).

WESTON HOSPITAL

629 Healthcare Way • SOMEWHERE, FL 32811 • 407-555-6541

PATIENT: HAWKINS, TYRONE

ACCOUNT/EHR #: HAWKTY001

Attending Physician: Renee O. Bracker, MD

(continued)

S: Patient is a 46-year-old male with insulin-dependent type 2 diabetic nephropathy and end-stage renal disease. He presents today for an arteriovenous shunt for dialysis. Tyrone complains of shortness of breath and extreme fatigue.

PE: H: 5′10″, Wt: 164, T: 99.2, R: 24, P: 106, BP: 175/63. Dr. Bracker notes some confusion and admits Tyrone for an emergency hemodialysis treatment. Once patient was stabilized, a Cimino-type direct arteriovenous anastomosis is performed by incising the skin of the left antecubital fossa. Vessel clamps are placed on the vein and adjacent artery. The vein is dissected free, and the downstream portion of the vein is sutured to an opening in the artery using an end-to-side technique. The skin incision is closed in layers.

Determine the most accurate ICD-10-CM code(s).

10

Coding Mental, Behavioral, and Neurologic Disorders

Key Terms

Abuse
Acute
Anxiety
Anxiolytic
Behavioral Disturbance
Chronic
Dependence
Depressive
Hypnotic
Manic
Phobia
Schizophrenia
Sedative
Somatoform Disorder
Use
Withdrawal

Learning Outcomes

After completing this chapter, the student should be able to:

LO 10.1 Determine underlying conditions that affect mental health.
LO 10.2 Distinguish mood and nonmood disorders.
LO 10.3 Apply the guidelines for reporting nonpsychotic mental conditions.
LO 10.4 Identify conditions affecting the central nervous system.
LO 10.5 Interpret details regarding peripheral nervous system conditions into accurate codes.
LO 10.6 Assess the diagnosis of pain and report it with accurate codes.

STOP! **Remember, you need to follow along in your ICD-10-CM code book for an optimal learning experience.**

10.1 Conditions That Affect Mental Health

Mental and behavioral disorders have long been a mystery to the average person, and the lack of understanding has fed fear of patients with these disorders. The dysfunction of a person's brain is often the result of many of the same things that cause other bodily health concerns, including genetics, congenital anomalies, traumatic injury, or the invasion of a pathogen. Any of these, along with other conditions and circumstances, have the ability to impact the health and function of the brain. Scientific research has evidenced shared signs and symptoms between psychiatric illness and neurologic illness.

The accepted understanding of mental illness is a condition that negatively affects an individual's thoughts, emotions, behaviors, ability to maintain effective social interactions, and ability to appropriately carry out the activities of daily living.

Mental Disorders Due to Known Physiological Conditions

In some cases, a mental disorder is caused by another condition in the body. The physiological condition may be any of various diagnoses, including an infarction of the brain, hypertensive cerebrovascular disease, or a disease such as Creutzfeldt-Jakob disease, Parkinson's disease, or trypanosomiasis (a condition commonly known as *sleeping sickness*). Moreover, some endocrine disorders, exogenous hormones, and toxic substances can cause cognitive and/or intellectual malfunction, including signs and symptoms of problematic memory, impaired judgment, and diminished intellect.

Dementia is included in this subsection of the ICD-10-CM code book's ***Chapter 5: Mental, Behavioral and Neurodevelopmental Disorders (F01–F99)***. This diagnosis can be identified by evidence of both neurologic and psychological signs and symptoms, such as differences in personality, altered thoughts and feelings, and behavioral changes.

When it comes to reporting diagnoses for mental disorders that are manifestations of physiological conditions, you need to identify from the documentation the specific known etiology in cerebral disease, brain injury, or other insult leading to this cerebral dysfunction.

Vascular Dementia

A patient may develop vascular dementia after having experienced an infarction of the brain that is known to be a manifestation of a previously existing vascular disease. In ICD-10-CM, code category F01 also includes a diagnosis of hypertensive cerebrovascular disease as well as arteriosclerotic dementia. A cerebrovascular disease and ischemic or hemorrhagic brain injury can often result in cognitive impairment known as vascular dementia.

EXAMPLE

At the code category F01, you can see the definition, along with some important notations:

✓4 **F01** **Vascular dementia**
Vascular dementia as a result of infarction of the brain due to vascular disease, including hypertensive cerebrovascular disease.
INCLUDES arteriosclerotic dementia
Code first **the underlying physiological condition or sequelae of cerebrovascular disease.**

Therefore, the notation to "*Code first* **the underlying physiological condition or sequelae of cerebrovascular disease**" logically supports your correct sequencing of codes that may be involved in the reporting of this diagnosis.

EXAMPLES

F01.50 Vascular dementia without behavioral disturbance

F01.51 Vascular dementia with behavior disturbance
Use additional code, **if applicable, to identify wandering in vascular dementia (Z91.83)**

Behavioral Disturbance
A type of common behavior that includes mood disorders (such as depression, apathy, and euphoria), sleep disorders (such as insomnia and hypersomnia), psychotic symptoms (such as delusions and hallucinations), and agitation (such as pacing, wandering, and aggression).

As you read down this code category listing, you can see that, in addition to identifying the underlying physiological condition, you also will need to identify whether or not the patient is documented as having **behavioral disturbance**. If so, has the patient also been documented as having episodes of "wandering"? These details will guide you toward the correct code or codes to accurately report this patient's condition.

Amnestic Disorder Due to Known Physiological Condition

Reporting amnestic disorder due to known physiological condition will take you to code category F04 Amnestic disorder, with the additional descriptions of Korsakov's psychosis and Syndrome, nonalcoholic. You can see that the *Code first* **underlying condition** notation requires that the underlying condition be physiological, thereby eliminating any psychological underlying conditions from qualifying for this code.

Note that ICD-10-CM reporting of this diagnosis has an EXCLUDES1 notation. An EXCLUDES1 notation identifies other diagnoses that are mutually exclusive to the diagnosis above the notation (in this case, F04). This is the absolute statement that the excluded code can never be used at the same time because the two conditions cannot occur together in one patient at one time.

EXCLUDES1 **amnesia NOS (R41.3)**
anterograde amnesia (R41.1)
dissociative amnesia (F44.0)
retrograde amnesia (R41.2)

F04 also carries an EXCLUDES2 notation identifying several amnestic disorders that are _not_ included in F04, therefore requiring either a different code or an additional code:

EXCLUDES2 **alcohol-induced or unspecified Korsakov's syndrome (F10.26, F10.96)**
Korsakov's syndrome induced by other psychoactive substances (F13.26, F13.96, F19.16, F19.26, F19.96)

Mood Disorder Due to Known Physiological Condition

A mood disorder is a daily issue of dealing with one's emotional state. This category of mental illnesses includes major depressive disorder, dysthymic disorder, and bipolar disorder. Code subcategory F06.3- differentiates itself from other diagnoses under "Mood [affective] disorders," which includes bipolar disorder (F30–F39), because this diagnosis (reported with F06.3-) includes a documented physiological underlying cause.

EXAMPLES

F06.30 Mood disorder due to known physiological condition, unspecified

F06.31 Mood disorder due to known physiological condition, with depressive features

F06.32 Mood disorder due to known physiological condition, with major depressive-like episode

F06.33 Mood disorder due to known physiological condition, with manic features

F06.34 Mood disorder due to known physiological condition, with mixed features

As you abstract documentation related to a mood disorder, you must be alert to mentions of any additional signs and symptoms.

Depressive features include decrease in interest in hobbies or favorite activities, hypersomnia, or insomnia virtually every day.

Manic features are identified by documented episodes of intensely disruptive and exaggerated behaviors of heightened mood.

Mixed features refer to documented and regular (virtually every day within 1 week) meeting of the criteria of both depressive and manic features. Also known as roller-coastering.

Beneath F06.3 is an EXCLUDES2 notation, indicating specific diagnoses that are not included in this subcategory:

EXCLUDES2 **mood disorders due to alcohol and other psychoactive substances (F10–F19 with .14, .24, .94)**
mood disorders, not due to known physiological condition or unspecified (F30–F39)

Personality and Behavioral Disorders Due to Known Physiological Condition

There have been known physiological conditions that manifest personality changes or behavioral disorders. Traumatic brain injury (TBI)–specifically, damage to the patient's frontal lobe–can be evidenced by apathy, a lack of ability to formulate plans, emotional bluntness, and inability to perform abstract thinking. In this code category, you will find a *Code first* **underlying physiological condition** notation applicable to all codes within.

Beneath F07.0 are two EXCLUDES notations, which further clarify which diagnoses are reported with this code and which require the coder to look elsewhere in the code set:

EXAMPLE

F07.0 Personality change due to known physiological condition (Frontal lobe syndrome) (Organic pseudopsychopathic personality) (Postleucotomy syndrome)
Code first **underlying physiological condition**

EXCLUDES1 **mild cognitive impairment (G31.84)**
postconcussional syndrome (F07.81)
postencephalitic syndrome (F07.89)
signs and symptoms involving emotional state (R45.-)

EXCLUDES2 **specific personality disorder (F60.-)**

EXAMPLE

F07.81 Postconcussion syndrome (Postcontusion syndrome or encephalopathy) (Posttraumatic brain syndrome, nonpsychotic)
Use additional code **to identify associated post-traumatic headache, if applicable (G44.3-)**

EXCLUDES1 **Current concussion (brain) (S06.0-) Postencephalitic syndrome (F07.89)**

Remember that an EXCLUDES1 notation in ICD-10-CM identifies diagnoses that are mutually exclusive–they cannot be reported for the same patient at the same time. Also, don't forget to read the notation at the top of this code category, directly beneath F07 . . . this applies to all codes within this code category.

Code first **underlying physiological condition**

LET'S CODE IT! SCENARIO

Eboni O'Neal, a 37-year-old female, came with her husband, Carl, to see Dr. Annikah, a psychiatrist, on a referral from her regular physician. She complains about unusual fatigue and problems remembering things. Her husband has complained that she has been unusually irritable. Carl stated that he has found Eboni wandering the neighborhood several times over the last few weeks. Eboni admitted to being on a new dairy-free, animal product–free diet. After a complete physical examination, Dr. Annikah performed a complete psychology exam and ordered blood work, which confirmed his diagnosis of dementia caused by vitamin B_{12} deficiency.

Let's Code It!

Dr. Annikah diagnosed Eboni with *dementia caused by vitamin B_{12} deficiency.* You also read that she did have incidents of *wandering.* When you turn to the Alphabetic Index, you see

Dementia (degenerative (primary)) (old age) (persisting) F03.90

in (due to)

vitamin B_{12} deficiency E53.8 *[F02.80]*

with behavioral disturbance E53.8 *[F02.81]*

You should remember from the chapter ***The Coding Process*** that the second code, in italicized brackets, tells you that you will need two codes for this diagnosis and in which order to report these two codes. Turn to the Tabular List to read the first suggested code:

✓4 **E53 Deficiency of other B group vitamins**

Read down and review all of the fourth-character choices to determine the most accurate code:

E53.8 Deficiency of other specified B group vitamins

Next, you know that you will need to follow this code with a code from F02—either F02.80 or F02.81. Let's take a look at both codes and see what exactly is meant by **behavioral disturbance**:

F02.80 Dementia in other diseases classified elsewhere without behavioral disturbance

F02.81 Dementia in other diseases classified elsewhere with behavioral disturbance

Did you notice the notation beneath F02.81?

Use additional code, **if applicable, to identify wandering in dementia in conditions classified elsewhere (Z91.83)**

(continued)

Aha! This tells you that "wandering" is considered a behavioral disturbance. Dr. Annikah documented that Eboni had been wandering, so you will need one more code:

Z91.83 Wandering in conditions classified elsewhere

Good job! You determined the three codes required to accurately report Dr. Annikah's encounter with Eboni.

Check the top of all three chapters in ICD-10-CM. Check them all for an INCLUDES notation, a ***Use additional code*** note, an EXCLUDES1 notation, and an EXCLUDES2 notation. Read carefully. Do any relate to Dr. Annikah's diagnosis of Eboni? No. Turn to the Official Guidelines and read Sections I.C.4, I.C.5, and I.C.21. There is nothing specifically applicable here either.

Now you can report these three codes with confidence.

E53.8 Deficiency of other specified B group vitamins

F02.81 Dementia in other diseases classified elsewhere with behavioral disturbance

Z91.83 Wandering in conditions classified elsewhere

Good coding!

Mental and Behavioral Disorders Due to Psychoactive Substance Use

Reporting Alcohol-Related and Drug-Related Disorders

When a patient is diagnosed with an alcohol- or drug-related disorder, the diagnosis is often more complex, as such conditions are susceptible to both psychological and physiological signs, symptoms, manifestations, and co-morbidities. Alcohol use doesn't damage the actual brain cells, but it does damage the ends of neurons, which are called *dendrites*. This results in problems conveying messages to the cell body.

Sedative
A tranquilizer; a drug used to calm or soothe.

Hypnotic
A drug that induces sleep.

Anxiolytic
A drug used to reduce anxiety.

EXAMPLES

NOTE: All codes in this example require additional characters.

F10.1	Alcohol abuse
F10.2	Alcohol dependence
F10.9	Alcohol use, unspecified
F11.1	Opioid abuse
F11.2	Opioid dependence
F11.9	Opioid use, unspecified
F12.1	Cannabis abuse
F12.2	Cannabis dependence
F12.9	Cannabis use, unspecified
F13.1	**Sedative**, **hypnotic** or **anxiolytic**-related abuse
F13.2	Sedative, hypnotic or anxiolytic-related dependence
F13.9	Sedative, hypnotic or anxiolytic-related use, unspecified
F14.1	Cocaine abuse
F14.2	Cocaine dependence
F14.9	Cocaine use, unspecified

Use
(1) The sharing of information between people working in the same health care facility for purposes of caring for the patient. (2) Occasional consumption of a substance without clinical manifestations.

Abuse
Regular consumption of a substance with manifestations.

Dependence
Ongoing, regular consumption of a substance with resulting significant clinical manifestations, and a dramatic decrease in the effect of the substance with continued use, therefore requiring an increased quantity of the substance to achieve intoxication.

Withdrawal
Abruptly stopping the use of a drug that has been used continuously prior to the cessation, which can result in both physical and psychological conditions.

The first thing you might notice about these codes is that details are required from the documentation to identify *use* of, *abuse* of, or *dependence* on the psychoactive substance. Also, there are codes for specifically reporting the *use* of alcohol and drugs that enable the tracking of the patient's behavior, which often will ultimately have a negative impact on their health. These details can give providers and researchers a great deal of useful information as they look for better ways to care for patients and their maladies.

What is the clinical difference between these terms?

Use: Consumption of a substance without significant clinical manifestations.

Abuse: Ongoing, regular consumption of a substance with resulting clinical manifestations.

Dependence: Ongoing, regular consumption of a substance with resulting significant clinical manifestations and a dramatic decrease in the effect of the substance with continued use, therefore requiring an increased quantity of the substance to achieve intoxication. In addition, the patient will require continued consumption of the substance to avoid withdrawal symptoms and other serious behavioral effects, occurring at any time in the same 12-month period.

Withdrawal: A psychological and/or physical condition that manifests after the sudden discontinuation of the use of a drug in an individual who has continually used the drug previously.

All of these codes require additional characters to identify details from the documentation about manifestations and co-morbidities. Let's take *alcohol abuse* as an example of what details you may need to abstract from the clinical documentation.

EXAMPLES

F10.1	Alcohol abuse
F10.10	Alcohol abuse, uncomplicated
F10.120	Alcohol abuse with intoxication, uncomplicated
F10.121	Alcohol abuse with intoxication delirium
F10.130	Alcohol abuse with withdrawal, uncomplicated
F10.131	Alcohol abuse with withdrawal delirium
F10.132	Alcohol abuse with withdrawal with perceptual disturbance
F10.14	Alcohol abuse with alcohol-induced mood disorder
F10.150	Alcohol abuse with alcohol-induced psychotic disorder with delusions
F10.180	Alcohol abuse with alcohol-induced anxiety disorder
F10.181	Alcohol abuse with alcohol-induced sexual dysfunction
F10.182	Alcohol abuse with alcohol-induced sleep disorder
F10.188	Alcohol abuse with other alcohol-induced disorder
F10.230	Alcohol dependence with withdrawal, uncomplicated

As you can see, ICD-10-CM requires an understanding of the psychological and behavioral impacts of the use, abuse, or dependence. Signs, symptoms, manifestations, and co-morbidities such as delirium, mood disorder, and hallucinations will be reported with one combination code from this subsection.

In the subcategories for alcohol use and dependence, you also will find codes including a state of withdrawal, again providing one combination code to report this condition.

EXAMPLE

F10.231 Alcohol dependence with withdrawal delirium

The extended descriptions and combination-code choices include those codes used to report the use of other nontherapeutic substances as well. Take, for example, caffeine use, hallucinogens, and inhalant use.

EXAMPLES

F15.120	Other stimulant abuse with intoxication, uncomplicated
F15.920	Other stimulant use, unspecified with intoxication, uncomplicated
F16.1-	Hallucinogen abuse
F16.2-	Hallucinogen dependence
F16.9-	Hallucinogen use, unspecified
F18.1-	Inhalant abuse
F18.9-	Inhalant use, unspecified

ICD-10-CM code descriptions separate inhalant abuse and dependence into its own specific code category (F18), and caffeine (yes, this is considered a substance) is included in the "Other" code category, now combined with amphetamine-related disorders.

As with the previous code categories in this subsection, the additional characters required for these ICD-10-CM codes include abstracting documentation for details on accompanying intoxication, delirium, perceptual disturbance, mood disorder, psychotic disorder with delusions or hallucinations, **anxiety** disorder, flashbacks, and other manifestations.

One more addition to this subsection of the ICD-10-CM code book's ***Chapter 5: Mental, Behavioral and Neurodevelopmental Disorders (F01–F99)*** is code category F17 Nicotine dependence. The EXCLUDES1 note reminds you that nicotine dependence is not the same diagnosis as tobacco use (Z72.0) or history of tobacco dependence (Z87.891). Therefore, the documentation will need to specifically discern between tobacco use and nicotine dependence.

CODING BITES

If the patient's blood alcohol level is documented, it should be reported using code category Y90 Evidence of alcohol involvement determined by blood alcohol level.

Anxiety
The feelings of apprehension and fear, sometimes manifested with physical manifestations such as sweating and palpitations.

EXAMPLES

F17.210	Nicotine dependence, cigarettes, uncomplicated
F17.211	Nicotine dependence, cigarettes, in remission
F17.213	Nicotine dependence, cigarettes, with withdrawal
F17.218	Nicotine dependence, cigarettes, with other nicotine-induced disorders
F17.220	Nicotine dependence, chewing tobacco, uncomplicated
F17.221	Nicotine dependence, chewing tobacco, in remission
F17.223	Nicotine dependence, chewing tobacco, with withdrawal
F17.228	Nicotine dependence, chewing tobacco, with other nicotine-induced disorders
F17.290	Nicotine dependence, other tobacco product, uncomplicated
F17.291	Nicotine dependence, other tobacco product, in remission
F17.293	Nicotine dependence, other tobacco product, with withdrawal
F17.298	Nicotine dependence, other tobacco product, with other nicotine-induced disorders

The bottom line is that ICD-10-CM has organized these codes in a logical and efficient order and provided you with many combination codes.

GUIDANCE CONNECTION

Read the ICD-10-CM Official Guidelines for Coding and Reporting, section **I. Conventions, General Coding Guidelines and Chapter-Specific Guidelines**, subsection **C. Chapter-Specific Coding Guidelines**, chapter **5. Mental, Behavioral and Neurodevelopmental Disorders (F01–F99)**, subsections **b. Mental and behavioral disorders due to psychoactive substance use, 2) Psychoactive substance use, abuse and dependence** and **3) Psychoactive substance use**.

LET'S CODE IT! SCENARIO

Jason Hurst, a 63-year-old male, has been a salesman for the last 30 years. He travels throughout the Midwest and has had a less-than-stellar career. Very often, he has come close to being fired for not making quota, but his supervisor takes pity on him because he has been with the company for so long. He is at the medical office today by court order after being arrested for his third DUI in the last 6 months. Seeking treatment is part of his plea deal so he doesn't lose his driver's license. He needs to be able to drive to see his customers.

Jason states he has tried to stop drinking but can't because it is part of his job. He must take customers out for a drink. And when he is back at his office, all the guys go out for drinks after work. When he is on the road, he finds nothing to do in the motel at night, so he drinks away the loneliness. The one time he tried to quit drinking, he got really sick. The only thing that helped him feel better was a little "hair of the dog."

He states that at times he is very sad and hopeless, while other times, especially when he is with clients, he is the life of the party and knows some of the best jokes. He pleads for help and begins to cry.

Dr. Walkowicz diagnoses Jason with alcohol dependence with alcohol-induced mood disorder.

Let's Code It!

Dr. Walkowicz diagnosed Jason with *alcohol dependence with alcohol-induced mood disorder.* Turn in the Alphabetic Index to find

Dependence (on) (syndrome) F19.20

alcohol (ethyl) (methyl) (without remission) F10.20

with

mood disorder F10.24

Now let's turn to find this suggested code in the Tabular List:

✓4 **F10 Alcohol related disorder**
Use additional code **for blood alcohol level, if applicable (Y90.-)**

This is not applicable in Jason's case, so continue reading to review all of the options for the required fourth character. Did you choose this code?

✓5 **F10.2 Alcohol dependence**

Don't skip over the EXCLUDES1 and EXCLUDES2 notations. You must read them all carefully, and then determine whether they apply to the specific case you are coding. In this case, they do not. Keep reading all of the fifth-character choices to determine the most accurate code. You can see the code that matches Dr. Walkowicz's notes perfectly!

F10.24 Alcohol dependence with alcohol-induced mood disorder

Good work!

In Remission

The determination of whether a patient who has been diagnosed with a mental or behavioral disorder due to the use of a psychoactive substance is in remission is in the judgment of the attending physician. Therefore, report the appropriate character identifying the state of remission only when the physician has specifically documented this condition.

EXAMPLES

F11.21 Opioid dependence, in remission
F14.21 Cocaine dependence, in remission

GUIDANCE CONNECTION

Read the ICD-10-CM Official Guidelines for Coding and Reporting, section **I. Conventions, General Coding Guidelines and Chapter-Specific Guidelines**, subsection **C. Chapter-Specific Coding Guidelines**, chapter **5. Mental, Behavioral and Neurodevelopmental Disorders (F01-F99)**, subsection **b. Mental and behavioral disorders due to psychoactive substance use, 1) In remission**.

10.2 Mood (Affective) and Nonmood (Psychotic) Disorders

Mood (Affective) Disorders

Bipolar Disorders

The etiology of bipolar disorders is uncertain and complex. The strongest evidence leads to the belief that many factors act together to activate the signs and symptoms. While some evidence exists that the condition tends to have familial connections, there have been studies of identical twins in which only one twin is affected.

Manic
An emotional state that includes elation, excitement, and exuberance.

Depressive
An emotional state that includes sadness, hopelessness, and gloom.

Bipolar disorder is categorized as a "mood disorder" identified by acute swings exhibited by the patient, ranging from euphoria and hyperactivity to depression and lethargy. An overly elated or overexcited state is called a **manic** episode, and an acute sad or hopeless state is known as a **depressive** episode. Bipolar disorder may also be present in a *mixed* state, during which the patient experiences both mania and depression simultaneously.

Bipolar disorder is a chronic illness, therefore requiring long-term, continuous treatment to control symptoms. Mood stabilizers (e.g., lithium carbonate), atypical antipsychotics (e.g., clozapine), and antidepressants are most commonly prescribed in combination.

This diagnosis is categorized into two types: Type I bipolar disorder is identified as alternating between manic episodes and depressive episodes, while type II bipolar patients deal with recurring depressive episodes with occasional mania.

EXAMPLES

F31	Bipolar disorder
F31.0	Bipolar disorder, current episode hypomanic
F31.11	Bipolar disorder, current episode, manic without psychotic features, mild
F31.12	Bipolar disorder, current episode, manic without psychotic features, moderate
F31.13	Bipolar disorder, current episode, manic without psychotic features, severe
F31.2	Bipolar disorder, current episode, manic, severe, with psychotic features
F31.31	Bipolar disorder, current episode, depressed, mild
F31.32	Bipolar disorder, current episode, depressed, moderate
F31.4	Bipolar disorder, current episode, depressed, severe, without psychotic features
F31.5	Bipolar disorder, current episode, depressed, severe, with psychotic features
F31.6-	Bipolar disorder, current episode, mixed
F31.81	Bipolar II disorder
F31.89	Other bipolar disorder (recurrent manic episodes NOS)

When you abstract the documentation regarding a current episode, you need to be on the lookout for details regarding the aspects:

- Manic means that the patient reports periods of high energy and an inability to sleep.
- Depressed mood regards periods of low energy, disinterest in favorite activities, and feeling sad for no apparent reason.
- Psychotic features include the patient experiencing either auditory or visual hallucinations.

The categorization of those patients in partial or full remission is also available, so you will need to check the documentation for this detail or query the physician.

EXAMPLES

F31.7-	Bipolar disorder, currently in remission
F31.71	Bipolar disorder, in partial remission, most recent episode hypomanic
F31.72	Bipolar disorder, in full remission, most recent episode hypomanic
F31.73	Bipolar disorder, in partial remission, most recent episode manic
F31.74	Bipolar disorder, in full remission, most recent episode manic
F31.75	Bipolar disorder, in partial remission, most recent episode depressed
F31.76	Bipolar disorder, in full remission, most recent episode depressed
F31.77	Bipolar disorder, in partial remission, most recent episode mixed
F31.78	Bipolar disorder, in full remission, most recent episode mixed

A patient in full remission has not experienced any significant mood fluctuation for at least 2 months, virtually always during treatment.

A patient in partial remission has experienced reduced episodes or has had no episodes for less than 60 days.

Major Depressive Disorder

Everyone feels sad or depressed at times. It is part of life. However, major depressive disorder causes patients to feel hopeless, guilty, and worthless. The typical activities of life (work, study, sleep, and fun) become difficult and, for some, nearly impossible. Some patients may experience ongoing (recurrent) episodes, while others suffer only a one-time (single) episode. Additional diagnostic terms used by some psychiatrists include *agitated depression*, *depressive reaction*, *major depression*, *psychogenic depression*, *reactive depression*, and *vital depression*.

Major depressive disorder may be mild, moderate, or severe and may be described as with or without psychotic features. Patients diagnosed with this illness also may experience partial or full remission. As the professional coding specialist, it is your job to ensure that your physician documents all of these details.

EXAMPLES

F32.-	Major depressive disorder, single episode
F33.-	Major depressive disorder, recurrent

You will need an additional character to identify the current episode as mild, moderate, severe without psychotic features, or severe with psychotic features.

F32.4	Major depressive disorder, single episode, in partial remission
F33.41	Major depressive disorder, recurrent, in partial remission

A patient in partial remission has experienced reduced episodes or has had no episodes for less than 60 days.

F32.5	Major depressive disorder, single episode, in full remission
F33.42	Major depressive disorder, recurrent, in full remission

A patient in full remission has not experienced any significant depressive symptoms for at least 2 months, virtually always during treatment.

ICD-10-CM

YOU CODE IT! CASE STUDY

Sherri L., a 23-year-old female, came in to see Dr. Keel, a psychiatrist. She has a very demanding and high-stress life, being a second-year law student. In addition, she is clerking for a judge, and she is planning her wedding for this coming summer. She states that she has always been highly motivated to achieve her goals. After graduating with top honors from college, she went on to achieve a 3.95 GPA in her first year in law school. She admits that she can be very self-critical when she is not able to achieve perfection, even though, intellectually, she knows that perfection is not necessary for success. Recently, she has been struggling with considerable feelings of worthlessness and shame due to her inability to perform as well as she has in the past.

For the past few weeks, Sherri has noticed that she is constantly feeling fatigued, no matter how much she has slept. She also states that it has been increasingly difficult to concentrate at work and pay attention in class. Her best friend, RaeAnn, who works with her at the courthouse, stated that, recently, Sherri is irritable and withdrawn, not at all her typical upbeat and friendly disposition. While she has always prided herself on perfect attendance at school and at work, Sherri has called in sick on several occasions. On those days she stayed in bed all day, watching TV and sleeping.

At home, Sherri's fiancé has noticed changes in her as well. He states that, in the last 6 months, it seems that she has lost interest in sex despite a very healthy sex life during the previous 2 years they had been together. He also has noticed that she has had difficulties falling asleep at night. Her tossing and turning for an hour or two after they go to bed has been keeping him awake. He confesses that he overheard her having tearful phone conversations with RaeAnn and her sister that have worried him. When he tries to get her to open up, she denies anything is wrong, emphatically stating, "I'm fine," and walking away.

Sherri states that she has found herself increasingly dissatisfied with her life. She admits to having frequent thoughts of wishing she was dead, yet denies ever considering suicide. She gets frustrated with herself because she feels that she has every reason to be happy yet can't seem to shake the sense of a heavy dark cloud enshrouding her. Dr. Keel diagnosed Sherri with major depressive disorder, single episode, moderate severity.

You Code It!

Go through the steps of coding, and determine the code or codes that should be reported for this encounter between Dr. Keel and Sherri.

Step #1: Read the case carefully and completely.
Step #2: Abstract the scenario. Which main words or terms describe why the physician cared for the patient during this encounter?
Step #3: Are there any details missing or incomplete for which you would need to query the physician? [If so, ask your instructor.]
Step #4: Check for any relevant guidance, including reading all of the symbols and notations in the Tabular List and the appropriate sections of the Official Guidelines.
Step #5: Determine the correct diagnosis code or codes to explain why this encounter was medically necessary.
Step #6: Double-check your work.

Answer:

Did you determine this to be the correct code?

F32.1 Major depressive disorder, single episode, moderate

Nonmood (Psychotic) Disorders

Schizophrenia

There is no known cause of **schizophrenia** (a psychotic disorder); however, evidence does exist that it may have an etiology of genetic, biological, cultural, and/or psychological foundations. The belief of a genetic predisposition is supported with statistical research showing that the close relatives of a schizophrenic are 50 times more likely to develop the condition.

Schizophrenia
A psychotic disorder with no known cause.

There is also a widely held belief of a biochemical imbalance, specifically excessive activity of dopaminergic synapses, encouraging the signs and symptoms of schizophrenia. Five types of schizophrenia are recognized by psychiatric professionals:

- *Paranoid*, also known as *paraphrenic schizophrenia* [F20.0]
- *Disorganized*, also known as *hebephrenic schizophrenia* or *hebephrenia* [F20.1]
- *Catatonic*, also known as *schizophrenic catalepsy*, *catatonia*, or *flexibilitas cerea* [F20.2]
- *Undifferentiated*, also known as *atypical schizophrenia* [F20.3]
- *Residual*, also known as *restzustand* [F20.5]

The signs and symptoms of schizophrenia are generally categorized into three groups: positive symptoms, negative symptoms, and cognitive symptoms. The specific behaviors related to this diagnosis will vary depending upon the type and phase of the disorder.

EXAMPLE

F20.0	Paranoid schizophrenia
F20.1	Disorganized schizophrenia
F20.2	Catatonic schizophrenia
F20.3	Undifferentiated schizophrenia (Atypical schizophrenia)
F20.5	Residual schizophrenia
F20.81	Schizophreniform disorder
F20.89	Other schizophrenia (Simple schizophrenia)
F21	Schizotypal disorder (Latent schizophrenia)
F25.0	Schizoaffective disorder, bipolar type
F25.1	Schizoaffective disorder, depressive type
F25.8	Other schizoaffective disorders

Coders working with health care professionals caring for patients diagnosed with schizophrenia should be aware of the known adverse effects of the antipsychotic drugs most often used to treat this condition. Also known as *neuroleptic drugs*, antipsychotics (such as haloperidol) are known to result in a high incident rate of extrapyramidal effects, including

- Drug-induced parkinsonism [G21.11] with signs of propulsive gait, stooped posture, muscle rigidity, tremors.
- Drug-induced acute dystonia [G24.02] showing signs of severe muscle contractions.
- Drug-induced akathisia [G25.71] showing signs of restlessness and pacing.

Some low-potency drugs in this category have been known to cause orthostatic hypotension [I95.2]–a sudden drop in blood pressure when the patient changes position quickly, such as standing up. A development of malignant neuroleptic syndrome [G21.0] has been reported in as many as 1% of patients taking antipsychotics.

Remember that when these adverse effects have been diagnosed, you will need to include an external cause code to identify the "drug taken for therapeutic purposes" as the reason for this condition. You would choose a code from category T43 Poisoning by, adverse effect of and underdosing of psychotropic drugs, not elsewhere classified in ICD-10-CM.

Schizoid Personality Disorder

There may appear to be some overlap in the signs and symptoms of schizophrenia (a psychotic disorder) and schizoid personality disorder; however, they are very different conditions.

Patients diagnosed with schizoid personality disorder exhibit a limited range of emotions and an aversion to social relationships and personal interactions. These patients have little to no interest in sex and are indifferent to both praise and criticism. Overall, these patients have a flat affect. Report this diagnosis with code F60.1 Schizoid personality disorder.

YOU CODE IT! CASE STUDY

Gary R., a 20-year-old male, is a junior at a state university. Over the past month, his parents have noticed that his behavior has become quite peculiar. Several times, his mother has overheard him speaking in a quiet yet angry tone, even though no one was in the room with him. Over the past 7 to 10 days, Gary has refused to answer or make calls on his cell phone, stating that he knows if he uses the phone, it will activate a deadly chip that has been implanted in his brain by evil men from space.

Gary's parents, as well as his brother and his best friend, have attempted to convince him to join them at an appointment with a psychiatrist for an evaluation, but he adamantly refused, until today. Several times, Gary has accused his parents of conspiring with the aliens to steal his brain. He no longer attends classes and will soon flunk out unless he can get some help.

Other than a few beers with his friends, Gary denies abusing alcohol or drugs. There is a family history of psychiatric illness; an estranged aunt has been in and out of psychiatric hospitals over the years due to erratic and bizarre behavior.

Dr. Zavakos diagnosed Gary with paranoid schizophrenia.

You Code It!

Go through the steps of coding, and determine the code or codes that should be reported for this encounter between Dr. Zavakos and Gary.

Step #1: Read the case carefully and completely.
Step #2: Abstract the scenario. Which main words or terms describe why the physician cared for the patient during this encounter?
Step #3: Are there any details missing or incomplete for which you would need to query the physician? [If so, ask your instructor.]
Step #4: Check for any relevant guidance, including reading all of the symbols and notations in the Tabular List and the appropriate sections of the Official Guidelines.
Step #5: Determine the correct diagnosis code or codes to explain why this encounter was medically necessary.
Step #6: Double-check your work.

Answer:

Did you determine this to be the correct code?

F20.0 Paranoid schizophrenia

10.3 Anxiety, Dissociative, Stress-Related, Somatoform, and Other Nonpsychotic Mental Disorders

Phobias

Are you terrified of something, with no real rationale? The definition of a **phobia** is the excessive and irrational fear of an object, activity, or situation. Of course, a slight fear of a spider or of flying would not typically result in a physician encounter or documented diagnosis. Therefore, for the most part, the code categories for phobias will be used to report the condition in which this fear has risen to the level at which it actually interferes with daily life and, therefore, requires treatment.

Phobia
Irrational and excessive fear of an object, activity, or situation.

EXAMPLES

F40.0-	Agoraphobia
F40.1-	Social phobia
F40.23-	Blood, injection, injury type phobia
F41.0	Panic disorder [episodic paroxysmal anxiety]
F41.1	Generalized anxiety disorder

Somatoform Disorders

Somatoform Disorder
The sincere belief that one is suffering an illness that is not present.

The term **somatoform disorders** may be new to you; however, you have probably heard of one type, *hypochondria (hypochondriacal disorder)*, in which patients have an ongoing belief that they have an illness that they do not have. This group of psychological disorders causes the patient to exhibit, or believe they exhibit, physical signs and symptoms.

EXAMPLES

F45.0	Somatization disorder (Multiple psychosomatic disorder)
F45.22	Body dysmorphic disorder
F45.41	Pain disorder exclusively related to psychological factors
F45.42	Pain disorder with related psychological factors ***Code also*** **associated acute or chronic pain (G89.-)**

GUIDANCE CONNECTION

Read the ICD-10-CM Official Guidelines for Coding and Reporting, section **I. Conventions, General Coding Guidelines and Chapter-Specific Guidelines**, subsection **C. Chapter-Specific Coding Guidelines**, chapter **5. Mental, Behavioral and Neurodevelopmental Disorders (F01-F99)**, subsection **a. Pain disorders related to psychological factors**.

YOU CODE IT! CASE STUDY

Brian B., a 52-year-old divorced father of two teenagers, states he has a successful, financially rewarding career. He has been with this company for the last 15 years, the last 5 as vice president of his division. Even though his job performance evaluations are good and he has been lauded by his boss, he is overwrought with worry constantly about losing his job and being unable to provide for his children. This worry has been troubling him for about the last 8 or 9 months. Despite really trying, he can't seem to shake the negative thoughts.

Over these last months, he noticed that he feels restless, tired, and stressed out. He often paces in his office when he's alone, especially when not deeply engaged in tasks. He's found difficulty in expressing himself and has been humiliated in a few meetings when this has occurred. At night, when attempting to go to sleep, he often finds that his brain won't shut off. Instead of resting, he finds himself obsessing over all the worst-case scenarios, including losing his job and ending up homeless.

Dr. Burnett diagnoses Brian with generalized anxiety disorder and discusses a treatment plan with him.

(continued)

You Code It!

Go through the steps of coding, and determine the code or codes that should be reported for this encounter between Dr. Burnett and Brian.

Step #1: Read the case carefully and completely.

Step #2: Abstract the scenario. Which main words or terms describe why the physician cared for the patient during this encounter?

Step #3: Are there any details missing or incomplete for which you would need to query the physician? [If so, ask your instructor.]

Step #4: Check for any relevant guidance, including reading all of the symbols and notations in the Tabular List and the appropriate sections of the Official Guidelines.

Step #5: Determine the correct diagnosis code or codes to explain why this encounter was medically necessary.

Step #6: Double-check your work.

Answer:

Did you determine this to be the correct code?

F41.1 Generalized anxiety disorder

Stress-Related Disorders

Post-traumatic stress disorder (PTSD) is a condition in which a horrible experience leaves a lasting imprint on the patient's sense of danger. Normally, when an individual senses danger, a "fight or flight" response initiates feelings of worry and fear. For those suffering from PTSD, the harmful or dangerous situation is gone, yet the sensation of fear continues.

Situations that may ignite PTSD can affect more individuals than just our wonderful military personnel returning from the horrors of war. Sadly, it has become far too typical to read about a shooting at a school or restaurant, rape, abuse (child, spouse, elder), transportation accidents (car, truck, train, airplane), natural disasters (hurricane, earthquake, flood), or other terrifying ordeals occurring in an all-American neighborhood. As health information management professionals and professional coding specialists, we should be aware, empathetic, and accurate. PTSD affects an estimated 7.5 million adults in the United States.

Signs and symptoms typically appear within 3 months of the event; however, in some cases, they can be internalized and take longer to recognize. Flashbacks, hyperarousal (overreactions), and avoidance are the most frequently experienced behaviors. When the symptoms are acute but then dissipate after a few weeks, this may be diagnosed as acute stress disorder (ASD), reported with ICD-10-CM code F43.0 Acute stress reaction, also known as crisis state or psychic shock.

When the patient experiences at least one flashback or "re-experiencing" symptom [including diaphoresis (sweating) and tachycardia (rapid heart rate)], at least two hyperarousal symptoms (patients may feel edgy, easily startled, or overly nervous), and at least three avoidance symptoms (avoid locations that are reminiscent of the event) that last longer than 1 month, it may be PTSD. Additionally, these patients often experience depression and anxiety as well as frequent attempts to self-medicate, resulting in substance abuse. PTSD is reported with one of these ICD-10-CM codes:

CODING BITES

NOTE: There is a difference between acute PTSD and chronic PTSD. If the documentation is ambiguous or unclear, query the physician.

F43.10 Post-traumatic stress disorder, unspecified

F43.11 Post-traumatic stress disorder, acute

F43.12 Post-traumatic stress disorder, chronic

When reporting PTSD, remember to include external cause codes to explain the specifics about the traumatic event. This is important to both treatment and reimbursement.

- *Cause of the injury*, such as an earthquake or a multicar accident.

EXAMPLES

All of these codes require additional characters to complete a valid code.

X34.XXX-	Earthquake
X37.0XX-	Hurricane (storm surge) (typhoon)
X96.3XX-	Assault by fertilizer bomb
X99.1XX-	Assault by knife
Y36.-	Operations of war
Y37.-	Military Operations

- *Place of the occurrence*, such as the park or the kitchen.

EXAMPLES

Y92.133	Barracks on military base as the place of occurrence of the external cause
Y92.212	Middle school as the place of occurrence of the external cause
Y92.26	Movie house or cinema as the place of occurrence of the external cause
Y92.821	Forest as the place of occurrence of the external cause

- *Activity during the occurrence*, such as almost drowning while SCUBA diving or being involved in a construction accident.

EXAMPLES

Y93.15	Activity, underwater diving and snorkeling
Y93.34	Activity, bungee jumping
Y93.H3	Activity, building and construction

- *Patient's status*, such as paid employment, on-duty military, or leisure activity.

The patient's status at the time also must be included in analysis for research purposes, in addition to the determination of financial liability for treatment. For example, reporting Y99.0 Civilian activity done for income or pay would connect to a workers' compensation liability, while Y99.1 Military activity would tie the diagnosis to military service.

Factitious Disorder

Factitious disorder is an adult personality and behavioral disorder that results in a patient reporting signs and symptoms that do not exist, or with that patient self-inflicting physical or psychological illness or injury. If you watch television, you are probably familiar with Munchausen's syndrome.

There are two expressions of factitious disorder: *imposed on* the individual him*self* or her*self*, and *by proxy*, during which the patient causes someone else to be ill or injured.

Code subcategory F68.1- Factitious disorder imposed on self requires a fifth character to describe the signs and symptoms as psychological, physical, or both psychological and physical.

Code F68.A Factitious disorder imposed on another is reported on the perpetrator's record–the individual diagnosed with, or suspected of having, Munchausen's. When reporting the condition of the victim of the individual suffering with Munchausen's syndrome by proxy (MSBP), report a code from category T74 Adult and child abuse, neglect and other maltreatment, confirmed or category T76 Adult and child abuse, neglect and other maltreatment, suspected in addition to the codes describing the illness or injury.

10.4 Physiological Conditions Affecting the Central Nervous System

Inflammatory Conditions of the Central Nervous System

Bacteria and viruses can invade the nervous system and cause infection, malfunction, and, in some cases, death. Examples include encephalitis (inflammation of the brain tissue), myelitis (inflammation of the spinal cord), intracranial abscess, and, probably the most well-known condition, meningitis.

Meningitis is an inflammatory disease of the CNS. However, as a professional coder, you must know more than the fact that the patient is diagnosed with meningitis. Meningitis can be caused by a virus or a bacterial invader that you will need to identify from the documentation; this may be a virus such as enterovirus, herpes zoster, or leptospira or a bacteria such as *Haemophilus influenzae*, streptococcus, pneumococcus, staphylococcus, or *E. coli*, to name just a few. Each specific detail may lead you to a different code or require a second code.

EXAMPLE

G00.1	Pneumococcal meningitis
G00.8	Other bacterial meningitis (Meningitis due to Escherichia coli)
G03.0	Nonpyogenic meningitis

LET'S CODE IT! SCENARIO

Lamonte Millwood went to see Dr. Vaughn after returning home from college on spring break. He stated that his new dorm room is a small suite and he has three roommates. He said that the last couple of days before he left to come home, two of his roommates were coughing and sneezing. Lamonte tells Dr. Vaughn that he has been nauseous and vomiting, he has become very sensitive to light, and he feels a bit confused, having trouble concentrating on his school work. Tests confirmed Dr. Vaughn's diagnosis of bacterial meningitis caused by Neisseria meningitidis.

Let's Code It!

Dr. Vaughn confirmed Lamonte's diagnosis of "*bacterial meningitis caused by* Neisseria meningitidis," so let's begin with the first part and turn to the Alphabetic Index to look up "Meningitis." You can see a long, long list of additional descriptors indented below this entry. Take a minute to review the elements listed to see if any of them match what the physician wrote in the documented diagnosis.

Meningitis

bacterial G00.9

Now, there is another indented list beneath the term "bacterial" that offers many different names of bacteria . . . except *Neisseria meningitidis (N. meningitidis)*. There are many possibilities, including gram-negative [G00.0] and specified organism NEC [G00.8]. Do you know if *N. meningitidis* is gram-negative or gram-positive?

According to the Centers for Disease Control and Prevention, *Neisseria meningitidis* is a gram-negative bacterium.

Let's go to the Tabular List and begin reading at the three-character code category suggested here:

✓4 **G00 Bacterial meningitis, not elsewhere classified**

(continued)

Read the INCLUDES and EXCLUDES1 notations directly below this code. You are good to continue reading down and review the two choices:

G00.8 **Other bacterial meningitis**
Use additional code **to further identify organism (B96.-)**

G00.9 **Bacterial meningitis, unspecified (Meningitis due to gram-negative bacteria, unspecified)**

Even though G00.9 includes gram-negative bacteria, which is accurate for Lamonte's diagnosis, it is not true that the bacterium is unspecified. It *was* specified as *Neisseria meningitidis*. So, you cannot honestly and accurately report G00.9.

Turn to B96 in your Tabular List to see if you can find a code to specify that *Neisseria meningitidis* is the specific bacterium involved. It appears that the only code that could be used truthfully would be

B96.89 **Other specified bacterial agents as the cause of diseases classified elsewhere**

This doesn't quite add any details, does it? Not really. Before you make a decision, check one more time in the Alphabetic Index under meningitis, only this time check for any mention of *Neisseria meningitidis*.

Meningitis

Neisseria A39.0

This points us to a code in the ICD-10-CM code book's ***Chapter 1: Certain Infectious and Parasitic Diseases (A00–B99)***. Let's take a look at it.

✓4 **A39** **Meningococcal infection**

A39.0 **Meningococcal meningitis**

Two choices to report this diagnosis: A39.0 or G00.8, B96.89

And still you are unable to provide the specific details you know are important. Therefore, you should append a special report, such as the pathology report, with this claim to provide these additional details.

Check the head of this chapter in ICD-10-CM. There is an EXCLUDES2 notation. Read carefully. Do any relate to Dr. Vaughn's diagnosis of Lamonte? No. Turn to the Official Guidelines and read Section I.C.6. There is nothing specifically applicable here either.

For this encounter between Dr. Vaughn and Lamonte, you can confidently report these codes:

G00.8 **Other bacterial meningitis**

B96.89 **Other specified bacterial agents as the cause of diseases classified elsewhere**

Great job!

Hereditary, Degenerative, and Demyelinating Diseases of the Central Nervous System

Some nervous system conditions that affect the function of the CNS are linked to genetics or degeneration but not trauma. The patient may have a condition that is well-known, such as Alzheimer's disease or dementia, or a lesser-known condition such as parkinsonism or Huntington's chorea.

As you have seen before, a diagnosis may seem to be complete but actually may not include enough information for a professional coder. For example, it is not enough to know the patient was diagnosed with dementia. To determine the most accurate code, you need more details, such as

Frontotemporal dementia (Pick's disease) G31.01

Dementia with Lewy bodies (Lewy body dementia) G31.83

You may remember we discussed coding some forms of dementia in the ***Conditions That Affect Mental Health*** section of this chapter. The good news here is that the coding process you learned will help you get to the correct ICD-10-CM chapter, know which specific descriptors to look for in the documentation, and then lead you directly to the most accurate code.

LET'S CODE IT! SCENARIO

Nate Mercado, an 81-year-old male, came to see Dr. Bronson with complaints of increasing forgetfulness and difficulty remembering new information. He states virtually no ability to focus or concentrate. His presentation confirms a deterioration in personal hygiene, and his appearance is somewhat disheveled. Nate's daughter insisted that he come to the physician. After a neurologic exam, psychometric testing, a PET scan, and an EEG, Dr. Bronson diagnosed Nate with late-onset Alzheimer's disease.

Let's Code It!

Dr. Bronson diagnosed Nate with *Alzheimer's disease*. Let's turn to the Alphabetic Index in the ICD-10-CM book and find

Disease
Alzheimer's G30.9 *[F02.80]*

Read the list of additional descriptors indented below this. The specific code to report will change on the basis of documentation of behavioral disturbance, early onset, and/or late onset. What did Dr. Bronson document?

Disease
Alzheimer's G30.9 *[F02.80]*
late onset G30.1 *[F02.80]*

Dr. Bronson stated nothing about behavioral disturbances, so this matches the notes. Let's turn to the Tabular List and begin reading at the three-character code:

✓4 **G30 Alzheimer's disease**

Take a look at the INCLUDES note here, which identifies Alzheimer's dementia senile and presenile forms, as well as the ***Use additional code*** notation, which directs you to the second code suggested in the Alphabetic Index listing, and an EXCLUDES1 note citing three diagnoses that are not reported from this code category. Do you see any of these diagnoses included in Dr. Bronson's documentation? No. Read all of the choices for the fourth character available in this code category and determine which one best matches what Dr. Bronson wrote in Nate's notes:

G30.1 Alzheimer's disease with late onset

This matches the documentation exactly! Good job! Now you must go and investigate the second code suggested by the Alphabetic Index: F02.80. Remember, even though the Alphabetic Index gave us five characters, you must always begin reading at the three-character level:

✓4 **F02 Dementia in other diseases classified elsewhere**

Directly below this entry, you can see a notation to ***Code first*** the underlying physiological condition, such as Alzheimer's disease. This is a great confirmation that you will need these two codes, and now you know the order in which to report them: G30.1 first, followed by the F02 code. Also, read carefully both the EXCLUDES1 and EXCLUDES2 notations. For Nate's encounter with Dr. Bronson, none of these apply. However, the next case you code may involve one of these diagnoses. Now is the best time to establish good coding habits.

Review the fourth-character choices. You will notice there is only one:

✓5 **F02.8 Dementia in other diseases classified elsewhere**

Now review the fifth-character choices. You have two. Which one matches Dr. Bronson's notes about Nate? Dr. Bronson makes no mention at all about any behavioral disturbance.

F02.80 Dementia in other diseases classified elsewhere without behavioral disturbance

You have done a great job determining the two codes to report for Dr. Bronson's diagnosis of Nate:

G30.1 Alzheimer's disease with late onset
F02.80 Dementia in other diseases classified elsewhere without behavioral disturbance

Multiple Sclerosis (MS)

Multiple sclerosis (MS) is a chronic, autoimmune, neurological disorder which begins to show signs and symptoms in adults aged 20 to 40 years old. Patients may suffer with: vision problems including optic neuritis (optic nerve inflammation); painful muscle spasms; concerns with their balance; and bladder control problems. Beginning in 2026, there are eight different codes from which to choose, so the specific type of MS can be clearly identified. These individualized diagnosis codes lead to a better alignment with the various treatment plans.

G35.A Relapsing-remitting multiple sclerosis

G35.B0 Primary progressive multiple sclerosis, unspecified

G35.B1 Active primary progressive multiple sclerosis

G35.B2 Non-active primary progressive multiple sclerosis

G35.C0 Secondary progressive multiple sclerosis, unspecified

G35.C1 Active secondary progressive multiple sclerosis

G35.C2 Non-active secondary progressive multiple sclerosis

G35.D Multiple sclerosis, unspecified

Hydrocephalus

When too much CSF accumulates in the ventricles of the brain, and the body cannot absorb it back into the vascular system fast enough, the brain tissues can be damaged and lose the ability to function properly. This can occur in infants (a congenital anomaly: ICD-10-CM code category Q03 Congenital hydrocephalus), or it can develop in adults (code category G91 Hydrocephalus).

You will find that, again, a diagnostic statement of "hydrocephalus" is insufficient to determine an accurate code, as there are several different types, each with its own specific code.

Communicating hydrocephalus, also referred to as secondary normal pressure hydrocephalus, is a condition in which the CSF is still able to flow out of the ventricles but then encounters an obstruction preventing it from moving further. This results in a flooding of the brain tissues in and around the ventricles. This is reported with code G91.0 Communicating hydrocephalus.

Noncommunicating hydrocephalus, also referred to as obstructive hydrocephalus, most commonly is caused by aqueductal stenosis, a narrowing of one or more of the aqueducts (narrow passageways) that connect the ventricles. This is reported with code G91.1 Obstructive hydrocephalus.

(Idiopathic) normal pressure hydrocephalus (NPH) is an abnormal increase in the quantity of CSF flowing into the ventricles. This is reported with code G91.2 (Idiopathic) normal pressure hydrocephalus.

Post-traumatic hydrocephalus, also known as hydrocephalus ex-vacuo, is the result of damage to the brain after a cerebrovascular accident (CVA) or a traumatic injury, such as TBI. This is reported with code G91.3 Post-traumatic hydrocephalus, unspecified.

Hydrocephalus also may occur as a manifestation of another condition, such as a neoplasm or congenital syphilis. As you have learned in these situations before, you will need to report that underlying condition's code first, followed by code G91.4 Hydrocephalus in diseases classified elsewhere.

LET'S CODE IT! SCENARIO

Jeffrey Himes was referred to Dr. Jonas, a neurosurgeon, after his last brain MRI came back showing signs of an abundance of cerebrospinal fluid (CSF) in the ventricles of his brain. After taking a full history and examination, Dr. Jonas determined that there was malabsorption of CSF in the brain—an official diagnosis of communicating hydrocephalus. Dr. Jonas discussed the treatment options with Jeffrey and his family.

(continued)

Let's Code It!

Dr. Jonas diagnosed Jeffrey with *hydrocephalus*. Let's turn to the Alphabetic Index in the ICD-10-CM book and find

Hydrocephalus (acquired) (external) (internal)
(malignant) (noncommunicating) (obstructive)
(recurrent) G91.9

This seems to match the notes, except included in the parenthetical nonessential modifiers is the term *noncommunicating*. When you look back at the notes, you can see that Dr. Jonas diagnosed Jeffrey with *communicating*—the opposite. So, you know that this code cannot be correct. There is still a long list of additional modifying terms indented below *hydrocephalus*. Read through all of the choices and see if you can determine which one matches the documentation. Did you find this?

Hydrocephalus

communicating G91.0

This matches the notes, so let's turn to the Tabular List and begin reading at the three-character code:

✓4 **G91 Hydrocephalus**

Carefully read the INCLUDES note that identifies acquired hydrocephalus and the EXCLUDES1 note citing three diagnoses that are not reported from this code category. Do you see any of these diagnoses included in Dr. Jonas's documentation? No. Read all of the choices for the fourth character available in this code category and determine which one best matches what Dr. Jonas wrote in Jeffrey's notes:

G91.0 Communicating hydrocephalus

This matches the documentation exactly! Good job!

Migraine Headaches

Medical researchers have been trying to determine the cause of migraine headaches for quite a long time. According to the U.S. National Library of Medicine, currently the theory is that genes related to the control of some brain cell function are the cause.

While the genetic potential for having migraines may be congenital, generally, this pain is not constant, but caused by specific actions or events in one's life. These are known as triggers, and they include

- Stress or anxiety.
- Insufficient sleep.
- Lack of food.
- Fluctuations in hormone levels (specifically in females).

There are several different types of migraine headaches, and these details should be available to you when you abstract the documentation.

Aura: The aura connected with a migraine is actually a sequence of neurologic symptoms that occur within the hour prior to the onset of the migraine itself (in adults). These experiences may affect their vision, such as the appearance of dark or colored spots; their physical sensations, such as tingling or numbness, possibly vertigo; or their senses, such as difficulty with speech or hearing.

Intractable: An intractable migraine also may be described in the documentation as pharmacologically resistant, treatment resistant, medically induced (refractory), and/or poorly controlled by treatment.

Status migrainosus: This term is used to identify that the patient's migraine headache has lasted more than 72 continuous hours.

Chronic: A diagnosis of chronic migraine is documented as the patient reporting more than 15 headache days within a 30-day period, with more than half of these described as migraines.

Other types of migraines: There are many more categories of migraine headaches that you may abstract from the documentation, such as cyclical vomiting, abdominal, or menstrual. Each of these has its own specific code within code category G43 Migraine.

Be alert to these terms, in connection with a migraine diagnosis. The absence of a term, such as aura or intractable, can be used as an indicator that the patient was "without" that aspect of the condition. What this means is that, if the physician does not specifically document that the patient *had* aura with their migraine, you are permitted to use a code that states, "without aura." It is not expected that the physician would necessarily document elements that are not present. However, if the detail is documented, a code that includes that detail must be reported.

10.5 Physiological Conditions Affecting the Peripheral Nervous System

Disorders that affect the peripheral nervous system may interfere with only one nerve, or multiple nerves. In an earlier chapter, you learned that conditions such as diabetes mellitus may cause the development of manifestations affecting the peripheral nervous system, such as diabetic neuropathy. There are various types of underlying causes, such as infection, compression, or injury.

Dominant and Nondominant Sides

Are you right-handed? If so, the right side of your body is considered your dominant side. Individuals who are left-handed have the left side of their bodies considered the dominant side. Then there are those who are ambidextrous (use both hands equally).

Patients suffering with *hemiplegia* (paralysis of one side of the body) or *hemiparesis* (weakness of one side of the body)–code category G81–will need documentation of whether the dominant side or nondominant side is affected. The same is required for a patient diagnosed with *monoplegia* (paralysis of one extremity, for example, one arm or one leg)–code category G83.

You may have no memory of a physician ever asking you whether you are right- or left-handed–I don't. While neurologists are trained to consider this, you may find this detail missing from the documentation. For such cases, querying the physician may not help because they may not know. ***ICD-10-CM Official Guidelines*** are here to help you determine the correct code when the affected (weakened or paralyzed) side is documented yet there is no indication of whether or not this is the patient's dominant side. Here is how the guidelines direct you:

- If the documentation states the right side is affected–report as dominant.
- If the documentation states the left side is affected–report as nondominant.

For those patients documented to be ambidextrous, whichever side is documented as affected should be reported as the patient's dominant side.

EXAMPLES

G81.12	Spastic hemiplegia affecting left dominant side
G83.14	Monoplegia of lower limb affecting left nondominant side

Remember that the laterality refers to the patient's right or left, not that of the writer of the documentation.

GUIDANCE CONNECTION

Read the ICD-10-CM Official Guidelines for Coding and Reporting, section **I. Conventions, General Coding Guidelines and Chapter-Specific Guidelines**, subsection **C. Chapter-Specific Coding Guidelines**, chapter **6. Diseases of the Nervous System**, subsection **a. Dominant/ nondominant side.**

Carpal Tunnel Syndrome

Many people know about carpal tunnel syndrome, when the nerve that feeds through the carpal tunnel within the wrist becomes painful, and sometimes incapacitating. The ligaments and tendons become swollen and compress the nerves threaded through the tunnel from the hand to the arm. In addition to having a confirmed diagnostic statement, you will need documentation of laterality to determine a specific code: G56.01 Carpal tunnel syndrome, right upper limb **or** G56.02 Carpal tunnel syndrome, left upper limb **or** G56.03 Carpal tunnel syndrome, bilateral upper limbs.

Plexus Disorders

Many plexus disorders are the result of a specific point in the peripheral neural pathway for that plexus becoming compressed. Typically, something causes the nerve to be pinched between muscle and bone, such as the thoracic outlet syndrome (brachial plexus disorder) occurring from the muscles of the neck and shoulder squeezing down on the nerve. See code G54.0 Brachial plexus disorders **or** G54.1 Lumbosacral plexus disorders.

Complex Regional Pain Syndrome

After a traumatic injury, complex regional pain syndrome (CRPS) may develop in the damaged extremity (arm/hand, leg/foot). Signs and symptoms include chronic (ongoing) pain; dramatic changes to the color, texture, or temperature of the epidural surface; a burning sensation; and edema and stiffness in involved joints, which often results in decreased mobility.

There are two types of CRPS: CRPS-I and CRPS-II.

CRPS-I used to be called reflex sympathetic dystrophy syndrome. Physicians classify this diagnosis when the patient denies the occurrence of any nerve injury.

G90.511 **Complex regional pain syndrome I of right upper limb**

G90.512 **Complex regional pain syndrome I of left upper limb**

G90.513 **Complex regional pain syndrome I of upper limb, bilateral**

G90.521 **Complex regional pain syndrome I of right lower limb**

G90.522 **Complex regional pain syndrome I of left lower limb**

G90.523 **Complex regional pain syndrome I of lower limb, bilateral**

CRPS-II has been previously documented as causalgia, for patients who have a confirmed nerve injury prior to this diagnosis.

G56.41 **Causalgia of right upper limb**

G56.42 **Causalgia of left upper limb**

G56.43 **Causalgia of bilateral upper limbs**

G57.71 **Causalgia of right lower limb**

G57.72 **Causalgia of left lower limb**

G57.73 **Causalgia of bilateral lower limbs**

CODING BITES

Four nerve plexuses branch from the spinal cord off into the peripheral nerve network:

- The **cervical plexus** branches nerves to the head, neck, and shoulder.
- The **brachial plexus** branches nerves to the chest, shoulders, upper arms, forearms, and hands.
- The **lumbar plexus** branches nerves to the back, abdomen, groin, thighs, knees, and calves.
- The **sacral plexus** branches nerves to the pelvis, buttocks, genitals, thighs, calves, and feet.

YOU CODE IT! CASE STUDY

ICD-10-CM

Simon Clossberg is a 37-year-old architect. While on a business trip to Los Angeles, Simon and guys on his team decided to have some fun and rented some motorcycles. Taking a turn too wide, Simon was involved in a one-vehicle motorcycle accident. In the accident, Simon was pinned and slid between the bike and the pavement, ultimately landing on his back. A police officer witnessed the accident and immediately called for medical assistance.

EMTs arrived within minutes and immediately immobilized Simon's neck and secured him to a rigid board prior to transporting him to the emergency department of the nearest hospital. Upon arrival at the ED, Simon was conscious and complained of pain in his lower back. ED physician Dr. NeJame examined Simon and found numerous abrasions and contusions, in addition to a loss of both sensation and motor control of his legs. After he was stabilized, Dr. NeJame admitted Simon and called for a neurologic consult. Dr. Cheslea completed the neurologic assessment.

The neurologic exam revealed the following: Simon demonstrated normal or near normal strength in flexing and extending his elbows, in extending his wrists, and when flexing his middle finger and abducting his little finger on both hands. However, he exhibited no movement when medical personnel tested his ability to flex his hips, extend his knees, and dorsiflex his ankles.

Stretch reflexes involving the biceps, brachioradialis, and triceps muscles were found to be normal, while those involving the patella and ankle were absent. In addition, Simon was found to have normal sensitivity to pin prick and light touch in areas of his body above the level of his inguinal (groin) region, but not below that region of the body.

Dr. Cheslea diagnosed Simon with lumbosacral plexus disorder.

(continued)

You Code It!

Go through the steps of coding, and determine the code or codes that should be reported for this encounter between Dr. Cheslea and Simon.

Step #1: Read the case carefully and completely.
Step #2: Abstract the scenario. Which main words or terms describe why the physician cared for the patient during this encounter?
Step #3: Are there any details missing or incomplete for which you would need to query the physician? [If so, ask your instructor.]
Step #4: Check for any relevant guidance, including reading all of the symbols and notations in the Tabular List and the appropriate sections of the Official Guidelines.
Step #5: Determine the correct diagnosis code or codes to explain why this encounter was medically necessary.
Step #6: Double-check your work.

Answer:

Did you determine this to be the correct code?

G54.1 Lumbosacral plexus disorder

Good work!

10.6 Pain Management

Acute
Severe; serious.

Chronic
Long duration; continuing over an extended period of time.

Neurologists are among the health care professionals who most often treat pain because neurologic conditions involve the nerve endings and electrical impulses within the nervous system. There are physicians who specialize in pain management, although specialized training is not mandatory. **Acute** pain is determined by the severity of the pain and its impact on the patient's ability to function. The most common types of **chronic** pain include headache, low back pain, cancer pain, arthritis pain, neurogenic pain, and psychogenic pain. There is no specific time measurement to determine chronic pain. Therefore, the judgment of the physician, as stated in the documentation, is what differentiates acute pain from chronic pain. You must be careful not to assume a diagnosis of *chronic pain syndrome*. This condition is different from chronic pain, and its diagnosis may be reported (code G89.4) only when the attending physician specifically documents this condition.

Pain can be a very difficult thing to deal with clinically because it is not the same for every patient. Medically speaking, pain is an unpleasant sensation often initiated by tissue damage that results in impulses being transmitted to the brain via specific nerve fibers. It can be challenging for the patient to describe the level of intensity, and each individual patient's ability to cope with pain will vary greatly. Clinically speaking, pain can be diagnosed as acute, chronic, or both acute and chronic.

Most health care facilities use some type of pain scale from 0 to 10 (see **Table 10-1**) to help improve communication with patients. The zero indicates no pain at all, and the scale increases up to the number 10, representing excruciating, intolerable pain. Some facilities use a scale that includes illustrations to help patients accurately communicate what they are feeling.

TABLE 10-1 Numeric Rating Scale for Pain

Numeric Rating	Meaning
0	No pain
1–3	Mild pain (nagging, annoying, interfering little with ADLs)
4–6	Moderate pain (interferes significantly with ADLs)
7–10	Severe pain (disabling; unable to perform ADLs)

Source: National Institutes of Health

Reporting Pain Separately

When the physician has documented a confirmed diagnosis and this condition is the underlying cause of the pain, pain should not be reported with a separate code. In these circumstances, the pain is considered to be an inclusive symptom. The exceptions to this guideline occur when

- The principal purpose of the encounter is pain management and the encounter does not include treatment or management of the underlying condition.
- The pain is noted as acute and/or chronic, documenting that the pain suffered by the patient is above and beyond the level typical of the underlying condition.

ICD-10-CM provides code category G89 Pain, not elsewhere classified, from which to choose an appropriate code.

EXAMPLES

1. Megan slipped during ice skating practice and broke her right ankle. After x-raying the ankle and applying the cast, Dr. Hustey gave her a prescription for pain medication. In this case, only the fractured ankle would be reported **(S82.64XA, Nondisplaced fracture of lateral malleolus of right fibula, initial encounter for closed fracture)**. The pain is an inclusive symptom of the fracture.
2. Megan came back to Dr. Hustey 10 days later complaining of unbearable pain and stating that the prescribed medication was not "doing the trick." Dr. Hustey discussed with Megan several management treatments for the acute pain, and she agreed to try a different medication. This encounter was only for pain management. Dr. Hustey did not attend to the fracture at all. Therefore, this encounter would be reported with two codes:

G89.11	Acute pain due to trauma
S82.64XD	Nondisplaced fracture of lateral malleolus of right fibula, subsequent encounter for fracture with routine healing

   A code from category G89 is reported to add details about the reason for this encounter with Dr. Hustey. The code for the fracture explains why Megan had pain.
3. Phillip is diagnosed with chronic tension headaches due to the extreme pressures of his job. He told the physician he could not stand the pain anymore and he needed help. This diagnosis would be reported with both of these codes:

G89.29	Other chronic pain
G44.229	Chronic tension-type headache, not intractable

The official guidelines state that if the pain is not specifically documented as acute or chronic, it should not be reported separately. The exceptions to this guideline include

- *Post-thoracotomy pain:* G89.12 Acute post-thoracotomy pain (post-thoracotomy pain NOS); G89.22 Chronic post-thoracotomy pain.
- *Postprocedural pain:* G89.18 Other acute postprocedural pain (postprocedural pain NOS); G89.28 Other chronic postprocedural pain.
- *Neoplasm-related pain:* G89.3 Neoplasm related pain (acute) (chronic).
- *Central pain syndrome:* G89.0 Central pain syndrome.

In these four situations, the code from category G89 should be reported in addition to any other conditions related to the encounter.

Postprocedural Pain

As stated above, postprocedural pain would be reported with either G89.18 or G89.28, depending upon the physician's documentation of the pain as either acute or chronic. One of these codes may be reported only when the pain is documented as

- More intense or lasting longer than the expected level of pain that is considered normal immediately after a surgical procedure.
- Not related to a detailed complication of the surgical procedure.

Site-Specific Pain Codes

There are many other code categories within ICD-10-CM used to report pain located in a specific anatomical site. Code category G89 Pain, not elsewhere classified, does not include any site-specific information. Anatomical site-specific code categories include

M54.5 **Low back pain (lumbago)**

M79.602 **Pain in left arm**

M79.672 **Pain in left foot**

Sequencing Pain Codes with Other Codes

To determine the proper sequencing of a code from category G89 with codes for site-specific pain or underlying conditions, the first question to be answered from the documentation is, "Why was this encounter necessary?" If the answer is for pain management, the code from category G89 should be first-listed or the principal diagnosis reported. If the encounter is for any other reason and the attention to pain management is secondary to the purpose for the encounter, then the first-listed or principal diagnosis code would report that other reason, and the code from category G89 would be reported afterward.

GUIDANCE CONNECTION

Read the ICD-10-CM Official Guidelines for Coding and Reporting, section **I. Conventions, General Coding Guidelines and Chapter-Specific Guidelines**, subsection **C. Chapter-Specific Coding Guidelines**, chapter **6. Diseases of the Nervous System**, subsection **b. Pain–category G89**.

LET'S CODE IT! SCENARIO

Patti Moscowicz came in to see Dr. Levine with complaints of extreme pain in her head. She stated that she was nauseous and irritable and that light made the pain even worse. Patti stated that these headaches seemed to happen every month, right before she got her menstrual period, and she couldn't take it anymore. She begged for something to help with the pain. After a full examination, Dr. Levine diagnosed her with chronic premenstrual migraine.

Let's Code It!

Dr. Levine diagnosed Patti with *premenstrual migraine headaches*, and pain management was the purpose of this visit to the physician. Let's turn to the ICD-10-CM Alphabetic Index and find

Migraine (idiopathic) G43.909

There is a list of additional descriptors indented below this. Go back to the physician's notes. Did he describe the migraine with more detail? Yes, he stated her migraine was premenstrual. So look down the list and see if you can find a suggested code:

Migraine (idiopathic) G43.909

menstrual G43.829

pre-menstrual—*see* Migraine, menstrual

Perfect! Now, let's turn to code category G43 in the Tabular List:

✓4 **G43** **Migraine**

Did you notice the notation below this code?

Use additional code **for adverse effect, if applicable, to identify drug (T36–T50 with fifth or sixth character 5)**

(continued)

There is no mention of any drugs or adverse reactions in Dr. Levine's documentation, so let's continue. Read the **EXCLUDES1** and **EXCLUDES2** notes. Nothing there matches the physician's notes, so continue down the column and review *all* of the choices for the mandatory fourth character. Which one matches what Dr. Levine wrote?

✓5 **G43.8 Other migraine**

There are fifth-character choices listed below this code, so you will have to look down the column and find the box containing the fifth-character choices. You will see the box directly below the three-character code category. Review the four choices. Which one matches?

✓6 **G43.82 Menstrual migraine, not intractable**

Good. There was no mention that Patti was having an intractable migraine. Read the notation beneath this code classification:

Code also associated premenstrual tension syndrome (N94.3)

There was no mention of this in Dr. Levine's notes on Patti. Review the choices for the sixth character:

G43.829 Menstrual migraine, not intractable, without mention of status migrainosus

Do you also need to include a code from the G89 code category? Check the Official Guidelines, specifically Section I.C.6.b.1)(b), **Use of category G89 codes in conjunction with site specific pain codes**. You will see that it states, *"If the code describes the site of the pain, but does not fully describe whether the pain is acute or chronic, then both codes should be assigned."* Terrific! Dr. Levine documented that Patti's pain was chronic, and code G43.829 does not include that specific detail. That's the answer to that question, so go and review all of the possible codes from code category G89 to determine the most accurate code to report:

G89.29 Other chronic pain

You have one last task to complete. Now that you have two codes to report Dr. Levine's reasons for caring for Patti during this encounter, you need to determine the correct sequence in which to report these codes. Refer again to that guideline, and the next part tells you, *"If the encounter is for pain control or pain management, assign the code from category G89 followed by the code identifying the specific site of pain."* You know from the notes that the reason for this encounter was pain management, so now you know the correct codes and the correct order in which to report the reason why Dr. Levine cared for Patti during this encounter:

G89.29 Other chronic pain

G43.829 Menstrual migraine, not intractable, without mention of status migrainosus

Good job!

Chapter Summary

Due to an increase in available care, more patients are receiving treatment for mental and behavioral disorders. Therefore, it is important for professional coding specialists to understand both psychological and physiological concerns. Through education and understanding, these patients can receive treatment and their providers can receive accurate reimbursement.

Many different circumstances and situations can be the cause of malfunction anywhere in the nervous system. As with any other organ system or diagnosis, professional coding specialists should never assume. Everything you need to report these conditions accurately is in the physician's documentation. If it is not, you must query the physician.

CODING BITES

Did you know there are hundreds of named phobias . . . such as

Acrophobia = fear of high places
Aerophobia = fear of air travel
Apiphobia = fear of bees
Bromidrosiphobia = fear of body odor

(continued)

Claustrophobia = fear of enclosed places
Gephyrophobia = fear of bridges
Haemophobia = fear of blood
Kakorrhaphiaphobia = fear of failure
Linonophobia = fear of string
Phasmophobia = fear of ghosts
Scotophobia = fear of the dark
Taphephobia = fear of being buried alive
Triskaidekaphobia = fear of the number 13

CHAPTER 10 REVIEW
Coding Mental, Behavioral, and Neurologic Disorders

Let's Check It! Terminology

Match each key term to the appropriate definition.

1. **LO 10.2** An emotional state that includes sadness, hopelessness, and gloom.
2. **LO 10.1** Ongoing, regular consumption of a substance with resulting significant clinical manifestations, and a dramatic decrease in the effect of the substance with continued use, therefore requiring an increased quantity of the substance to achieve intoxication.
3. **LO 10.2** An emotional state that includes elation, excitement, and exuberance.
4. **LO 10.1** The feelings of apprehension and fear, sometimes manifested with physical manifestations such as sweating and palpitations.
5. **LO 10.3** The sincere belief that one is suffering an illness that is not present.
6. **LO 10.1** Consumption of a substance without significant clinical manifestations.
7. **LO 10.1** Common behaviors include mood disorders, sleep disorders, psychotic symptoms, and agitation.
8. **LO 10.3** Irrational and excessive fear of an object, activity, or situation.
9. **LO 10.1** Ongoing, regular consumption of a substance with resulting clinical manifestations.
10. **LO 10.2** A psychotic disorder with no known cause.

A. Abuse
B. Anxiety
C. Behavioral Disturbance
D. Dependence
E. Depressive
F. Manic
G. Phobia
H. Schizophrenia
I. Somatoform Disorders
J. Use

Let's Check It! Concepts

Choose the most appropriate answer for each of the following questions.

1. **LO 10.1** When a patient is diagnosed with an alcohol- or drug-related disorder, such condition is susceptible to ________________ signs, symptoms, manifestations, and co-morbidities.
   a. psychological **b.** physiological
   c. psychological and physiological **d.** none of these
2. **LO 10.2** All of the following are mood disorders *except*
   a. depression. **b.** apathy. **c.** euphoria. **d.** hallucinations.
3. **LO 10.1** Pete smokes marijuana on a regular basis, and it takes a little more each time to achieve the full effect. Pete is beginning to have some problems with his memory and gets irritable when he doesn't smoke pot. Pete is _____ marijuana.
   a. using **b.** abusing **c.** dependent on **d.** withdrawing from

4. **LO 10.3** Which of the following is a somatoform disorder?
   a. panic disorder
   b. bipolar disorder
   c. hypochondriacal disorder
   d. schizophreniform disorder

5. **LO 10.2** The patient has been diagnosed with bipolar disorder, current episode, manic, severe, with psychotic features. The correct code is
   a. F31.
   b. F31.2.
   c. F31.4.
   d. F31.5.

6. **LO 10.4** Huntington's chorea is an example of a(n)
   a. inflammatory disease of the CNS.
   b. trauma of the CNS.
   c. hereditary disease of the CNS.
   d. disease of the PNS.

7. **LO 10.4** The Official Guidelines state that if the pain is not specifically documented as acute or chronic, it should not be reported separately. The exceptions to this guideline include all of the following *except*
   a. neoplasm-related pain.
   b. tension headaches.
   c. central pain syndrome.
   d. post-thoracotomy pain.

8. **LO 10.3** ____________ is a condition in which a horrible experience leaves a lasting imprint on the patient's sense of danger.
   a. Fear
   b. Anxiety
   c. Post-traumatic stress disorder
   d. Reactive depression

9. **LO 10.5** The _____ plexus branches nerves to the chest, shoulders, upper arms, forearms, and hands.
   a. brachial
   b. cervical
   c. lumbar
   d. sacral

10. **LO 10.6** To determine the proper sequencing of a code from category G89 with codes for site-specific pain or underlying conditions, the first question to be answered from the documentation is
   a. Where did the encounter take place?
   b. How was the service provided?
   c. When did the encounter take place?
   d. Why was the encounter necessary?

Let's Check It! Guidelines

Refer to the Official Guidelines and fill in the blanks according to Chapter 5, Mental, Behavioral, and Neurodevelopmental Disorders, and Chapter 6, Diseases of the Nervous System, Chapter-Specific Coding Guidelines.

G89	default	G89.2	cancer	psychological
relationship	one	acute	pain	associated
G89.4	G89.0	F45.41	G89.3	only
documentation	F45.42	substance related	in remission	

1. Assign code _____, for pain that is exclusively related to _____ disorders. As indicated by the Excludes 1 note under category G89, a code from category G89 should not be assigned with code F45.41.
2. Code _____, Pain disorders with related psychological factors, should be used with a code from category _____, Pain, not elsewhere classified, if there is documentation of a psychological component for a patient with acute or chronic pain.
3. Selection of codes describing _____ for categories F10–F19, Mental and behavioral disorders due to psychoactive substance use (categories F10–F19 with -.11, -.21, -.91) requires the provider's clinical judgment and are assigned only on the basis of provider _____ (as defined in the Official Guidelines for Coding and Reporting), unless otherwise instructed by the classification.
4. When the provider documentation refers to use, abuse, and dependence of the same substance, only _____ code should be assigned to identify the pattern of use.
5. These codes are to be used only when the psychoactive substance use is _____ with a _____ disorder (Chapter 5 disorders such as sexual dysfunction, sleep disorder, or a mental or behavioral disorder) or medical condition, and such a _____ is documented by the provider.

6. Codes in category G89, Pain, not elsewhere classified, may be used in conjunction with codes from other categories and chapters to provide more detail about acute or chronic ______ and neoplasm-related pain, unless otherwise indicated below.
7. The ______ for post-thoracotomy and other postoperative pain not specified as acute or chronic is the code for the ______ form.
8. Chronic pain is classified to subcategory ______.
9. Code ______ is assigned to pain documented as being related, associated or due to ______, primary or secondary malignancy, or tumor.
10. Central pain syndrome ______ and chronic pain syndrome ______ are different from the term "chronic pain," and therefore codes should ______ be used when the provider has specifically documented this condition.

Let's Check It! Rules and Regulations

Please answer the following questions from the knowledge you have gained after reading this chapter.

1. **LO 10.1** What is the clinical difference between use, abuse, and dependence?
2. **LO 10.2** Explain schizoid personality disorder.
3. **LO 10.3** What is a phobia?
4. **LO 10.4** Differentiate between an inflammatory and a hereditary/degenerative type of disease of the nervous system. Give an example of each type.
5. **LO 10.5** Why is it important to know which side is dominant when coding weakness or paralysis? How do the guidelines help us if the dominant side is not documented in the patient's chart? How do the guidelines direct the coder for a patient who has been documented as being ambidextrous?

YOU CODE IT! Basics

First, identify the main term in the following diagnoses; then code the diagnosis.

Example: Korsakoff's alcoholic psychosis

a. main term: *psychosis* b. diagnosis *F10.96*

1. Nicotine dependence:
   a. main term: ______ b. diagnosis: ______
2. Generalized anxiety disorder:
   a. main term: ______ b. diagnosis: ______
3. Vascular dementia:
   a. main term: ______ b. diagnosis: ______
4. Mild cognitive impairment:
   a. main term: ______ b. diagnosis: ______
5. Cocaine abuse:
   a. main term: ______ b. diagnosis: ______
6. Schizoaffective manic type disorder:
   a. main term: ______ b. diagnosis: ______
7. Delirium with multiple etiologies:
   a. main term: ______ b. diagnosis: ______
8. Infantile autism:
   a. main term: ______ b. diagnosis: ______
9. Bacterial meningitis, *E. coli*:
   a. main term: ______ b. diagnosis: ______
10. Acute disseminated encephalitis:
    a. main term: ______ b. diagnosis: ______
11. Early-onset cerebellar ataxia:
    a. main term: ______ b. diagnosis: ______
12. Amyotrophic lateral sclerosis:
    a. main term: ______ b. diagnosis: ______
13. Postencephalitic parkinsonism:
    a. main term: ______ b. diagnosis: ______
14. Generalized idiopathic epilepsy:
    a. main term: ______ b. diagnosis: ______
15. Congenital dystonic cerebral palsy:
    a. main term: ______ b. diagnosis: ______

YOU CODE IT! Practice

Using the techniques described in this chapter, carefully read through the case studies and determine the most accurate ICD-10-CM code(s) and external cause code(s), if appropriate, for each case study.

1. Albert Goings, a 54-year-old male, presents today with abdominal cramping and diarrhea. Albert had knee surgery 6 months ago, and the surgeon prescribed oxycodone for pain control. Albert has stopped taking the medication but is having difficulty. Dr. Kenneth documents dilated pupils as well as goose bumps. Albert is diagnosed with oxycodone dependence, uncomplicated.
2. Charles Homer, a 6-year-old male, is brought in by his parents to see his pediatrician, Dr. Freibert. Mrs. Homer is concerned because Charles has been eating dirt and sand and he has tried to eat paper for approximately 1 month. Dr. Freibert completes a thorough examination and notes paleness and failure to thrive. Charles is admitted to Weston Hospital for a full workup. After reviewing the laboratory and developmental test results, Charles is diagnosed with pica.
3. Kelley Dumont, a 19-year-old female, comes in to see Dr. Molusky. Kelley complains that she feels powerless and depressed. Kelley is accompanied by her mother. Mrs. Dumont states that Kelley has given up activities and has become fearful. Dr. Molusky completes a psychological examination and diagnoses Kelley with chronic paranoid reaction.
4. Kevin Genutis, a 24-year-old male, presents with the complaint of experiencing early orgasm and ejaculation, usually a minute or two after beginning sexual activity. Dr. Fox completes an examination and diagnoses Kevin with premature ejaculation.
5. April Carter, a 56-year-old female, was brought to the emergency department by a friend who found her in a stupor. After Dr. Hoogenboom completed a thorough examination and after documenting posturing, echolalia, and echopraxia, April is admitted for further psychological testing. After reviewing the test results, Dr. Hoogenboom diagnoses April with schizophrenic catatonia.
6. Brent Brooke, an 18-year-old male, presents for immunizations before joining the army. Brent passes out when given an injection. Dr. Meetze diagnoses Brent with fear of injections.
7. Melissa Roxburgh, a 21-year-old female, presents for a checkup. Melissa states she is deliberately trying to lose weight, exercises strenuously, and uses appetite suppressants. Dr. Fritz documents a BMI of 16.5, hypotension, and tachycardia as well as Melissa's inability to concentrate. Dr. Fritz decides to admit Melissa. After reviewing the laboratory results and a psychological evaluation, Melissa is diagnosed with anorexia nervosa, restricting type.
8. Gregory Abreu, a 37-year-old male, was previously diagnosed with African rhodesiense trypanosomiasis infection due to *Trypanosoma bruceri*. Greg presents today with the complaint of a severe headache and a stiff neck. Greg says he feels so bad that it actually hurts to walk. Dr. Crumpler notes a fever of 102 F and shivering. Greg is admitted to Weston Hospital, where the results of a lumbar puncture confirm an elevated CSF pressure of 24 cm H_2O. Gregory is diagnosed with meningitis.
9. Carol Abuelo, a 39-year-old female, presents today with general restlessness. Dr. Sabbagha documents unintentional and uncontrollable movements as well as slowed saccadic eye movements. Carol is admitted. An MRI scan reveals atrophy of the caudate nuclei and genetic tests confirmed the diagnosis of Huntington's chorea.
10. Harold Darden, a 5-month-old male, is brought in by his parents for a checkup. Dr. Hottel notes muscle weakness and a weak cry. Mrs. Darden says that Harold seems to have some difficulty swallowing. Harold is admitted to Weston Hospital. The genetic blood tests, EMG, and NCV all confirm a diagnosis of infantile spinal muscular atrophy, type I.
11. Ruby Jenkins, a 26-year-old female, presents with popping or clicking sounds in her ears. After a thorough examination and the appropriate tests, Dr. Thompson diagnoses Ruby with palatal myoclonus.
12. Joe Frances, a 47-year-old male, presents with weakness and a numb feeling in his legs. Dr. Wigley notes hypertonia and orders an MRI, which reveals a thoracic spinal cord lesion. Joe is diagnosed with acute transverse myelitis.
13. Daniela Wiebenga, an 11-year-old female, is brought in by her mother. Mrs. Wiebenga is concerned because Daniela is starting to knock over objects and drop things, mostly in the morning. Daniela says it's hardest in the morning and seems to get better as the day progresses. Dr. Jefferson orders an EEG, which reveals spikes and waves, and admits Daniela. After a full workup, Daniela is diagnosed with juvenile absence epilepsy.

(continued)

14. Eric Lewter, a 56-year-old male, presents with the feeling of tiredness but has been sleeping a lot over the last 3 to 4 months. Eric is accompanied by his wife, Peggy, who states she has noticed some mild mood changes as well. Dr. Shealy completes a thorough examination and the appropriate tests and diagnoses Eric with Kleine-Levin syndrome (KLS).

15. Paige Henderson, a 42-year-old female, comes in today with the complaint of numbness in her left little finger. Dr. McKenna notes Paige has difficulty performing fine motor movements with her left hand and fingers. After an examination and the appropriate tests, Dr. McKenna diagnoses Paige with tardy ulnar nerve palsy, left arm.

YOU CODE IT! Application

The following exercises provide practice in abstracting physicians' notes and learning to work with documentation from our health care facility, Prader, Bracker, & Associates. These case studies are modeled on real patient encounters. Using the techniques described in this chapter, carefully read through the case studies and determine the most accurate ICD-10-CM code(s) and external cause code(s), if appropriate, for each case study.

PRADER, BRACKER, & ASSOCIATES

A Complete Health Care Facility

159 Healthcare Way • SOMEWHERE, FL 32811 • 407-555-6789

PATIENT: PORTER, KELSEY

ACCOUNT/EHR #: PORTKE001

Attending Physician: Oscar R. Prader, MD

Kelsey is a straight "A" student at the state university. He is well liked and respected, handsome, tall, and personable. However, he is finding it increasingly difficult to socialize with his friends without the need to, unobtrusively, wash his hands for fear of contamination. He began carrying antibacterial wipes for those occasions when he could not get to a sink. He had difficulty tolerating medication to help defuse these feelings, and he has found talk therapy to be of little benefit. He stated that he came to my office with his parents, desperately hoping to get some relief.

After a thorough 2½-hour evaluation, I diagnosed Kelsey with OCD.

Diagnosis: Obsessive-compulsive disorder (OCD)

Determine the most accurate ICD-10-CM code(s).

PRADER, BRACKER, & ASSOCIATES

A Complete Health Care Facility

159 Healthcare Way • SOMEWHERE, FL 32811 • 407-555-6789

PATIENT: MYRICK, JULIE

ACCOUNT/EHR #: MYRIJU001

Attending Physician: Oscar R. Prader, MD

S: Julie, a 47-year-old female, came to see me because her youngest son was getting married, leaving her alone. She stated that, over the last several weeks, she had begun having panic attacks whenever she thought about the upcoming separation. Patient has tried cognitive behavioral therapy and different medications without success.

O: CBC results showed the size of her red blood cells (MCV) was slightly abnormal. The range was 80–100, and she was 101. Evidence-based medicine has documented an elevated MCV could indicate a B_{12} deficiency, so I had Julie do a Schilling test, which was positive.

(continued)

A: Panic disorder without agoraphobia, vitamin B_{12} deficiency.

P: Rx B_{12} injections; patient to return in 10–14 days.

Determine the most accurate ICD-10-CM code(s).

PRADER, BRACKER, & ASSOCIATES

A Complete Health Care Facility

159 Healthcare Way • SOMEWHERE, FL 32811 • 407-555-6789

PATIENT: FALCONE, ANTONIO

ACCOUNT/EHR #: FALANT001

Attending Physician: Renee O. Bracker, MD

Antonio, a 43-year-old male, was referred by his therapist of 3 years, Ms. Benton, for psychiatric evaluation and consideration of medication to treat worsening depression. At the initial interview, Antonio's wife, Marie, an attorney, was present to provide some history and perceptions. She was quite cooperative yet strangely detached. She answered all of the questions that I asked in a genuine manner. All pathological causes of sadness have been ruled out. A complete workup is performed.

It gradually became clear that the source of Antonio's persistent depression was his wife's lack of accountability and responsibility in the marriage. She was frequently late for sessions, with no notice. Antonio always wanted to be a family man. Marie refuses to work at the marriage, crushing Antonio's expectations of a satisfying marriage.

Antonio checked into a hotel 500 miles away from home and threatened suicide 2 days ago. When Antonio returned, he came directly to my office. This episode was due to his wife's lack of therapy participation. Antonio stated he feels like a failure because he can't make the marriage work. Suicide seemed to be a viable exit strategy from the pain.

My recommendations were that an environment change was needed to recover from the suicidal ideation. Antonio was experiencing continued depression caused by this environment in which his level of control over the outcome was minimal. This led to more severe and frequent depression. I advised him to stay out of the house.

Diagnosis: Major depressive disorder, recurrent, moderate

Determine the most accurate ICD-10-CM code(s).

WESTON HOSPITAL

629 Healthcare Way • SOMEWHERE, FL 32811 • 407-555-6541

PATIENT: LYNCH, VICTOR

ACCOUNT/EHR #: LYNVIC001

Attending Physician: Renee O. Bracker, MD

S: This is a 3-year-old male who is recovering from a mild case of the flu and suddenly began vomiting. The babysitter may have given him aspirin by accident instead of acetaminophen. Victor's mother brought him to the ED for unexplained irritability and restlessness. He later develops convulsions, which are treated with anticonvulsants. He is admitted to PICU.

O: T: 36.7, P: 102, R 48, BP 115/69, oxygen saturation 99% in room air. Height, weight, and head circumference are all at the 50th percentile. PERRLA. No signs of external trauma. Sclera nonicteric. EOMs cannot be fully tested, but they are conjugate. TMs are normal. Neck reveals no adenopathy. He is agitated and uncooperative. Heart regular without murmurs or gallops. Lungs are clear. Abdomen—normal bowel sounds. No definite tenderness. No inguinal hernias are present. He moves all extremities.

(continued)

LABS: Serum bilirubin: normal. Serum AST and ALT: increased. Serum ammonia: increased. Prothrombin time: prolonged. A CT scan of the brain shows cerebral edema. Neurologic symptoms rapidly deteriorate and he becomes unresponsive. Patient is intubated and put on mechanical ventilation and IV fluid is started. A liver biopsy reveals diffuse, small lipid deposits in the hepatocytes (microvesicular steatosis) without significant necrosis or inflammation.

A: Reye's syndrome

P: Continue to follow and treat.

Determine the most accurate ICD-10-CM code(s).

WESTON HOSPITAL

629 Healthcare Way • SOMEWHERE, FL 32811 • 407-555-6541

PATIENT: YAN, MARANDA

ACCOUNT/EHR #: YANMAR001

Attending Physician: Oscar R. Prader, MD

S: This is a 23-year-old female who presents with a chief complaint of clumsiness and blurred vision. Patient states she had been feeling fine until about 10 days ago when she noticed some numbness and weakness in her right leg, and suddenly her vision became blurry.

O: VS are normal. She is alert but subdued, afebrile with some ataxia noted. HEENT exam is notable for severe visual loss and pale optic discs on funduscopy. Her heart, lungs, and abdomen are normal. She is noted to have a hyporeflexive paraparesis noted on the right.

I decided to admit her to the hospital. An MRI scan shows multiple lesions in the periventricular white matter and cerebellum. Pattern visual evoked responses showed markedly delayed latencies. Corticosteroids are prescribed. Prognosis—a full recovery within 10–14 days.

A: Relapsing-remitting multiple sclerosis (RRMS)

P: Continue to follow and treat with traditional medication.

Determine the most accurate ICD-10-CM code(s).

11

Coding Dysfunction of the Optical and Auditory Systems

Key Terms

Accommodation
Blepharitis
Bulbar Conjunctiva
Cataract
Choroid
Ciliary Body
Cone
Conjunctivitis
Cornea
Corneal Dystrophy
Dacryocystitis
Extraocular Muscles
Glands of Zeis
Glaucoma
Iris
Keratitis
Lacrimal Apparatus
Lens
Meibomian Glands
Moll's Glands
Orbit
Palpebrae
Palpebral Conjunctiva
Proptosis
Pupil
Retina
Retinal Detachment
Retinopathy
Rod
Sclera
Uveal Tract
Vitreous Chamber

Learning Outcomes

After completing this chapter, the student should be able to:

LO 11.1 Identify conditions affecting the external eye.
LO 11.2 Interpret the details documented about diseases of the internal optical system to report the accurate code.
LO 11.3 Determine the accurate code to report other conditions of the eye.
LO 11.4 Abstract documentation accurately to report conditions affecting the auditory system.
LO 11.5 Enumerate the causes, signs, and symptoms of hearing loss.

STOP! Remember, you need to follow along in your ICD-10-CM code book for an optimal learning experience.

11.1 Diseases of the External Optical System

The Exterior of the Eye

The **palpebrae** (eyelids) cover the eyeballs to protect them from injury and environmental invaders as well as to maintain the proper level of moisture. Some people think eyelids are made of epidermis, like regular skin; however, they are really composed of connective tissue. The *levator palpebrae muscle superioris* (*levator* = lift; *palpebrae* = eyelids; muscle; *superioris* = above) is responsible for opening and closing the upper eyelid, while the fascia behind the orbicularis oculi muscle (the orbital septum) creates a barrier between the lids and the **orbit**. There is a thin mucous membrane that lines the inside of the eyelid, known as the **palpebral conjunctiva**; this lines the eyelid internally, creasing over at the fornix, and covers the surface of the eyeball. At that point, it becomes known as the **bulbar conjunctiva** (see **Figure 11-1**).

Within the palpebrae (eyelids), there are three types of glands:

- **Moll's glands**: ordinary sweat glands.
- **Meibomian glands**: sebaceous glands that secrete a tear film component that prevents tears from evaporating so that the area stays moist.
- **Glands of Zeis**: altered sebaceous glands that are connected to the eyelash follicles.

Palpebrae
The eyelids [singular: palpebra].

Orbit
The bony cavity in the skull that houses the eye and its ancillary parts (muscles, nerves, blood vessels).

Palpebral Conjunctiva
A mucous membrane that lines the palpebrae.

Bulbar Conjunctiva
A mucous membrane on the surface of the eyeball.

Moll's Glands
Ordinary sweat glands.

Meibomian Glands
Sebaceous glands that secrete a tear film component that prevents tears from evaporating so that the area stays moist.

Glands of Zeis
Altered sebaceous glands that are connected to the eyelash follicles.

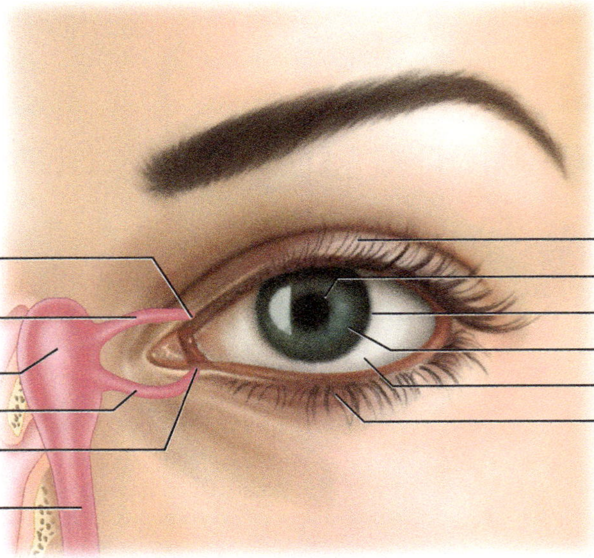

FIGURE 11-1 The anatomical components of the external eyes

EXAMPLES

H00.024	Hordeolum internum left upper eyelid
H00.15	Chalazion left lower eyelid
H01.112	Allergic dermatitis of right lower eyelid
H02.031	Senile entropion of right upper eyelid
H02.131	Senile ectropion of right upper eyelid

You may be thinking, "*Hey, wait a minute. You just taught us that palpebra is the medical term for eyelid. And yet here in the code descriptions, they each state 'eyelid,' the English word.*" That's very true. However, the reason you need to learn that the term *palpebra* means eyelid is because when your physician is writing operative notes or procedure notes, they may use the term *palpebra*, and if you're not familiar with that and you don't know what it means, you won't know how to code this.

Blepharitis

Blepharitis
Inflammation of the eyelid.

Staphylococcal blepharitis, also known as ulcerative **blepharitis**, is a condition in which the rims of the eyelids become inflamed and appear red. Most often, this condition is chronic and affects bilaterally, as well as simultaneously to the upper and lower lids. In addition to the redness, dry scales and ulcerations may form.

Squamous blepharitis is similar, with inflammation of the glands of Zeis. Signs and symptoms include itching, burning, photophobia, mucous discharge, and a crusty formation on the eyelids.

As you abstract documentation with a confirmed diagnosis of blepharitis, you will need to confirm the specific eye involved (right or left) as well as the specific lid (upper or lower). Code subcategory H01.0- Blepharitis.

YOU CODE IT! CASE STUDY

Rosemary Seaborn, a 25-year-old female, came to see Dr. Spencer, an ophthalmologist, with complaints of itching and a burning sensation in both of her eyes. She stated her upper eyelids looked like they had "dandruff" with a crusty appearance, and she noted an increased sensitivity to light. After examinations and testing, Dr. Spencer documented a confirmed case of bilateral squamous blepharitis on her upper palpebrae.

You Code It!

Review the details of this documentation, and determine the accurate code or codes to report Dr. Spencer's diagnosis for Rosemary.

Step #1: Read the case carefully and completely.
Step #2: Abstract the scenario. Which main words or terms describe why the physician cared for the patient during this encounter?
Step #3: Are there any details missing or incomplete for which you would need to query the physician? [If so, ask your instructor.]
Step #4: Check for any relevant guidance, including reading all of the symbols and notations in the Tabular List and the appropriate sections of the Official Guidelines.
Step #5: Determine the correct diagnosis code or codes to explain why this encounter was medically necessary.
Step #6: Double-check your work.

Answer:

Did you determine these to be the correct codes?

H01.021 Squamous blepharitis right upper eyelid
H01.024 Squamous blepharitis left upper eyelid

Exophthalmic Conditions

Exophthalmos, also known as **proptosis**, is an abnormal displacement of the eyeball. Most often, ophthalmic Graves' disease is the underlying condition that results in the eyeball bulging outward while the eyelids retract backward, bilaterally. Trauma, such as ethmoid bone fracture, may cause a unilateral diagnosis. Edema, hemorrhage, thrombosis, or varicosities also may cause exophthalmos, either unilaterally or bilaterally.

Proptosis
Bulging out of the eye; also known as *exophthalmos*.

As you abstract the documentation, note the difference between the displacement of the orbit, or eyeball, and whether or not the exophthalmos is constant, intermittent, or pulsating so you can determine the accurate code:

H05.21- Displacement (lateral) of globe
H05.24- Constant exophthalmos
H05.25- Intermittent exophthalmos
H05.26- Pulsating exophthalmos

CODING BITES

NOTE: All of these codes [in the H05 code category] require a sixth character to specify right eye, left eye, or bilateral (both eyes) involved.

Disorders of the Lacrimal Apparatus

The *lacrimal glands*, the *upper canaliculi*, the *lower canaliculi*, the *lacrimal sac*, and the *nasolacrimal duct* are together known as the **lacrimal apparatus**. Tears are created in the main lacrimal gland and then flow through several excretory ducts, pass through the canaliculi and the lacrimal sac, and continue down the nasolacrimal duct into the nasal cavity–the nose. This is why when you cry, your nose runs.

Lacrimal Apparatus
A system in the eye that consists of the lacrimal glands, the upper canaliculi, the lower canaliculi, the lacrimal sac, and the nasolacrimal duct.

Signs and symptoms of an obstructed lacrimal apparatus include recurring conjunctivitis (pink eye), discharge of pus or mucus from the eyelids and/or the conjunctiva, blurred vision, and excessive tearing.

Congenital nasolacrimal duct anomalies: a neonate may be born with a duct abnormality, an obstruction, or a lacrimal apparatus that is not fully developed. This is reported with one of these codes:

Q10.4 Absence and agenesis of lacrimal apparatus

or

Q10.5 Congenital stenosis and stricture of lacrimal duct

or

Q10.6 Other congenital malformations of lacrimal apparatus

Neonatal lacrimal duct (passages) obstruction: an infant born with a healthy lacrimal apparatus may still develop an obstruction of the nasolacrimal duct. As you are abstracting the documentation, confirm that this condition is acquired and not congenital so you can determine the accurate code:

H04.531 Neonatal obstruction of right nasolacrimal duct

or

H04.532 Neonatal obstruction of left nasolacrimal duct

or

H04.533 Neonatal obstruction of bilateral nasolacrimal ducts

Dacryops, also known as lacrimal gland cyst or lacrimal duct cyst, is reported with one of these codes:

H04.111 Dacryops of right lacrimal gland

or

H04.112 Dacryops of left lacrimal gland

or

H04.113 Dacryops of bilateral lacrimal glands

Dacryocystitis

Dacryocystitis
Lacrimal gland inflammation.

Dacryocystitis is lacrimal gland inflammation (*dacryo* = lacrimal sac or duct + *cyst* = sac + *itis* = inflammation). This may be a manifestation of a nasolacrimal duct obstruction and can be acute and/or chronic. Research shows that *Staphylococcus aureus*—or, on occasion, beta-hemolytic streptococci—is the pathogen responsible for acute dacryocystitis inflammation, whereas the chronic condition is more often caused by *Streptococcus pneumoniae* or, on occasion, a fungal infection such as *Actinomyces* or *Candida albicans.*

Signs and symptoms include pain, redness, and swelling over the inner aspect of the lower eyelid and epiphora. As you are abstracting the documentation, confirm whether the patient is a neonate or not, so you can determine the accurate code:

H04.321 Acute dacryocystitis of right lacrimal passage

or

H04.322 Acute dacryocystitis of left lacrimal passage

or

H04.323 Acute dacryocystitis of bilateral lacrimal passages

or

P39.1 Neonatal conjunctivitis and dacryocystitis

ICD-10-CM

YOU CODE IT! CASE STUDY

Raven Mercado, a 27-year-old female, came in to see Dr. Garner complaining of swelling, pain, and redness on her left eyelid. She was pretty certain it was a stye, but it was so painful, she had to ask for help. Dr. Garner examined her and confirmed a diagnosis of hordeolum externum of the left lower eyelid (commonly known as a stye).

You Code It!

Go through the steps of coding, and determine the code or codes that should be reported for this encounter between Dr. Garner and Raven.

Step #1: Read the case carefully and completely.

Step #2: Abstract the scenario. Which main words or terms describe why the physician cared for the patient during this encounter?

Step #3: Are there any details missing or incomplete for which you would need to query the physician? [If so, ask your instructor.]

Step #4: Check for any relevant guidance, including reading all of the symbols and notations in the Tabular List and the appropriate sections of the Official Guidelines.

Step #5: Determine the correct diagnosis code or codes to explain why this encounter was medically necessary.

Step #6: Double-check your work.

Answer:

Did you determine this to be the correct code?

H00.015 Hordeolum externum left lower eyelid

11.2 Diseases of the Internal Optical System

Interior of the Eye

The organ that is commonly referred to as the *eye* (see **Figure 11-2**) consists of the eyeball, the optic nerves, the **extraocular muscles**, the cranial nerves, the blood vessels, orbital adipose (fat), and the lacrimal system.

Extraocular Muscles
The muscles that control the eye.

Disorders of the Conjunctiva

Conjunctivitis, commonly known as *pink eye*, actually refers to an inflammation of the conjunctiva of the eye. The most common signs and symptoms include swelling, itching, burning, and redness of the conjunctiva as well as the palpebral conjunctiva (lining of the eyelids).

Conjunctivitis
Inflammation of the conjunctiva.

A pathogen (bacterium or virus), allergic reactions, environmental irritants, a contact lens product, eye drops, or eye ointments may all be an underlying cause of conjunctivitis. This condition is highly contagious (easily spread from one person to another). Viral conjunctivitis is reported from the infectious disease chapter of the ICD-10-CM code book, ***Chapter 1: Certain Infectious and Parasitic Diseases (A00–B99)***. You will need to check the pathology report to determine an accurate code:

B00.53 Herpesviral conjunctivitis

B30.1 Conjunctivitis due to adenovirus

B30.3 Acute epidemic hemorrhagic conjunctivitis (enteroviral)

Conjunctivitis due to coxsackievirus 24

Conjunctivitis due to enterovirus 70

Hemorrhagic conjunctivitis (acute) (epidemic)

B30.8 **Other viral conjunctivitis**
Newcastle conjunctivitis

Mucopurulent conjunctivitis is evident by mucus and pus produced by the inflammation, whereas *atopic conjunctivitis* is most often caused by allergies. Yet, be careful: *Vernal conjunctivitis* is the result of an allergic reaction to seasonal allergens, such as pollen or mold. Abstract the specific details about the conjunctivitis, as well as the laterality for the eye involved (right, left, or bilateral), from the documentation.

H10.01- **Acute follicular conjunctivitis**

H10.02- **Other mucopurulent conjunctivitis**

H10.1- **Acute atopic conjunctivitis**
Acute papillary conjunctivitis

H10.21- **Acute toxic conjunctivitis**

H10.22- **Pseudomembranous conjunctivitis**

H10.23- **Serous conjunctivitis, except viral**

NOTE: All of the codes in code category H10 Conjunctivitis require a fifth or sixth character to report laterality.

Disorders of the Sclera, Cornea, Iris, and Ciliary Body

Sclera
The membranous tissue that covers all of the eyeball (except the cornea); also known as *the white of the eye*.

Cornea
Transparent tissue covering the eyeball; responsible for focusing light into the eye and transmitting light.

The portion of the **sclera** at the medial anterior aspect (the middle of the front) of the eyeball is called the **cornea**. It is a curved, multilayer, transparent, and avascular (no blood vessels) segment of this structure (see **Figure 11-3**). The cornea's only function within the eye is to refract light rays. There are five layers that make up the cornea:

- *Epithelium:* the location of sensory nerves.
- *Bowman's membrane:* the location of epithelial cells.
- *Stroma:* the supporting tissue that makes up 90% of the corneal structure.
- *Descemet's membrane:* elastic fibers.
- *Endothelium:* cells that help to maintain proper hydration of the cornea to keep it moist.

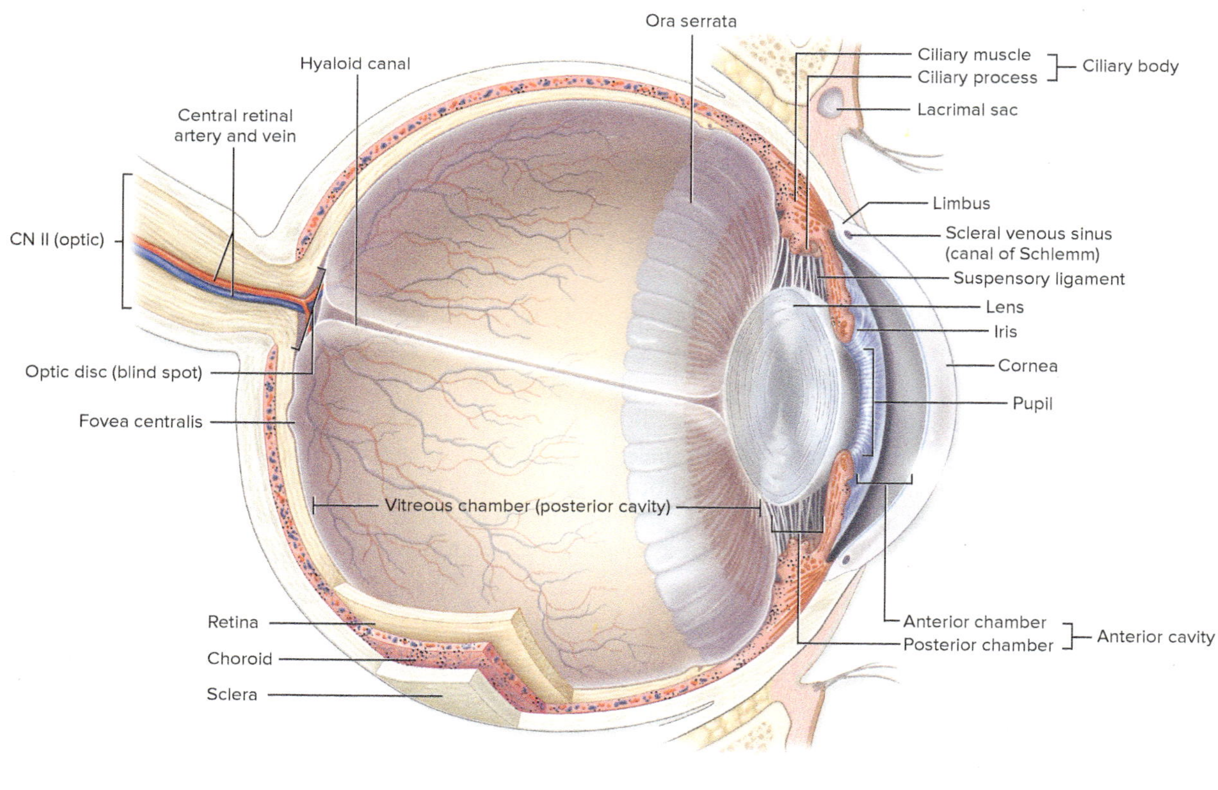

FIGURE 11-2 The anatomical components of the orbital septum (view from the right side)

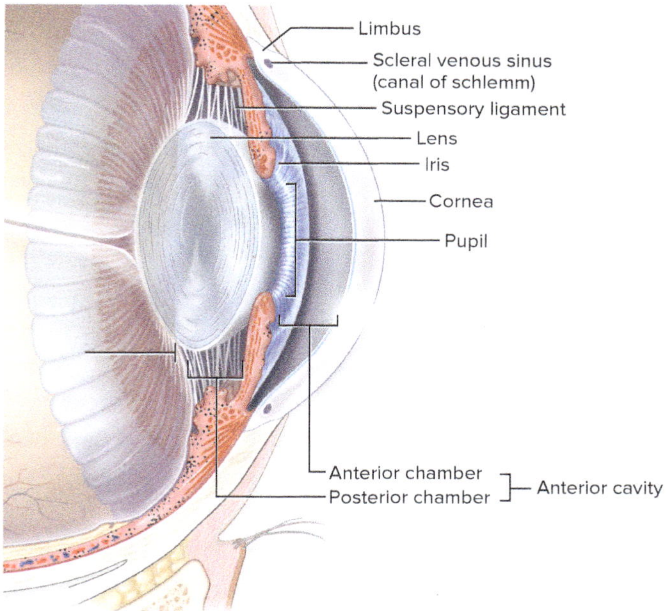

FIGURE 11-3 An illustration showing the sclera, iris, and cornea

The posterior (back) surface of the cornea is coated in an aqueous humor that keeps intraocular pressure at a consistent volume and rate of outflow.

Keratitis, an inflammation and ulceration of the cornea, may be instigated by any type of pathogen: bacterium, virus, or fungus. You will need to abstract two additional details from the documentation: the location of the ulcer on the cornea, as well as the laterality affected (right, left, bilateral).

> **Keratitis**
> An inflammation of the cornea, typically accompanied by an ulceration.

H16.11-	**Macular keratitis**
H16.12-	**Filamentary keratitis**
H16.13-	**Photokeratitis**
H16.14-	**Punctate keratitis**

NOTE: All of the codes in code subcategory H16.1 Other and unspecified superficial keratitis without conjunctivitis require a fifth or sixth character to report laterality.

When reporting a corneal ulcer, you will need to abstract two additional details from the documentation: the location of the ulcer on the cornea, as well as the laterality affected (right, left, bilateral).

> **CODING BITES**
>
> Hypopyon is an inflammation in the anterior chamber of the eye.
>
> Mooren's ulcer is also known as peripheral ulcerative keratitis.
>
> Mycotic corneal ulcer is also known as fungal ulcerative keratitis.

H16.01-	**Central corneal ulcer**
H16.02-	**Ring corneal ulcer**
H16.03-	**Corneal ulcer with hypopyon**
H16.04-	**Marginal corneal ulcer**
H16.05-	**Mooren's corneal ulcer**
H16.06-	**Mycotic corneal ulcer**
H16.07-	**Perforated corneal ulcer**

NOTE: All of the codes in code subcategory H16.0 Corneal ulcer require a fifth or sixth character to report laterality.

When caused by herpes simplex virus, type 1, the diagnosis is dendritic corneal ulcer (herpesviral keratitis). Typically, it is a unilateral condition, and initial signs and symptoms include reduced visual clarity, tearing, photophobia, and varying levels of pain (anywhere from mild discomfort to acute pain). As you can see, there are several different viruses that cause keratitis. You should find this detail in the documentation and the pathology report.

B00.52 Herpesviral keratitis

B01.81 Varicella keratitis

B02.33 Zoster keratitis

> **Corneal Dystrophy**
> Growth of abnormal tissue on the cornea, often related to a nutritional deficiency.

Corneal dystrophy occurs when one or more parts of the cornea develop an accumulation of cloudy material, resulting in the loss of normal clarity. There are over 20 varieties of corneal dystrophies, all of which share several characteristics:

- Genetic (inherited).
- Bilateral.
- Not the result of external causes, such as injury or diet.
- Develop gradually.
- Onset limited to a single layer of the cornea, with the disorder spreading later to the others.

Some of the most common corneal dystrophies include Fuchs' dystrophy (endothelial corneal dystrophy), keratoconus, lattice dystrophy, and map-dot-fingerprint (epithelial corneal) dystrophy.

H18.51 Endothelial corneal dystrophy

Fuchs' dystrophy

H18.52 Epithelial (juvenile) corneal dystrophy

H18.53 Granular corneal dystrophy

H18.54 Lattice corneal dystrophy

H18.55 Macular corneal dystrophy

LET'S CODE IT! SCENARIO

Jessica Harvey, a 41-year-old female, came in to see Dr. Loughlin with complaints of pain in her left eye upon blinking, photophobia, and increased tearing. She also has noticed some blurring. She states she hasn't been able to put her contact lenses in for several days. Dr. Loughlin examined Jessica and dropped fluorescein dye into the conjunctival sac, which stained the outline of the ulcer, the entire outer rim of the cornea. Dr. Loughlin diagnosed Jessica with a ring corneal ulcer of the left eye.

Let's Code It!

Dr. Loughlin diagnosed Jessica with a *ring corneal ulcer* of the *left eye*. In the Alphabetic Index, let's look at the main term—*ulcer*.

Ulcer, ulcerated, ulcerating, ulceration, ulcerative

Find the term *cornea* in the long list below. Then, in the list indented beneath *cornea*, determine the most accurate match to Dr. Loughlin's notes:

Ulcer, ulcerated, ulcerating, ulceration, ulcerative

cornea H16.00-

ring H16.02-

Now to the Tabular List—let's check out the top of the code category:

✓4 **H16 Keratitis**

Are you in the wrong place? Remember that earlier, when you learned about keratitis, you learned it is an inflammation and ulceration of the cornea. Double-check, though, to be certain. Do you see a confirmation that you are in the correct location?

(continued)

✓5 **H16.0 Corneal ulcer**

Whew! Now review the options for the fifth and sixth characters to see if you can determine an accurate code:

H16.022 Ring corneal ulcer, left eye

That matches perfectly!

Check the top of this subsection and the head of this chapter in ICD-10-CM. There are notations at the beginning of this chapter: a **NOTE** and an EXCLUDES2 notation. Read carefully. Do any relate to Dr. Loughlin's diagnosis of Jessica? No. Turn to the Official Guidelines and read Section I.C.7. There is nothing specifically applicable here either.

Now you can report H16.022 for Jessica's diagnosis with confidence.

Good coding!

Disorders of the Lens

The **lens** of the eye is located at the anterior of the **vitreous chamber** (see **Figure 11-3**). The lens is a semipermeable membrane that is transparent, avascular (contains no blood vessels), and biconvex. The lens goes through what's called **accommodation**, which is the process of changing shape to accomplish seeing objects both near and far. To view objects that are close (near vision), the lens reshapes to a spherical body, the **pupil** contracts, and the eyes converge (come toward the middle). When looking at something at a distance (far vision), the lens flattens out, the eyes straighten, and the pupils dilate (open wider). As individuals get older, the lens gets tired of accommodating and is not as flexible as it used to be. This makes it more likely the lens may get stuck in the near-vision shape, meaning the individual is nearsighted and may need corrective lenses (eyeglasses or contact lenses) to enable them to see far away. When somebody is farsighted, the lens gets stuck in the flattened position and the individual will need corrective lenses to see close up.

Lens
A transparent, crystalline segment of the eye, situated directly behind the pupil, that is responsible for focusing light rays as they enter the eye and travel back to the retina.

Vitreous Chamber
The interior segment of the eye that contains the vitreous body.

Accommodation
Adaptation of the eye's lens to adjust for varying focal distances.

Pupil
The opening in the center of the iris that permits light to enter and continue on to the lens and retina.

Cataract
Clouding of the lens or lens capsule of the eye.

A **cataract** is the gradual opacity (clouding) of the lens or lens capsule of the eye, which causes a reduction of vision. Many individuals perceive this to be a condition of the elderly; however, cataracts can occur at any age, including being present at birth. Patients with diabetes mellitus are especially prone to developing cataracts. Complicated cataracts are most often an idiopathic condition, caused by a preexisting condition such as diabetes mellitus or hypoparathyroidism. However, this condition also can be caused by trauma, especially after a foreign body has injured the lens.

Ophthalmoscopy examination, or a slit-lamp exam, can be used to confirm the presence of a cataract by enabling the observation of a dark area in the normally consistent red reflex of the lens.

H25.11 Age-related nuclear cataract, right eye

H26.012 Infantile and juvenile cortical, lamellar, or zonular cataract, left eye

Q12.0 Congenital cataract

ICD-10-CM

YOU CODE IT! CASE STUDY

Nicholas McCord, a 45-year-old male, was tightening the rope holding a load on the bed of his pickup truck when the rope broke suddenly. His fist, clenching the rope, snapped backward, hitting him in the right eye. The pain was difficult for him to deal with, so his friends brought him to the emergency department. After examination, Dr. Espinal diagnosed Nicholas with an anterior dislocation of his right eye lens. He was taken up to the procedure room.

(continued)

You Code It!

Go through the steps of coding, and determine the code or codes that should be reported for this encounter between Dr. Espinal and Nicholas.

Step #1: Read the case carefully and completely.

Step #2: Abstract the scenario. Which main words or terms describe why the physician cared for the patient during this encounter?

Step #3: Are there any details missing or incomplete for which you would need to query the physician? [If so, ask your instructor.]

Step #4: Check for any relevant guidance, including reading all of the symbols and notations in the Tabular List and the appropriate sections of the Official Guidelines.

Step #5: Determine the correct diagnosis code or codes to explain why this encounter was medically necessary.

Step #6: Double-check your work.

Answer:

Did you determine this to be the correct code?

H27.121 Anterior dislocation of lens, right eye

Disorders of the Choroid and Retina

The Uveal Tract

The **uveal tract** is the middle layer of the eye; it has three sections: the **iris** (in the anterior), followed by the **ciliary body**, and the **choroid** in the posterior. Together, the parts of the uvea improve the contrast of the image created by the retina. The uvea accomplishes this by reducing the light reflected within the eye while absorbing outside light as it is transmitted. The uvea is also responsible for providing nutrition to the eye structure and exchanging gases (see **Figure 11-4**).

Uveal Tract
The middle layer of the eye, consisting of the iris, ciliary body, and choroid.

Iris
The round, pigmented muscular curtain in the eye.

Ciliary Body
The vascular layer of the eye that lies between the sclera and the crystalline lens.

Choroid
The vascular layer of the eye that lies between the retina and the sclera.

The Retina

The **retina**, the area of the eye that contains nerve endings, is responsible for receiving visual images and forwarding these images to the brain for analysis (see **Figure 11-4**). The choroid is lightly attached to the retinal pigment epithelium (RPE) and is adjacent to the rods and cones that function as light receptors. The **rods** are located throughout the retina and are responsible for detecting movement so that you can see when something in front of you is moving. There are three types of **cones** that, together, provide designation for up to 150 shades of color: one type of cone reacts to red light, one to blue-violet light, and the third to green light. Isn't it amazing that you can go into a paint store and see 500 different colors, yet the eye can really only interpret up to 150? The eye combines the light wavelengths to enable perception of a multitude of colors.

Retinal detachment is the separation of the outer RPE from the neural retina, creating a space immediately beneath the retina. This subretinal space then fills with fluid (liquid vitreous) and obstructs the flow of choroidal blood (which supplies oxygen and nutrients to the retina). Signs and symptoms include floaters (floating black spots) as well as photopsia (recurring flashes of light).

Retina
A membrane in the back of the eye that is sensitive to light and functions as the sensory end of the optic nerve.

Rod
An elongated, cylindrical cell within the retina that is photosensitive in low light.

Cone
A receptor in the retina that is responsible for light and color.

Retinal Detachment
A break in the connection between the retinal pigment epithelium layer and the neural retina.

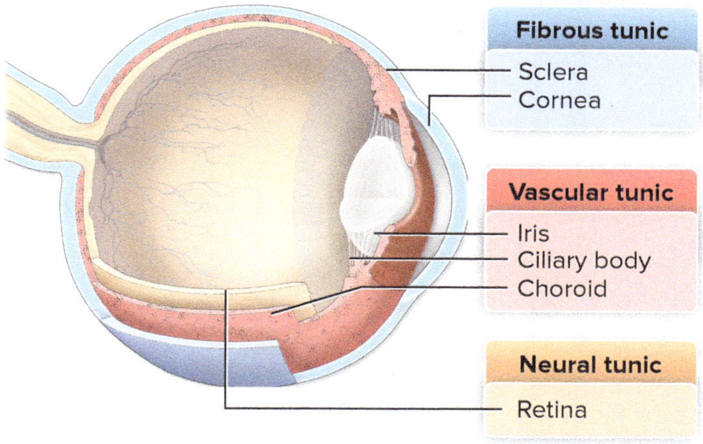

FIGURE 11-4 The anatomical components of the interior of the eye

H33.012 **Retinal detachment with single break, left eye**

H33.021 **Retinal detachment with multiple breaks, right eye**

H33.21 **Serous retinal detachment, right eye**

11.3 Other Conditions Affecting the Eyes

Glaucoma

Glaucoma is a malfunction of the fluid pressure within the eye; the pressure rises to a level that can cause damage to the optic disc and nerve. Glaucoma is essentially categorized as either open angle or closed angle:

Glaucoma
The condition that results when poor draining of fluid causes an abnormal increase in pressure within the eye, damaging the optic nerve.

- *Open angle:* a slowly developing, chronic condition that typically has no signs or symptoms until very advanced.
- *Closed angle:* a painful condition with a sudden onset and rapidly progressing vision loss.

In addition to abstracting the documented diagnosis of glaucoma, you will need to confirm the current stage of development of this condition to accurately report the seventh character:

- *mild* stage (evidence of changes in the aqueous outflow system of the eye).
- *moderate* stage (elevated intraocular pressure).
- *severe* stage (atrophy of the optic nerve and loss of the visual field).
- *indeterminate* stage (for unusual circumstances, when the physician documented being unable to determine the stage; this is *not* the same as unspecified).

H40.1113 **Primary open-angle glaucoma, right eye, severe stage**

H40.2221 **Chronic angle-closure glaucoma, left eye, mild stage**

GUIDANCE CONNECTION

Read the ICD-10-CM Official Guidelines for Coding and Reporting, section **I. Conventions, General Coding Guidelines and Chapter-Specific Guidelines**, subsection **C. Chapter-Specific Coding Guidelines**, chapter **7. Diseases of the Eye and Adnexa**, subsection **a. Glaucoma**.

YOU CODE IT! CASE STUDY

ICD-10-CM

PATIENT NAME: Peter Calvern

PREOPERATIVE DIAGNOSIS: Narrow-angle glaucoma, right eye.

POSTOPERATIVE DIAGNOSIS: Narrow-angle glaucoma, right eye.

OPERATION PERFORMED: Laser iridotomy, right eye.

SURGEON: JoAnn Hannigan, MD

ANESTHESIA: Topical proparacaine.

INDICATIONS FOR PROCEDURE: The patient is a 67-year-old male with a history of narrow-angle glaucoma, at high risk for blindness or angle-closure glaucoma, diagnosed on physical examination by gonioscopy. Risks, benefits, and alternatives of laser iridotomy were discussed with the patient preoperatively. The patient agreed and signed appropriate consent preoperatively.

DESCRIPTION OF PROCEDURE: On the day of the procedure, the right eye was identified as the operative eye. The patient received three sets q5min of the following drops: proparacaine, pilocarpine, and Iopidine. Appropriate constriction and anesthesia were achieved. The patient was then brought back to the laser suite, where first the argon laser was used to pretreat the iris superiorly in an area that was covered by the lid with the following settings: 800 milliwatts, 0.06 second duration and 50 micron spot size. Then, the YAG laser was used to complete the iridotomy with the following settings: 5 millijoules, 2 pulses and a total of 2 pulses applied. Good flow of aqueous was noted from the posterior chamber to the anterior chamber and a patent iridotomy was obtained. The patient was given the following postoperative instructions: no bending, coughing, lifting, straining, or sneezing. Return to the clinic for further follow-up care, and the patient is to use prednisolone acetate 1 drop, left eye, 4 times a day for 1 week.

You Code It!

Review this documentation about the procedure that Dr. Hannigan performed on Peter, and determine the correct code or codes to report the reason why this procedure was medically necessary.

Step #1: Read the case carefully and completely.

Step #2: Abstract the scenario. Which main words or terms describe why the physician cared for the patient during this encounter?

Step #3: Are there any details missing or incomplete for which you would need to query the physician? [If so, ask your instructor.]

Step #4: Check for any relevant guidance, including reading all of the symbols and notations in the Tabular List and the appropriate sections of the Official Guidelines.

Step #5: Determine the correct diagnosis code or codes to explain why this encounter was medically necessary.

Step #6: Double-check your work.

Answer:

Did you determine this to be the correct code?

H40.031 Anatomical narrow angle, right eye

Good work!

Diabetic Retinopathy

Retinopathy
Degenerative condition of the retina.

Patients diagnosed with diabetes mellitus are at risk for ophthalmic manifestations of their improper glucose levels. Diabetic **retinopathy** is the most common; it is a condition that causes damage to the tiny blood vessels inside the retina (*retina* + *-pathy* = disease). Signs and symptoms include

- Blurry or double vision.
- Rings around lights.
- Flashing lights.
- Blank spots.
- Dark or floating spots (commonly known as *floaters*).
- Pain in one or both eyes.
- Sensation of pressure in one or both eyes.
- Difficulty in seeing things peripherally (out of the corners of the eyes).
- Macular edema, which occurs when fluid and protein deposits collect on or beneath the macula (a central area of the retina), resulting in swelling (edema). The swelling then causes the macula to thicken, distorting the person's central vision.

Diabetic retinopathy progresses through four stages of development:

1. Mild nonproliferative retinopathy (microaneurysms).
2. Moderate nonproliferative retinopathy (blockage in some retinal vessels).
3. Severe nonproliferative retinopathy (more vessels are blocked, depriving the retina of blood supply).
4. Proliferative retinopathy (most advanced stage).

When diagnosis and treatment are implemented in the early stages, vision loss can be reduced. Therefore, individuals with diabetes mellitus are encouraged to get regular eye exams. Diabetic retinopathy is one of the leading causes of blindness in U.S. adults, affecting more than 4 million Americans.

EXAMPLES

E10.321	Type 1 diabetes mellitus with mild nonproliferative diabetic retinopathy with macular edema
E11.36	Type 2 diabetes mellitus with diabetic cataract

Remember, whenever a combination code is available that includes the underlying condition and the manifestation in one code, you must use this to report the diagnosis. If no combination code is accurate, then you will probably need to report multiple codes to provide the whole picture.

Hypertensive Retinopathy

Patients with hypertension (high blood pressure) can develop damage to the retina because of the unusually high pressure of the blood traveling through the vessels. This condition is known as *hypertensive retinopathy*. The higher the pressure and the longer this condition has been ongoing, the more severely the retina may be harmed. Signs and symptoms most evident for those with hypertensive retinopathy include

- Double vision
- Dimmed vision
- Blindness (vision loss)
- Headaches

EXAMPLES

H35.031	Hypertensive retinopathy, right eye
H35.032	Hypertensive retinopathy, left eye

Did you notice that, with diabetic retinopathy, the combination codes are available to you in the subsection for the underlying condition, diabetes mellitus? However, with hypertensive retinopathy, these combination codes are with the ophthalmic codes—the manifestation. You always need to read carefully and completely.

GUIDANCE CONNECTION

Read the ICD-10-CM Official Guidelines for Coding and Reporting, section **I. Conventions, General Coding Guidelines and Chapter-Specific Guidelines**, subsection **C. Chapter-Specific Coding Guidelines**, chapter **9. Diseases of the Circulatory System**, subsection **a. 5) Hypertensive Retinopathy**.

LET'S CODE IT! SCENARIO

PATIENT'S NAME: Arlene Masconetti

MRN: ALMAS0122

PRE/POSTOPERATIVE DIAGNOSIS: Cataract, traumatic and mature, right eye.

PROCEDURE PERFORMED: Phacoemulsification and implantation of intraocular lens, right eye.

SURGEON: Jason Britemann, MD

ANESTHESIA: MAC with retrobulbar.

PREPROCEDURE: Patient is a 37-year-old female who had been playing softball with coworkers and got hit by a ball in the right eye, causing a total traumatic cataract. She tried to ignore the discomfort, but it was interfering with her doing her work, and she was afraid to drive. Patient was given the complete information on this procedure, possible outcomes, and projected outcomes, and she signed consent. Prior to bringing the patient to the operating room, the patient received three sets of topical dilating, antibiotic drops.

DESCRIPTION OF OPERATION: The patient was brought to the procedure room and placed in a supine position on the operating table, and was prepped and draped in a sterile manner. She was sedated and retrobulbar injection of 0.75% Marcaine and 1% lidocaine was made. No complications were evident. A lid speculum was inserted to part the eyelid. A paracentesis was made infratemporally. The anterior chamber was filled with air and then indocyanine green to stain the anterior capsule. The cataract was noted to be extremely mature. A small capsulorrhexis was initiated. Immediately, milky white fluid extruded from the capsulorrhexis opening. A 27-gauge cannula was then used to aspirate this fluid. The cystotome was then used to complete the capsulorrhexis. The nucleus was gently rocked to facilitate mobility. The phacoemulsification apparatus was introduced into the eye. The nucleus was phacoemulsified and removed without any complications. The remaining cortex was removed with irrigation and aspiration. An SA60 AC 21-diopter lens was placed in the bag and the remaining viscoelastic was removed. One interrupted 10-0 nylon suture was placed in the cornea. The patient tolerated the procedure well. The lid speculum was removed. One drop of Betadine, one drop of Ciloxan, and bacitracin ointment were placed into the eye and patch and shield were applied. The patient was returned to postanesthesia care in satisfactory condition. The patient was instructed to take the eye patch off at 6 p.m. and use the topical Vigamox and Pred Forte eye drops every 2 hours until bedtime.

Let's Code It!

Dr. Britemann performed cataract surgery on Arlene to treat her traumatic and mature cataract of her right eye. Open your ICD-10-CM code book to the Alphabetic Index and find

Cataract (cortical) (immature) (incipient) H26.9

Hmm. The first thing you might notice is that this included a nonessential modifier of "immature," and Dr. Britemann documented that Arlene's cataract is mature. What is the difference? This is why it is always such a great idea to have a medical dictionary nearby. A *mature cataract* is one that produces swelling and opacity of the entire lens. In this case, mature is not the same as senile (an age-related cataract). As you look down the indented list, notice there is no specific listing for Cataract, mature. However, keep reading and you will find:

Cataract (cortical) (immature) (incipient) H26.9

traumatic H26.10-

Let's take a look at this code and see what additional information the Tabular List might offer. You can always come back here to the Alphabetic Index.

(continued)

✓4 H26 Other cataract
EXCLUDES1 *congenital cataract (Q12.0)*

Before you review the fourth character options, scan this entire subsection, code categories H25, H26, H27, and H28. Do you see any description that suits Dr. Britemann's diagnosis of Arlene? Neither do I, so continue investigating the options available within H26.

✓5 H26.1 Traumatic cataract
Use additional code **(Chapter 20) to identify external cause**

The required fifth character will explain if the trauma was localized, partially resolved, or total. Go back to the documentation and determine which is the accurate character:

✓6 H26.13 Total traumatic cataract

You are making good progress. The sixth character will report which eye or whether both eyes are injured.

H26.131 Total traumatic cataract, right eye

Check the top of this subsection and the head of this chapter in ICD-10-CM. A **NOTE** and an **EXCLUDES2** notation are at the head of this chapter. Read carefully. Do any relate to Dr. Britemann's diagnosis of Arlene? No. Turn to the Official Guidelines and read Section I.C.7. There is nothing specifically applicable here, either.

Now you can report H26.131 for Arlene's diagnosis with confidence.

H26.131 Total traumatic cataract, right eye

Wait a minute. You are not done yet. Remember the *Use Additional Code* notation? External cause codes are required. Turn to the Index to External Causes. Arlene was hit, or struck, by a ball. So, find

Struck (accidentally) **by**

ball (hit) (thrown) W21.00-

softball W21.07-

Now, turn in the Tabular List, to find:

✓4 **W21** **Striking against or struck by sports equipment**

EXCLUDES1 assault with sports equipment (Y08.0-)

striking against or struck by sports equipment with subsequent fall (W18.01)

✓5 W21.0 Struck by hit or thrown ball

✓xx7 W21.07 Struck by softball

You will learn more about external cause codes in this book's chapter ***Coding Injury, Poisoning, and External Causes****.*

H26.131	**Total traumatic cataract, right eye**
W21.07XXA	**Struck by softball**
Y93.64	**Activity, baseball (activity, softball)**
Y99.8	**Other external cause status**

Good coding!

11.4 Dysfunctions of the Auditory System

Auditory Diseases

Otitis media is the inflammation of the middle ear. There are various types of this condition: suppurative and nonsuppurative, acute and chronic. While otitis media is common in children, it is not exclusively a childhood condition. Interestingly, the cases of this diagnosis increase during the winter, while there is an increase of otitis externa (inflammation of the external ear) in the summer. ICD-10-CM code category H66.- Suppurative and unspecified otitis media requires additional characters to report details including acute or chronic, suppurative or nonsuppurative, and with or without rupture of the eardrum, as well as laterality.

Endolymphatic hydrops (Ménière's disease) is a dysfunction of the labyrinth (semicircular canals). Signs and symptoms include vertigo, sensorineural hearing loss, and tinnitus. A feeling of fullness within the ear is not uncommon. Report this diagnosis with ICD-10-CM code H81.0- Ménière's disease, with an additional character to identify laterality.

ICD-10-CM

LET'S CODE IT! SCENARIO

Kaitlyn Logan, a 27-year-old female, was at a club and met a guy doing ear piercings. She got a piercing through the cartilage of her upper left ear. Now, 3 days later, her ear is erythematous (red), swollen, and painful to the touch. Dr. Sweeting examined her ear and diagnosed her with acute perichondritis of the left pinna. He prescribed fluoroquinoline with a semisynthetic penicillin and told her to come back in 2 weeks.

Let's Code It!

Dr. Sweeting diagnosed Kaitlyn with *acute perichondritis of the left pinna.* Let's turn in the Alphabetic Index to find

Perichondritis

Read down the indented list, and you will see that *pinna* is listed:

Perichondritis

pinna —*see* Perichondritis, ear

However, this is giving us a directive, not a code, to look back up the list to

Perichondritis

ear (external) H61.00

acute H61.01-

chronic H61.02-

OK, now we have a suggested code to get us started. Turn to the three-digit code category suggested here:

✓4 **H61 Other disorders of external ear**

You remember from earlier in this chapter that the pinna is a part of the external ear, so this may be the correct code category. Go ahead and review the fourth and fifth characters available and see if any match Dr. Sweeting's diagnosis.

✓5 **H61.0 Chondritis and perichondritis of external ear**

✓6 **H61.01 Acute perichondritis of external ear**

That is great. Now review the choices for the sixth character, and determine the complete code to report for Dr. Sweeting's encounter with Kaitlyn.

H61.012 Acute perichondritis of left external ear

Good job!

Otosclerosis is a condition of increasing growth of spongy bone in the otic capsule. This growth interferes with the travel of sound vibrations from the tympanic membrane to the cochlea, causing a progressive deterioration of hearing. This condition is seen most frequently in adults between the ages of 18 and 35, and it is more prevalent in females. Report this condition with ICD-10-CM code category H80.- Otosclerosis, with additional characters to identify the specific location within the ear as well as laterality.

LET'S CODE IT! SCENARIO

Alexis Acosta, a 33-year-old female, was having a terrible time with dizziness. She states that she has also had a problem keeping her balance. A complete examination by Dr. McQuaig confirmed a diagnosis of bilateral aural vertigo.

Let's Code It!

Dr. McQuaig confirmed a diagnosis of *bilateral aural vertigo.* Turn to the Alphabetic Index and find

Vertigo R42

Wait. Before you turn to the Tabular List, review the additional terms shown in the indented list.

Vertigo R42

aural H81.31-

This matches the diagnosis documented by Dr. McQuaig much closer, doesn't it? Let's check this out in the Tabular List, of course, beginning at the code category:

✓4 **H81 Disorders of vestibular function**

Directly below this is an EXCLUDES1 notation. Does either of these diagnoses relate to Dr. McQuaig's notes about Alexis? No. Good. Continue reading to review the available choices for the fourth and fifth characters. Did you find this?

✓6 **H81.31 Aural vertigo**

Perfect! Just one more thing: Take a look at Dr. McQuaig's documentation and determine which ear or ears are affected. Now you can report with confidence that Alexis's diagnosis is

H81.313 Aural vertigo, bilateral

Good work!

Tumors of the ear canal include osteomas and sebaceous cysts and can grow large enough to interfere with hearing. Should the growth become infected, the patient may develop a fever and other signs of inflammation, including pain. While these tumors rarely become malignant, pain might indicate a malignancy. Examination with an otoscope can typically confirm this diagnosis, although a biopsy would be required to confirm benign or malignant status.

EXAMPLES

C30.1	Malignant neoplasm of middle ear (malignant neoplasm of inner ear)
C44.212	Basal cell carcinoma of skin of right ear and external auricular canal
D14.0	Benign neoplasm of middle ear, nasal cavity, and accessory sinuses
D23.22	Other benign neoplasm of skin of left ear and external auricular canal

Labyrinthitis is an infection within the inner ear's labyrinth. The most evident symptom is incapacitating vertigo that may last as long as 5 days. Sensorineural hearing loss also may occur. Viral labyrinthitis can be a manifestation of some upper respiratory tract infections, or caused by trauma or toxic drug ingestion. In some cases, cholesteatoma may form on the bone of the labyrinth and erode it. Labyrinthitis may be described as circumscribed, destructive, diffused, latent, purulent, or suppurative. Report H83.0- Labyrinthitis with an additional character to identify laterality.

ICD-10-CM

YOU CODE IT! CASE STUDY

Rebekka Keith, a 9-year-old female, was brought to her pediatrician, Dr. Granberry, because her right ear was very painful and inflamed, and there was presence of both blood and fluid in her ear canal. She had suffered with the flu (upper respiratory infection), which had resolved last week. Physical examination revealed blebs and evidence that one or two had ruptured spontaneously, causing the presence of fluid and blood. Culture identified the pathogen as Haemophilus influenzae. *Dr. Granberry diagnosed Rebekka with acute infectious bullous myringitis of the right ear and prescribed antibiotic ear drops.*

You Code It!

Go through the steps of coding, and determine the diagnosis code or codes that should be reported for this encounter between Dr. Granberry and Rebekka.

Step #1: Read the case carefully and completely.

Step #2: Abstract the scenario. Which main words or terms describe why the physician cared for the patient during this encounter?

Step #3: Are there any details missing or incomplete for which you would need to query the physician? [If so, ask your instructor.]

Step #4: Check for any relevant guidance, including reading all of the symbols and notations in the Tabular List and the appropriate sections of the Official Guidelines.

Step #5: Determine the correct diagnosis code or codes to explain why this encounter was medically necessary.

Step #6: Double-check your work.

Answer:

Did you determine these to be the correct codes?

H73.011 **Acute bullous myringitis, right ear**

B96.3 **Hemophilus influenzae (H. influenzae) as the cause of diseases classified elsewhere**

11.5 Causes, Signs, and Symptoms of Hearing Loss

There are several things that might contribute to loss of hearing: genetics and congenital anomalies, pathogens, and external causes that may be traumatic or environmental.

Signs and Symptoms of Hearing Loss

While each individual will notice loss of hearing in a different way, these are the most common complaints:

- Hearing speech and other sounds as muffled.
- Having difficulty understanding conversations, particularly when in a crowd or in a noisy place (e.g., a restaurant).
- Frequently asking others to speak more slowly, clearly, and loudly.
- Turning up the volume of the television or radio.
- No longer engaging in conversation.
- Avoiding some social settings.

The degrees of hearing loss are measured in decibels (dB). This part of the assessment identifies the volume heard–from soft sounds to loud. The horizontal lines of the audiogram track the patient's acknowledged sounds. Audiologists tend to measure volumes from zero dB (soft sounds) up to 120 dB (extremely loud sounds). Hearing loss is classified in degrees of hearing from normal to profound. This determination is evaluated using the standard hearing thresholds–the softest a sound was heard at a specific frequency (see **Table 11-1**).

TABLE 11-1 Degrees of Hearing Loss

Indication of Hearing Loss	Hearing Threshold (dB)
Normal hearing	0–20
Mild hearing loss	21–40
Moderate hearing loss	41–55
Moderately severe hearing loss	56–70
Severe hearing loss	71–90
Profound hearing loss	91 and above

The website of Johns Hopkins Medicine. The landing page provides an overview of audiograms, explaining how to understand the results of hearing tests and the significance of various components of the audiogram.
Source: "Understanding Your Audiogram," *Johns Hopkins Medicine*, The Johns Hopkins University, hopkinsmedicine.org

EXAMPLES

Z01.10 Encounter for examination of ears and hearing without abnormal findings
Z13.5 Encounter for screening for eye and ear disorders

Here are two examples of code you might report to explain the reason *why* the physician or audiologist met with the patient for this encounter.

Genetics and Congenital Anomalies Causing Hearing Loss

During gestation, some infections, such as rubella, herpes, or toxoplasmosis, are known to possibly cause deafness in the fetus. In addition, congenital anomalies may cause a malformation of any of the ear structures, and there are over 400 genetic conditions that have been identified as causing genetic hearing loss. Most often, these circumstances result in sensorineural hearing loss.

EXAMPLES

P00.2 Newborn (suspected to be) affected by maternal infectious and parasitic diseases
Q16.5 Congenital malformation of inner ear
H91.1- Presbycusis
H93.25 Central auditory processing disorder (congenital auditory imperception)

Psychogenic (Hysterical) Hearing Loss

Sometimes a traumatic event can be so upsetting to an individual that it results in neurologic symptoms that have no organic cause. This is a psychiatric disorder that was formerly called "hysteria."

EXAMPLE

F44.6 Conversion disorder with sensory symptom or deficit (psychogenic deafness)

Idiopathic Causes of Hearing Loss

Cerumen (earwax) serves an important function within the ear canal. It protects the skin of the ear canal; protects the middle ear from bacteria, fungi, insects, and water; and enables cleaning and lubrication. However, too much cerumen can build up in the canal and form an obstruction, blocking the entrance of sound waves and causing sudden conductive hearing loss. Recurrent ear infections can result in scarring of the tympanic membrane, reducing its ability to transmit sounds into the middle ear.

Presbycusis is the deterioration of the ability to hear that naturally occurs for about a third of adults as they get into their late 60s to mid 70s. Report this diagnosis from code category H91.1 Presbycusis with a fifth character to report laterality.

EXAMPLES

H61.22	Impacted cerumen, left ear
H91.21	Sudden idiopathic hearing loss, right ear

YOU CODE IT! CASE STUDY

Tatiana Clayton, a 39-year-old female, felt something in her ear. She was having problems hearing in her left ear and felt very uncomfortable. When Dr. Silver asked her, she stated that it felt like something was inside her ear. Upon inspection with the otoscope, Dr. Silver diagnosed a polyp in her middle ear.

You Code It!

Go through the steps of coding, and determine the code or codes that should be reported for this encounter between Dr. Silver and Tatiana.

Step #1: Read the case carefully and completely.

Step #2: Abstract the scenario. Which main words or terms describe why the physician cared for the patient during this encounter?

Step #3: Are there any details missing or incomplete for which you would need to query the physician? [If so, ask your instructor.]

Step #4: Check for any relevant guidance, including reading all of the symbols and notations in the Tabular List and the appropriate sections of the Official Guidelines.

Step #5: Determine the correct diagnosis code or codes to explain why this encounter was medically necessary.

Step #6: Double-check your work.

Answer:

Did you determine this to be the correct code?

H74.42 Polyp of left middle ear

Terrific!

Traumatic (External) Causes of Hearing Loss

The ear is well protected, for the most part, by the skull; however, trauma can still damage it and interfere with the proper transmission of sound. Fireworks set off too close to a person's ear, explosions, and even standing too close to the amplifiers at a rock concert can result in a loss of hearing. A skull fracture also might cause injury to the ear structures or nerves. While you might not have thought about this, some medications and drugs can result in ototoxic hearing loss. Ototoxic medications–including gentamicin (an aminoglycoside antibiotic) and cisplatin and carboplatin (both cancer chemotherapy drugs)–may cause permanent hearing loss. Others–such as aspirin and other salicylate pain relievers, quinine (which is used to treat malaria), and some loop diuretics–are known to result in temporary hearing loss.

EXAMPLES

H83.3X1	Noise effects on right inner ear
H91.03	Ototoxic hearing loss, bilateral
S09.21XA	Traumatic rupture of right ear drum

Remember, whenever an external cause is documented, you must include the additional codes to explain how the injury or poisoning occurred.

EXAMPLES

T36.8X5A Adverse effect of other systemic antibiotics, initial encounter
W36.1XXA Explosion and rupture of aerosol can, initial encounter

Sound Levels Causing Hearing Loss

Walk down the street and you can hear construction equipment or the siren from a passing ambulance that may cause you to cover your ears to lessen the discomfort. Your neighbor revs his motorcycle as he drives past your house, or you go to the airport to see your parents off on a flight for vacation and you wait as the jet takes off into the sky. What is "loud"? And what is so loud that it could damage your hearing? Take a look at **Table 11-2** to see the decibel (dB) levels of some of the sounds of everyday life.

TABLE 11-2 Common Sounds

Sound	Noise Level (dB)	Effect
Boom cars	145	
Jet engines (near)	140	
Shotgun firing Jet takeoff (100–200 ft.)	130	
Rock concerts (varies)	110–140	Threshold of pain begins around 125 dB.
Oxygen torch	121	
Discotheque/boom box Thunderclap (near)	120	Threshold of sensation begins around 120 dB.
Stereos (over 100 watts)	110–125	
Symphony orchestra Power saw (chainsaw) Pneumatic drill/jackhammer	110	**Regular exposure to sound over 100 dB for more than 1 minute risks permanent hearing loss.**
Snowmobile	105	
Jet flyover (1,000 ft.)	103	
Electric furnace area Garbage truck/cement mixer	100	No more than 15 minutes of unprotected exposure recommended for sounds between 90 and 100 dB.
Farm tractor	98	
Newspaper press	97	
Subway, motorcycle (25 ft.)	88	Very annoying.
Lawn mower, food blender Recreational vehicles, TV	85–90 70–90	**85 dB is the level at which hearing damage (8 hr) begins.**
Diesel truck (40 mph, 50 ft.)	84	
Average city traffic Garbage disposal	80	Annoying; interferes with conversation; constant exposure may cause damage.
Washing machine	78	
Dishwasher	75	
Vacuum cleaner, hair dryer	70	Intrusive; interferes with telephone conversation.
Normal conversation	50–65	

Source: Decibel table developed by the National Institute on Deafness and Other Communication Disorders, National Institutes of Health. January 1990. nidcd.nih.gov

EXAMPLE

When the physician documents that sound has caused the patient's hearing loss, you may report an external cause code from the ✓4 **W42 Exposure to noise** code category.

GUIDANCE CONNECTION

Read the ICD-10-CM Official Guidelines for Coding and Reporting, section **I. Conventions, General Coding Guidelines and Chapter-Specific Guidelines**, subsection **C. Chapter-Specific Coding Guidelines**, chapter **20. External Causes of Morbidity**.

Chapter Summary

One of the five senses, vision is involved in virtually every aspect of one's life. This incredible complex organ system captures light and transmits it via interactive anatomical sites to the optic nerve and into the brain for evaluation and interpretation. Even though it is protected by the skull, the optical system is still susceptible to the invasions of pathogens (bacteria, viruses, fungi); can be damaged by trauma; and can be impacted by other environmental issues, such as UV light rays from the sun.

The auditory (hearing) system enables the human body to hear–one of only two senses that have their own organ systems. The auditory system passes along sound vibrations captured by the external ear, through the middle ear and the inner ear, to the cerebellum for interpretation.

CODING BITES

There are many abbreviations related directly to the optical and auditory systems that may be used by your health care providers in their documentation. Some of the most common abbreviations are shown below:

Optical System–Related Abbreviations

OD = right eye

OS = left eye

OU = each eye

ACC = accommodation

PERRLA = pupils equal, round, reactive to light and accommodation

VA = visual acuity

VF = visual field

REM = rapid eye movements

ARMD = age-related macular degeneration

Audiology-Related Abbreviations

AD = right ear

AS = left ear

AC audiometry = air conduction audiometry

BC audiometry = bone conduction audiometry

dB = decibel

dBHL = decibel hearing level

dBSPL = decibel sound pressure level

dBHTL = decibel hearing threshold level

HF = high frequency

HL = hearing level

Hz = hertz (and kHz: kilohertz)

LF = low frequency

PTA = pure tone audiometry

CHAPTER 11 REVIEW
Coding Dysfunction of the Optical and Auditory Systems

Enhance your learning by completing these exercises and more at mcgrawhillconnect.com!

Let's Check It! Terminology

Match each key term to the appropriate definition.

Part I

1. **LO 11.2** A membrane in the back of the eye that is sensitive to light and functions as the sensory end of the optic nerve.
2. **LO 11.2** An elongated, cylindrical cell within the retina that is photosensitive in low light.
3. **LO 11.2** A receptor in the retina that is responsible for light and color.
4. **LO 11.2** The membranous tissue that covers the entire eyeball (except the cornea); also known as *the white of the eye.*
5. **LO 11.2** Transparent tissue covering the eyeball; responsible for focusing light into the eye and transmitting light.
6. **LO 11.2** The vascular layer of the eye that lies between the retina and the sclera.
7. **LO 11.1** A transparent, crystalline segment of the eye, situated directly behind the pupil, that is responsible for focusing light rays as they enter the eye and travel back to the retina.
8. **LO 11.2** The opening in the center of the iris that permits light to enter and continue on to the lens and retina.
9. **LO 11.1** The bony cavity in the skull that houses the eye and its ancillary parts (muscles, nerves, and blood vessels).
10. **LO 11.2** The round, pigmented muscular curtain in the eye.

A. Choroid
B. Cones
C. Cornea
D. Iris
E. Lens
F. Orbit
G. Pupil
H. Retina
I. Rod
J. Sclera

Part II

1. **LO 11.1** The eyelids.
2. **LO 11.1** Sebaceous glands that secrete a tear film component that prevents tears from evaporating so that the area stays moist.
3. **LO 11.2** The vascular layer of the eye that lies between the sclera and the crystalline lens.
4. **LO 11.2** The interior segment of the eye that contains the vitreous body.
5. **LO 11.1** Altered sebaceous glands that are connected to the eyelash follicles.
6. **LO 11.1** A system in the eye that consists of the lacrimal glands, the upper canaliculi, the lower canaliculi, the lacrimal sac, and the nasolacrimal duct.
7. **LO 11.1** A mucous membrane that lines the palpebrae.
8. **LO 11.1** Adaptation of the eye's lens to adjust for varying focal distances.
9. **LO 11.1** Ordinary sweat glands.
10. **LO 11.2** The muscles that control the eye.
11. **LO 11.1** A mucous membrane on the surface of the eyeball.
12. **LO 11.2** The middle layer of the eye, consisting of the iris, ciliary body, and choroid.

A. Accommodation
B. Bulbar Conjunctiva
C. Ciliary Body
D. Extraocular Muscles
E. Glands of Zeis
F. Lacrimal Apparatus
G. Meibomian Glands
H. Moll's Glands
I. Palpebral Conjunctiva
J. Palpebrae
K. Uveal Tract
L. Vitreous Chamber

Part III

1.	**LO 11.1** Inflammation of the eyelid.	**A.**	Blepharitis
2.	**LO 11.3** Degenerative condition of the retina.	**B.**	Conjunctivitis
3.	**LO 11.2** A break in the connection between the retinal pigment epithelium layer and the neural retina.	**C.**	Corneal Dystrophy
4.	**LO 11.2** An inflammation of the cornea, typically accompanied by an ulceration.	**D.**	Dacryocystitis
5.	**LO 11.1** Bulging out of the eye; also known as *exophthalmos*.	**E.**	Glaucoma
6.	**LO 11.2** Inflammation of the conjunctiva.	**F.**	Keratitis
7.	**LO 11.1** Lacrimal gland inflammation.	**G.**	Proptosis
8.	**LO 11.3** The condition that results when poor draining of fluid causes an abnormal increase in pressure within the eye, damaging the optic nerve.	**H.**	Retinal Detachment
9.	**LO 11.2** Growth of abnormal tissue on the cornea, often related to a nutritional deficiency.	**I.**	Retinopathy

Let's Check It! Concepts

Choose the most appropriate answer for each of the following questions.

1. **LO 11.1** All of the following are layers of the cornea *except*
   a. epithelium. **b.** conjunctiva. **c.** stroma. **d.** endothelium.
2. **LO 11.1** Tears are created in the main
   a. lacrimal gland. **b.** upper canaliculi. **c.** lacrimal sac. **d.** lower canaliculi.
3. **LO 11.2** ______ is commonly known as *pink eye*.
   a. Keratitis **b.** Dacryocystitis **c.** Conjunctivitis **d.** Blepharitis
4. **LO 11.2** The muscles that control the eye are known as
   a. intraocular. **b.** palpebrae. **c.** vitreous. **d.** extraocular.
5. **LO 11.3** What is the correct diagnosis code for intermittent angle-closure glaucoma, left eye?
   a. H40.23 **b.** H40.231 **c.** H40.232 **d.** H40.233
6. **LO 11.3** Signs and symptoms of diabetic retinopathy include all of the following *except*
   a. double vision. **b.** flashing lights. **c.** rings around lights. **d.** headaches.
7. **LO 11.4** Auditory dysfunction of the labyrinth is known as
   a. otitis media. **b.** otosclerosis.
   c. endolymphatic hydrops. **d.** tumors of the ear canal.
8. **LO 11.4** ________ is an infection within the inner ear's labyrinth.
   a. Labyrinthitis **b.** Otitis media **c.** Chondritis **d.** Perichondritis
9. **LO 11.5** Too much cerumen can build up in the canal and form an obstruction, blocking the entrance of sound waves and causing sudden
   a. inner ear hearing loss. **b.** sensorineural hearing loss.
   c. organ of Corti hearing loss. **d.** conductive hearing loss.
10. **LO 11.5** The hearing threshold for moderately severe hearing loss is
    a. 20 dB and below. **b.** 40 to 55 dB. **c.** 56 to 70 dB. **d.** 90 dB and above.

Let's Check It! Guidelines

*Refer to the Official Guidelines and fill in the blanks according to **Chapter** 7, Diseases of the Eye and Adnexa, Chapter-Specific Coding Guidelines.*

glaucoma	different	seventh	one
highest	each	admitted	
laterality	H40	clinical	
4	bilateral	progresses	
stage	both	type	

1. Assign as many codes from category _____, Glaucoma, as needed to identify the type of _____, the affected eye, and the glaucoma stage.
2. When a patient has _____ glaucoma and both eyes are documented as being the same type and _____, and there is a code for bilateral glaucoma, report only the code for the type of glaucoma, bilateral, with the seventh character for the stage.
3. When a patient has bilateral glaucoma and _____ eyes are documented as being the same _____ and stage, and the classification does not provide a code for bilateral glaucoma report only ____ code for the type of glaucoma with the appropriate seventh character for the stage.
4. When a patient has bilateral glaucoma and each eye is documented as having a _____ type or stage, and the classification distinguishes _____, assign the appropriate code for _____ eye rather than the code for bilateral glaucoma.
5. If a patient is _____ with glaucoma and the stage _____ during the admission, assign the code for ______ stage documented.
6. Assignment of the _____ character "_____" for "indeterminate stage" should be based on the _____ documentation.

Let's Check It! Rules and Regulations

Please answer the following questions from the knowledge you have gained after reading this chapter.

1. **LO 11.1** What are the three types of glands within the palpebrae, including their function?
2. **LO 11.2** Explain the difference between rods and cones.
3. **LO 11.3** What is hypertensive retinopathy? Include some of the most common signs and symptoms.
4. **LO 11.4** Explain otosclerosis, including the ICD-10-CM category code.
5. **LO 11.5** List five signs and symptoms of hearing loss.

YOU CODE IT! Basics

First, identify the condition in the following diagnoses; then code the diagnosis.

Example: Hordeolum externum, left upper eye

a. main term: *Hordeolum* **b.** diagnosis: *H00.014*

1. Stenosis of lacrimal sac, bilateral:
   a. main term: ______ **b.** diagnosis: ______
2. Transient ischemic deafness, bilateral:
   a. main term: ______ **b.** diagnosis: ______
3. Retinal telangiectasis, bilateral:
   a. main term: ______ **b.** diagnosis: ______
4. Ulcerative blepharitis, right upper eyelid:
   a. main term: ______ **b.** diagnosis: ______
5. Cholesteatoma of attic, left ear:
   a. main term: ______ **b.** diagnosis: ______
6. Subluxation of lens, left eye:
   a. main term: ______ **b.** diagnosis: ______
7. Granuloma of right orbit:
   a. main term: ______ **b.** diagnosis: ______

(continued)

8. Chronic perichondritis of external ear, left:
   a. main term: ______ b. diagnosis: ______
9. Labyrinthine dysfunction, right ear:
   a. main term: ______ b. diagnosis: ______
10. Bullous keratopathy, left eye:
   a. main term: ______ b. diagnosis: ______
11. Mechanical entropion of eyelid, right lower:
   a. main term ______ b. diagnosis: ______
12. Total attic perforation of tympanic membrane, right ear:
   a. main term: ______ b. diagnosis: ______
13. Recurrent bilateral mastoiditis:
   a. main term: ______ b. diagnosis: ______
14. Senile ectropion of eyelid, left lower:
   a. main term: ______ b. diagnosis: ______
15. Vestibular neuronitis, left ear:
   a. main term: ______ b. diagnosis: ______

YOU CODE IT! Practice

Using the techniques described in this chapter, carefully read through the case studies and determine the most accurate ICD-10-CM code(s) and external cause code(s), if appropriate, for each case study.

1. George McKeown, a 65-year-old male, presents with pain around his right eye and sensitivity to bright light. Dr. Zabawa notes redness of the eye and sagging skin around the lower eyelid. George is diagnosed with entropion of the right eye, lower eyelid.
2. Sheila Friday, a 17-year-old female, presents with the complaint that her left upper eyelid is swollen but doesn't hurt. This is the third time it has happened. Dr. Moss completes a thorough examination and diagnoses Sheila with blepharochalasis, left upper eyelid.
3. John Di Toma, a 10-month-old male, was diagnosed with congenital bilateral cataracts several weeks ago. John is admitted today for the surgical removal of the cataracts.
4. Robert Gould, a 42-year-old male, presents today complaining of pain and lack of vision in his left eye. Robert states that he was playing in a baseball game at the local baseball field and was accidentally struck in the face by the ball. Dr. Beck notes visual acuity of 20/200 (OS), a protruding eyeball, and an intraocular pressure of 42 mmHg. Normal right eye exam. Robert is admitted, where the CT scan confirms the diagnosis of subarachnoid hematoma.
5. Fred Grossman, a 36-year-old male, presents with the complaint of blurred vision and difficulty seeing at night. Dr. Cole, an ophthalmologist, takes a complete medical history and completes a thorough examination. The results of the slit lamp examination of the cornea confirm a diagnosis of stable keratoconus, right eye.
6. Jill Pruitt, a 9-year-old female, is brought in today by her mother. Jill was jumping on her bed in her bedroom at home when she fell off and struck her head on the floor; now she is seeing double. Dr. Browder completes an examination and decides to admit Jill for observation. After CT scan results were reviewed, Jill is diagnosed with temporary diplopia.
7. Donald McShane, a 32-year-old male, presents with the complaints of headaches, blurred vision, and eye pain. Dr. Clayton notes redness of the eyes and irregular pupils. Don has been having recurrent episodes and his condition has worsened. The oral steroid treatment does not seem to be effective. After an examination, Dr. Clayton makes the decision to admit Don for a complete workup. Don is diagnosed with acute recurrent iridocyclitis, bilaterally.
8. Streeta Frederick, a 31-year-old female, presents with the complaints of headaches, hearing loss, and dizziness. Dr. Molair completes an examination and admits Streeta. The MRI confirms a diagnosis of primary malignant neoplasm of inner ear, left.
9. Micah Fullmore, a 17-year-old male, comes in today with a swollen left ear lobe that is painful. Dr. Wiccetta notes a red pus-filled lump and, after an examination, Micah is diagnosed with furuncle of external left ear.
10. Rosa Fuller, a 24-year-old female, presents with ear pain. Dr. Rider documents a thick greyish-white matter. After a thorough examination, Rosa is diagnosed with diffuse otomycosis, external ear.

(continued)

11. Mark Gamble, a 57-year-old male, presents with a low fever and right ear pain. Dr. Martin completes an examination with otoscope, which confirmed a moderately bulging, nonperforated, right tympanic membrane; left tympanic membrane is noted to be within normal limits. Dr. Martin also notes this is the third bout this year. Mark is diagnosed with acute suppurative otitis media, recurrent, right ear.
12. Latoya Simpkins, a 36-year-old female, presents with the complaint of right ear pain. Dr. Herauf also documents a low-grade fever, cough, and nasal drainage. Dr. Herauf completes an examination with otoscope, which visualizes a cloudy bulging eardrum with blisters. Latoya is diagnosed with bullous myringitis.
13. Ken Medlock, a 37-year-old male, presents today with the complaint of ringing in his ears and the feeling of being unbalanced. Ken also states he is having difficulty with his hearing and has pressure in both ears. Dr. Burgos completes an examination and decides to admit Ken for a full workup. Sensorineural hearing loss is verified by audiometry; MRI scan and electrocochleography confirm the final diagnosis of bilateral Ménière's disease.
14. Tamika Robinson, a 12-year-old female, is having difficulty hearing at school. Dr. Zaprzalka uses an otoscope to visualize the tympanic membrane, noting left and right are within normal range without indication of inflammation. The results of audiometry suggest conductive hearing loss. The CT scan confirms the diagnosis of cochlear otosclerosis, right ear.
15. Rodney Sabido, a 49-year-old male, is suddenly having difficulty with his hearing. Rod describes it as the pitch is higher in one ear than the other. Dr. Butterfield completes an examination and the audiometry confirms a diagnosis of diplacusis, right ear.

ICD-10-CM

YOU CODE IT! Application

The following exercises provide practice in abstracting physicians' notes and learning to work with documentation from our health care facility, Prader, Bracker, & Associates. These case studies are modeled on real patient encounters. Using the techniques described in this chapter, carefully read through the case studies and determine the most accurate ICD-10-CM code(s) and external cause code(s), if appropriate, for each case study.

WESTON EYE CENTER

629 Healthcare Way • SOMEWHERE, FL 32811 • 407-555-6541

PATIENT: OLDENBERG, KYLE

ACCOUNT/EHR #: OLDEKY001

Attending Physician: Renee O. Bracker, MD

Kyle Oldenberg, 65-year-old male, presents today with the complaints of gradual loss of vision OD of a 2-month duration. Kyle states it doesn't hurt, "just getting to where I can't see." Kyle saw his ophthalmologist and was diagnosed with angle closure glaucoma and was referred to us for treatment.

PMH: Healthy, no medications

FH: Noncontributory with no history of glaucoma

SH: Drinks alcohol socially and denies use of tobacco

Eye Exam:

- Best corrected visual acuities: 20/20 OS, barely hand motion vision OD.
- Pupils: >2.9 LU RAPD OD
- EOM: full OU
- IOP: 17 mmHg OS, 66 mmHg OD
- DFE: retina exam—normal macula, vessels, and periphery OU. Optic nerves: 0.3 C/D OS, complete cup OD.

Gonioscopy: moderately open angles OD. (+) Sampaolesi's line OD.

Dx: Pseudoexfoliation glaucoma, moderate stage

P: Selective laser trabeculoplasty (ALT or SLT)

Determine the most accurate ICD-10-CM code(s).

(continued)

PRADER, BRACKER, & ASSOCIATES

A Complete Health Care Facility

159 Healthcare Way • SOMEWHERE, FL 32811 • 407-555-6789

PATIENT: TRUDELL, LEONARD

ACCOUNT/EHR #: TRUDLE001

Attending Physician: Renee O. Bracker, MD

S: Leonard presents today with a red, irritated right eye and decreased vision.

O: History of Present Illness: A 69-year-old male presented to our office with a 1-day history of conjunctival infection and mild discomfort in his right eye (OD). He had a known history of pigmentary glaucoma that was treated with PCIOL and trabeculectomy with mitomycin C in the right eye 5 years earlier. His visual acuity had decreased from 20/120 to 20/250 OD.

Past Ocular History: Pigmentary glaucoma (OD), age-related macular degeneration in both eyes (OU). The patient had suffered a severe retinal detachment in the left eye (OS).

Medical History: Hypertension, thyroidectomy.

Medications: Latanoprost OD qhs, Synthroid, and Buspar.

Family History: Noncontributory.

Social History: The patient denies alcohol and tobacco use.

Exam, Ocular:

- Visual acuity, with correction: OD—20/250; OS—Light perception.
- Intraocular pressure: OD—8 mmHg.
- External and anterior segment examination, OD: Conjunctival hyperemia with papillary reaction. There were 4+ cells (per high-power field) visible in the anterior chamber with a small (0.75-mm) hypopyon. The right eye had an elevated, thin avascular bleb with a small infiltrate visible within the bleb. The bleb had a positive Seidel test.
- Dilated fundus exam (DFE), OD: 3+ vitreous cell with a hazy view. Visible retina appeared to be normal.

Course: Performed aqueous and vitreous taps; administered intravitreal vancomycin and ceftazidime; and prescribed hourly topical, fortified gentamycin and vancomycin drops.

The patient responded well to treatment. His visual acuity has returned to baseline, and the bleb leak resolved in 6 weeks.

A: Bleb-related endophthalmitis

P: Next appointment 2 months or earlier prn

Determine the most accurate ICD-10-CM code(s).

WESTON HOSPITAL

629 Healthcare Way • SOMEWHERE, FL 32811 • 407-555-6541

PATIENT: SIMONSON-WALKER, SIERRA

ACCOUNT/EHR #: SIMOSI001

Attending Physician: Oscar R. Prader, MD

S: Sierra Simonson-Walker, a 61-year-old woman, presented with left ear discharge with some bleeding. Sierra has a 4-year history of progressive hearing loss in the left ear. She denied any pain, numbness, or weakness.

O: Upon examination, her right ear is within normal limits and the left ear canal is completely blocked with skin debris not consistent with cerumen. An attempt was made to remove the debris in the office, but the patient could not tolerate the severe discomfort.

(continued)

Medical History: Progressive hearing loss, no ear surgery, no recurring ear infections, no prolonged exposure to sun, no head and neck malignancies.

Family History: Noncontributory

Social History: The patient denies alcohol and tobacco use.

Maximum conductive hearing loss on the left and normal hearing on the right is verified by the audiometry.

CT scan showed opacification of the external ear canal with no evidence of bone erosion.

The patient is admitted and taken to the operating room; the debris is visualized to be flaky and keratinaceous. A portion of this was traced back to the anterior portion of the cartilaginous ear canal, where it appeared to be adherent to the skin. This lesion was removed en block and sent to frozen pathology, resulting in no identified carcinoma. There was also some irregular-appearing tissue along the tympanic membrane, which also was removed and sent with the specimen. The patient underwent a tympanoplasty without complication.

Final pathology, however, shows squamous cell carcinoma. The patient was then taken for a lateral temporal bone resection and external ear canal closure.

A: Squamous cell carcinoma of the external ear canal, left

P: Will continue to follow patient closely

Determine the most accurate ICD-10-CM code(s).

WESTON HOSPITAL

629 Healthcare Way • SOMEWHERE, FL 32811 • 407-555-6541

PATIENT: RIVERA, WALTER

ACCOUNT/EHR #: RIVEWA001

Attending Physician: Renee O. Bracker, MD

S: Walter Rivera, a 57-year-old male, presents today with ear pain and loss of hearing. Dr. Wiccetta, his primary care physician, noted some facial paralysis and slurred speech. Walter is admitted for a full workup.

O: H: 5′10″, Wt: 176, T: 97.3 F, HR: 86, R: 25, BP: 176/92. Patient is in obvious pain. Right pupil is 2.6 mm and left is 3.1 mm. Left auricle shows erythematous and is tender and swollen; tympanic membrane is not visible. Chest is clear; heart is regular without murmurs, rubs, or gallops; abdomen is soft and nontender; normal bowel sounds; no hepatosplenomegaly. Extremities are within normal range; skin is clear. Patient is alert and oriented.

Laboratory results:

Sodium 135 mEq/L, potassium 4.6 mEq/L, chloride 91 mEq/L, creatinine 0.6 mg/dL, glucose 274 mg/dL, calcium 9.3 mg/dL, total protein 6.7 g/dL, albumin 3.6 g/dL, total bilirubin 0.7 mg/dL, hemoglobin 15.3 g/dL, WBC 22.4 × 10^3/μL, hematocrit 48.0, platelet count 288 × 10^3/μL.

CT scan shows thickened tissue of the external auditory canal. Brain appears normal from MRI scan.

A: Diabetes, type 2, and malignant otitis externa, right

P: Antipseudomonal therapy

Determine the most accurate ICD-10-CM code(s).

PRADER, BRACKER, & ASSOCIATES

A Complete Health Care Facility

159 Healthcare Way • SOMEWHERE, FL 32811 • 407-555-6789

PATIENT: BARDARO, LYNNE

ACCOUNT/EHR #: BARDLY001

(continued)

Attending Physician: Renee O. Bracker, MD

S: Lynne, a 37-year-old female, presents today with the complaint that her right ear is throbbing.

O: T: 101, BP: 137/83, R: 21, P: 78. PERRLA. Lynne is in moderate discomfort. She admits to a pain level of 4 on a scale of 0–10.

Past medical history: Noncontributory.

Review of systems: Negative.

Medications: None.

Ear exam: Left is within normal range. Right pinna: a lump is noted, as well as swelling and inflammation. It appears to be a localized pool of blood. Dr. Bracker evacuates the blood and applies a pressure bandage.

A: Auricle hematoma

P: Rx: antibiotics

Follow up with patient in 10–14 days.

Determine the most accurate ICD-10-CM code(s).

12

Coding Cardiovascular Conditions

Key Terms

- **Angina Pectoris**
- **Atherosclerosis**
- **Atrium**
- **Cerebral Infarction**
- **Cerebrovascular Accident (CVA)**
- **Edema**
- **Elevated Blood Pressure**
- **Embolus**
- **Gestational Hypertension**
- **Hypertension**
- **Hypotension**
- **Infarction**
- **Myocardial Infarction (MI)**
- **NSTEMI**
- **Secondary Hypertension**
- **STEMI**
- **Thrombus**
- **Vascular**
- **Ventricle**

Learning Outcomes

After completing this chapter, the student should be able to:

LO 12.1 Abstract the documentation accurately to report heart dysfunction.
LO 12.2 Discern the specifics of cardiovascular disease.
LO 12.3 Evaluate documentation to determine details about abnormal blood pressure diagnoses.
LO 12.4 Identify known manifestations of hypertension.
LO 12.5 Interpret the details of cerebrovascular disease.
LO 12.6 Distinguish the sequelae of cerebrovascular disease and report them accurately.

STOP! Remember, you need to follow along in your ICD-10-CM code book for an optimal learning experience.

12.1 Heart Conditions

At the center of your body is the heart. Like the engine in a car, this small organ pumps oxygen-rich blood through your arteries to every cell in your body, from your head to your toes. The heart beats approximately once every second (60 beats per minute). Each beat is a compression—the heart contracting to force blood through it and out through the aorta to travel through the body delivering oxygen (see **Figure 12-1**).

Heart Disorders

Cardiac Arrest

Cardiac arrest means the heart actually stops beating. Typically, this happens suddenly. The key factor that you need to know about this condition is that it must be caused by something else. Possible causes of cardiac arrest include an underlying condition such as a myocardial infarction (dead tissue within the heart), an arrhythmia (abnormal heartbeat), electric shock (such as from wiring or lightning), a drug interaction, a drug overdose, a medical procedure, or a trauma. Therefore, along with abstracting this specific diagnosis, you will also need to look for the underlying cause (**Figure 12-2**).

There are several codes available to report this condition, specifying the underlying cause; here are some of the codes shown in the Tabular List:

I46.2 Cardiac arrest due to underlying cardiac condition
Code first **underlying cardiac condition**

I46.8 Cardiac arrest due to other underlying condition
Code first **underlying condition**

I97.710 Intraoperative cardiac arrest during cardiac surgery

I97.711 Intraoperative cardiac arrest during other surgery

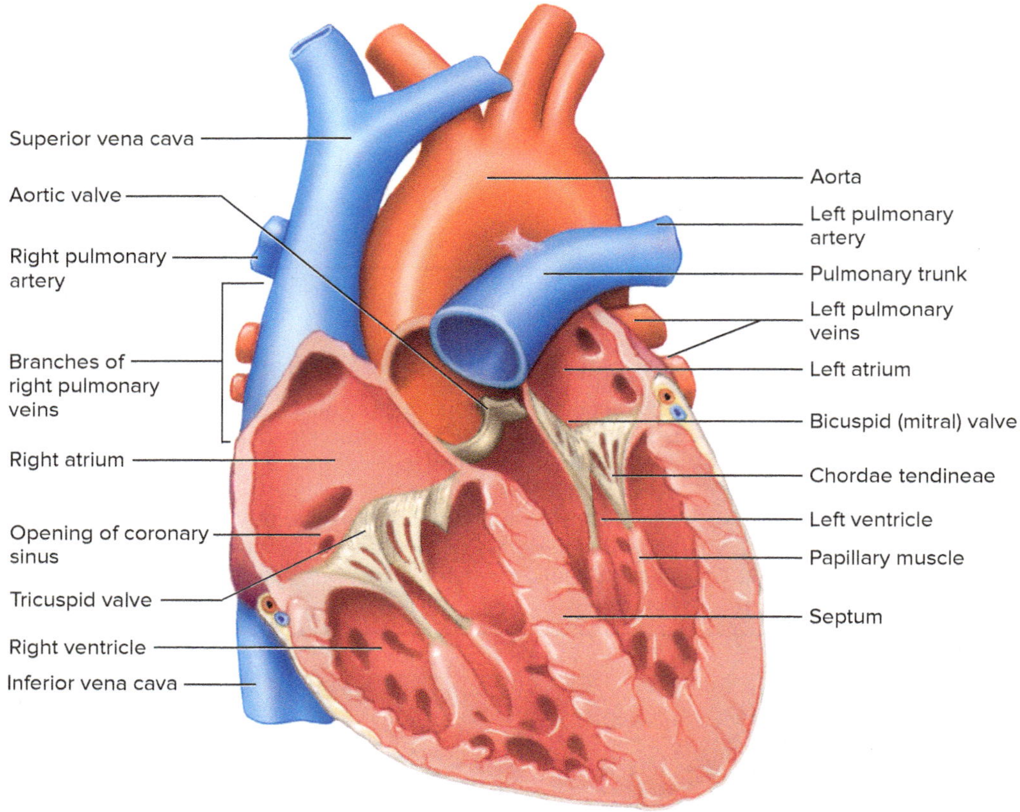

FIGURE 12-1 The anatomical components of the heart

Arrest, arrested

- cardiac I46.9

-- complicating

--- abortion — *see* Abortion, by type, complicated by, cardiac arrest

--- anesthesia (general) (local) or other sedation — *see* Table of Drugs and Chemicals, by drug

---- in labor and delivery O74.2

---- in pregnancy O29.11-

---- postpartum, puerperal O89.1

--- delivery (cesarean) (instrumental) O75.4

-- due to

--- cardiac condition I46.2

--- specified condition NEC I46.8

-- intraoperative I97.71-

FIGURE 12-2 ICD-10-CM, Alphabetic Index, partial, from Cardiac Arrest to Intraoperative Arrest

Source: *ICD-10-CM Official Guidelines for Coding and Reporting*, The Centers for Medicare and Medicaid Services (CMS) and the National Center for Health Statistics (NCHS)

I97.120	Postprocedural cardiac arrest during cardiac surgery
I97.121	Postprocedural cardiac arrest during other surgery
O75.4	Other complications of obstetric surgery and procedures

As you can interpret from these code descriptions, you would have to go back to the physician's documentation and specifically identify the underlying condition (that caused the cardiac arrest). You need this information so you can determine which of these two codes to report, and so you will know what that other (principal) diagnosis code should be.

CODING BITES

In reality, there is a code available with no specific underlying cause:

I46.9 Cardiac arrest, cause unspecified

As you learned in *Abstracting Clinical Documentation*, you are required to query the physician to obtain the details about the cause of this patient's cardiac arrest to be added to the documentation so the code you report is accurate.

GUIDANCE CONNECTION

Read the ICD-10-CM Official Guidelines for Coding and Reporting, section **II. Selection of Principal Diagnosis**, as well as section **III. Reporting Additional Diagnoses**.

Dysrhythmia/Arrhythmia

Dysrhythmia, or *arrhythmia*, refers to an irregular heartbeat. Signs include *tachycardia* (rapid heartbeat, more than 100 beats per minute) or *bradycardia* (abnormally slow heartbeat, less than 60 beats per minute). A short-term version of tachycardia may be *palpitations*, a condition in which the patient feels a very rapid heartbeat that lasts only a few minutes. Palpitations are a temporary condition that may be caused by another condition, such as anxiety, whereas tachycardia is an ongoing malfunction of the heart.

R00.0 Tachycardia, unspecified

R00.1 Bradycardia, unspecified

I49.8 Other specified cardiac arrhythmias

I49.9 Cardiac arrhythmia, unspecified

I97.89 Other postprocedural complications and disorders of the circulatory system, not elsewhere classified

When you search for dysrhythmia or arrhythmia, the ICD-10-CM Alphabetic Index directs you to I49.9. You can see that there are no codes specific to dysrhythmia. Notice that other codes are suggested when this condition is diagnosed in a newborn or occurring postoperatively. These details are a tip for you to go back to the documentation and check the patient's age or if the patient was in the postoperative period when the dysrhythmia occurred. Essentially, this diagnosis is vague, as it expresses what is wrong (irregular heartbeat) but does not relate the reason or reasons why the heartbeat is abnormal. You will need more specific information about the patient's condition, from either the documentation or the physician, to determine the correct code(s).

Mitral Valve Prolapse

Mitral valve prolapse is a rather common abnormality that prevents the mitral valve from closing properly (the mitral valve is the gateway between the left **atrium** and the left **ventricle**). A prolapse may develop or be influenced by other conditions, including hyperthyroidism, congenital heart lesions, or Marfan syndrome.

Atrium
A chamber that is located in the top half of the heart and receives blood.

Ventricle
A chamber that is located in the bottom half of the heart and receives blood from the atrium.

In the Alphabetic Index, find

Prolapse, prolapsed

mitral (valve) I34.1

When you turn to the code category in the Tabular List, you will see

✓4 **I34 Nonrheumatic mitral valve disorders**

I34.1 Nonrheumatic mitral (valve) prolapse

The inclusion of the term "nonrheumatic" is a tip to go back into the documentation to ensure that the physician did not state that the patient's condition was caused by rheumatic fever. Rheumatic fever can manifest heart inflammation as well as affect joints and other parts of the body. Rheumatic fever with heart involvement as well as chronic rheumatic heart diseases are reported from code categories I01–I09.

Atrial Fibrillation

Atrial fibrillation is a condition in which atria shudder or tremble in the heart instead of contracting to push blood through to the ventricles. This results in incomplete emptying of the atria, leaving blood to collect and sometimes clot. Episodes of paroxysmal atrial tachycardia (PAT), a rapid heart rate that can go as high as 150 or 200 beats per minute, can occur. Anticoagulants (drugs that prevent clotting) and/or thrombolytics (clot-dissolving drugs) are often prescribed.

I48.21 **Permanent atrial fibrillation**

I47.11 **Inappropriate sinus tachycardia, so stated**

Z79.01 **Long term (current) use of anticoagulants**

Z79.02 **Long term (current) use of antithrombotics/antiplatelets**

Z79.82 **Long term (current) use of aspirin**

And when the reason, or one of the reasons, for the encounter is regular blood testing, you also will need to report:

Z51.81 **Encounter for therapeutic drug level monitoring**

LET'S CODE IT! SCENARIO

Sara Cohen, a 73-year-old woman, was brought to the ED via ambulance after a witnessed cardiac arrest at the local airport.

Past medical history included hypertension, elevated cholesterol, and obstructive sleep apnea. She wore CPAP nightly but continued to experience daytime somnolence. She has smoked half a pack of cigarettes a day for the past 40 years and drank no alcohol. She had a chronic daily cough. She walked 2 miles daily without dyspnea or other limitation. She had never experienced chest pain, palpitations, presyncope, or syncope and had no known history of CAD. Current medications included nifedipine 30 mg orally once daily and simvastatin 20 mg orally once daily.

On the day of presentation, she was at the airport waiting for a flight to visit her grandchildren. Bystanders at the airport reported that they saw her suddenly drop to the floor while walking in the terminal. At a subsequent interview, the first lay responder described that the woman collapsed abruptly without any vocalization and was found to be unresponsive, pulseless, and without respirations. This lay responder, along with another bystander who was a nurse without formal training in advanced resuscitation, began CPR. This particular airport had recently instituted a policy of providing public access defibrillators in the terminals. Bystanders notified airport security staff, who brought a defibrillator to the scene and also called the EMTs. The woman was revived and brought to the hospital.

After examination, Dr. Troy diagnosed Sara with sudden cardiac arrest. He admitted her to the hospital for further testing to determine the cause of this event.

Let's Code It!

Dr. Troy diagnosed Sara with *sudden cardiac arrest*. Turn in your ICD-10-CM Alphabetic Index and find

Arrest, arrested

cardiac I46.9

There is no mention of "sudden," but the rest matches, so let's turn in the Tabular List to find this code, and we can read from there.

✓4 I46 Cardiac arrest

EXCLUDES1 Cardiogenic shock (R57.0)

I46.2 Cardiac arrest due to underlying cardiac condition
Code first underlying cardiac condition

I46.8 Cardiac arrest due to other underlying condition
Code first underlying condition

I46.9 Cardiac arrest, cause unspecified

(continued)

Let's go back and read Dr. Troy's documentation carefully. Did he identify the cause of Sara's cardiac arrest? No, actually he specifically stated that he was admitting Sara with the express purpose of determining the underlying condition. Therefore, this is the code you must report:

I46.9 Cardiac arrest, cause unspecified

Good work!

Heart Failure

A diagnosis of heart failure is serious; however, it does not mean the heart has totally "failed" to function. This condition, also known as *congestive heart failure (CHF)*, is characterized by the inability of an individual's heart to pump a sufficient quantity of blood throughout the body. CHF can cause fluid to back up into the lungs, resulting in respiratory problems such as shortness of breath and fatigue. In addition, fluid might build up in the lower extremities, causing edema (swelling) in the feet, ankles, and legs. In some patients, the edema can become so acute (severe) that they may have pain and trouble walking.

The National Heart, Lung, and Blood Institute reported in November 2015 that approximately 5.7 million people in the United States currently have a diagnosis of heart failure. The institute estimates that this condition contributes to as many as 30,000 deaths each year.

> **CODING BITES**
>
> To determine the diagnosis code for heart failure, you need to know:
>
> - What type of heart failure?
> - Is it acute or chronic?

The Types of Heart Failure

Left heart failure, also known as *pulmonary edema* or cardiac asthma, indicates an insufficiency of the heart's left ventricle. This malfunction results in the accumulation of fluid in the lungs. When this happens, patients also may develop respiratory problems.

I50.1 Left ventricular failure, unspecified

Right heart failure, secondary to left heart failure, is diagnosed when the heart cannot pump and circulate the blood needed throughout the body. Patients with this diagnosis may develop hypertension, congestion, edema, and fluid collection in the lungs.

I50.814 Right heart failure (due to left heart failure)

Systolic heart failure occurs when the contractions of the ventricles are too weak to push the blood through the heart. The documentation should include the specific detail that the condition is acute, chronic, or acute on chronic.

I50.21 Acute systolic (congestive) heart failure

I50.22 Chronic systolic (congestive) heart failure

I50.23 Acute on chronic systolic (congestive) heart failure

Diastolic heart failure is the result of a ventricle of the heart being unable to fill as it should. The documentation should include the specific detail that the condition is acute, chronic, or acute on chronic.

I50.31 Acute diastolic (congestive) heart failure

I50.32 Chronic diastolic (congestive) heart failure

I50.33 Acute on chronic diastolic (congestive) heart failure

Combined systolic and diastolic heart failure means that the function of the heart is weak and unable to process blood properly. The documentation should include the specific detail that the condition is acute, chronic, or acute on chronic.

I50.41 Acute combined systolic (congestive) and diastolic (congestive) heart failure

I50.42 Chronic combined systolic (congestive) and diastolic (congestive) heart failure

I50.43 Acute on chronic combined systolic (congestive) and diastolic (congestive) heart failure

Secondary Hypertension
The condition of hypertension caused by another condition or illness.

CODING BITES

When a condition, such as right heart failure, causes the patient to develop another condition, such as hypertension, that other condition may be referred to as a *secondary* condition.

For example, if Ralph developed hypertension due to his right heart failure, you would report the hypertension as **secondary hypertension**.

YOU CODE IT! CASE STUDY

Judith Patriko, a 78-year-old female, came to see her cardiologist, Dr. Fillmari, to follow up on her CHF. The edema (swelling) of her legs has improved, but she continues to have dyspnea (shortness of breath) with mild exertion. No syncope (fainting) at this time. Dx: Chronic diastolic congestive heart failure.

You Code It!

Look at Dr. Fillmari's notes for Judith Patriko, and determine the best, most appropriate code or codes.

Step #1: Read the case carefully and completely.
Step #2: Abstract the scenario. Which main words or terms describe why the physician cared for the patient during this encounter?
Step #3: Are there any details missing or incomplete for which you would need to query the physician? [If so, ask your instructor.]
Step #4: Check for any relevant guidance, including reading all of the symbols and notations in the Tabular List and the appropriate sections of the Official Guidelines.
Step #5: Determine the correct diagnosis code or codes to explain why this encounter was medically necessary.
Step #6: Double-check your work.

Answer:

Did you determine this to be the diagnosis code?

I50.32 Chronic diastolic (congestive) heart failure

Good job!

Myocardial Infarction

Myocardial Infarction (MI)
Malfunction of the heart due to necrosis or deterioration of a portion of the heart muscle; also known as a *heart attack*.

When a part of the heart muscle deteriorates, or actually dies, that muscle can no longer function properly. This malfunction within a person's heart, known as a **myocardial infarction (MI)**, will cause persistent pain in the chest, left arm, jaw, and neck; fatigue; nausea; vomiting; and shortness of breath. A preliminary diagnosis of MI, based on these signs and symptoms, can be confirmed by an electrocardiogram (EKG or ECG), blood tests measuring the serial serum enzyme levels, and/or an echocardiogram.

GUIDANCE CONNECTION

Read the ICD-10-CM Official Guidelines for Coding and Reporting, section **I. Conventions, General Coding Guidelines and Chapter-Specific Guidelines**, subsection **C. Chapter-Specific Coding Guidelines**, chapter **9. Diseases of the Circulatory System**, subsection **e. Acute myocardial infarction (AMI).**

An ST elevation myocardial infarction (**STEMI**) is a heart event during which the coronary artery is completely blocked by a **thrombus** or **embolus**. The ST segment is a specific range seen in an EKG (ECG). A nontransmural ST elevation myocardial infarction (**NSTEMI**) indicates that only a portion of the artery is occluded (blocked).

To determine the code for a diagnosis of MI, you will need to know

- What specific part of the heart was affected by the infarction?
- Has this patient been treated for an MI before? If so, how long ago?
- Is this infarction a STEMI or an NSTEMI?

Anatomical Site of the AMI

An infarction can occur in almost any location within the heart, and it is important that you identify the specific site from the documentation to support the accurate code to report. You will see that the individual codes in the code category for STEMI infarctions include different locations, specifically identified by the fourth character:

I21.01 **ST elevation (STEMI) myocardial infarction involving left main coronary artery**

I21.02 **ST elevation (STEMI) myocardial infarction involving left anterior descending coronary artery**

I21.11 **ST elevation (STEMI) myocardial infarction involving right coronary artery**

I21.21 **ST elevation (STEMI) myocardial infarction involving left circumflex coronary artery**

Subsequent MI

Another important aspect of a diagnosis of MI is whether or not this is the first time a patient has experienced this event. When a patient is documented as having had an acute myocardial infarction (AMI) of the same type (type 1 or unspecified type) within the last 4 weeks (28 days) and is at your facility for a second event, this current MI is reported with a code describing a "subsequent" MI:

I22.0 **Subsequent ST elevation (STEMI) myocardial infarction of anterior wall**

I22.1 **Subsequent ST elevation (STEMI) myocardial infarction of inferior wall**

I22.2 **Subsequent non-ST elevation (NSTEMI) myocardial infarction**

I22.8 **Subsequent ST elevation (STEMI) myocardial infarction of other sites**

If the subsequent MI is a different type than the previous MI, the appropriate code from I21 should be reported, not a code from I22.

When the previous MI is documented either as a "healed MI" or as a past MI without any current signs or symptoms, it is reported with this code:

I25.2 **Old myocardial infarction**

GUIDANCE CONNECTION

Read the ICD-10-CM Official Guidelines for Coding and Reporting, section **I. Conventions, General Coding Guidelines and Chapter-Specific Guidelines**, subsection **C. Chapter-Specific Coding Guidelines**, chapter **9. Diseases of the Circulatory System**, subsection **e. Acute myocardial infarction (AMI), 4) Subsequent acute myocardial infarction.**

STEMI
An ST elevation myocardial infarction—a heart event during which the coronary artery is completely blocked by a thrombus or embolus.

Thrombus
A blood clot in a blood vessel [plural: thrombi].

Embolus
A thrombus that has broken free from the vessel wall and is traveling freely within the vascular system.

NSTEMI
A nontransmural elevation myocardial infarction—a heart event during which the coronary artery is partially occluded (blocked).

CODING BITES

A thrombus is a blood clot that has attached itself to the wall of a blood vessel. If left untreated, it may cause a blockage, preventing blood from flowing through the artery or vein. In addition, there is always concern that the clot will detach and float through the vessel and pass through an organ. A detached clot is known as an *embolus*; it can get stuck as it passes through an organ and can completely prevent blood from moving through. The greatest danger occurs when an embolus travels into the lung or the heart, potentially causing death.

CODING BITES

If the physician documents this encounter has focused on the patient's subsequent or second MI and the . . .

- Previous MI was within the last 4 weeks = code from category I22
- Previous MI was more than 4 weeks ago = code I25.2

YOU CODE IT! CASE STUDY

Mark is sitting in the stands watching his son play softball when all of a sudden he feels a severe pain in his chest. He is having difficulty taking a breath, and the pain is radiating down his left arm. He arrives at the ED via ambulance, and Dr. Constantine and nurses work on him, taking blood and doing an EKG. Dr. Constantine determines that Mark had an ST elevation myocardial infarction (STEMI) of the inferolateral wall. Once he is stabilized, Mark is admitted into the hospital and transferred to the ICU.

You Code It!

Go through the steps of coding, and determine the code or codes that should be reported for this encounter between Dr. Constantine and Mark.

Step #1: Read the case carefully and completely.
Step #2: Abstract the scenario. Which main words or terms describe why the physician cared for the patient during this encounter?
Step #3: Are there any details missing or incomplete for which you would need to query the physician? [If so, ask your instructor.]
Step #4: Check for any relevant guidance, including reading all of the symbols and notations in the Tabular List and the appropriate sections of the Official Guidelines.
Step #5: Determine the correct diagnosis code or codes to explain why this encounter was medically necessary.
Step #6: Double-check your work.

Answer:

Did you determine this to be the correct code?

I21.19 ST elevation (STEMI) myocardial infarction involving other coronary artery of inferior wall (Inferolateral transmural [Q wave] infarction [acute])

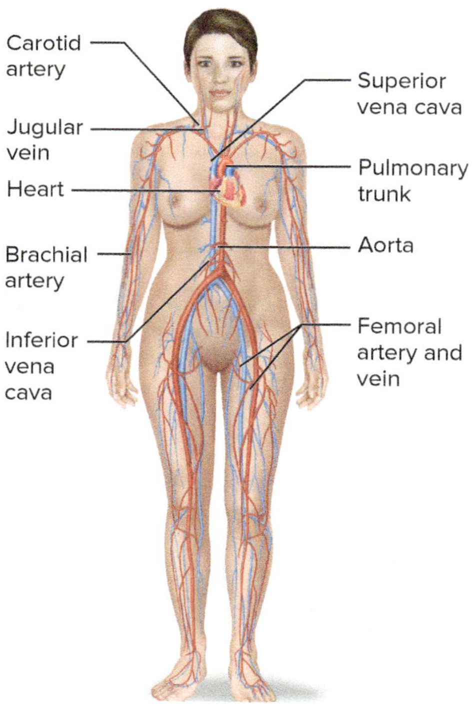

FIGURE 12-3 The cardiovascular system, highlighting major vessels

12.2 Cardiovascular Conditions

The circulatory (cardiovascular) system (**Figure 12-3**) includes the heart, arteries, and veins. It has the job of circulating blood to carry oxygen to cells throughout the body and to move waste products away from those cells. The circulatory network touches and affects every area of the body, from hair and tissues to organ function.

CODING BITES

Cardiovascular: ***cardio*** = heart + ***-vascular*** = vessels (veins and arteries)

Arteries = blood vessels that carry oxygenated blood from the heart to the tissues and cells throughout the body.

Veins = blood vessels that carry deoxygenated blood, along with carbon dioxide and cell waste, away from the tissues and cells throughout the body and back to the heart.

Circulatory conditions are very serious because they affect the flow of blood and, therefore, the delivery of oxygen. While problems with circulation can affect a patient of any age, older individuals are more susceptible to such conditions. As the body ages, the strength and elasticity of blood vessels decrease and they become less efficient. In addition, long-term poor nutrition and insufficient cardiovascular exercise take their toll and contribute to the circulatory system's inability to do its job.

Deep Vein Thrombosis

Earlier in this chapter, you learned about thrombi and emboli–blood clots that develop within the blood vessels. Deep vein thrombi can block the blood flow, causing venous insufficiency and affecting the ability of oxygen to get to the tissues throughout the body. A lack, or reduction, of blood flow can cause edema, congestion, necrosis, and pain. In addition, there is the danger that the blood clot can break loose and travel within the veins and arteries (embolism), causing damage to internal organs, blocking oxygen from the lungs (pulmonary embolism), or blocking off blood flow through the heart.

Reporting a diagnosis of deep vein thrombosis (DVT) [the presence of a blood clot attached to the wall of an interior vein] will require you to know a few specifics to determine the most accurate code:

- Is the condition identified as acute or chronic?
- Where (the specific anatomical site) has the thrombus been located?

I82.412 Acute embolism and thrombosis of left femoral vein

I82.543 Chronic embolism and thrombosis of tibial vein, bilateral

YOU CODE IT! CASE STUDY

Dr. Victorelli examined Carter Franchez and diagnosed him with a chronic thrombosis of the right popliteal vein.

You Code It!

Review the notes about why Dr. Victorelli provided care to Carter Franchez and determine the accurate diagnosis code or codes.

Step #1: Read the case carefully and completely.
Step #2: Abstract the scenario. Which main words or terms describe why the physician cared for the patient during this encounter?
Step #3: Are there any details missing or incomplete for which you would need to query the physician? [If so, ask your instructor.]
Step #4: Check for any relevant guidance, including reading all of the symbols and notations in the Tabular List and the appropriate sections of the Official Guidelines.
Step #5: Determine the correct diagnosis code or codes to explain why this encounter was medically necessary.
Step #6: Double-check your work.

Answer:

Did you determine this to be the accurate code?

I82.531 Chronic embolism and thrombosis of right popliteal vein

Good job!

Atherosclerosis and Coronary Artery Disease (CAD)

Atherosclerosis, also known as *arteriosclerosis*, is a stricture or stenosis of an artery (e.g., code I70.0 Atherosclerosis of aorta) that may require the placement of a stent (a wire mesh tube inserted to support the walls of the artery and to keep them open). You have probably heard about this in some commercials on television that talk about the buildup of plaque in the arteries and the damage that may result. Atherosclerosis (*athero* = artery + *sclerosis* = hardening) is the medical term for plaque-lined arteries. You also may see the abbreviation ASHD (arteriosclerotic heart disease). The plaque builds up on the inner walls of the arteries, thereby narrowing the passageway and reducing the flow of blood. Remember that arteries carry oxygenated blood from the heart to the tissues and cells throughout the body.

Atherosclerosis
A condition resulting from plaque buildup on the interior walls of the arteries, causing reduced blood flow; also known as *arteriosclerosis*.

In coronary artery disease (CAD), plaque collects specifically within the coronary arteries (arteries within the heart); the heart itself becomes oxygen-deprived. This means there will be a greater potential for a stroke (cerebrovascular accident [CVA]), a heart attack, or death. According to the National Heart, Lung, and Blood Institute, CAD is the number-one cause of death in the United States.

When you look in the ICD-10-CM Alphabetic Index, you will read:

Disease, diseased

- coronary (artery) — *see* Disease, heart, ischemic, atherosclerotic

- heart (organic) I51.9

-- ischemic (chronic or with a stated duration of over 4 weeks) I25.9

--- atherosclerotic (of) I25.10

---- with angina pectoris — *see* Arteriosclerosis, coronary (artery)

---- coronary artery bypass graft — *see* Arteriosclerosis, coronary (artery)

> **Angina Pectoris**
> Chest pain.

A patient may first be alerted to reduced flow of blood to the heart muscle by angina. **Angina pectoris** is an event of acute chest pain caused by an insufficient supply of oxygen to an area of the heart. This condition may be treated with drugs categorized as vasodilators, such as Isordil or Nitrostat (sublingual nitroglycerin), that dilate arterial walls, making it easier for blood to flow smoothly. When hypertension is also present, a calcium channel blocker, such as Norvasc or Vascor, may be prescribed instead. Report angina pectoris with a code from category I20.- Angina pectoris, with a required additional character for the specific type of angina, and be certain to pay attention to the notation directly above this code category that applies to this whole range of codes I20–I25:

Use additional code **to identify presence of hypertension (I10–I16)**

GUIDANCE CONNECTION

Read the ICD-10-CM Official Guidelines for Coding and Reporting, section **I. Conventions, General Coding Guidelines and Chapter-Specific Guidelines**, subsection **C. Chapter-Specific Coding Guidelines**, chapter **9. Diseases of the Circulatory System**, subsection **b. Atherosclerotic coronary artery disease with angina.**

In addition to diet and exercise modification, antilipemic drugs, such as Lipitor or Zocor, may be prescribed to decrease the lipid (fat) blood level. If these actions are not sufficient, a percutaneous transluminal coronary angioplasty (PTCA) may be performed. During a PTCA, a catheter is threaded through the artery to the site of the plaque buildup. A balloon on the tip of the catheter is expanded, compacting the plaque against the walls of the artery, thereby reducing the blockage.

YOU CODE IT! CASE STUDY

PATIENT: Basti, Carl

REASON FOR CONSULTATION: Surgical evaluation for coronary artery disease.

HISTORY OF PRESENT ILLNESS: The patient is a 47-year-old male who has a known history of coronary artery disease. He underwent previous PTCA and stenting procedures in December and most recently in August. Since that time, he has been relatively stable with medical management. However, in the past several weeks, he started to notice some exertional dyspnea with chest pain.

For the most part, the pain subsides with rest. For this reason, he was reevaluated with a cardiac catheterization. This demonstrated 3-vessel coronary artery disease with a 70% lesion to the right coronary artery; this was a proximal lesion. The left main had a 70% stenosis. The circumflex also had a 99% stenosis. Overall left ventricular function was mildly reduced with an ejection fraction of about 45%. The left ventriculogram did note some apical hypokinesis. In view of these findings, surgical consultation was requested and the patient was seen and evaluated by Dr. Isaacson.

(continued)

PAST MEDICAL HISTORY:

1. Coronary artery disease as described above with previous PTCA and stenting procedures.
2. Dyslipidemia.
3. Hypertension.

ALLERGIES: None.

MEDICATIONS: Aspirin 81 mg daily, Plavix 75 mg daily, Altace 2.5 mg daily, metoprolol 50 mg b.i.d., and Lipitor 10 mg q.h.s.

SOCIAL HISTORY: He quit smoking approximately 8 months ago. Prior to that time, he had about a 35- to 40-pack-per-year history. He does not abuse alcohol.

FAMILY MEDICAL HISTORY: Mother died prematurely of breast cancer. His father died prematurely of gastric carcinoma.

REVIEW OF SYSTEMS: There is no history of any CVAs, TIAs, or seizures. No chronic headaches. No asthma, TB, hemoptysis, or productive cough. There is no congenital heart abnormality or rheumatic fever history. He has no palpitations. He notes no nausea, vomiting, constipation, diarrhea, but immediately prior to admission, he did develop some diffuse abdominal discomfort. He says that since then, this has resolved. No diabetes or thyroid problem. There is no depression or psychiatric problems. There are no musculoskeletal disorders or history of gout; no hematologic problems or blood dyscrasias; no bleeding tendencies; and no recent fevers, malaise, changes in appetite, or changes in weight.

PHYSICAL EXAMINATION: His blood pressure is 120/70; pulse is 80. He is in a sinus rhythm on the EKG monitor. Respirations are 18 and unlabored. Temperature is 98.2 degrees Fahrenheit. He weighs 260 pounds and is 5 feet 10 inches. In general, this was a pleasant male who currently is not in acute distress. Skin color and turgor are good. Pupils were equal and reactive to light. Conjunctivae clear. Throat is benign. Mucosa was moist and noncyanotic. Neck veins not distended at 90 degrees. Carotids had 2+ upstrokes bilaterally without bruits. No lymphadenopathy was appreciated. Chest had a normal AP diameter. The lungs were clear in the apices and bases; no wheezing or egophony appreciated. The heart had a normal S1, S2. No murmurs, clicks, or gallops. The abdomen was soft, nontender, nondistended. Good bowel sounds present. No hepatosplenomegaly was appreciated. No pulsatile masses were felt. No abdominal bruits were heard. His pulses are 2+ and equal bilaterally in the upper and lower extremities. No clubbing is appreciated. He is oriented x3. Demonstrated a good amount of strength in the upper and lower extremities. Face was symmetrical. He had a normal gait.

IMPRESSION: This is a 47-year-old male with significant multivessel coronary artery disease. The patient also has a left main lesion. He has undergone several PTCA and stenting procedures within the last year to year and a half. At this point, in order to reduce the risk of any possible ischemia in the future, surgical myocardial revascularization is recommended.

PLAN: We will plan to proceed with surgical myocardial revascularization. The risks and benefits of this procedure were explained to the patient. All questions pertaining to this procedure were answered.

Vaughn Pronder, MD

You Code It!

Carefully review Dr. Pronder's documentation after his evaluation of Carl Basti, and determine the correct diagnosis code or codes to report.

Step #1: Read the case carefully and completely.
Step #2: Abstract the scenario. Which main words or terms describe why the physician cared for the patient during this encounter?
Step #3: Are there any details missing or incomplete for which you would need to query the physician? [If so, ask your instructor.]
Step #4: Check for any relevant guidance, including reading all of the symbols and notations in the Tabular List and the appropriate sections of the Official Guidelines.
Step #5: Determine the correct diagnosis code or codes to explain why this encounter was medically necessary.
Step #6: Double-check your work.

(continued)

Answer:

Did you determine these to be the correct codes?

I25.10	**Atherosclerotic heart disease of native coronary artery without angina pectoris**
I10	**Essential (primary) Hypertension**
Z87.891	**Personal history of nicotine dependence**
Z79.82	**Long-term (current) use of aspirin**

Good work!

12.3 Hypertension

The average adult has approximately 10 pints (5 liters) of blood in their cardiovascular system. Together, the components of the cardiovascular system will pump these 10 pints through the body every minute. The level of pressure at which the blood travels through the vessels is very important.

Blood Pressure

Hypotension
Low blood pressure; systolic blood pressure below 90 mmHg and/or diastolic measurements of lower than 60 mmHg.

The force with which blood travels through your veins and arteries must create enough pressure to ensure the cycle of oxygenation and carbon dioxide is maintained properly. Blood pressure that is too low—a condition known as **hypotension** (*hypo* = low or under + *tension* = pressure)—can result in organs and tissue cells being unable to function. In hypotension, the patient has lower-than-normal blood pressure. Low blood pressure indicates an inadequate flow of blood and, therefore, inadequate oxygen to the brain, heart, and other vital organs. Lightheadedness and dizziness can occur in a person with hypotension. Some medications, such as antianxiety drugs and diuretics, can cause hypotension, as can alcohol and narcotics. Conditions such as advanced diabetes, dehydration, or arrhythmia also can result in a patient suffering from hypotension. Code category I95 will provide you with the details you will need to abstract from the documentation about this diagnosis:

I95.0	Idiopathic hypotension
I95.1	Orthostatic hypotension
I95.2	Hypotension due to drugs ***Use additional code*** **for adverse effect, if applicable, to identify drug**
I95.3	Hypotension of hemodialysis
I95.81	Postprocedural hypotension
I95.89	Other hypotension

Hypertension
High blood pressure, usually a chronic condition; often identified by a systolic blood pressure above 140 mmHg and/or a diastolic blood pressure above 90 mmHg.

Hypertension (*hyper* = high or over + *tension* = pressure) is a condition when blood pressure is too high. The increased force of the blood's pressure moving through the vessels can actually damage organs and tissues as the blood rushes through.

A health care professional will use a sphygmomanometer (blood pressure machine) to measure a patient's blood pressure and will document the results in two numbers. For example: A patient's blood pressure is documented in the chart as 125/85. The number 125 represents the systolic pressure and the number 85 is the diastolic pressure (see **Table 12-1**).

Systolic pressure (SP) is the measure of the maximum push of blood being forced into an artery from the ventricle during a cardiac contraction. This is the top number of a reported blood pressure.

Diastolic pressure (DP) is the measure of the pressure of blood left in the arteries in between ventricular contractions. This is the bottom number of a reported blood pressure.

Hypertension is a condition that millions of people must deal with every day and is a major cause of death. According to the Centers for Disease Control and Prevention (CDC), 29% of all American adults—70 million people—have high blood pressure. These numbers include more women than men and a greater prevalence in individuals over 65 years of age. There are estimates

TABLE 12-1 Blood Pressure Levels

Systolic/Diastolic Measurement (mmHg)	Diagnosis
< 120/< 80	Normal
120–129/< 80	Elevated
130–139 or 80–89	Hypertension stage 1
140 or higher/90 or higher	Hypertension stage 2
Higher than 180 and/or higher than 120	Hypertensive Crisis

Source: *Harvard Health*, April 2018, https://www.health.harvard.edu/heart-health/reading-the-new-blood-pressure-guidelines

that only about one-third of hypertensive people have been officially diagnosed and are getting treatment. It is believed that as many as 50% of all people over age 60 are included in these numbers.

The CDC also determined that high blood pressure was a primary or contributing cause of death for more than 360,000 people in the United States in 2013. The risk of heart disease is increased 300% by the presence of hypertension, and the risk of stroke is increased 700%. Research also proves that African Americans are at a much higher risk of hypertension and its effects than any other racial or ethnic group.

Elevated Blood Pressure

Elevated blood pressure is not the same as a diagnosis of *hypertension*. Almost anyone might have a single measure above the norm. Some individuals get nervous when visiting a health care facility, while others may have just eaten something with a great deal of salt, causing an unusual measure one time. For their own reasons, the physician may want to document a reading of elevated blood pressure and therefore include this as a diagnosis to be reported.

> **Elevated Blood Pressure**
> An occurrence of high blood pressure; an isolated or infrequent reading of a systolic blood pressure above 120 mmHg and/or a diastolic blood pressure above 80 mmHg.

R03.0 Elevated blood-pressure reading, without diagnosis of hypertension

Hypertension is a chronic state of elevated blood pressure. Therefore, without the specific diagnosis of hypertension, you, as the professional coder, cannot report a code for hypertension.

Primary Hypertension

Hypertension frequently shows no signs and symptoms, other than continuous high blood pressure measurements, until the condition alters **vascular** function in the heart, brain, and/or kidneys. This effect is similar to what would happen if the pressure level at which water flows through the pipes in your home increased: high pressure can break a dish in your kitchen sink and make a mess. Patients with high blood pressure specifically diagnosed as *hypertension* are known to suffer manifestations of this condition, including damage to the heart and kidneys. Hypertension causes the heart to work harder than normal and can result in left ventricular hypertrophy, which can subsequently cause left-sided heart failure or right-sided heart failure as well as pulmonary **edema** (excess fluid in the tissues).

> **Vascular**
> Referring to the vessels (arteries and veins).

> **Edema**
> An overaccumulation of fluid in the cells of the tissues.

There are many risk factors that promote the development of hypertension. Here are a few of the most common:

- An underlying disorder such as renal disease or Cushing's syndrome.
- Chronic emotional stress.
- A sedentary lifestyle.
- Excessive sodium in the diet.
- Family history of hypertension.
- Postmenopausal state.
- Advancing age.
- Excessive use of alcohol.
- Obesity.
- African American ancestry.

CODING BITES

Hypertension is a systemic disease, meaning it can affect every part of the body, throughout the patient's entire system. With this in mind, a diagnosis of hypertension will affect treatment of almost any other condition, disease, or injury. Therefore, a code for the hypertension is almost always included, regardless of the reason for the encounter and even if treatment of the hypertension is not performed directly.

A diagnosis will typically come from trending–charting the blood pressure readings over time (an excellent tool in most electronic health record software programs). In addition, a physician can support a diagnosis of hypertension with other data derived from a variety of sources:

- *Auscultation* (listening to sounds with a stethoscope) over the abdominal aorta as well as the carotid, renal, and femoral arteries may reveal bruits (an abnormal sound created by blood flowing past an obstruction; also known as *turbulent flow*).
- *Ophthalmoscopy* (examination of the interior of the eye) may reveal arteriovenous nicking.
- *Patient history* may include a family history of hypertension.
- *Chest x-ray* may reveal cardiomegaly (enlargement of the heart).
- *Echocardiography* may show left ventricular hypertrophy (*hyper* = high or over + *-trophy* = growth).
- *Electrocardiogram* (ECG or EKG) may show ischemia (shortage of oxygen due to reduced or restricted blood flow).

When the documentation includes a specific diagnosis of hypertension, you, the coder, will need more information to accurately report this diagnosis.

Essential Hypertension

Essential (primary) hypertension is the usual type of hypertension. Code category I10 is used for any diagnosis written by the physician that is stated as high blood pressure, arterial hypertension, benign hypertension, malignant hypertension, primary hypertension, or systemic hypertension.

Most often, essential hypertension can be kept under control with diet (including avoiding high-sodium foods) and medication (e.g., angiotensin-converting enzyme, or ACE inhibitors, diuretics, and beta-blockers).

ICD-10-CM

LET'S CODE IT! SCENARIO

Anna Epstein, a 63-year-old female, came to see Dr. Tanner. She was complaining of occasional dizziness and a headache. After a complete examination, Dr. Tanner diagnosed Anna with idiopathic systemic hypertension.

Let's Code It!

Dr. Tanner diagnosed Anna with *idiopathic systemic hypertension*. Let's turn to the Alphabetic Index and find the main term *hypertension* and begin reading. If you look down the alphabetic listing under *hypertension*, you will see no listing for *idiopathic* or *systemic*. So go back to the very first entry for this key term, "Hypertension, hypertensive," and read the words shown in parentheses following that entry.

Do you see the words *(idiopathic)* and *(systemic)* included? Both of the adjectives used by Dr. Tanner in his diagnostic statement are in the listing. Therefore, the diagnosis code for Anna's current diagnosis is I10. Turn to the Tabular List to double-check.

One more stop: Let's turn to the ICD-10-CM Official Guidelines and check **Chapter 9: Diseases of the Circulatory System (I00–I99)**, subsection **a. Hypertension**. There don't seem to be any guidelines that relate to Dr. Tanner's diagnosis for Anna.

I10 Essential (primary) hypertension

INCLUDES **high blood pressure**

hypertension (arterial) (benign) (essential) (malignant) (primary) (systemic)

Perfect!

Secondary Hypertension

There are occasions when another condition or a medication may cause hypertension instead of hypertension causing other conditions (manifestations) in the patient. Medications such as corticosteroids (e.g., prednisone), antidepressants (e.g., Sinequan), and hormones (e.g., Estrace) or diseases such as Cushing's syndrome or scleroderma may trigger a hypertensive condition. When the hypertensive condition is generated by, or secondary to, another disease or medication, the condition is called secondary hypertension.

The involvement of renal disease as an underlying cause of hypertension, also known as *renovascular hypertension*, may be diagnosed as a result of testing including:

- *Urinalysis*, which shows protein levels and red and white blood cells indicating glomerulonephritis (inflammation of small blood vessels in the kidneys).
- *Excretory urography*, which reveals renal atrophy (wasting away of a kidney), pointing to chronic renal disease, or a shortening of one kidney, which may indicate unilateral renal disease.
- *Blood tests for serum potassium levels* (measuring the levels of potassium in the blood), which show levels below the normal measure of 3.5 mEq/L, which can indicate primary hyperaldosteronism (*hyper* = high or over + *aldosterone* = a hormone produced by the adrenal cortex that prompts the kidney to preserve sodium and water).

Hypertension is coded as secondary when the physician uses terms such as "due to" an underlying disease, "resulting from" another condition, or other descriptors that point to another disease or condition. In such cases, you will need two codes:

1. The underlying condition.
2. The type of secondary hypertension (I15.*x*).

There is a notation to "***Code also underlying condition***." Note that sequencing is not identified in this notation. Therefore, you will need to report the two codes based on the sequencing guidelines in the ICD-10-CM Official Guidelines, section II, which will guide you in determining the principal diagnosis code. So the order in which you will list the two codes is determined by the answer to the question, "Why did the patient come to see the physician today?"

GUIDANCE CONNECTION

Read the ICD-10-CM Official Guidelines for Coding and Reporting, section **I. Conventions, General Coding Guidelines and Chapter-Specific Guidelines**, subsection **C. Chapter-Specific Coding Guidelines**, chapter **9. Diseases of the Circulatory System**, subsection **a.6) Hypertension, secondary**.

EXAMPLES

I15.0	Renovascular hypertension
I15.1	Hypertension secondary to other renal disorders
I15.2	Hypertension secondary to endocrine disorders
I15.8	Other secondary hypertension
I15.9	Secondary hypertension, unspecified

LET'S CODE IT! SCENARIO

Breanna Payne, a 67-year-old female, came to see Dr. Lebonna in his office. She was having headaches and bouts of dizziness. After a physical examination, a urinalysis, and blood work, he diagnosed her with benign hypertension. Dr. Lebonna's notes stated that Breanna's hypertension was the result of her existing diagnosis of pituitary-dependent Cushing's disease.

Let's Code It!

Dr. Lebonna diagnosed Breanna with *benign hypertension due to pituitary-dependent Cushing's disease*. This means that Cushing's disease caused Breanna's hypertension. First, go to the Alphabetic Index and look under *hypertension*. Look down the indented column until you see "due to" (which is the same as "result of" stated in the physician's notes).

(continued)

Now, look at the indented listing under "due to"; you will see no listing for "Cushing's disease." So "specified disease" is a strong consideration. You can also keep looking down the column until you see "secondary" specified disease NEC I15.8. Both paths take you to the same suggested code:

Hypertension

due to

endocrine disorders I15.2

Now let's check this code in the Tabular List:

I15.2 Hypertension secondary to endocrine disorders

Did you remember that the pituitary gland is a component of the endocrine system? Now, one more thing: is there a notation beneath I15 alerting you that something is missing?

Code also underlying condition

That's right—a code for the Cushing's disease. In the Alphabetic Index, you see the following under *Cushing's*:

Cushing's

syndrome or disease E24.9

pituitary-dependent E24.0

In the Tabular List, you will see

✓4 **E24 Cushing's syndrome**

Next, there is an EXCLUDES1 note:

EXCLUDES1 *congenital adrenal hyperplasia (E25.0)*

Just because Breanna is 67 years old does not mean this isn't a congenital condition. However, Dr. Lebonna provides no documentation stating that her Cushing's disease is congenital, so this EXCLUDES1 note does not apply to this patient for this encounter.

E24.0 Pituitary-dependent Cushing's disease

Check for any relevant guidance, including reading all of the symbols and notations in the Tabular List and the appropriate sections of the Official Guidelines. Nothing is directed to this specific case, so you will report these two codes for this encounter between Dr. Lebonna and Breanna:

I15.2 Hypertension secondary to endocrine disorders

E24.0 Pituitary-dependent Cushing's disease

How should these codes be sequenced? List the hypertension first (I15.2) because the symptoms of the hypertension (headaches, dizziness) are what brought Breanna to Dr. Lebonna's office for this encounter.

Hypertensive Crisis

Code category I16 provides three codes for reporting a hypertensive crisis. This is when a patient suffers an acute and dramatic increase in blood pressure, measuring approximately 180/120. This situation can result in blood vessels becoming damaged and leaking, as well as dysfunction of the heart's ability to pump blood through the body.

A hypertensive crisis is categorized as either urgent or emergency.

- I16.0 Hypertensive urgency identifies a patient with an extremely high spike of blood pressure, with the belief that the vessels have not yet been damaged.
- I16.1 Hypertensive emergency documents that the patient's extraordinarily high blood pressure has caused damage to blood vessels and/or organs. This diagnosis can be associated with life-threatening complications. Reporting this code also requires an additional code, when applicable, as per the Use Additional code notation, so be certain to read the documentation carefully for mention of any organ dysfunction involvement.

CODING BITES

Code category I16 includes a notation applicable to all codes in this category:

Code also **any identified hypertensive disease (I10–I15)**

Use Additional code, if applicable, to identify specific organ dysfunction, such as:
acute kidney injury (N17.-)
acute myocardial infarction (I21.-)
acute pulmonary edema (left and/or right ventricular failure) (J81.0, I50.-)
aortic dissection (I71.0-)
cerebral hemorrhage (I60.-. I61.-, I62.-)
cerebral infarction (I63.-)
eclampsia (O15.-)
hypertensive encephalopathy (I67.4)
seizure (R56.9)

- I16.9 Hypertensive crisis, unspecified is a code that should rarely be reported. Instead, as you have learned, you should query the physician to determine what type of crisis it is and have the documentation amended.

Resistant Hypertension

For some patients, the prescribed treatment for their hypertension is not effective. For these patients, documented as having resistant hypertension, code I1A.0 must be reported after the existing hypertension code.

Example: Dr. Rosen documented that, after 6 months, the antihypertensive medication was not lowering Tanya's essential hypertension numbers, as intended. Therefore, additional recommendations are provided. You will report this as:

I10 **Essential (primary) hypertension**
I1A.0 **Resistant hypertension**

NOTE: There is no code for long-term use of an antihypertensive, so you don't need to worry about adding a third code.

Hypertension and Pregnancy

When a pregnant woman has a diagnosis of hypertension, you will first need to determine from the documentation whether she developed hypertension before or after conception.

Gestational Hypertension
Hypertension that develops during pregnancy and typically goes away once the pregnancy has ended.

A woman with a preexisting diagnosis of hypertension who then becomes pregnant will be reported with the appropriate code from the O10 Pre-existing hypertension complicating pregnancy, childbirth, and the puerperium code category. A code from the O10 code category reports this situation clearly with additional details, provided by the fourth character, to report the specific hypertensive manifestation, if any:

O10.0- **Pre-existing essential hypertension complicating pregnancy, childbirth, and the puerperium**
O10.1- **Pre-existing hypertensive heart disease complicating pregnancy, childbirth, and the puerperium**
O10.2- **Pre-existing hypertensive chronic kidney disease complicating pregnancy, childbirth, and the puerperium**
O10.3- **Pre-existing hypertensive heart and chronic kidney disease complicating pregnancy, childbirth, and the puerperium**
O10.4- **Pre-existing secondary hypertension complicating pregnancy, childbirth, and the puerperium**

However, if the hypertension is diagnosed as **gestational hypertension**, or transient hypertension, you will report a code from O13 Gestational [pregnancy-induced] hypertension without significant proteinuria. This is not unusual and generally means that the hypertension will go away after the baby is born.

GUIDANCE CONNECTION

Read the ICD-10-CM Official Guidelines for Coding and Reporting, section **I. Conventions, General Coding Guidelines and Chapter-Specific Guidelines**, subsection **C. Chapter-Specific Coding Guidelines**, chapter **9. Diseases of the Circulatory System**, subsection **a.7) Hypertension, transient**.

O13.1 **Gestational [pregnancy-induced] hypertension without significant proteinuria, first trimester**
O13.2 **Gestational [pregnancy-induced] hypertension without significant proteinuria, second trimester**
O13.3 **Gestational [pregnancy-induced] hypertension without significant proteinuria, third trimester**

Should the woman's diagnosed hypertension cause problems directly related to the pregnancy or complicating the pregnancy, you will choose the best, most appropriate code from the ICD-10-CM code book's ***Chapter 15: Pregnancy, Childbirth and the Puerperium (O00–O9A)***.

LET'S CODE IT! SCENARIO

Zena Browning, a 23-year-old female, is 20 weeks pregnant. Dr. Shinto diagnoses her with gestational hypertension. Even though there is no evidence of proteinuria, he is concerned about the effect of the condition on her pregnancy and writes a prescription.

Let's Code It!

Zena Browning has *gestational hypertension.* Her hypertensive condition is complicating her pregnancy. Turn to the term *hypertension* in the Alphabetic Index and look down the column of adjectives below the primary term *hypertension.* You see

Hypertension

complicating

pregnancy

gestational (pregnancy-induced) (transient) (without proteinuria) O13.-

That matches Dr. Shinto's notes. Now you must turn to the Tabular List to confirm the code *and* determine the correct fourth character:

O13 Gestational [pregnancy-induced] hypertension without significant proteinuria

Now turn to the first page of the ICD-10-CM code book's ***Chapter 15: Pregnancy, Childbirth and the Puerperium (O00–O9A)*** to see the definitions of the trimesters. You can see the information:

1st trimester—less than 14 weeks, 0 days

2nd trimester—14 weeks, 0 days to less than 28 weeks, 0 days

3rd trimester—28 weeks, 0 days until delivery

Zena is in her 20th week, so she is in her 2nd trimester. This points us to the correct fourth character of 2. The code to be used for this visit between Dr. Shinto and Zena Browning is

O13.2 Gestational [pregnancy-induced] hypertension without significant proteinuria, second trimester

Before you report this code, be certain to carefully check for any relevant guidance, including reading all of the symbols and notations in the Tabular List and the appropriate sections of the Official Guidelines. Confirmed! Good job!

12.4 Manifestations of Hypertension

GUIDANCE CONNECTION

Read the ICD-10-CM Official Guidelines for Coding and Reporting, section **I. Conventions, General Coding Guidelines and Chapter-Specific Guidelines**, subsection **C. Chapter-Specific Coding Guidelines**, chapter **9. Diseases of the Circulatory System**, subsection **a.1) Hypertensive with heart disease.**

Hypertensive Heart Disease

When a patient has heart disease or heart failure and also has hypertension, you must carefully examine the words used by the physician in the description.

1. Heart condition *due to* hypertension
2. *Hypertensive* heart condition
3. Heart condition *with* hypertension

If the physician states that the patient has both hypertension and heart disease, a combination code from code category I11 Hypertensive heart disease must be recorded.

I11.0 Hypertensive heart disease with heart failure
Use additional code **to identify type of heart failure (I50.-)**

I11.9 Hypertensive heart disease without heart failure

Hypertensive Heart Disease with Heart Failure

In cases where a physician states that a patient has heart failure due to hypertension, you will need to

1. Use the appropriate fourth character, as shown in the Tabular List under category I11.
2. *Use additional code* to specify the type of heart failure from category I50.-.

ICD-10-CM includes a notation directing you to *Use additional code* **to identify type of heart failure (I50.-)** to remind you.

EXAMPLE

Acute congestive heart failure due to benign hypertension

You will report two codes, in this sequence: I11.0, I50.31

I11.0 Hypertensive heart disease with heart failure

I50.31 Acute diastolic (congestive) heart failure

CODING BITES

Determine what type of heart failure the patient has so you can report it with an additional code. You learned about the different types of heart failure earlier in this chapter.

LET'S CODE IT! SCENARIO

Colin Fahey, a 53-year-old male, was diagnosed with chronic diastolic congestive heart failure due to benign hypertension. Dr. Engman wrote a prescription for medication and scheduled follow-up tests.

Let's Code It!

Colin was diagnosed with *congestive heart failure due to benign hypertension.*

Turn in the Alphabetic Index to find

Failure, failed

heart (acute) (senile) (sudden) I50.9

hypertensive—*see* Hypertension, heart

OK, turn to . . .

Hypertension, hypertensive (accelerated) (benign) (essential) (idiopathic) (malignant) (systemic) I10

heart (disease) (conditions in I51.4-I51.9 due to hypertension) I11.9

Remember from earlier in this chapter that when the diagnostic statement is written "heart condition *due to* hypertension," the guidelines state that only one code, from category I11, is used. Turn to the Tabular List for I11:

I11 Hypertensive heart disease
INCLUDES **any condition in I51.4–I51.9 due to hypertension**

This description fits perfectly. Now we must look at the fourth character. Dr. Engman wrote "congestive heart failure," bringing us to

I11.0 Hypertensive heart disease with heart failure
Use additional code **to identify type of heart failure (I50.-)**

Does the documentation identify the specific type of heart failure? Yes, Dr. Engman indicated that Colin has congestive heart failure. Let's turn to

I50 Heart failure

Read the notation under the code:

Code first:

heart failure due to hypertension (I11.0)

(continued)

This is the book's way of reinforcing the guideline as well as the notation that you found beneath I11. Continue reading, and you see that the second code you need to include for Colin's diagnosis is this:

I50.32 Chronic diastolic (congestive) heart failure

Be certain to check for any relevant guidance, including reading all of the symbols and notations in the Tabular List and Section I.C.9 of the Official Guidelines. There is nothing that alters the determination of these codes.

You need to show both codes for the visit between Colin and Dr. Engman:

I11.0 Hypertensive heart disease with heart failure
I50.32 Chronic diastolic (congestive) heart failure

Good work!

Hypertensive Chronic Kidney Disease

When a diagnosis of hypertensive chronic kidney disease is documented, you will report a combination code, as appropriate. In such cases, a cause-and-effect relationship between the hypertension and the kidney disease does *not* need to be specifically stated by the physician. The mere existence of both conditions in the same body at the same time is enough to report them together. You will need the documentation to specify the stage of the chronic kidney disease to determine the correct code in ICD-10-CM. Code category I12 is to be used for reporting a patient with a diagnosis of hypertensive chronic kidney disease.

✓4 **I12 Hypertensive chronic kidney disease**

The fourth-character choices are

I12.0 Hypertensive chronic kidney disease with stage 5 chronic kidney disease or end stage renal disease
Use additional code **to identify the stage of chronic kidney disease (N18.5, N18.6)**

I12.9 Hypertensive chronic kidney disease with stage 1 through stage 4 chronic kidney disease or unspecified chronic kidney disease
Use additional code **to identify the stage of chronic kidney disease (N18.1–N18.4, N18.9)**

You can see that beneath each of these codes is a notation:

- Beneath I12.0:

  Use additional code **to identify the stage of chronic kidney disease (N18.5, N18.6)**

- Beneath I12.9:

  Use additional code **to identify the stage of chronic kidney disease (N18.1–N18.4, N18.9)**

Should you see that the physician has documented both hypertensive chronic kidney disease *and* acute renal failure, you will need to report the acute renal failure in addition, with a code from category N17.

CODING BITES

If you can't find the information in the documentation as to what stage of kidney disease the patient has, query the physician.

GUIDANCE CONNECTION

Read the ICD-10-CM Official Guidelines for Coding and Reporting, section **I. Conventions, General Coding Guidelines and Chapter-Specific Guidelines**, subsection **C. Chapter-Specific Coding Guidelines**, chapter **9. Diseases of the Circulatory System**, subsection **a.2) Hypertensive chronic kidney disease**.

YOU CODE IT! CASE STUDY

ICD-10-CM

Matthew Spencer, a 69-year-old male, is admitted to Franklin General Hospital for observation with a diagnosis of stage 3 chronic renal disease due to benign hypertension.

(continued)

You Code It!

Go through the steps of coding, and determine the code or codes that should be reported for Matthew Spencer's admission into the hospital.

Step #1: Read the case carefully and completely.

Step #2: Abstract the scenario. Which main words or terms describe why the physician cared for the patient during this encounter?

Step #3: Are there any details missing or incomplete for which you would need to query the physician? [If so, ask your instructor.]

Step #4: Check for any relevant guidance, including reading all of the symbols and notations in the Tabular List and the appropriate sections of the Official Guidelines.

Step #5: Determine the correct diagnosis code or codes to explain why this encounter was medically necessary.

Step #6: Double-check your work.

Answer:

Did you determine these to be the diagnosis codes?

I12.9 Hypertensive chronic kidney disease with stage 1 through stage 4 chronic kidney disease or unspecified chronic kidney disease

N18.3 Chronic kidney disease, stage 3 (moderate)

Hypertensive Heart and Chronic Kidney Disease

If the patient is diagnosed with both hypertensive heart disease and hypertensive chronic kidney disease, you will choose one combination code from category I13. Now, great emphasis has been placed on the fact that you should never assume. You are permitted to code only what you know for a fact from the documentation. But, as you know, every rule has an exception, and this is it. The Official Guidelines state that you "*may assume the relationship between the hypertensive heart disease and hypertensive renal disease even if the physician does not state this relationship in the diagnosis.*"

You will still need to confirm that a cause-and-effect relationship is specified for the hypertension and the heart condition, even though the cause-and-effect relationship between the hypertension and the kidney disease does not have to be specified. The additional-character choices for code I13 will identify whether the patient is documented to have

- Heart failure or not.
- Stage 1, 2, 3, or 4 chronic kidney disease or unspecified stage.
- Stage 5 chronic kidney disease, or ESRD.

In addition to using this code, you also will need a code for the specific type of heart failure and another to report the stage of the kidney disease. ICD-10-CM includes notations under code I13 to remind you of the additional coding:

Use additional code **to identify type of heart failure (I50.-)**

Use additional code **to identify stage of chronic kidney disease (N18.-)**

GUIDANCE CONNECTION

Read the ICD-10-CM Official Guidelines for Coding and Reporting, section **I. Conventions, General Coding Guidelines and Chapter-Specific Guidelines**, subsection **C. Chapter-Specific Coding Guidelines**, chapter **9. Diseases of the Circulatory System**, subsection **a.3) Hypertensive heart and chronic kidney disease**.

YOU CODE IT! CASE STUDY

Clarissa Bennelli, a 71-year-old female, is seen at Weston Hospital with a diagnosis of acute systolic congestive heart failure due to hypertensive heart disease. Ms. Bennelli responds positively to Lasix therapy. She is also diagnosed with stage 1 chronic renal disease.

You Code It!

Go through the steps of coding, and determine the code or codes that should be reported for Clarissa Bennelli's admission into the hospital.

Step #1: Read the case carefully and completely.
Step #2: Abstract the scenario. Which main words or terms describe why the physician cared for the patient during this encounter?
Step #3: Are there any details missing or incomplete for which you would need to query the physician? [If so, ask your instructor.]
Step #4: Check for any relevant guidance, including reading all of the symbols and notations in the Tabular List and the appropriate sections of the Official Guidelines.
Step #5: Determine the correct diagnosis code or codes to explain why this encounter was medically necessary.
Step #6: Double-check your work.

Answer:

Did you determine these to be the diagnosis codes?

I13.0 **Hypertensive heart and chronic kidney disease with heart failure and stage 1 through stage 4 chronic kidney disease or unspecified chronic kidney disease**

I50.21 **Acute systolic (congestive) heart failure**

N18.1 **Chronic kidney disease, stage 1**

Good job!

Hypertensive Retinopathy

Retinopathy is a degenerative disease of the eye, most specifically the retina. The condition can be caused by diabetes, hypertension, or other circumstances. In cases where the patient is diagnosed with hypertensive retinopathy due to hypertension, you will need two codes to thoroughly report the patient's condition.

GUIDANCE CONNECTION

Read the ICD-10-CM Official Guidelines for Coding and Reporting, section **I. Conventions, General Coding Guidelines and Chapter-Specific Guidelines**, subsection **C. Chapter-Specific Coding Guidelines**, chapter **9. Diseases of the Circulatory System**, subsection **a.5) Hypertensive retinopathy**.

Your first code is from the subcategory H35.03- Hypertensive retinopathy. This code requires a sixth character to identify which eye is affected:

H35.031 **Hypertensive retinopathy, right eye**

H35.032 **Hypertensive retinopathy, left eye**

H35.033 **Hypertensive retinopathy, bilateral**

Then you will need an additional code to identify the type of hypertension that caused the retinopathy. Choose that code from the I10–I15 range. There is a reminder notation for you, shown beneath code H35.0:

Code also **any associated hypertension (I10.-)**

Hypertensive Cerebrovascular Disease

Patients diagnosed with cerebrovascular disease due to hypertension will have two codes assigned. The first code will report the cerebrovascular disease, a code from the I60–I69 range. The second code will identify the hypertension, using the appropriate code from the I10–I15 range. Both the guidelines and a notation under the category heading shown directly above code I60 remind you of the necessity for a second code. You can see that the notation also instructs you as to in which order to place the codes:

Use additional code **to identify presence of hypertension (I10–I15)**

GUIDANCE CONNECTION

Read the ICD-10-CM Official Guidelines for Coding and Reporting, section **I. Conventions, General Coding Guidelines and Chapter-Specific Guidelines**, subsection **C. Chapter-Specific Coding Guidelines**, chapter **9. Diseases of the Circulatory System**, subsection **a.4) Hypertensive cerebrovascular disease**.

YOU CODE IT! CASE STUDY

Denise Argudin, a 53-year-old female, came to see Dr. Fenwick because she was experiencing headaches and problems with her vision. Denise was diagnosed with essential benign hypertension 3 years ago. After a thorough physical examination and further questioning about her visual disturbances, Dr. Fenwick ordered a CT scan of her head and a few other tests. The test results indicate that Denise has hypertensive encephalopathy.

You Code It!

Carefully review Dr. Fenwick's notes on his visit with Denise, along with the test results. Determine the best, most appropriate diagnosis code or codes.

Step #1: Read the case carefully and completely.

Step #2: Abstract the scenario. Which main words or terms describe why the physician cared for the patient during this encounter?

Step #3: Are there any details missing or incomplete for which you would need to query the physician? [If so, ask your instructor.]

Step #4: Check for any relevant guidance, including reading all of the symbols and notations in the Tabular List and the appropriate sections of the Official Guidelines.

Step #5: Determine the correct diagnosis code or codes to explain why this encounter was medically necessary.

Step #6: Double-check your work.

Answer:

Did you determine these to be the diagnosis codes?

I67.4 Hypertensive encephalopathy

I10 Essential hypertension

Good job!

12.5 CVA and Cerebral Infarction

While arteries and veins run through the entire body, special attention is paid to those that service the brain—the cerebellum—the cerebrovascular system.

CODING BITES

Cerebrovascular = ***cerebro*** = cerebellum (brain)

+

-vascular = blood vessels

Cerebrovascular Accident (CVA)
Rupture of a blood vessel causing hemorrhaging in the brain or an embolus in a blood vessel in the brain causing a loss of blood flow; also known as *stroke.*

A **cerebrovascular accident (CVA)** is technically considered a condition of the neurologic system, yet this diagnosis is reported with codes included in this subsection (codes I60–I67) because a CVA is the result of an obstruction in a cerebral blood vessel. A CVA, also referred to as a *stroke*, is the result of a thrombus or embolism getting lodged in a cerebral vessel and preventing blood from flowing through the area.

There are times when the blockage (occlusion) resolves quickly, either on its own or from the administration of blood-thinning/clot-busting medication (tPA), making the event short-lived. This is known as an *ischemic* attack (code categories I63, I65, and I66) (**Figure 12-4**).

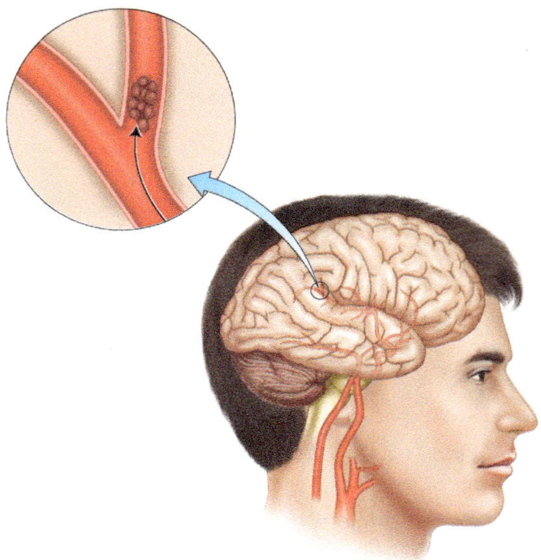

FIGURE 12-4 Illustration highlighting the position of an embolus causing an ischemic stroke

In some cases, the obstruction causes a backup of blood that subsequently bursts through the vessel wall, and a hemorrhage floods the area of the brain. This is known as a *hemorrhagic* attack (code categories I60, I61, I67) (see **Figure 12-5**).

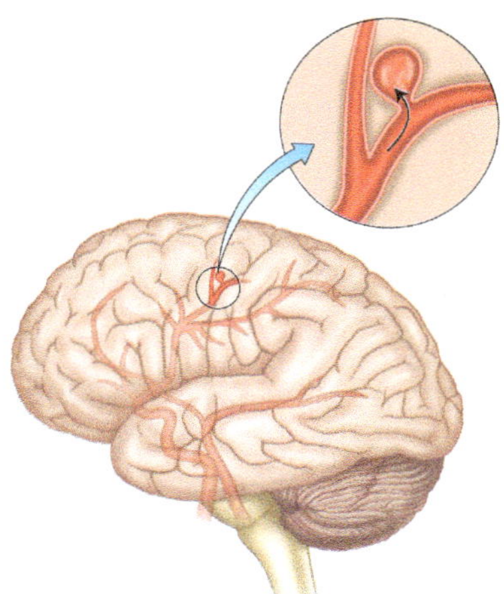

FIGURE 12-5 Illustration highlighting an aneurysm causing a hemorrhagic stroke

While a CVA is not technically the same as a **cerebral infarction**, the term *CVA* is frequently used to indicate a cerebral infarction. An **infarction** occurs when the occlusion created by the thrombus deprives surrounding tissue of oxygen and the cells die (necrosis).

Cerebral Infarction
An area of dead tissue (necrosis) in the brain caused by a blocked or ruptured blood vessel.

Infarction
Tissue or muscle that has deteriorated or died (necrotic).

You will need specific details about the patient's condition, abstracted from the documentation, to determine the correct code category, and then the correct code to report:

- Was the attack a result of a hemorrhage from a cerebral aneurysm or an obstruction from a thrombus or embolism?
- What is the specific anatomical site of the attack?

I61.- **Nontraumatic intracerebral hemorrhage**

I63.- **Cerebral infarction (occlusion and stenosis of cerebral arteries, resulting in cerebral infarction)**

I65.- **Occlusion and stenosis of precerebral arteries, not resulting in cerebral infarction**

I66.- **Occlusion and stenosis of cerebral arteries, not resulting in cerebral infarction**

It can happen that a cerebrovascular hemorrhage or infarction is brought about by a medical procedure, most typically surgery. When the procedure is plainly identified as the cause of the infarction, you have to use two codes. The first code will be

I97.810 **Intraoperative cerebrovascular infarction during cardiac surgery**

I97.811 **Intraoperative cerebrovascular infarction during other surgery**

I97.820 **Postprocedural cerebrovascular infarction following cardiac surgery**

I97.821 **Postprocedural cerebrovascular infarction following other surgery**

As noted below code I97.8, you will need an additional code to identify the exact complication. The second code will identify the exact nature of the infarction, and you will choose it from the I60–I67 range, as appropriate, according to the documentation.

GUIDANCE CONNECTION

Read the ICD-10-CM Official Guidelines for Coding and Reporting, section **I. Conventions, General Coding Guidelines and Chapter-Specific Guidelines**, subsection **C. Chapter-Specific Coding Guidelines**, chapter **9. Diseases of the Circulatory System**, subsection **c. Intraoperative and postprocedural cerebrovascular accident.**

NIH Stroke Scale

The National Institutes of Health Stroke Scale (NIHSS) is used to assess a patient's cerebral activity and function after a cerebrovascular accident (CVA–also known as a stroke). The assessment tool provides health care professionals with a numeric (quantifiable) way to measure impairment.

Code category R29.7 National Institutes of Health Stroke Scale (NIHSS) score provides you with 43 codes from which to choose to accurately report the score. Notice that this code is reported after the code to report the type of cerebral infarction (code category I63).

GUIDANCE CONNECTION

Read the ICD-10-CM Official Guidelines for Coding and Reporting, section **I. Conventions, General Coding Guidelines and Chapter-Specific Guidelines**, subsection **C. Chapter-Specific Coding Guidelines**, chapter **18. Symptoms, signs, and abnormal clinical and laboratory findings, not elsewhere classified**, subsection **i. NIHSS Stroke Scale.**

YOU CODE IT! CASE STUDY

Ruben Sackheim, a 55-year-old male, was brought into the recovery room after having a craniectomy for the drainage of an intracranial abscess. Dr. Turner's notes indicate that Ruben had a postoperative cerebrovascular infarction with intracranial hemorrhage and an acute subdural hematoma.

You Code It!

Look at Dr. Turner's notes for Ruben, and determine the best, most appropriate code or codes.

Step #1: Read the case carefully and completely.
Step #2: Abstract the scenario. Which main words or terms describe why the physician cared for the patient during this encounter?
Step #3: Are there any details missing or incomplete for which you would need to query the physician? [If so, ask your instructor.]
Step #4: Check for any relevant guidance, including reading all of the symbols and notations in the Tabular List and the appropriate sections of the Official Guidelines.
Step #5: Determine the correct diagnosis code or codes to explain why this encounter was medically necessary.
Step #6: Double-check your work.

Answer:

Did you determine these to be the diagnosis codes?

I97.821 Postprocedural cerebrovascular infarction following other surgery

I62.01 Nontraumatic acute subdural hemorrhage

Good job!

12.6 Sequelae of Cerebrovascular Disease

The sequelae, or late effects, of cerebrovascular disease are coded differently from other sequelae.

ICD-10-CM provides a series of combination codes in category I69 Sequela of cerebrovascular disease. It is not unusual for patients who are status post CVA to suffer with neurologic deficits that last past the initial onset of the condition. In such cases, the physician must connect the dots and specifically identify the current condition as a sequela, or late effect, of the cerebrovascular issue.

Should the patient be diagnosed with neurologic deficits from both a previous cerebrovascular condition *and* a current CVA, you are permitted to use both a code from the I60–I67 range *and* a code from the I69 category.

EXAMPLES

Sometimes a deficit, known as a sequela from a CVA, includes:

- Cognitive deficit.
- Speech and language deficit including aphasia, dysphasia, dysarthria, and fluency disorders.
- Monoplegia (paralysis) of a limb (arm or leg).
- Hemiplegia and hemiparesis (paralysis of one side of the body).

When there are no neurologic deficits present and the patient has a personal history of cerebrovascular disease, you should use a code from subcategory Z86.7- Personal history of diseases of the circulatory system, and not code I69. Remember, you will only code that history when it has been documented that the physician addressed the condition during the current encounter.

You will see similar notes in other locations as well. Sometimes, they can be confusing to understand. What the note above means is this: when you read in the patient's chart that they were previously diagnosed with a condition that was originally reported with any of the codes in the range I60–I67 and, during this visit, the physician documents that the patient currently has a neurologic deficit, such as paralysis or dysphasia, that is a result of that earlier condition, you will use a code from category I69 to report the new condition—the neurologic deficit.

CODING BITES

There is a **NOTE** in the Tabular List, directly under code I69, that reads:

NOTE: Category I69 is to be used to indicate conditions in I60–I67 as the cause of sequelae. The "sequelae" include conditions specified as such or as residuals which may occur at any time after the onset of the causal condition.

GUIDANCE CONNECTION

Read the ICD-10-CM Official Guidelines for Coding and Reporting, section **I. Conventions, General Coding Guidelines and Chapter-Specific Guidelines**, subsection **C. Chapter-Specific Coding Guidelines**, chapter **9. Diseases of the Circulatory System**, subsection **d. Sequelae of cerebrovascular disease.**

LET'S CODE IT! SCENARIO

ICD-10-CM

Arlene Williams goes to see Dr. McGovern. She was diagnosed with a cerebral embolism 3 months ago that has now been resolved. She explains that she has been having difficulty putting words together to make a sentence and it seems to be getting worse. After examination, Dr. McGovern diagnoses her with post-cerebral embolic dysphasia.

Let's Code It!

Arlene has been diagnosed with *post-cerebral embolic dysphasia*. This is one way the physician may state that the dysphasia is a late effect of the cerebral embolism she had before.

Turn to the ICD-10-CM Alphabetic Index and look up the term *dysphasia*.

There is one code suggested: R47.02. In the Tabular List, find the beginning of this code category:

✓4 **R47 Speech disturbances, not elsewhere classified**

Dysphasia is a speech disturbance—a problem speaking—so that is OK, so far. There is nothing in the EXCLUDES1 note that relates to this patient. As you read down, you see that fourth and fifth characters are required, so continue reading the column until you get to

R47.0 Dysphasia and aphasia

R47.02 Dysphasia

This is where the Alphabetic Index pointed you, so look closely at this code. Below it is another EXCLUDES1 note, which tells you that this code does not include a diagnosis of *dysphasia due to a late effect of cerebrovascular accident* and directs you to the codes in the I69 code category.

EXCLUDES1 ***dysphasia following cerebrovascular disease (I69. with final characters -21)***

Go back to the physician's notes (the scenario). The documentation doesn't state that Arlene had cerebrovascular disease; it states that she had a cerebral embolism. Is this the same thing, or is it unrelated to this notation?

This is the same thing: A cerebral embolism is a type of CVA. When you look it up, you will see that a cerebral embolism is reported with code I66.9, clearly in the range of I60–I67. This means you will report the dysphasia from a code in the I69 category.

Therefore, this EXCLUDES1 note applies to this encounter, and you must turn to code I69 to determine the correct code to report Arlene's diagnosis. The notation directly under **I69 Sequelae of cerebrovascular disease** confirms that you are in the right place now. Read down and determine the code:

I69.821 Dysphasia following other cerebrovascular disease

(continued)

Before you report this code, remember to check for any relevant guidance, including reading all of the symbols and notations in the Tabular List and the appropriate sections of the Official Guidelines. No additional direction is there, and you can now report this code with confidence!

Good work!

CODING BITES

Read carefully! *Dysphasia* (ending in "sia") means impaired speech and *dysphagia* (ending in "gia") means difficulty swallowing. Another word that is close is *dysplasia,* which means abnormal cell growth. Big difference!

Chapter Summary

Cardiovascular conditions may initially be treated within the specialty of a cardiologist. However, the manifestations of heart failure and heart disease can affect the patient anywhere in the body—from the brain to the feet. Blood vessels extend throughout the body, from the large aorta to the tiny capillaries, delivering oxygen and transporting carbon dioxide back to the lungs so it can be released. When something goes awry, the health of the entire body, as well as the patient's quality of life, can be negatively affected.

Hypertension is a condition that you may encounter as a professional coder while working for a family physician, an internist, a gerontologist, or a cardiologist. It can be a very dangerous condition and can cause many co-morbidities and manifestations. As complex as the condition is, so is the coding of the diagnosis. As with all other situations, it must be diagnosed and documented by the attending physician. Read the notes carefully, and query the physician when necessary to get all the specifics that you need to code accurately.

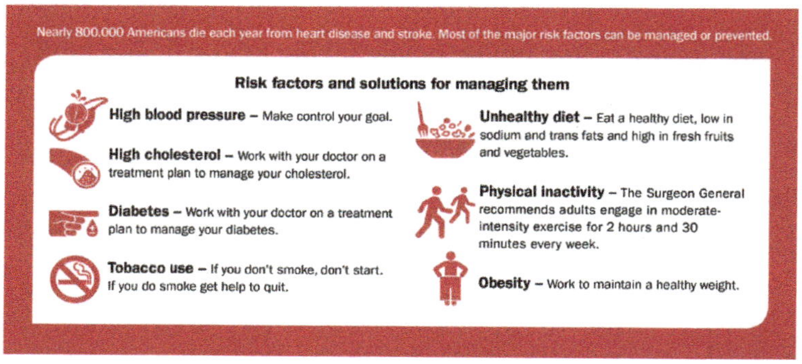

Source: http://www.cdc.gov/vitalsigns/heartdisease-stroke/infographic.html

CHAPTER 12 REVIEW
Coding Cardiovascular Conditions

Enhance your learning by completing these exercises and more at mcgrawhillconnect.com!

Let's Check It! Terminology

Match each key term to the appropriate definition.

Part I

1. **LO 12.2** Chest pain.
2. **LO 12.3** An occurrence of high blood pressure; an isolated or infrequent reading of a systolic blood pressure above 120 mmHg and/or a diastolic blood pressure above 80 mmHg.

A. Angina Pectoris
B. Atherosclerosis
C. Atrium

3. **LO 12.5** A stroke.
4. **LO 12.5** An area of dead tissue (necrosis) in the brain caused by a blocked or ruptured blood vessel.
5. **LO 12.2** A condition resulting from plaque buildup on the interior walls of the arteries, causing reduced blood flow.
6. **LO 12.1** A thrombus that has broken free and is traveling freely within the vascular system.
7. **LO 12.1** A chamber that is located in the top half of the heart and receives blood.
8. **LO 12.3** An overaccumulation of fluid in the cells of the tissues.

D. Cerebral Infarction
E. Cerebrovascular Accident (CVA)
F. Edema
G. Elevated Blood Pressure
H. Embolus

Part II

1. **LO 12.1** A chamber that is located in the bottom half of the heart and receives blood from the atrium.
2. **LO 12.3** High blood pressure, usually a chronic condition; often identified by a systolic blood pressure above 140 mmHg and/or a diastolic blood pressure above 90 mmHg.
3. **LO 12.3** Hypertension that develops during pregnancy and typically goes away once the pregnancy has ended.
4. **LO 12.1** A heart event during which the coronary artery is partially occluded (blocked).
5. **LO 12.1** A heart event during which the coronary artery is completely blocked by a thrombus or embolus.
6. **LO 12.1** A blood clot in a blood vessel.
7. **LO 12.1** A heart attack.
8. **LO 12.3** The condition of hypertension caused by another condition or illness.
9. **LO 12.5** Tissue or muscle that has deteriorated or died (necrotic).
10. **LO 12.3** Referring to the vessels (arteries and veins).
11. **LO 12.3** Low blood pressure; systolic blood pressure below 90 mmHg and/or diastolic measurements of lower than 60 mmHg.

A. Gestational Hypertension
B. Hypertension
C. Hypotension
D. Infarction
E. Myocardial Infarction (MI)
F. NSTEMI
G. Secondary Hypertension
H. STEMI
I. Thrombus
J. Vascular
K. Ventricle

Let's Check It! Concepts

Choose the most appropriate answer for each of the following questions.

1. **LO 12.2** ____ are blood vessels that carry oxygenated blood from the heart to the tissues and cells throughout the body.
   a. Arteries **b.** Veins **c.** Venules **d.** Cardiovascular
2. **LO 12.5** The patient is diagnosed with a cerebral infarction due to thrombosis of left anterior cerebral artery. How is this coded?
   a. I63.321 **b.** I63.322 **c.** I63.323 **d.** I63.329
3. **LO 12.1** ____ refers to an irregular heartbeat.
   a. Angina **b.** Dyspnea **c.** Dysrhythmia **d.** Edema
4. **LO 12.4** If the patient has a diagnosis of heart failure due to hypertension, you will need to
   a. use the appropriate fourth character, as shown in the Tabular List under category I11.
   b. use an additional code to specify the type of heart failure from category I50.
   c. use code I10.
   d. use both the appropriate fourth character, as shown in the Tabular List under category I11, and an additional code to specify the type of heart failure from category I50.
5. **LO 12.1** A heart event during which the coronary artery is completely blocked by a thrombus or embolus is called a(n)
   a. myocardial infarction. **b.** thrombus.
   c. nontransmural myocardial infarction. **d.** ST elevation myocardial infarction.

6. **LO 12.3** A diagnosis of secondary hypertension means you will code
   - **a.** the underlying condition only.
   - **b.** the hypertension only.
   - **c.** the underlying condition code and the hypertension code.
   - **d.** the hypertension code first and then the underlying condition code.
7. **LO 12.3** When a pregnant woman is diagnosed with hypertension, you must determine
   - **a.** if it is gestational hypertension.
   - **b.** if it is an infarction.
   - **c.** if it is transient hypertension.
   - **d.** if it is familial.
8. **LO 12.6** The code for a patient with no neurologic deficits and who had a previous diagnosis of cerebrovascular disease (which has since resolved) should be reported from
   - **a.** the I60–I69 range.
   - **b.** the I69 code category.
   - **c.** the Z86.7- code subcategory.
   - **d.** none of these.
9. **LO 12.3** According to ICD-10-CM Official Guidelines section I.C.9.a.7, "Assign code ____, Elevated blood pressure reading without diagnosis of hypertension, unless patient has an established diagnosis of hypertension."
   - **a.** R03.1
   - **b.** I15.1
   - **c.** R03.0
   - **d.** I10
10. **LO 12.3** A physician can support a diagnosis of hypertension with all of the following data *except*
    - **a.** auscultation over the abdominal aorta.
    - **b.** EKG.
    - **c.** chest x-ray.
    - **d.** ACE.

Let's Check It! Guidelines

Refer to the Official Guidelines and fill in the blanks according to the Chapter 9, Diseases of the Circulatory System, Chapter-Specific Coding Guidelines.

I13	current	Two
site	I60-I69	AMI
I69	STEMI	before
hypertension	secondary	deficits
evolves	admitted	underlying
subendocardial	first	N18
combination	I15	Uncontrolled

1. The appropriate code from category ____ should be used as a ____ code with a code from category I12 to identify the stage of chronic kidney disease.
2. The codes in category ____, Hypertensive heart and chronic kidney disease, are ____ codes that include hypertension, heart disease, and chronic kidney disease.
3. For hypertensive cerebrovascular disease, ____ assign the appropriate code from categories ____, followed by the appropriate ____ code.
4. Secondary hypertension is due to an underlying condition. ____ codes are required: one to identify the ____ etiology and one from category ____ to identify the hypertension. Sequencing of codes is determined by the reason for admission/encounter.
5. ____ hypertension may refer to untreated hypertension or hypertension not responding to current therapeutic regimen.
6. If a patient with coronary artery disease is ____ due to an acute myocardial infarction (AMI), the AMI should be sequenced ____ the coronary artery disease.
7. Codes from category ____ may be assigned on a health care record with codes from I60–I67, if the patient has a ____ cerebrovascular disease and ____ from an old cerebrovascular disease.
8. The ICD-10-CM codes for acute myocardial infarction (AMI) identify the ____, such as anterolateral wall or true posterior wall.
9. If NSTEMI ____ to STEMI, assign the ____ code.
10. If an____ is documented as nontransmural or subendocardial, but the site is provided, it is still coded as a ____ AMI.

Let's Check It! Rules and Regulations

Please answer the following questions from the knowledge you have gained after reading this chapter.

1. **LO 12.3** Differentiate between systolic pressure and diastolic pressure.
2. **LO 12.3** What is the difference between hypertension and elevated blood pressure?
3. **LO 12.3** What is gestational hypertension?
4. **LO 12.1** Explain the difference between STEMI and NSTEMI.
5. **LO 12.4** Read the ICD-10-CM Official Guidelines for Coding and Reporting, section I. Conventions, General Coding Guidelines and Chapter-Specific Guidelines, subsection C. Chapter-Specific Coding Guidelines, chapter 9. Diseases of the Circulatory System, subsection a.1) Hypertensive with heart disease. Explain the coding guideline.

ICD-10-CM

YOU CODE IT! Basics

First, identify the main term in the following diagnoses; then code the diagnosis.

Example: Acute rheumatic myocarditis:

a. main term: *myocarditis* b. diagnosis: *I01.2*

1. Acute diastolic (congestive) heart failure:
   a. main term: ______ **b.** diagnosis:______
2. Secondary hypertension due to pheochromocytoma:
   a. main term: ______ **b.** diagnosis:______
3. Left posterior fascicular block:
   a. main term: ______ **b.** diagnosis:______
4. Aneurysm of heart, 6-week duration:
   a. main term:______ **b.** diagnosis:______
5. Ischemic cardiomyopathy:
   a. main term: ______ **b.** diagnosis:______
6. Chronic total occlusion of coronary artery:
   a. main term: ______ **b.** diagnosis:______
7. Atherosclerosis of bypass graft of coronary artery of transplanted heart:
   a. main term: ______ **b.** diagnosis:______
8. Chronic embolism of superior vena cava:
   a. main term: ______ **b.** diagnosis:______
9. Rupture of pulmonary vessels:
   a. main term: ______ **b.** diagnosis:______
10. Nonrheumatic pulmonary valve stenosis:
    a. main term: ______ **b.** diagnosis:______
11. Arteriosclerotic endocarditis:
    a. main term: ______ **b.** diagnosis:______
12. Giant cell myocarditis:
    a. main term: ______ **b.** diagnosis:______
13. Cardiac arrest due to cardiac condition:
    a. main term:______ **b.** diagnosis:______
14. Ventricular fibrillation:
    a. main term: ______ **b.** diagnosis:______
15. Neurogenic orthostatic hypotension:
    a. main term:______ **b.** diagnosis:______

ICD-10-CM

YOU CODE IT! Practice

Using the techniques described in this chapter, carefully read through the case studies and determine the most accurate ICD-10-CM code(s) and external cause code(s), if appropriate, for each case study.

1. Kitty Hearn, a 63-year-old female, presents today with the complaint of chest tightness. She also states that her left jaw and shoulder hurt. Dr. Kickey notes diaphoresis. Kitty has smoked cigarettes for 40 years. Dr. Kickey completes an examination and reviews blood test results, which reveal a high level of creatine phosphokinase (CPK). Kitty is admitted to the hospital, where a coronary angiography confirms the diagnosis of crescendo angina.

(continued)

2. Calvin Ballew, an 8-year-old male, is brought in by his parents with the complaint that Calvin has been "out of sorts" for the last day or two and has not been eating well. Dr. Barfield notes a cough and labored breathing. After a thorough examination, Dr. Barfield decides to admit Calvin to Weston Hospital. The blood tests reveal an increased erythrocyte sedimentation rate (ESR), and ECG confirms a diagnosis of chronic rheumatic myocarditis.
3. Judith Raj, a 49-year-old female, has been diagnosed with hypertension heart disease and stage II chronic kidney disease. Dr. Bennett documents the fact that Judith is not in heart failure at this time.
4. Kay Risinger, a 57-year-old female, presents today with chest pain and shortness of breath on exertion. Kay also admits that it is difficult to breathe at night when lying in bed. Dr. Tate notes a cough and completes a thorough examination. The echocardiogram confirms a diagnosis of rheumatic aortic regurgitation with mitral valve disease.
5. Johnette Barrett, a 27-year-old female, is brought in by her husband, who is concerned because Johnette has been very confused. Johnette says her chest hurts and it feels like her heart is racing. Dr. Bakker notes labored breathing. Patient is admitted to the hospital, where test results confirm the diagnosis of paroxysmal atrial fibrillation.
6. Richard Grimm, a 57-year-old male, suffered a cerebral infarction 3 months ago due to an occlusion of the left anterior cerebral artery. Richard is having difficulty with his speech and is finding it hard to write. Dr. McManus diagnoses Richard with aphasia due to the cerebral infarction.
7. Vanessa Dostoimov, a 67-year-old female, had a pericardiotomy 6 weeks ago. Dr. Baker last saw Vanessa 2 weeks ago for a fever and chest pain. Today, Dr. Baker notes patient is experiencing similar symptoms and documents a pericardial rub, tachycardia, and hepatomegaly. Vanessa is admitted to the hospital for a possible pericardiocentesis. After a thorough examination and review of the test results, Vanessa was diagnosed with postcardiotomy syndrome.
8. Jessie Jacobs, a 48-year-old female, presents today with the complaint of shortness of breath and weakness. During the examination, Jessie experiences severe chest pain. Dr. Raley completes an ECG, which confirms a diagnosis of acute transmural myocardial infarction ST elevated inferior diaphragmatic wall. Jessie is admitted to Weston Hospital for stabilization and treatment.
9. Ben Jamison, a 51-year-old obese male, was diagnosed with a chronic embolism of the left subclavian vein.
10. James Tedder, a 62-year-old male, complains of chest tightness with physical activity. James also says he has a funny feeling in his neck. Dr. Franklin notes tachycardia and admits him to Weston Hospital. A cardiac CT scan and stress ECG confirm a diagnosis of silent myocardial ischemia.
11. Shirley Hatfield, a 59-year-old female, presents today with the complaint of a tender swollen left leg. Dr. Neal documents a nonpressure ulceration left ankle limited to skin breakdown. After an examination and a Doppler sonography were completed, Shirley was diagnosed with chronic total arterial occlusion of left extremity with atherosclerosis of arteries of the left extremity.
12. Gary Allen, a 59-year-old male, presents today with chest pain and cough. Upon examination, Dr. Rogers documents a low-grade fever, dyspnea, tachypnea, and a pleural friction rub. The decision is made to admit Gary to Weston Hospital, where he is diagnosed with a saddle embolus of pulmonary artery with acute cor pulmonale.
13. Earline Hodges, a 57-year-old female, has a sharp sudden chest pain. Dr. Harper notes a pericardial rub. The laboratory results confirm infective pericarditis due to retrovirus.
14. Donald Ross, a 49-year-old male, presents today with numbness in his fingers and toes. Dr. Jones notes pale coloration in the ring finger of his right hand. Don also states that the numbness is worse with temperature changes. Dr. Jones completes a thorough examination and reviews the laboratory results, which confirm a diagnosis of Raynaud's syndrome without gangrene.
15. Dedrick Andrews, a 43-year-old male, presents today with a cough, fever, and night sweats. Dr. Jamerson completes an examination, the appropriate laboratory tests, and a chest x-ray. Dedrick is diagnosed with septic arterial embolism of thoracic aorta with lung abscess due to MSSA.

ICD-10-CM

YOU CODE IT! Application

The following exercises provide practice in abstracting physicians' notes and learning to work with documentation from our health care facility, Prader, Bracker, & Associates. These case studies are modeled on real patient encounters. Using the techniques described in this chapter, carefully read through the case studies and determine the most accurate ICD-10-CM code(s) and external cause code(s), if appropriate, for each case study.

(continued)

PRADER, BRACKER, & ASSOCIATES

A Complete Health Care Facility

159 Healthcare Way • SOMEWHERE, FL 32811 • 407-555-6789

PATIENT: PETERS, CHARLENE

ACCOUNT/EHR #: PETECH001

Attending Physician: Renee O. Bracker, MD

S: Pt is a 68-year-old female who suffered a cerebral infarction 3 weeks ago. Her son is concerned about the patient's dysarthria, which doesn't seem to be getting any better. The patient understands but is having difficultly pronouncing her words. Dr. Bracker also notes a low degree of audibility.

O: Ht. 5′4″, Wt. 146 lb., R 18, T 99.6, BP 138/95. Physical examination: unremarkable.

A: Dysarthria, following a cerebral infarction.

P: 1. Pt to return PRN

2. Referral to speech therapist

Determine the most accurate ICD-10-CM code(s).

WESTON HOSPITAL

629 Healthcare Way • SOMEWHERE, FL 32811 • 407-555-6541

PATIENT: CROWDER, CHRISTOPHER

ACCOUNT/EHR #: CROWCH001

Attending Physician: Oscar R. Prader, MD

ADMITTING DIAGNOSES: Deep venous thrombosis (DVT) left leg

Urinary tract infection (UTI)

Parkinson's disease

FINAL DIAGNOSES: Acute DVT, left

UTI

Parkinson's disease

HOSPITAL COURSE: The patient presented to the office with left leg pain, and uneasiness as well as cloudy urine. He was evaluated, and Doppler studies of the leg confirmed DVT. Urinalysis reveals infection and the patient was started on Levaquin and Lovenox subcu 1 mg per kg twice a day; after 3 days patient asymptomatic for both his urinary symptoms and calf pain. Patient's vital signs are stable. He is afebrile. Lungs clear. Heart rhythm regular.

Neurologic examination: Tremors and rigidity secondary to Parkinson's disease. Rest is unremarkable. His Doppler studies were positive for left popliteal vein thrombosis and flow abnormalities in superficial femoral vein. The results of the pelvic sonogram reveal an enlarged prostate and questionable intraluminal. Right kidney, normal. Left kidney, cyst lower pole.

PT, INR on the day of discharge was 13.5 and 0.9. His UA was positive for blood, negative for leukocyte esterase, nitrites, and WBC. His CHEM-7 showed sodium of 135, potassium 3.8, chloride 98, CO_2 29, sugar 126, BUN 18 mg/dL, and creatinine 1.1. WBC 6,500, H&H 17.2 and 52. Platelets 150,000. He was discharged home.

DISPOSITION: Arrange for home health.

Follow-up with his primary physician in 7 to 10 days. Arrange for patient evaluation for repeat urinalysis and urology consultation for possible BPH and bladder mass.

Determine the most accurate ICD-10-CM code(s).

(continued)

PRADER, BRACKER, & ASSOCIATES

A Complete Health Care Facility

159 Healthcare Way • SOMEWHERE, FL 32811 • 407-555-6789

PATIENT: NOLAN, SHERYESSE

ACCOUNT/EHR #: NOLASH001

Attending Physician: Oscar R. Prader, MD

S: Pt is a 53-year-old female who comes in today complaining of fainting, chest pain, and difficulty breathing of approximately 1-week duration. Patient was diagnosed 3 years ago with hypertension. Hypertension has been under control with diet and exercise.

O: Ht. 5′5″, Wt. 153 lb., R 19, T 98.4, BP 148/89. Results of blood tests, UA, CBC, ECG, and echocardiogram indicate the development of renal sclerosis (stage 4) with benign hypertension. Tests also reveal left ventricular failure and acute systolic heart failure.

A: Renal sclerosis with benign hypertension; left ventricular failure and acute systolic heart failure

P: 1. Pt to return PRN

2. Referral for renal dialysis evaluation

Determine the most accurate ICD-10-CM code(s).

PRADER, BRACKER, & ASSOCIATES

A Complete Health Care Facility

159 Healthcare Way • SOMEWHERE, FL 32811 • 407-555-6789

PATIENT: GUZMANN, EVAN

ACCOUNT/EHR #: GUZMEV001

Attending Physician: Renee O. Bracker, MD

S: Pt is a 68-year-old male returning to discuss test results done 2 days ago at our imaging center. Patient is accompanied by his wife, Angie.

O: Ht. 5′10″, Wt. 184 lb., R 20, T 98.9, BP 134/86. I explain to the patient and his wife that the test results show a narrowing of the basilar, carotid, and vertebral arteries on his left side, which we believe to be the cause of the symptoms experienced by Mr. Guzmann that we discussed in our last encounter. These arterial strictures account for the headaches, dizziness, and reduced mental acuity. There is currently no cerebral infarction. We discussed a variety of treatment options, and they both agreed to a surgical consultation referral to explore the possibility of a shunt insertion.

A: Stenosis of precerebral arteries, including the basilar, carotid, and vertebral arteries

P: 1. Pt to return PRN

2. Referral for surgical consult for shunt placement

Determine the most accurate ICD-10-CM code(s).

WESTON HOSPITAL

629 Healthcare Way • SOMEWHERE, FL 32811 • 407-555-6541

PATIENT: WEINER, PHILLIP

ACCOUNT/EHR #: WEINPH001

(continued)

Attending Physician: Oscar R. Prader, MD

Pt is a 73-year-old male who was admitted to the hospital because of asthenia, xerostomia, fatigue. The patient states he is very weak, drinks a lot of water, but has not been urinating much. His blood pressure was 165/91, and he has been having pain in the left jaw and neck.

PMH: 2003 he had bladder suspension operation and has a history of PVCs.

The patient has had trouble with some edema of the ankles and feet.

The electrocardiogram shows a sinus rhythm with premature ventricular contractions.

FH: Father died of CVA. Mother died of stomach cancer.

CURRENT MEDICATIONS: Inderal; Ativan; Zestril

ALLERGIES: NKA

FINAL DIAGNOSES:

1. Acute myocardial infarction—anterior wall
2. Systemic arterial hypertension
3. Cardiomegaly with chronic systolic CHF
4. Cardiac arrhythmia

Determine the most accurate ICD-10-CM code(s).

13

Coding Respiratory Conditions

Key Terms

Chronic Obstructive Pulmonary Disease (COPD)
Exacerbation
Influenza
Pneumonia
Pneumothorax
Respiratory Disorder
Status Asthmaticus

Learning Outcomes

After completing this chapter, the student should be able to:

LO 13.1 Discern the various underlying causes of respiratory disorders.
LO 13.2 Report the different types of respiratory disorders.
LO 13.3 Determine the correct way to report cases of pneumonia and influenza.
LO 13.4 Analyze the details required to report chronic respiratory conditions.
LO 13.5 Accurately code any involvement of tobacco in the patient's respiratory disorder.
LO 13.6 Identify the appropriate use of external cause codes when applicable to respiratory conditions.

STOP! Remember, you need to follow along in your ICD-10-CM code book for an optimal learning experience.

13.1 Underlying Causes of Respiratory Disease

Respiratory Disorder
A malfunction of the organ system relating to respiration.

Respiratory disorders can be caused by many things, including trauma, genetics, environmental concerns, congenital anomalies, and infection. Regardless of the underlying cause, having difficulty bringing oxygen into the lungs and getting carbon dioxide out of the body can interfere with the patient's quality of life—and, actually, the ability to live life at all.

Congenital Anomalies

Respiratory distress and cyanosis are the two most frequent manifestations of congenital anomalies of the lungs and are usually identified within the child's first 24 months. The most common congenital respiratory disorder is *pulmonary hypoplasia*, a situation in which the lung does not form completely or forms improperly. When you are reporting this condition, ICD-10-CM requires you to determine from the documentation whether the pulmonary hypoplasia is a result of short gestation (i.e., prematurity) or not. If the gestation is short, it is reported with code P28.0 Primary atelectasis of newborn (pulmonary hypoplasia associated with short gestation). If it is not, it is reported with code Q33.6 Congenital hypoplasia and dysplasia of lung.

The most common cause of neonate mortality is respiratory distress syndrome (RDS), and it is seen most often in premature births. RDS can be fatal within 72 hours if not treated. Mechanical ventilation improves patient outcomes. Idiopathic RDS is reported with code P22.0 for a *newborn* or code J80 for *acute RDS in a child or adult patient*. Remember, the definition of a neonate (newborn) is one who is age 28 days or younger.

CODING BITES

Congenital anomalies occur during gestation. However, the problem may not be diagnosed until later on in the patient's life.

Genetic Disorders

Alpha-1 antitrypsin deficiency is a genetic condition that may cause respiratory dysfunction as well as liver disease. Individuals with an alpha-1 antitrypsin deficiency often will develop emphysema, with the first signs and symptoms appearing in adulthood (between ages 20 and 50). Cystic fibrosis is another genetic condition that causes malfunction of the mucous glands and results in progressive damage to the lungs. A mutation of the BMPR2 gene causes pulmonary arterial hypertension, a genetic condition with extremely high hypertension specifically in the pulmonary artery. Dyspnea and fainting are symptoms of this condition. *Primary pulmonary arterial hypertension* is reported with code I27.0, while *secondary pulmonary arterial hypertension* is reported with code I27.21.

Manifestations of Another Disease

Measles, as well as the adenovirus, may cause obliterative bronchiolitis (J44.9). Left-sided heart failure can cause pulmonary edema (J81.0 or J81.1), an accumulation of fluid in the lung. The administration of diuretics will help reduce the fluid, while vasodilators are given to decrease vascular resistance. High concentrations of oxygen, via cannula or face mask, will help improve the delivery of oxygen into the tissues.

Pleurisy, an inflammation of the parietal and visceral pleurae, is usually a complication of another condition, such as pneumonia, lupus erythematosus, pulmonary infarction, trauma to the chest, or tuberculosis (TB). *Tuberculous pleurisy*, for example, is reported with combination code A15.6.

Trauma

Car accidents and other activities can result in trauma to the chest, throat, or nose that can interfere with a patient's ability to breathe. Traumatic pneumothorax (S27.0XX-) may result from a penetrating chest wound or can occur due to a medical misadventure during the insertion of a central venous line or during thoracic surgery. During a pneumothorax, air accumulates between the parietal and visceral pleurae, reducing the space in the chest cavity and thereby limiting the room the lungs have to expand during inhalation. When the lungs cannot expand properly, oxygen cannot be brought down into the lungs far enough, so breathing becomes difficult and the exchange of gases (oxygen and carbon dioxide) is hindered. Blunt trauma to the chest, or a penetrating wound, can also cause hemothorax, in which blood (instead of air, as in pneumothorax) fills the pleural cavity. Report this condition with code J94.2 Hemothorax.

ICD-10-CM

LET'S CODE IT! SCENARIO

Vincent Perdimo, a 17-year-old male, decided he wanted to audition for the State Fair. After watching some videos online, he decided that he could do a fire-eating act. As he was practicing in his backyard, he accidentally aspirated some of the isopropyl alcohol he poured in his mouth. After he began having problems breathing, his parents took him to the ED. Dr. Van Hooven documented that Vincent had severe pulmonary complications and appeared to have pneumonitis with partial respiratory insufficiency. After a workup and testing, Vincent was admitted into the hospital with a diagnosis of acute respiratory distress syndrome.

Let's Code It!

Dr. Van Hooven diagnosed Vincent with acute respiratory distress syndrome.

In your ICD-10-CM code book, turn to the Alphabetic Index, and find

Syndrome

Read all the way down this long list and find

Syndrome
    respiratory
        distress
            acute J80
                adult J80

This is a great start. Turn to J80 in the Tabular List.

J80 Acute respiratory distress syndrome

EXCLUDES1 respiratory distress syndrome in newborn (perinatal) (P22.0)

(continued)

This code's description matches Dr. Van Hooven's documentation perfectly. And the EXCLUDES1 note does not apply because Vincent is not a newborn.

Check the top of this subsection and the head of this chapter in ICD-10-CM. There are no notations at the beginning of this subsection; however, there are notations at the beginning of this chapter: a **NOTE**, a ***Use additional code*** note, and an EXCLUDES2 notation. Read carefully. Do any relate to Dr. Van Hooten's diagnosis of Vincent? No. Turn to the Official Guidelines and read Section I.C.10. There is nothing specifically applicable here, either.

Now you can report J80 for Vincent's diagnosis with confidence. Hold it! Vincent's respiratory distress syndrome did not just occur; it was the result of an external cause. Turn to the ICD-10-CM *Index to External Causes*. What should you look up? Do you think it has a listing for fire-eating? You never know, so take a look. Nope. Dr. Van Hooten documented that this happened because Vincent "aspirated" isopropyl alcohol. Try looking up Aspiration. Isopropyl alcohol is definitely not food, not a foreign body, and not vomitus. Hmm. What now?

As you think about what actually happened to Vincent, it was the isopropyl alcohol in his lungs that caused the problem. Perhaps this should be reported as a poisoning because this is a chemical. Turn in the Table of Drugs and Chemicals and find

Alcohol

isopropyl

Look across on this line to the first column. It is documented that this was an accident, so the code T51.2X1 is suggested. Turn to the Tabular List to this code category:

✓4 **T51 Toxic effect of alcohol**

Read all of the fourth character options and you will see:

✓5 **T51.2 Toxic effect of 2-Propanol (Toxic effect of isopropyl alcohol)**

✓6 **T51.2X Toxic effect of 2-Propanol (Toxic effect of isopropyl alcohol)**

✓7 **T51.2X1 Toxic effect of 2-Propanol (Toxic effect of isopropyl alcohol), accidental (unintentional)**

Look back up to the top of this code category. There is a box containing the options for the seventh character. This was the first time Dr. Van Hooven cared for Vincent for this respiratory condition, so use the seventh character A = Initial encounter.

Now you know, with confidence, what codes to report for Vincent's diagnosis:

J80 **Acute respiratory distress syndrome**

T51.2X1A **Toxic effect of 2-Propanol (Toxic effect of isopropyl alcohol), accidental (unintentional), initial encounter**

Good coding!

Environment

Respiratory dysfunction can be caused by elements in the world around us. Those elements can be natural, like volcanic dust from an erupting volcano or dander from cats, or human-made, such as asbestos in the ceiling (J61). Legionnaires' disease, an aerobic Gram-negative bacillus, is transmitted through the air—for example, through air-conditioning systems (J67.7). Men are more susceptible than women. Administration of antibiotics, specifically erythromycin, is the primary treatment, along with fluid replacement and oxygen administration, if necessary. When a patient is diagnosed with coal worker's pneumoconiosis, another environmentally caused lung disease, this is reported with code J60 Coal worker's pneumoconiosis, along with code Y92.64 Mine or pit as the place of occurrence of the external cause and Y99.0 Civilian activity done for income or pay.

Some patients may suffer respiratory problems from air contaminants at work, which would be reported with a subsequent code; for example: Z57.31 Occupational exposure to environmental tobacco smoke; Z57.39 Occupational exposure to other air contaminants; Z77.110 Contact with and (suspected) exposure to air pollution; or Z77.22 Contact with and (exposure to) environmental tobacco smoke (acute) (chronic).

Lung Infections

Both bacteria and viruses can cause respiratory disorders. Bacterial pneumonia (J15.-), community-acquired pneumonia, nosocomial (originating in a hospital) pneumonia, viral pneumonia (J12.-), and opportunistic pneumonia (affecting individuals with compromised immunities) are common examples of respiratory infection. In addition, bronchitis (inflammation of the bronchi) (J20.-) and influenza (J09.- or J10.-) also are frequently seen, particularly in children and the elderly. Viruses affecting the pulmonary parenchyma result in interstitial pneumonia (J84.9). *Mycobacterium tuberculosis*, acquired by inhaling aerosols, has been seen more often in the last several years, especially in patients who are HIV-positive and have developed AIDS. When an HIV-positive patient is diagnosed with TB affecting the lungs, this condition would be reported with code B20 HIV, followed by code A15.0 Tuberculosis of the lung.

Lifestyle Behaviors

Smoking cigars and cigarettes is known to cause respiratory disorders, including lung cancer. In addition, sedentary lifestyles can encourage the creation of thrombi in the legs. What does that have to do with the lungs? A dislodged thrombus becomes an embolus that can travel through the pulmonary artery into the lungs, becoming a pulmonary embolus. An acute pulmonary embolism NOS is reported with code I26.99; however, several other details are required for a complete code.

GUIDANCE CONNECTION

At the very beginning of this chapter in ICD-10-CM, there is a ***Use additional code*** notation. It states:

Use additional code**, where applicable, to identify:**

exposure to environmental tobacco smoke (Z77.22)

exposure to tobacco smoke in the perinatal period (P96.81)

history of tobacco use (Z87.891)

occupational exposure to environmental tobacco smoke (Z57.31)

tobacco dependence (F17.-)

tobacco use (Z72.0)

This applies to all codes in this chapter of ICD-10-CM, which makes sense, right? It has been proven that inhaling tobacco has a negative effect on the pulmonary system. If the physician's documentation is not clear on this detail, you must query the physician to have it added, if applicable, so you can report this code, as well as the specific respiratory diagnosis.

See more details about this later in this chapter, in the section **Reporting Tobacco Involvement**.

Similar to smoking is a lifestyle behavior known as vaping. Using an electronic cigarette to simulate tobacco smoking began as a healthier alternative. However, individuals using this method have developed specific respiratory conditions. When the documentation identifies vaping-related disorder, report code U07.0 as the principal diagnosis code. Report manifestations separately, using the appropriate codes, such as acute respiratory failure with a code from J96.0- .

YOU CODE IT! CASE STUDY

Baby boy Luciano was born vaginally at 33 weeks. Complete physical exam performed. No anomalies were noted with the exception of a perforated nasal septum. He is admitted into the NICU (Neonatal Intensive Care Unit). Dr. Aronson, a pediatrician specializing in congenital respiratory disorders, was called in for a consultation.

You Code It!

What ICD-10-CM code or codes will you use to report baby boy Luciano's diagnosis?

Step #1: Read the case carefully and completely.

Step #2: Abstract the scenario. Which main words or terms describe why the physician cared for the patient during this encounter?

Step #3: Are there any details missing or incomplete for which you would need to query the physician? [If so, ask your instructor.]

(continued)

Step #4: Check for any relevant guidance, including reading all of the symbols and notations in the Tabular List and the appropriate sections of the Official Guidelines.

Step #5: Determine the correct diagnosis code or codes to explain why this encounter was medically necessary.

Step #6: Double-check your work.

Answer:

Did you determine this to be the code?

Q30.3 Congenital perforated nasal septum

13.2 Disorders of the Respiratory System

Pleural Disorders

The pleura is made up of two membranes: the visceral pleura, a thin membrane that coats the outside of the lung, and the parietal pleura, a membrane that lines the inside of the thoracic (chest) cavity. *Pleurisy*, also known as *pleuritis*, identifies the presence of inflammation on one or both of the pleural membranes. This condition can cause pain to the patient with each breath. A virus is most often the cause. To report pleurisy, the Alphabetic Index provides a long list of possibilities that lead to a surprisingly short number of codes:

A15.6	**Tuberculous pleurisy**
J10.1	**Influenza due to other identified influenza virus with other respiratory manifestations**
R09.1	**Pleurisy**
J90	**Pleurisy with effusion, not elsewhere classified**
S27.63XA	**Injury to the pleura, laceration of pleura, initial encounter**

(*NOTE:* Of course, you remember that with code S27.63XA, an external cause code should be reported to identify how the injury happened, as well as the place of occurrence.)

The very narrow space between the two pleural membranes is referred to as the *pleural space* or *pleural cavity*. Normally, this space contains a tiny amount of fluid, just enough to enable the visceral pleura and the parietal pleura to move and function without irritation. If excess air or fluid gets into this space, it can cause pressure on the lung and prevent the patient from inhaling because the lung does not have the room required to expand as the oxygen is brought in. Pleural space disorders include pleural effusion, pneumothorax, and hemothorax:

- *Pleural effusion:* the presence of excess fluid in the pleural cavity, frequently a manifestation of congestive heart failure.

J91.0	**Malignant pleural effusion**
J94.0	**Chylous effusion**
P28.89	**Newborn pleural effusion**

> **Pneumothorax**
> A condition in which air or gas is present within the chest cavity but outside the lungs.

- ***Pneumothorax:*** the presence of excess air or gases in the pleural space, typically caused by respiratory disease such as chronic obstructive pulmonary disorder (COPD) or tuberculosis (TB).

J86.9	**Pyothorax without fistula (empyema) [an infection within the pleural space]**
J93.81	**Chronic pneumothorax**

- *Hemothorax*: an accumulation of blood in the pleural cavity, most often caused by an injury to the thoracic cavity (the chest).

J94.2 Hemothorax

Pulmonary Embolism

As you probably remember, an embolus is the medical term for a blood clot (thrombus) or other tiny piece of bone marrow fat (most often created by high cholesterol) that travels within the bloodstream. During its passage through the body, this embolus can get stuck in an artery and block the flow of blood through that area. When this occurs in the lungs, it is called a *pulmonary embolism*.

The presence of a pulmonary embolism can create serious problems for the patient, including dyspnea (shortness of breath), pain, and/or hemoptysis (coughing up blood). Over the course of time, a pulmonary embolism can result in permanent damage to the lung as well as damage to the organs being denied oxygen because of the blockage. A pulmonary embolism also can cause an infarction (necrotic tissue) due to the lack of oxygen to the cells. A large clot, or cluster of several clots, can result in the patient's death.

CODING BITES

Why is a hemothorax coded as a type of pleural effusion? Remember that a pleural effusion is the accumulation of excessive fluid in the pleural space. Blood is a type of fluid.

I26.02 Saddle embolus of pulmonary artery with acute cor pulmonale

I27.82 Chronic pulmonary embolism

LET'S CODE IT! SCENARIO

ICD-10-CM

Fawn Springwater, a 3-year-old female, was brought to her pediatrician, Dr. Canterberg, with an odd-sounding cough and chest congestion. She had the measles just a short time prior. After a complete PE and the appropriate tests, Dr. Canterberg diagnosed Fawn with the croup.

Let's Code It!

Fawn was diagnosed with *the croup*. Let's turn to the Alphabetic Index:

Croup, croupous (catarrhal) (infective) (inflammatory) (nondiphtheritic) J05.0

The Tabular List confirms:

✓4 J05 Acute obstructive laryngitis [croup] and epiglottitis

You can see a ***Use additional code*** notation beneath this code category directing you to "*identify the infectious agent.*" Notice that *croup* is included, in brackets. This is the common term for the medical diagnosis of acute obstructive laryngitis. However, this is not what Fawn was diagnosed with, so keep reading down the column to review the choices for the required fourth character:

J05.0 Acute obstructive laryngitis

Good job!

Respiratory Syncytial Virus Infections

While most adults and teenagers suffer only mild symptoms (similar to a cold), respiratory syncytial virus infection (RSV) can cause serious problems for infants. Similar to other infectious diseases, RSV can be spread from person to person by touching an infected person or by coming in contact with an infected object like a toy or a tabletop. Upon infection, infants can have difficulty breathing, stuffy noses, and fever. RSV is actually the pathogen that causes respiratory illness in young children such as pneumonia or acute bronchitis.

✓4 B97 Viral agents as the cause of diseases classified elsewhere

Read down the column to review your choices for the required fourth character.

B97.4 Respiratory syncytial virus (RSV) as the cause of diseases classified elsewhere

This code looks perfect except for one thing. Did you read the note directly above code B95 that states:

NOTE: These categories are provided for use as supplementary or additional codes to identify the infection agent(s) in diseases classified elsewhere.

So, if the notes state that the child has pneumonia due to RSV, you would first list the pneumonia followed by B97.4.

Pulmonary Fibrosis

Fibrosis is the creation of extra fibrous tissue (also known as *scar tissue*) in response to inflammation or irritation. When this abnormal process occurs in the lungs, it is called *pulmonary fibrosis*. This development of thickened tissue reduces the flexibility of the lung sac, making it harder for the lungs to expand with inspiration and contract for expiration. Idiopathic pulmonary fibrosis may also be referred to as cryptogenic fibrosing alveolitis, diffuse interstitial fibrosis, idiopathic interstitial pneumonitis, and Hamman-Rich syndrome.

Pulmonary fibrosis may be caused by another disease, such as TB, or develop as a result of debris inhaled from an environment, such as the dust that may be breathed in by sand blasters or coal miners during their work. Pulmonary fibrosis is also associated as a side effect of certain medications.

J84.10 Pulmonary fibrosis, unspecified

YOU CODE IT! CASE STUDY

Hans Surgesson, a 47-year-old male, has been suffering with chronic inflammation of his left bronchus. He admits to previous crack cocaine use but denies current use. He complains of a dry, hacking, paroxysmal cough and occasional dyspnea lasting at least 5 months. Chest x-ray and pulmonary function tests lead Dr. Mellville to diagnose Hans with idiopathic pulmonary fibrosis due to mucopurulent chronic bronchitis. Hans is placed on oxygen therapy immediately.

You Code It!

Go through the steps of coding, and determine the diagnosis code or codes that should be reported for this encounter between Dr. Mellville and Hans.

Step #1: Read the case carefully and completely.
Step #2: Abstract the scenario. Which main words or terms describe why the physician cared for the patient during this encounter?
Step #3: Are there any details missing or incomplete for which you would need to query the physician? [If so, ask your instructor.]
Step #4: Check for any relevant guidance, including reading all of the symbols and notations in the Tabular List and the appropriate sections of the Official Guidelines.
Step #5: Determine the correct diagnosis code or codes to explain why this encounter was medically necessary.
Step #6: Double-check your work.

Answer:

Did you determine these to be the correct codes?

J84.112 Idiopathic pulmonary fibrosis

J41.1 Mucopurulent chronic bronchitis

Terrific!

Respiratory Failure

Respiratory failure identifies that a patient's lungs are not working efficiently. The result may be a reduced intake of oxygen or an excess of carbon dioxide that is not thoroughly being expelled from the lungs, or both. You have learned throughout this chapter about the problems that can occur in the body when it does not get enough oxygen, a condition called *hypoxemic respiratory failure*, or when there is too much carbon dioxide, a condition called *hypercapnic respiratory failure*.

Respiratory failure can be a manifestation of a respiratory disease, such as COPD. In addition, certain injuries can affect a patient's ability to breathe. For example, a spinal cord injury may involve damage to the nerves that control breathing. A drug or alcohol overdose also can have an impact on the nervous system in a manner that affects the nervous system's ability to properly control respiration. Code choices include

J96.0- **Acute respiratory failure**

J96.1- **Chronic respiratory failure**

J96.2- **Acute and chronic respiratory failure**

GUIDANCE CONNECTION

Read the ICD-10-CM Official Guidelines for Coding and Reporting, section **I. Conventions, General Coding Guidelines and Chapter-Specific Guidelines**, subsection **C. Chapter-Specific Coding Guidelines**, chapter **10. Diseases of the Respiratory System**, subsection **b. Acute Respiratory Failure**.

The physician may diagnose the patient with acute respiratory failure as a primary diagnosis when it meets the requirements to be first-listed as directed in the Official Guidelines. More typically, you will find that respiratory failure will be a secondary diagnosis, as mentioned previously.

13.3 Pneumonia and Influenza

Pneumonia

Pneumonia is a serious infection of the lung parenchyma (tissue) and typically hinders the exchange of gases. When an individual with normal, healthy lungs contracts pneumonia, the expectation of a complete recovery is good. However, early treatment is important. Even with this good news, pneumonia is one of the top 10 leading causes of death in the United States. A virus, bacterium, fungus, or other type of protozoan can cause pneumonia. You have to know which type of pneumonia the patient has contracted in order to code it accurately.

> **Pneumonia**
> An inflammation of the lungs.

Viral Pneumonia

- Influenza
- Adenovirus
- Respiratory syncytial virus
- Measles (rubeola)
- Chickenpox (varicella)
- Cytomegalovirus

Bacterial Pneumonia

- Streptococcus (*Streptococcus pneumoniae*)
- *Klebsiella*
- Staphylococcus

GUIDANCE CONNECTION

Read the ICD-10-CM Official Guidelines for Coding and Reporting, section **I. Conventions, General Coding Guidelines and Chapter-Specific Guidelines**, subsection **C. Chapter-Specific Coding Guidelines**, chapter **10. Diseases of the Respiratory System**, subsection **c. Influenza due to certain identified influenza viruses**.

Protozoan Pneumonia

- *Pneumocystis carinii*

Aspiration pneumonia is a specific type of condition that results from the patient vomiting and then inhaling gastric or oropharyngeal contents into the trachea and/or lungs.

EXAMPLES

J12.0 Adenoviral pneumonia

J15.0 Pneumonia due to Klebsiella pneumoniae

Note that these examples of pneumonia codes are both combination codes, reporting both the condition (pneumonia) and the pathogen (adenovirus or *Klebsiella*). Not all pneumonia codes are combination codes, so you may need to remember to use an additional code to identify the pathogen.

Pneumonia as a Manifestation of HIV

In some cases, pneumonia *may be* a manifestation of HIV infection. Therefore, if the notes report that the patient has also been diagnosed with HIV-positive status, you have to include

B20 Human immunodeficiency virus (HIV) disease

Code B20 should be listed first, followed by the appropriate pneumonia code. There are other types of pneumonia that may have other underlying diseases. Read the notations carefully.

ICD-10-CM

LET'S CODE IT! SCENARIO

Craig Alaksar, a 13-year-old male, came to see Dr. Winston with a complaint of a sore throat, fever, cough, chills, and malaise. Dr. Winston examined Craig, took a chest x-ray, and did a WBC count. After reviewing the results of the exam and tests, Dr. Winston diagnosed Craig with adenovirus pneumonia.

Let's Code It!

Dr. Winston identified Craig's health concern as *adenovirus pneumonia*. The Alphabetic Index will direct you to

Pneumonia

adenoviral J12.0

Will the Tabular List confirm that it is the correct code? Turn to

✓4 **J12 Viral pneumonia, not elsewhere classified**

There are no notations or directions, so keep reading to review all of the choices for the required fourth character:

J12.0 Adenoviral pneumonia

You will remember that when there is an infectious organism involved, you must code it. Dr. Winston's notes identify it as the adenovirus. Should you use an additional code or not?

Professional coding specialists are responsible for relating the entire story with all specific details applicable to the diagnosis. This one combination code tells both the condition *and* the infectious organism. There is no reason to provide a second code to repeat the same information. Therefore, the code on Craig's claim form will be J12.0 alone.

Ventilator-Associated Pneumonia

When a patient needs help breathing because of a malfunction in the respiratory system, they may be placed on a ventilator, a machine that will essentially complete respiration. While the patient is hooked up to the machine, which uses a tube placed into the patient's throat, pathogens can travel directly into the patient's lungs, potentially resulting in the development of ventilator-associated pneumonia (VAP). The attending physician must specifically document the diagnosis of VAP before you can report code J95.851. Only the physician can link the ventilator with the infection. If the documentation is not clear, you must query the physician for clarification.

Beneath this code is a ***Use additional code*** notation reminding you that you will need to report a second code to identify the specific organism responsible for this infection. Also, an **EXCLUDES1** notation directs you to report code P27.8 instead if the patient is a newborn.

> **GUIDANCE CONNECTION**
>
> Read the ICD-10-CM Official Guidelines for Coding and Reporting, section **I. Conventions, General Coding Guidelines and Chapter-Specific Guidelines**, subsection **C. Chapter-Specific Coding Guidelines**, chapter **10. Diseases of the Respiratory System**, subsection **d. Ventilator associated Pneumonia**.

Influenza

Influenza, the formal term for what is commonly known as the *flu* or the *grippe*, is a highly contagious and serious illness. It is a respiratory tract infection that can affect individuals of all ages, but it is most dangerous to young children, the elderly, and those who have chronic diseases because these individuals have immune systems that are more sensitive and more susceptible.

> **Influenza**
> An acute infection of the respiratory tract caused by the influenza virus.

The signs and symptoms that are inclusive in a diagnosis of influenza include

- Achy feeling in the muscles, or overall body ache
- Chills
- Fever
- Headache
- Cough
- Sore throat

To code a diagnosis of influenza correctly, you have to know what virus is involved:

J09.X- **Influenza due to identified novel influenza A viruses [Avian influenza] [Bird influenza] [Swine influenza]**

J10.- **Influenza due to other identified influenza virus**

J11.- **Influenza due to unidentified influenza virus**

> **CODING BITES**
>
> Do you know the difference between a cold and the flu? Colds rarely cause a fever or headaches.
>
> Do you know that what is commonly known as the "stomach flu" is actually gastroenteritis—inflammation in the stomach and small intestines?

As you abstract the documentation, you will need to look for mention of any manifestations, such as respiratory, gastrointestinal, encephalopathy, myocarditis, or otitis media, for example. You will need these details to determine the fifth character.

YOU CODE IT! CASE STUDY

ICD-10-CM

Andrea Ignitto, a 21-year-old female, came into the University Clinic with complaints of nasal congestion, cough, sore throat, fatigue, and overall aches. She states that she has had bouts of mild diarrhea for the last 2 days. She indicates that her roommate and about five others on her dorm floor were sick with similar symptoms. She has a low-grade fever, chills, and nausea but denies vomiting. She claims loss of appetite and feeling weak with generalized aches and pains. Her cough is mostly nonproductive. She denies chest pain or shortness of breath.

PAST MEDICAL HISTORY: Right knee surgery. [She is a soccer captain.]

CURRENT MEDICATIONS: Birth control pills

(continued)

ALLERGIES: Sulfa

SOCIAL HISTORY: The patient drinks a couple of beers per week.

REVIEW OF SYSTEMS: Essentially as in the HPI

OBJECTIVE:

VITAL SIGNS: Blood pressure 116/82, pulse 100, temperature 100.4 F, respiratory rate is 18. Pain is 7/10. Saturation is 97% on room air.

GENERAL: The patient is looking unwell, but in no acute distress.

HEENT: Atraumatic and normocephalic. Pupils are equal, round, reactive to light, and accommodation. Extraocular movements are intact. There is no icterus, cyanosis, or pallor of the conjunctivae. Tympanic membranes are dull but not inflamed bilaterally. Nasal turbinates are congested with clear exudates. Sinuses are uncomfortable to percussion. Posterior pharynx is minimally erythematous. No exudates are noted.

CHEST: Air entry is adequate bilaterally with occasional scattered rhonchi. No crackles are appreciated.

HEART: Sounds 1 and 2 are heard and are normal. Regular rate and rhythm, somewhat tachycardic, but no murmurs, gallops, or rubs.

ABDOMEN: Soft and nontender. Bowel sounds are present but somewhat hyperactive. There is no hepatosplenomegaly.

SKIN: Clear, slight pallor.

EXTREMITIES: Without edema, cyanosis, or clubbing.

Specimen taken and tested in our office lab. Novel A influenza virus is confirmed.

ASSESSMENT: Influenza with gastrointestinal manifestations.

PLAN:

1. The patient will be put on Phenergan with Codeine 5 mL p.o. t.i.d. for 7 days.
2. Zyrtec 10 mg p.o. daily for 10 to 14 days.
3. She is instructed to take Tylenol p.r.n. for aches and pains, to drink a lot of liquids, and to stay in the dorm, in bed if possible, and rest.
4. She has been given a note for her coach and any professors.
5. If she does not get any better, she will come back.

Gary H. Mulder, MD

You Code It!

Read carefully about Dr. Mulder's diagnosis of Andrea and determine the correct diagnosis code or codes.

Step #1: Read the case carefully and completely.
Step #2: Abstract the scenario. Which main words or terms describe why the physician cared for the patient during this encounter?
Step #3: Are there any details missing or incomplete for which you would need to query the physician? [If so, ask your instructor.]
Step #4: Check for any relevant guidance, including reading all of the symbols and notations in the Tabular List and the appropriate sections of the Official Guidelines.
Step #5: Determine the correct diagnosis code or codes to explain why this encounter was medically necessary.
Step #6: Double-check your work.

Answer:

Did you determine this to be the code?

J09.X3 Influenza due to identified novel influenza A virus with gastrointestinal manifestations

13.4 Chronic Respiratory Disorders

Chronic Obstructive Pulmonary Disease

One of the most common respiratory disorders that you may code is **chronic obstructive pulmonary disease (COPD)**. It is estimated that as much as 10% of the world population over age 40 has a lung disorder that is on a par with COPD. COPD is distinguished by restricted airflow. It is not fully reversible and, therefore, is a leading cause of disability and death. Clinically, there are three types of COPD:

- Chronic bronchitis
- Emphysema
- Asthma

Chronic Obstructive Pulmonary Disease (COPD)
An ongoing obstruction of the airway.

EXAMPLES

J40	Bronchitis, not specified as acute or chronic
J41.-	Simple and mucopurulent chronic bronchitis
J42	Unspecified chronic bronchitis
J43.-	Emphysema
J44.-	Other chronic obstructive pulmonary disease
J45.-	Asthma

Diagnoses in the COPD section can be particularly complex. You will need to be very diligent as you read the terms in the physician's notes and those included in the code descriptions. It is, as always, crucial that you refer to the index and then verify the code in the Tabular List.

Let's look at some of the diagnostic statements that might be used in the documentation, by reading through the INCLUDES note under J44.

✓4 **J44 Other chronic obstructive pulmonary disease**

INCLUDES **asthma with chronic obstructive pulmonary disease**
chronic asthmatic (obstructive) bronchitis
chronic bronchitis with airways obstruction
chronic bronchitis with emphysema
chronic emphysematous bronchitis
chronic obstructive asthma
chronic obstructive bronchitis
chronic obstructive tracheobronchitis

There is also an EXCLUDES1 note that will remind you to read very carefully. You can see that chronic *obstructive* bronchitis is INCLUDED in the J44 code category, while chronic bronchitis is EXCLUDED. This is the ICD-10-CM code book's way of reminding you that one word–"obstructive"–makes a big difference as to which code to report.

CODING BITES

Never, never, never, never code out of the Alphabetic Index. *Always* confirm the code by reading the complete description in the Tabular List.

LET'S CODE IT! SCENARIO

Tiffany Burnstein, a 57-year-old female, quit smoking 2 years ago after a two-pack-a-day habit that lasted 40 years. She came to see Dr. Mercado with an insidious onset of dyspnea, tachypnea, and malaise. PE showed use of her accessory muscles for respiration. Dr. Mercado took a chest x-ray, EKG, RBC count, and pulmonary function test. The results directed a diagnosis of panlobular emphysema.

Let's Code It!

Dr. Mercado diagnosed Tiffany with *panlobular emphysema*. The Alphabetic Index shows

Emphysema

panlobular J43.1

Go to the Tabular List to confirm this code:

✓4 **J43 Emphysema**

Read the ***Use additional code*** notation carefully, as well as the EXCLUDES1 note. Does either of them relate to Tiffany's condition? Yes, the note to ***Use additional code*** for "history of tobacco use" applies. First, keep reading and review all of the choices for the required fourth character:

J43.1 Panlobular emphysema

Now let's follow the lead to the code for "history of tobacco use." Turn to code Z87:

✓4 **Z87 Personal history of other diseases and conditions**

Z87.891 Personal history of nicotine dependence

Now you have two codes to report the story of why Dr. Mercado cared for Tiffany:

J43.1 Panlobular emphysema

Z87.891 Personal history of nicotine dependence

Exacerbation and Status Asthmaticus

Exacerbation
An increase in the severity of a disease or its symptoms.

Status Asthmaticus
The condition of asthma that is life-threatening and does not respond to therapeutic treatments.

CODING BITES

If both diagnoses are included in the notes—status asthmaticus *and* acute exacerbation of asthma—use only one asthma code, for status asthmaticus. Do not use two asthma codes.

You may notice that some of the codes in this section have the designation for acute **exacerbation** of asthma, COPD, or other related condition. It is a clinical term and can be assigned only by the attending physician.

Acute exacerbation of asthma indicates an increase in the severe nature of a patient's asthmatic condition. The patient may be suffering from wheezing or shortness of breath, commonly called an *asthma attack*. **Status asthmaticus**, however, is a life-threatening condition and is a diagnosis indicating that the patient is not responding to therapeutic procedures. If a patient is diagnosed with status asthmaticus *and* COPD or acute bronchitis, the status asthmaticus should be the first-listed code. As a life-threatening condition, it is considered to be the diagnosis with the greatest severity and follows the sequencing rules that you learned earlier. In addition, status asthmaticus, being the more severe condition, will override an additional diagnosis of acute exacerbation of asthma.

GUIDANCE CONNECTION

Read the ICD-10-CM Official Guidelines for Coding and Reporting, section **I. Conventions, General Coding Guidelines and Chapter-Specific Guidelines**, subsection **C. Chapter-Specific Coding Guidelines**, chapter **10. Diseases of the Respiratory System**, subsection **a. Chronic Obstructive Pulmonary Disease [COPD] and Asthma.**

LET'S CODE IT! SCENARIO

Isabella LaVelle, a 41-year-old female, has a history of intermittent dyspnea and wheezing. She comes today to see Dr. Slater with complaints of tachypnea, chest tightness, and a cough with thick mucus. The results of Dr. Slater's PE, the chest x-ray, sputum culture, EKG, pulmonary function tests, and an arterial blood gas analysis indicate moderate, persistent asthma with COPD, with exacerbation.

Let's Code It!

Dr. Slater's diagnosis of Isabella's condition is *moderate, persistent asthma with COPD, with exacerbation*. This is also referred to as *chronic obstructive asthma*. Let's turn to the Alphabetic Index and look up

Asthma

with

chronic obstructive pulmonary disease J44.9

with

exacerbation (acute) J44.1

That's great, it matches perfectly. Turn in the Tabular List to

✓4 **J44 Other chronic obstructive pulmonary disease**

You can see "chronic obstructive asthma" in the INCLUDES list. Also notice the instruction to ***Code also*** type of asthma, if applicable (J45.-).

J44.0 Chronic obstructive pulmonary disease with acute lower respiratory infection

J44.1 Chronic obstructive pulmonary disease with (acute) exacerbation

J44.9 Chronic obstructive pulmonary disease, unspecified

You can see that J44.1 matches. Terrific! Now let's turn to J45 to determine the additional code for the asthma.

Go back to Dr. Slater's notes and determine if Isabella's asthma is documented as mild, moderate, or severe and if her condition is intermittent or persistent. Then match all of the options within code category J45 to determine which code is accurate:

J45.41 Moderate persistent asthma with (acute) exacerbation

One more detail to address: certainly you saw the ***Use additional code*** notation regarding tobacco exposure, use, dependence, or history. Is there documentation that Isabella was a smoker? No! Good for her (and good for you). Now you have the codes to report this encounter:

J44.1 Chronic obstructive pulmonary disease with (acute) exacerbation

J45.41 Moderate persistent asthma with (acute) exacerbation

Good job!

YOU CODE IT! CASE STUDY

Oliver Rockwell, a 61-year-old male, was brought into the emergency department (ED) by ambulance because he was having a severe asthma attack. His wife, Karolyn, stated that he was diagnosed with asthma about 2 years prior. This attack began 5 days ago and has not responded to his inhaler, his regular asthma pills, or any other treatment. Dr. Pressman diagnosed Oliver with acute exacerbation of late-onset severe, persistent asthma with status asthmaticus.

You Code It!

Go through the steps of coding, and determine the diagnosis code or codes that should be reported for this encounter between Dr. Pressman and Oliver.

Step #1: Read the case carefully and completely.
Step #2: Abstract the scenario. Which main words or terms describe why the physician cared for the patient during this encounter?
Step #3: Are there any details missing or incomplete for which you would need to query the physician? [If so, ask your instructor.]
Step #4: Check for any relevant guidance, including reading all of the symbols and notations in the Tabular List and the appropriate sections of the Official Guidelines.
Step #5: Determine the correct diagnosis code or codes to explain why this encounter was medically necessary.
Step #6: Double-check your work.

Answer:

Did you determine this to be the correct code?

J45.52 Severe persistent asthma with status asthmaticus

You are really getting good at this!

13.5 Reporting Tobacco Involvement

One set of elements that has become required is the reporting of tobacco use, abuse, and/or dependence. For example, at the start of the ICD-10-CM code book's *Chapter 10: Diseases of the Respiratory System (J00–J99)*, there is a notation that applies to all codes within:

Use additional code, **where applicable, to identify:**

Exposure to environmental tobacco smoke (Z77.22)

Exposure to tobacco smoke in the perinatal period (P96.81)

History of tobacco use (Z87.891)

Occupational exposure to environmental tobacco smoke (Z57.31)

Tobacco dependence (F17.-)

Tobacco use (Z72.0)

Surely you know that tobacco use can be a risk factor to the development of respiratory illness. ICD-10-CM makes it easier to collect data on tobacco use. To do so, you need to understand what the terms *exposure*, *use*, *abuse*, *dependence*, and *history* really mean.

- *Exposure* means that the patient has been in contact with, or in close proximity to, a source of tobacco smoke in such a way that the harmful effects of this agent may impact the patient. When it comes to health care issues, this would apply to an individual who does not use tobacco products but lives or works with someone who smokes, resulting in the patient's breathing in secondhand tobacco smoke on an ongoing basis. If this individual develops a respiratory disease as a result of this environment, you would include a code to report this exposure.

EXAMPLE

Z77.22 Contact with and (suspected) exposure to environmental tobacco smoke (acute) (chronic) [Exposure to second hand tobacco smoke]

- *Use* is the term that identifies that the patient smokes tobacco on a regular basis, taken by their own initiative, even though the substance is known to be a detriment to one's health. There are no obvious clinical manifestations.

EXAMPLE

V72.0 Tobacco use

- *Abuse* describes the patient's habitual smoking of tobacco, taken by their own initiative, even though the substance is known to be a detriment to one's health. Clinical manifestations are evident as signs and symptoms develop. The patient deals with a daily fixation on obtaining and smoking tobacco with virtually everything else in life becoming secondary.

EXAMPLE

F17.218 Nicotine dependence, cigarettes, with other nicotine-induced disorders

- *Dependence* indicates the patient's compulsive, continuous smoking of tobacco that has resulted in significant clinical manifestations as well as the physiological need for the substance to function normally. Any interruption results in signs and symptoms of withdrawal, occurring within a continuous 12-month time frame.

EXAMPLE

F17.220 Nicotine dependence, chewing tobacco, uncomplicated

- *History* describes a patient who has successfully quit using tobacco products.

EXAMPLE

Z87.891 Personal history of tobacco dependence

ICD-10-CM

YOU CODE IT! CASE STUDY

Evan Pattison has been smoking cigarettes for more than 10 years. He has tried to quit several times, unsuccessfully. Evan tells the physician that he has been very stressed and smoking much more than usual and now his throat hurts and his voice is hoarse. Dr. Dieter evaluates Evan and determines acute laryngitis due to tobacco dependence.

(continued)

You Code It!

Read the scenario and determine what code or codes you need to report why Dr. Dieter cared for Evan.

Step #1: Read the case carefully and completely.
Step #2: Abstract the scenario. Which main words or terms describe why the physician cared for the patient during this encounter?
Step #3: Are there any details missing or incomplete for which you would need to query the physician? [If so, ask your instructor.]
Step #4: Check for any relevant guidance, including reading all of the symbols and notations in the Tabular List and the appropriate sections of the Official Guidelines.
Step #5: Determine the correct diagnosis code or codes to explain why this encounter was medically necessary.
Step #6: Double-check your work.

Answer:

Did you determine these to be the codes?

J04.0 **Acute laryngitis**

F17.210 **Nicotine dependence, cigarettes, uncomplicated**

13.6 Respiratory Conditions Requiring External Cause Codes

Earlier in this text, you learned about external cause codes and how to determine whether they are necessary. There are respiratory conditions that may require external cause codes to explain how, and sometimes where, an external condition was involved in causing this health problem. Some of these conditions are

J39.8: **Cicatrix of trachea might need an external cause code to identify it as a late effect of an injury or poisoning.**

J67.0: **Farmer's lung might need an external cause code for a workers' compensation claim.**

J68.-: **Respiratory conditions due to inhalation of chemicals, gases, fumes, and vapors would need an external cause code to identify the chemical.**

J70.-: **Respiratory conditions due to other external agents would need an external cause code to identify the external cause of the condition.**

J95.811: **Postprocedural pneumothorax would need an external cause code to identify that it was a postoperative condition.**

External Cause Codes

When a patient has been injured traumatically, has been poisoned, has had an adverse reaction, has been abused or neglected, or has experienced other harm as a result of an external cause, you will need to report the details of the event so that you tell the whole story. In addition to reporting the other codes, you also will need to report codes that explain

- *Cause of the injury*, such as a car accident or a fall off a ladder.
- *Place of the occurrence*, such as the park or the kitchen.
- *Activity during the occurrence*, such as playing basketball or gardening.
- *Patient's status*, such as paid employment, on-duty military, or leisure activity.

CODING BITES

Refer back to the ***Abstracting Clinical Documentation*** chapter to remind yourself about reporting external cause codes whenever you are reporting an injury or poisoning.

GUIDANCE CONNECTION

Read the ICD-10-CM Official Guidelines for Coding and Reporting, section **I. Conventions, General Coding Guidelines and Chapter-Specific Guidelines**, subsection **C. Chapter-Specific Coding Guidelines**, chapter **20. External Causes of Morbidity**.

ICD-10-CM

LET'S CODE IT! SCENARIO

Amanda Bleigh, a 33-year-old female, works in a veterinary clinic. After a very sick stray animal was brought in, she was instructed by her boss to disinfect the floor of the clinic by mopping it with straight bleach. It was cold outside, so all the doors and windows were closed tightly. Amanda began to have trouble breathing. She went immediately to Dr. Litzkom's office, where, after examination and tests, he diagnosed her with acute chemical bronchitis.

Let's Code It!

Dr. Litzkom diagnosed Amanda with *acute chemical bronchitis*. In the Alphabetic Index:

Bronchitis

acute

chemical (due to gases, fumes, or vapors) J68.0

Will the Tabular List confirm this suggested code?

✓4 **J68** **Respiratory conditions due to inhalation of chemicals, gases, fumes, and vapors**

Did you notice that there are two notations: ***Code first*** (T51–T65) to identify cause and ***Use additional code*** to report the associated respiratory condition. Keep reading down the column to

J68.0 **Bronchitis and pneumonitis due to chemicals, gases, fumes, and vapors (chemical bronchitis [acute])**

Next, you must report how and where Amanda was exposed to the chemical. Let's go to the Alphabetic Index for external cause codes and look up how Amanda was injured by the bleach—she inhaled the chemical:

Inhalation

gases, fumes, or vapors NEC T59.9- specified agent — see Table of Drugs and Chemicals, by substance

Turn to the Table of Drugs and Chemicals and look down the first column to find *bleach*:

Bleach NEC

Reading across this line, in the column titled "Poisoning, Accidental," you will see the suggested poisoning code. Remember: If the condition was not an adverse reaction to properly prescribed and taken medication, it is reported as a poisoning. The code suggested on the line for bleach is T54.91.

Now turn to the Tabular List to confirm the most accurate code. Let's begin with the poisoning code:

✓4 **T54** **Toxic effect of corrosive substances**

There are no notations or directives, so keep reading to find the most accurate fourth, fifth, and sixth characters:

T54.91XA **Toxic effect of unspecified corrosive substance, accidental (unintentional), initial encounter**

This does look like the best choice.

In addition, Amanda was at work when the exposure happened, so you will need an external cause code to report where she was at the time of her injury. The External Cause Code Alphabetic Index will direct you:

Place of occurrence

hospital Y92.239

cafeteria Y92.233

corridor Y92.232

(continued)

There is no specific listing for *veterinary clinic*. However, *hospital* does come the closest. Let's turn to the code in the Tabular List and check the description:

Y92.232 Corridor of hospital as the place of occurrence of the external cause

Well, that really does hit the target. Remember, the code is being included to explain that Amanda was hurt at work; such information is most often required to support a workers' compensation claim.

These are the three codes on Amanda's report:

J68.0	**Bronchitis and pneumonitis due to chemicals, gases, fumes and vapors (chemical bronchitis [acute])**
T54.91XA	**Toxic effect of unspecified corrosive substance, accidental (unintentional), initial encounter**
Y92.232	**Corridor of hospital as the place of occurrence of the external cause**

Chapter Summary

Sadly, most people take breathing for granted . . . until they cannot do it without difficulty or pain. You have to know how to code respiratory conditions accurately whether you are working for a family physician, a pediatrician, a respiratory therapist, or a pulmonologist. In addition, respiratory conditions might be present in a patient of an immunologist; allergist; or ear, nose, and throat (ENT) specialist.

CODING BITES

Did you know . . . ?

- The average healthy adult's respiration rate is 12 to 15 per minute. Adult men breathe more slowly than adult women. Neonates breathe 30 to 60 times per minute.
- The entire surface area of both lungs combined is approximately the same surface area as a tennis court.
- Expiration (breathing out) not only expels carbon dioxide from the body, but water as well—an estimated 12 ounces a day.
- A yawn is an autonomic response when your brain determines the body needs more oxygen.
- The left lung is smaller than the right lung to accommodate the placement of the heart in the thoracic cavity.

CHAPTER 13 REVIEW
Coding Respiratory Conditions

McGraw Hill connect

Enhance your learning by completing these exercises and more at mcgrawhillconnect.com!

Let's Check It! Terminology

Match each key term to the appropriate definition.

1. **LO 13.4** An increase in the severity of a disease or its symptoms.
2. **LO 13.3** An acute infection of the respiratory tract caused by the influenza virus.
3. **LO 13.4** An ongoing obstruction of the airway.
4. **LO 13.1** A malfunction of the organ system relating to respiration.
5. **LO 13.3** An inflammation of the lungs.

A. Chronic Obstructive Pulmonary Disease (COPD)

B. Exacerbation

C. Influenza

6. **LO 13.4** The condition of asthma that is life-threatening and does not respond to therapeutic treatments.
7. **LO 13.2** A condition in which air or gas is present within the chest cavity but outside the lungs.

D. Pneumonia
E. Pneumothorax
F. Respiratory Disorder
G. Status Asthmaticus

Let's Check It! Concepts

Choose the most appropriate answer for each of the following questions.

1. **LO 13.4** COPD stands for
   a. chronic obstructive pneumonia dyspnea.
   b. chronic olfactory pharyngitis disease.
   c. chronic other pneumonic disease.
   d. chronic obstructive pulmonary disease.
2. **LO 13.4** One of the three types of COPD is
   a. sinusitis. **b.** pneumonia. **c.** emphysema. **d.** pharyngitis.
3. **LO 13.3** When the cause of pneumonia is an underlying disease such as HIV, the codes should be sequenced
   a. pneumonia first, underlying disease second.
   b. pneumonia only.
   c. underlying disease only.
   d. underlying disease first, pneumonia second.
4. **LO 13.1** Respiratory disorders can be
   a. genetic. **b.** environmental. **c.** congenital. **d.** all of these.
5. **LO 13.3** When a known infectious organism is involved in a respiratory condition,
   a. code only the infectious organism.
   b. code both the known organism and the respiratory condition.
   c. code only the respiratory condition.
   d. use a personal history code.
6. **LO 13.4** If the diagnostic statement includes both status asthmaticus and acute exacerbation of asthma,
   a. code only the status asthmaticus.
   b. code only the acute exacerbation of asthma.
   c. code both status asthmaticus and acute exacerbation with two codes.
   d. these two diagnoses cannot be in the same patient at the same time.
7. **LO 13.2** Jake Phillipson, a 59-year-old male, presents with dyspnea, tachypnea, and chest pain. After an examination, Jake is diagnosed with a saddle embolus of pulmonary artery with acute cor pulmonale. How would this be coded?
   a. I26.09 **b.** Z86.711 **c.** I26.92 **d.** I26.02
8. **LO 13.6** Respiratory conditions need external cause codes
   a. never.
   b. sometimes.
   c. always.
   d. only if there is an external cause for the condition.
9. **LO 13.5** ____ is the term that identifies that the patient smokes tobacco on a regular basis, taken by their own initiative, even though the substance is known to be a detriment to one's health. There are no obvious clinical manifestations.
   a. Exposure **b.** Use **c.** Abuse **d.** Dependence
10. **LO 13.3** Code the diagnosis of pneumonitis due to inhalation of lubricating oil, unintentional, initial encounter.
   a. T52.0X1A **b.** J69.1 **c.** T52.0X1A, J69.1 **d.** J69.1, T52.0X1A

Let's Check It! Guidelines

Refer to the Official Guidelines and fill in the blanks according to Chapter 10, Diseases of the Respiratory System, Chapter-Specific Coding Guidelines.

secondary	principal	documentation	mechanical
all	J95.851	not	J96.0
J96.2	exacerbation	confirmed	one
admission			

1. An acute _____ is a worsening or a decompensation of a chronic condition.
2. A code from subcategory _____, Acute respiratory failure, or subcategory _____, Acute and chronic respiratory failure, may be assigned as a principal diagnosis when it is the condition established after study to be chiefly responsible for occasioning the admission to the hospital, and the selection is supported by the Alphabetic Index and Tabular List.
3. Respiratory failure may be listed as a _____ diagnosis if it occurs after admission, or if it is present on admission, but does not meet the definition of _____ diagnosis.
4. Code only _____ cases of influenza due to certain identified influenza viruses (category J09), and due to other identified influenza virus (category J10).
5. As with _____ procedural or postprocedural complications, code assignment is based on the provider's _____ of the relationship between the condition and the procedure.
6. Code _____, Ventilator-associated pneumonia, should be assigned only when the provider has documented ventilator-associated pneumonia (VAP).
7. Code J95.851 should _____ be assigned for cases where the patient has pneumonia and is on a _____ ventilator and the provider has not specifically stated that the pneumonia is ventilator-associated pneumonia.
8. A patient may be admitted with _____ type of pneumonia (e.g., code J13, Pneumonia due to Streptococcus pneumonia) and subsequently develop VAP. In this instance, the principal diagnosis would be the appropriate code from categories J12–J18 for the pneumonia diagnosed at the time of _____.

Let's Check It! Rules and Regulations

Please answer the following questions from the knowledge you have gained after reading this chapter.

1. **LO 13.2** What is pleural effusion? What is the correct ICD-10-CM code for malignant pleural effusion?
2. **LO 13.3** Explain what ventilator-associated pneumonia is. Include the correct ICD-10-CM code you would use to report VAP.
3. **LO 13.4** Differentiate between exacerbation and status asthmaticus.
4. **LO 13.5** In relation to tobacco involvement, explain the difference between *exposure*, *use*, *abuse*, *dependence*, and *history*.
5. **LO 13.6** Explain why a respiratory condition might require an external cause code. Include an example.

ICD-10-CM

YOU CODE IT! Basics

First, identify the condition in the following diagnoses; then code the diagnosis.

Example: Acute nasopharyngitis:

a. main term: *Nasopharyngitis* b. diagnosis: *J00*

1. Vasomotor rhinitis:
   a. main term: ______ b. diagnosis:______
2. Nasal catarrh, chronic:
   a. main term:______ b. diagnosis:______
3. Acute recurrent empyema of sphenoidal sinus:
   a. main term:______ b. diagnosis:______
4. Hypertrophy of tonsils:
   a. main term:______ b. diagnosis:______

(continued)

5. Obstructive laryngitis:
   a. main term:______ b. diagnosis:______
6. Chronic laryngotracheitis:
   a. main term: ______ b. diagnosis:______
7. Aspiration pneumonia due to solids and liquids:
   a. main term:______ b. diagnosis:______
8. Bronchitis due to rhinovirus:
   a. main term:______ b. diagnosis:______
9. Cellulitis of nose:
   a. main term:______ b. diagnosis:______
10. Polypoid sinus degeneration:
   a. main term:______ b. diagnosis:______
11. Adenoid vegetations:
   a. main term:______ b. diagnosis:______
12. Abscess of lung:
   a. main term:______ b. diagnosis:______
13. Bronchiectasis with exacerbation:
   a. main term:______ b. diagnosis:______
14. Seropurulent pleurisy with fistula:
   a. main term:______ b. diagnosis:______
15. Pulmonary gangrene:
   a. main term:______ b. diagnosis:______

ICD-10-CM

YOU CODE IT! Practice

Using the techniques described in this chapter, carefully read through the case studies and determine the most accurate ICD-10-CM code(s) and external cause codes, if appropriate, for each case study.

1. Fred Draper, a 39-year-old male, is HIV-positive, asymptomatic. Fred was just admitted with organic pneumonia.
2. Rebecca Key, a 21-year-old female, presents with a fever and sore throat. Dr. Brice notes large lymph nodes. The throat culture confirms a diagnosis of streptococcal pharyngitis.
3. Larry Ligon, a 58-year-old male, presents today with severe chest congestion. Dr. Snell also notes difficulty breathing and wheezing. Larry is admitted to the hospital, where further laboratory tests confirm the diagnosis of streptococcus, group B, pneumonia.
4. Sally Griffith, a 13-year-old female, was brought to the ED by her mother. Sally had a cough and fever, and her eyes were tearing. She was complaining that her eyes were itchy and burning. After a thorough examination and chest x-ray, Dr. Minister diagnosed her with an upper respiratory infection with bilateral acute conjunctivitis.
5. Chris Fravel, a 13-year-old male, is brought in by his mother with the complaints of sore throat, fever, and that it hurts when he swallows. Dr. Dennis documents white pus-filled spots on the tonsils and large lymph nodes. After completing an examination and an optical fiber endoscopy, Chris is diagnosed with chronic tonsillitis and adenoiditis.
6. Allison Mabry, a 6-year-old female, is brought in by her parents with a fever and hoarseness. Allison says it hurts when she swallows and it's hard to breathe. Dr. Macon completes an examination noting drooling; culture is positive for haemophilus influenza. Allison is diagnosed with acute epiglottitis.
7. Benjamin Fulkenbury, a 46-year-old male, comes in today with cough, runny nose, sneezing, and body aches. Dr. Pruessner completes a thorough examination and notes a temperature of 104 F. Ben is admitted, where a CXR and laboratory tests confirm the diagnosis of influenza virus A/H5N1 with pleural effusion.
8. Sandra Busbee, a 43-year-old female, comes in today with a cough and chest pain. Dr. Lindsey completes a thorough examination, the appropriate tests, and a chest x-ray. Sandra is diagnosed with acute bronchitis due to parainfluenza virus.
9. Dale Hunter, a 52-year-old male, was diagnosed with chronic bronchitis 3 months ago and is on medication. This morning, he came to see Dr. Teasdale because he began to cough and is having difficulty breathing. Dr. Teasdale admitted him into the hospital with a diagnosis of chronic obstructive pulmonary disease with acute exacerbation.

(continued)

10. Monica Adams, a 65-year-old female, comes in today with hoarseness and neck pain. Dr. Fazio completes a thorough examination and the appropriate tests and notes that Monica smokes cigarettes. Monica undergoes a laryngoscopy, which confirms the diagnosis of vocal cord nodules.
11. Caitlyn Joy, a 12-year-old female, comes in today with a nosebleed. She was playing a pickup game of basketball at the local sports area and was struck in the face by the basketball. After an examination, Dr. Jordan diagnoses Caitlyn with a deviated nasal septum.
12. Randy Prescott, a 56-year-old male, presents today with a cough and shortness of breath. Dr. Holden documents notable weight loss from Randy's last visit 6 months ago. Randy admits to joint aches and some chest pain. After a thorough examination and the appropriate tests, Dr. Holden diagnoses Randy with berylliosis.
13. Larry Crosstree, a 29-year-old male, presents today concerned about vocal pitch changes he has been experiencing for approximately 2 weeks. Dr. Leonard notes the frequent need for breath while Larry is speaking as well as hoarseness. Larry is admitted to the hospital, where an MRI scan of the neck and chest confirms a diagnosis of complete bilateral paralysis of the laryngeal nerve.
14. Nakeisha Dittman, a 27-year-old female, presents today with a cough, fever, shortness of breath, and night sweats, 2-week duration. Dr. Mokeba completes a thorough examination and decides to admit Nakeisha to the hospital. Further laboratory tests confirm the diagnosis of acute eosinophilic pneumonia with secondary spontaneous pneumothorax.
15. Beth Northing, a 25-year-old female, was diagnosed 6 months ago with asthma. She presents today with the complaint of shortness of breath and a tight chest. Dr. Hayden completes an examination, noting cyanosis of the lips and confusion. Dr. Hayden diagnoses Beth with a severe, persistent asthma attack with status asthmaticus and admits her into the hospital.

YOU CODE IT! Application

The following exercises provide practice in abstracting physicians' notes and learning to work with documentation from our health care facility, Prader, Bracker, & Associates. These case studies are modeled on real patient encounters. Using the techniques described in this chapter, carefully read through the case studies and determine the most accurate ICD-10-CM code(s) and external cause code(s), if appropriate, for each case study.

WESTON HOSPITAL

629 Healthcare Way • SOMEWHERE, FL 32811 • 407-555-6541

PATIENT: YOUNG, ELIAS

ACCOUNT/EHR #: YOUNEL001

Attending Physician: Oscar R. Prader, MD

Elias Young, a 71-year-old male, is brought to the ED by EMS. Elias is on ACUD mode on ventilator with a respiration of 11 breaths per minute. No cyanosis is noted. Pt is currently alert and oriented and able to answer some questions. Dr. Prader notes as time progresses patient is showing signs of confusion and disorientation. He is admitted to the hospital.

The patient's blood gases showed a compensated respiratory acidosis, VS are stable, and patient is afebrile. BP: 148/83. Sinus tachycardia on the monitor at about 131 beats per minute. Lung fields are clear to auscultation and percussion.

DIAGNOSES: 1. Respiratory failure, chronic

2. Sinus tachycardia

PLAN/RECOMMENDATIONS:

1. 100% ventilator support for the time being
2. Nutrition with PulmoCare at 60 cc an hour
3. Follow up laboratory

Determine the most accurate ICD-10-CM code(s).

(continued)

PRADER, BRACKER, & ASSOCIATES

A Complete Health Care Facility

159 Healthcare Way • SOMEWHERE, FL 32811 • 407-555-6789

PATIENT: NADER, ERICK

ACCOUNT/EHR #: NADEER001

Attending Physician: Oscar R. Prader, MD

S: Erick Nader, an 18-month-old male, is brought in today by his parents because of shortness of breath and a cough that has grown worse over the last 24 hours.

O: H: 32.5″, W: 25 lb., T: 103 F, P: 138, R: 37, SpO2: 96% on room air, BP: 95/62. A "bark-like" cough is noted and upon auscultation stridor is heard. A lateral neck x-ray is taken.

A: Stridulous croup

P: 0.5 mL of racemic epinephrine via small volume nebulizer is administered

Determine the most accurate ICD-10-CM code(s).

WESTON HOSPITAL

629 Healthcare Way • SOMEWHERE, FL 32811 • 407-555-6541

PATIENT: SMUTH, SARAH

ACCOUNT/EHR #: SMUTSA001

Attending Physician: Renee O. Bracker, MD

Sarah Smuth, a 52-year-old female, underwent total knee replacement surgery 5 days ago. Patient is alert and oriented, but began to complain of chest pain and dyspnea 3 days after surgery. Laboratory tests reveal a WBC of 15, HR: 101, R: 20 and shallow, P: 56, BP: 135/85, T: 98.9 F, SpO2 is 95% receiving oxygen via nasal cannula at 2 Lpm. VS have remained stable. Diminished sounds and fine crackles are noted on auscultation. Post-op day 3—CXR confirms atelectasis; pneumonia is ruled out. Post-op day 4—patient has not improved; a repeat CXR shows no improvement of atelectasis and a bronchoscopy was performed and mucus plugs were removed. Post-op day 5—patient begins to show improvement and full resolution is expected.

A: Atelectasis, post-op complication

P: Albuterol nebulizer every 4 hours and prn

Deep breathing exercises and coughing. Monitor via continuous capnography.

Determine the most accurate ICD-10-CM code(s).

WESTON HOSPITAL

629 Healthcare Way • SOMEWHERE, FL 32811 • 407-555-6541

PATIENT: ALBERTSON, JONAH

ACCOUNT/EHR #: ALBEJO001

Attending Physician: Renee O. Bracker, MD

Jonah Albertson, a 62-year-old male, was transported to the ED by EMS after an MVA. Patient was involved in a three-car accident while driving home. Patient does not appear to have any injuries. Patient denies any pain or discomfort at this time. Patient is alert and oriented, but appears anxious.

VS: H: 6′1″, W: 192 lb., P: 94, R: 24, T: 99.1 F, BP: 90/60, SpO2 100% on room air.

(continued)

Laboratory results 25 minutes after arrival:

pH: 7.5

PaO_2: 195 mmHg

$PaCO_2$: 32 mmHg

SaO_2: 90%

HCO_3: 20 mEq

Hgb: 13.9 gms

COHgb: 11.2%

With the level of carbon monoxide on the hemoglobin, the patient is placed on a nonrebreathing mask. COHgb has decreased to 7.1% and patient is breathing comfortably 4 hours after arrival. Patient is admitted for observation.

Three hours later, respiration becomes more rapid and labored. Patient shows extreme fatigue. Auscultation reveals fine crackles throughout both lungs. CXR shows bilateral infiltrates extending into all four lung quadrants.

Arterial blood gases are rechecked:

pH: 7.31

PaO_2: 71 mmHg

$PaCO_2$: 43 mmHg

SaO_2: 89%

HCO_3: 22 mEq

COHgb: 3.9%

Heart Rate: 79

Blood Pressure: 88/57

Dx: ARDS

P: Intubation and mechanical ventilation

Determine the most accurate ICD-10-CM code(s).

PRADER, BRACKER, & ASSOCIATES

A Complete Health Care Facility

159 Healthcare Way • SOMEWHERE, FL 32811 • 407-555-6789

PATIENT: MASHEN, CYRUS

ACCOUNT/EHR #: MASHCY001

Attending Physician: Oscar R. Prader, MD

S: This new Pt is a 57-year-old male complaining of a stabbing chest pain and shortness of breath. Patient states the pain is worse when he breathes in.

PMH: Noncontributory

PFH: Noncontributory

O: VS: within normal range. Chest: Pleural rub on auscultation. Dullness upon percussion. Chest x-ray shows approximately 2.75 liters of fluid in the pleural space.

A: Interlobar pleurisy

P: Schedule aspiration of pleural fluid

Determine the most accurate ICD-10-CM code(s).

14

Coding Digestive System Conditions

Key Terms

Accessory Organs
Anus
Ascending Colon
Cecum
Cholelithiasis
Common Bile Duct
Descending Colon
Duodenum
Edentulism
Esophagus
Fundus
Gallbladder
Gangrene
Hemorrhage
Hernia
Ileum
Jejunum
Liver
Mesentery
Obstruction
Oral Cavity
Pancreas
Pancreatic Islets
Perforation
Rectum
Salivary Glands
Sigmoid Colon
Sphincter
Stomach
Teeth
Transverse Colon
Vermiform Appendix

Learning Outcomes

After completing this chapter, the student should be able to:

LO 14.1 Analyze the documentation for applicable details needed to report diseases affecting the mouth and salivary glands accurately.

LO 14.2 Interpret documentation to determine necessary details to report conditions affecting the esophagus and stomach correctly.

LO 14.3 Apply your knowledge to identify main terms relating to intestinal disorders.

LO 14.4 Evaluate the specifics from the documentation related to digestive accessory organs and malabsorption disorders accurately.

LO 14.5 Determine when additional codes are required to report the involvement of alcohol.

STOP! Remember, you need to follow along in your ICD-10-CM code book for an optimal learning experience.

14.1 Diseases of Oral Cavity and Salivary Glands

Oral Cavity

Virtually all nourishment enters the body at the mouth, also referred to as the **oral cavity**. The components within this area include the lips, cheeks, tongue, lingual tonsils, hard and soft palates, uvula, palatine tonsils, pharyngeal tonsils, and teeth (**Figure 14-1**).

Teeth are components of the mouth, required for proper digestion. Typically, as you probably know from your own experiences, they have their very own specialists, dentists, to care for them. Teeth are small, calcified protrusions consisting of multiple tissues of varying density and hardness. Rooted in the jaws (maxillary [upper jaw] and mandibular [lower jaw]), the bases of the teeth are protected and secured by the gums. Their job is to grind and crush food and food particles so they can combine with saliva for easier movement through the rest of the digestive system.

Oral Cavity
The opening in the face that begins the alimentary canal and is used for the input of nutrition; also known as the *mouth*.

Teeth
Small, calcified protrusions with roots in the jaw [singular: tooth].

EXAMPLE

Perry brought his 8-month-old son, Benjamin, to Dr. Reddington, his pediatrician, because he had been crying all night long. It seemed nothing he or his wife did calmed him. After examination, Dr. Reddington diagnosed Benjamin with teething syndrome and provided Perry with several ways to help the family through this experience. This diagnosis is reported with the following code:

K00.7 Teething syndrome

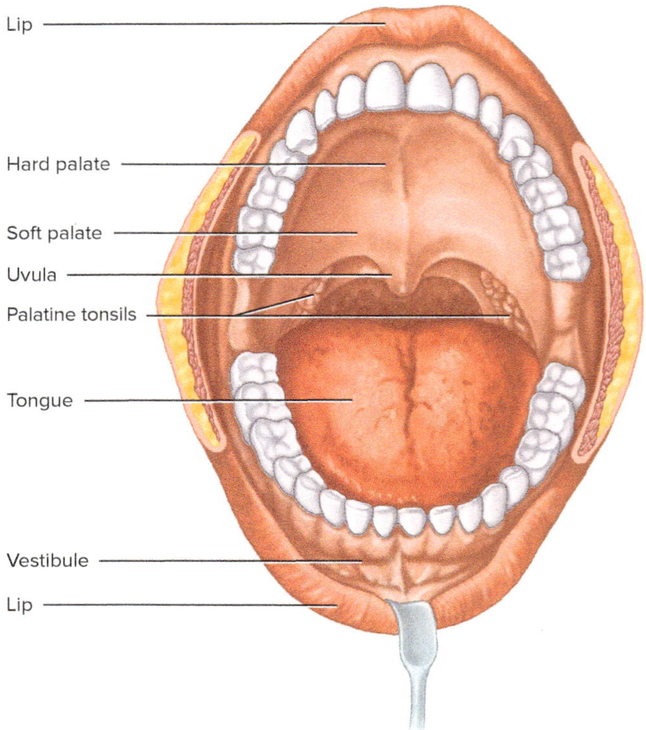

FIGURE 14-1 An illustration of the anatomical components of the oral cavity (human mouth)

> **Edentulism**
> Absence of teeth.

Diagnoses, related to the teeth, range from everything from baby's first tooth to dental caries (commonly known as a dental cavity) to issues of the surrounding tissue, such as gingivitis and other periodontal diseases, to **edentulism** (tooth loss).

When you are abstracting the documentation regarding acquired loss of teeth, you will need to identify three specified details from the notes:

1. **Is the loss complete or partial?**

   ✓4 K08.1 Complete loss of teeth

   ✓4 K08.4 Partial loss of teeth

2. **What is the cause of this loss?**

   ✓4 K08.11 Complete loss of teeth due to trauma

   ✓4 K08.12 Complete loss of teeth due to periodontal diseases

   ✓4 K08.13 Complete loss of teeth due to caries

   ✓4 K08.41 Partial loss of teeth due to trauma

   ✓4 K08.42 Partial loss of teeth due to periodontal diseases

   ✓4 K08.43 Partial loss of teeth due to caries

3. **What class classification is documented?**
   - *Class I* describes the stage of edentulism believed to have the best prognosis to have successful treatment using conventional prosthodontic techniques.
   - *Class II* identifies a patient with deterioration of the gums and other supporting structures, along with systemic disease interactions, soft tissue concerns, as well as patient management and/or lifestyle considerations affecting the prognosis of the treatment.
   - *Class III* establishes the existence of other factors significantly affecting the outcomes of treatment and the need for surgical revision of the supporting structures (gums and bone) to create an opportunity for prosthodontics.
   - *Class IV* reports a severely compromised condition of the supporting structures requiring surgical reconstruction. If due to the patient's health, personal preferences, past dental history, along with financial considerations, a customized prosthodontic technique may need to be created for an acceptable outcome.

Remember that ICD-10-CM diagnosis codes provide the explanation of why a particular procedure, treatment, or service is provided. You can see that the descriptions of each of these class classifications provides the justification for the treatment plan.

LET'S CODE IT! SCENARIO

Hannah Kim, a 49-year-old female, comes in to see her dentist, Dr. Morrison. She knew that she had periodontitis for a while, but now the teeth on the lower right side of her mouth are really bothering her. Dr. Morrison did a full evaluation and found that five teeth on the lower right were so loose that they came out with little encouragement. Dr. Morrison determined that Hannah has partial loss (edentulism) of teeth due to periodontal disease, class I.

Let's Code It!

Hannah lost five teeth due to periodontal disease. Let's turn to the Alphabetic Index and find the key term of the diagnosis:

Edentulism — see Absence, teeth, acquired

Turn to:

Absence

teeth, tooth (congenital) K00.0

acquired (complete) K08.109

partial K08.409

class I K08.401

class II K08.402

class III K08.403

class IV K08.404

Also take note of the listings within this long list for the loss of teeth due to caries (dental cavities), periodontal disease, trauma, or another specified cause. These will take you to other specific codes.

Refer to the physician's documentation and read that Hannah was diagnosed with *partial class I edentulism*, so let's turn to the Tabular List and find

✓4 **K08 Other disorders of teeth and supporting structures**

Read the EXCLUDES2 notation carefully. Does it have anything to do with this encounter? No! Great, so now review all the choices for the required fourth character and determine which one most accurately reports the diagnosis:

✓5 **K08.4 Partial loss of teeth**

There are EXCLUDES1 and EXCLUDES2 notes here. Read them carefully, and reread Dr. Morrison's documentation. Nothing there matches. Next, you must review the options for the fifth character.

✓6 **K08.42 Partial loss of teeth due to periodontal diseases**

Check the documentation. Dr. Morrison wrote that Hannah's loss of teeth was caused by the periodontitis, and it was class I. Review all of the choices, and determine the most accurate code:

K08.421 Partial loss of teeth due to periodontal diseases, class I

Good work!

Salivary Glands

> **Salivary Glands**
> Three sets of bilateral exocrine glands that secrete saliva: parotid glands, submaxillary glands, and sublingual glands.

As the teeth and tongue are breaking down food in preparation for the journey down the alimentary canal, three sets of major **salivary glands** (the parotid, submandibular, and sublingual glands) secrete saliva to moisten and bind the food particles. This begins the chemical digestion of carbohydrates, dissolves foods so their flavor can be appreciated, and helps enable swallowing of the food particles. In addition, saliva helps to clean the teeth and mouth after the particles leave the oral cavity.

As with almost any other part of the body, these glands can become infected. The salivary glands may be negatively impacted by either a bacterium or a virus, so be alert to check the pathology report.

Sialoadenitis, also known as parotitis, is described as acute, acute recurrent, or chronic. Note that *chronic* means ongoing (typically lasting more than 3 months), whereas *acute recurrent* means that the condition is severe, it clears up, and everything is fine for a while, but then it comes back again.

K11.21 Acute sialoadenitis

K11.22 Acute recurrent sialoadenitis

K11.23 Chronic sialoadenitis

YOU CODE IT! CASE STUDY

Isaac McNealy, a 37-year-old male, came in with complaints of pain in his face and mouth. He states that the pain becomes worse just before and during meals. He also claims that he has trouble swallowing and when he went to the dentist, he couldn't open his mouth very wide at all. Dr. Randolph did an ultrasound of Isaac's face and neck and confirmed that he was suffering with calculus of the salivary duct.

You Code It!

Read this documentation, and determine the correct ICD-10-CM diagnosis code or codes to report Dr. Randolph's diagnosis of Isaac's condition.

Step #1: Read the case carefully and completely.

Step #2: Abstract the scenario. Which main words or terms describe why the physician cared for the patient during this encounter?

Step #3: Are there any details missing or incomplete for which you would need to query the physician? [If so, ask your instructor.]

Step #4: Check for any relevant guidance, including reading all of the symbols and notations in the Tabular List and the appropriate sections of the Official Guidelines.

Step #5: Determine the correct diagnosis code or codes to explain why this encounter was medically necessary.

Step #6: Double-check your work.

Answer:

Did you determine this to be the code?

K11.5 Sialolithiasis

(Calculus of salivary gland or duct)

14.2 Conditions of the Esophagus and Stomach

Esophagus
The tubular organ that connects the pharynx to the stomach for the passage of nourishment.

Sphincter
A circular muscle that contracts to prevent passage of liquids or solids.

Esophagus

The tubelike structure that connects the hypopharynx to the stomach is known as the **esophagus**. As you can see in **Figure 14-2**, the esophagus lies parallel and posterior to the trachea. Just as the epiglottis blocks food and liquid from entering the trachea, the esophagus has its own gateway, called the *upper esophageal sphincter*, to restrict the entrance of air into the stomach. A **sphincter** is a circular muscle that can open or close an opening. There are several sphincters along the alimentary canal.

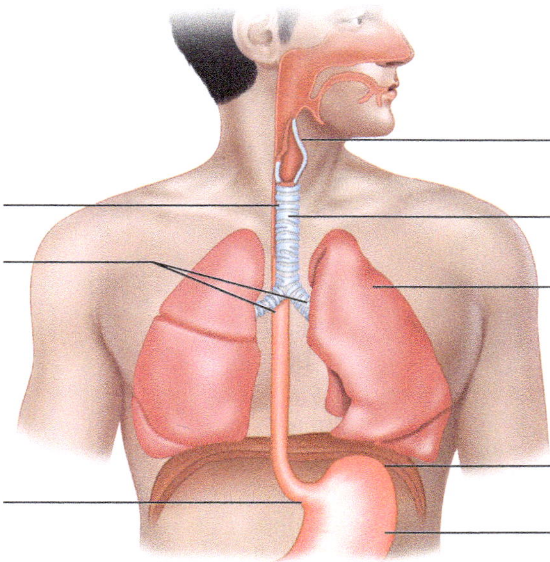

FIGURE 14-2 An illustration showing the anatomical sites from the epiglottis to the gastroesophageal junction

A second esophageal sphincter is located at the juncture between the esophagus and the stomach (the lower esophageal sphincter). This sphincter is designed to prevent the contents of the stomach from splashing back up into the esophagus. When this sphincter does not function properly, the patient might experience chronic heartburn, nausea, and possibly a sore throat. This may lead to a diagnosis of gastroesophageal reflux disease (GERD).

Gastroesophageal Reflux Disease (GERD)

Heartburn may not seem like a big concern; however, for many patients with persistent heartburn, one of the first symptoms of GERD is an increased intensity of that burning or painful sensation when bending down, lying down, or vigorously exercising. Dysphagia (difficulty with swallowing) and/or esophagitis also may occur.

GERD may be caused by a slacking lower esophageal sphincter, which separates the stomach from the esophagus and is designed to prevent backflow from the stomach upward.

EXAMPLES

K21.00	Gastroesophageal reflux disease with esophagitis without bleeding
K21.9	Gastroesophageal reflux disease without esophagitis

Stomach
A saclike organ within the alimentary canal designed to contain nourishment during the initial phase of the digestive process.

Fundus
The domed section of an organ farthest from its opening.

Stomach

The next organ along the alimentary canal is the **stomach**. As stated earlier, the stomach connects to the esophagus at the lower esophageal sphincter in the cardiac region of the stomach, also known as the *cardia*. To the left, the stomach curves upward, creating the fundic region, or **fundus**. A fundus is defined as a domed portion of a hollow organ that sits the farthest from, above, or opposite an opening. As you can see in **Figure 14-3**, the fundus of the stomach is located superior to (above) the opening to the esophagus.

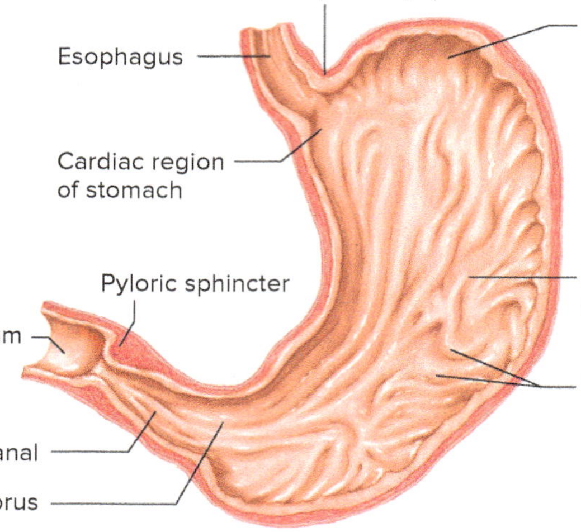

FIGURE 14-3 An illustration identifying the specific anatomical sites of the stomach

The lining of the stomach, a mucous membrane, contains gastric glands that secrete gastric juices. As with the function of saliva in the processing of food in the mouth, the gastric juices support the extraction of nutritional elements in the contents that entered from the esophagus. Mucous cells coat the internal wall of the stomach to prevent the gastric juices from digesting it. When this coating is flawed, the patient might develop a gastric (peptic) ulcer, a condition in which the acids in the stomach actually eat a hole in the lining and wall of the stomach. This diagnosis is reported with code K25.9 Gastric ulcer, unspecified as acute or chronic, without hemorrhage or perforation.

As the shape of the stomach's body curves downward, the inside of the curve on the side of the cardia is referred to as the *lesser curvature*, and the outside curve, coming down from the fundus, is referred to as the *greater curvature*. The lower portion of the stomach narrows as it nears the duodenum and connects to the small intestine. The pyloric sphincter is located here to control the emptying of the contents of the stomach into the lower half of the digestive system.

EXAMPLES

K31.1 Adult hypertrophic pyloric stenosis

K31.3 Pylorospasm, not elsewhere classified

Ulcers

An ulcer is a sore or hole in the tissue. Ulcers can occur externally, such as a decubitus ulcer, or they can form internally. The terms used to document an internal ulcer in the digestive system may include

- Ulcer of esophagus.
- Gastric ulcer (in the lining of the stomach).
- Duodenal ulcer.
- Gastrojejunal ulcer.

You will notice that these descriptors identify the location of the ulcer, such as the esophagus, the stomach, or the jejunum.

Further description of these ulcers may include known complications resulting from an ulcer in this segment of the upper digestive system: **perforation** and **hemorrhage**.

Perforation
An atypical hole in the wall of an organ or anatomical site.

Hemorrhage
Excessive or severe bleeding.

CODING BITES

If a medication caused the ulcer, an external cause code will be required to identify the specific drug and whether or not it was taken for therapeutic purposes.

LET'S CODE IT! SCENARIO

Pauline Ochoa had been taking aspirin several times a day every day for pain in her knees. Her husband, John, came home and found her lying on the kitchen floor. Emergency medical services (EMS) brought her to the ED. Tests revealed an acute perforated, hemorrhaging peptic ulcer due to chronic use of aspirin.

Let's Code It!

Pauline was diagnosed with an *acute perforated, hemorrhaging peptic ulcer*, so let's turn to the Alphabetic Index of ICD-10-CM and find

Ulcer, ulcerated, ulcerating, ulceration, ulcerative

There is a very long list of additional terms indented beneath this main listing, so read through it and find

Ulcer, ulcerated, ulcerating, ulceration, ulcerative
  peptic (site unspecified) K27.9

Beneath *peptic* is another indented list. Is there anything here that matches the physician's notes?

Ulcer, ulcerated, ulcerating, ulceration, ulcerative
  peptic (site unspecified) K27.9
    with
    hemorrhage K27.4
    and perforation K27.6
  acute K27.3
    with
    hemorrhage K27.0
    and perforation K27.2

Hmmm. The good news is that all of these choices are within one code category, K27, so let's turn to the Tabular List and begin reading at

✓4 **K27 Peptic ulcer, site unspecified**
Use additional code **to identify alcohol abuse and dependence (F10.-)**

Read the INCLUDES and EXCLUDES1 notes, as well as the *Use additional code* notation. Then read down and review all of the choices for the required fourth character. Which one matches the physician's notes the best?

K27.2 Acute peptic ulcer, site unspecified, with both hemorrhage and perforation

Excellent!

Are you done? No. Remember that notation beneath the code category?

Use additional code **to identify alcohol abuse and dependence (F10.-)**

(continued)

Was there any mention of alcohol abuse or alcohol dependence in the documentation? No. However, you do know that aspirin caused this ulcer. There is no notation, but remember that your job is to tell the *whole* story. So you will need to find an external cause code to report which drug caused Pauline's peptic ulcer. Aspirin is a drug, so let's turn to the *Table of Drugs and Chemicals* and find the name of the drug that caused Pauline's peptic ulcer in the first column ("Substance"): aspirin. Look across the line to the code listed in the column under "Adverse Effect." Remember that Pauline was taking the aspirin for therapeutic use—a medical reason. This shows code T39.015.

Let's turn to the T codes in the Tabular List and begin reading at

✓4 T39 Poisoning by, adverse effect of and underdosing of nonopioid analgesics, antipyretics, and antirheumatics

Notice that beneath this code category is a notation:

The appropriate 7th character is to be added to each code from category T39

A initial encounter

D subsequent encounter

S sequela

Remember, this is here for reference later. But first you need the fourth, fifth, and sixth characters. Read down and review all of the choices. Which one matches most accurately?

✓7 T39.015- Adverse effect of aspirin

Great! Now you need that seventh character. Go back to the documentation. Is this the first time that Pauline is being treated by this physician for this diagnosis? She is in the emergency department, so, yes, this is the initial encounter. Now you have two codes to report Pauline's condition:

K27.2 Acute peptic ulcer, site unspecified, with both hemorrhage and perforation

T39.015A Adverse effect of aspirin, initial encounter

Hernias

Hernia
A condition in which one anatomical structure pushes through a perforation in the wall of the anatomical site that normally contains that structure.

Gangrene
Necrotic tissue resulting from a loss of blood supply.

Obstruction
A blockage or closing.

A **hernia** is a condition that is created when a tear or opening in a muscle permits a part of an internal organ to push through. Due to the nature of one anatomical part squeezing through a hole in another site, the blood supply can be cut off to the section stuck in that opening. When that happens, the tissue might become necrotic (deteriorate and die) and/or develop **gangrene**. In addition, this condition can create an **obstruction** in the structure or organ, preventing the normal flow of material.

There are several types of hernias or anatomical sites that can be susceptible to herniation:

- *Hiatal* (esophageal) hernia may occur when a portion of the stomach pokes through an opening in the diaphragm; congenital diaphragmatic hernias are considered birth defects and reported from the congenital malformations section of ICD-10-CM.
- *Umbilical* hernia may occur when the muscle around the navel (belly button) does not close completely, permitting an internal organ to protrude.
- *Incisional* hernia is a defect that may occur at the site of a previous abdominal surgical opening (scar tissue).
- *Inguinal* hernias, more common in men, appear in the groin area.
- *Femoral* hernias, more common in women, appear in the upper thigh.

CODING BITES

If an activity, such as lifting something very heavy, causes an inguinal hernia, or if a surgical procedure causes an incisional hernia, additional codes may be required to tell the whole story.

YOU CODE IT! CASE STUDY

Jeffrey Gilberts, a 3-hours-old male, is brought in for Dr. Gensin to surgically repair his diaphragmatic hernia. He was born with this abnormal fistula in the diaphragm, diagnosed at 28 weeks gestation, but it was determined that he was not a candidate for in utero surgery.

You Code It!

Go through the steps of coding, and determine the code or codes that should be reported for this encounter between Dr. Gensin and Jeffrey Gilberts.

Step #1: Read the case carefully and completely.

Step #2: Abstract the scenario. Which main words or terms describe why the physician cared for the patient during this encounter?

Step #3: Are there any details missing or incomplete for which you would need to query the physician? [If so, ask your instructor.]

Step #4: Check for any relevant guidance, including reading all of the symbols and notations in the Tabular List and the appropriate sections of the Official Guidelines.

Step #5: Determine the correct diagnosis code or codes to explain why this encounter was medically necessary.

Step #6: Double-check your work.

Answer:

Did you determine this to be the correct code?

Q79.0 Congenital diaphragmatic hernia

Good job!

14.3 Conditions Affecting the Intestines

Small Intestine

The inferior aspect of the pyloric sphincter is the **duodenum**, the first segment of the small intestine. The duodenum curves around like the letter "C," with the pancreas tucked in the center. The hepatopancreatic sphincter, also called the *sphincter of Oddi*, is the connection point between the duodenum, the pancreatic duct, and the common bile duct that comes from the gallbladder and the liver.

Duodenum
The first segment of the small intestine, connecting the stomach to the jejunum.

Jejunum
The segment of the small intestine that connects the duodenum to the ileum.

Mesentery
A fold of a membrane that carries blood to the small intestine and connects it to the posterior wall of the abdominal cavity.

EXAMPLES

K29.80 Duodenitis without bleeding

K31.5 Obstruction of duodenum

As the duodenum trails into that last portion, at the bottom of the "C," it curves around and becomes the **jejunum**, the segment of the small intestine that twists and turns throughout the abdomen (see **Figure 14-4**). The **mesentery** is a membrane that connects to the jejunum like a spider web filled with blood vessels, nerves, and lymphatic vessels to provide nourishment to the intestine. On the anterior side of the abdominal cavity, coming from the greater curvature of the stomach down to the anterior of the jejunum like a protective curtain, is a double fold of the peritoneum called the *greater omentum*.

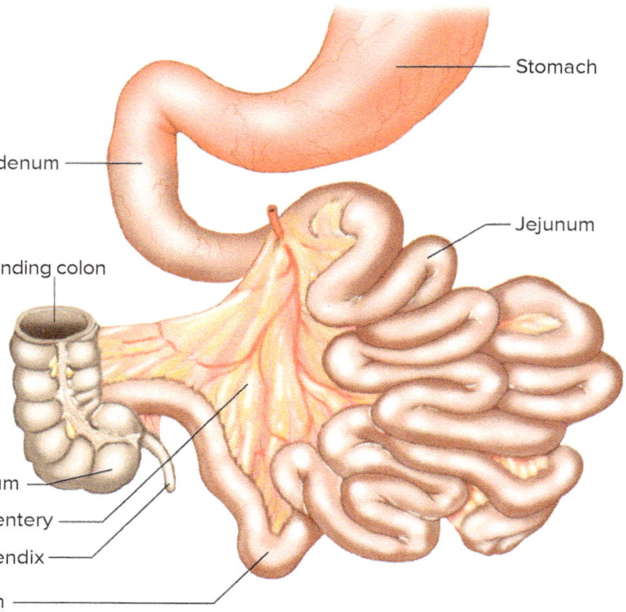

FIGURE 14-4 An illustration identifying the anatomical sites of the lower alimentary canal from the stomach to the cecum

> **Ileum**
> The last segment of the small intestine.

> **Cecum**
> A pouchlike organ that connects the ileum with the large intestine; the point of connection for the vermiform appendix.

> **CODING BITES**
>
> Be careful to not confuse il*e*um (with an *e*), the end of the small intestine, with il*i*um (with an *i*), the widest portion of the pelvic bones.
>
> - il*e*um is the end of the small intestine. Connect *il*e*um* with *e*nd.
> - il*i*um is a portion of the hip bone. Think of the *i* in *hi*p.

The last segment of the small intestine is the **ileum**. The ileum connects to the **cecum**, the bridge to the large intestine via the ileocecal sphincter. This sphincter controls the passage of material from the small intestine into the large intestine.

Gastrojejunal Ulcer

A lesion that develops in the small intestine can be quite problematic because it may interfere with the absorption of nutrients in the digestive process. As you review documentation for a diagnosis of a gastrojejunal ulcer, you will need to abstract some key details:

1. **Is the ulcer identified as acute or chronic?**

   K28.0–K28.3 Acute gastrojejunal ulcer . . .

   K28.4–K28.7 Chronic gastrojejunal ulcer . . .

2. **Is the ulcer hemorrhaging?**

   K28.0 Acute gastrojejunal ulcer with hemorrhage

   K28.4 Chronic or unspecified gastrojejunal ulcer with hemorrhage

3. **Has the ulcer perforated the wall of the small intestine?**

   K28.1 Acute gastrojejunal ulcer with perforation

   K28.5 Chronic or unspecified gastrojejunal ulcer with perforation

4. **Are hemorrhage and perforation both documented?**

   K28.2 Acute gastrojejunal ulcer with both hemorrhage and perforation

   K28.6 Chronic or unspecified gastrojejunal ulcer with both hemorrhage and perforation

5. **Has either hemorrhage or perforation been documented individually? If not . . .**

   K28.3 Acute gastrojejunal ulcer without hemorrhage or perforation

   K28.7 Chronic or unspecified gastrojejunal ulcer without hemorrhage or perforation

Of course, be certain to read the notations at the top of this code category:

Use additional code **to identify alcohol abuse and dependence (F10.-)**

EXCLUDES1 *primary ulcer of small intestine (K63.3)*

Read the documentation carefully, again, to determine if the physician noted whether the patient suffers with alcohol abuse or alcohol dependence. If so, you will need to code this, as well.

The jejunum is one specific part of the small intestine. The small intestine includes the duodenum, jejunum, mesentery, ileum, and cecum.

YOU CODE IT! CASE STUDY

Bernadette Bowers, a 29-year-old female, came to see Dr. Grandem with symptoms of persistent diarrhea and ongoing right lower quadrant (RLQ) abdominal pain. Lab work showed an increased white blood cell count and erythrocyte sedimentation rate. A barium enema showed string sign. A biopsy confirmed a diagnosis of Crohn's disease of the jejunum.

You Code It!

Go through the steps of coding, and determine the code or codes that should be reported for this encounter between Dr. Grandem and Bernadette.

Step #1: Read the case carefully and completely.
Step #2: Abstract the scenario. Which key words or terms describe why the physician cared for the patient during this encounter?
Step #3: Are there any details missing or incomplete for which you would need to query the physician? [If so, ask your instructor.]
Step #4: Check for any relevant guidance, including reading all of the symbols and notations in the Tabular List and the appropriate sections of the Official Guidelines.
Step #5: Determine the correct diagnosis code or codes to explain why this encounter was medically necessary.
Step #6: Double-check your work.

Answer:

Did you determine this to be the correct code?

K50.00 Crohn's disease of the small intestine without complications

Good job!

The Appendix

In the area between the end of the small intestine and the beginning of the large intestine is a small finger-like appendage known as the **vermiform appendix**, also called the *appendix*. Located in the lower right area of the abdomen, the reason for this tiny organ is a mystery because it has no known function.

Vermiform Appendix
A long, narrow mass of tissue attached to the cecum; also called *appendix*.

If a blockage develops within the appendix, this blockage can cause pressure to increase inside, interrupting blood flow, and becoming inflamed. This condition is known as *appendicitis*, and physicians can describe this diagnosis as: acute, chronic, or recurrent.

K36 Other appendicitis
Chronic appendicitis
Recurrent appendicitis

When treatment is not provided in a short time, the infected appendix is at risk for developing gangrene. As the coder, it is important to look for how the condition is described in the documentation to determine which one of the available combination codes might be accurate.

K35.00 Unspecified acute appendicitis

K35.890 Other acute appendicitis without perforation or gangrene

K35.891 Other acute appendicitis without perforation, with gangrene

If the blockage is not treated, the appendix can rupture (burst) and allow the infection to spread into the abdomen. This is known as *peritonitis*. When identified and treated quickly, the peritonitis can be limited to the immediate area (localized). However, after time, the infection can spread throughout the abdomen affecting other organs. Risk for an abscess and/or gangrene can increase, as well.

EXAMPLES

Codes used to report acute appendicitis with peritonitis:

K35.20	Acute appendicitis with generalized peritonitis, without perforation, with abscess
K35.31	Acute appendicitis with localized peritonitis and gangrene, without perforation
K35.33	Acute appendicitis with perforation and localized peritonitis, with abscess

Large Intestine

The colon is also known as the large intestine. As you look at the illustration (see **Figure 14-5**), you might wonder why it is considered large when the small intestine seems to be so much longer. This distinction has nothing to do with length; the large intestine has a larger diameter.

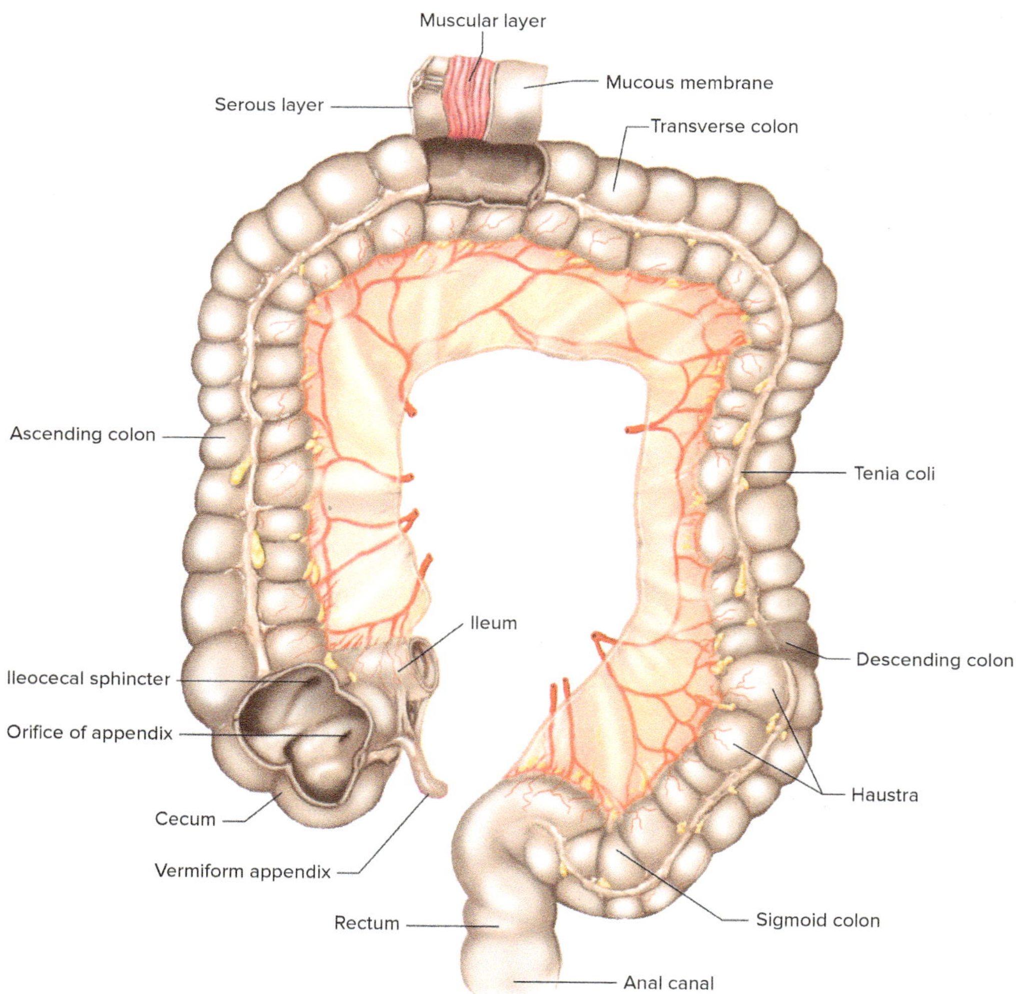

FIGURE 14-5 An illustration identifying the anatomical sites of the large intestine

You may notice that the two terms *colon* and *large intestine* are used almost interchangeably. In reality, they are technically not the same thing. The large intestine consists of the cecum, the vermiform appendix, the colon, the rectum, and the anus. The colon represents the majority of the large intestine. Let's take a look at the parts of the large intestine.

Starting at the cecum, the colon frames the abdomen almost like the beltway around Washington, D.C., and is referred to in four segments.

The ileum of the small intestine connects to the **ascending colon** on the right side of the large intestine at the cecum. The *vermiform appendix,* a rounded tubular appendage, protrudes from the end of the cecum. The ascending colon stretches upward from the cecum to just below the liver in the superior aspect of the abdomen. At this point, this tubular structure makes a sharp left turn, known as the *hepatic flexure* (named because of the proximity to the liver) and runs across to the left side. This section is known as the **transverse colon** because it traverses across the abdomen (*transverse* = across). On the left side, the colon turns downward at a curve known as the *splenic flexure* (named because of the proximity to the spleen), becoming the **descending colon**. It continues down until it slightly curves, just above the pelvis, and becomes the **sigmoid colon**.

The large intestine turns again, downward. This area is called the **rectum** (rectal vault), and it leads directly into the anal canal. At the distal end of the anal canal, the *internal and external anal sphincters* form the **anus**—the opening to the outside.

Ascending Colon
The portion of the large intestine that connects the cecum to the hepatic flexure.

Transverse Colon
The portion of the large intestine that connects the hepatic flexure to the splenic flexure.

Descending Colon
The segment of the large intestine that connects the splenic flexure to the sigmoid colon.

Sigmoid Colon
The dual-curved segment of the colon that connects the descending colon to the rectum; also referred to as the *sigmoid flexure.*

Rectum
The last segment of the large intestine, connecting the sigmoid colon to the anus.

Anus
The portion of the large intestine that leads outside the body.

EXAMPLES

K51.20 Ulcerative (chronic) proctitis without complications

K56.41 Fecal impaction of the intestine

YOU CODE IT! CASE STUDY

Gerald Candahar, a 51-year-old male, was brought into the procedure room so Dr. Avalino could remove his anal polyps.

You Code It!

Go through the steps of coding, and determine the code or codes that should be reported for this encounter between Dr. Avalino and Gerald.

Step #1: Read the case carefully and completely.
Step #2: Abstract the scenario. Which key words or terms describe why the physician cared for the patient during this encounter?
Step #3: Are there any details missing or incomplete for which you would need to query the physician? [If so, ask your instructor.]
Step #4: Check for any relevant guidance, including reading all of the symbols and notations in the Tabular List and the appropriate sections of the Official Guidelines.
Step #5: Determine the correct diagnosis code or codes to explain why this encounter was medically necessary.
Step #6: Double-check your work.

Answer:

Did you determine this to be the correct code?

K62.0 Anal polyp

Good job!

Ulcerative Colitis

An inflammation of the lining of the colon is known as ulcerative colitis. This is often a chronic illness and believed to be a malfunction in the immune response within the mucosa. Studies have shown a familial tendency. Signs and symptoms include bloody diarrhea with asymptomatic periods of time between attacks. Abdominal pain, irritability, weight loss, weakness, nausea, and vomiting are also indicators.

Manifestations, such as pancolitis, proctitis, rectosigmoiditis, and inflammatory polyps in the colon are not uncommon. In addition, the presence of rectal bleeding, obstruction within the intestinal tract, fistulae, and abscesses must be included in the code or codes, as documented.

The terms you need to abstract from the documentation will lead you to the correct fourth character to identify the manifestations:

✓5	K51.0	Ulcerative (chronic) pancolitis
✓5	K51.2	Ulcerative (chronic) proctitis
✓5	K51.3	Ulcerative (chronic) rectosigmoiditis
✓5	K51.4	Inflammatory polyps of colon
✓5	K51.5	Left sided colitis
✓5	K51.8	Other ulcerative colitis

Then, fifth and sixth characters will identify the presence of rectal bleeding, intestinal obstruction, fistula, abscess, or other complication.

Diverticular Disease of the Intestine

Since the first page of this book, you have learned that you must read carefully and completely, and this habit will be especially important when determining the code for a patient diagnosed with diverticular disease. There are two conditions, which are very different, reported from code category ✓4 K57 Diverticular disease of intestine:

- *Diverticulosis:* small pouches develop and protrude outward through the intestine.
- *Diverticulitis:* when these pouches become inflamed or infected.

While abstracting the documentation, you also will need to determine:

1. Is the small intestine, the large intestine, or both affected?
2. Is there mention of perforation, abscess, or bleeding?

YOU CODE IT! CASE STUDY

Lisa Begas, a 63-year-old female, came in complaining of a low-grade fever with chills for 3 days, nausea and vomiting, and cramps. Dr. Allendale did a CT scan of her abdomen and pelvis, and determined that she had diverticulitis without perforation or bleeding of the colon.

You Code It!

Read the scenario of Dr. Allendale's encounter with Lisa, and determine the accurate diagnosis code or codes.

Step #1: Read the case carefully and completely.
Step #2: Abstract the scenario. Which main words or terms describe why the physician cared for the patient during this encounter?
Step #3: Are there any details missing or incomplete for which you would need to query the physician? [If so, ask your instructor.]

(continued)

Step #4: Check for any relevant guidance, including reading all of the symbols and notations in the Tabular List and the appropriate sections of the Official Guidelines.

Step #5: Determine the correct diagnosis code or codes to explain why this encounter was medically necessary.

Step #6: Double-check your work.

Answer:

Did you determine this to be the code?

K57.32 Diverticulitis of large intestine without perforation or abscess without bleeding

Fissures and Fistula of Anal and Rectal Regions

When a narrow tunnel forms between the anal canal and the external aspect of the skin near the buttocks it is known as a fistula. For 2025, there are 27 new codes each identifying a location of a fistula [anal, rectal, or anorectal], its complexity [simple or complex], as well as frequency [initial, persistent, or recurrent].

K60.3- **-Anal fistula**

K60.4- **-Rectal fistula**

K60.5- **-Anorectal fistula**

14.4 Dysfunction of the Digestive Accessory Organs and Malabsorption

The digestive **accessory organs** play a role in the way the body processes food and water so that each tissue and organ system has the fuel to function. These organs secrete enzymes, alkalis, and other substances that are required for the process of digestion, and they include the gallbladder, liver, and pancreas. The accessory organs connect to the alimentary canal and support it, but they are not a part of it.

Accessory Organs
Organs that assist the digestive process and are adjacent to the alimentary canal: the gallbladder, liver, and pancreas.

Gallbladder
A pear-shaped organ that stores bile until it is required to aid the digestive process.

Common Bile Duct
The juncture of the cystic duct of the gallbladder and the hepatic duct from the liver.

Gallbladder

In the top left corner of **Figure 14-6**, the pear-shaped pouch is the **gallbladder**. This sac is a storage tank for bile, a yellow-green liquid created by the liver and used by the body to assist in the digestive process. When required, the gallbladder contracts to release bile into the duodenum via the **common bile duct** and the hepatopancreatic ampulla. The common bile duct is the juncture where the *hepatic duct* (which comes from the liver) meets the *cystic duct* (which comes from the gallbladder). At the *hepatopancreatic sphincter*, both the common bile duct and the pancreatic duct meet to continue into the duodenum.

CODING BITES

Due to the interactive nature of the anatomical organs in this small area of the body, you may notice long, complex medical terms used in diagnostic statements. Don't be intimidated; just use your knowledge from medical terminology class and parse the terms. For example: choledocholithiasis: *chole* = bile + *docho* = common bile duct + *lith* = calculus + *iasis* = pathologic condition.

EXAMPLES

K81.0 Acute cholecystitis

K82.3 Fistula of gallbladder

Cholecystitis

Cholecystitis is the medical term for inflammation of the gallbladder (*chole* = bile + *cyst* = fluid-filled sac + *-itis* = inflammation). In cases where the disease affects the bile duct rather than the gallbladder, the diagnosis is cholangitis.

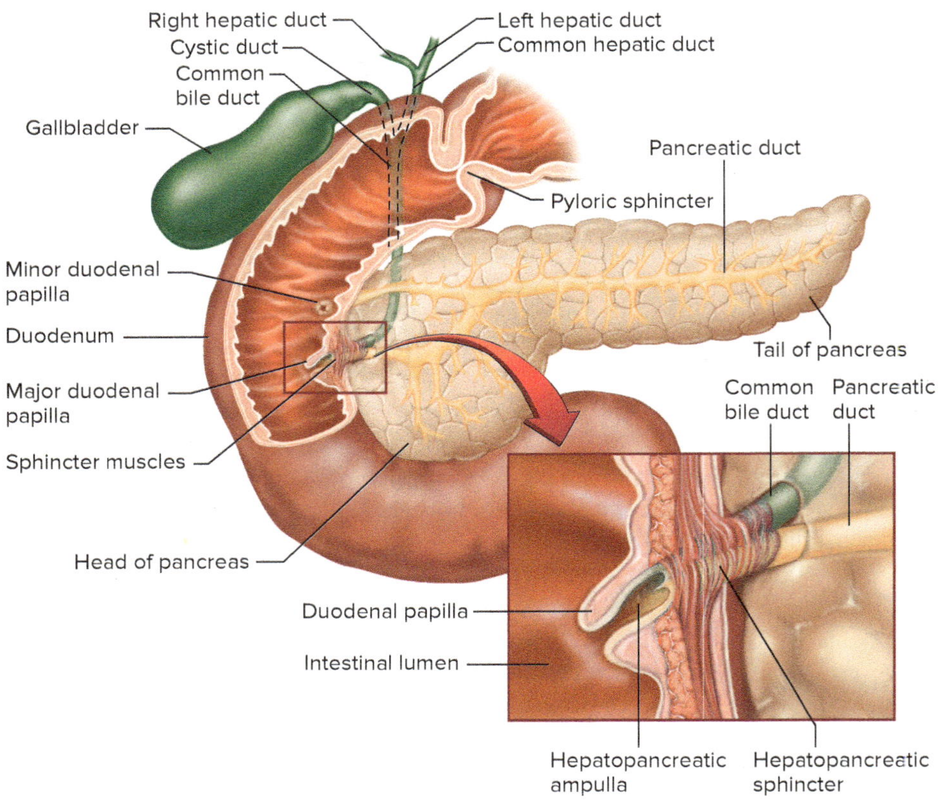

FIGURE 14-6 An illustration identifying the anatomical sites within the accessory organs

> **Cholelithiasis**
> Gallstones.

Calculi can accumulate in this area and harden into small rocks (stones) that may block the flow of bile from the gallbladder. This condition is known as **cholelithiasis**. This may occur with or without cholecystitis, changing the code used to report the condition.

EXAMPLES

K80.70	Calculus of gallbladder and bile duct without cholecystitis without obstruction
K81.1	Chronic cholecystitis

Pancreas

> **Pancreas**
> A gland that secretes insulin and other hormones from the islet cells into the bloodstream and manufactures digestive enzymes that are secreted into the duodenum.

> **Pancreatic Islets**
> Cells within the pancreas that secrete insulin and other hormones into the bloodstream.

Situated posterior to the stomach, tucked inside a curve of the duodenum, is the **pancreas**. The section of the pancreas adjacent to the duodenum, called the *head of the pancreas*, extends to the center section (the body of the pancreas), and then further extends to the tail of the pancreas, which forms almost a fingerlike shape. The **pancreatic islets** (the islets of Langerhans) create glucagon and insulin, as well as other hormones, and secrete them into the bloodstream. Similar to the gallbladder, the pancreas manufactures certain digestive enzymes that pass into the duodenum via the pancreatic duct (see **Figure 14-6**).

Malfunction of the pancreas may lead to various health problems, including pancreatic cancer, pancreatitis, cystic fibrosis, and diabetes mellitus. One of the most dangerous concerns about the impact on the body of conditions of the pancreas is that signs and symptoms are few and nonspecific, making diagnosis difficult. For example, there is actually a treatment for pancreatic cancer. However, due to lack of signs and symptoms that typically promote early identification and treatment, diagnosis is not often realized until the malignancy has metastasized to other organs and cannot be halted.

Pancreatitis

Acute pancreatitis occurs suddenly and usually goes away in a few days with treatment. However, when you are determining the correct code for this diagnosis, you must abstract the underlying cause of the pancreatitis:

K85.0- **Idiopathic acute pancreatitis**

K85.1- **Biliary acute pancreatitis**

K85.2- **Alcohol-induced acute pancreatitis**

K85.3- **Drug-induced acute pancreatitis**

Note that alcohol-induced acute pancreatitis and alcohol-induced chronic pancreatitis are reported from different code categories.

K86.0 **Alcohol-induced chronic pancreatitis**

Liver

The **liver** is an almost triangular-shaped organ (see **Figure 14-7**) located in the right upper quadrant (RUQ) of the abdominal cavity, beneath the diaphragm, anterior to the stomach and pancreas. As the largest gland in the body, it performs many functions, including regulating blood sugar levels and aiding the digestive process by secreting bile to the gallbladder. The liver cleans the blood of toxins; metabolizes proteins, fats, and carbohydrates; and manufactures some blood proteins.

Liver
The organ, located in the upper right area of the abdominal cavity, that is responsible for regulating blood sugar levels; secreting bile for the gallbladder; metabolizing fats, proteins, and carbohydrates; manufacturing some blood proteins; and removing toxins from the blood.

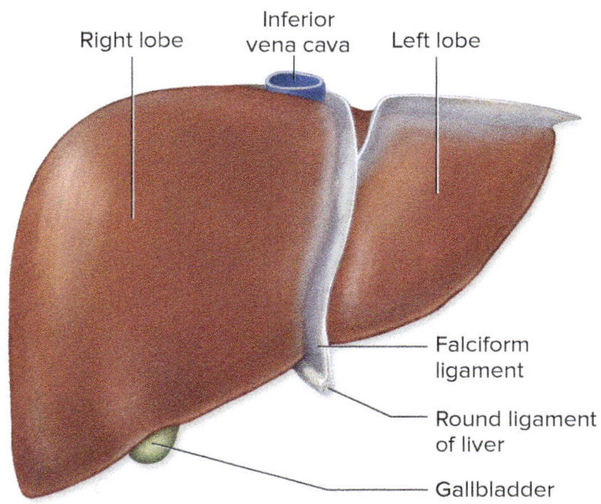

FIGURE 14-7 An illustration identifying the anatomical sites of the liver (anterior view)

CODING BITES

The medical root *hepa-* or *hepat-* is used in most diagnoses and other descriptive terms to refer to the liver as the anatomical site involved. For example, the term *hepatic failure* identifies a condition that has rendered the liver ineffective.

Hepatitis

Hepatitis (*hepa-* = liver + *-itis* = inflammation or disease) is a swelling of the liver that causes a reduction in function. Most often, hepatitis is caused by a virus, resulting in a diagnosis that includes the specific type of inflammation, such as hepatitis A, hepatitis B, and so on. (For more details on this condition, see the chapter ***Coding Infectious Diseases***.)

There are cases when drugs and alcohol can lead to this same diagnosis. Identified as acute or chronic nonviral hepatitis, most patients will exhibit signs and symptoms very similar to viral hepatitis, including nausea, vomiting, and jaundice (yellowing of the skin). Take a look at the *Use additional code* notation beneath code category K70:

K70 **Alcohol liver disease**

Use additional code **to identify:**

alcohol abuse and dependence (F10.-)

CODING BITES

You will need to determine from the documentation if the use (abuse) of alcohol has contributed to the diagnosis because this may affect the determination of the correct code or the need for an additional code. At code category K70 Alcoholic liver disease is a notation to remind you:

> ***Use additional code*** **to identify: alcohol abuse and dependence (F10.-)**

EXAMPLES

B18.2	Chronic viral hepatitis C
K70.10	Alcoholic hepatitis without ascites
K76.4	Peliosis hepatis

Cirrhosis

After a person suffers with chronic hepatic disease, fibrotic tissue may form on hepatic cells causing scarring, known as *cirrhosis of the liver*. This condition may be caused by injury as well. The scar tissue impairs the normal function of the liver and can result in easy bruising or bleeding, abdominal swelling, lower extremity edema, and possibly kidney failure. There is evidence that approximately 5% of patients suffering with cirrhosis will develop liver cancer.

EXAMPLES

K74.3	Primary biliary cirrhosis
K74.69	Other cirrhosis of liver

YOU CODE IT! CASE STUDY

After struggling to deal with a sharp pain that went from his stomach area straight through to his back, Saul Braverman went to see Dr. Spiegel. After a full examination and an ultrasound, Dr. Spiegel confirmed Saul's cholelithiasis and they discussed plans for surgery.

You Code It!

Abstract this documentation about the encounter between Dr. Spiegel and Saul.

Step #1: Read the case carefully and completely.
Step #2: Abstract the scenario. Which main words or terms describe why the physician cared for the patient during this encounter?
Step #3: Are there any details missing or incomplete for which you would need to query the physician? [If so, ask your instructor.]
Step #4: Check for any relevant guidance, including reading all of the symbols and notations in the Tabular List and the appropriate sections of the Official Guidelines.
Step #5: Determine the correct diagnosis code or codes to explain why this encounter was medically necessary.
Step #6: Double-check your work.

Answer:

Did you determine this to be the code?

K80.20 Calculus of gallbladder without cholecystitis without obstruction

Celiac Disease

While you may see a great deal in the news and advertisements about gluten-free products, the facts support that celiac disease, also known as gluten enteropathy, is uncommon. This condition is suffered by twice as many women than men, and has been seen to be familial (common in families).

Recurrent attacks of diarrhea, abdominal distention due to flatulence, stomach cramps, and weakness are some of the most frequently experienced signs and symptoms. When diagnosed in adults, celiac disease may be the underlying cause of multiple ulcers forming within the lining of the small intestine. Biopsies from the small bowel, identifying histologic changes, would confirm this diagnosis.

EXAMPLE

K90.0 Celiac disease

Use additional code **for associated disorders including:**

dermatitis herpetiformis (L13.0)

gluten ataxia (G32.81)

Code also **exocrine pancreatic insufficiency (K86.81)**

14.5 Reporting the Involvement of Alcohol in Digestive Disorders

Alcohol abuse can increase the risk of developing several serious disorders of the digestive system. When the documentation includes a connection of alcohol abuse in the diagnosis, you will need to report this with an additional code.

When reading the documentation for digestive system disorders, be aware of these diagnoses that are known to be connected to alcohol abuse. If there is any indication, you might need to query the physician.

- *Mouth cancer and gum disease:* alcohol abuse increases the risk, second only to tobacco abuse.
- *GERD and gastritis:* excessive use of alcohol can damage the sphincter between the esophagus and the stomach, permitting stomach acids to backwash into the esophagus. The lining of the stomach also can become irritated.
- *Malabsorption and malnutrition:* the consistent and excessive intake of alcohol can interfere with the body's ability to absorb nutrients.
- *Pancreatitis:* alcohol abuse can cause inflammation in the pancreas and interfere with the proper function of the digestive process.
- *Alcoholic liver disease:* alcohol abuse can cause this condition, a precursor to cirrhosis.

CODING BITES

In some cases, throughout the ICD-10-CM, the Tabular List will remind you that the involvement of alcohol abuse also must be reported:

✓4 **K05 Gingivitis and periodontal diseases**

Use additional code **to identify: alcohol abuse and dependence (F10.-)**

YOU CODE IT! CASE STUDY

Noel Cooper, a 43-year-old male, came to see Dr. Briscow with complaints of epigastric discomfort, nausea, and indigestion over the last several days. He admits to drinking alcohol at lunch and dinner daily. He states he often has a couple in the evening as well. A gastroscopy was performed, and Dr. Briscow confirmed a diagnosis of acute gastritis due to alcohol abuse.

(continued)

You Code It!

Review the details of this encounter between Dr. Briscow and Noel Cooper.

Step #1: Read the case carefully and completely.
Step #2: Abstract the scenario. Which main words or terms describe why the physician cared for the patient during this encounter?
Step #3: Are there any details missing or incomplete for which you would need to query the physician? [If so, ask your instructor.]
Step #4: Check for any relevant guidance, including reading all of the symbols and notations in the Tabular List and the appropriate sections of the Official Guidelines.
Step #5: Determine the correct diagnosis code or codes to explain why this encounter was medically necessary.
Step #6: Double-check your work.

Answer:

Did you determine these to be the codes?

K29.00 Acute gastritis without bleeding

F10.188 Alcohol abuse with other alcohol-induced disorder

Good job!!

Chapter Summary

The organs included in the digestive system run from the head to the bottom of the torso. Therefore, several different health care specialists may be involved in caring for patients with digestive disorders, depending upon where the abnormality is located. Health care issues within the digestive system can occur as the result of a congenital anomaly, a traumatic event, or dietary influence. This means that there may be times when an external cause code is required to be included so that you can tell the whole story about the reasons why (the medical necessity) this patient was cared for.

CODING BITES

Health Conditions Connected to Poor Oral Hygiene	
Disease of the gums of the mouth, known as *periodontal disease*, has been shown to affect the health of other organs throughout the body. Some examples include:	
Cardiovascular system	• Increased risk of stroke • Increased risk of fatal heart attack • Increased risk of cardiovascular disease • Increased risk of clotting disorder
Respiratory system	Bacteria from mouth, dental plaque buildup, and throat can contribute to pneumonia and other lung diseases.
Musculoskeletal system	Increased risk of osteopenia.
Endocrine system	Interference with control of diabetes mellitus.
Reproductive system	• During gestation, mothers with advanced periodontitis are at increased risk for premature and/or underweight neonates. • Microbes from periodontitis can cross through the placenta and expose the fetus to infection.

CHAPTER 14 REVIEW
Coding Digestive System Conditions

Let's Check It! Terminology

Match each key term to the appropriate definition.

Part I

1. **LO 14.1** Small, calcified protrusions with roots in the jaw.
2. **LO 14.4** Cells within the pancreas that secrete insulin and other hormones into the bloodstream.
3. **LO 14.4** A large gland responsible for creating digestive enzymes.
4. **LO 14.3** The last segment of the small intestine.
5. **LO 14.2** A saclike organ within the alimentary canal designed to contain nourishment during the initial phase of the digestive process.
6. **LO 14.3** A long, narrow mass of tissue attached to the cecum; also called *appendix*.
7. **LO 14.3** The last segment of the large intestine, connecting the sigmoid colon to the anus.
8. **LO 14.2** The tubular organ that connects the pharynx to the stomach for the passage of nourishment.
9. **LO 14.4** The organ, located in the upper right area of the abdominal cavity, that is responsible for regulating blood sugar levels; secreting bile for the gallbladder; metabolizing fats, proteins, and carbohydrates; manufacturing some blood proteins; and removing toxins from the blood.
10. **LO 14.3** The portion of the large intestine that leads outside the body.
11. **LO 14.3** The first segment of the small intestine, connecting the stomach to the jejunum.
12. **LO 14.3** The segment of the small intestine that connects the duodenum to the ileum.

- **A.** Anus
- **B.** Duodenum
- **C.** Esophagus
- **D.** Ileum
- **E.** Jejunum
- **F.** Liver
- **G.** Pancreas
- **H.** Pancreatic Islets
- **I.** Rectum
- **J.** Stomach
- **K.** Teeth
- **L.** Vermiform Appendix

Part II

1. **LO 14.3** A pouchlike organ that connects the ileum with the large intestine; the point of connection for the vermiform appendix.
2. **LO 14.3** The segment of the large intestine that connects the splenic flexure to the sigmoid colon.
3. **LO 14.3** The portion of the large intestine that connects the hepatic flexure to the splenic flexure.
4. **LO 14.4** The juncture of the cystic duct of the gallbladder and the hepatic duct from the liver.
5. **LO 14.3** The portion of the large intestine that connects the cecum to the hepatic flexure.
6. **LO 14.3** The dual-curved segment of the colon that connects the descending colon to the rectum.
7. **LO 14.1** The opening in the face that begins the alimentary canal and is used for the input of nutrition; also known as the *mouth*.
8. **LO 14.1** Three sets of bilateral exocrine glands that secrete saliva: parotid glands, submaxillary glands, and the sublingual glands.

- **A.** Ascending Colon
- **B.** Cecum
- **C.** Common Bile Duct
- **D.** Descending Colon
- **E.** Oral Cavity
- **F.** Salivary Glands
- **G.** Sigmoid Colon
- **H.** Transverse Colon

Part III

1. **LO 14.2** A blockage or closing.
2. **LO 14.2** An atypical hole in the wall of an organ or anatomical site.
3. **LO 14.4** Organs that assist the digestive process and are adjacent to the alimentary canal: the gallbladder, liver, and pancreas.
4. **LO 14.4** Gallstones.
5. **LO 14.3** A fold of a membrane that carries blood to the small intestine and connects it to the posterior wall of the abdominal cavity.
6. **LO 14.2** A circular muscle that contracts to prevent passage of liquids or solids.
7. **LO 14.4** A pear-shaped organ that stores bile until it is required to aid the digestive process.
8. **LO 14.2** The domed section of an organ farthest from its opening.
9. **LO 14.1** Absence of teeth.
10. **LO 14.2** A condition in which one anatomical structure pushes through a perforation in the wall of the anatomical site that normally contains that structure.
11. **LO 14.2** Necrotic tissue resulting from a loss of blood supply.
12. **LO 14.2** Excessive or severe bleeding.

A. Accessory Organs
B. Cholelithiasis
C. Edentulism
D. Fundus
E. Gallbladder
F. Gangrene
G. Hemorrhage
H. Hernia
I. Mesentery
J. Obstruction
K. Perforation
L. Sphincter

Let's Check It! Concepts

Choose the most appropriate answer for each of the following questions.

1. **LO 14.2** The correct code for a diaphragmatic hernia with obstruction without gangrene is
   a. K44. **b.** K44.0. **c.** K44.1. **d.** K44.9.
2. **LO 14.3** The duodenum, jejunum, and ileum are all parts of the
   a. esophagus. **b.** liver. **c.** small intestine. **d.** large intestine.
3. **LO 14.1** When you are abstracting the documentation regarding acquired loss of teeth: Class _____ establishes the existence of other factors significantly affecting the outcomes of treatment and the need for surgical revision of the supporting structures (gums and bone) to create an opportunity for prosthodontics.
   a. I **b.** II **c.** III **d.** IV
4. **LO 14.4** Cirrhosis of the liver can be caused by
   a. abuse of alcohol. **b.** trauma. **c.** disease. **d.** all of these.
5. **LO 14.2** A hiatal hernia occurs at the
   a. esophagus. **b.** small intestine. **c.** surgical site. **d.** groin.
6. **LO 14.3** What is the correct code for an acute appendicitis with peritonitis?
   a. K35.200 **b.** K35.30 **c.** K35.80 **d.** K35.891
7. **LO 14.3** The transverse colon lies between the
   a. ascending colon and the hepatic flexure. **b.** hepatic flexure and the splenic flexure.
   c. splenic flexure and the sigmoid colon. **d.** sigmoid colon and the anus.
8. **LO 14.4** Cholelithiasis is commonly known as
   a. disease of the liver. **b.** disease of the colon. **c.** gallstones. **d.** pancreatic cancer.
9. **LO 14.2** Necrotic tissue resulting from a loss of blood supply is known as
   a. obstruction. **b.** hemorrhage. **c.** perforation. **d.** gangrene.
10. **LO 14.5** All of the following are known to be diagnoses that could be connected to alcohol abuse *except*
    a. GERD. **b.** pancreatitis.
    c. malabsorption and malnutrition. **d.** all of these could be connected to alcohol abuse.

Let's Check It! Rules and Regulations

Please answer the following questions from the knowledge you have gained after reading this chapter.

1. **LO 14.1** When you are abstracting the documentation regarding acquired loss of teeth, you will need to identify three specified details from the notes. What are the three details?
2. **LO 14.2** Explain the condition of GERD.
3. **LO 14.3** What are the key details you need to abstract from the documentation for coding a gastrojejunal ulcer?
4. **LO 14.4** Which is the largest gland in the body? Where is it located, and what is its function?
5. **LO 14.5** Discuss how alcohol abuse can affect the digestive system.

ICD-10-CM

YOU CODE IT! Basics

First, identify the condition in the following diagnoses; then code the diagnosis.

Example: Acute pulpitis

a. main term: *Pulpitis* **b.** diagnosis: *K04.0*

1. Dental caries on pit and fissure surface, penetrating into dentin:
   a. main term:______ **b.** diagnosis:______
2. Acute generalized periodontitis severe:
   a. main term:______ **b.** diagnosis:______
3. Odontogenic cyst:
   a. main term:______ **b.** diagnosis:______
4. Exfoliative cheilitis:
   a. main term:______ **b.** diagnosis:______
5. Leukoplakia of oral mucosa:
   a. main term:______ **b.** diagnosis:______
6. Hypertrophy of tongue papillae:
   a. main term:______ **b.** diagnosis:______
7. Eosinophilic esophagitis:
   a. main term:______ **b.** diagnosis:______
8. Acute gastric ulcer:
   a. main term:______ **b.** diagnosis:______
9. Alcoholic gastritis:
   a. main term:______ **b.** diagnosis:______
10. Hyperplasia of the appendix:
    a. main term:______ **b.** diagnosis:______
11. Inguinal hernia with gangrene:
    a. main term:______ **b.** diagnosis:______
12. Inflammatory polyps of colon with abscess:
    a. main term:______ **b.** diagnosis:______
13. Chronic ischemic colitis:
    a. main term:______ **b.** diagnosis:______
14. Rectal prolapse:
    a. main term:______ **b.** diagnosis:______
15. Radiation proctitis:
    a. main term:______ **b.** diagnosis:______

ICD-10-CM

YOU CODE IT! Practice

Using the techniques described in this chapter, carefully read through the case studies and determine the most accurate ICD-10-CM code(s) and external cause code(s), if appropriate, for each case study.

1. Dorothea Greig, a 26-year-old female, presents with the complaint of persistent pain in her lower left abdomen, 1-week duration. Dorothea says she has also experienced nausea and vomiting. Dr. Hendrix notes weakness and a temperature of 102.2 F. The decision is made to admit the patient. Following a review of the laboratory tests, liver function tests, and the CT scan, Dorothea is diagnosed with diverticulitis of both the small and large intestines; abscess is noted.

(continued)

2. Kent Rhodes, a 28-month-old male, is brought in by his parents for a checkup. Dr. Washington notes Kent's deciduous teeth are smaller than normal and widely spaced with notches on the biting surface. Kent is diagnosed with Hutchinson's teeth.
3. Leigh Norman, a 37-year-old female, comes in today with the complaint of shortness of breath. Dr. Schimek notes tachypnea, tachycardia, and cyanosis. Upon auscultation, bowel sounds are heard in the chest area. Leigh is admitted to Weston Hospital. After reviewing the arterial blood gases, laboratory results, and CT scan, Leigh is diagnosed with a diaphragmatic hernia with obstruction. Surgery is scheduled.
4. John Bandings, a 53-year-old male, presents today with fever and jaundice. John admits to drinking alcohol for decades. After reviewing the test results, Dr. Fong diagnoses John with alcoholic cirrhosis of the liver with ascites.
5. Maxine Weber, a 42-year-old female, comes in today with the complaint of severe pain in the right side of her lower abdomen. Maxine also says she has vomited. Dr. Jefferson documents a temperature of 101 F. Maxine is admitted to the hospital, where a CT scan confirms the diagnosis of acute appendicitis with localized peritonitis.
6. Archie Blume, a 41-year-old male, presents with the complaint of swollen tender gums and bleeding after he brushes his teeth. Dr. Day notes Archie uses tobacco. After an examination and x-rays, Archie is diagnosed with acute gingivitis, nonplaque induced.
7. Allen Klebb, a 36-year-old male, comes in today complaining of diarrhea and vomiting. Allen just finished his radiation treatments for his hand malignancy. Dr. Ard diagnoses Allen with gastroenteritis due to radiation.
8. Paula Dent, a 3-year-old female, is diagnosed with a congenital trachea-esophageal fistula with atresia of the esophagus. Paula is admitted to Weston Hospital for surgical repair.
9. Walter Logan, a 59-year-old male, presents today with a yellow-brownish tongue. Walter admits to a bad taste in his mouth. Dr. Roche completes an examination, noting hypertrophy of the central dorsal tongue papillae. The biopsy confirms a diagnosis of black hairy tongue.
10. Robert Thomas, an 82-year-old male, presents today with severe epigastric pain. Robert also has been experiencing sharp chest pain that radiated to the left side of the neck and arm. Robert is admitted to the hospital, where an upper GI series confirms the diagnosis of volvulus of the colon with perforation.
11. Michelle Toatley, a 51-year-old female, presents with the complaints of stomach pain and bloating. Michelle admits to vomiting. Dr. Mobley notes patient has a history of heartburn and current alcohol abuse. The EGD confirms a diagnosis of acute gastric ulcer.
12. Harry Wisemann, a 46-year-old male, comes in today with the complaint of long-lasting heartburn and pain under his breastbone. Harry admits to taking aspirin several times a day for many years. Dr. Camut diagnoses Harry with an ulcer of the esophagus due to ingestion of aspirin.
13. C.E. Molyneaux, a 34-year-old male, comes in today with the complaint of a lump in his groin area. Dr. Williams completes a physical examination of the groin region and notes a bulge on the right side when C.E. is standing erect. A CT scan confirms a diagnosis of a femoral hernia, unilateral. C.E. is admitted to the hospital for surgical repair.
14. Carla Jett, a 45-year-old female, presents today with bloody diarrhea and weakness. Carla states this has been going on over the last few weeks. Dr. Edenton completes a thorough examination, noting a small ulcer on Carla's left leg and a temperature of 102.1 F. Carla is admitted to the hospital for a full workup. After reviewing the laboratory tests and the MRI scan, Carla is diagnosed with ulcerative pancolitis with rectal bleeding and pyoderma gangrenosum.
15. Jonathan Stutts, a 41-year-old male, comes in today with the complaint of abdominal pain with some diarrhea and bloating. Dr. Dresdner completes a thorough examination with the appropriate laboratory tests. Jonathan is diagnosed with idiopathic sclerosing mesenteric fibrosis.

YOU CODE IT! Application

The following exercises provide practice in abstracting physicians' notes and learning to work with documentation from our health care facility, Prader, Bracker, & Associates. These case studies are modeled on real patient encounters. Using the techniques described in this chapter, carefully read through the case studies and determine the most accurate ICD-10-CM code(s) and external cause code(s), if appropriate, for each case study.

(continued)

WESTON HOSPITAL

629 Healthcare Way • SOMEWHERE, FL 32811 • 407-555-6541

PATIENT: UMBRELL, MORGAN

ACCOUNT/EHR #: UMBRMO001

Attending Physician: Renee O. Bracker, MD

S: Patient is a 41-year-old female complaining of localized pain in the upper right quadrant radiating to the right scapular tip. Pain usually begins postprandial and is intense for approximately a 5-hour duration and then subsides. Pain is not relieved by emesis, flatus, or position change.

O: H: 5′3″, Wt: 146 lb., R: 19, HR: 125, BP: 135/73, T: 102.4 F. Dr. Bracker notes diaphoresis, slight jaundice, as well as hypoactive bowel sound. CT scan confirms a bile duct calculus. Morgan is admitted for surgery.

A: Choledocholithiasis, acute with cholangitis, and obstruction

P: Laparoscopic cholecystectomy

Determine the most accurate ICD-10-CM code(s).

PRADER, BRACKER, & ASSOCIATES

A Complete Health Care Facility

159 Healthcare Way • SOMEWHERE, FL 32811 • 407-555-6789

PATIENT: SEQUEN, EUGENE

ACCOUNT/EHR #: SEQUEU001

Attending Physician: Oscar R. Prader, MD

Patient is a 49-year-old male diagnosed with chronic acid reflux. Barium swallow fluoroscopy, esophageal pH probe, esophageal manometry, and esophagoscopy were completed. He presents today to discuss the results of those tests.

I explain that the test results indicate that he has GERD. The first course of treatment is to adopt a low-fat, high-fiber diet. The second course would be surgical repair. Patient was instructed not to eat at least 2 hours before going to bed, and the head of the bed should be elevated 6 to 8 inches while in supine position.

Patient was informed that surgery may be necessary if diet and positioning do not relieve symptoms.

Determine the most accurate ICD-10-CM code(s).

PRADER, BRACKER, & ASSOCIATES

A Complete Health Care Facility

159 Healthcare Way • SOMEWHERE, FL 32811 • 407-555-6789

PATIENT: HERMAN, CONNIE

ACCOUNT/EHR #: HERMCO001

Attending Physician: Oscar R. Prader, MD

S: This 43-year-old female comes in with complaints of hematemesis and epigastric pain.

O: Esophageal tears are visualized during a fiberoptic endoscopy.

(continued)

A: Mallory-Weiss syndrome, confirmed.

P: The options of electrocoagulation therapy for hemostasis and surgery to suture the esophageal lacerations if the condition did not resolve itself were discussed.

Determine the most accurate ICD-10-CM code(s).

PRADER, BRACKER, & ASSOCIATES

A Complete Health Care Facility

159 Healthcare Way • SOMEWHERE, FL 32811 • 407-555-6789

PATIENT: GRAILLE, VAN

ACCOUNT/EHR #: GRAIVA001

Attending Physician: Oscar R. Prader, MD

S: Patient is a 27-year-old male complaining of abdominal pain with alternating diarrhea and constipation. Abdominal distention is evident.

O: Complete history is obtained, including psychological profile. Sigmoidoscopy is completed.

A: Irritable bowel syndrome with diarrhea, confirmed.

P: Patient is asked to keep a food diary in order to identify foods that aggravate the condition.

Follow-up appointment 10–14 days

Determine the most accurate ICD-10-CM code(s).

PRADER, BRACKER, & ASSOCIATES

A Complete Health Care Facility

159 Healthcare Way • SOMEWHERE, FL 32811 • 407-555-6789

PATIENT: ELLISON, THERESA

ACCOUNT/EHR #: ELLITH001

Attending Physician: Renee O. Bracker, MD

S: Patient is a 36-year-old female complaining of regular epigastric pain beginning in the umbilical region and radiating toward her spine. Last night the pain was so severe she vomited.

O: Examination reveals crackles in lower lobe at the base of the lung, tachycardia, and a temperature of 102 F. Lab results show increased serum lipase levels and increased polymorphonuclear leukocytes. Ultrasound shows enlarged pancreas.

A: Acute pancreatitis

P: Admit to hospital.

Determine the most accurate ICD-10-CM code(s).

15

Coding Integumentary Conditions

Key Terms

Blister
Bulla
Carbuncle
Cyst
Decubitus Ulcer
Dermis
Epidermis
Furuncle
Gangrene
Hair
Hair Follicle
Macule
Nevus
Nodule
Papule
Patch
Phalanges
Pressure Ulcer
Pustule
Scale
Skin
Subcutaneous
Ulcer

Learning Outcomes

After completing this chapter, the student should be able to:

LO 15.1 Apply the guidelines for reporting conditions of the skin.
LO 15.2 Analyze disorders of the nails, hair, glands, and sensory nerves.
LO 15.3 Determine the specific characteristics of a lesion as they relate to coding.
LO 15.4 Abstract the reasons for preventive care and report them accurately to support medical necessity.

STOP! Remember, you need to follow along in your ICD-10-CM code book for an optimal learning experience.

15.1 Disorders of the Skin

The Skin

The average person has roughly 2 square yards (5,184 inches) of **skin** surface area. As the largest organ in the human body, the skin does so much more than just keep all your internal organs covered. Each of its layers, the **epidermis** and the **dermis**, plays an important role in protecting the body.

The dermis is a sturdy collagenous layer that connects the epidermis to the fatty tissue layer. Blood vessels, nerves, glands, hair follicles, and lymph channels are all located in this stratum of the skin. In **Figure 15-1**, you can see how all of the components of the integumentary system work together—the skin (epidermis and dermis) along with the accessory structures (hair, nails, glands, and sensory receptors). Notice how the line between the epidermis and the dermis has hills and ridges, known as *dermal papillae*. Fingerprints are formed by these genetically prompted elevations and valleys, which are then altered further during formation as a fetus presses against the wall of the uterus. This explains why no two people have the same fingerprints, not even identical twins.

Fastening the skin to the underlying elements of the anatomy is the fatty tissue, also known as the *hypodermis* (*hypo* = below + *dermis* = dermal) or the **subcutaneous** layer.

Skin
The external membranous covering of the body.

Epidermis
The external layer of the skin, the majority of which is squamous cells.

Dermis
The internal layer of the skin; the location of blood vessels, lymph vessels, hair follicles, sweat glands, and sebum.

Subcutaneous
The layer beneath the dermis; also known as the *hypodermis*.

Dermatitis

Dermatitis is technically an inflammation of the skin (*derma* = skin + *-itis* = inflammation). However, it is not as simple as this; there are several types of dermatitis.

Atopic dermatitis (category L20) includes Besnier's prurigo, flexural eczema, infantile eczema, and intrinsic (allergic) eczema. Most often, this chronic inflammation affects infants (1 month to 1 year of age) with family histories of atopic conditions such as allergic rhinitis and bronchial asthma. Signs and symptoms include erythematous areas on extremely dry skin, appearing as lesions on the forehead, cheeks, arms, and legs. The pruritus nature of this condition results in scratching that induces scaling and edema.

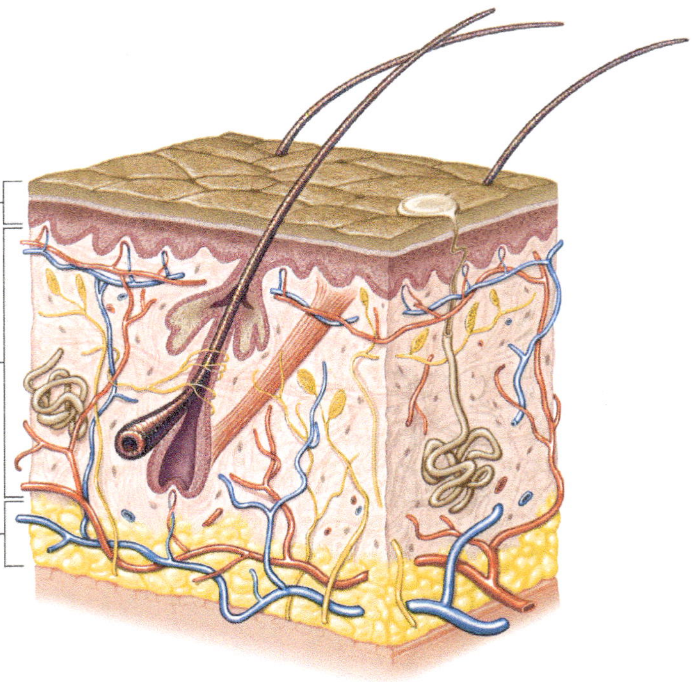

FIGURE 15-1 An illustration identifying the layers of the skin

Seborrheic dermatitis (category L21) includes seborrhea capitis and seborrheic infantile dermatitis, commonly affecting the scalp and face. Symptoms include itching, erythematous areas, and inflammation, characterized by lesions covered with brownish gray or yellow scales in areas in which sebaceous glands are plentiful.

Diaper dermatitis (category L22), commonly referred to as *diaper rash*, is caused by continuously wet skin. Often, this develops when diapers are not changed frequently enough to permit the area to dry out.

Allergic contact dermatitis (category L23) is the result of the skin touching a material or substance to which the patient is sensitive. In addition to erythematous areas, vesicles develop that itch, scale, and may ooze.

Irritant contact dermatitis (category L24) is caused by exposure of the skin to detergents, solvents, acids, or alkalis. Blisters and/or ulcerations may appear in the area that came in contact with the chemical. The 2022 code set adds several more codes to identify the specific cause of the irritant contact dermatitis. Be certain documentation includes these details.

Exfoliative dermatitis (category L26) is an acute and chronic inflammation with widespread erythema and scales. The loss of the stratum corneum (the outermost layer of the epidermis) is at the heart of this condition, along with hair loss, fever, and shivering.

Dermatitis due to substances taken internally (category L27) would include an inflammatory eruption of the epidermis in reaction to medications, drugs, ingested food, or other substances. It may be easy to think that this might be limited to a response only to oral medicines, but, technically, a drug injected, infused, or delivered via subcutaneous patch also places the pharmaceutical internally. Keep a watchful eye on the ***Use additional code*** notations within this code category, which remind you to include an external cause code.

Psoriasis

Identified by epidermal erythematous papules and plaques covered with silvery scales, psoriasis is a chronic illness. Exacerbations (flare-ups) can be treated to relieve the symptoms. Patients can inherit the tendency to develop psoriasis because it is genetically passed from parent to child. Its pruritic nature can sometimes result in pain along with itching in the areas covered with dry, cracked, encrusted lesions appearing on the scalp, chest, elbows, knees, shins, back, and buttocks. The silver scales may flake away easily or create a thickened cover over the lesion. There are several types of psoriasis, including the following:

Psoriasis vulgaris, also known as *nummular psoriasis* or *plaque psoriasis*, is the most common type of psoriasis. It usually causes dry, red skin lesions (plaques) covered with silvery scales. Reported with code L40.0 Psoriasis vulgaris.

Guttate psoriasis appears more often in young adults (under the age of 30) as well as children. Lesions covered by a fine scale will typically develop as small, teardrop-shaped sores on the scalp, arms, trunk, and legs. Reported with code L40.4 Guttate psoriasis.

Psoriatic arthritis mutilans presents with pain, edema, and/or loss of flexibility in at least one joint. When affecting the fingers or toes, the nails may show pitting or begin to separate from the nail bed. Reported with code L40.52 Psoriatic arthritis mutilans.

Pressure Ulcers

A **pressure ulcer** can be created in an area of skin when tissue breaks down. Also known as a *bedsore, plaster ulcer, pressure sore,* or **decubitus ulcer**, it can occur if the patient is unable to move or shift their own weight, such as when an individual is confined to a wheelchair or bed, even for a short period of time. The constant pressure against the skin reduces the blood supply to that particular area, and the affected tissue becomes necrotic (dies). You might have experienced this yourself with a pebble in your shoe or a simple fold of your sock within a tight shoe. The area where the pressure impacted your foot became more and more painful. If you took your shoe right off, you might have noticed a red area. If you waited a length of time before removing your shoe, you found a painful **blister**. The longer the pressure and irritation are maintained, the worse the damage to the skin (see **Figure 15-2**).

Pressure Ulcer
An open wound or sore caused by pressure, infection, or inflammation.

Decubitus Ulcer
A bedsore or wound created by lying in the same position, on the same irritant without relief.

Blister
A bubble or sac formed on the surface of the skin, typically filled with a watery fluid or serum.

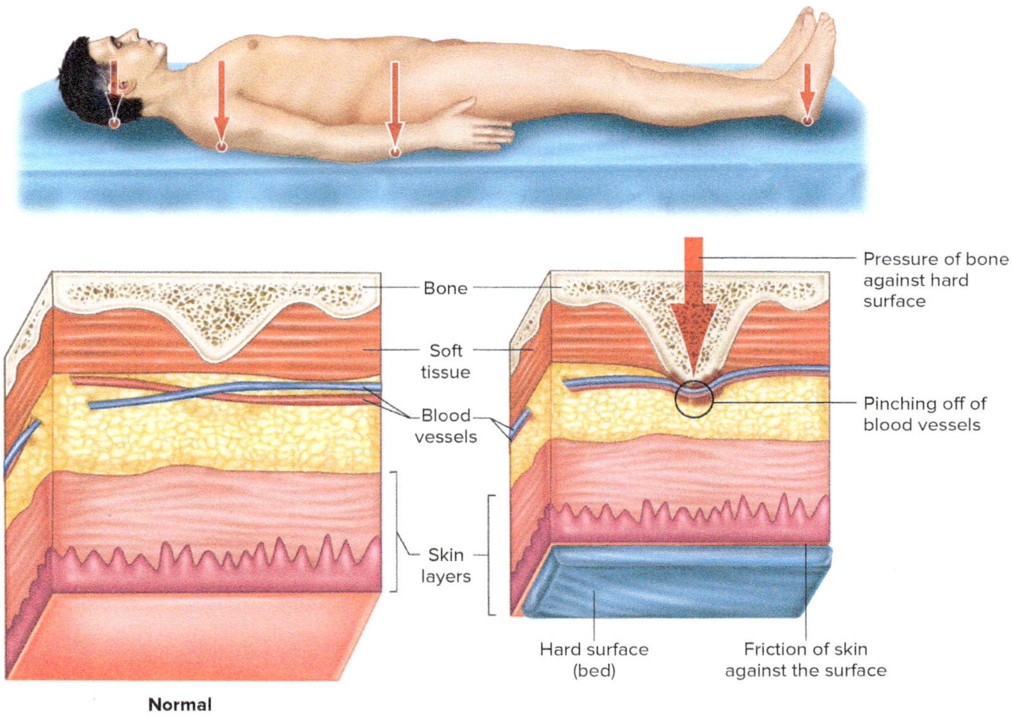

FIGURE 15-2 An illustration identifying the etiology of pressure ulcers including the layers of the skin affected

The National Pressure Ulcer Advisory Panel (NPUAP) defines a pressure ulcer as "a localized injury to the skin and/or underlying tissue, usually over a bony prominence, as a result of pressure, or pressure in combination with shear and/or friction."

As a professional coding specialist, you will need to know two factors to determine the correct codes for a diagnosed pressure ulcer:

- Anatomical location (where on the body the ulcer is).
- Depth of the lesion (also known as the *stage of ulcer*).

There are five codeable stages of pressure ulcers (see **Figure 15-3**):

- *Stage 1* affects the epidermal layer and is recognized by persistent erythema (redness). A stage 1 pressure ulcer is visualized as a reddened area on the skin that, when pressed with the finger, is nonblanchable (does not turn white).

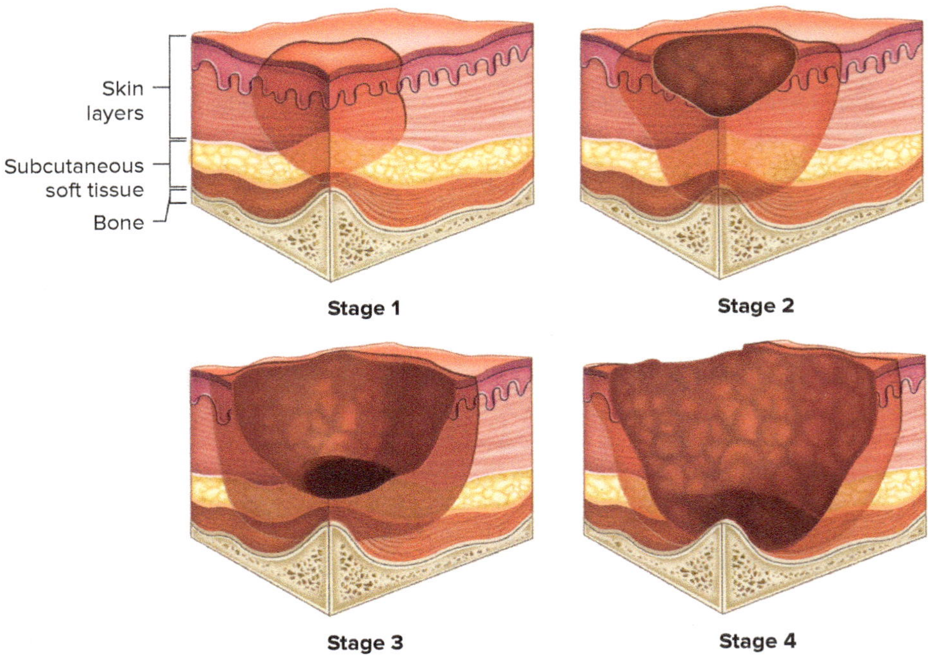

FIGURE 15-3 An illustration showing each of the four pressure ulcer stages

- *Stage 2* is a partial-thickness loss involving both the epidermis and the dermis; sometimes a fluid-filled blister is evident. A stage 2 pressure ulcer shows visible blisters or forms an open sore. The tissue surrounding the sore may be red and irritated like an abrasion, blister, or shallow crater with a red-pink wound bed.
- *Stage 3* pressure ulcer involves skin loss through and including the subcutaneous tissue. A stage 3 pressure ulcer looks like a crater with visible damage to the tissue below the skin. Full-thickness tissue loss may expose subcutaneous fatty tissue but not bone, tendon, or muscle.
- *Stage 4* indicates the skin layers are necrotic and the ulcer reaches down into muscle and possibly bone. Stage 4 pressure ulcers have become so deep that there is damage to the muscle and bone, sometimes along with tendon and joint damage. While the depth of the ulcer varies on the basis of the anatomical site, there is full-thickness tissue loss with bone, tendon, or muscle exposed.
- An *unstageable ulcer* is *not* an unspecified stage. There are times when slough and eschar must be removed to reveal the base of the wound before the true depth, or stage, can be accurately determined. The lesion may be inaccessible–because it is covered by a wound dressing that has not been removed or by a sterile blister or because of some other documented reason.

Should an unstageable pressure ulcer become stageable after debridement, code for the stage identified and documented after that debridement only.

GUIDANCE CONNECTION

Read the ICD-10-CM Official Guidelines for Coding and Reporting, section **I. Conventions, General Coding Guidelines and Chapter-Specific Guidelines**, subsection **C. Chapter-Specific Coding Guidelines**, chapter **12. Diseases of the Skin and Subcutaneous Tissue**, subsection **a. Pressure ulcer stage codes.**

ICD-10-CM has created combination codes, therefore requiring only one code to identify both the anatomical site and the stage of the ulcer.

EXAMPLE

Holder Pronce has a stage 3 pressure ulcer on his left hip.

L89.223 Pressure ulcer of left hip, stage 3

Healing Pressure Ulcers

It is logical that a patient will be attended to by a health care professional during the time the pressure ulcer is healing. Typically, the documentation will identify the original stage and describe the ulcer as "healing." For example, "Harvey Rhoden was seen today by Dr. Steelman to follow up on his stage 2 pressure ulcer. Dr. Steelman documented that the ulcer is healing nicely." In this case, you would continue to code this as a stage 2 pressure ulcer.

At the time of discharge, if the patient's pressure ulcer has healed, and is documented as healed, you will need to report the stage and site of this ulcer as described in the admissions documentation. This will provide the medical necessity for the treatment of this condition while the patient was in the facility and resulted in the healed outcome.

Evolving Pressure Ulcers

Sadly, there are occasions when a patient is admitted into the hospital with a pressure ulcer that, during their stay, gets worse and progresses into a higher stage of ulcer. Should this happen, you will need to report two codes at discharge:

1. Code for the site and stage of the pressure ulcer as documented when the patient was admitted into the hospital.
2. Report an additional code for the site and stage of the ulcer as documented when the patient is discharged.

Presence of Gangrene

Notice the *Code first* notation beneath the code category L89 Pressure ulcer to report the code for any gangrenous condition associated with the ulcer by using code I96 Gangrene, not elsewhere classified (Gangrenous cellulitis). You are directed by this notation to list the gangrene code first, followed by the pressure ulcer code.

Did you notice that the code for gangrene is in the chapter of codes used to report diseases of the circulatory system? This makes sense because **gangrene** is necrosis, cell death, and decay caused by insufficient blood supply to the affected cells. Remember that pressure ulcers are caused by the ongoing compression of the skin, often resulting in the prevention of blood flow into the area. Look again at **Figure 15-3**.

GUIDANCE CONNECTION

Read the ICD-10-CM Official Guidelines for Coding and Reporting, section **I. Conventions, General Coding Guidelines and Chapter-Specific Guidelines**, subsection **C. Chapter-Specific Coding Guidelines**, chapter **12. Diseases of the Skin and Subcutaneous Tissue**, subsection **a.5) Patients admitted with pressure ulcers documented as healing**.

GUIDANCE CONNECTION

Read the ICD-10-CM Official Guidelines for Coding and Reporting, section **I. Conventions, General Coding Guidelines and Chapter-Specific Guidelines**, subsection **C. Chapter-Specific Coding Guidelines**, chapter **12. Diseases of the Skin and Subcutaneous Tissue**, subsection **a.6) Patients admitted with pressure ulcer evolving into another stage during the admission**.

Gangrene
Necrotic tissue resulting from a loss of blood supply.

LET'S CODE IT! SCENARIO

ICD-10-CM

After attempting to jump his motorcycle over five barrels and crashing on the other side, Hunter Massler ended up in the hospital for 6 weeks with a left, closed, transverse fractured femoral shaft; a right, closed, oblique fractured femoral shaft; and three fractured ribs, left side. He was unable to move without extreme pain, so he lay in bed virtually motionless, except with help from the nurse. After several weeks, while changing the sheets, Nurse Kenesson identified a pressure ulcer on each of his hips. Dr. Weiner staged the ulcers bilaterally as stage 2 and ordered wound care immediately. While there, Dr. Weiner also checked Hunter's progress on the healing of his fractures.

Let's Code It!

Dr. Weiner came in to stage and treat Hunter's pressure ulcers: *bilateral hip pressure ulcers*, both documented as stage 2. Let's turn to the Alphabetic Index and find

Ulcer, ulcerated, ulcerating, ulceration, ulcerative

pressure (pressure area) L89.9-

hip L89.2-

(continued)

Perfect! Now let's turn to L89 in the Tabular List and read completely.

✓4 **L89 Pressure ulcer**

Read the INCLUDES, *Code first*, and EXCLUDES2 notations. There is nothing here to direct you elsewhere, so continue reading and review *all* of the required fourth-character choices to determine the one that matches the physician's notes:

✓5 **L89.2 Pressure ulcer of hip**

This matches the notes, so you know you are in the right place. Next, you must determine the required fifth character for this ulcer code. Check the documentation; is the pressure ulcer on his right hip or left hip? Both, actually, so you will need two codes, one for each hip:

✓6 **L89.21 Pressure ulcer of right hip**

✓6 **L89.22 Pressure ulcer of left hip**

To identify the sixth characters, you will need to abstract from the documentation regarding the stage of each ulcer. The documentation states stage 2 for both.

L89.212 Pressure ulcer of right hip, stage 2

L89.222 Pressure ulcer of left hip, stage 2

These pressure ulcer codes will be reported first because the ulcers are the principal reason Dr. Weiner came to see Hunter for this encounter. Then follow these steps with the codes to report Hunter's fractures, and you will have the diagnosis codes to report this encounter:

L89.212 Pressure ulcer of right hip, stage 2

L89.222 Pressure ulcer of left hip, stage 2

S72.325D Nondisplaced transverse fracture of shaft of left femur, subsequent encounter for closed fracture with routine healing

S72.334D Nondisplaced oblique fracture of shaft of right femur, subsequent encounter for closed fracture with routine healing

S22.42XD Multiple fractures of ribs, left side, subsequent encounter for closed fracture with routine healing

Good work!

Non-Pressure Ulcers

A non-pressure skin ulcer is an open sore, an intrusion into and beyond the epidermis layer. Signs and symptoms include edema (swelling), erythema (redness), and tenderness. Some may secrete a clear fluid or blood; when an infection is present, pus can be seen.

Generally, non-pressure ulcers of the skin are reported from code categories L97 *Non-pressure chronic ulcer of lower limb, not elsewhere classified* and L98 *Other disorders of skin and subcutaneous tissue, not elsewhere classified.* In the 2026 code set, more than a dozen new codes have been added to report non-pressure chronic ulcers, each specific to the anatomical location of the sore in combination with documented complications. For example:

L98.A224 Non-pressure chronic ulcer of left forearm with necrosis of bone

> **GUIDANCE CONNECTION**
>
> Read the ICD-10-CM Official Guidelines for Coding and Reporting subsection **C. Chapter-Specific Coding Guidelines,** chapter **12. Diseases of the Skin and Subcutaneous Tissue,** subsection **b. Non-Pressure Chronic Ulcers**

Due to the fact that a non-pressure chronic ulcer may be caused by a variety of factors, you, as the medical coder must check the documentation to ensure accurate reporting. For example, the CODE FIRST notation beneath code category L97 requiring a code for any associated or contributing underlying condition. For example, it is not unusual for non-pressure ulcerations to appear on those patients diagnosed with diabetes mellitus. Others with chronic venous hypertension and peripheral artery disease (PAD) often develop these sores. In these cases, the principal diagnosis code or first-reported code must be, such as:

E11.621 Type 2 diabetes mellitus with foot ulcer

15.2 Disorders of the Nails, Hair, Glands, and Sensory Nerves

Nails

> **Phalanges**
> Fingers and toes [singular: phalange or phalanx].

As you can see in **Figure 15-4**, there are several components of nails–those hard, protective layers at the ends of your **phalanges** (fingers and toes). The most well-known part of the nail is the *nail plate*, the main part of the nail, which lies upon a layer of skin (nail bed). At the point where the nail plate goes beneath the skin [*eponychium* = nail fold + cuticle (lunula)] of the finger (or toe) is the *lunula*, a white area shaped like a crescent moon (therefore, the term *lunula*, from *luna*, meaning moon). As the nail grows over the tip of the phalange, the area of epidermis beneath is called the *hyponychium*.

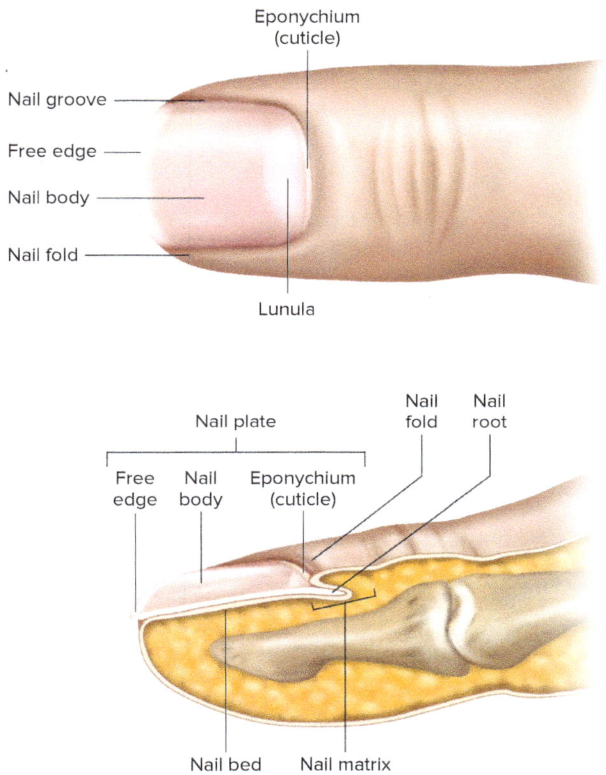

FIGURE 15-4 An illustration identifying the anatomical sites of the basic parts of a human nail: nail plate, lunula, root, nail matrix, nail bed, free edge

Nail Disorders

The human body has 20 nails–10 fingernails and 10 toenails–and as with any other anatomical site, things can go wrong.

- *Onycholysis:* this is a detachment of the nail from the bed of the nail. Onset occurs at either the distal or lateral attachment. Patients previously diagnosed with psoriasis or thyrotoxicosis are most often seen with this condition. Reported with code L60.1 Onycholysis.
- *Beau's lines:* these are deeply grooved, horizontal lines (from side to side) on either a fingernail or a toenail. Previous infection, injury, or other disruption to the nail fold, the location of nail formation, may be the cause. Reported with code L60.4 Beau's lines.
- *Yellow nail syndrome:* a thickened nail that has become yellowed is typically seen in patients previously diagnosed with a systemic disease, such as lymphedema or bronchiectasis. This is reported with code L60.5 Yellow nail syndrome.

You have learned, with many diseases in various body systems, that a disease in one location of the body may negatively impact another part of the body. This can happen with the nails as well, so ICD-10-CM provides a specific code to report this:

L62 **Nail disorders in diseases classified elsewhere**

Code first **underlying disease, such as: pachydermoperiostosis (M89.4-)**

LET'S CODE IT! SCENARIO

Priscilla Ablerts, an 83-year-old female, was brought in with toenails that had grown out of normal shape. It had gotten to the point that she could no longer wear closed shoes, and her daughter was concerned. After examination, Dr. Terranzo diagnosed Priscilla with onychogryphosis.

Let's Code It!

Dr. Terranzo diagnosed Priscilla with *onychogryphosis*. Turn in the ICD-10-CM Alphabetic Index to find

Onychogryphosis, onychogryposis L60.2

Let's turn in the Tabular List to the code category:

✓4 **L60 Nail disorders**

EXCLUDES2 *clubbing of nails (R68.3)*

onychia and paronychia (L03.0-)

Neither of these conditions applies to Priscilla's reason for seeing Dr. Terranzo for this encounter, so keep reading down to evaluate all of the fourth-character options. Which is the most accurate?

L60.2 Onychogryphosis

This matches Dr. Terranzo's documentation. However, you know that before you can report this code, you need to check the EXCLUDES1 note for this subsection (right above L60). This does not relate to this case. Now, check the EXCLUDES2 note at the very beginning of this chapter in the ICD-10-CM Tabular List. Last stop is at the Official Guidelines, section I.C.12. There seem to be no guidelines here that relate to Dr. Terranzo's care for Priscilla, so you can now report this code with confidence:

L60.2 Onychogryphosis

Good job!

Hair
A pigmented, cylindrical filament that grows out from the hair follicle within the epidermis.

Hair Follicle
A saclike bulb containing the hair root.

Hair

Hair is a pigmented (colored), hard keratin that grows from the **hair follicle**—the location of the hair root. As you can see in **Figure 15-5**, the follicle is embedded in the dermis and fatty tissue of the skin layers. As you probably know from your own body, hair may grow externally, such as on your scalp, as well as internally, such as inside the nasal or ear cavity. The hairs in the nose help to prevent certain particles from entering the respiratory system.

Disorders of the Hair

For some patients, a bad hair day can be much more serious than a cowlick or frizz.

- *Alopecia mucinosa:* this skin disorder may first be identified by erythematous plaqueing of the skin without any hair growth. The flat patches of hairlessness may occur on the scalp, face, or legs. Reported with code L65.2 Alopecia mucinosa.
- *Trichorrhexis nodosa:* evidenced by a hair shaft defect that causes weak spots, this disorder results in hair that easily breaks. Most often, this condition is caused by environmental factors such as blow drying, permanent waves, or excessive chemical exposure. Reported with code L67.0 Trichorrhexis nodosa.
- *Hirsutism:* women with this condition have excessive hair growth on anatomical sites where hair does not typically occur, such as the chest or chin. It is believed to be caused by an abnormal hormonal level, particularly male hormones such as testosterone. Reported with code L68.0 Hirsutism.

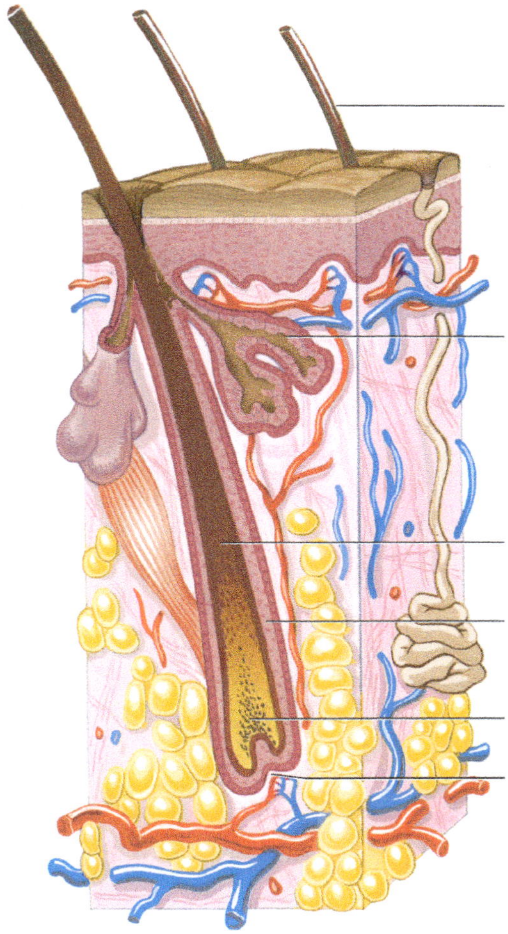

FIGURE 15-5 An illustration identifying the anatomical parts of a hair; from papilla to shaft

Glands

Three different types of glands are located within the skin:

- *Sebaceous glands* produce an oil-rich element, known as *sebum*, that lies on the outer surface of the epidermis and along the hair. The substance has a waterproofing effect. Individuals with oily skin may have overly active sebaceous glands.
- *Eccrine glands* are sweat glands that are responsible for maintaining proper body temperature by excreting sweat (water, salt, and wastes) via the pores in the skin. Production of more sweat is the reaction to cool an overheated body (see **Figure 15-6**).
- *Apocrine glands* release a discharge that is high in protein. Located in the axilla (armpits), anal, and genital areas, bacteria interact with the protein and create an odor.

Eccrine Sweat Disorders

As with any other anatomical site, the eccrine sweat glands can malfunction. One condition is known as *focal hyperhidrosis* (excessive sweating). This is reported with a specific character to identify the region of the body affected (i.e., axillae, face, palms, or soles). Primary hyperhidrosis is an idiopathic condition (no known etiology), whereas secondary focal hyperhidrosis (also known as *Frey's syndrome*) is often caused by damage to the parotid glands, resulting in excessive salivation. Hypohidrosis (code L74.4), also known as *anhidrosis*, is a condition in which the glands do not produce enough perspiration. This may lead to hyperthermia, heat stroke, or heat exhaustion.

You can see that the ICD-10-CM code descriptions use the term *miliaria*, which is the medical term for a skin disorder–the appearance of red bumps or blisters–caused by blocked sweat ducts and trapped sweat beneath the skin. Laypeople call this *heat rash*.

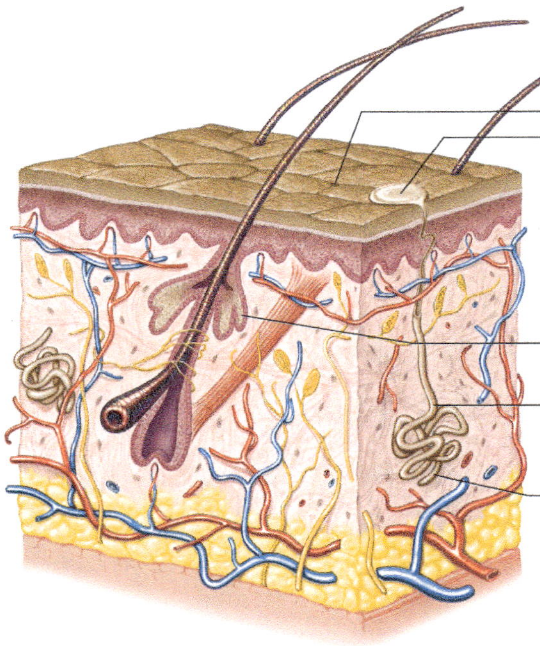

FIGURE 15-6 An illustration identifying the anatomical sites of sweat glands

L74.0	**Miliaria rubra**
L74.1	**Miliaria crystallina**
L74.2	**Miliaria profunda**
L74.4	**Anhidrosis (Hypohidrosis)**

Apocrine Sweat Disorders

One of the challenges in dealing with an apocrine sweat disorder is the potential for embarrassment due to the increase in body odor. Natural odors can be a natural attraction between humans; however, when body odor is out of balance, this can cause both physiological and psychological problems. Bromhidrosis (foul-smelling perspiration, code L75.0) or chromhidrosis (pigmented perspiration, code L75.1) can be publicly humiliating to any adult.

L75.0	**Bromhidrosis**
L75.1	**Chromhidrosis**
L75.2	**Apocrine miliaria (Fox-Fordyce disease)**
L75.8	**Other apocrine sweat disorders**

ICD-10-CM

YOU CODE IT! CASE STUDY

Ellyn Pacard, a 41-year-old female, presents to Dr. Grall with what she believes to be nonscarring male-pattern alopecia. Examination reveals small patches of scalp, with some limited mild erythema. "Exclamation point" hairs are located on the periphery with some indication of new patches and regrowth. Explained to patient that complete regrowth is possible in this diagnosis.

Diagnosis: alopecia capitis

Treatment plan: intralesional corticosteroid injections followed by minoxidil applications.

(continued)

You Code It!

Read Dr. Grall's notes on his encounter with Ellyn carefully, and code the visit.

Step #1: Read the case carefully and completely.
Step #2: Abstract the scenario. Which main words or terms describe why the physician cared for the patient during this encounter?
Step #3: Are there any details missing or incomplete for which you would need to query the physician? [If so, ask your instructor.]
Step #4: Check for any relevant guidance, including reading all of the symbols and notations in the Tabular List and the appropriate sections of the Official Guidelines.
Step #5: Determine the correct diagnosis code or codes to explain why this encounter was medically necessary.
Step #6: Double-check your work.

Answer:

Did you determine this to be the correct code?

L63.0 Alopecia (capitis) totalis

Good work!

Sensory Nerves

In a part of the nervous system known as the *somatic* (relating to the body) *sensory system*, sensory nerve endings are located in the layers of the skin to provide sensory feedback–the sense of touch. These nerves enable you to feel pressure, pain, temperature (hot and cold), textures (rough and smooth), and more.

There is more about the nervous system in this book's chapter titled ***Coding Mental, Behavioral, and Neurological Disorders***.

LET'S CODE IT! SCENARIO

Serena Brynner is a 19-year-old female who came in to see Dr. Trenton with thickened, hardened skin and subcutaneous tissue on her forearms, bilaterally. Examination shows Addison's keloid present. She is given a referral to a plastic surgeon.

Let's Code It!

Dr. Trenton diagnosed Serena with *Addison's keloid* on both of her forearms. Let's begin by finding this key term in the Alphabetic Index:

Keloid, cheloid L91.0

Addison's L94.0

Let's find this code category in the Tabular List:

✓4 **L94 Other localized connective tissue disorders**

The terms here don't match exactly. Let's check a medical encyclopedia to find out exactly what an Addison's keloid is:

Addison's keloid is a skin disease consisting of patches of yellowish or ivory-colored hard, dry, smooth skin. It is more common in females. Also known as morphea or circumscribed scleroderma.

This helps a great deal. Read the complete code descriptions in this code category. Did you connect to this code?

L94.0 Localized scleroderma [morphea] (Circumscribed scleroderma)

Fantastic!

15.3 Lesions

Cyst
A fluid-filled or gas-filled bubble in the skin.

Furuncle
A staphylococcal infection in the subcutaneous tissue; commonly known as a *boil.*

Papule
A raised lesion with a diameter of less than 5 mm.

Nodule
A tissue mass or papule larger than 5 mm.

Macule
A flat lesion with a different pigmentation (color) when compared with the surrounding skin.

Nevus
An abnormally pigmented area of skin. A birthmark is an example.

Patch
A flat, small area of differently colored or textured skin; a large macule.

Bulla
A large vesicle that is filled with fluid.

Pustule
A swollen area of skin; a vesicle filled with pus.

Scale
Flaky exfoliated epidermis; a flake of skin.

Ulcer
An erosion or loss of the full thickness of the epidermis.

Many people believe a lesion is a sore on the epidermis; however, lesions also might occur internally. Skin lesions are categorized as primary or secondary and are pathologically determined to be benign or malignant. Even though the majority of lesions are external, reporting them is not confined to the codes in the ICD-10-CM code book's ***Chapter 12: Diseases of the Skin and Subcutaneous Tissue (L00–L99)***. Essentially, lesion codes are located throughout the code set; they are most often found in the section related to the anatomical location or by a specific term. Many skin lesions (see **Figure 15-7**) are identified by name or type, including

- **Cyst:** a fluid-filled or gas-filled bubble in the skin.
- **Furuncle:** a staphylococcal infection in the subcutaneous tissue; commonly known as a *boil.*
- **Papule:** a raised lesion with a diameter of less than 5 mm.
- **Nodule:** a tissue mass or papule larger than 5 mm.
- **Macule:** a flat lesion with a different pigmentation (color) when compared with the surrounding skin. An *ephelidis* (freckle) is a small macule.
- **Nevus:** an abnormally pigmented area of skin. A birthmark is an example.
- **Patch:** a flat, small area of differently colored or textured skin; a large macule.
- **Bulla:** a large vesicle that is filled with fluid.
- **Pustule:** a swollen area of skin; a vesicle filled with pus.
- **Scale:** flaky exfoliated epidermis; a flake of skin.
- **Ulcer:** an erosion or loss of the full thickness of the epidermis.

EXAMPLE

L02.32 Furuncle of buttock

Let's turn to the Alphabetic Index and find the key term *lesion*. Review the terms shown in the indented list that follows, providing additional description for the type of lesion documented. For the most part, these lesions are directly described by their anatomical location, with no additional clinical terminology.

EXAMPLES

Lesion, aortic (valve) I35.9 (an internal lesion)

Lesion, lip K13.0 (an external lesion)

Lesion, basal ganglion G25.9 (an internal lesion)

Lesion, eyelid H00.03- (an external lesion)

Carbuncle
A painful, pus-filled boil due to infection of the epidermis and underlying tissues, often caused by Staphylococcus.

Often, a skin lesion is diagnosed with a specific name or by type. Therefore, the most effective way to find the codes in the Alphabetic Index is to look up the exact term that the physician used in the diagnostic statement first, before trying to generalize by interpreting *lesion* and using that term. For example, **carbuncles** and furuncles, also known as *boils* (a type of pustule caused by an infection), are listed by the terms *carbuncle* and *furuncle*, rather than under the main term of *lesion*, with the fourth character identifying the anatomical location of the skin condition.

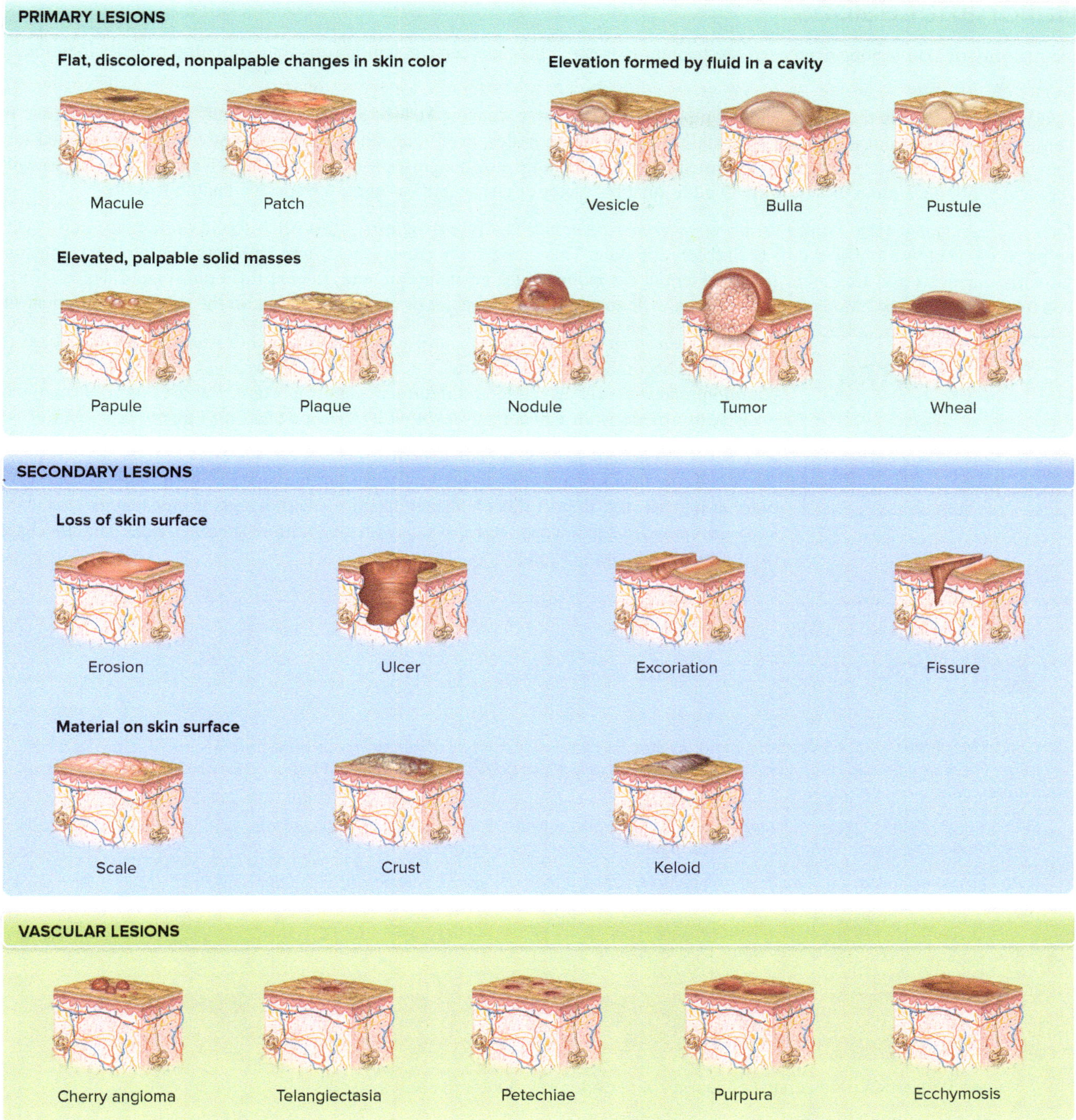

FIGURE 15-7 An illustration showing the various types of skin lesions

EXAMPLES

Carbuncle, chin L02.03

Carbuncle, hand L02.53-

Carbuncle, scalp L02.831

Malignant Lesions

The majority of skin lesions diagnosed are benign. However, there are certain skin lesions that are pathologically identified as malignant.

Malignant melanoma is the most deadly type of skin malignancy, causing 80% of all skin malignancy fatalities. The most frequently identified sites of melanoma metastases are the lymph nodes, liver, lung, and brain. The ABCDE method is used most often to evaluate a possible site, then confirmed by a biopsy. Confirmed diagnoses will be reported with a code from the category C43.- Malignant melanoma of skin, with an additional character or characters based on the specific anatomical site.

Merkel cell carcinoma (also known as *neuroendocrine carcinoma*) is a rare diagnosis. Most often found on the face and neck, it can be recognized by a bluish-red or flesh-colored nodule. This malignancy grows quickly and will metastasize quickly, meaning that early diagnosis and treatment are an essential component of a positive outcome. Report this confirmed diagnosis with a code from category C4A.- Merkel cell carcinoma with an additional character or characters based on the specific anatomical site.

> **CODING BITES**
>
> For more information on malignant neoplasms, refer to the chapter titled ***Coding Neoplasms*** in this text.

Squamous cell carcinoma is often pink and scaly with notched or irregular borders. It has the potential to become erythematous (reddened) or ulcerated with easy bleeding. Metastasis is common, making early detection and treatment very important. Report this confirmed diagnosis with a code from category C44.-Other and unspecified malignant melanoma of skin with an additional character or characters based on the specific anatomical site.

Basal cell carcinoma is the most frequently seen skin malignancy, with patients aged 80 or older at highest risk. Report this confirmed diagnosis with a code from category C44.-Other and unspecified malignant melanoma of skin with an additional character or characters based on the specific anatomical site.

YOU CODE IT! CASE STUDY

ICD-10-CM

Carlos Monteverde, a 63-year-old male, comes in to see Dr. Harris, complaining of an extremely painful spot on his thigh. He states he has been very tired lately, especially since he noticed this bump. Patient history reveals a preexistent furunculosis.

Examination shows deep follicular abscess of several follicles with several draining points. CBC shows an elevated white blood cell count. Wound culture identifies Staphylococcus aureus.

Area is cleaned thoroughly. Instructions given to patient to apply warm, wet compresses at home.

A: Carbuncle of the thigh, left

P: Rx for erythromycin, q8h, and mupirocin ointment

You Code It!

Read Dr. Harris's notes on his encounter with Carlos carefully, and code the visit.

Step #1: Read the case carefully and completely.
Step #2: Abstract the scenario. Which main words or terms describe why the physician cared for the patient during this encounter?
Step #3: Are there any details missing or incomplete for which you would need to query the physician? [If so, ask your instructor.]
Step #4: Check for any relevant guidance, including reading all of the symbols and notations in the Tabular List and the appropriate sections of the Official Guidelines.
Step #5: Determine the correct diagnosis code or codes to explain why this encounter was medically necessary.
Step #6: Double-check your work.

(continued)

Answer:

Did you determine these to be the correct codes?

L02.436	**Carbuncle of left lower limb**
B95.61	**Methicillin susceptible Staphylococcus aureus infection as the cause of diseases classified elsewhere**

Good job!

15.4 Prevention and Screenings

The most frequently diagnosed malignancy in the United States is skin cancer. While some individuals have a higher risk of developing this type of malignant neoplasm, the truth is that anyone can find himself or herself with this diagnosis.

The best way to prevent skin lesions is to avoid known causes. Of course, some suggest staying out of the sun altogether, but this could decrease a patient's exercise and outdoor activities, which are also good for one's health. Therefore, protective clothing and use of sunscreen with a sun protection factor (SPF) of 15 or higher is strongly recommended prior to going out into the sun. Tanning beds also may cause an increased risk.

The Centers for Disease Control and Prevention (CDC) suggests ways to protect yourself from UV rays that can cause harm:

- Stay in the shade as much as possible, especially during the hours of 10 a.m. through 4 p.m.
- Keep your extremities (arms and legs) covered with clothing.
- Use a wide-brimmed hat to shade and protect your head, face, neck, and ears.
- Wear sunglasses to protect your eyes (and reduce your risk for cataracts).
- Apply sunscreen with an SPF of 15 or higher.
- Avoid the use of any indoor tanning beds or booths including sunlamps.

Physicians are encouraged by the CDC to perform an annual exam of all patients, especially those who are older and higher at risk. The scalp, ears, nasolabial folds, and wrinkles are key points.

EXAMPLES

There can be other reasons for a healthy patient to see a physician about skin-related issues:

Z12.83	**Encounter for screening for malignant neoplasm of skin**
Z20.7	**Contact with and (suspected) exposure to pediculosis, acariasis, and other infestations**
Z52.11	**Skin donor, autologous**
Z52.19	**Skin donor, other**
Z84.0	**Family history of diseases of the skin and subcutaneous tissue**
Z86.31	**Personal history of diabetic foot ulcer**
Z87.2	**Personal history of disease of the skin and subcutaneous tissue**
Z94.5	**Skin transplant status**
Z96.81	**Presence of artificial skin**

YOU CODE IT! CASE STUDY

PATIENT NAME: Christopher Flemming

SUBJECTIVE: The patient is a 54-year-old male who presents for his annual preventive screening of moles. He has no particular lesions he is concerned about, although he states his wife has told him that he has a lot of moles on his back. He does not think any of them are changing. He did have an atypical nevus removed from one of the toes on his left foot about 3 years ago. He did not require re-excision after the biopsy. He was told to have annual skin exams and he just has not followed through with it. His other complaint is acne on his chest and back.

PAST MEDICAL HISTORY: Negative for skin cancer.

MEDICATIONS: None.

ALLERGIES: NKDA.

FAMILY HISTORY: Negative for melanoma.

SOCIAL HISTORY: Moderate sun exposure. He does use sunscreen, when he remembers.

OBJECTIVE: Alert and oriented x3. Normal mood. Normal body habitus. Examined his face, neck, chest, abdomen, back, upper extremities and lower extremities, hands and feet bilaterally. There were no lesions anywhere worrisome for cutaneous malignancy; however, he does have an above-average number of pigmented macular nevi. These range from 2–6 mm in diameter. The lesions appear similar to each other and are widely distributed on his chest, abdomen, and back; few on his upper and lower extremities and face. On his upper back, there are scattered 2.5 mm inflammatory papules and pustules.

ASSESSMENT:

1. Mild truncal acne.
2. Multiple nevi.
3. History of solitary atypical nevus.

PLAN:

1. Reviewed ABCDs of pigmented lesions, sun protection. Discussed self-exam. Advised he return for skin examination annually as the mole pattern he has does put him at a higher lifetime risk of development of melanoma.
2. He was given erythromycin solution to use b.i.d. for acne.
3. Follow-up is scheduled in 1 year.

You Code It!

Review this documentation from Dr. Stirpe's evaluation of Christopher, and determine the correct code or codes to report the medical necessity for this encounter.

Step #1: Read the case carefully and completely.

Step #2: Abstract the scenario. Which main words or terms describe why the physician cared for the patient during this encounter?

Step #3: Are there any details missing or incomplete for which you would need to query the physician? [If so, ask your instructor.]

Step #4: Check for any relevant guidance, including reading all of the symbols and notations in the Tabular List and the appropriate sections of the Official Guidelines.

Step #5: Determine the correct diagnosis code or codes to explain why this encounter was medically necessary.

Step #6: Double-check your work.

Answer:

Did you determine these to be the correct codes?

Z12.83 **Encounter for screening for malignant neoplasm of skin**

D22.5 **Melanocytic nevi of trunk**

L70.8 **Other acne**

Chapter Summary

With all the advertising about lotions to preserve youthful skin, shampoos and conditioners for soft hair, and manicures and pedicures for nails, you may forget that the elements of the integumentary system (skin, hair, nails) are not just cosmetic or decorative elements of our bodies. In addition, the glands embedded in the skin support the ongoing proper function of the body.

CODING BITES

Early detection is the best, most effective way to deal with any malignancy, including skin cancer. This means that a regular habit of self-examination is wise. The CDC developed a five-point checklist to help you check yourself for melanoma.

"A" stands for Asymmetrical. Does the mole or spot have an irregular shape with two parts that look very different?

"B" stands for Border. Is the border irregular or jagged?

"C" is for Color. Is the color uneven? Do you see variations of brown, black, blue, or white?

"D" is for Diameter. Is the mole or spot larger than the size of a pea (6 mm)?

"E" is for Evolving. Has the mole or spot changed during the past few weeks or months?

If the answer to any of these steps is Yes, the patient should contact a dermatologist for a complete screening.

CHAPTER 15 REVIEW
Coding Integumentary Conditions

Let's Check It! Terminology

Match each key term to the appropriate definition.

Part I

1. **LO 15.1** A bubble or sac formed on the surface of the skin, typically filled with a watery fluid or serum.
2. **LO 15.1** An open wound or sore caused by pressure, infection, or inflammation.
3. **LO 15.2** Death and decay of tissue due to inadequate blood supply.
4. **LO 15.1** The layer beneath the dermis; also known as the *hypodermis*.
5. **LO 15.3** A painful, pus-filled boil due to infection of the epidermis and underlying tissues, often caused by Staphylococcus.
6. **LO 15.1** A skin lesion caused by continuous pressure on one spot, particularly on a bony prominence.
7. **LO 15.2** A saclike bulb containing the hair root.
8. **LO 15.2** A pigmented, cylindrical filament that grows out from the hair follicle within the epidermis.
9. **LO 15.2** Fingers and toes.
10. **LO 15.1** The external layer of the skin, the majority of which is squamous cells.
11. **LO 15.1** The internal layer of the skin; the location of blood vessels, lymph vessels, hair follicles, sweat glands, and sebum.
12. **LO 15.1** The external membranous covering of the body.

A. Blister
B. Carbuncle
C. Decubitus Ulcer
D. Dermis
E. Epidermis
F. Gangrene
G. Hair
H. Hair Follicle
I. Phalanges
J. Skin
K. Subcutaneous
L. Pressure Ulcer

Part II

1.	**LO 15.3** An erosion or loss of the full thickness of the epidermis.	**A.**	Bulla
2.	**LO 15.3** A large macule.	**B.**	Cyst
3.	**LO 15.3** A raised lesion with a diameter of less than 5 mm.	**C.**	Furuncle
4.	**LO 15.3** An abnormally pigmented area of skin. A birthmark is an example.	**D.**	Macule
5.	**LO 15.3** A flat lesion with a different pigmentation (color) when compared with the surrounding skin.	**E.**	Nevus
6.	**LO 15.3** A papule larger than 5 mm.	**F.**	Nodule
7.	**LO 15.3** A fluid-filled or gas-filled bubble in the skin.	**G.**	Papule
8.	**LO 15.3** A boil.	**H.**	Patch
9.	**LO 15.3** Flaky exfoliated epidermis.	**I.**	Pustule
10.	**LO 15.3** A large vesicle that is filled with fluid.	**J.**	Scale
11.	**LO 15.3** A vesicle filled with pus.	**K.**	Ulcer

Let's Check It! Concepts

Choose the most appropriate answer for each of the following questions.

1. **LO 15.1** The _____ is a sturdy collagenous layer that connects the _____ to the fatty tissue layer.
   - **a.** epidermis, dermis
   - **b.** dermis, epidermis
   - **c.** fatty tissue, dermis
   - **d.** subcutaneous, epidermis
2. **LO 15.1** Seborrheic dermatitis is coded from category _____.
   - **a.** L20
   - **b.** L21
   - **c.** L22
   - **d.** L23
3. **LO 15.3** Latoya Gregson was diagnosed with a left hand nevus. The correct code would be
   - **a.** D22.6.
   - **b.** D22.60.
   - **c.** D22.61.
   - **d.** D22.62.
4. **LO 15.2** Women with this condition have excessive hair growth on anatomical sites where hair does not typically occur, such as the chest or chin. This condition is known as
   - **a.** trichotillomania.
   - **b.** hirsutism.
   - **c.** alopecia.
   - **d.** cilia.
5. **LO 15.1** Kathy Harrington, a 17-year-old female, comes in today complaining of red, tender skin and having chills. Kathy admits to sun bathing all day yesterday. After an examination, Dr. Dills diagnoses Kathy with a second-degree sunburn. What is the correct code?
   - **a.** L55.9
   - **b.** L55.0
   - **c.** L55.1
   - **d.** L55.2
6. **LO 15.2** _____ are sweat glands that are responsible for maintaining proper body temperature by excreting sweat (water, salt, and wastes) via the pores in the skin.
   - **a.** Sebaceous glands
   - **b.** Eccrine glands
   - **c.** Apocrine glands
   - **d.** Holocrine glands
7. **LO 15.3** _____ is recognized by a bluish-red or flesh-colored nodule.
   - **a.** Basal cell carcinoma
   - **b.** Malignant melanoma
   - **c.** Merkel cell carcinoma
   - **d.** Squamous cell carcinoma
8. **LO 15.1** When skin layers are lost through and including the subcutaneous tissue, this is a _____ pressure ulcer.
   - **a.** stage 1
   - **b.** stage 2
   - **c.** stage 3
   - **d.** stage 4
9. **LO 15.1** _____ presents with pain, edema, and/or loss of flexibility in at least one joint. When affecting the fingers or toes, the nails may show pitting or begin to separate from the nail bed.
   - **a.** Psoriatic arthritis mutilans
   - **b.** Psoriasis vulgaris
   - **c.** Guttate psoriasis
   - **d.** Plaque psoriasis

10. LO 15.4 All of the following are ways to protect yourself from UV rays that can cause harm *except*

   a. keep your extremities covered with clothing.
   b. use indoor tanning beds regularly.
   c. use a wide-brimmed hat to shade and protect your head, face, neck, and ears.
   d. wear sunglasses to protect your eyes (and reduce your risk for cataracts).

Let's Check It! Guidelines

Refer to the Official Guidelines and fill in the blanks according to Chapter 12, Diseases of the Skin and Subcutaneous Tissue, Chapter-Specific Coding Guidelines.

all	site	clinical	documentation	no
completely	highest	progresses	ulcer	admitted
terms	L89	healing	stage	two

1. Codes from category L89, Pressure _____, identify the _____ of the pressure ulcer as well as the stage of the ulcer.
2. Assign as many codes from category _____ as needed to identify _____ the pressure ulcers the patient has, if applicable.
3. When there is _____ documentation regarding the _____ of the pressure ulcer, assign the appropriate code for unspecified stage (L89.-9).
4. Assignment of the pressure ulcer stage code should be guided by _____ documentation of the stage or documentation of the _____ found in the Alphabetic Index.
5. No code is assigned if the documentation states that the pressure ulcer is _____ healed.
6. Pressure ulcers described as _____ should be assigned the appropriate pressure ulcer stage code based on the _____ in the medical record.
7. If a patient is _____ with a pressure ulcer at one stage and it _____ to a higher stage, _____ separate codes should be assigned: one code for the site and stage of the ulcer on admission and a second code for the same ulcer site and the _____ stage reported during the stay.

Let's Check It! Rules and Regulations

Please answer the following questions from the knowledge you have gained after reading this chapter.

1. **LO 15.1** What are two factors a professional coding specialist needs to know to determine the correct code(s) for a diagnosed pressure ulcer?
2. **LO 15.1** List the stages of pressure ulcers, and explain how you differentiate among the stages.
3. **LO 15.1** Read the ICD-10-CM Official Guidelines for Coding and Reporting, section I. Conventions, General Coding Guidelines and Chapter-Specific Guidelines, subsection C. Chapter-Specific Coding Guidelines, chapter 12. Diseases of the Skin and Subcutaneous Tissue, subsection a.2) Unstageable pressure ulcers. Explain the guideline, including instructions concerning clinical documentation.
4. **LO 15.2** Explain the different types of glands that are located within the skin. What is the function of each?
5. **LO 15.3** List two types of malignant lesions; describe each one, including the category code.

ICD-10-CM

YOU CODE IT! Basics

First, identify the condition in the following diagnoses; then code the diagnosis.

Example: Bullous impetigo

a. main term: *impetigo* **b.** diagnosis: *L01.03*

1. Carbuncle of perineum:

   a. main term: _____ **b.** diagnosis: _____

(continued)

2. Acute lymphangitis:
   a. main term: ______ b. diagnosis:______
3. Coccygeal fistula with abscess:
   a. main term: ______ b. diagnosis:______
4. Pemphigus vulgaris:
   a. main term:______ b. diagnosis:______
5. Flexural eczema:
   a. main term:______ b. diagnosis:______
6. Seborrhea capitis:
   a. main term:______ b. diagnosis:______
7. Irritant contact dermatitis due to cosmetics:
   a. main term:______ b. diagnosis:______
8. Psoriasis vulgaris:
   a. main term:______ b. diagnosis:______
9. Psoriatic arthritis mutilans:
   a. main term:______ b. diagnosis:______
10. Lichen nitidus:
   a. main term:______ b. diagnosis:______
11. Telogen effluvium:
   a. main term:______ b. diagnosis:______
12. Alopecia universalis:
   a. main term:______ b. diagnosis:______
13. Acne conglobata:
   a. main term:______ b. diagnosis:______
14. Pilar cyst:
   a. main term:______ b. diagnosis:______
15. Livedoid vasculitis:
   a. main term:______ b. diagnosis:______

ICD-10-CM

YOU CODE IT! Practice

Using the techniques described in this chapter, carefully read through the case studies and determine the most accurate ICD-10-CM code(s) and external cause code(s), if appropriate, for each case study.

1. Angie Ullman, a 7-year-old female, is brought into the ER by her parents due to a painful rash on her legs. The ER physician documents a temperature of 101 F and admits Angie to the hospital with the diagnosis of severe poison ivy. Angie's mother admitted she was walking their dog at the local park this morning and must have come in contact with the poison ivy there.
2. Anna Morris, a 22-year-old female, presents today with a blister on her left elbow. Her elbow is painful and warm to the touch. After an examination, Dr. Lane diagnoses Anna with a pressure ulcer of the elbow, stage 2.
3. A.G. Harrison, a 62-year-old male, complains of a deep sore on his right heel. After an examination, Dr. Miles notes that the subcutaneous tissue is visible with necrosis and admits A.G. to the hospital. Dr. Miles diagnoses A.G. with a decubitus ulcer of the heel, stage 3.
4. George Bowden, a 34-year-old male, presents today with a painful pus-filled lump on the nape of his neck. After an examination, Dr. Harris diagnoses George with a neck carbuncle.
5. Maechearda McConico, a 23-year-old female, presents with a bleeding mole on her left eyebrow. After a thorough examination and the appropriate tests, Dr. Ardis diagnoses Maechearda with a malignant melanoma in situ.
6. Matt Kicklighter, an 18-year-old male, presents today with fluid-filled blisters on his back. Matt states that the blisters are easily broken. After an examination and testing, Dr. Gardener diagnoses Matt with staphylococcal scalded skin syndrome with 14% exfoliation due to erythematous.
7. Judy Shirer, a 48-year-old female, comes in today with swollen, red, and painful skin on her face. Judy says she also feels nauseous. Dr. Lee notes red streaking around the cheeks and eyes and a temperature of 103 F. After examining Judy, Dr. Lee admits her to the hospital, where further laboratory test results confirm the diagnosis of facial cellulitis, MRSA.
8. Aaron Ragin, a 17-year-old male, presents today with a painful red lump on his chest. Dr. Godwin completes an examination and the appropriate laboratory tests. Aaron is diagnosed with a furuncle due to Staphylococcus.
9. Harriett Mooney, a 6-year-old female, is brought in by her parents. Harriett has dry scaly skin. Dr. Lebrun completes an examination and a patch test, which confirms the diagnosis of infantile eczema.

(continued)

10. Kathy Neal, a 56-year-old female, presents today with an itchy purple-colored lower lip. Dr. Grimsley notes flat-topped papules intermingled with lacy white lines. Kathy is diagnosed with bullous lichen planus.
11. Brenda Mets, a 32-year-old female, was diagnosed with basal cell carcinoma on her nose 10 days ago. Brenda is admitted to the hospital today for electrodesiccation and curettage by Dr. Dease.
12. Donald Ross, a 33-year-old male, presents today with raised bumps on his back. Dr. Margroff notes pustules. Don admits to skin tenderness. Dr. Margroff completes an examination and diagnoses Donald with generalized pustular psoriasis.
13. Beth Whitman, an 81-year-old female, presents with a sore on the medial side of her right calf. After examining the area and documenting edema and ulceration, Dr. Sanoski decides to admit Beth to the hospital. After a workup, Beth is diagnosed with a venous stasis ulcer with muscle necrosis, right calf. A possible skin graft is discussed with the patient.
14. Eugene Sanford, a 49-year-old male, comes in today with the complaint of a small red prickly rash under his scrotum. Dr. Kimrey completes an examination and the appropriate tests. Eugene is diagnosed with apocrine miliaria.
15. Gary Sanders, a 78-year-old male, comes in today with the complaint that the mole on his right ankle has begun to rapidly change in shape and color. Dr. Jones completes an examination noting ABCD: asymmetry, elevation above skin surface with an irregular border, blue-grey in color, firm to the touch, and a diameter of 8 mm and thickness of 1.63 mm. Gary is admitted to Weston Hospital. Skin and lymph node biopsies were ordered as well as imaging studies and blood tests. After reviewing the results of the pathology report and other tests, Gary is diagnosed with a malignant nodular melanoma. Excision of lesion is scheduled.

YOU CODE IT! Application

The following exercises provide practice in abstracting physicians' notes and learning to work with documentation from our health care facility, Prader, Bracker, & Associates. These case studies are modeled on real patient encounters. Using the techniques described in this chapter, carefully read through the case studies and determine the most accurate ICD-10-CM code(s) and external cause code(s), if appropriate, for each case study.

PRADER, BRACKER, & ASSOCIATES

A Complete Health Care Facility

159 Healthcare Way • SOMEWHERE, FL 32811 • 407-555-6789

PATIENT: CHILDERS, AARON

ACCOUNT/EHR #: CHILAA001

Attending Physician: Oscar R. Prader, MD

This 59-year-old male presents today with a rash on the bottom of his feet. Patient admits he is also having trouble with his vision and has dysuria.

VS normal; on visual foot examination, rash has a cobblestone appearance. After a thorough examination and testing, patient is diagnosed with acquired keratoderma due to reactive arthritis of the foot joint (Reiter's disease).

Patient is given 5 mg IM, methotrexate

Rx: Methotrexate, 2.5 mg tab, PO, once a day, x 10 days

P: Return PRN

(continued)

Determine the most accurate ICD-10-CM code(s).

PRADER, BRACKER, & ASSOCIATES

A Complete Health Care Facility

159 Healthcare Way • SOMEWHERE, FL 32811 • 407-555-6789

PATIENT: STEEVANG, BRANDON

ACCOUNT/EHR #: STEEBR001

Attending Physician: Oscar R. Prader, MD

S: This is a 39-year-old male with advanced human immunodeficiency virus infection who has presented to the emergency department with severe itching with a duration of approximately 10 days. On a scale of 1 to 10, he rates the itching as 10 of 10 in severity. Patient states he has been compliant with his antiretroviral therapy. He has been drinking excessively and taking diphenhydramine every 4 hours for the last several days.

O: H: 6′1″, Wt: 176, T: 98.9, R: 19, P: 66, BP: 132/76. On examination, he is constantly scratching his skin. There are spots of blood on his clothing. Xerosis is noted as well as several brown patches on his extremities. The scrotum appears leathery and thickened. A skin scraping for scabies mite is performed and sent to the lab for analysis.

A: Scabies, HIV

Rx: Permethrin, 5% cream, apply to all skin surfaces. Leave on for at least 9 hours, then wash off with warm water.

P: Follow-up appointment with PCP

Determine the most accurate ICD-10-CM code(s).

PRADER, BRACKER, & ASSOCIATES

A Complete Health Care Facility

159 Healthcare Way • SOMEWHERE, FL 32811 • 407-555-6789

PATIENT: CHARLES, RICHARD

ACCOUNT/EHR #: CHARRI001

Attending Physician: Renee O. Bracker, MD

S: This 35-year-old male came in after experiencing a severe episode with a prodrome of tingling of his lip before the appearance of lesions. He has been diagnosed with recurrent herpes simplex labialis. These episodes typically last between 1 and 2 weeks. He has no other medical problems and would like some easy-to-follow recommendations to manage this chronic illness.

O: VS normal. On visual examination, a small blister/sore on the lower lip is documented.

A: Recurrent herpes simplex labialis

Rx: Valacyclovir 2g, PO, followed by 2g in 12 hours

P: Return PRN

Determine the most accurate ICD-10-CM code(s).

WESTON HOSPITAL

629 Healthcare Way • SOMEWHERE, FL 32811 • 407-555-6541

PATIENT: MEDINA, LEAH

ACCOUNT/EHR #: MEDILE001

(continued)

Attending Physician: Renee O. Bracker, MD

S: Leah Medina, a 6-year-old female, was at home helping her father clean out the attic when she was bitten by a black spider. Her father, Jacob, thought quickly and captured the spider in an old jar. Leah began to run a fever and vomited several hours later, so her father rushed her to the ED.

O: H: 50.5″, Wt: 58.0 lbs., T: 102 F, R: 22, P: 90, BP: 127/88. Leah says she feels really tired and hurts all over. She has constantly scratched the bite area since arriving at the ED. She appears lethargic; rash is noted over body; heart is regular with no gallops or murmurs; lungs are clear; a dark blue/purple wound is noted on the right thigh. PMH and FH are both noncontributory. Dr. Bracker was able to identify the spider as a black widow spider and admits Leah to the hospital.

A: Black widow spider bite

P: Anitvenom 6,000 units IV in 50 mL of normal saline over 15 minutes

Determine the most accurate ICD-10-CM code(s).

WESTON HOPSITAL

629 Healthcare Way • SOMEWHERE, FL 32811 • 407-555-6541

PATIENT: CHABANNI, LORI

ACCOUNT/EHR #: CHABLO001

Attending Physician: Renee O. Bracker, MD

S: This 46-year-old female with a 3-month history of ulcerations and abscesses involving both breasts was admitted today. Patient states the ulcerations began to appear after breast reduction surgery, approximately 2 weeks postop. The patient had no history of ulcerations before the breast reduction surgery. She also states that her muscles and joints ache.

O: VS: T: 102 F, all other VS are within normal range; patient is in obvious distress. PMH: remarkable for hypertension and quiescent ulcerative colitis. FH: Noncontributory. Deep ulcers under breast, bilaterally, are noted with well-defined borders. Ulcer edges are worn and surrounding skin is red. Coloration of ulcers is violet to blue. Incision and drainage of breast abscesses is scheduled.

A: Pyoderma gangrenosum

P: Pulse IV methylprednisolone, 500 mg daily for 3 consecutive days

Determine the most accurate ICD-10-CM code(s).

16

Coding Muscular and Skeletal Conditions

Key Terms

Arthropathy
Articulation
Chondropathy
Dorsopathy
Intervertebral Disc
Laterality
Myopathy
Site
Spondylopathy
Vertebra

Learning Outcomes

After completing this chapter, the student should be able to:

LO 16.1 Code accurately arthropathic conditions of the muscles.
LO 16.2 Determine the proper way to report dorsopathies and spondylopathies.
LO 16.3 Interpret the details required to report soft tissue disorders.
LO 16.4 Identify the specifics of diseases that affect the musculoskeletal system reported from other areas of ICD-10-CM.
LO 16.5 Report diagnoses related to pathological fractures accurately.

STOP! Remember, you need to follow along in your ICD-10-CM code book for an optimal learning experience.

16.1 Arthropathies

As you can see in **Figure 16-1**, the entire skeleton appears to be wrapped with muscles from top to bottom and all the way around. Each muscle has a specific function.

Myopathy
Disease of a muscle [plural: myopathies].

Arthropathy
Disease or dysfunction of a joint [plural: arthropathies].

Chondropathy
Disease affecting the cartilage [plural: chondropathies].

Dorsopathy
Disease affecting the back of the torso [plural: dorsopathies].

Spondylopathy
Disease affecting the vertebrae [plural: spondylopathies].

Injuries are not the only concern that can affect an individual's musculoskeletal health. Diseases, infections, and other problems can occur. There are pathogens (bacteria, viruses, and fungi) that directly attack the muscles of the body. The physician's notes might identify the patient's condition as **myopathy**, **arthropathy**, **chondropathy**, **dorsopathy**, or **spondylopathy**. Some of these conditions are described in this list:

CODING BITES

Myopathy: *myo* = muscle + *-pathy* = disease.

Arthropathy: *arthro* = joint + *-pathy* = disease.

Chondropathy: *chondro* = cartilage + *-pathy* = disease.

Dorsopathy: *dorso* = back + *-pathy* = disease.

Spondylopathy: *spondylo* = vertebra + *-pathy* = disease.

Rheumatoid arthritis (RA) is an autoimmune systemic inflammatory disease that affects joints as well as the surrounding muscles, tendons, and ligaments. Report a code from category M05 Rheumatoid arthritis with rheumatoid factor or M06 Other rheumatoid arthritis. To determine the complete valid code, you will need to identify, from the documentation, the specific anatomical site. Be alert because more than one anatomical site may be involved, and ICD-10-CM provides you with combination codes to report the complete story of this patient's condition.

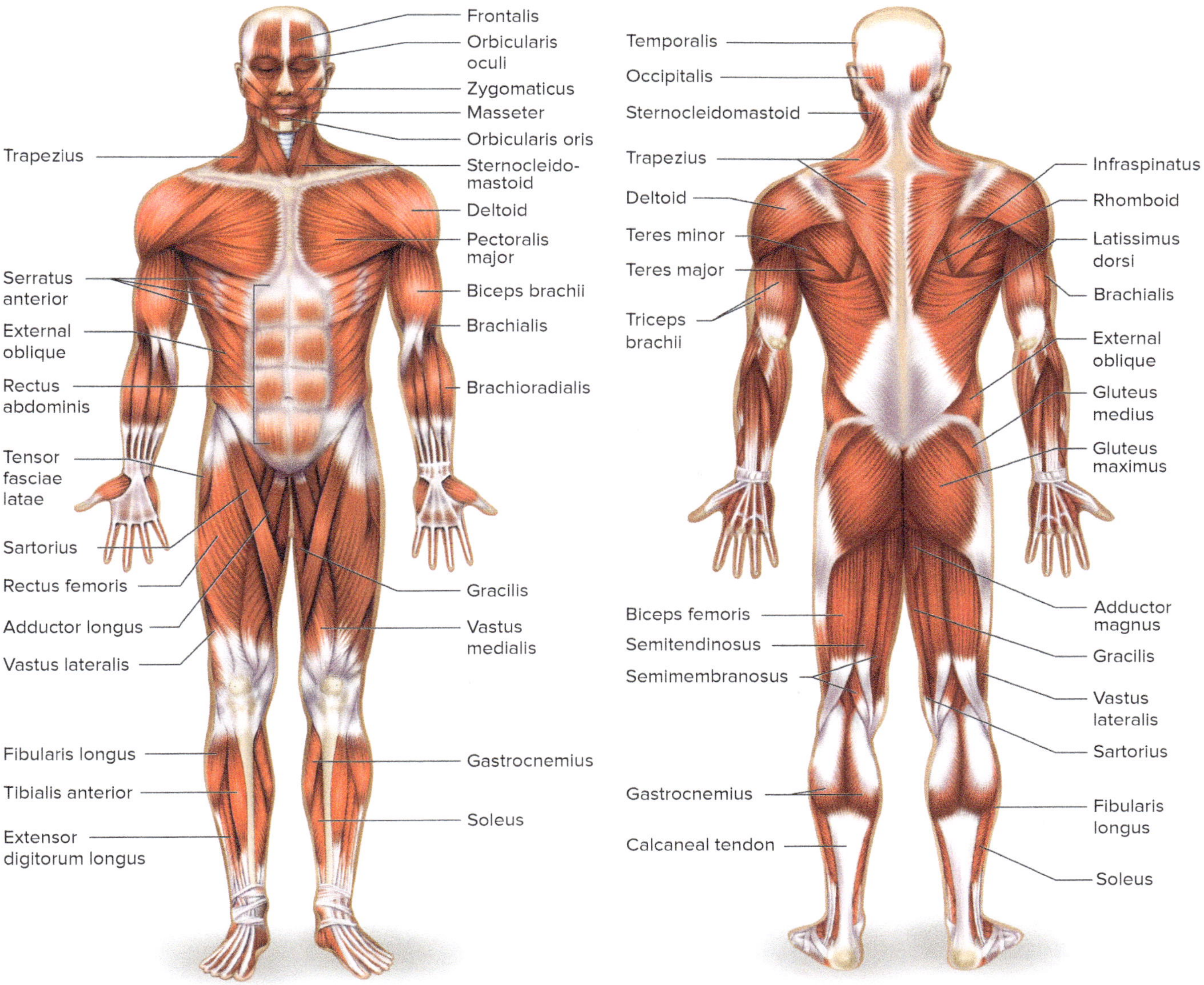

FIGURE 16-1 An illustration identifying the muscles of the body: anterior and posterior

EXAMPLES

M05.151	Rheumatoid lung disease with rheumatoid arthritis of right hip
M05.242	Rheumatoid vasculitis with rheumatoid arthritis of the left hand
M05.361	Rheumatoid heart disease with rheumatoid arthritis of right knee
M06.022	Rheumatoid arthritis without rheumatoid factor, left elbow
M06.071	Rheumatoid arthritis without rheumatoid factor, right ankle and foot

Rheumatoid factor (RF) is a test that quantifies the amount of the RF antibodies in the blood. A positive RF is the abnormal result indicating a higher number of antibodies have been detected—confirmation of the autoimmune response mechanism. You would find the data on the pathology report.

CODING BITES

Many people confuse RA (rheumatoid arthritis) with OA (osteoarthritis). RA is a condition that affects the muscles, joints, and/or connective tissue, whereas OA is the deterioration of cartilage within joints as well as spinal vertebrae.

ICD-10-CM

YOU CODE IT! CASE STUDY

Gary Simmons, a 19-year-old male, came in with complaints of intense pain and swelling of his left elbow. Vital signs evidence a low-grade fever. Gary states that he injured his forearm in hockey practice and it got infected, but he was too busy with classes and practice to go to the medical clinic on campus. Now, all of a sudden, he has pain in his elbow that he cannot ignore. Dr. Lannahan applied a local anesthetic and used fine needle aspiration to extract some synovial fluid. Analysis shows gross pus and testing shows a high white blood cell count. The synovial fluid glucose is 55 mg/dL. This confirmed a diagnosis of acute septic arthritis, due to gram-positive Staphylococcus aureus.

You Code It!

Go through the steps of coding, and determine the code or codes that should be reported for this encounter between Dr. Lannahan and Gary.

Step #1: Read the case carefully and completely.
Step #2: Abstract the scenario. Which main words or terms describe why the physician cared for the patient during this encounter?
Step #3: Are there any details missing or incomplete for which you would need to query the physician? [If so, ask your instructor.]
Step #4: Check for any relevant guidance, including reading all of the symbols and notations in the Tabular List and the appropriate sections of the Official Guidelines.
Step #5: Determine the correct diagnosis code or codes to explain why this encounter was medically necessary.
Step #6: Double-check your work.

Answer:

Did you determine these to be the correct codes?

M00.022 **Staphylococcal arthritis, left elbow**

B95.61 **Methicillin susceptible Staphylococcus aureus infection as the cause of diseases classified elsewhere**
(Staphylococcus aureus infection NOS as the cause of diseases classified elsewhere)

Genu recurvatum, the backward curving of the knee joint, as well as other bowing of the long bones of the leg, may be treated with braces, casting, and/or orthotics. Congenital genu recurvatum is reported with code Q68.2 Congenital deformity of knee. When this condition is the sequela (late effect) of rickets, it is reported with M21.26- Flexion deformity, knee, followed by code E64.3 Sequela of rickets.

Gout, also known as *gouty arthritis*, is the result of the buildup of uric acid in the body, caused by either a malfunction that produces too much uric acid or an anomaly that makes it difficult for the body to get rid of uric acid. The specific underlying cause may be idiopathic or secondary, as a manifestation of renal impairment, adverse reaction to a drug, or a toxic effect. Gout presents in the joints, most often a toe, knee, or ankle, and begins with a throbbing or extreme pain in the middle of the night. The joint will be tender, warm to the touch, and erythematous (red). The most common treatment is a prescription for nonsteroidal anti-inflammatory drugs (NSAIDs). In ICD-10-CM, gout is reported from code category M10- Gout or from code category M1A- Chronic gout, with additional characters required to report the underlying cause (i.e., drug-induced, idiopathic, etc.) as well as the specific anatomical location (i.e., ankle, elbow, foot, etc.).

Osteoarthritis is a chronic degeneration of the articular cartilage simultaneous with the formation of bone spurs on the underlying bone within a joint. The cause of the osteoarthritis might be an idiomatic condition (such as code M17.11 Unilateral primary osteoarthritis, right knee); secondary to another underlying condition (such as code M18.52 Other unilateral secondary osteoarthritis of first carpometacarpal joint, left hand); or post-traumatic (such as code M19.172 Post-traumatic osteoarthritis, left ankle and foot). Treatments typically begin with NSAIDs and/or corticosteroid injections. In some cases, a brace or crutches may be helpful.

LET'S CODE IT! SCENARIO

Timothy Metrosky, a 55-year-old male, came to see Dr. Weingard with complaints of acute pain in his left hip. He had been diagnosed with stage 1 chronic kidney disease about 1 year ago, but it has been under control with medication. Dr. Weingard aspirated synovial fluid from his hip, and the pathology report confirmed that Timothy had developed secondary gout in his hip.

Let's Code It!

Dr. Weingard diagnosed Timothy with gout in his left hip, secondary to his renal impairment. Turn to the Alphabetic Index, look up *Gout*, and read down the list. Hmmm.

Gout, gouty (acute) (attack) (flare) (*see also* Gout, chronic) M10.9

Was Timothy diagnosed with chronic gout? Check the notes. No. So, look down the indented list to find "secondary," or something similar . . .

Gout, gouty

in (due to) renal impairment M10.30

hip M10.35-

Great! The terms "*due to*" and "*secondary*" both indicate the condition [gout] was caused by another condition [kidney disease]. Now turn to the Tabular List and confirm the code.

Start reading at the code category

✓4 **M10 Gout**

Read the ***Use additional code*** notation carefully to see if it applies. None are applicable. Now check the **EXCLUDES2** note. You have already confirmed that the patient does not have chronic gout; therefore, this does not apply either.

Continue reading to find the accurate fourth character:

✓5 **M10.3 Gout due to renal impairment**

There is a ***Code first*** notation that states you need to report Timothy's renal impairment as the first code, followed by this code for the gout. But, as long as you are here, keep reading down the column to review the fifth-character and sixth-character options and determine which matches Dr. Weingard's documentation:

M10.352 Gout due to renal impairment, left hip

Very good! Now go back to the Alphabetic Index and find

Disease, kidney, chronic, stage 1 N18.1

Double-check this code in the Tabular List.

✓4 **N18 Chronic kidney disease (CKD)**

Read the ***Code first*** and ***Use additional code*** notations carefully. Do they apply to this case? No. So, continue down to find the accurate fourth character.

N18.1 Chronic kidney disease, stage 1

(continued)

You have the two codes required to report Dr. Weingard's diagnosis for Timothy. And remember that the ***Code first*** notation directed you to the correct sequencing of these two codes.

N18.1 Chronic kidney disease, stage 1

M10.352 Gout due to renal impairment, left hip

Make certain to check the top of both subsections and the head of both chapters in ICD-10-CM. There are notations at the beginning: an INCLUDES notation, a ***Code first*** notation, a ***Use additional code*** notation, **NOTE**s at the head of both chapters, and EXCLUDES2 notations. Read carefully. Do any relate to Dr. Weingard's diagnosis of Timothy? No. Turn to the Official Guidelines and read Section I.C.13 (for the musculoskeletal system) and I.C.14 (for the renal disease). There is nothing specifically applicable here, either. Now you can report N18.1, M10.352 for Timothy's diagnosis with confidence. Good coding!

Systemic lupus erythematosus (SLE) is an autoimmune disease affecting the joints, kidneys, brain, skin, and other organs. Interestingly, ICD-10-CM places this code category within the musculoskeletal system chapter. SLE may be an adverse effect of certain drugs. When this is documented, you will code M32.0 Drug-induced systemic lupus erythematosus, as well as an additional external cause code to identify the specific drug involved. If the etiology of the SLE is unknown, you will need to abstract from the physician's notes if any organ or organ system is specifically affected. When this is documented, use a combination code from subcategory M32.1- Systemic lupus erythematosus with organ or system involvement, with the fifth character naming that system or issue, such as

M32.11 Endocarditis in systemic lupus erythematosus

M32.13 Lung involvement in systemic lupus erythematosus

LET'S CODE IT! SCENARIO

Manuel Daniels, a 43-year-old male, came to see Dr. Biehl complaining of pain and stiffness in his lower jaw. Upon examination, Dr. Biehl noted swelling and erythema at the temporomandibular joint. Dr. Biehl diagnosed Manuel with arthralgia of temporomandibular joint, right side.

Let's Code It!

Dr. Biehl diagnosed Manuel with *arthralgia of temporomandibular joint.* In the Alphabetic Index, find

Arthralgia

temporomandibular M26.62

Let's turn to the Tabular List and locate the beginning of the code category:

✓4 **M26 Dentofacial anomalies (including malocclusion)**

Beginning at the code category was a good idea. There is an EXCLUDES1 notation. Read it carefully and determine whether any of this guidance is applicable to this specific encounter. There is nothing here that relates to Manuel's condition, so review all of the choices for the fourth character to determine what matches Dr. Biehl's documentation about Manuel's diagnosis:

✓5 **M26.6 Temporomandibular joint disorders**

There is an EXCLUDES2 notation with two temporomandibular conditions listed. Again, read it carefully and determine whether any of this guidance is applicable to this specific encounter. There is nothing here that relates to Manuel's condition, so review all of the choices for the fifth character to determine what matches Dr. Biehl's documentation about Manuel's diagnosis. This part of the coding process is very important to determining the correct code to report.

(continued)

Review the list of fifth characters. The documentation will bring you to this code:

✓6 **M26.62 Arthralgia of temporomandibular joint**

Very good. Now, a sixth character is required to report the laterality. Check the documentation; which side of Manuel's jaw was affected? The right side. Read through all of the sixth-character options and determine the correct code to report:

M26.621 Arthralgia of right temporomandibular joint

Good job!

16.2 Dorsopathies and Spondylopathies (Conditions Affecting the Joints of the Spine)

Components of the Spine

From the neck, where the *atlas* (C1–the first cervical vertebra) articulates with the skull, and all the way down the column to the *coccyx*, the spine is a long stack of individual bones called **vertebrae**, separated by **intervertebral discs**.

Vertebra
A bone that is a part of the construction of the spinal column [plural: vertebrae].

Intervertebral Disc
A fibrocartilage segment that lies between vertebrae of the spinal column and provides cushioning and support.

Vertebrae

An individual vertebra is more than just a bone–it is actually a complex segment of the anatomical structure. In each of the sections of the vertebral column, the size and shape of the vertebrae change. The cervical, thoracic, and lumbar vertebrae are shaped slightly differently as the bones reconfigure on the basis of their position in the column and the support that is necessary. The cervical vertebrae are the smallest of all, and the lumbar vertebrae are the largest. The various aspects of all the vertebrae, however, are the same. As you can see in **Figure 16-2**, the vertebral body protects the spinal cord anteriorly, while the spinous process and pedicle protect it posteriorly.

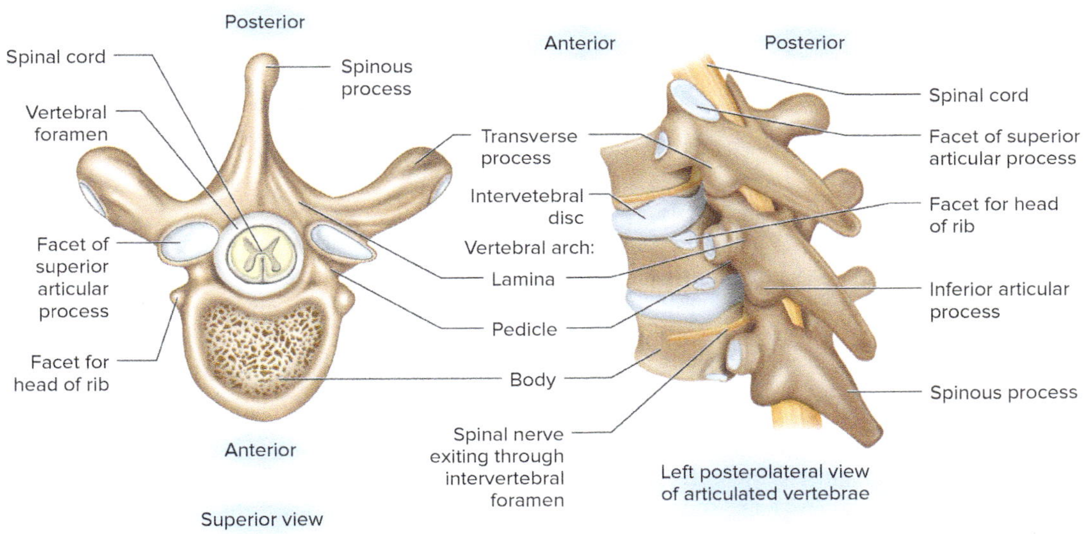

FIGURE 16-2 An illustration identifying the aspects of the vertebrae: anterior and posterior

Vertebrae are identified by their location and position in each section of the spinal column (see **Figure 16-3**):

- *Cervical vertebrae:* there are seven cervical vertebrae–beginning with the atlas (the first cervical vertebra) followed by the axis (the second cervical vertebra)–that run down the posterior (back) of the neck to the top of the shoulder area. These vertebrae are identified as C1, C2, C3, C4, C5, C6, and C7.

- *Thoracic vertebrae*: there are 12 thoracic vertebrae that run along the posterior segment of the torso (the thoracic cavity). The rib cage connects at these points. These vertebrae are identified as T1, T2, T3, T4, T5, T6, T7, T8, T9, T10, T11, and T12.
- *Lumbar vertebrae*: the five lumbar vertebrae are located at approximately the waist/hips area and are identified as L1, L2, L3, L4, and L5.
- *Sacrum:* this is a triangular-shaped bone that begins as five individual vertebrae, which fuse together by the time the average person is in their mid-twenties. The sacrum vertebrae may be identified as S1, S2, S3, S4, and S5.
- *Coccyx:* also known as the *tailbone*, this bottommost tip of the spinal column begins as three to five individual vertebrae, which fuse together in adulthood. For the average person, this fusion begins in the mid-twenties, and the vertebrae have completely fused into one bone by middle age.

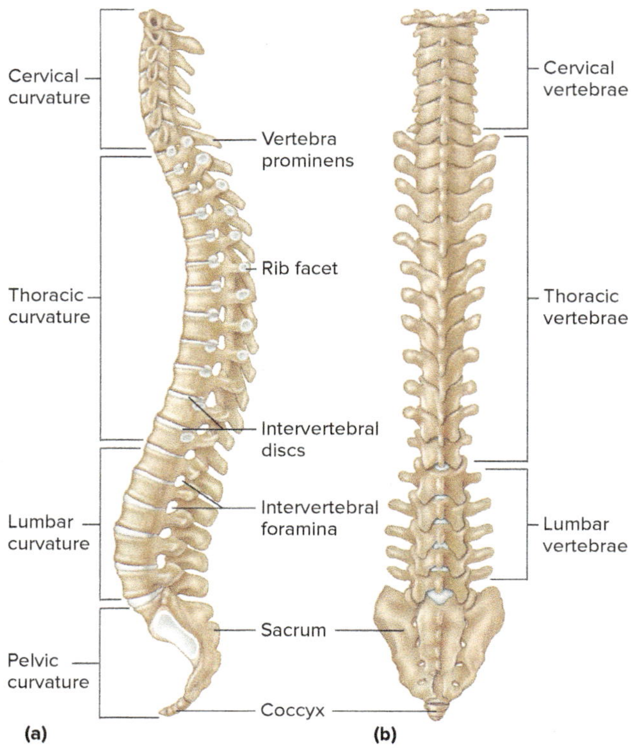

FIGURE 16-3 An illustration identifying the anatomical sites of the spinal column

Conditions Affecting the Spine

Kyphosis is a bending forward of the vertebral column, most often at the thoracic vertebrae. This condition may be congenital or may be caused by poor posture or other spinal disorder. Kyphosis used to be commonly referred to as "dowager's hump." A brace and exercise are often the first course of treatment. Spinal arthrodesis may relieve symptoms, and surgery may be done when neurologic function is impaired. This condition is reported with code M40.04 Postural kyphosis, thoracic region. However, multiple codes are available for kyphosis determined by section of the spine as well as underlying cause.

Scoliosis is similar to kyphosis, in that it results in a bending of the spinal column; however, with scoliosis, the bend is sideways rather than forward. The spine might resemble the letter S or C. Scoliosis is most often diagnosed in children aged 0–18, and more likely in females than males. Uneven gait and unbalanced hips and/or shoulders are signs that initiate further investigation.

Infantile idiopathic scoliosis is identified prior to the age of 4, equally in boys and girls, and more than 90% of these cases resolve without medical treatment.

Juvenile idiopathic scoliosis is diagnosed in children between the ages of 4 and 10, and is found more frequently in males than females. The curve in these children is often left-sided.

Adolescent idiopathic scoliosis is seen in patients aged 10–18 and may be evidenced in as high as 4% of this portion of the population. Researchers believe there may be a genetic connection; however, this has not yet been proven.

EXAMPLE

In all scoliosis diagnoses, you will need to abstract the specific region of the spine affected.

M41.02 Infantile idiopathic scoliosis, cervical region

M41.115 Juvenile idiopathic scoliosis, thoracolumbar region

M41.127 Adolescent idiopathic scoliosis, lumbosacral region

YOU CODE IT! CASE STUDY

Marci Wakefield started having pain in her back, after completing a full course of radiation treatments for a malignant tumor. Dr. Diaz diagnosed her with scoliosis of the thoracic region as a result of the radiation.

You Code It!

Go through the steps of coding, and determine the code or codes that should be reported for this encounter between Dr. Diaz and Marci.

Step #1: Read the case carefully and completely.
Step #2: Abstract the scenario. Which key words or terms describe why the physician cared for the patient during this encounter?
Step #3: Are there any details missing or incomplete for which you would need to query the physician? [If so, ask your instructor.]
Step #4: Check for any relevant guidance, including reading all of the symbols and notations in the Tabular List and the appropriate sections of the Official Guidelines.
Step #5: Determine the correct diagnosis code or codes to explain why this encounter was medically necessary.
Step #6: Double-check your work.

Answer:

M96.5 Postradiation scoliosis

Did you determine these to be the correct codes?

CODING BITES

Why is Marci's condition coded as *secondary scoliosis* and not . . .

M41.24 Other idiopathic scoliosis, thoracic region

Idiopathic means with no known cause. But the notes *do* state a cause of her scoliosis–the radiation. So this cannot be correct.

What about this code:

Q67.5 Congenital deformity of spine (Congenital scoliosis)

Congenital means present at birth. But Marci was not born with scoliosis–it developed as a result of her having radiation treatments.

Secondary means that something else (other than nature or something unknown) caused this condition. In this case, the radiation caused the scoliosis. The radiation came first, and the scoliosis came second.

Spinal ankylosis is the fusion within a vertebral joint caused by disease. This is not a procedure where the physician may fuse a joint. Code subcategory M43.2 Fusion of spine requires a fifth character to report the specific region affected.

Ankylosing spondylitis (AS) is actually a type of inflammation within the vertebral joint (arthritis). This also may be seen in the joints between the spine and the pelvic girdle. AS affects men more than women. Code category M45 Ankylosing spondylitis is used to report AS, with a fourth character to specify the region affected.

Intervertebral disc infection is caused by a pathogen and is different from the inflammation of arthritis because it is suppurative (produces pus). Code subcategory M46.3 Infection of intervertebral disc (pyogenic) requires a fifth character to identify the specific region where the infection is located, as well as an additional code from B95–B97 to identify the pathogen.

LET'S CODE IT! SCENARIO

George Cornelius came to see Dr. Rymer with complaints of sudden-onset, severe lower back pain. He states that the pain is in the left side of his buttocks, his left leg, and sometimes his left foot. At times, he states that his leg seems weak as well. Dr. Rymer takes a complete patient history, including specific times and actions that intensify the pain. Then x-rays, followed by an MRI, are taken of George's spine, showing a herniated (intervertebral) disc at L3–L4.

Let's Code It!

Dr. Rymer diagnosed George with a *herniated (intervertebral) disc*. Turn to the Alphabetic Index, look up *herniated*, and read down the list to find *disc*. Hmmm. It is not there. Try looking for *intervertebral*. Look down and see

Hernia, hernial (acquired) (recurrent) K46.9

intervertebral cartilage or disc — *see* Displacement, intervertebral disc

OK, let's turn to that in the Alphabetic Index:

Displacement, displaced

intervertebral disc NEC

lumbar region M51.26

You might ask, How do we know that it is the lumbar region? Look back at Dr. Rymer's notes. He wrote that the herniated disk is at L3–L4. The "L" means the lumbar vertebrae, and the notation L3–L4 indicates that the affected intervertebral disc is between the third and fourth lumbar vertebrae. Now turn to the Tabular List and confirm the code.

Start reading at

✓4 **M51 Thoracic, thoracolumbar, and lumbosacral intervertebral disc disorders**

There is an EXCLUDES2 note that mentions disorders of the cervical and sacral discs. However, George's lumbar disc is what is dislocated, so you can keep reading down the column to review the fourth-character and fifth-character options and determine which matches Dr. Rymer's documentation:

✓5 **M51.2 Other thoracic, thoracolumbar, and lumbosacral intervertebral disc displacement**

M51.26 Other intervertebral disc displacement, lumbar region

Go back to Dr. Rymer's notes and see that while this doesn't match exactly, it does tell the story of why Dr. Rymer cared for George. Terrific!

This code tells the whole story about George's specific injury. Now ask yourself, Do I need to find the external cause code(s) to explain how George's injury happened? No. A herniated disc is not necessarily the result of a traumatic event. Therefore, there is no need to report any external cause.

Good work!

16.3 Soft Tissue Disorders

Fibromyalgia, also known as myofibrositis, or fibromyositis, causes the patient to experience tenderness on their extremities, as well as their neck and shoulders, back, and hips. In addition, the patient will suffer headaches, trouble sleeping, and sometimes forgetfulness and difficulties thinking. Code M79.7 Fibromyalgia.

Myositis identifies the inflammation of a muscle caused by a muscle strain. When a diagnosis of infective myositis is documented, you will need to report a code from subcategory M60.0 Infective myositis, with a fifth character to identify the specific anatomical site (shoulder, upper arm, hand, thigh, etc.) and a sixth character to report laterality. In addition to the M60.0– code, you will need *an additional code* from B95–B97 to report the specific pathogen.

Polymyositis is a systemic rheumatic disorder evidenced by inflammatory and degenerative changes in the muscles. The signs and symptoms of muscle weakness, discomfort, and tenderness appear suddenly, most often in the proximal muscles. These symptoms interrupt the patient's ability to perform activities of daily living (ADL). To report this diagnosis accurately, you will need to abstract from the documentation the involvement of the respiratory system (M33.21), myopathy (M33.22), or other specific organs being hampered by this condition (M33.29).

Dermatopolymyositis is a systemic rheumatic disorder characterized by inflammatory and degenerative changes in the skin and muscles. The first sign is often an erythematous rash that appears on the face, neck, torso (front and back), and upper extremities. In addition, there may be a heliotropic rash on the eyelids along with periorbital edema. To report this diagnosis accurately, you will need to abstract from the documentation the involvement of the respiratory system (M33.11), myopathy (M33.12), or other specific organs being hampered by this condition (M33.19).

Juvenile dermatomyositis (JDM) is a systemic, autoimmune, inflammatory muscle condition that often appears with vasculopathy in children 18 years of age or younger. To report this diagnosis accurately, you will need to abstract from the documentation the involvement of the respiratory system (M33.01), myopathy (M33.02), or other specific organs being hampered by this condition (M33.09).

Bursitis is a painful inflammation of a bursa, most often the result of recurring trauma. Once you make your way to code category M71 Other bursopathies, you will need to abstract from the physician's notes the type of problem: Is there an abscess or infection? If so, in addition to identifying the specific anatomical site (shoulder, elbow, hand, etc.) and laterality, you will need to find the confirmation of the pathogen, so you can accurately add a second code from B95.- or B96.- to report this detail as well.

Epicondylitis is an inflammation of the elbow joint that typically begins as a small tear in the muscle and then is aggravated by activities. *Lateral epicondylitis* is commonly known as "tennis elbow," while *medial epicondylitis* is commonly known as "golfer's elbow," reported by codes M77.1 Lateral epicondylitis and M77.0 Medial epicondylitis, respectively. Both codes require a fifth character to identify the right or left elbow.

Achilles tendon contracture is a shortening of the tendocalcaneus (heel cord), which is caused by chronic poor posture, continual wearing of high-heeled shoes, or landing on the ball of the foot rather than the heel while jogging or is a manifestation of cerebral palsy or poliomyelitis. Use code M67.0 Short Achilles tendon (acquired), with a fifth character to identify the right or left ankle, or Q66.89 Other specified congenital deformities of feet.

Torticollis is a condition in which the sternocleidomastoid muscle becomes spasmed (shortened), causing the head to bend to one side and the chin to the opposite side. This condition may be acquired, reported with code M43.6 Torticollis, unless the documentation states Q68.0 Congenital deformity of sternocleidomastoid muscle, F45.8 Other somatoform disorders, G24.3 Spasmodic torticollis, or other diagnosis shown in the **EXCLUDES1** notation beneath M43.6.

Muscle spasms, commonly known as *muscle cramps*, are involuntary twitches and are often caused by myositis or fibromyositis. Sometimes these spasms are caused by metabolic or mineral imbalances. Abstract the documentation to identify the anatomical site. Use code M62.830 Muscle spasm of back, M62.831 Muscle spasm of calf (Charley-horse), M62.838 Other muscle spasm, or R25.2 Cramp and spasm.

Type III traumatic spondylolisthesis of the axis (C2) is a displacement of the vertebra anteriorly over the vertebra below it. An open reduction of the C2 vertebra followed by a posterior spinal fusion with a pedicle lag screw is used to repair the injury. Report this with code M43.12 Spondylolisthesis, cervical region.

LET'S CODE IT! SCENARIO

Elliott Carlyle, a 17-year-old male, is believed to be an up-and-coming star on the golf course. He explains to Dr. Carole that the pain in his left elbow has become severe and his ability to grasp the club is weakened. Physical exam included flexion and pronation, confirming medial epicondylitis.

Let's Code It!

Dr. Carole diagnosed Elliott with *medial epicondylitis*. In the ICD-10-CM Alphabetic Index, let's turn to find the documented term. . . . Find

Epicondylitis (elbow)

There are only two items on the indented list:

Epicondylitis (elbow)

lateral M77.1-

medial M77.0-

Check the scenario to confirm which diagnosis was documented. Let's go to the Tabular List to check this code category. Find

✓4 **M77 Other enthesopathies**

Check the diagnoses shown in the EXCLUDES1 and EXCLUDES2 notations. Do either of them relate to Elliott's diagnosis? No, good. Now, read down and review all of the fourth-character options. Which matches the documentation?

✓5 **M77.0 Medial epicondylitis**

M77.01 Medial epicondylitis, right elbow

M77.02 Medial epicondylitis, left elbow

Therefore, the most accurate code is

M77.02 Medial epicondylitis, left elbow

Check the top of this subsection and the head of this chapter in ICD-10-CM. Both a **NOTE** and an EXCLUDES2 notation appear at the beginning of this ICD-10-CM chapter. Read carefully. Do any relate to Dr. Carole's diagnosis of Elliott? No. Turn to the Official Guidelines and read Section I.C.13. There is nothing specifically applicable here, either.

Now you can report M77.02 for Elliott's diagnosis with confidence.

Good coding! Good work!

Osteochondrosis, also known as *osteochondropathy* or *Osgood-Schlatter disease*, is a painful separation of the epiphysis of the tibial tubercle from the tibial shaft. This condition most often affects preteen and early teenage boys after a traumatic event. Treatments include immobilization of the knee and rest. In severe cases, surgical repair may be required. One code example is M93.1 Kienbock's disease of adults (adult osteochondrosis of carpal lunates).

Osteitis deformans, also known as *Paget's disease*, may cause severe and chronic pain as well as impaired movement due to abnormal bone growth on the spinal cord. The preferred first phase of treatment is pharmaceutical. Report this from code category M88 Osteitis deformans (Paget's disease of bone), with additional characters to report the specific bone affected as well as laterality.

Osteoporosis is a disease that is believed to be the manifestation of slowing bone formation that occurs simultaneously with an increase in the body's reabsorption of bone. One exception is *post-traumatic osteoporosis*, also known as *Sudeck's atrophy*. The existence of osteoporosis increases the patient's susceptibility to fractures. The presence of a pathological fracture will change the code determination in ICD-10-CM. Code category M80 reports osteoporosis *with* a current pathological fracture, while code category M81 reports osteoporosis *without* a current pathological fracture.

GUIDANCE CONNECTION

Read the ICD-10-CM Official Guidelines for Coding and Reporting, section **I. Conventions, General Coding Guidelines and Chapter-Specific Guidelines**, subsection **C. Chapter-Specific Coding Guidelines**, **chapter 13. Diseases of the Musculoskeletal System and Connective Tissue**, subsection **d. Osteoporosis**.

LET'S CODE IT! SCENARIO

Everett Rotarine, a 43-year-old male, was having pain in his left thigh, which his orthopedist, Dr. Nixon, identified as excessive bone resorption, the osteoclastic phase of Paget's disease. X-rays and a urinalysis showing elevated levels of hydroxyproline confirmed the osteoclastic hyperactivity. Everett comes in today to discuss the test findings and treatment options.

Let's Code It!

Dr. Nixon diagnosed Everett with *Paget's disease*. You may remember that this is an eponym and will be shown in the ICD-10-CM Alphabetic Index, so let's turn to find the suggested code. Find

Paget's disease

Notice the long list of additional descriptors of this condition indented beneath this listing. Look at the scenario again.

Paget's disease
  bone M88.9
    femur M88.85-

Let's go to the Tabular List to check this code category. Find

✓4 **M88 Osteitis deformans (Paget's disease of bone)**

Let's keep reading:

✓5 **M88.8 Osteitis deformans of other bones**
✓6 **M88.85 Osteitis deformans of thigh**
M88.852 Osteitis deformans of left thigh

Therefore, the most accurate code is

M88.852 Osteitis deformans of left thigh

Good work!

16.4 Musculoskeletal Disorders from Other Body Systems

Acquired Conditions

Muscle tumors do not occur frequently and can often be malignant. Use code categories C49 Malignant neoplasm of other connective and soft tissue, C79.89 Secondary malignant neoplasms of other specified sites, or D21 Other benign neoplasms of connective and other soft tissue.

Duchenne's muscular dystrophy (DMD) is caused by a mutation of the DMD gene within the X chromosome, resulting in the body's inability to create the dystrophin protein within the muscles. Due to this, males are more likely to contract the condition because females have an additional X chromosome that may counteract the mutated gene, as long as the second X chromosome is not damaged as well. Initial signs and symptoms of DMD include leg muscle weakness followed by weakness of the shoulder muscles. DMD is most often diagnosed in early childhood and may be terminal by age 21 should the weakness spread to either heart or respiratory muscles. New trials using gene therapy are hopeful. Use code G71.0 Muscular dystrophy.

Myasthenia gravis is a chronic autoimmune condition that causes muscle weakness, primarily in the face and neck, due to the immune system incorrectly attacking the muscle cells in the body. It may progress and involve additional weakness in the muscles of the extremities (arms and legs). Use code G70.00 Myasthenia gravis without (acute) exacerbation or G70.01 Myasthenia gravis with (acute) exacerbation.

Paralytic syndromes are conditions in which muscle control is reduced or nonexistent. Cerebral palsy (code category G80), hemiplegia and hemiparesis (code category G81), and paraplegia (paraparesis) and quadriplegia (quadriparesis) (code category G82) are some of the conditions that may interfere with the ADL.

CODING BITES

NOTICE that these conditions–*congenital myopathies, muscular dystrophy, myasthenia gravis,* and *paralytic syndromes*–are reported with codes from the ICD-10-CM code book's ***Chapter 6: Diseases of the Nervous System (G00–G99).*** Remember that the nerves signal the muscles to function. Therefore, paralysis is actually a dysfunction of the nerves that communicate with the affected specific muscles.

ICD-10-CM

YOU CODE IT! CASE STUDY

Theda Granddura, a 37-year-old female, came to see Dr. Lyndon complaining of weakness in her arms and hands. She stated that sometimes she is unsteady on her feet, and her right eyelid was droopy. Two days ago, she tried to pick up a glass and could not get her fingers to "work right." An EMG was performed in the office, confirming a diagnosis of myasthenia gravis.

You Code It!

Review the details in Dr. Lyndon's documentation of this encounter with Theda to determine the accurate ICD-10-CM code or codes to report her diagnosis.

Step #1: Read the case carefully and completely.
Step #2: Abstract the scenario. Which main words or terms describe why the physician cared for the patient during this encounter?
Step #3: Are there any details missing or incomplete for which you would need to query the physician? [If so, ask your instructor.]
Step #4: Check for any relevant guidance, including reading all of the symbols and notations in the Tabular List and the appropriate sections of the Official Guidelines.
Step #5: Determine the correct diagnosis code or codes to explain why this encounter was medically necessary.
Step #6: Double-check your work.

Answer:

Did you determine this to be the correct code?

G70.00 Myasthenia gravis without (acute) exacerbation

Congenital Disorders

Congenital myopathies include minicore disease, nemaline myopathy, and fiber-type disproportion. One code, G71.2, reports several muscle abnormalities diagnosed in a neonate or infant. Most often, the infant will not meet normal developmental milestones, particularly those involving muscular actions, such as sitting up or rolling over. Such babies also may have problems feeding.

Developmental dysplasia of the hip (DDH), also known as *congenital hip dysplasia*, is most common in a baby born breech, a large neonate, or a multiparity baby. DDH is a condition in which the head of the femur is displaced from the acetabulum. Use code Q65.89 Other specified congenital deformities of hip (congenital acetabular dysplasia).

Ectromelia or *hemimelia* can occur in either the upper or lower limb. Ectromelia is the congenital absence or imperfection of one or more limbs. Hemimelia is a congenital abnormality affecting only the distal segment of either the upper or lower limb. This condition is reported with code Q73.8 Other reduction defects of unspecified limb (ectromelia of limb NOS) (hemimelia of limb NOS).

Klippel-Feil syndrome is a condition characterized by the development of a short, wide neck due to either an abnormal number of cervical vertebrae or fused hemivertebrae (the incomplete development of one side of a vertebra). Use code Q76.1 Klippel-Feil syndrome (cervical fusion syndrome).

Spina bifida is a condition in which the bony encasement of the spinal cord fails to close. Surgical repair is done as soon as possible in an effort to reduce serious disabilities. There have been some successful cases of in utero surgical repair. This condition is reported from code category Q05- Spina bifida, with an additional character to identify the specific area of the spine that is affected.

16.5 Pathological Fractures

The skeleton of the human body (see **Figure 16-4**) provides the structure for both form and function. The 206 bones in the adult body comprise a framework hinged together at the **articulations** (joints) that is stabilized by muscles and connective tissues.

Articulation
A joint.

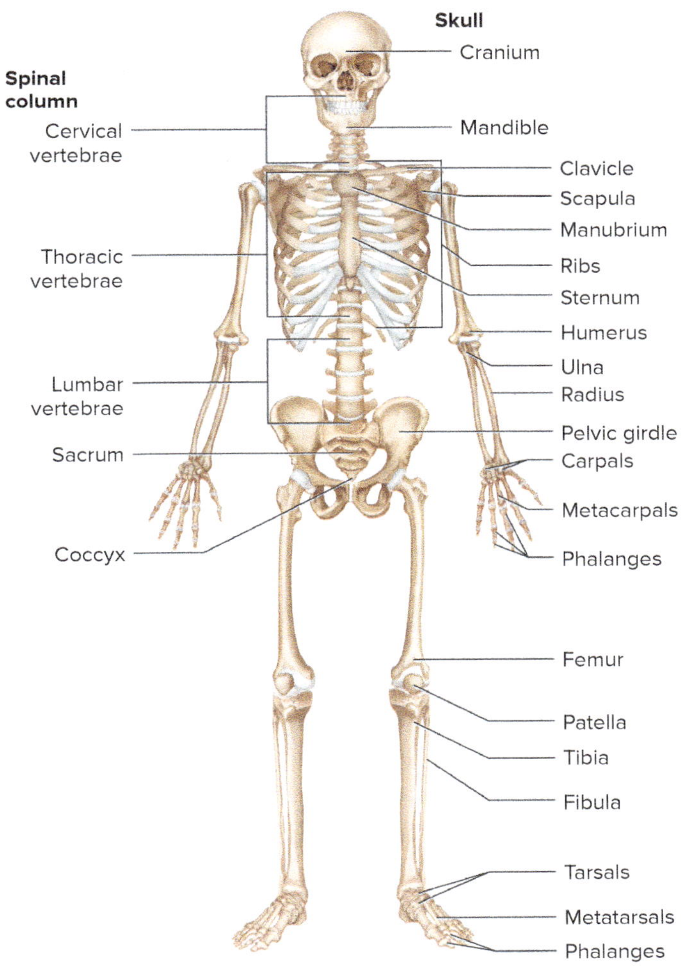

FIGURE 16-4 An illustration identifying the major bones of the human skeleton

Site
The specific anatomical location of the disease or injury.

Laterality
The right or left side of anatomical sites that have locations on both sides of the body; e.g., right arm or left arm; *unilateral* means one side and *bilateral* means both sides.

GUIDANCE CONNECTION

Read the ICD-10-CM Official Guidelines for Coding and Reporting, section **I. Conventions, General Coding Guidelines and Chapter-Specific Guidelines**, subsection **C. Chapter-Specific Coding Guidelines**, chapter **13. Diseases of the Musculoskeletal System and Connective Tissue**, subsection **a. Site and laterality**.

In your job as a professional coding specialist, it is important to abstract from the documentation details regarding the **site** of the disease or injury (the specific bone) as well as the **laterality** (right side or left side), when applicable.

Some conditions may affect any part of the skeletal system and therefore require that the specific anatomical location be documented. For instance, when a long bone, such as an ulna or femur, is affected, you might find that knowing the name of the bone is insufficient; you also will need to know the part of the bone, such as the shaft. When the segment of the bone that is diseased leads into, and participates in, the formation of a joint (articulation), read the documentation carefully. Even if the part of the bone affected is *at the joint*, you must report the bone as the diseased anatomical site.

GUIDANCE CONNECTION

Read the ICD-10-CM Official Guidelines for Coding and Reporting, section **I. Conventions, General Coding Guidelines and Chapter-Specific Guidelines**, subsection **C. Chapter-Specific Coding Guidelines**, chapter **13. Diseases of the Musculoskeletal System and Connective Tissue**, subsection **a.1) Bone versus joint**.

Diseases and other conditions can create problems with the bones and may be caused by a congenital malformation, pathology, or a traumatic event. As always, these are important details for coders to know.

The bones are, typically, the strongest parts of our bodies. However, in some cases, disease can deteriorate the structure of a bone so much that it breaks under the slightest pressure. Even normal activity can result in the weakened part of the bone breaking (fracture). When this happens, it is known as a pathological fracture.

GUIDANCE CONNECTION

Read the ICD-10-CM Official Guidelines for Coding and Reporting, section **I. Conventions, General Coding Guidelines and Chapter-Specific Guidelines**, subsection **C. Chapter-Specific Coding Guidelines**, chapter **13. Diseases of the Musculoskeletal System and Connective Tissue**, subsection **c. Coding of Pathologic Fractures**.

The most common underlying cause of a pathological fracture is osteoporosis. However, other health conditions, such as a bone cyst, an infection, genetic disorders, and malignancy, may do just as much harm.

Treatment for pathological fractures may be similar to that for a traumatic fracture. However, not always. In virtually all cases, the underlying condition is treated as well.

EXAMPLES

Pathological fractures are reported from these code subcategories:

M84.4- **Pathological fracture, not elsewhere classified**

M84.5- **Pathological fracture in neoplastic disease**

M84.6- **Pathological fracture in other diseases**

When reporting a code for a pathological fracture, you will need to assign a seventh character to identify the point in the treatment for this condition.

A Use the seventh character A for the entire scope of time that the patient is receiving active treatment for this fracture. This seventh character reports the status of "active treatment," not the relationship between physician and patient (new patient).

D Once the patient has completed active treatment, this character should be reported to identify follow-up for routine healing.

G The seventh character G would be reported for subsequent care for a pathological fracture with delayed healing.

K Subsequent care provided for a nonunion would be identified with a seventh character of K.

P When a malunion occurs, the subsequent care would be reported with a seventh character of P.

S Care for any sequela (late effect) of the original pathological fracture is identified with a seventh character of S.

GUIDANCE CONNECTION

Read the ICD-10-CM Official Guidelines for Coding and Reporting, section **I. Conventions, General Coding Guidelines and Chapter-Specific Guidelines**, subsection **C. Chapter-Specific Coding Guidelines**, chapter **13. Diseases of the Musculoskeletal System and Connective Tissue**, subsection **c. Coding of Pathologic Fractures**, and chapter **2. Neoplasms**, subsection **1.6) Pathologic fracture due to a neoplasm.**

ICD-10-CM

YOU CODE IT! CASE STUDY

Deliah Livingston, a 49-year-old female, was diagnosed with breast cancer a year ago. She had a double mastectomy 6 months ago. She came to see Dr. Wells for a checkup and he discovered that Deliah's malignancy had metastasized to the proximal portion of her right femur. Dr. Wells suggested surgery to insert a metal rod to support the bone. She told him she would think about it. Yesterday, she was walking down her driveway and all of a sudden her thighbone splintered and she fell. In the Emergency Department, Dr. Travers diagnosed Deliah with a pathological fracture of the proximal femur, just below the hip joint, due to metastatic malignancy.

You Code It!

Abstract the documentation about this ED encounter between Deliah and Dr. Travers and determine how to report the reasons for this visit.

HINT: You will need some of what you learned from the ***Coding Neoplasms*** *chapter here.*

Step #1: Read the case carefully and completely.
Step #2: Abstract the scenario. Which main words or terms describe why the physician cared for the patient during this encounter?
Step #3: Are there any details missing or incomplete for which you would need to query the physician? [If so, ask your instructor.]
Step #4: Check for any relevant guidance, including reading all of the symbols and notations in the Tabular List and the appropriate sections of the Official Guidelines.
Step #5: Determine the correct diagnosis code or codes to explain why this encounter was medically necessary.
Step #6: Double-check your work.

Answer:

Did you determine these to be the correct codes?

M84.551A **Pathological fracture in neoplastic disease, right femur, initial encounter for fracture**

C79.51 **Secondary malignant neoplasm of bone**

Z85.3 **Personal history of malignant neoplasm of breast**

Chapter Summary

The entire body is wrapped from head to toe and all the way around by muscles: voluntary muscles that assist movement of the skeleton and involuntary muscles that are controlled by the nervous system. Each muscle has its specific function, and they are all susceptible to injury, inflammation, and disease.

The 206 bones of the adult human skeleton provide the foundational structure for the components of the body. These bones protect internal organs as well as enable certain functions. Each bone is categorized by its shape: long bones, flat bones, short bones, irregularly shaped bones, and sesamoid bones. Any of these bones can be afflicted by malformation during gestation (congenital conditions), disease (pathological conditions), or injury (traumatic conditions).

CODING BITES

INTERESTING FACTS ABOUT HUMAN MUSCLES

Longest muscle = Sartorius (thigh) muscle

Smallest muscle = Stapedius (in the ear)

Largest muscle = Gluteus maximus (buttocks)

Strongest muscle = Masseter (chewing)

Busiest muscles = Eye muscles

Goosebump muscles = Tiny muscles in the hair root

Smiling requires 17 facial muscles.

Frowns require 42 facial muscles.

CHAPTER 16 REVIEW
Coding Muscular and Skeletal Conditions

Let's Check It! Terminology

Match each key term to the appropriate definition.

1. **LO 16.2** A fibrocartilage segment that lies between vertebrae of the spinal column and provides cushioning and support.
2. **LO 16.5** A joint.
3. **LO 16.5** The specific anatomical location of the disease or injury.
4. **LO 16.2** A bone that is a part of the construction of the spinal column.
5. **LO 16.5** The right or left side of anatomical sites that have locations on both sides of the body.

A. Articulation
B. Intervertebral Disc
C. Laterality
D. Site
E. Vertebra

Let's Check It! Concepts

Choose the most appropriate answer for each of the following questions.

1. **LO 16.2** Jane Timmerman was diagnosed with lower back strain, subsequent encounter. What is the correct code?
   a. S39.002A **b.** S39.012D **c.** S39.022D **d.** S39.092S

2. **LO 16.1** _____ is an autoimmune systemic inflammatory disease that affects joints as well as the surrounding muscles, tendons, and ligaments.
   - **a.** Duchenne's muscular dystrophy
   - **b.** Nemaline myopathy
   - **c.** Rheumatoid arthritis
   - **d.** Myasthenia gravis
3. **LO 16.1** A chronic degeneration of the articular cartilage simultaneous with the formation of bone spurs on the underlying bone within a joint is known as
   - **a.** rheumatoid arthritis.
   - **b.** gout.
   - **c.** genu recurvatum.
   - **d.** osteoarthritis.
4. **LO 16.3** _____ is a condition in which the sternocleidomastoid muscles become spasmed (shortened), causing the head to bend to one side and the chin to the opposite side.
   - **a.** Bursitis
   - **b.** Epicondylitis
   - **c.** Achilles tendon contracture
   - **d.** Torticollis
5. **LO 16.2** Sammie Blane was diagnosed with cervicothoracic postural kyphosis. How is this coded?
   - **a.** M40.209
   - **b.** M40.202
   - **c.** M40.03
   - **d.** M40.12
6. **LO 16.3** A systemic rheumatic disorder characterized by inflammatory and degenerative changes in the skin and muscles is known as
   - **a.** myositis.
   - **b.** juvenile dermatomyositis.
   - **c.** osteochondrosis.
   - **d.** dermatopolymyositis.
7. **LO 16.4** Myotonic muscular dystrophy is coded _____.
   - **a.** G71.11
   - **b.** G71.00
   - **c.** G71.12
   - **d.** G71.13
8. **LO 16.4** _____ is a chronic autoimmune condition that causes muscle weakness, primarily in the face and neck, due to the immune system incorrectly attacking the muscle cells in the body.
   - **a.** Duchenne's muscular dystrophy
   - **b.** Myasthenia gravis
   - **c.** Ectromelia
   - **d.** Paralytic syndromes
9. **LO 16.5** Ben Watson is diagnosed with a malunion. It will be reported with which seventh character?
   - **a.** A
   - **b.** G
   - **c.** P
   - **d.** K
10. **LO 16.5** When disease deteriorates the structure of a bone so much that it breaks under the slightest pressure, this is known as a _____ fracture.
    - **a.** malformation
    - **b.** traumatic
    - **c.** congenital
    - **d.** pathological

Let's Check It! Guidelines

Refer to the Official Guidelines and fill in the blanks according to the Chapter 13, Diseases of the Musculoskeletal System and Connective Tissue, Chapter-Specific Coding Guidelines.

no	laterality	joint	Z87.310	without
systemic	history	active	A	multiple
healed	not	site	bone	time
fracture	affected	current	known	musculoskeletal
represents	traumatic	one		

1. Most of the codes within **Chapter 13** have _____ and _____ designations. The site _____ the bone, joint, or the muscle involved.
2. For categories where _____ multiple site code is provided and more than _____ bone, joint, or muscle is involved, _____ codes should be used to indicate the different sites involved.
3. For certain conditions, the bone may be affected at the upper or lower end (e.g., avascular necrosis of bone, M87, Osteoporosis, M80, M81). Though the portion of the bone _____ may be at the _____, the site designation will be the _____, not the joint.
4. Bone, joint, or muscle conditions that are the result of a _____ injury are usually found in **Chapter 13**.
5. 7th character _____ is for use as long as the patient is receiving _____ treatment for the fracture.

6. Osteoporosis is a ____ condition, meaning that all bones of the ____ system are affected.
7. Category M81, Osteoporosis ____ current pathological fracture, is for use for patients with osteoporosis who do ____ currently have a pathological fracture due to the osteoporosis, even if they have had a ____ in the past.
8. For patients with a ____ of osteoporosis fractures, status code ____ , Personal history of (healed) osteoporosis fracture, should follow the code from M81.
9. Category M80, Osteoporosis with ____ pathological fracture, is for patients who have a current pathological fracture at the ____ of an encounter.
10. A code from category M80, not a ____ fracture code, should be used for any patient with ____ osteoporosis who suffers a fracture, even if the patient had a minor fall or trauma, if that fall or trauma would not usually break a normal, healthy bone.

Let's Check It! Rules and Regulations

Please answer the following questions from the knowledge you have gained after reading this chapter.

1. **LO 16.1** What is arthropathy? Include ways that the physician might identify the patient's condition; also include an example of an arthropathic condition.
2. **LO 16.2** List two conditions that affect the spine and explain each one.
3. **LO 16.3** Explain the difference between osteochondrosis and osteoporosis.
4. **LO 16.4** List an acquired musculoskeletal disorder and a congenital disorder and discuss each.
5. **LO 16.5** Explain the difference between a traumatic fracture and a pathological fracture. Why is it important to know the difference?

ICD-10-CM

YOU CODE IT! Basics

First, identify the condition in the following diagnoses; then code the diagnosis.

Example: Trigger thumb, right:

a. main term: *Trigger* **b.** diagnosis: *M65.311*

1. Infective myositis, left foot:
   a. main term:______ **b.** diagnosis:______
2. Pyogenic, bacterial, arthritis, left knee:
   a. main term:______ **b.** diagnosis:______
3. Foreign body granuloma of soft tissue, right thigh:
   a. main term:______ **b.** diagnosis:______
4. Juxtaphalangeal distal osteoarthritis:
   a. main term:______ **b.** diagnosis:______
5. Nontraumatic rupture of muscle, left shoulder:
   a. main term:______ **b.** diagnosis:______
6. Hallux valgus, left foot:
   a. main term:______ **b.** diagnosis:______
7. Ischemic infarction of muscle, left hand:
   a. main term:______ **b.** diagnosis:______
8. Osteomyelitis neonatal jaw:
   a. main term:______ **b.** diagnosis:______
9. Infantile idiopathic scoliosis, lumbosacral:
   a. main term:______ **b.** diagnosis:______
10. Contracture of right ankle:
    a. main term:______ **b.** diagnosis:______
11. Atrophy of left lower leg:
    a. main term:______ **b.** diagnosis:______
12. Ankylosis of right wrist:
    a. main term:______ **b.** diagnosis:______
13. Abscess of tendon sheath, right forearm:
    a. main term:______ **b.** diagnosis:______
14. Spinal stenosis, cervicothoracic region:
    a. main term:______ **b.** diagnosis:______
15. Calcific tendinitis, left pelvic region:
    a. main term:______ **b.** diagnosis:______

ICD-10-CM

YOU CODE IT! Practice

Using the techniques described in this chapter, carefully read through the case studies and determine the most accurate ICD-10-CM code(s) and external cause code(s), if appropriate, for each case study.

1. Nancy Nottingham, a 52-year-old female, presents today with a severe burning pain and swelling in her upper right arm and fingers. Dr. Olden notes edema and allodynia. After a thorough examination, Nancy is diagnosed with reflex sympathetic dystrophy (RSD).
2. Arturo Garwood, a 57-year-old male, comes in today with left shoulder pain and weakness. Arturo admits that he struggles to raise his left arm above his head. Dr. Dow completes an examination and orders an MRI scan. The MRI results confirm the diagnosis of incomplete rotator cuff tear.
3. Sharron Webster, a 3-year-old female, was brought in by her parents to see her pediatrician, Dr. Surrant, 4 days ago. Sharron had a boil on her left thigh that Dr. Surrant incised and drained. Sharron is now running a fever of 102 F. Dr. Surrant decides to admit Sharron to Weston Hospital. The MRI scan revealed abscess of the vastus intermedius muscle. A wound culture grew *Staphylococcus aureus*. Sharron is diagnosed with pyomyositis.
4. Tamara Gibbons, a 37-year-old female, presents today with pain on the inside of her right knee. Dr. Booker completes a history and physical examination. After reviewing the MRI results, Tamara is diagnosed with Plica syndrome.
5. Jay Lawson, a 13-year-old male, is brought in by his parents to see Dr. Bouknight, his pediatrician. Jay is complaining of left hip pain and stiffness. Dr. Bouknight completes a physical examination and notes limited left hip motion as well as soft tissue swelling. Jay is admitted to Weston Hospital. Aspiration of synovial fluid reveals an elevated cell count of 136 cells/mL with 52% being polymorphonuclear leukocytes. Jay is diagnosed with intermittent hydrarthrosis.
6. Terrell Meddy, a 58-year-old male, comes in today to see Dr. McNair with the complaint his left elbow is stiff and painful and feels warm. Terrell doesn't remember hitting his elbow on anything. After an examination, Dr. McNair diagnosed Terrell with olecranon bursitis of the elbow.
7. Shirley Moody, an 11-year-old female, is brought in by her mother. Mrs. Moody states that Shirley is experiencing severe muscle weakness. Dr. Bernstein completes a physical examination and notes heart arrhythmias, aphasia, and dyspnea. Shirley says that the weakness seems to last about 4 hours and comes and goes. Dr. Bernstein admits Shirley into the hospital and orders an electromyographic (EMG) test. The results of the ECG, EMG, and muscle biopsy confirm the diagnosis of hypokalemic periodic paralysis.
8. Angie Dawson, a 4-year-old female, is brought in by her parents. Angie is having difficulty chewing her food as well as having some speech problems. Dr. Hunt notes misalignment between the teeth of the dental arches as Angie's jaw closes. Dr. Hunt completes a thorough examination and the appropriate tests. Angie is diagnosed with malocclusion, Angle's class II.
9. Ned Taylor, a 33-year-old male, presents today with severe weakness in his left hip. Dr. Louthan notes enlarged neck lymph node, a rash, and high fever. Ned admits to some eye and chest pain with general lethargy. After a thorough examination, Dr. Louthan decides to admit Ned to the hospital. The laboratory test and MRI confirmed the diagnosis of arthritis of the hip due to O'nyong-nyong fever.
10. Rykia Huffman, a 21-year-old female, presents today with the complaint of uneven hips and leg length. Dr. Gamble completes a physical examination and orders a weight-bearing, full-length spine x-ray, AP, which confirms the diagnosis of idiopathic scoliosis, lumbosacral region.
11. Kendall Everett, a 41-year-old female, comes in today with the complaint her right hand aches and itches. Kendall also admits it has become harder to hold objects in her right hand. Dr. Inabinet completes an examination and a table top test, which was positive for Dupuytren's disease.
12. Jason Okoro, a 46-year-old male, presents with pain in his right foot. Jason admits it hurts to walk. Dr. Denka completes an examination and after reviewing the results of the MRI, Jason is diagnosed with a synovial cyst rupture between the second and third metatarsal bones.
13. Valerie Halsey, a 51-year-old female, complains of lower back pain and numbness. Valerie also admits it is sometimes difficult to control her left leg. Dr. Spratt completes a physical examination and history of the symptoms. Dr. Spratt has Valerie perform the straight leg raise test, which was positive for Lasegue's sign. Valerie is diagnosed with wallet sciatica, left side.

(continued)

14. James Ard, a 31-year-old male, comes in today to see Dr. Smyth. Jim complains his head is tilting and he can't control it. He also admits to neck spasms, and it seems to him that it is worse after he has taken his afternoon run. After a thorough examination and testing, Dr. Smyth diagnoses Jim with spasmodic torticollis.

15. Marygrace Fuller, a 16-year-old female, participated in rhythmic gymnastics yesterday at the local gym. When she woke up this morning, her left ankle was stiff and ached. After an examination, Dr. Jefferson diagnosed Marygrace with Achilles tendinitis.

YOU CODE IT! Application

The following exercises provide practice in abstracting physicians' notes and learning to work with documentation from our health care facility, Prader, Bracker, & Associates. These case studies are modeled on real patient encounters. Using the techniques described in this chapter, carefully read through the case studies and determine the most accurate ICD-10-CM code(s) and external cause code(s), if appropriate, for each case study.

PRADER, BRACKER, & ASSOCIATES

A Complete Health Care Facility

159 Healthcare Way • SOMEWHERE, FL 32811 • 407-555-6789

PATIENT: LOPEZ, JUANA

ACCOUNT/EHR #: LOPEJU001

Attending Physician: Oscar R. Prader, MD

S: Patient is a 15-year-old female with complaints of dysphagia and occasional problems speaking. She complains of dyspnea and finds it painful to raise her arms over her head. In the last couple of days, she states that climbing stairs and even getting up from a chair are painful and challenging.

O: ROM indicates weakness in the proximal muscles, specifically shoulders and hips. Both MRI and electromyography indicate polymyositis with myopathy. This was confirmed by autoimmune antibody testing.

A: Polymyositis with myopathy

P: Rx: Prednisone

Rx: Methotrexate

Determine the most accurate ICD-10-CM code(s).

PRADER, BRACKER, & ASSOCIATES

A Complete Health Care Facility

159 Healthcare Way • SOMEWHERE, FL 32811 • 407-555-6789

PATIENT: MARCHEON, GABRIELLA

ACCOUNT/EHR #: MARCGA001

Attending Physician: Renee O. Bracker, MD

Assessment: Derangement of anterior horn medial meniscus due to old tear, right knee.

Order for physical therapy:

Moist heat, cryotherapy, muscle stimulation, whirlpool, massage

ROM: active, active assistive, passive

(continued)

Exercise: isometric, isotonic ambulation training, as tolerated

3 a week for 6 weeks.

Session # 3/6: Pain Level: 4/10

Pt states pain shooting down right medial lower leg and numbness in toes.

Total time: 35 minutes

10 min. Cold pack/right knee

25 min. Therapeutic exercise . . . to increase strength and ROM

Symptoms began to return in right lower leg toward the end of the exercise. No new exercises added.

Donata R. Chen, MPT

Determine the most accurate ICD-10-CM code(s).

PRADER, BRACKER, & ASSOCIATES

A Complete Health Care Facility

159 Healthcare Way • SOMEWHERE, FL 32811 • 407-555-6789

PATIENT: STRICK, JOSEPH

ACCOUNT/EHR #: STRIJO001

Attending Physician: Oscar R. Prader, MD

On Sept. 10, the patient's daughter noticed him walking on his toes, in obvious pain, and having trouble moving his left foot. She insisted on him coming here to have me check because she was worried.

PE: Patient states sharp pain is experienced during dorsiflexion of the left foot. ROM is limited. Circulation good.

DX: Achilles tendon contracture, left

PLAN: Referral for physical therapy

Rx for specialized series of shoes

Determine the most accurate ICD-10-CM code(s).

PRADER, BRACKER, & ASSOCIATES

A Complete Health Care Facility

159 Healthcare Way • SOMEWHERE, FL 32811 • 407-555-6789

PATIENT: LAO, HANNAH

ACCOUNT/EHR #: LAOHAN001

Attending Physician: Oscar R. Prader, MD

Hannah Lao, a 59-year-old female, came to see Dr. Prader with pain, swelling, and erythema in her left foot and ankle. She stated that she was diagnosed with open-angle glaucoma and prescribed acetazolamide (a diuretic) by Dr. Carson, her ophthalmologist. She stated she never mentioned she was using a topical lotion of urea (a diuretic) prescribed by her dermatologist to hydrate her dry skin. Hannah stated she didn't think a lotion would count when asked about current medications.

Dr. Prader realized the combination of the two diuretics lowered her serum uric acid too quickly, causing drug-induced gout.

Determine the most accurate ICD-10-CM code(s).

(continued)

PRADER, BRACKER, & ASSOCIATES

A Complete Health Care Facility

159 Healthcare Way • SOMEWHERE, FL 32811 • 407-555-6789

PATIENT: BRACKSLEY, NATASHA

ACCOUNT/EHR #: BRACNA001

Attending Physician: Renee O. Bracker, MD

It has been 8 months since I saw this 67-year-old female. She states experiencing terrible "knee pain" in both legs. Patient states taking extra-strength Tylenol around the clock (two tablets every 4 hours) with little or no relief.

PE: She has Heberden's and Bouchard's nodes and deformity of the knee joints with decreased range of motion. On the basis of the patient's history and this examination, osteoarthritis is suspected. Patient is taken to x-ray. AP, 2 views, x-rays of each knee confirm diagnosis of osteoarthritis. There are no other findings.

DX: Osteoarthritis, bilateral

Rx: Tripod cane

Patient is advised to begin taking OTC glucosamine plus chondroitin sulfate. Patient to return prn.

Determine the most accurate ICD-10-CM code(s).

17

Coding Injury, Poisoning, and External Causes

Key Terms

Abuse
Avulsion
Burn
Corrosion
Dislocation
Extent
First-Degree Burn
Fracture
Laceration
Malunion
Myalgia
Nonunion
***Physicians' Desk Reference* (PDR)**
Rule of Nines
Second-Degree Burn
Severity
Site
Third-Degree Burn

Learning Outcomes

After completing this chapter, the student should be able to:

LO 17.1 Analyze the documentation to determine when external cause codes are required.
LO 17.2 Apply guidelines for coding traumatic injuries.
LO 17.3 Determine seventh characters for injury codes accurately.
LO 17.4 Identify a suggested code from the Table of Drugs and Chemicals.
LO 17.5 Distinguish between poisonings and adverse effects.
LO 17.6 Abstract documentation to accurately report burns.
LO 17.7 Demonstrate coding protocols for reporting abuse and neglect.
LO 17.8 Evaluate documented complications of care to report them accurately.

STOP! Remember, you need to follow along in your ICD-10-CM code book for an optimal learning experience.

17.1 Reporting External Causes of Injuries

When a patient has been injured traumatically, the first code or codes you need to report will explain the specific injury, such as a fractured arm or a burned foot. We will discuss those details as you move through this chapter. There are more codes required for these circumstances to tell the whole story. This means that you also need to report codes that explain the:

- *Cause of the injury*, such as a car accident or a fall off a ladder.
- *Place of the occurrence*, such as the park or the kitchen.
- *Activity during the occurrence*, such as playing basketball or gardening.
- *Patient's status*, such as paid employment, on-duty military, or leisure activity.

CODING BITES

An external cause code can *never* be a first-listed code, and it can *never* be the only code reported. External cause codes are reported secondary to the codes that report the injury itself.

That's a lot of information. However, think of how important these details are to the reimbursement process as well as to research studies. When you report that the patient's status was "civilian activity done for income or pay," it will be clear that this is a workers' compensation case and not a claim to be sent to the patient's health insurance carrier. If the cause of the injury was "driver of pickup truck or van injured in collision with heavy transport vehicle or bus in nontraffic accident," this information may direct the claim to the auto insurance company (not the health insurance carrier), and there may be the possibility that the information can support any legal action. Including a code to report a "fall into swimming pool" may help with getting improved fencing and saving others.

To begin the process of determining the appropriate external cause codes for a specific encounter, you will start in the Alphabetic Index. However, these codes have a separate index. You will not use the *Alphabetic Index to Diseases*, which you have been using in previous chapters and cases. Instead, you will use the *Alphabetic Index to External Causes*, often located after the *Alphabetic Index to Diseases*, after the *Table of Drugs and Chemicals*, and before the *Tabular List*.

GUIDANCE CONNECTION

Read the ICD-10-CM Official Guidelines for Coding and Reporting, section **I. Conventions, General Coding Guidelines and Chapter-Specific Guidelines**, subsection **C. Chapter-Specific Coding Guidelines**, chapter **20. External Causes of Morbidity,** subsection **a. General external cause coding guidelines.**

Cause of the Injury Code

Dislocation
The movement of a muscle away from its normal position.

When a part of the body meets with an external object and the result is injury, you must explain what that external object or force was, along with the code or codes for the injury itself. The cause may be anything from being stepped on by a cow (W55.29X-) to falling from scaffolding (W12.XXX-) to the forced landing of a (hot air) balloon injuring the occupant (V96.02X-). Domestic violence, child abuse, and elder abuse are considered assault and may be the cause of a physical injury (code category Y07). Whatever it may have been, you need to determine from the documentation what it was that caused the fracture, **dislocation**, sprain, or strain and report it with the appropriate code or codes.

Place of the Occurrence Code

Where was the patient when they were injured? Code category Y92 Place of occurrence of the external cause provides you with many options so you can report, for example, that the swimming pool at which the patient slipped and tore his deltoid muscle was at a single-family (private) house, a mobile home, a boarding house, a nursing home, or another noninstitutional or institutional location. The codes are quite specific, so you need to ensure that your physicians understand the need to be equally specific in their documentation.

GUIDANCE CONNECTION

Read the ICD-10-CM Official Guidelines for Coding and Reporting, section **I. Conventions, General Coding Guidelines and Chapter-Specific Guidelines**, subsection **C. Chapter-Specific Coding Guidelines**, chapter **20. External Causes of Morbidity,** subsection **b. Place of occurrence guideline**.

Activity Code

Code category Y93 Activity codes provides you with many activities from which to choose to identify what exactly the patient was doing when they became injured. Dancing, yoga, gymnastics, trampolining, cheerleading . . . each has its own code, and this is just one subcategory!

GUIDANCE CONNECTION

Read the ICD-10-CM Official Guidelines for Coding and Reporting, section **I. Conventions, General Coding Guidelines and Chapter-Specific Guidelines**, subsection **C. Chapter-Specific Coding Guidelines**, chapter **20. External Causes of Morbidity**, subsection **c. Activity code.**

Patient's Status

This sounds a bit obscure, certainly. What was the patient's status at the time the injury occurred? There are four options within code category Y99 External cause status:

- *Civilian activity done for income or pay*—in other words, on the job for pay or other compensation, excluding on-duty military or volunteers.
- *Military activity*, excluding off-duty status at the time.
- *Volunteer activity.*
- *Other external cause status*, which includes leisure activities, student activities, and working on a hobby.

As we discussed earlier in this section, this detail is important to the entire process, including reimbursement as well as continuity of care.

GUIDANCE CONNECTION

Read the ICD-10-CM Official Guidelines for Coding and Reporting, section **I. Conventions, General Coding Guidelines and Chapter-Specific Guidelines**, subsection **C. Chapter-Specific Coding Guidelines**, chapter **20. External Causes of Morbidity**, subsection **k. External cause status**.

LET'S CODE IT! SCENARIO

Phyllis Bush, a 27-year-old female, was learning to rock climb at her gym. As she was scaling the wall, her foot slipped and Phyllis grabbed on with her right hand, pulling something in her shoulder. The severe pain caused her to stop by her physician's office on her way home. Dr. Dellin took x-rays and determined that she had an inferior dislocation of the humerus, right side. Dr. Dellin put Phyllis's arm into a sling and gave her a prescription for a pain reliever.

Let's Code It!

Dr. Dellin diagnosed Phyllis with an *inferior dislocation of the humerus, right side*. Turn to the Alphabetic Index and look up *dislocation, humerus*. Read down the list and see

Dislocation, humerus, proximal end — *see* Dislocation, shoulder

Even though Dr. Dellin's notes didn't specify proximal, that was necessary to get to inferior—anatomically:

Dislocation, shoulder

humerus S43.00-

inferior S43.03-

Perfect! Now, turn to the Tabular List and confirm the code. Start reading at

✓4 **S43 Dislocation and sprain of joints and ligaments of shoulder girdle**

There is a ***Code also*** note reminding you to also report a code for any associated open wound. Phyllis does not have an open wound, so this does not apply. There is also an EXCLUDES2 note that mentions a strain of muscle, fascia, and tendon of the shoulder and upper arm (S46.-). However, Phyllis dislocated her humerus, so you can keep reading down the column to review the fourth-character and fifth-character options and determine which matches Dr. Dellin's documentation:

✓5 **S43.0 Subluxation and dislocation of shoulder joint**

✓6 **S43.03 Inferior subluxation and dislocation of humerus**

Go back to Dr. Dellin's notes and see that this matches exactly. Terrific! Now a sixth character is required. Review the options, check the documentation again, and determine

✓7 **S43.034- Inferior dislocation of right humerus**

Fantastic! A seventh character is required to explain where in the treatment path this encounter is. You can see the options directly under the code category S43. This is the first time that Dr. Dellin is treating Phyllis's dislocation. Great! This leads you to the complete, most accurate code to report Phyllis's injury:

S43.034A Inferior dislocation of right humerus, initial encounter

This code tells the whole story about Phyllis's specific injury.

(continued)

Now you need to find the external cause code(s) to explain how Phyllis's injury happened. Turn to the *External Cause Code* Alphabetic Index. *Climb*—no; *exercise*—no; *fall*—possibly. None of these listings really describes how Phyllis got hurt. Actually, she was involved in an "activity," so let's take a look:

Activity (involving) (of victim at time of event) Y93.9

Keep reading down the long indented list below until you get to

climbing NEC Y93.39
  mountain Y93.31
  rock Y93.31
  wall climbing Y93.31

Perfect! That is exactly what she was doing. Let's take a look in the Tabular List:

✓4 **Y93** **Activity codes**

✓5 **Y93.3** **Activities involving climbing, rappelling, and jumping off**

The EXCLUDES1 note lists activities not related to Phyllis's injury, so keep reading down the list:

Y93.31 **Activity, mountain climbing, rock climbing, and wall climbing**

A code is needed to report the place of occurrence. Where was Phyllis when she got injured? At her gym.

✓4 **Y92** **Place of occurrence of the external cause**

Y92.39 **Other specific sports and athletic area as the place of occurrence of the external cause (Gymnasium)**

One more thing: What was Phyllis's status, which you can describe using the codes within **Y99 External cause status**? The wall climbing was a leisure activity for Phyllis, so you will report

Y99.8 **Other external cause status (hobby not done for income)**

Now you have all of the codes you need to tell the *whole story* about Phyllis's injury and why Dr. Dellin treated her:

S43.034A	**Inferior dislocation of right humerus, initial encounter**
Y93.31	**Activity, mountain climbing, rock climbing, and wall climbing**
Y92.39	**Other specific sports and athletic area as the place of occurrence of the external cause (Gymnasium)**
Y99.8	**Other external cause status (hobby not done for income)**

Good work!

17.2 Traumatic Injuries

The term *injury* refers to traumatic damage to some aspect of the body, virtually always caused by a fall, crash, weapon, or some other external cause. The damage may be minor (superficial), or it may be life-threatening. It may occur during time at work or while playing. It may be the result of an automobile accident or a fight. Or it may occur during an indoor or outdoor activity.

Traumatic Fractures

Fracture
Broken cartilage or bone.

Both bone and cartilage can break—that is, become fractured. **Fractures** can be the result of trauma, such as a fall or car accident, or they can be the result of a pathological condition (underlying disease), such as osteoporosis, that causes the bone to weaken so much that it breaks. This is important information for you to abstract from the physician's documentation because traumatic fractures and pathological fractures are coded differently. Actually, they have separate listings in the Alphabetic Index: Fracture, pathological, and Fracture, traumatic.

When a fracture of a bone occurs, the coder must identify the segment of the bone that was affected. For example: the sternal end of the clavicle is called this because it is the end that connects to the sternum (ICD-10-CM code S42.011 Anterior displaced fracture of sternal end of right clavicle). The acromial or lateral end of the clavicle connects to the acromioclavicular joint (ICD-10-CM code S42.031 Displaced fracture of lateral end of right clavicle).

Types of Fractures

One of the first factors needed for accurate coding of a fracture is whether the fracture is *open* or *closed* (see **Figure 17-1**).

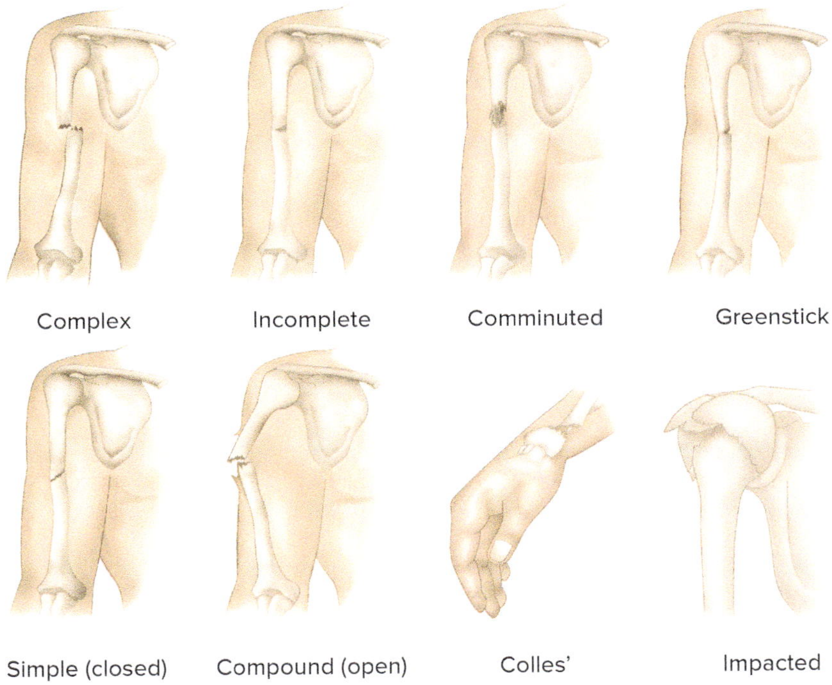

FIGURE 17-1 Illustrations of several different types of fractures

An open fractured bone is found in conjunction with an open wound through which the bone may or may not extend. A closed, or simple, fracture has no accompanying wound and remains within the confines of the body. Some types of fractures are explained in the following paragraphs.

Avulsion fractures happen when a tiny bone piece breaks off at the point where a ligament or tendon attaches to the bone. This is an occurrence of a piece of bone that has broken away at a tubercle. When the fracture is not displaced, treatment is similar to that for a soft tissue injury. In severe cases, surgery may be required to realign and stabilize an affected growth plate.

Burst fractures occur when a vertebra has been crushed in all directions. This fracture may be described as stable or unstable. Imaging (x-rays, CT scan, or MRI), as well as physical and neurologic exams, typically will support a diagnosis. Stable burst fractures may be treated with a molded turtle shell brace or a body cast. If neurologic damage is identified, then the fracture is considered unstable and will require surgery. An anterior or posterior approach may be used to insert internal fixation, a bone graft, and/or fusion. The specific bone affected will determine the code.

Comminuted fracture identifies the breaking of the bone into several pieces. A closed reduction may be required prior to immobilization by cast or splint. Internal fixation may be necessary to correct an impacted fracture with an open reduction.

Depressed fracture indicates that the bone has been displaced inward.

Fatigue fractures occur most often in the second or third metatarsal shaft and are typically the result of continuous weight-bearing activities such as long-distance running, ballet dancing, or sports. An example is M48.4- Fatigue fracture of vertebra. Additional names for this type of fracture include march fracture, Deutschlander's disease, and stress fracture–reported from subcategory M84.3- Stress fracture (fatigue fracture) (march fracture).

Fissured (linear) fracture is a break that runs along the length of a long bone.

CODING BITES

Open fractures also may be documented as infected, missile, puncture, compound, or with a foreign body.

Closed fractures also may be documented as comminuted, depressed, elevated, fissured, greenstick, impacted, linear, simple, slipped epiphysis, or spiral.

Greenstick fracture is one in which the fracture exists on one side of the bone while the other side is not broken but bent. Example: S42.311A Greenstick fracture of shaft of humerus, right arm, initial encounter for closed fracture.

Impacted fracture occurs when a fragment from the broken bone embeds itself into the body of another.

Infected fracture documents that there is presence of an infection at the fracture site. This often will require additional codes to report the underlying bacterium or virus, as well as the infection itself.

Lateral mass fracture of the atlas (C1), as the name implies, involves the lateral masses. These are the sturdiest sections of the C1 vertebra and include a superior facet and an inferior facet. This fracture occurs at the point where the spine meets the base of the cranium. A stable fracture means the transverse ligament is still intact, and a cervical collar or cervicothoracic brace is the first course of treatment. For unstable fractures, cranial traction will support a reduction of the displaced bone. After time, a halo vest can be used. Fusion of C1–C3 may be required for more severe subluxation. Use code S12.040 Displaced lateral mass fracture of first cervical vertebra or S12.041 Nondisplaced lateral mass fracture of first cervical vertebra.

Maisonneuve's fracture is a spiral fracture of the proximal portion of the fibula. This type of fracture includes a disruption of ligaments. Stable fractures can be treated with a long leg cast. Internal fixation may be required in more severe cases.

Oblique fracture is a fracture line that runs at an angle to the axis of the bone. Casting is the typical first course of treatment. In severe cases, an open reduction and possibly internal fixation will be used. Repair to surrounding ligaments may be required as well.

Periosteal fractures occur below the periosteum (membrane covering the bone surface) and are usually not displaced.

Pilon fracture is an oblique, comminuted fracture of the distal tibia. Treatment may begin with stabilization, using external traction to permit the soft tissue injuries to heal prior to surgical intervention. Open reduction with internal fixation, as well as external fixation and percutaneous plating, may be used once the soft tissue has recovered.

Puncture fracture can identify that a puncture from outside the body penetrated to cause the fracture or that the broken bone has punctured the skin after the fracture occurred. Example: S91.231A Puncture wound without foreign body of right great toe with damage to nail, initial encounter.

Salter-Harris physeal fracture is a fracture of the epiphyseal plate (a thin layer of bone; a growth plate, an area near the end of a long bone that contains growing tissue, also known as the *physis*), and it is commonly found in children. ICD-10-CM separately codes four of the nine types of Salter-Harris fracture: Salter-Harris type I is a transverse fracture of the growth plate; type II is a fracture of the growth plate and the metaphysis; type III is a fracture of the growth plate and the epiphysis; and type IV is a fracture line that travels through all three: the growth plate, metaphysis, and epiphysis. Closed reductions and traction can be used for less severe cases. Types III and IV more often will require surgical intervention using open reduction and internal fixation. Example: S79.011A Salter-Harris type I physeal fracture of upper end of right femur, initial encounter for closed fracture.

Segmental fracture is similar to the comminuted fracture; however, the broken pieces of the bone separate. Internal fixation with open reduction is used to prevent misalignment of the bone fragments. In some cases, bone cement is included in the repair. Some surgical procedures also include attachment of external fixation.

Spiral fracture happens when a twisting force causes the bone to break around a long bone in a spiral direction. Example: S52.244A Nondisplaced spiral fracture of shaft of ulna, right arm, initial encounter for closed fracture.

Torus fracture is also known as a *buckle fracture*; it is a compression of one side of a bone's protrusion, also known as the *torus*, while the other side is bent. This fracture is typically nondisplaced and, therefore, is correctable with a cast or splint.

Transcondylar fracture is a fracture that runs through a condyle (a rounded knoblike prominence at the end of a bone). Such fractures are categorized as flexion or extension fractures. Treatment can begin with immobilization for nondisplaced injury. However, treatment for this type of fracture can be difficult due to the break's location and the lack of bone available for successful union. Example: S42.431A Displaced fracture (avulsion) of lateral epicondyle of right humerus, initial encounter for closed fracture.

Transverse fracture is a fracture line that runs across the bone; it may be an open or closed fracture. An open reduction with internal fixation may be required if the bone has separated. A closed reduction might alternatively be employed. Casting is typical.

Wedge compression fracture occurs when only the anterior portion of a vertebra is crushed, which causes the vertebra to take on a wedge shape. Vertebroplasty will stabilize the fracture and prevent further damage. Example: A wedge compression fracture of L3 would be reported with code S32.030A Wedge compression fracture of third lumbar vertebra, initial encounter for closed fracture.

GUIDANCE CONNECTION

Read the ICD-10-CM Official Guidelines for Coding and Reporting, section **I. Conventions, General Coding Guidelines and Chapter-Specific Guidelines**, subsection **C. Chapter-Specific Guidelines**, chapter **19. Injury, Poisoning, and Certain Other Consequences of External Causes**, subsection **c. Coding of traumatic fractures.**

Skull Fracture

A skull fracture will first be qualified by the area injured, such as the vault of the skull (frontal or parietal bone–code S02.0XXA) or the base of the skull (sphenoid or temporal bone–code S02.19XA). *NOTE:* A second code would report any intracranial injury, if applicable.

Fractures of the skull are characterized differently than others throughout the body and include the following:

- *Basal skull fracture* is a break in the floor of the skull.
- *Blowout fracture* indicates a break in the floor of the orbit that is typically caused by a severe blow to the eye.
- *Depressed skull fracture* identifies an inward displacement of one of the bones of the skull.
- *Stellate fracture* is one with a clear central point of the fracture and with break lines radiating from this central spot.

CODING BITES

The Tabular List categorizes the codes used to report injuries first by anatomical site (the location of the injury) and then by the specific injury (contusion, insect bite, etc.).

YOU CODE IT! CASE STUDY

Sally was knelt down, putting in some new plants by the fence, when something touched her ankle. She looked down to see a garter snake. Even though garter snakes are nonvenomous, she was frightened, screamed, and began to run toward the house. She kept running as fast as she could, looking over her shoulder to keep an eye on the snake when she tripped over her own foot on the flat patio surface and fell into the door, banging her head with great force. Sally's husband took her to the ED where an MRI revealed a closed, linear fracture, of the right temporal bone of the skull.

You Code It!

Go through the steps of coding, and determine the code or codes that should be reported for Sally's injury. [HINT: Don't forget the External Cause codes]

Step #1: Read the case carefully and completely.

Step #2: Abstract the scenario. Which main words or terms describe why the physician cared for the patient during this encounter?

Step #3: Are there any details missing or incomplete for which you would need to query the physician? [If so, ask your instructor.]

Step #4: Check for any relevant guidance, including reading all of the symbols and notations in the Tabular List and the appropriate sections of the Official Guidelines.

Step #5: Determine the correct diagnosis code or codes to explain why this encounter was medically necessary.

Step #6: Double-check your work.

(continued)

Answer:

Did you determine these to be the correct codes?

S02.19XA	**Other fracture of the base of skull [fracture of temporal bone]**
W01.198A	**Fall on same level from slipping, tripping and stumbling with subsequent striking against other object**
W59.19XA	**Other contact with nonvenomous snake**
Y92.017	**Garden or yard in single-family (private) house as the place of occurrence of the external cause**
Y93.H2	**Activity, gardening and landscaping**
Y99.8	**Other external cause status (leisure activity)**

Maxillary Fracture

Facial trauma might result in a LeFort fracture, which is a bilateral maxillary fracture with involvement of the surrounding bone, including the zygomatic bones. Such fractures are identified by type: a LeFort I fracture (code S02.411-) is a downward horizontal facial fracture and typically involves the maxillary alveolar rim and inferior nasal aperture. A LeFort II fracture (code S02.412-) is more triangular, involving the inferior orbital rim, the nasal bridge, and the frontal processes of the maxilla. A LeFort III fracture (code S02.413-) is a transverse fracture, sometimes referred to as a *craniofacial dissociation*. This fracture involves the zygomatic arch, the nasal bridge, and the upper maxilla and extends along the orbit floor (posteriorly).

EXAMPLES

S02.402A	Zygomatic fracture, unspecified side, initial encounter for closed fracture
S02.413D	LeFort III fracture, subsequent encounter for fracture with routine healing

Sequelae (Late Effects) of Fractures

Malunion
A fractured bone that did not heal correctly; healing of bone that was not in proper position or alignment.

Nonunion
A fractured bone that did not heal back together; no mending or joining together of the broken segments.

Once a bone has been given the opportunity to heal, it may not heal properly. The most common types of late effects of fractures are **malunion** and **nonunion**. A malunion (*mal* = bad + *union* = together) of a fractured bone means that the pieces of the bone healed back together but not in an effective way. Unfortunately, the most common treatment for a malunion is for the physician to rebreak the bone and set it again, hoping that it will heal properly the second time. When the parts of a broken bone do not heal back together at all, despite the proper treatment and time allotment, this is known as a nonunion (*non* = not + *union* = together).

In ICD-10-CM's Alphabetic Index, when you look up *Fracture, malunion*, you will see the notation "*See* Fracture, by site." When you look up *Fracture, nonunion*, you will see the notation "*See* Nonunion, fracture." At *Nonunion, fracture*, the notation states, "*See* Fracture, by site."

Traumatic Wounds

Lacerations (Superficial Wounds)

Laceration
Damage to the epidermal and dermal layers of the skin made by a sharp object.

Each one of us has had a laceration at some time or another. Perhaps it was a paper cut or a cut from a knife while chopping vegetables. This smooth slit or opening in the epidermal layer is typically superficial and does not bleed. A **laceration** caused by a sharp object is generally a ragged wound (see **Figure 17-2**). Unlike a superficial cut, a laceration is deeper, damaging the dermal layer of the skin. It penetrates the blood vessels, resulting in bleeding. These more severe injuries also may be vulnerable to infection and pain. Depending upon the specific object or event that caused the laceration, the physician may order an x-ray to determine whether any foreign bodies, such as shards of glass or splinters from wood, are lodged within the wound.

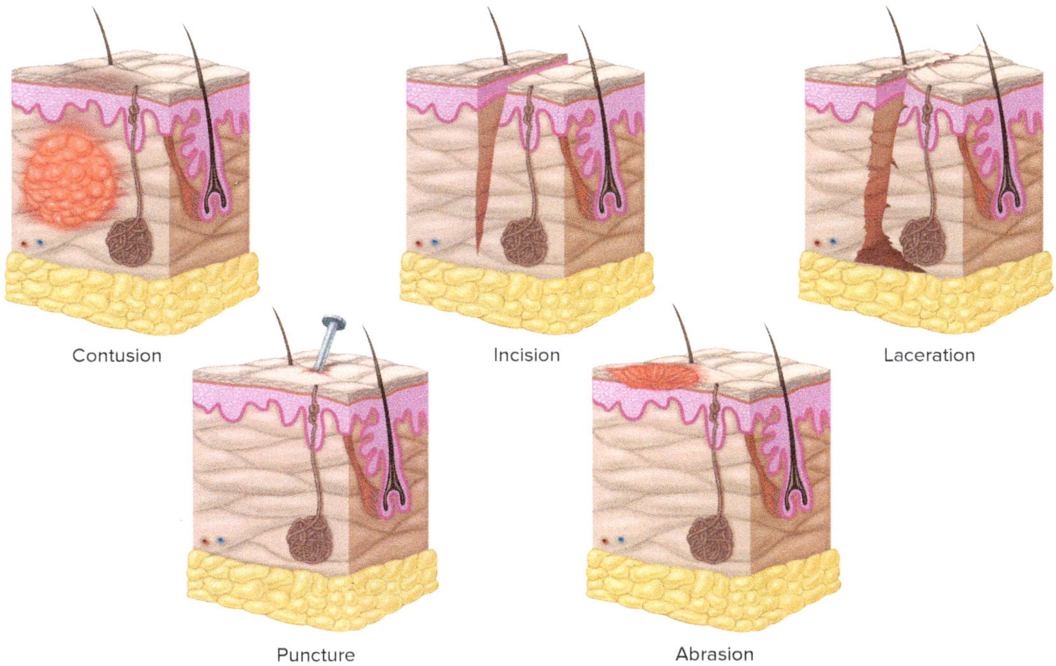

FIGURE 17-2 Illustrations of different types of wounds, including lacerations and puncture wounds

Contusions and Hematomas

A *contusion*, commonly known as a *bruise* or "black-and-blue mark," is an injury to the body that typically does not break the skin but that does damage to the underlying blood vessels. The bleeding in the dermal layer is seen only through the epidermis as a dark color. As the contusion heals, the colors change until the collected blood is dissipated and everything has healed. When the bleeding coagulates into a blood clot, this is called a *hematoma*. The seriousness of these injuries largely depends on the anatomical site where the bleeding and/or clot is located. A contusion or hematoma on the leg or arm is typically a minor event that rarely requires a physician's skill, whereas a contusion to the brain or a subdural hematoma could be life-threatening.

Puncture Wounds

When a pointed, narrow object enters deeply into the visceral (inside) aspects of the body, the injury is known as a *puncture wound* (see **Figure 17-2**). A carpenter's nail, a knife, scissors, and a fishhook are just a few items that can cause an injury of this nature. Due to the characteristics of this type of wound, infection and internal damage are possible. The physician may check for dirt, debris, or foreign objects within the wound. They also may order blood tests to check for a pathogen that might cause an infection. Stitches and possible surgery may be required, depending upon the specific depth and location of the injury.

Avulsions

The medical term **avulsion** describes a situation in which all layers of the skin (epidermis and dermis) are forcibly torn away from the body, typically a surface trauma. Due to the pulling off of the dermal layers, the underlying structures, including adipose tissue, muscles, tendons, and bone, become open to the outside. Rock climbers may suffer "flappers," an avulsion of the fingertip pad. When this occurs to a fingernail or toenail, it is known as a *nail avulsion*–the nail plate is torn off the nail bed. Unlike the case with avulsions at other anatomical sites, in nail avulsions the nail is not reattached. Instead, the fingertip and nail bed are covered to protect the area until the keratin has formed a new nail.

> **Avulsion**
> Injury in which layers of skin are traumatically torn away from the body.

Animal, Insect, or Human Bites

Animal bites and human bites can be a particular concern due to the potential spread of bacteria and viruses via saliva transference. Insects may transmit their own fluids and sometimes venom.

ICD-10-CM

LET'S CODE IT! SCENARIO

Nathan Kirchner, an 8-year-old male, was hiking in a public park with his Boy Scout troop when they came to a clearing and he saw a foal and its mother looking over the fence in a corral in the northeast edge of the park. He reached out his left hand to pet the foal, and the mother horse bit his thumb. His scout leader took him to the emergency room. After examination and some tests, Dr. Clifton cleaned the wound, applied a sterile dressing, and gave Nathan an antibiotic.

Let's Code It!

Dr. Clifton's notes state that Nathan had been bitten on the thumb by a horse. When you turn to the Alphabetic Index, you see

Bite(s) (animal) (human)

thumb S61.05

Remember the Coding Tip from the beginning of this chapter? These codes are first categorized by the anatomical site and then by the specific injury.

When you turn to the Tabular List, you confirm

✓4 **S61 Open wound of wrist, hand and fingers**

Before you continue reading, be certain to pay attention to the notations here. There is a ***Code also*** if a wound infection is documented; there is an EXCLUDES1 notation with two diagnoses that do not relate to Nathan's case; and there are options for the required seventh character. You will need to come back to this after you determine the correct code. So keep reading to determine the correct fourth character:

✓5 **S61.0 Open wound of thumb without damage to nail**

There is another EXCLUDES1 notation. Has Dr. Clifton documented that the nail was also damaged? No. So continue reading to determine the correct fifth character:

✓6 **S61.05 Open bite of thumb without damage to nail**

There is another detail you need to abstract from the documentation: Nathan's right or left thumb?

✓7 **S61.052 Open bite of left thumb without damage to nail**

Now you need to determine the correct seventh character. Go back to the beginning of this code category and review your choices.

S61.052A Open bite of left thumb without damage to nail, initial encounter

Perfect! Yet you have not explained the whole story about why Dr. Clifton cared for Nathan. This code states he was bitten on the left thumb, but not by whom or what. To report how Nathan got bitten and by what, you will need external cause codes. Turn to the Alphabetic Index to External Causes and look up

Bite

horse W55.11

Turn in the Tabular List to

✓4 **W55 Contact with other mammals**

(continued)

Of course, you are going to read this code's EXCLUDES1 notation carefully. None of the exclusions apply to this case. And there are your options for the seventh character. But, first, read down to determine the correct fourth, fifth, and sixth characters:

✓5 **W55.1** **Contact with horse**

✓7 **W55.11X** **Bitten by horse**

And now, go back up for the seventh character:

W55.11XA **Bitten by horse, initial encounter**

Terrific! You also will need to determine the codes to report the place of occurrence, activity, and the external cause status. Try this on your own. Did you determine that these are the codes?

Y92.830 **Public park as the place of occurrence of the external cause**

Y93.01 **Activity, walking, marching, and hiking**

Y99.8 **Other external cause status**

You are really getting to be a great coder!

Traumatic Injury to the Muscles

A muscle injury is most often the result of some type of trauma or overexertion during exercise or sports. Traumatic injuries to muscles may be described in a number of ways:

- *Strain* is a tearing of the fibers of the muscle involved, most often the result of overstretching the muscle during movement.
- *Sprain* is a partially torn or overstretched ligament.
- *Contusion* is usually the result of a minor trauma to a muscle, causing a bruise.
- *Tear* (muscle tear) is a separation within the muscle fibers. A bowstring tear, also known as a *bucket-handle tear*, occurs longitudinally in the meniscus.
- **Myalgia** is the medical term for muscle pain.
- *Rupture* is the tear in an organ or tissue.

Myalgia
Pain in a muscle.

EXAMPLES

S53.21XA Traumatic rupture of right radial collateral ligament, initial encounter

S76.122A Laceration of left quadriceps muscle, fascia, and tendon, initial encounter

S83.211A Bucket-handle tear of medial meniscus, current injury, right knee, initial encounter

GUIDANCE CONNECTION

Review the ICD-10-CM Official Guidelines for Coding and Reporting, section **I. Conventions, General Coding Guidelines and Chapter-Specific Guidelines**, subsection **C. Chapter-Specific Coding Guidelines**, chapter **13. Diseases of the Musculoskeletal System and Connective Tissue**, subsection **b**, **Acute traumatic versus chronic or recurrent musculoskeletal conditions**, in addition to chapter **19. Injury, Poisoning, and Certain Other Consequences of External Causes**, subsection **b. Coding of injuries**.

YOU CODE IT! CASE STUDY

Theresa Flores experienced her first parachute jump with her boyfriend 3 months ago. She loved it and is now working on her certification for parachute jumping. On her last jump, she sprained the lateral collateral ligament of her left knee after landing the wrong way. Dr. Hadden confirmed the injury and treated it.

You Code It!

Go through the steps of coding, and determine the code or codes that should be reported for this encounter between Dr. Hadden and Theresa.

Step #1: Read the case carefully and completely.
Step #2: Abstract the scenario. Which main words or terms describe why the physician cared for the patient during this encounter?
Step #3: Are there any details missing or incomplete for which you would need to query the physician? [If so, ask your instructor.]
Step #4: Check for any relevant guidance, including reading all of the symbols and notations in the Tabular List and the appropriate sections of the Official Guidelines.
Step #5: Determine the correct diagnosis code or codes to explain why this encounter was medically necessary.
Step #6: Double-check your work.

Answer:

Did you determine these to be the correct codes?

S83.422A **Sprain of lateral collateral ligament of left knee, initial encounter**

V97.22XA **Parachutist injured on landing, initial encounter**

Y99.8 **Other external cause status (leisure activity)**

17.3 Using Seventh Characters to Report Status of Care

Throughout the long list of codes available to report traumatic injury, you will see that a majority require seventh (7th) characters. These characters report where the patient is, at this encounter, in the treatment plan.

Character	Description	Meaning
A	Initial encounter	Patient is receiving active treatment including evaluation and continuing treatment by any physician.
D	Subsequent encounter	Patient has completed active treatment and is receiving routine care for the condition during the healing process or the recovery phase.
S	Sequela	Late effects, also known as residual effects, of another condition, such as scar formation after a burn.

CODING BITES

Remember that whenever you are reporting an injury, you also will need to report external cause codes to explain how the patient got injured and identify the place of occurrence. To learn more, see the section ***Reporting External Causes of Injuries*** in this chapter. Also, many of the codes from the ICD-10-CM code book's *Chapter 19: Injury, Poisoning, and Certain Other Consequences of External Causes (S00–T88)* require seventh characters for reporting the type of encounter.

CODING BITES

When reporting an encounter for *sequela* care, the principal (first-listed) code is the one identifying the specific sequela (i.e., scar, malunion of fractured bone, etc.), followed by the code that reports the original injury or poisoning with a seventh character of S.

GUIDANCE CONNECTION

Read the ICD-10-CM Official Guidelines for Coding and Reporting, section **I. Conventions, General Coding Guidelines and Chapter-Specific Guidelines**, subsection **C. Chapter-Specific Coding Guidelines**, chapter **19. Injury, Poisoning, and Certain Other Consequences of External Causes**, subsection **a. Application of 7th characters in Chapter 19**.

Seventh Characters for Fracture Care

When reporting a code identifying that the patient has a fracture (more about this in the section ***Traumatic Injuries*** in this chapter), the definitions of the seventh characters change a bit to provide more details about the specific fracture.

Skeletal Fractures

Character	Description
A	Initial encounter for closed fracture
B	Initial encounter for open fracture
D	Subsequent encounter for fracture with routine healing
G	Subsequent encounter for fracture with delayed healing
K	Subsequent encounter for fracture with nonunion
P	Subsequent encounter for fracture with malunion
S	Sequela

CODING BITES

Example of a *subsequent encounter* for fracture care might include a cast change, removal of a cast, x-ray to evaluate healing of a fracture, or adjusting a patient's medication.

Fracture of Forearm, Femur, and Lower Leg (Including Ankle)

Character	Description
A	Initial encounter for closed fracture
B	Initial encounter for open fracture type I or II (or NOS)
C	Initial encounter for open fracture type IIIA, IIIB, or IIIC
D	Subsequent encounter for closed fracture with routine healing
E	Subsequent encounter for open fracture type I or II with routine healing
F	Subsequent encounter for open fracture type IIIA, IIIB, or IIIC with routine healing
G	Subsequent encounter for closed fracture with delayed healing
H	Subsequent encounter for open fracture type I or II with delayed healing
J	Subsequent encounter for open fracture type IIIA, IIIB, or IIIC with delayed healing
K	Subsequent encounter for closed fracture with nonunion
M	Subsequent encounter for open fracture type I or II with nonunion
N	Subsequent encounter for open fracture type IIIA, IIIB, or IIIC with nonunion
P	Subsequent encounter for closed fracture with malunion
Q	Subsequent encounter for open fracture type I or II with malunion
R	Subsequent encounter for open fracture type IIIA, IIIB, or IIIC with malunion
S	Sequela

CODING BITES

Aftercare codes from the ICD-10-CM code book's Chapter 21 (Z codes) should *NOT* be reported when the injury or poisoning code uses a seventh character.

GUIDANCE CONNECTION

Read the ICD-10-CM Official Guidelines for Coding and Reporting, section **I. Conventions, General Coding Guidelines and Chapter-Specific Guidelines**, subsection **C. Chapter-Specific Coding Guidelines**, chapter **19. Injury, Poisoning, and Certain Other Consequences of External Causes**, subsection **c.1) Initial vs. subsequent encounter for fractures**.

17.4 Using the Table of Drugs and Chemicals

Often located directly after the alphabetical listing is the Table of Drugs and Chemicals (see **Figure 17-3**). (*NOTE:* Different published versions of the ICD-10-CM book may place sections in a different order.) The Table of Drugs and Chemicals is used when a drug or chemical caused an adverse reaction, poisoned the patient, or caused a toxic effect. Similar to the Neoplasm Table, the Table of Drugs and Chemicals is organized in columns.

Substance	Poisoning, Accidental (unintentional)	Poisoning, Intentional self-harm	Poisoning, Assault	Poisoning, Undetermined	Adverse Effect	Underdosing
		#				
1-propanol	T51.3X1	T51.3X2	T51.3X3	T51.3X4	--	--
2-propanol	T51.2X1	T51.2X2	T51.2X3	T51.2X4	--	--
2,4-D (dichlorophen-oxyacetic acid)	T60.3X1	T60.3X2	T60.3X3	T60.3X4	--	--
2,4-toluene dilsocyanate	T65.0X1	T65.0X2	T65.0X3	T65.0X4	--	--
2,4,5-T (trichloro-phenoxyacetic acid)	T60.1X1	T60.1X2	T60.1X3	T60.1X4	--	--
14-hydroxydihydro-morphinone	T40.2X1	T40.2X2	T40.2X3	T40.2X4	T40.2X5	T40.2X6
		A				
ABOB	T37.5X1	T37.5X2	T37.5X3	T37.5X4	T37.5X5	T37.5X6
Abrine	T62.2X1	T62.2X2	T62.2X3	T62.2X4	--	--
Abrus(seed)	T62.2X1	T62.2X2	T62.2X3	T62.2X4	--	--
Absinthe	T51.0X1	T51.0X2	T51.0X3	T51.0X4	--	--
- beverage	T51.0X1	T51.0X2	T51.0X3	T51.0X4	--	--
Acaricide	T60.8X1	T60.8X2	T60.8X3	T60.8X4	--	--
Acebutolol	T44.7X1	T44.7X2	T44.7X3	T44.7X4	T44.7X5	T44.7X6
Acecarbromal	T42.6X1	T42.6X2	T42.6X3	T42.6X4	T42.6X5	T42.6X6
Aceclidine	T44.1X1	T44.1X2	T44.1X3	T44.1X4	T44.1X5	T44.1X6
Acedapsone	T37.0X1	T37.0X2	T37.0X3	T37.0X4	T37.0X5	T37.0X6
Acetylline piperazine	T48.6X1	T48.6X2	T48.6X3	T48.6X4	T48.6X5	T48.6X6
Acemorphan	T40.2X1	T40.2X2	T40.2X3	T40.2X4	T40.2X5	T40.2X6
Acenocoumarin	T45.511	T45.512	T45.513	T45.514	T45.515	T45.516
Acenocoumarol	T45.511	T45.512	T45.513	T45.514	T45.515	T45.516
Acepifylline	T48.6X1	T48.6X2	T48.6X3	T48.6X4	T48.6X5	T48.6X6
Acepromazine	T43.3X1	T43.3X2	T43.3X3	T43.3X4	T43.3X5	T43.3X6
Acesulfamethoxypyridazine	T37.0X1	T37.0X2	T37.0X3	T37.0X4	T37.0X5	T37.0X6
Acetal	T52.8X1	T52.8X2	T52.8X3	T52.8X4	--	--
Acetaldehyde (vapor)	T52.8X1	T52.8X2	T52.8X3	T52.8X4	--	--
- liquid	T65.891	T65.892	T65.893	T65.894	--	--
P-Acetamidophenol	T39.1X1	T39.1X2	T39.1X3	T39.1X4	T39.1X5	T39.1X6
Acetaminophen	T39.1X1	T39.1X2	T39.1X3	T39.1X4	T39.1X5	T39.1X6
Acetalminosalol	T39.1X1	T39.1X2	T39.1X3	T39.1X4	T39.1X5	T39.1X6
Acetanilide	T39.1X1	T39.1X2	T39.1X3	T39.1X4	T39.1X5	T39.1X6

(continued)

Substance	Poisoning, Accidental (unintentional)	Poisoning, Intentional self-harm	Poisoning, Assault	Poisoning, Undetermined	Adverse Effect	Underdosing
Acetarsol	T37.3X1	T37.3X2	T37.3X3	T37.3X4	T37.3X5	T37.3X6
Acetazolamide	T50.2X1	T50.2X2	T50.2X3	T50.2X4	T50.2X5	T50.2X6
Acetiamine	T45.2X1	T45.2X2	T45.2X3	T45.2X4	T45.2X5	T45.2X6
Acetic						
- acid	T54.2X1	T54.2X2	T54.2X3	T54.2X4	--	--
-- with sodium acetate (ointment)	T49.3X1	T49.3X2	T49.3X3	T49.3X4	T49.3X5	T49.3X6
-- ester (solvent) (vapor)	T52.8X1	T52.8X2	T52.8X3	T52.8X4	--	--
-- irrigating solution	T50.3X1	T50.3X2	T50.3X3	T50.3X4	T50.3X5	T50.3X6
-- medicinal (lotion)	T49.2X1	T49.2X2	T49.2X3	T49.2X4	T49.2X5	T49.2X6
- anhydride	T65.891	T65.892	T65.893	T65.894	--	--

FIGURE 17-3 ICD-10-CM Table of Drugs and Chemicals, in part, from 1-propanol through acetic anhydride

Source: *ICD-10-CM Official Guidelines for Coding and Reporting*, The Centers for Medicare and Medicaid Services (CMS) and the National Center for Health Statistics (NCHS)

GUIDANCE CONNECTION

Read the ICD-10-CM Official Guidelines for Coding and Reporting, section **I. Conventions, General Coding Guidelines and Chapter-Specific Guidelines**, subsection **C. Chapter-Specific Coding Guidelines**, chapter **19. Injury, Poisoning, and Certain Other Consequences of External Causes**, subsections **e. Adverse effects, poisoning, underdosing and toxic effects** and **e.1) Do not code directly from the Table of Drugs**.

Drug and Chemical Names

The first column of the table lists the names of drugs and chemicals, in alphabetic order. The list includes prescription medications, over-the-counter medications, household and industrial chemicals, and many other items with a chemical basis. Aspirin, indigestion relief medication, drugstore-brand allergy relievers, alcohol (for drinking or sterilization), window cleaner, battery acid, and lots of other similar substances are included, as well as medications prescribed by a physician.

Sometimes, it is easy to find what you're looking for. For example, Giselle had a bad reaction to Nytol. Even though *Nytol* is the brand name of an over-the-counter sleep medication, you will find it easily in the list of substances in the first column of the Table of Drugs and Chemicals.

Other times, it may not be this easy, and the name–whether brand name, generic name, or chemical name–that is documented in the physician's notes may not be in the table. If you don't find it, you may have to do some research. Some of the drugs and chemicals are listed by their brand or common names, such as Metamucil or Nytol. Others are listed by their chemical or generic names, such as barbiturates (sedatives). If you are not certain, consult a ***Physicians' Desk Reference*** **(PDR)**, a group of books that list all the approved drugs, herbal remedies, and over-the-counter medications by brand name, chemical name, generic name, and drug category.

Physicians' Desk Reference **(PDR)** A series of reference books identifying all aspects of prescription and over-the-counter medications, as well as herbal remedies.

EXAMPLE

Vesicare—the brand name.

Solifenacin succinate—the generic or chemical name.

Muscarinic receptor antagonist—the drug category.

Anticholinergic—the general drug category.

In our example, you can see Vesicare is shown as the trade or brand name. The generic or chemical name is solifenacin succinate. If a physician prescribed it for a patient, who then had an adverse reaction or took an overdose, you would most likely see one or the other of those names in the notes. However, you will find neither of them listed in the Table of Drugs and Chemicals. The next piece of information given to you by the PDR is found in the description of the drug: muscarinic receptor antagonist. Unfortunately, there is nothing in the table under *muscarinic* either. Because the patient either had an adverse reaction or had taken an overdose, take a look at the following paragraphs from the PDR:

> **ADVERSE REACTIONS**
>
> **. . . Expected side effects of antimuscarinic agents . . .**
>
> **OVERDOSAGE**
>
> **. . . Overdosage with Vesicare can potentially result in severe *anticholinergic* effects . . .**

The two paragraphs provide us with two new descriptors for the drug: *antimuscarinic* and *anticholinergic*. Both of them are shown in the Table of Drugs and Chemicals and, interestingly, lead you to the same codes.

ICD-10-CM

LET'S CODE IT! SCENARIO

Kurt Hershey found an unmarked barrel in the back of the warehouse where he works. He opened the top and leaned over to see what was inside. Vapors from the benzene solvent being stored in that barrel overcame Kurt. He had difficulty breathing because he accidentally inhaled the chemical. He was taken to the physician immediately. Dr. Blanchard diagnosed Kurt with respiratory distress syndrome, a toxic effect from inhaling the benzene.

Let's Code It!

Kurt had *a toxic effect from inhaling the benzene*. The notes also state that Kurt had *respiratory distress*. You learned that you need at least two codes: toxic effect + external cause code.

The first code identifies the chemical or substance and intent. In Kurt's case, the substance was the vapor from a barrel of benzene solvent. Turn to the Alphabetic Index's Table of Drugs and Chemicals. Look down the first column and find *benzene*:

Benzene

homologues (acetyl) (dimethyl) (methyl) (solvent)

You know from the documentation that this was an accidental poisoning, so look across the line to the first column titled "Poisoning, Accidental (Unintentional)":

Benzene T52.1X1

homologues (acetyl) (dimethyl) (methyl) (solvent) T52.2X1

Hmm. It can be difficult to know what was in that barrel. You can get more information from the Tabular List and see if that helps. Start at the three-character number and be certain to check any notations or directives:

✓4 **T52 Toxic effect of organic solvents**

Be sure to read the **EXCLUDES1** notation. Does it relate to Kurt's diagnosis? No. Good! There are the seventh-character options for later, but first you must determine the rest of the code, so keep reading down the column:

✓5 **T52.1 Toxic effects of benzene**

✓5 **T52.2 Toxic effects of homologues of benzene**

Homologues are not mentioned in the documentation, so review the options for the fifth and sixth characters under T52.1:

✓7 **T52.1X1 Toxic effects of benzene, accidental (unintentional)**

(continued)

Remember, you need to include the seventh character.

T52.1X1A Toxic effects of benzene, accidental (unintentional), initial encounter

Great! You now have the first-listed code for Kurt's encounter.

The next code reports the *effect* that the benzene vapors had on Kurt.

The notes state he had respiratory distress. In the main section of the Alphabetic Index, find

Distress

respiratory (adult) (child) R06.03

Look up the code in the Tabular List

R06.03 Acute respiratory distress

This matches!

Two more codes—remember, you also need external cause codes to report where the accident occurred and Kurt's status (why he was doing this). In the Index to External Causes, turn to "Place of occurrence." The notes state that Kurt was in a warehouse when this accident happened, so read down the list, and you will see

Place of occurrence

warehouse Y92.59

Go to the Tabular List, beginning with the code category:

✓4 **Y92 Place of occurrence of the external cause**

Read down the column to review your choices for the required fourth and fifth characters.

Y92.59 Other trade areas as the place of occurrence of the external cause (warehouse as the place of occurrence of the external cause)

Your last code will report Kurt's status. You know he was at work, so you will use this code:

Y99.0 Civilian activity done for income or pay

This completes the report.

T52.1X1A Toxic effects of benzene, accidental (unintentional), initial encounter

R06.03 Acute respiratory distress

Y92.59 Other trade areas as the place of occurrence of the external cause (warehouse as the place of occurrence of the external cause)

Y99.0 Civilian activity done for income or pay

You are really becoming a great coder!

17.5 Adverse Effects, Poisoning, Underdosing, and Toxic Effects

When an individual comes in contact with a drug or a chemical that has an unhealthy impact, it must be coded. The person might have had an unusual reaction to a medication prescribed by a health care professional or might have been exposed to something noxious.

The first step is for you to determine whether the patient was poisoned, suffering an adverse effect (or reaction), or experiencing a toxic effect.

GUIDANCE CONNECTION

Read the ICD-10-CM Official Guidelines for Coding and Reporting, section **I. Conventions, General Coding Guidelines and Chapter-Specific Guidelines**, subsection **C. Chapter-Specific Coding Guidelines**, chapter **19. Injury, Poisoning, and Certain Other Consequences of External Causes**, subsection **e. Adverse effects, poisoning, underdosing and toxic effects.**

Adverse Reaction

When health care providers determine that a pharmaceutical substance may improve an individual's health status, they will typically prescribe that medication for therapeutic use. A patient is diagnosed with an adverse effect, or reaction, when *all* of the following occur and the patient has a negative outcome anyway:

- A health care professional correctly *prescribes* a drug for a patient.
- The correct patient receives the correct *drug*.
- The correct dosage is given to the patient (or taken by the patient). [The correct dosage includes the correct *amount* in the correct *frequency*.]
- The correct *route* of administration is used.

EXAMPLE

Dr. Levinson prescribed 10 mg of Lexapro, bid, po, for Terence Romulles for anxiety.

Lexapro is the brand name of an anti-anxiety medication.

10 mg is the quantity (amount) of the dosage.

bid is the abbreviation meaning twice per day—the frequency.

po is the abbreviation meaning "by mouth"—the route of administration.

The patient then has an unexpected bad reaction to that drug. There may have been no way to know the patient was allergic to this medication because he had never taken it before. Unpredictable reactions to drugs can be prompted by genetic factors, other conditions or diseases, allergies, or other issues.

When an adverse reaction has occurred, you will need a minimum of two codes.

First, code for the effect. The code or codes will report exactly what the reaction was, such as a rash, vomiting, or unconsciousness. When you abstract the physician's documentation, you may find this is a confirmed diagnosis, or signs and symptoms experienced by the patient as a result of taking the medication.

Second, code for the external cause. The external cause code will explain that the patient took the drug for therapeutic use. You can find this code in the Table of Drugs and Chemicals by first locating the name of the drug (either the brand name or the generic name) in the first column and then reading across that row to the column under the heading "Adverse Effect."

CODING BITES

You might need more than one code to report the negative effect of this medication on this patient. Remember, you need to tell the whole story in codes.

EXAMPLE

Giana Roman took her prescription for amoxicillin exactly as the physician and the pharmacist instructed. She broke out in a rash because it turned out she was allergic to this antibiotic and no one knew.

The "effect" is the rash "dermatitis due to drugs taken internally" = **L27.0 Generalized skin eruption due to drugs and medicaments taken internally**

+

The external cause code explains "therapeutic use of amoxicillin" = **T36.0X5A Adverse effect of penicillins, initial encounter**

Poisoning

Most people think of poisoning as something from a great detective novel or movie; however, a poisoning can happen under many different circumstances. In reality, when a person comes in contact with a drug (not prescribed by a physician or not taken as prescribed) or a chemical and a health problem results, it is called a poisoning.

The drug or substance might have been ingested, inhaled, absorbed through the skin, injected, or taken by some other method. Remember that this may be a drug, or it may be a chemical, such as cleaning supplies, gasoline, or other type of poison or toxic substance. Your first step is to abstract the name of the substance that poisoned the patient so you can look it up on the Table of Drugs and Chemicals.

Next, you will need to discover the circumstances under which this patient came to be poisoned. Was it . . .

- *An accident (unintentional).* Things happen, such as a child finding a bottle of medication and thinking it's candy or finding cleaning spray and thinking it would be fun to wash his face with it. A patient mistakenly took the wrong amount of a medication, or the clinician mistakenly administered the wrong quantity to the wrong patient (if this was a drug). Two substances could also be taken that contradicted each other.
- *A suicide attempt (intentional self-harm).* Sadly, a person might take an overdose while trying to harm himself or herself, intentionally.
- *An assault.* This occurs when someone tries to cause intentional harm to someone else. It sounds like a scene from that detective movie, but it does happen in real life.
- *Underdosing.* Most often, this occurs when the patient cannot afford the medication, so they take less each time so one prescription will last longer. Or this may occur because a label is misread or an implanted medication pump malfunctions. In any of these situations, the patient is not receiving the quantity necessary for therapeutic value and thus does not improve as expected due to the medication's ineffectiveness.

GUIDANCE CONNECTION

Read the ICD-10-CM Official Guidelines for Coding and Reporting, section **I. Conventions, General Coding Guidelines and Chapter-Specific Guidelines**, subsection **C. Chapter-Specific Coding Guidelines**, chapter **19. Injury, Poisoning, and Certain Other Consequences of External Causes**, subsection **e.5)(b) Poisoning**.

CODING BITES

Think P.E. for Poison

P = poison code is reported first [the code suggested by the appropriate column of the Table of Drugs and Chemicals]

E = effect of the poisoning is reported next [the bad reaction the patient had to the substance, such as a rash, vomiting, or unconsciousness]

The effect of the poisoning might be a confirmed diagnosis or documentation of signs and/or symptoms. You may need more than one code to tell the whole story about how this poisoning has affected the patient.

GUIDANCE CONNECTION

The ICD-10-CM guidelines reduce the number of codes you will need to report some conditions. Codes in categories T36–T65 are combination codes that include the substances related to adverse effects, poisonings, toxic effects, and underdosing, as well as the external cause.

Underdosing and Patient Noncompliance

Sometimes, a patient has an adverse effect because they did not take the medication as ordered by the physician or didn't take the drugs at all. Some patients forget, some are resistant to needing a drug, and some cannot afford the required number of pills. When taking too little of the quantity prescribed (underdosing) is the patient's action, rather than an error on the part of a health care professional, this is considered noncompliance and is reported with an additional code to explain:

Z91.120 **Patient's intentional underdosing of medication regimen due to financial hardship**

Z91.128 **Patient's intentional underdosing of medication regimen for other reason**

Z91.130 **Patient's unintentional underdosing of medication regimen due to age-related debility**

Z91.138 **Patient's unintentional underdosing of medication regimen for other reason**

Z91.14 **Patient's other noncompliance with medication regimen**

CODING BITES

Code subcategories Z91.12- and Z91.13- both have a *Code first* notation, so you don't have to wonder about proper sequencing.

Toxic Effects

A toxic effect, such as irritation or carcinogenicity, may result from a part of the human body interacting with a chemical or other nonmedicinal substance. When an individual comes in contact with a toxic substance, whether ingested (such as liquid window cleaner), inhaled (such as asbestos), or touched (such as acid), you will report this using the same coding process as reporting a poisoning. The external cause code will come from a different range of codes, that's all.

T51–T65 Toxic effects of substances chiefly nonmedicinal as to source

As per the Official Guidelines, when reporting a toxic effect, the toxic effect code is reported first, followed by the code or codes to report the manifested effects of that toxin.

CODING BITES

The difference between a poisoning and a toxic effect is the substance. A poisoning or adverse effect is a reaction to a natural or medicinal substance, whereas a toxic effect is a reaction to a harmful substance.

ICD-10-CM

LET'S CODE IT! SCENARIO

Dr. Barry, a pediatrician, was called in to see Abigail Scanter, a 3-year-old female, brought in by her mother after she discovered Abigail on the floor with part of a detergent pod in her mouth, half empty. Abigail was having difficulty breathing; she had vomited; and her mouth, throat, and esophagus were erythematous, swollen, and irritated. Dr. Barry ordered blood tests and immediately began to pump Abigail's stomach based on his diagnosis of a toxic effect of the accidental ingestion of detergent.

Let's Code It!

Dr. Barry confirmed that Abigail was ill due to the toxic effects of ingesting the detergent.

Turn to the Table of Drugs and Chemicals to find **Detergent** in the first column, **Substance**:

Detergent

external medication

local

medicinal

nonmedicinal

specified NEC

Were you surprised to see so many different options? I was. Which fits this diagnosis? Let's think this through:

Detergent

external medication — *the problem here was not external*

local — *she swallowed the detergent, so it was not local*

medicinal — *definitely not*

nonmedicinal — *this fits!*

specified NEC — *possibly*

Look across the row where *nonmedicinal* is listed to the first column to the right, the column **Poisoning, Accidental (unintentional)** . . . you will see code T55.1X1 suggested. This is the same code suggested on the next row for "*specified NEC*" so that will save some time.

(continued)

Turn in the ICD-10-CM Tabular List to the code category

✓4 **T55 Toxic effect of soaps and detergents**

The fourth character requires you to determine if Abigail was affected by soap or detergent, leading you to

✓5 **T55.1 Toxic effect of detergents**

✓6 **T55.1X Toxic effect of detergents**

✓7 **T55.1X1 Toxic effect of detergents, accidental (unintentional)**

You will find the seventh-character options in the box immediately below the code category. You can tell this is the first time Dr. Barry is caring for Abigail for this reason, and this is the first time Abigail is receiving care for this event, leading you to confirm this code:

T55.1X1A Toxic effect of detergents, accidental (unintentional), initial encounter

In this case, the codes for Abigail's difficulty in breathing, vomiting, and irritated mouth and esophagus would follow.

Good job!

Substance Interactions

When the cause of the poisoning or toxic effect is the interaction between two substances (e.g., drugs and alcohol), then you will need to report both substances involved. You will need one poisoning code for each substance causing the reaction, as well as one or more codes to accurately report the effect of the interaction.

Interactions can occur between two or more drugs, drugs and alcohol or other drinks, drugs and food, or many other combinations. For example, you might notice a warning "*Don't take this drug with milk or other dairy products.*" This is a warning provided to prevent an interaction—the mixture of two or more substances that changes the effect of any of the individual substances.

ICD-10-CM

LET'S CODE IT! SCENARIO

Meryl Brighton was prescribed Zyprexa (olanzapine), a psychotropic, by her psychiatrist, Dr. Cauldwell, for treatment of her bipolar disorder. Meryl mentioned that her family physician, Dr. Wall, had her on Norvasc (amlodipine), an antihypertensive, for her high blood pressure. Dr. Cauldwell told Meryl to stop taking the Norvasc while on the Zyprexa. Meryl forgot and took both medicines at the same time. Meryl suffered a dangerous case of severe hypotension and was rushed to the ED by ambulance.

Let's Code It!

Meryl was diagnosed with severe hypotension as a result of taking both Zyprexa and Norvasc. She was told not to take both medications, but she forgot and took them both anyway. This means that this was an accidental drug interaction.

First, you will need to determine the codes for the substances and intent. Open your ICD-10-CM code book to the Table of Drugs and Chemicals and look for

Zyprexa

Move across the row to find the suggested code in the first column for **Poisoning, Accidental (Unintentional)** . . . T43.591

Turn in the Tabular List to code category

✓4 **T43 Poisoning by, adverse effect of and underdosing of psychotropic drugs, not elsewhere classified**

(continued)

Carefully read the EXCLUDES1 and EXCLUDES2 notes. Do they have any connection to Meryl's diagnosis? Not this time, so read down and review all of the fourth-character options.

✓5 **T43.5 Poisoning by, adverse effect of and underdosing of other and unspecified antipsychotics and neuroleptics**

Carefully read the EXCLUDES1 note. Meryl did not become poisoned by rauwolfia, so continue reading to find the appropriate fifth character.

✓6 **T43.59 Poisoning by, adverse effect of and underdosing of other antipsychotics and neuroleptics**

Next, find the appropriate sixth character for Meryl's accidental ingestion of Zyprexa.

✓7 **T43.591 Poisoning by other antipsychotics and neuroleptics, accidental (unintentional)**

Almost done; find the appropriate seventh character. You will find the box with the options at the top of this subsection, right under the T43 code.

T43.591A Poisoning by other antipsychotics and neuroleptics, accidental (unintentional), initial encounter

Good job! Now, you need to go back to the Table of Drugs and Chemicals, and look for

Norvasc

It is not listed. So, use a PDR (*Physicians' Desk Reference*) or the website [www.pdr.net] and learn that the generic name for Norvasc is amlodipine besylate and it is an antihypertensive.

Antihypertensive drug NEC

Move across the row to find the suggested code in the first column for **Poisoning, Accidental (Unintentional)** . . . T46.5X1

Turn in the Tabular List to code category

✓4 **T46 Poisoning by, adverse effect of and underdosing of agents primarily affecting the cardiovascular system**

Carefully read the EXCLUDES1 note. Meryl did not become poisoned by metaraminol, so continue reading to find the appropriate fourth character.

✓5 **T46.5 Poisoning by, adverse effect of and underdosing of other antihypertensive drugs**

Carefully read the EXCLUDES2 notes. Meryl did not become poisoned by any of these, so continue reading to find the appropriate fifth character.

✓6 **T46.5X Poisoning by, adverse effect of and underdosing of other antihypertensive drugs**

Next, find the appropriate sixth character for Meryl's accidental ingestion of Norvasc.

✓7 **T46.5X1 Poisoning by other antihypertensive drugs accidental (unintentional)**

Almost done, find the appropriate seventh character. You will find the box with the options at the top of this subsection, right under the T46 code.

T46.5X1A Poisoning by other antihypertensive drugs accidental (unintentional), initial encounter

Good job! One more code to go. You need to report the effect that this interaction had on Meryl. Turn to the Alphabetic Index and find:

Hypotension (arterial) (constitutional) I95.9

with a list indented beneath. Stop and review the scenario again. What exactly caused Meryl's hypotension? The interaction of the two drugs. Therefore, it was drug-induced. Read down and find

Hypotension (arterial) (constitutional) I95.9

drug-induced I95.2

(continued)

Turn to the Tabular List, and begin at the code category . . .

✓4 **I95 Hypotension**

Carefully read the **EXCLUDES1** note. None of these apply to this encounter with Meryl, so continue reading to find the appropriate fourth character.

I95.2 Hypotension due to drugs

Use additional code **for adverse effect, if applicable, to identify drug (T36–T50 with fifth or sixth character 5)**

Does this turn your sequencing upside down? No. Read this carefully. In this case, for Meryl's current issue, she did not have an adverse effect. It was a poisoning. Great!

Now you can report, with confidence . . .

T43.591A **Poisoning by other antipsychotics and neuroleptics, accidental (unintentional), initial encounter**

T46.5X1A **Poisoning by other antihypertensive drugs accidental (unintentional), initial encounter**

I95.2 **Hypotension due to drugs**

Good coding!

YOU INTERPRET IT!

Identify if this is an accidental poisoning, an adverse effect, a suicide attempt, or an assault.

1. The EMTs brought Katherine into the ER. Her roommate found her unconscious with an empty pill bottle by her side, along with a suicide note. ____________
2. Harrison rushed his 3-year-old son into the ER. He had found him sitting on the bathroom floor with his bottle of Synthroid, half empty. ____________
3. Roger picked up his new prescription at the drug store. Within 30 minutes of taking the first tablet, he began to break out in a rash. ____________
4. Ellen was brought into the Urgent Care late one night by her friends. They were out at a club and she suddenly lost consciousness. The blood tests showed that someone at the club had put something in her drink. ____________

17.6 Reporting Burns

A patient can sustain a **burn** or **corrosion** to any part of the body in many different ways. It can be the result of the skin coming near to or in actual contact with a flame, such as a candle or the flame on a gas stove. A burn can happen when contact is made with a hot object, such as a hot plate or curling iron. Chemicals, such as lye or acid, can cause a corrosion upon contact with a person's skin. As a professional coding specialist, you may need to code the diagnosis of a burn or corrosion.

Burn
Injury by heat or fire.

Corrosion
A burn caused by a chemical; chemical destruction of the skin.

When a patient has suffered a burn, virtually every case will require multiple codes to tell the whole story. So, we came up with a memory tip to help you remember the details you need, the minimum number of codes you need, and the sequencing of (the order in which to report) the codes. To report these diagnoses correctly, you have to ***S/S.E.E.*** the burn. You need at least three codes to properly report the diagnosis of a burn:

First-listed code(s): S/S = site and severity (from categories T20–T25)

Next-listed code: E = extent (from code category T31)

Last-listed code(s): E = external cause code(s)

CODING BITES

A burn is caused by fire or heat, while a corrosion is caused by a chemical.

Let's look at these components and what they mean.

> **GUIDANCE CONNECTION**
>
> Read the ICD-10-CM Official Guidelines for Coding and Reporting, section **I. Conventions, General Coding Guidelines and Chapter-Specific Guidelines**, subsection **C. Chapter-Specific Coding Guidelines**, chapter **19. Injury, Poisoning, and Certain Other Consequences of External Causes**, subsection **d. Coding of burns and corrosions**.

Site and Severity

Site

Site
The specific anatomical location of the disease or injury.

Severity
The level of seriousness.

Your first-listed code or codes will be combination codes that report both the **site** and **severity** of the injury. *Site* refers to the anatomical site that is affected by the burn. When you look at the descriptions for the codes in range T20–T28, you see that each code category is first defined by a general part or section of the human body:

T20	**Burn and corrosion of head, face, and neck**
T21	**Burn and corrosion of trunk**
T22	**Burn and corrosion of shoulder and upper limb, except wrist and hand**
T23	**Burn and corrosion of wrist and hand**
T24	**Burn and corrosion of lower limb, except ankle and foot**
T25	**Burn and corrosion of ankle and foot**
T26	**Burn and corrosion confined to eye and adnexa**
T27	**Burn and corrosion of respiratory tract**
T28	**Burn and corrosion of other internal organs**

> **GUIDANCE CONNECTION**
>
> Read the ICD-10-CM Official Guidelines for Coding and Reporting, section **I. Conventions, General Coding Guidelines and Chapter-Specific Guidelines**, subsection **C. Chapter-Specific Coding Guidelines**, chapter **19. Injury, Poisoning, and Certain Other Consequences of External Causes**, subsections **d.2) Burns of the same local site** and **d.5) Assign separate codes for each burn site**.

> **EXAMPLE**
>
> Hope Rockfield suffered a burn to her left knee. Lower limb is the general anatomical site, and knee is the specific site of the burn.

First-Degree Burn
Redness of the epidermis (skin).

Second-Degree Burn
Blisters on the skin; involvement of the epidermis and the dermis layers.

Third-Degree Burn
Destruction of all layers of the skin, with possible involvement of the subcutaneous fat, muscle, and bone.

Severity

The fourth character for each category (except categories T26–T28) identifies the severity. Using the layers of the skin, the severity of a burn is identified by degree (see **Figure 17-4**):

- **First-degree burns** are evident by erythema (redness of the epidural layer).
- **Second-degree burns** are identified by fluid-filled blisters in addition to the erythema.
- **Third-degree burns** have damage evident in the epidermis, dermis, and fatty tissue layers and can involve the muscles and nerves below.
- *Deep third-degree burned* skin will show necrosis (death of the tissue) and at times may result in the loss (amputation) of a body part.

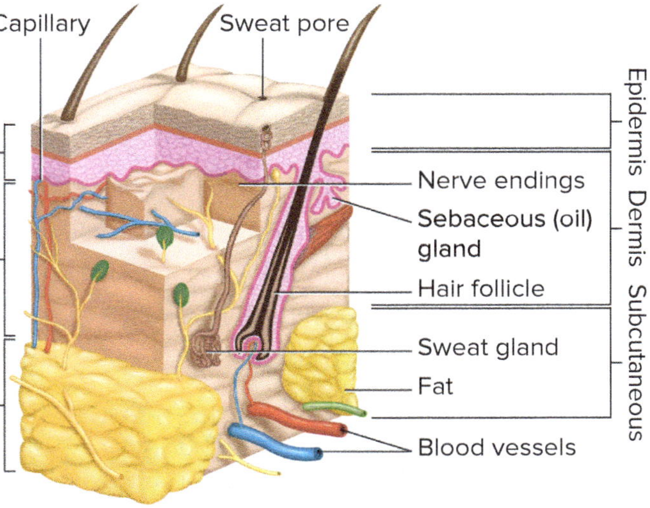

FIGURE 17-4 An illustration identifying the impact on the layers of skin for the different degrees of burns

The fourth characters available in this section give you the ability to report the documented severity of the burn or corrosion:

.0 Unspecified degree

.1 Erythema (first degree)

.2 Blisters, epidermal loss (second degree)

.3 Full-thickness skin loss (third degree NOS)

.4 Corrosion of unspecified degree

.5 Corrosion of first degree

.6 Corrosion of second degree

.7 Corrosion of the third degree

CODING BITES

The code descriptions in this section all include both the medical terms (such as *blisters*) and the degree (such as *second degree*), so you can match either to the documentation.

Specific Site

The fifth character gives you the opportunity to report additional details regarding the anatomical site of the burn. Of course, these details will change in accordance with the anatomical region of the code category. Let's take a look at samples from code category T23 Burn and corrosion of wrist and hand:

T23.-1 Burn . . . of thumb (nail)

T23.-2 Burn . . . of single finger (nail) except thumb

T23.-3 Burn . . . of multiple fingers (nail), not including thumb

T23.-4 Burn . . . of multiple fingers (nail), including thumb

T23.-5 Burn . . . of palm

T23.-6 Burn . . . of back of hand

T23.-7 Burn . . . of wrist

T23.-9 Burn . . . of multiple sites of wrist and hand

CODING BITES

The description of the fifth character 0 (zero) states "unspecified site." Use this character *very, very* rarely. Think about it: How can a physician diagnose and treat a burn and not know exactly where it is?

EXAMPLE

Troy was talking to his buddy and stepped back, hitting the back of his right calf on the hot tailpipe of his motorcycle. The physician at the emergency room documented second-degree burns.

The first three characters = **T24 Burn and corrosion of lower limb, except ankle and foot**.

The fourth character = **T24.2 Burn of second degree of lower limb, except ankle and foot**.

The fifth character = **T24.23 Burn of second degree of lower leg**.

The sixth character = **T24.231 Burn of second degree of right lower leg**.

The seventh character = **T24.231A Burn of second degree of right lower leg, initial encounter**.

And there you have the complete code to report Troy's injury. Of course, as you remember, you also will need to report an external cause code to explain how Troy's leg became burned.

ICD-10-CM

LET'S CODE IT! SCENARIO

Anthony, a 15-year-old male, was working on a school project in the basement and accidentally released the hot glue gun onto the palm of his left hand. Dr. Clermont treated him for third-degree burns of the palm of his hand.

Let's Code It!

Anthony was diagnosed with *third-degree burns of the palm*. Let's turn to the Alphabetic Index and look up *burns*:

Burn

palm(s) T23.059

Turn to the Tabular List, and read

✓4 **T23 Burn and corrosion of wrist and hand**

Notice the available seventh-character options listed directly beneath this code. You will need that information later. First, you need to determine the other characters, so read through your choices for the fourth character:

✓5 **T23.3 Burn of third degree of wrist and hand**

That is much more specific and accurate. Now you have to review the fifth-character choices for code T23.3. Did you notice that there is a character to specify that the burn was on his palm?

✓6 **T23.35 Burn of third degree of palm**

The choices for the sixth character clearly identify which palm:

✓7 **T23.352 Burn of third degree of left palm**

One more character—remember, the options for the seventh character for this code are shown directly beneath the three-character code category. Is this the first time Dr. Clermont is seeing Anthony for this burn? Yes.

T23.352A Burn of third degree of left palm, initial encounter

This code tells the complete story, doesn't it? Of course, you will need to also report the external cause code.

Multiple Sites Fall into the Same Code Category

When various sites fall into the same code category (the first three characters of the code), you will report all of these sites with just one code. If the burns are of different severity, use the fourth character that reports the most severe burn (determined by severity), the highest degree.

Then identify that more than one specific site has been burned by using the fifth character that reports "multiple sites," such as T25.19- Burn of first degree of multiple sites of ankle and foot.

LET'S CODE IT! SCENARIO

Damien Connell opened the cover of the bar-b-que to see how the coals were doing. He decided to add some lighter fluid to hurry it along, and the flames roared up into his face. Gina, his wife, rushed him to the emergency department. After an exam, Dr. Hawks diagnosed Damien with a third-degree burn on his chin and second-degree burns on his nose and cheek.

Let's Code It!

Let's begin by abstracting Damien's condition. He has

Third-degree burn on his chin

Second-degree burn on his nose

Second-degree burn on his cheek

In the Alphabetic Index, turn to the term *burn*. You will notice that the long, long list of terms indented beneath this main term all identify anatomical sites, the location on the body that has been burned. Find the suggested codes for all three of Damien's burns:

Burn, chin, third-degree T20.33

Burn, nose, second-degree T20.24

Burn, cheek, second-degree T20.26

Notice that the code category T20 is the same for all three sites: chin, nose, and cheek. Therefore, you use only one code to report these burn sites. Turn to code T20 in the Tabular List:

✓4 **T20 Burn and corrosion of head, face, and neck**

Read carefully the EXCLUDES2 listed diagnoses. None of them apply to Damien's condition. Remember that your seventh-character options are listed here as well, for later.

Go ahead and read down the column to review all of the choices for the required fourth character. Now you need to determine which fourth character to use. The burn on his chin is a third-degree burn (fourth character 3), but the burns on his nose and cheek are only second-degree burns (fourth character 2). Should you report both? The guidelines direct you to report only one code, with the fourth character that reports the *most severe* of all the burns, so you need to use the fourth character of 3:

✓5 **T20.3 Burn of third degree of head, face, and neck**

Notice that the ***Use additional external cause code*** notation is here to remind you that you need to do this next, after you determine all of the appropriate codes to report the injury itself.

Review the fifth-character options in this subcategory:

The fifth character 3 reports his chin was burned.

The fifth character 4 reports his nose was burned.

The fifth character 6 reports his cheek was burned.

Again, the guidelines tell you that you must combine all of these into one accurate code. Take a look at the fifth character 9, which reports multiple sites of face, head, and neck. Perfect!

(continued)

Put it all together and get the most accurate code that tells the whole story:

✓x7 **T20.39 Burn of third degree of multiple sites of head, face, and neck**

Look back up to the beginning of the code category to review your options for the seventh character. This is the first time Dr. Hawks is caring for Damien's burns. Now you have the complete code to report:

T20.39XA Burn of third degree of multiple sites of head, face, and neck, initial encounter

Excellent!

Extent

Extent
The percentage of the body that has been affected by the burn or corrosion.

The next code you have to report indicates the **extent**, or percentage, of the body involved. The three-character category for reporting the extent of a burn is T31 and the extent of a corrosion is T32. Either of these codes requires a total of five characters to be valid, no matter what the extent of the burn or corrosion.

T31 Burns classified according to extent of body surface involved

T32 Corrosions classified according to extent of body surface involved

Turn to code T31 in the Tabular List. The required fourth character will identify the percentage of the patient's *entire body* that is affected by any and all burns, of all degrees (severity). The code descriptions refer to this as *percentage of body surface*, also known as *total body surface area (TBSA).*

Rule of Nines
A general division of the whole body into sections that each represents 9%; used for estimating the extent of a burn.

The physician may specify the percentages directly in their notes. A statement like "third-degree burns over 10% of the body" or "7% of the body burned" will give you the information you need to find the correct fourth character for code T31 or T32. However, other times, the physician may not use a number, and you will have to calculate the percentage yourself. To calculate, you can use the **rule of nines**.

GUIDANCE CONNECTION

Read the ICD-10-CM Official Guidelines for Coding and Reporting, section **I. Conventions, General Coding Guidelines and Chapter-Specific Guidelines,** subsection **C. Chapter-Specific Coding Guidelines,** chapter **19. Injury, Poisoning, and Certain Other Consequences of External Causes,** subsection **d.6) Burns and corrosions classified according to extent of body surface involved.**

The rule of nines is used to estimate the TBSA that has been affected by the burns. The body is divided into sections, each section representing 9% of the human body (see **Figure 17-5**):

Head and neck 9%

Arm, right 9%

Arm, left 9%

Chest 9%

Abdomen 9%

Upper back 9%

Lower back 9%

Leg, right, anterior (front) 9%

Leg, right, posterior (back) 9%

Leg, left, anterior (front) 9%

Leg, left, posterior (back) 9%

Genitalia 1%

As you read through the physician's notes, be aware of the anatomical site, not only for your site code but also for your calculation of the extent of the body involved in the burns.

Next, you must determine the most accurate fifth character for this code. The fifth character identifies the percentage of the patient's body that is *suffering with third-degree burns* only. You also can use the rule of nines to calculate the percentage of area affected by third-degree burns to find the best fifth character.

Of course, these percentages are general—to be used for estimation purposes. As you look at the code descriptions for the fourth and the fifth characters, you will see that the choices for codes T31 and T32 all have descriptors that require you to know the percentage of the body involved only within a 10% range. Therefore, you don't have to worry too much about narrowing down the number.

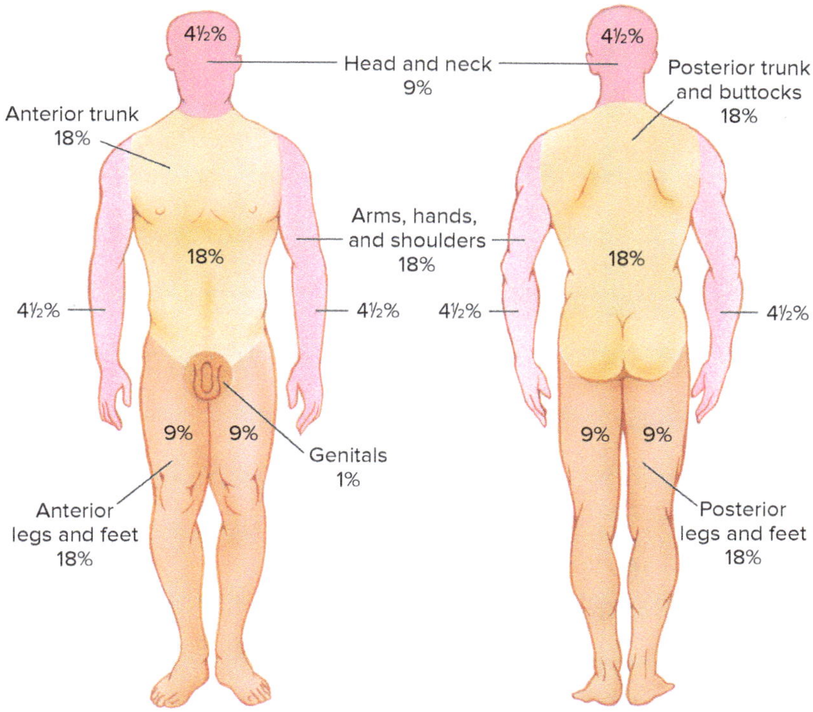

FIGURE 17-5 An illustration identifying the rule of nines, which can be used to estimate the extent of burns

When you are determining the fourth and fifth characters for code T31 or T32, you may have to add the percentages for several anatomical sites together.

While everyone knows that the rule of nines provides an estimate and is not expected to be precise, it is a professional coder's job to be as specific as possible. Therefore, you want to adjust the percentage as appropriate.

GUIDANCE CONNECTION

Read the ICD-10-CM Official Guidelines for Coding and Reporting, section **I. Conventions, General Coding Guidelines and Chapter-Specific Guidelines**, subsection **C. Chapter-Specific Coding Guidelines**, chapter **19. Injury, Poisoning, and Certain Other Consequences of External Causes,** subsection **d.1) Sequencing of burn and related condition codes**.

EXAMPLE

Celia suffered third-degree burns on her lower back and the back of her left leg and second-degree burns on her anterior forearm, wrist, and hand:

Lower back (9%) + left leg, back (9%) + anterior forearm (2%) + wrist and hand (1%) = total body surface (21%)

✓5 T31.2 Burns involving 20%–29% of body surface

Only her back and leg had *third*-degree burns:

Lower back (9%) + left leg, back (9%) = 18%

T31.21 Burns involving 20%–29% of body surface with 10%–19% third-degree burns

ICD-10-CM

LET'S CODE IT! SCENARIO

Eli Glosyck, a 28-year-old male, was trying to start a campfire when the flames flared and burned him on the back of his right hand, right forearm, and right elbow. He was rushed to the emergency room, where Dr. Compton determined that he had third-degree burns on his hand and forearm and second-degree burns on his elbow.

Let's Code It!

Dr. Compton diagnosed Eli with *third-degree burns on his hand and forearm* and *second-degree burns on his elbow*. Go to the Alphabetic Index and look up *burn, hand*. Find that listing and the others:

Burn, hand, third-degree T23.309

Burn, forearm, third-degree T22.319

Burn, elbow, second-degree T22.229

Does the Tabular List confirm the codes? Let's check each one:

✓4 **T23 Burn and corrosion of wrist and hand**

You can see that a fourth character is required, so read down the column to

✓5 **T23.3 Burn of third degree of wrist and hand**

The burns on Eli's hand were documented as third-degree, so that is correct. Now you need to determine the required fifth and sixth characters. Read all of the choices and determine which is the most accurate.

✓6 **T23.36 Burn of third degree of back of hand**

✓7 **T23.361 Burn of third degree of back of right hand**

Don't forget the seventh character. The options are at the beginning of this code category.

T23.361A Burn of third degree of back of right hand, initial encounter

This code tells the whole story about the burn to Eli's hand. Now look at the other codes suggested by the Alphabetic Index:

Burn, forearm, third-degree T22.319

Burn, elbow, second-degree T22.229

Did you notice that both of these burns are reported using the same three-character code category, T22?

✓4 **T22 Burn and corrosion of shoulder and upper limb, except wrist and hand**

You have two codes with the same three-character code category. The guidelines state that you must combine these into one code, T22, but which fourth character should you use? Remember, the guidelines also direct you to use the character that reports the greatest severity (the highest degree) of the burn. Third degree is more severe than second degree, so you will use

✓5 **T22.3 Burn of third degree of shoulder and upper limb, except wrist and hand**

Read the fifth-character choices for this code category. Which one code can report the burn to both Eli's forearm and his elbow?

✓6 **T22.39 Burn of third degree of multiple sites of shoulder and upper limb, except wrist and hand**

The sixth character will report which forearm and elbow were burned:

✓7 **T22.391 Burn of third degree of multiple sites of right shoulder and upper limb, except wrist and hand**

(continued)

And the seventh character will report which encounter this is:

T22.391A Burn of third degree of multiple sites of right shoulder and upper limb, except wrist and hand, initial encounter

Good! Next, you need a code to report the extent of the burns. Eli was burned on the following sites:

Hand (part of the arm), 9%
Forearm (part of the same arm), 9%
Elbow (also part of the same arm), 9%

The rule of nines states that one arm represents 9%. Eli had burns on his hand, forearm, and elbow of the same arm. You can see that it would not make sense to add 9% for each of these injuries, as it is still only one arm, so you get a TBSA of 9%. Of this 9%, you must note that only an estimated 4% of his body (his hand and forearm) suffered third-degree burns. Therefore, the next code on Eli's chart will be:

T31.0 Burns involving less than 10% of body surface

The codes you have for Eli's burns are T23.361A, T22.391A, and T31.0 (plus the external cause codes, of course!).

Good work!

Infection in the Burn Site

If not treated properly, a burn site can become infected. This can happen because the inner layers of the tissue are exposed, and it might be difficult to keep the wound clean and sterile. If an infection occurs, you should add a code for the specific pathogen. Sequence the infection code after the burn code but before the T31 or T32 code.

GUIDANCE CONNECTION

Read the ICD-10-CM Official Guidelines for Coding and Reporting, section **I. Conventions, General Coding Guidelines and Chapter-Specific Guidelines**, subsection **C. Chapter-Specific Coding Guidelines**, chapter **19. Injury, Poisoning, and Certain Other Consequences of External Causes**, subsection **d.4) Infected burn**.

Solar and Radiation Burns

When a patient has been burned not by fire or chemicals but by some kind of radiation, the injuries are not reported with codes from the T20–T28 range.

Even with all the ads promoting sunblock lotions and ointments to protect the skin, individuals still manage to get sunburns. These burns also are identified in three degrees to report damage to the skin as a result of overexposure to the natural sun, and each degree has its own code:

L55.0 Sunburn of first degree

L55.1 Sunburn of second degree

L55.2 Sunburn of third degree

Some individuals have a hypersensitivity to the sun, similar to an allergic reaction. Actually, this can be diagnosed as a photoallergic or a phototoxic response to the sun. This type of severe reaction can be determined to be an effect of solar radiation and is reported with one of the following codes:

L56.0 Drug phototoxic response

L56.1 Drug photoallergic response

L56.2 Photocontact dermatitis (berloque dermatitis)

L56.3 Solar urticaria

In addition to physiological sensitivity to the sun, certain medications can cause a patient to develop a sensitivity to the sun. When this is the case, you will need to add an external cause code to report the specific drug that caused this situation.

Sequelae (Late Effects) of Burns and Corrosions

Often, a scar or contracture develops at the site of a healed burn or corrosion. There are times when this lasting condition requires treatment or a procedure. In these cases, you will report the original burn or corrosion code using the seventh character "S," for sequela, to identify that the care and treatment are directed at the late effect of the burn or corrosion.

GUIDANCE CONNECTION

Read the ICD-10-CM Official Guidelines for Coding and Reporting, section **I. Conventions, General Coding Guidelines and Chapter-Specific Guidelines**, subsection **C. Chapter-Specific Coding Guidelines**, chapter **19. Injury, Poisoning, and Certain Other Consequences of External Causes**, subsections **d.7) Encounters for treatment of late effects of burns** and **d.8) Sequelae with a late effect code and current burn**.

17.7 Abuse, Neglect, and Maltreatment

> **Abuse**
> This term is used in different manners: (a) extreme use of a drug or chemical; (b) violent and/or inappropriate treatment of another person (child, adult, elder); (c) Regular consumption of a substance with manifestations.

Some people treat other people terribly. Such treatment may be physical or sexual **abuse**, neglect, or abandonment. Often, people consider unacceptable behavior as being directed toward a child, yet adults also are abused, neglected, and maltreated. As our elder population increases, these adults also are vulnerable and need health care professionals to watch out for them and protect them.

T74-	**Adult and child abuse, neglect, and other maltreatment, confirmed**
T76-	**Adult and child abuse, neglect, and other maltreatment, suspected**
O9A.3-	**Physical abuse complicating pregnancy, childbirth and the puerperium**
O9A.4-	**Sexual abuse complicating pregnancy, childbirth and the puerperium**
O9A.5-	**Psychological abuse complicating pregnancy, childbirth and the puerperium**
Z04.4-	**Encounter for examination and observation following alleged rape**
Z04.7-	**Encounter for examination and observation following alleged physical abuse**

GUIDANCE CONNECTION

Read the ICD-10-CM Official Guidelines for Coding and Reporting, section **I. Conventions, General Coding Guidelines and Chapter-Specific Guidelines**, subsection **C. Chapter-Specific Coding Guidelines**, chapter **19. Injury, Poisoning, and Certain Other Consequences of External Causes**, subsection **f. Adult and child abuse, neglect and other maltreatment**, and chapter **20. External Causes of Morbidity**, subsection **g. Child and adult abuse guidelines**.

The difference between categories T74 and T76 is important and is determined by the documentation: category T74 reports that the physician knows (confirms) this situation; category T76 records a suspicion. You know that suspected conditions are generally not coded and reported. However, most states require health care professionals to report any instances of abuse or neglect, even if it is just a suspicion at this point.

When applicable, the code from T74 or T76 should be the first-listed or principal diagnosis, followed by the injury code and/or mental health code. For cases in which the circumstances have been confirmed, a code to report the specific cause of the injury should be included, most often from code range X92–Y08. In any case of abuse, neglect, or maltreatment, if the perpetrator is known, an additional code from category Y07 should be included.

YOU CODE IT! CASE STUDY

Judah Messner, a 5-month-old male, was brought into the ED with third-degree burns on all five fingers of his left hand and both second-degree and third-degree burns on the back of his left hand. His aunt brought him in after visiting the home and seeing her sister's boyfriend stick the baby's hand into a pot of boiling water on the stove. She states she quickly grabbed the baby from this man and rushed him here. She stated that she did not want to risk staying on the premises awaiting the ambulance. When asked about the baby's mother, the aunt stated she just stood there, crying, and did not come with the child. The child was taken into treatment and the police were notified.

You Code It!

Read this scenario, and determine the correct codes to report Judah's injuries.

Step #1: Read the case carefully and completely.
Step #2: Abstract the scenario. Which main words or terms describe why the physician cared for the patient during this encounter?
Step #3: Are there any details missing or incomplete for which you would need to query the physician? [If so, ask your instructor.]
Step #4: Check for any relevant guidance, including reading all of the symbols and notations in the Tabular List and the appropriate sections of the Official Guidelines.
Step #5: Determine the correct diagnosis code or codes to explain why this encounter was medically necessary.
Step #6: Double-check your work.

Answer:

Did you determine these to be the codes?

T23.342A **Burn of third degree of multiple left fingers (nail), including thumb, initial encounter**

T23.362A **Burn of third degree of back of left hand, initial encounter**

T74.12XA **Child physical abuse, confirmed, initial encounter**

X12.XXXA **Contact with other hot fluids, initial encounter**

17.8 Complications of Care

Even though medical procedures and the standards of care are heavily researched and tested, things can go wrong. Complications can occur for any number of reasons. Before a condition can be coded as a "complication of care," the documentation must specifically identify the cause-and-effect relationship between the health care procedure, service, or treatment and the current condition that is noted as a complication.

Pain caused by medical devices and grafts previously implanted is reported with a code from categories T80–T88 (such as T82.847A Pain from cardiac prosthetic devices, implants and grafts, initial encounter), along with either code G89.18 Other acute postprocedural pain or G89.28 Other chronic postprocedural pain, as appropriate.

As you might imagine, transplanting an organ from one individual to another is a complex surgical accomplishment and saves thousands of lives. When a complication of the transplantation has been documented, a code from category T86 Complications of transplanted organs and tissue should be reported, followed by a second code to specify the complication itself.

Not all intraprocedural or postprocedural complications are reported from code categories T80–T88. They may be reported with codes from any chapter of the code set. The Alphabetic Index will guide you.

GUIDANCE CONNECTION

Read the ICD-10-CM Official Guidelines for Coding and Reporting, section **I. Conventions, General Coding Guidelines and Chapter-Specific Guidelines**, subsection **B. General Coding Guidelines**, paragraph **16. Documentation of Complications of Care**, as well as subsection **C. Chapter-Specific Coding Guidelines**, chapter **19. Injury, Poisoning, and Certain Other Consequences of External Causes**, subsection **g. Complications of care**.

EXAMPLES

J95.2	Acute pulmonary insufficiency following nonthoracic surgery
K91.840	Postprocedural hemorrhage of a digestive system organ or structure following a digestive system procedure

YOU CODE IT! CASE STUDY

Dr. Prentiss ordered 1 pint of A+ blood to be transfused into Sami Yariz in the postoperative area. The nurse was in a hurry and did not read carefully when she grabbed the blood and hung it on the IV pole. A few hours later, the patient began to complain of feeling very hot (temperature of 103 F) and pain in his back. At that time, one of the assistants noticed that the patient was given AB+ blood. The patient was treated immediately for ABO incompatibility. Hemolytic transfusion reaction was confirmed.

You Code It!

Review this scenario, and determine the correct ICD-10-CM code or codes to report.

Step #1: Read the case carefully and completely.
Step #2: Abstract the scenario. Which main words or terms describe why the physician cared for the patient during this encounter?
Step #3: Are there any details missing or incomplete for which you would need to query the physician? [If so, ask your instructor.]
Step #4: Check for any relevant guidance, including reading all of the symbols and notations in the Tabular List and the appropriate sections of the Official Guidelines.
Step #5: Determine the correct diagnosis code or codes to explain why this encounter was medically necessary.
Step #6: Double-check your work.

Answer:

Did you determine this to be the correct code?

T80.310A ABO incompatibility with acute hemolytic transfusion reaction, initial encounter

CODING BITES

External cause codes explain

- *Cause of the injury*, such as a car accident or a fall off a ladder.
- *Place of the occurrence*, such as the park or the kitchen.
- *Activity during the occurrence*, such as playing basketball or gardening.
- *Patient's status*, such as paid employment, on-duty military, or leisure activity.

Chapter Summary

People injure themselves in many different ways under many different circumstances, or others may harm someone—by accident or on purpose. Some patients may try to hurt themselves. Whether a fractured bone, a third-degree burn, a pulled muscle, or an adverse effect of a medication, when something like this happens, those of us working in health care help them.

As professional coding specialists, you must remember that, in these situations, you not only need to determine the code or codes to explain *why* the patient needs health care services, you also must explain how the patient got hurt and where the injury occurred.

You Interpret It! Answers

1. Attempted suicide, **2.** Accidental poisoning, **3.** Adverse effect, **4.** Assault

CHAPTER 17 REVIEW
Coding Injury, Poisoning, and External Causes

Let's Check It! Terminology

Match each key term to the appropriate definition.

Part I

1. **LO 17.2** Layers of skin traumatically torn away from the body.
2. **LO 17.5** Redness of the epidermis (skin).
3. **LO 17.5** A burn caused by a chemical; chemical destruction of the skin.
4. **LO 17.5** Destruction of all layers of the skin, with possible involvement of the subcutaneous fat, muscle, and bone.
5. **LO 17.5** Injury by heat or fire.
6. **LO 17.5** The level of seriousness.
7. **LO 17.5** Blisters on the skin; involvement of the epidermis and the dermis layers.
8. **LO 17.5** A general division of the whole body portioned out to each represent 9%; used for estimating the extent of a burn.
9. **LO 17.2** Damage to the epidermal and dermal layers of the skin made by a sharp object.
10. **LO 17.5** The location on or in the human body; the anatomical part of the body.

A. Avulsion
B. Burn
C. Corrosion
D. First-Degree Burn
E. Laceration
F. Rule of Nines
G. Second-Degree Burn
H. Severity
I. Site
J. Third-Degree Burn

Part II

1. **LO 17.6** This term is used in different manners: (a) extreme use of a drug or chemical; (b) violent and/or inappropriate treatment of another person.
2. **LO 17.5** The percentage of the body that has been affected by the burn or corrosion.
3. **LO 17.2** A fractured bone that did not heal correctly; healing of bone that was not in proper position or alignment.
4. **LO 17.1** The displacement of a limb, bone, or organ from its customary position.
5. **LO 17.2** Broken cartilage or bone.
6. **LO 17.2** Pain in a muscle.
7. **LO 17.3** A series of reference books identifying all aspects of prescription and over-the-counter medications, as well as herbal remedies.
8. **LO 17.2** A fractured bone that did not heal back together; no mending or joining together of the broken segments.

A. Abuse
B. Dislocation
C. Extent
D. Fracture
E. Malunion
F. Myalgia
G. Nonunion
H. *Physicians' Desk Reference* (PDR)

Let's Check It! Concepts

Choose the most appropriate answer for each of the following questions.

1. **LO 17.1** Karen Graysen, a 31-year-old female, lives in a mobile home. This morning she was working in her garden and was injured. What is the correct external cause code for the place of occurrence?

   a. Y92.015 **b.** Y92.046 **c.** Y92.027 **d.** Y92.096

2. **LO 17.2** _____ fracture identifies the breaking of the bone into several pieces.

   a. Burst **b.** Depressed **c.** Comminuted **d.** Fatigue

3. **LO 17.2** A bruise or black-and-blue mark is known as a(n)

   a. contusion. **b.** avulsion. **c.** puncture. **d.** bite.

4. **LO 17.2** How would you code an avulsion of the left eye, initial encounter?

   a. S05.02XA **b.** S05.72XA **c.** S05.52XA **d.** S05.92XA

5. **LO 17.3** Drugs and chemicals are listed in the Table of Drugs and Chemicals in all of these manners except

   a. the brand name. **b.** the chemical name. **c.** the drug category. **d.** the size of the dose.

6. **LO 17.3** The Table of Drugs and Chemicals does not include a specific listing for

   a. adhesives. **b.** lettuce opium. **c.** marsh gas. **d.** vodka.

7. **LO 17.4** The columns in the ICD-10-CM Table of Drugs and Chemicals include

   a. Intentional Self-Harm. **b.** Malignant. **c.** Toxin. **d.** Ca in situ.

8. **LO 17.5** An example of a late effect of a burn is

   a. malunion. **b.** contracture. **c.** infection. **d.** epidermal loss.

9. **LO 17.5** A third-degree burn of the chin, subsequent encounter, would be coded _____.

   a. T20.33XD **b.** S01.411A **c.** S00.83XD **d.** T20.33XS

10. **LO 17.6** Jennie James, a 28-year-old female, is pregnant and in her third trimester. Jennie presents today with the complaint that her right forearm hurts. Upon examination, bruises are noted. When asked how she got the bruises, Jennie stated that her husband came home upset and twisted her arm because dinner was not ready. What is the correct code for the physical abuse complicating the pregnancy?

    a. O9A.311 **b.** O9A.312 **c.** O9A.313 **d.** O9A.319

Let's Check It! Guidelines

Part I

Refer to the Official Guidelines and fill in the blanks according to ***Chapter 19****, Injury, Poisoning, and Certain Other Consequences of External Causes, Chapter-Specific Coding Guidelines.*

aftercare	highest	active	anatomic
extent	Superficial	separate	first
primary	acute	7th	T32
degree	minor	external	severity
Z	initial	late	subsequent
	T31	"S"	

1. Most categories in chapter 19 have a _____ character requirement for each applicable code.
2. The aftercare _____ codes should not be used for _____ for conditions such as injuries or poisonings, where 7th characters are provided to identify _____ care.
3. _____ injuries such as abrasions or contusions are not coded when associated with more severe injuries of the same site.
4. When a primary injury results in _____ damage to peripheral nerves or blood vessels, the _____ injury is sequenced _____ with additional code(s) for injuries to nerves and spinal cord (such as category S04), and/or injury to blood vessels (such as category S15).
5. Traumatic fractures are coded using the appropriate 7th character for _____ encounter (A, B, C) for each encounter where the patient is receiving _____ treatment for the fracture.
6. Multiple fractures are sequenced in accordance with the _____ of the fracture.
7. When the reason for the admission or encounter is for treatment of _____ multiple burns, sequence first the code that reflects the burn of the _____ degree.
8. Classify burns of the same _____ site and on the same side but of different _____ to the subcategory identifying the highest degree recorded in the diagnosis.
9. Nonhealing burns are coded as _____ burns.

10. When coding burns, assign _____ codes for each burn site.
11. Assign codes from category _____ , Burns classified according to extent of body surface involved, or _____ , Corrosions classified according to _____ of body surface involved, when the site of the burn is not specified or when there is a need for additional data.
12. Encounters for the treatment of the _____ effects of burns or corrosions (i.e., scars or joint contractures) should be coded with a burn or corrosion code with the 7th character _____ for sequela.

Part II

Refer to the Official Guidelines and fill in the blanks according to ***Chapter 19****, Injury, Poisoning, and Certain Other Consequences of External Causes, Chapter-Specific Coding Guidelines.*

external	adverse	many	assault	properly	sequelae
improper	toxic	current	Underdosing	Z04.71	complication
confirmed	correctly	individually	suspected	source	T36-T50

1. When appropriate, both a code for a _____burn or corrosion with seventh character "A" or "D" and a burn or corrosion code with 7th character "S" may be assigned on the same record (when both a current burn and _____ of an old burn exist).
2. An _____ cause code should be used with burns and corrosions to identify the _____ and intent of the burn, as well as the place where it occurred.
3. Use as _____ codes as necessary to describe completely all drugs, medicinal or biological substances.
4. If two or more drugs, medicinal or biological substances are reported, code each _____ unless a combination code is listed in the Table of Drugs and Chemicals.
5. When coding an _____ effect of a drug that has been _____ prescribed and _____ administered, assign the appropriate code for the nature of the adverse effect followed by the appropriate code for the adverse effect of the drug (T36–T50).
6. When coding a poisoning or reaction to the _____ use of a medication (e.g., overdose, wrong substance given or taken in error, wrong route of administration), first assign the appropriate code from categories _____ .
7. _____ refers to taking less of a medication than is prescribed by a provider or a manufacturer's instruction.
8. When a harmful substance is ingested or comes in contact with a person, this is classified as a _____ effect.
9. For cases of _____abuse or neglect an external cause code from the _____ section (X92–Y09) should be added to identify the cause of any physical injuries.
10. If a _____ case of abuse, neglect, or mistreatment is ruled out during an encounter code _____, Encounter for examination and observation following alleged physical adult abuse, ruled out, or code Z04.72, Encounter for examination and observation following alleged child physical abuse, ruled out, should be used, not a code from T76.
11. Intraoperative and postprocedural _____ codes are found within the body system chapters with codes specific to the organs and structures of that body system.

Part III

Refer to the Official Guidelines and fill in the blanks according to ***Chapter 20****, External Causes of Morbidity, Chapter-Specific Coding Guidelines.*

A00.0-T88.9	never	Y92	encounter
secondary	assault	data	Y38.9
Y93	"S"	full	initial
completely	Y99	once	status

1. External cause codes are intended to provide _____ for injury research and evaluation of injury prevention strategies.
2. An external cause code may be used with any code in the range of _____ , Z00–Z99, classification that is a health condition due to an external cause.
3. Assign the external cause code, with the appropriate 7th character (initial encounter, subsequent encounter, or sequela) for each _____ for which the injury or condition is being treated.

4. Use the ____ range of external cause codes to ____ describe the cause, the intent, the place of occurrence, and if applicable, the activity of the patient at the time of the event, and the patient's status, for all injuries, and other health conditions due to an external cause.
5. An external cause code can ____ be a principal (first-listed) diagnosis.
6. Codes from category ____ , Place of occurrence of the external cause, are secondary codes for use after other external cause codes to identify the location of the patient at the time of injury or other condition.
7. Generally, a place of occurrence code is assigned only ____ , at the ____ encounter for treatment.
8. Assign a code from category ____ , Activity code, to describe the activity of the patient at the time the injury or other health condition occurred.
9. Adult and child abuse, neglect, and maltreatment are classified as ____ .
10. Sequela are reported using the external cause code with the 7th character ____ for sequela.
11. Assign code ____ , Terrorism, ____ effects, for conditions occurring subsequent to the terrorist event.
12. Assign a code from category ____ , External cause status, to indicate the work ____ of the person at the time the event occurred.

Let's Check It! Rules and Regulations

Please answer the following questions from the knowledge you have gained after reading this chapter.

1. **LO 17.2** Explain the difference between a traumatic fracture and a pathological fracture. Why is it important to know the difference?
2. **LO 17.5** What does the acronym *S/S.E.E.* mean in relation to a burn? What details does it help you remember?
3. **LO 17.5** How do you identify the severity of burns? Include the description of each stage.
4. **LO 17.6** Turn to the Official Guidelines for Chapter 19. Injury, poisoning, and certain other consequences of external causes–I.C.19.f. Discuss adult and child abuse, neglect, and other maltreatment as outlined in the Chapter 19 guidelines; include reference to *Abuse in a pregnant patient*.
5. **LO 17.4** Explain patient noncompliance and the different codes that represent noncompliance.

YOU CODE IT! Basics

ICD-10-CM

First, identify the condition in the following diagnoses; then code the diagnosis.

Example: Abrasion of scalp, initial encounter:

a. main term: *Abrasion* b. diagnosis: *S00.01XA*

1. Underdosing of succinimides, initial encounter:
   a. main term: ______ b. diagnosis: ______
2. External constriction of left eyelid, initial encounter:
   a. main term: ______ b. diagnosis: ______
3. Laceration without foreign body of nose, initial encounter:
   a. main term: ______ b. diagnosis: ______
4. Open bite of left cheek, subsequent encounter:
   a. main term: ______ b. diagnosis: ______
5. Corrosion of trachea, sequela:
   a. main term: ______ b. diagnosis: ______
6. Toxic effect of ethanol, assault, subsequent encounter:
   a. main term: ______ b. diagnosis: ______
7. Puncture wound with foreign body of scalp, initial encounter:
   a. main term: ______ b. diagnosis: ______
8. Second-degree burn of the right axilla, initial encounter:
   a. main term: ______ b. diagnosis: ______
9. Displaced shaft fracture of the left clavicle (traumatic), subsequent encounter for fracture with malunion:
   a. main term: ______ b. diagnosis: ______

(continued)

10. Concussion with loss of consciousness of 28 minutes, initial encounter:
    a. main term: ______ b. diagnosis: ______
11. Contusion of left ear, subsequent encounter:
    a. main term: ______ b. diagnosis: ______
12. Crushing injury of larynx:
    a. main term: ______ b. diagnosis: ______
13. Corrosion of third degree of left shoulder, initial encounter:
    a. main term: ______ b. diagnosis: ______
14. Adverse effect of antimycobacterial drugs, combination:
    a. main term: ______ b. diagnosis: ______
15. Pathological fracture of right tibia due to neoplastic disease, delayed healing:
    a. main term: ______ b. diagnosis: ______

YOU CODE IT! Practice

Using the techniques described in this chapter, carefully read through the case studies and determine the most accurate ICD-10-CM code(s) and external cause code(s), if appropriate, for each case study.

1. Richard Pittmon, a 22-year-old male, was playing baseball with some friends at the local park and as he was crossing home plate, he was struck on his right leg by the baseball. The ED physician, Dr. Bonneville, took a history of the injury and completed an examination and the appropriate tests. Richard is diagnosed with an open shaft fracture type I, oblique, of the tibia.
2. Jamie McIntyre, a 43-year-old female, presents today with a painful blister on her right hand. Jamie is trying to get in shape and has begun to play handball. Dr. Brown completes an examination and diagnoses Jamie with a superficial blister on the palm of her hand between the third and fourth metacarpals.
3. Billy Ugro, a 7-year-old male, was brought in by his mother. Billy was playing this afternoon in his backyard on the sliding board and fell, scraping his left cheek. Dr. Tucker, his pediatrician, examines the area and cleans and dresses the wound. Billy is diagnosed with a second-degree abrasion.
4. Janie Walters, a 27-year-old female, presents today with burns on her left hand. Over the weekend, Janie was at a campout and, while toasting marshmallows over a bonfire, got too close to the flame, burning her left fingers. Dr. Platzs thoroughly examines Janie's hand and fingers, noting redness with blisters on the second, third, and fourth phalanges. Janie is diagnosed with second-degree burns of the fingers, multiple sites.
5. Jerry Ard, a 31-year-old male, presents today with a cut to his thigh. Jerry was dressing a piece of venison when the knife slipped and cut his left thigh accidentally. Dr. Phillips examines the incised wound and cleans the area, then closes with sutures. Jerry is diagnosed with a laceration to the thigh.
6. Grace Fuller, a 16-year-old female, was brought into the ED by her parents. They found Grace extremely drowsy. Dr. Rowell, the ED physician, notes slow heart rate and breathing. Dr. Rowell also notes constricted pupils. Grace's parents state she has been diagnosed with bipolar depression and has been taking cyclazocine. Grace is drowsy; however, she will not respond to Dr. Rowell. Dr. Rowell completes a thorough examination with the appropriate laboratory tests, which confirm an overdose of cyclazocine. Grace is admitted to Weston Hospital for a full workup.
7. Patricia Neil, a 34-year-old female, presents today with a painful left foot. Patricia accidentally hit her foot on a desk this morning and is concerned she might have broken it. Dr. Dickerson examines Patricia's foot and notes swelling and discoloration. Dr. Dickerson orders an x-ray, which confirms no fractures. Patricia is diagnosed with a contusion, bruise harm score 1.
8. Michael George, a 28-year-old male, presents today with a wound to his lower right leg. Michael stated this morning at home he accidentally stepped on his cat's tail and the cat bit him. The cat has been vaccinated for rabies. Dr. Coleman examines, cleans, and dresses the area and prescribes a round of antibiotics as a precaution.
9. Kim Horton, a 4-year-old female, is brought in today by her father. Kim was playing with her father's pocket change and swallowed a nickel. Dr. Grebner, her pediatrician, notes labored breathing and orders an x-ray, which shows the nickel is lodged in the oropharynx. Dr. Grebner is able to remove the nickel without difficulty.

(continued)

10. Dean Williams, a 5-year-old male, is brought into the ED by ambulance. Dean's grandmother stated he was playing in the yard where she has ornamental plants. One plant has mezereon berries and the birds were eating them, so Dean ate one too. Dean began to have a choking sensation. Dr. Adams completes a thorough examination and the laboratory results confirmed the diagnosis of accidental poisoning.

11. Annie Froster, an 8-year-old female, was brought in by her mother to see her pediatrician, Dr. Benton. Annie has been having difficulty swallowing. After an examination and the appropriate tests, Dr. Lukenson diagnoses Annie with a lye stricture of the esophagus. Annie admitted that her stepfather forced her to drink lye, confirmed by local police.

12. Carolina Tanner, an 18-year-old female, came into the emergency department with a wrist sprain where a baseball had hit her. She is on her school baseball team and was at a practice game being played on the school baseball field and got hit by the ball. She was in obvious pain, and the wrist was swollen and too painful upon attempts to flex. After Dr. Rodgers reviewed the x-ray, Carolina is diagnosed with a Salter-Harris, type II fracture of the distal radius, left.

13. Tricia Thornwell, a 68-year-old female, was going walking when she fell down the icy front steps of her house; now she can't bear weight on her right leg. She is brought into the ER by ambulance. After the ER physician completed a thorough exam and reviewed the x-ray, he diagnosed her with a femoral neck base fracture, nondisplaced.

14. Paula Caine, a 41-year-old female, was deep-frying fish and the kettle fell over and burned her right thigh. Paula was rushed to the ER by her husband, where the ER physician, Dr. Dinkins, diagnosed her with a second-degree burn on her right thigh. Dr. Dinkins dressed the wounds and sent her to the burn unit.

15. Helen Carrizo, an 18-year-old female, presents to the ED with a painful left ankle. Helen is accompanied by her mother. Helen had been rollerblading and tripped, falling on the sidewalk. Helen is unable to flex her ankle, which has begun to swell. Dr. Webber gathered a brief history of the incident that caused the injury, as well as any history relating to her legs and feet. He then performed a limited examination of her left leg, ankle, and foot. The imaging confirmed a sprained calcaneofibular ligament and a sprained anterior tibiofibular ligament.

ICD-10-CM

YOU CODE IT! Application

The following exercises provide practice in abstracting physicians' notes and learning to work with documentation from our health care facility, Prader, Bracker, & Associates. These case studies are modeled on real patient encounters. Using the techniques described in this chapter, carefully read through the case studies and determine the most accurate ICD-10-CM code(s) and external cause code(s), if appropriate, for each case study.

WESTON HOSPITAL

629 Healthcare Way • SOMEWHERE, FL 32811 • 407-555-6541

PATIENT: TRUMAN, HERBERT

ACCOUNT/EHR #: TRUMHE001

Attending Physician: Oscar R. Prader, MD

S: Pt is a 47-year-old male brought in by ambulance accompanied by his wife. Wife states he has been confused, dizzy, and vomiting all morning.

O: Ht. 5′11″, Wt. 187 lb., R 16. During the physical examination, the patient has a dramatic drop in vital sign measurements and suffers cardiac arrest. The crash team takes over and patient is successfully resuscitated. Blood work reveals overdose of digoxin. After Pt is stabilized, he states he was rushing to get to work this morning and couldn't remember if he had taken his medication, so he took it again.

A: Cardiac arrest due to overdose of digoxin, accidental

P: Admit for stabilization

Oxygenation

Hydration IV fluids

Monitor electrolyte balance

(continued)

PRADER, BRACKER, & ASSOCIATES

A Complete Health Care Facility

159 Healthcare Way • SOMEWHERE, FL 32811 • 407-555-6789

PATIENT: JANKOWSKI, HILDA

ACCOUNT/EHR #: JANKHI001

Attending Physician: Renee O. Bracker, MD

S: Patient, a 9-year-old female, was brought in by her mother. She had just returned from a school hiking trip in the mountains when her parents noticed a problem with her right shoulder. The patient states that her shoulder started bothering her early Sunday morning, but by the time she arrived home Sunday evening, it was much worse. Her mother called a nurse hotline and the nurse suggested an anti-inflammatory, so the parents gave her 250 mg of Tylenol.

The patient is right-handed and noticed, upon waking this morning, that she could not move her arm without a great deal of pain and that her hand was tingling, particularly her fingers. She denies any fall or accident during the trip.

O: Exam revealed some muscle wasting, observed around the right scapula. Movements of the elbow and wrist were both within normal range. However, abduction of her right arm was difficult. She denies being able to extend the arm without support, and she required movement of her entire upper arm to accomplish abduction of this arm.

Additional specific history about activities during the trip revealed that throughout the weekend, she carried a heavy backpack. The left strap had broken, so the entire weight was supported by her right shoulder and arm, creating a traction-countertraction force centered on the axilla and neck area, which produced a stretching force. She stated that each day she carried this on her right shoulder for as long as 10 or 12 hours.

A: Dislocation of the inferior acromioclavicular joint

P: Sling

Rest and ice packs

Rx: Nonsteroidal anti-inflammatory

Determine the most accurate ICD-10-CM code(s).

PRADER, BRACKER, & ASSOCIATES

A Complete Health Care Facility

159 Healthcare Way • SOMEWHERE, FL 32811 • 407-555-6789

PATIENT: ZIMMER, CYRUS

ACCOUNT/EHR #: ZIMMCY001

Attending Physician: Oscar R. Prader, MD

S: This new Pt is a 56-year-old male who was involved in an accident when the motorcycle he was driving was struck by a car on a street near his house. Cyrus admits to riding motorcycles for recreation. He is complaining about some neck pain. He has tingling into his hands and feet. He states that his left arm hurts when he tries to pull it overhead. PMH is remarkable for kidney trouble. Past bronchoscopy, laparoscopy, and kidney stone surgery, otherwise noncontributory as per the medical history form completed by the patient and reviewed this encounter.

O: Ht. 5′9″, Wt. 181 lb., R 18. On exam, the left shoulder demonstrates full passive motion. He has normal strength testing. He has no deformity. He has some tenderness over the trapezial area. The reflexes are brisk and symmetric. X-rays of his chest 2 views and C spine AP/LAT are relatively benign, as are complete x-rays of the shoulder.

A: Anterior displaced type II dens fracture of the second cervical vertebra, and an anterior dislocation of the proximal end of the left humerus.

P: 1. Rx Naprosyn

2. Referral to PT

3. Referral to orthopedist

Determine the most accurate ICD-10-CM code(s).

(continued)

PRADER, BRACKER, & ASSOCIATES

A Complete Health Care Facility

159 Healthcare Way • SOMEWHERE, FL 32811 • 407-555-6789

PATIENT: KIM, LINDA

ACCOUNT/EHR #: KIMLI001

Attending Physician: Oscar R. Prader, MD

S: This new Pt is a 29-year-old female who presents with splatter burns on the back of her right hand and her right cheek. She stated that she was deep-frying shrimp for a dinner party at her home in the kitchen and the grease splattered unexpectedly.

O: Ht. 5′6″, Wt. 152 lb., R 20. Skin is red and blistered on both sites. There is some epidermal loss. Area was cleansed with antiseptic, and ointment was applied before a clean gauze bandage was put on the hand. The facial area was also cleansed and bandaged.

A: Second-degree burns to back of hand and face.

P: 1. Rx: Aspirin for pain, prn

2. Return in 1 week for dressing change.

Determine the most accurate ICD-10-CM code(s).

WESTON HOSPITAL

629 Healthcare Way • SOMEWHERE, FL 32811 • 407-555-6541

PATIENT: O'MALLEY, REGINA

ACCOUNT/EHR #: OMALRE001

Attending Physician: Renee O. Bracker, MD

S: Pt is a 6-year-old female seen in our emergency facility. She was brought in by ambulance, accompanied by her mother. Mother states that they were baking cookies when the phone rang; she turned to answer it and when she returned, the child was unconscious on the kitchen (apartment) floor, a bottle of wintergreen oil found empty next to the patient.

O: Pt is listless and unresponsive. Respiration labored, BP 80/65, P slow and erratic. Skin is pale and moist. Stomach pumped. Pt responding to treatment.

A: Poisoning by overdose of wintergreen oil, accidental

P: Admit to pediatric unit.

Determine the most accurate ICD-10-CM code(s).

18

Coding Genitourinary, Gynecology, Obstetrics, Congenital, and Pediatrics Conditions

Key Terms

Abortion
Anemic
Anomaly
Benign Prostatic Hyperplasia (BPH)
Bladder Cancer
Chronic Kidney Disease (CKD)
Clinically Significant
Congenital
Deformity
Genetic Abnormality
Gestation
Glomerular Filtration Rate (GFR)
Gynecologist (GYN)
Low Birth Weight (LBW)
Malformation
Morbidity
Mortality
Obstetrics (OB)
Perinatal
Prematurity
Prenatal
Prostatitis
Puerperium
Urea
Urinary System
Urinary Tract Infection (UTI)

Learning Outcomes

After completing this chapter, the student should be able to:

LO 18.1 Identify the details required to accurately report renal and urologic malfunctions.
LO 18.2 Explain the conditions affecting the male genital system.
LO 18.3 Abstract the components for reporting sexually transmitted diseases accurately.
LO 18.4 Enumerate the reasons for gynecologic care.
LO 18.5 Apply the guidelines for coding routine obstetrics care.
LO 18.6 Determine the correct codes for reporting complications of pregnancy.
LO 18.7 Utilize the official guidelines for well-baby encounters and congenital anomalies.

STOP! **Remember, you need to follow along in your ICD-10-CM code book for an optimal learning experience.**

18.1 Renal and Urologic Malfunctions

Components of the Urinary System

The components of the **urinary system** (see **Figure 18-1**) are the same in both men and women. This organ system is responsible for removing waste products (known as **urea**) that are left behind by protein (food), excessive water, disproportionate amounts of electrolytes, and other nitrogenous compounds from the blood and the body. A failure to eliminate these wastes from the body in a timely fashion may actually result in the body poisoning itself. The organ components of the urinary system include

- *Kidney* (right and left), each leading to a
- *Ureter* (right and left), each leading to the
- *Urinary bladder*, which then passes urine through the
- *Urethra*, to travel outside the body.

As with many body systems, diseases and illnesses, congenital anomalies, medications, and pathogens can cause havoc within the urinary system. These problems may require straightforward treatments, such as using antibiotics for a **urinary tract infection (UTI)**, or more complex treatments, such as dialysis or transplantation.

Renal malfunction affects every organ and body system, so physical examination may alert the physician to a concern in this area. The skin's color and texture can change, periorbital edema can modify vision, or the patient may develop difficulty with muscle function, including gait and posture. Mental status also can be influenced. Electrolyte imbalance can alter hypertension levels, while metabolic acidosis can result in hyperventilation.

Urinary System
The organ system responsible for removing waste products that are left behind in the blood and the body.

Urea
A compound that is excreted in urine.

Urinary Tract Infection (UTI)
Inflammation of any part of the urinary tract: kidney, ureter, bladder, or urethra.

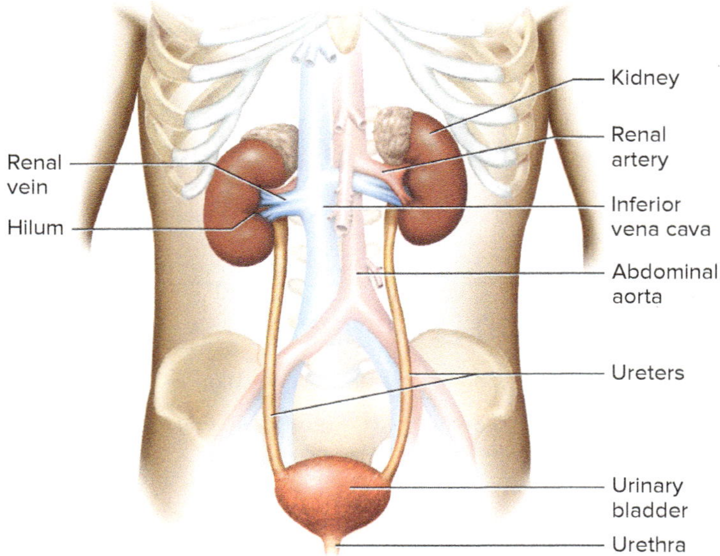

FIGURE 18-1 An illustration identifying the anatomical sites of the urinary system

Diagnostic Tools

A patient history of hypertension, diabetes mellitus, and/or bladder infections also may be indicative of urinary system conditions. Genetic predispositions can be identified with family histories that include glomerulonephritis or polycystic kidney disease. Nephrotoxicity can be caused by the patient's abuse of antibiotics or analgesics.

Blood tests can measure the levels of uric acid, creatinine, and blood urea nitrogen (BUN), providing insight into kidney function. Of course, urinalysis can add data about pH as well as clarity, color, and odor of the specimen. Measurement of urine output may require 24-hour specimen collection. Checking levels of antidiuretic hormone (ADH), produced by the pituitary gland, and/or levels of aldosterone, a hormone produced by the adrenal cortex, also may indicate kidney concerns.

Kidney-ureter-bladder (KUB) radiography can measure the size, shape, and position of these organs, as well as identify any possible areas of calcification.

Ultrasonography, fluoroscopy, computerized tomography (CT) scans, and/or magnetic resonance imaging (MRI) of the urinary system also may be appropriate to support the confirmation of a diagnosis.

An intravenous pyelogram (IVP) records a series of x-ray images, taken rapidly, as contrast material injected intravenously passes through the urinary tract. A retrograde pyelogram also uses contrast material; however, this iodine-based fluid is injected through the ureters to investigate a suspicion of an obstruction, such as kidney stones (calculi).

ICD-10-CM

LET'S CODE IT! SCENARIO

Nila Taglia, a 33-year-old female, just returned from her honeymoon in the islands. She is feeling a burning sensation and some pain on urination, so she came to see Dr. Slater. After exam and urinalysis, Nila was diagnosed with acute cystitis due to E. coli.

Let's Code It!

Dr. Slater's notes state that Nila has *acute cystitis.* When you turn to the Alphabetic Index, you see

Cystitis (exudative) (hemorrhagic) (septic) (suppurative) N30.90

acute N30.00

(continued)

When you turn to the Tabular List, you confirm

✓4 **N30 Cystitis**

Take a second to read the ***Use additional code*** and EXCLUDES1 notations carefully. Do you know what the infectious agent is so you can code it? Yes, you do. Dr. Slater included this detail *(E. coli)* in his notes. And Nila does not have prostatocystitis. Great! But first, we must determine the code for the cystitis. Did you find

✓5 **N30.0 Acute cystitis**

There is an EXCLUDES1 notation listing two diagnoses. Take a minute to review them and determine whether either one applies to Nila's condition. No, neither of them does, so continue down and review all of the fifth-character choices. Which matches Dr. Slater's notes?

N30.00 Acute cystitis without hematuria

Wait, you are not done yet. You still need to report the infectious agent. The ***Use additional code*** notation referred you to code range B95–B97. Let's turn to B95 in the Tabular List. Review all of the code descriptions in this subsection. Did you find

✓5 **B96.2 Escherichia coli [E. coli] as the cause of diseases classified elsewhere**

That's good. However, you need more information to determine the accurate fifth character. Did you realize there was more than one type of *E. coli*? Hmm. Even though you have documentation that the infectious agent is *E. coli*, it is not enough information. For this exercise, you will need to report the unspecified version. Once you get on the job, you will need to double-check the pathology report to be more specific.

N30.00 Acute cystitis without hematuria

B96.20 Unspecified Escherichia coli [E. coli] as the cause of diseases classified elsewhere

Chronic Kidney Disease

The kidneys are so important to the extraction of waste within the body. Therefore, when one or both malfunction, toxicity can form, and the patient can become very ill. Chronic kidney disease (CKD) can be caused by disease, trauma, or an adverse reaction to medication.

In the section about the kidneys, you learned that glomerular filtration is an important process in removing wastes (creatinine) from the blood as it flows through the kidneys. The **glomerular filtration rate (GFR)** is measured by blood tests to check the creatinine level. When kidney function is not at an optimum level, creatinine continues to amass in the blood because it is not being removed as necessary. The National Kidney Foundation identifies a normal GFR range as 90–120 mL/min. GFR decreases with age, so geriatric patients are likely to have lower levels. Actually, a 90-year-old patient may have kidney function at 50% solely due to age-related changes.

> **Glomerular Filtration Rate (GFR)**
> The measurement of kidney function; used to determine the stage of kidney disease. GFR is calculated by the physician using the results of a creatinine test in a formula with the patient's gender, age, race, and other factors; normal GFR is 90 and above.

Monthly tests would be performed to identify a chronic condition. **Chronic kidney disease (CKD)** may be indicated by the following lab results:

> **Chronic Kidney Disease (CKD)**
> Ongoing malfunction of one or both kidneys.

- *Normal GFR:* Kidney damage may exist even with a normal GFR–CKD stage 1, code N18.1
- *GFR of 60–89:* CKD stage 2 (mild renal disease), code N18.2
- *GFR of 30–59:* CKD stage 3 (moderate renal disease), code N18.3
- *GFR of 15–29:* CKD stage 4 (severe renal disease), code N18.4
- *GFR below 15:* CKD stage 5, code N18.5
- *End-stage renal disease (ESRD):* CKD stage 5 requiring ongoing dialysis or transplantation, code N18.6

YOU CODE IT! CASE STUDY

Shane Moyet, a 41-year-old male, was tested as part of his annual physical. He came in today with his wife to get his test results. Dr. Contreras diagnosed him with moderate chronic kidney disease. She sat and discussed treatment options with Shane and his wife.

You Code It!

Go through the steps of coding, and determine the code or codes that should be reported for this encounter between Dr. Contreras and Shane Moyet.

Step #1: Read the case carefully and completely.
Step #2: Abstract the scenario. Which key words or terms describe why the physician cared for the patient during this encounter?
Step #3: Are there any details missing or incomplete for which you would need to query the physician? [If so, ask your instructor.]
Step #4: Check for any relevant guidance, including reading all of the symbols and notations in the Tabular List and the appropriate sections of the Official Guidelines.
Step #5: Determine the correct diagnosis code or codes to explain why this encounter was medically necessary.
Step #6: Double-check your work.

Answer:

Did you determine this to be the correct code?

N18.30 Chronic kidney disease, stage 3 (moderate)

CKD with Other Conditions

CKD can be caused by hypertension, diabetic neuropathy (diabetes mellitus), untreated obstruction such as renal calculi (kidney stones), or a congenital anomaly such as polycystic kidneys. CKD progresses slowly; therefore, early diagnosis and treatment provide the best prognosis.

Hypertensive Chronic Kidney Disease

When a patient is documented to have both hypertension and CKD, you are to assume that there is a cause-and-effect relationship between the two conditions. The physician does not have to specifically state that one caused the other in the documentation. Report this with a code from category I12 Hypertensive chronic kidney disease.

Diabetes with Renal Manifestations

A patient who has been diagnosed with diabetes may develop problems with their kidneys, such as CKD, diabetic nephropathy, or Kimmelstiel-Wilson syndrome. When this is documented, regardless of the specific reason for the encounter, you will report a code from one of the following code categories, depending upon the type of diabetes mellitus:

E08.2- Diabetes mellitus due to underlying condition with kidney complications

E09.2- Drug or chemical induced diabetes mellitus with kidney complications

E10.2- Type 1 diabetes mellitus with kidney complications

E11.2- Type 2 diabetes mellitus with kidney complications

E13.2- Other specified diabetes mellitus with kidney complications

In all of these code categories, if the patient's kidney complication is CKD, you will need to report an additional code to identify the stage of the disease. You will see the *Use additional code* notation.

LET'S CODE IT! SCENARIO

Sergio Prisma, a 21-year-old male, was diagnosed with type 1 diabetes mellitus when he was 7 years old. He has been lax about testing his glucose and giving himself his insulin shots because he has been so busy with his courses and activities at Hillgraw University. After a complete HPI and exam, Dr. Allenson performed a glucose test and a urinalysis. The results showed the early signs of type 1 diabetic nephrosis.

Let's Code It!

Dr. Allenson's notes state that Sergio has *type 1 diabetic nephrosis*. When you turn to the Alphabetic Index, you see

Diabetes, diabetic (mellitus) (sugar) E11.9

The word *nephrosis* is not there, but "kidney complications" is shown, suggesting code E11.29. Let's take a look in the Tabular List:

✓4 **E11 Type 2 diabetes mellitus**

Oh, wait a minute. This code category is for type 2 diabetes. Dr. Allenson's notes document that Sergio has type 1 diabetes. Turn the pages and review this whole section to see if you can determine a more accurate code category. Did you find this code category:

✓4 **E10 Type 1 diabetes mellitus**

There is an INCLUDES note as well as an EXCLUDES1 notation listing several diagnoses. Take a minute to review them and determine whether any apply to Sergio's condition. No, none of them do, so continue down and review all of the fourth-character choices. Which matches Dr. Allenson's notes?

✓5 **E10.2 Type 1 diabetes mellitus with kidney complications**

You remember that *nephrosis* is an abnormal condition of the kidney. Review the three potential fifth-character options. Which do you believe most accurately reports Sergio's condition?

E10.21 Type 1 diabetes mellitus with diabetic nephropathy

Nephropathy (*nephro* = kidney + *-pathy* = disease) means the same as *nephrosis*, so you have found the correct code. Good job!

Anemia in CKD

The malfunction of the kidneys as they attempt to filter out the impurities in the body may trigger an **anemic** condition in the body. This condition can leave the patient weak, fatigued, and potentially short of breath because there is less oxygen carried through the bloodstream to the cells. When the patient is documented with these two conditions, you will need to

> **Anemic**
> Any of various conditions marked by deficiency in red blood cells or hemoglobin.

- *Code first* the underlying chronic kidney disease (CKD) (N18.-).
- Follow this with code D63.1 Anemia in chronic kidney disease.

Dialysis

There are two types of dialysis that may be used to treat a patient with renal malfunction: peritoneal dialysis and hemodialysis.

Peritoneal dialysis infuses a dialysate solution into the peritoneal cavity. Subsequently, the solution passes through the peritoneal membrane (which lines the abdominal cavity), collecting waste. The solution is then drained and thereby removes the waste.

Hemodialysis draws blood out of the body via an intravenous tube and passes the blood through a machine that removes waste products and returns clean blood to the body via a second intravenous connection.

When the patient is preparing for the dialysis treatments, you will need to know which type of dialysis the patient will be receiving:

Z49.01 Encounter for fitting and adjustment of extracorporeal dialysis catheter

or

Z49.02 Encounter for fitting and adjustment of peritoneal dialysis catheter

Plus, note the reminder directly beneath the code category:

Code also **associated end stage renal disease (N18.6)**

Within the first few weeks after beginning the series of dialysis treatments, the physician will want to have the patient come in for an efficiency or adequacy test. The purpose of the test is to measure the exchanges to ensure that the treatments are removing enough urea. The test results enable the health care professionals to adjust the dose, or amount, of the dialysis in each treatment. To report the reason for the encounter, report one of these codes:

Z49.31 Encounter for adequacy testing for hemodialysis

or

Z49.32 Encounter for adequacy testing for peritoneal dialysis

Most patients will need to receive dialysis several times each week, usually until a transplant is available. For each of these encounters, the diagnosis codes to report will include this code:

Z99.2 Dependence on renal dialysis (hemodialysis status) (peritoneal dialysis status) (presence of arteriovenous shunt for dialysis)

Sadly, some patients cannot deal with an ongoing need for treatment and may not come in for their sessions. As you learned, this can have a negative impact on their health, and it must be documented. The diagnosis codes to report will include this:

Z91.15 Patient's noncompliance with renal dialysis

Transplantation

At the point when the kidney is so severely damaged that it cannot be rehabilitated, a transplant may be the only solution to improve the patient's health and possibly save their life. A patient receiving a transplant must deal with the challenge of needing lifelong medication as well as follow-up care. However, great success has been achieved in increasing transplant patients' quality of life. Of course, there is always the possibility that the patient's body might reject the new organ, but the greatest roadblock for these patients is the long wait for a donor:

Z76.82 Awaiting organ transplant status

GUIDANCE CONNECTION

Read the ICD-10-CM Official Guidelines for Coding and Reporting, section **I. Conventions, General Coding Guidelines and Chapter-Specific Guidelines**, subsection **C. Chapter-Specific Coding Guidelines, chapter 15. Diseases of Genitourinary System**, subsection **a.2) Chronic kidney disease and kidney transplant status.**

Of course, a donor is needed. With kidney transplants, the donor may be either a live individual or a cadaver. If the donor is live, the individual will need this diagnosis code to support medical necessity for the preoperative testing, the procedure itself to remove the donated organ, and the postoperative care:

Z52.4 Kidney donor

Organ transplantation is an incredible health care procedural accomplishment, giving thousands of individuals with previously terminal conditions a second chance to live a normal and productive life. Patients who have received an organ transplant will typically need to take antirejection medication and receive regular checkups. Therefore, after the transplant has taken place, the patient's post-transplant status may need to be reported:

Z94.0 Kidney transplant status

Transplanting an organ from one person into another person is not always a perfect cure. There may be several issues that may require additional treatment. In some cases, the transplant does not eliminate all of the kidney disease. One kidney may have a milder case of CKD and not need transplantation, whereas the other kidney does. Therefore, it is acceptable to report both post-transplant status and current CKD in the same patient at the same time when the physician documents both conditions concurrently.

When a transplanted organ begins to show signs of rejection, failure, infection, or other complication, this will need to be treated and, in some cases, the transplanted organ will need to be removed.

T86.11 Kidney transplant rejection

T86.12 Kidney transplant failure

T86.13 Kidney transplant infection (use additional code to report specific infection)

T86.19 Other complication of kidney transplant

Z98.85 Transplanted organ removal status

CODING BITES

Code category **T86 Complications of transplanted organs and tissue** has a *Use additional code* notation to remind you to also report any other transplant complications, such as

Graft-versus-host disease (D89.81-)

Malignancy associated with organ transplant (C80.2-)

Post-transplant lymphoproliferative disorders (PTLD) (D47.Z1)

Acute Renal Failure

Acute renal failure (ARF) is a sudden malfunction of the kidney often caused by an obstruction, a circulatory problem, or possible renal parenchymal disease. This condition is often reversible with medical treatment.

The most typical cause of ARF in critically ill patients and the cause of approximately 75% of all cases of ARF is a condition known as *acute tubular necrosis (ATN)*, also called *acute tubulointerstitial nephritis (ATIN)*–code N10. Nephrotoxic injury, such as that caused by the ingestion of certain chemicals, can cause ATN but is reversible when diagnosed and treated early. Ischemic ATN may be the result of an injury to the glomerular epithelial cells causing cellular collapse or injury to the vascular endothelium, resulting in cellular swelling and therefore obstruction.

Report this condition with a code from category N17 Acute kidney failure, with an additional character to identify accompanying tubular necrosis, acute cortical necrosis, or medullary necrosis.

Treatment typically includes the provision of diuretics and fluids to flush the system. Electrolyte and fluid balances must be maintained to avoid fluid overload. Some cases require peritoneal dialysis.

ICD-10-CM

YOU CODE IT! CASE STUDY

Frieda Sacks, an 81-year-old female, has been having problems with her kidneys for a while, with two kidney infections over the last 5 years. Dr. Cannon diagnosed her with acute renal insufficiency.

You Code It!

Go through the steps of coding, and determine the code or codes that should be reported for this encounter between Dr. Cannon and Frieda.

Step #1: Read the case carefully and completely.

Step #2: Abstract the scenario. Which key words or terms describe why the physician cared for the patient during this encounter?

(continued)

Step #3: Are there any details missing or incomplete for which you would need to query the physician? [If so, ask your instructor.]

Step #4: Check for any relevant guidance, including reading all of the symbols and notations in the Tabular List and the appropriate sections of the Official Guidelines.

Step #5: Determine the correct diagnosis code or codes to explain why this encounter was medically necessary.

Step #6: Double-check your work.

Answer:

Did you determine this to be the correct code?

N28.9 Disorder of kidney and ureter, unspecified (renal insufficiency (acute))

Urinary Tract Infection

CODING BITES

Infections can occur commonly, particularly in an organ system that is open to the outside of the body. Conditions such as a kidney infection, cystitis (bladder infection), or a urinary tract infection (UTI) are certainly not exotic infectious conditions. In these cases, you will need to

Use additional code **to identify organism.**

You may have to check the pathology report to determine what the organism is if it is not specified in the physician's notes.

Cystitis and urethritis are both lower urinary tract infections (UTIs), which are often resolved easily with treatment. Ten times more women than men are affected by one of these conditions. In the elderly, a weakening of the bladder muscles may create a foundation for bladder infections (cystitis). Children with a confirmed UTI should be examined for a urinary tract abnormality. This condition would not only predispose them to UTIs but may also present a greater likelihood for renal damage in the future. Report this with a code from category N30 Cystitis, with an additional character to report specifics.

Most UTIs are caused by a Gram-negative enteric bacterium. The pathology report will identify which one. This is important to know because there is a *Use additional code* notation to identify the infectious agent. Additionally, a urinary catheter, a neurogenic (neuromuscular dysfunction) bladder, or a fistula between the intestine and the bladder might cause a UTI. Medicare may consider a UTI caused by a urinary catheter to be a nonreimbursable hospital-acquired condition (HAC).

Urinalysis of a clean-catch midstream void will confirm this diagnosis and will provide the specific name of the pathogen for coding.

Renal Calculi

Renal calculi, commonly known as *kidney stones*, might actually form anywhere within the urinary system; however, formation in the renal pelvis or the calyces of the kidneys is most common. While the precise cause of these uncomfortable formations is not known, decreased urine production, infection, urinary stasis, and metabolic conditions, such as gout, are considered predispositions. Code category N20 Calculus of kidney and ureter, N21 Calculus of lower urinary tract, or N22 Calculus of urinary tract in diseases classified elsewhere would be appropriate for reporting this diagnosis.

When the individual stones are small, hydration is prescribed to enable natural passage of the calculi. Larger stones may need to be removed surgically, most often using a cystoscope or using lithotripsy to break up the larger pieces to permit natural passage.

ICD-10-CM

YOU CODE IT! CASE STUDY

Brandon Markinson, a 51-year-old male, was in so much pain that he was doubled over. He went to the emergency department at the hospital near his house. Dr. Deitz took an x-ray and determined that Brandon had nephrolithiasis. She discussed treatment options with him.

(continued)

You Code It!

Go through the steps of coding, and determine the code or codes that should be reported for this encounter between Dr. Deitz and Brandon.

Step #1: Read the case carefully and completely.
Step #2: Abstract the scenario. Which key words or terms describe why the physician cared for the patient during this encounter?
Step #3: Are there any details missing or incomplete for which you would need to query the physician? [If so, ask your instructor.]
Step #4: Check for any relevant guidance, including reading all of the symbols and notations in the Tabular List and the appropriate sections of the Official Guidelines.
Step #5: Determine the correct diagnosis code or codes to explain why this encounter was medically necessary.
Step #6: Double-check your work.

Answer:

Did you determine this to be the correct code?

N20.0 Calculus of kidney (Nephrolithiasis)

Malignant Neoplasm of the Bladder

Bladder Cancer
Malignancy of the urinary bladder.

Malignant neoplasm of the bladder, commonly known as **bladder cancer**, is the fourth most frequently diagnosed cancer in men and the eighth most frequent in women. While various types of malignant cells can invade this organ, transitional cell carcinoma is seen most often and develops in the lining of the urinary bladder. This would be reported with a code from category C67 Malignant neoplasm of the bladder, with an additional character to report the specific location of the tumor (trigone, dome, etc.). The definitive test to confirm this condition is a cystoscopy with biopsy.

YOU CODE IT! CASE STUDY

Corneilus St. Augusteine contracted syphilis of his kidney, and now Dr. Acosta determines that an anterior urethral stricture has developed as a result.

You Code It!

Go through the steps of coding, and determine the code or codes that should be reported for this encounter between Dr. Acosta and Corneilus.

Step #1: Read the case carefully and completely.
Step #2: Abstract the scenario. Which key words or terms describe why the physician cared for the patient during this encounter?
Step #3: Are there any details missing or incomplete for which you would need to query the physician? [If so, ask your instructor.]
Step #4: Check for any relevant guidance, including reading all of the symbols and notations in the Tabular List and the appropriate sections of the Official Guidelines.
Step #5: Determine the correct diagnosis code or codes to explain why this encounter was medically necessary.
Step #6: Double-check your work.

Answer:

Did you determine these to be the correct codes?

N35.114 Post-infective anterior urethral stricture, not elsewhere classified, male

A52.75 Syphilis of kidney and ureter

18.2 Diseases of the Male Genital Organs

> **Prostatitis**
> Inflammation of the prostate.

Due to the proximity of the prostate to the urethra and bladder (see **Figure 18-2**), the most common underlying condition promoting UTI is **prostatitis**. In men, the prostate is a gland that sits inferior to (below) the urinary bladder. It is shaped like a chestnut and wraps around the urethra as the urethra descends from the bladder to the outside of the body. *E. coli* is the pathogen causing approximately 80% of these cases. A urine culture of specimens collected using a four-step process known as the *Meares and Stamey technique* provides the best data for a confirmed diagnosis. Antibiotics are the standard-of-care treatment. Code category N41 Inflammatory diseases of the prostate requires a fourth character to identify whether the inflammation is acute, chronic, an abscess, or another issue.

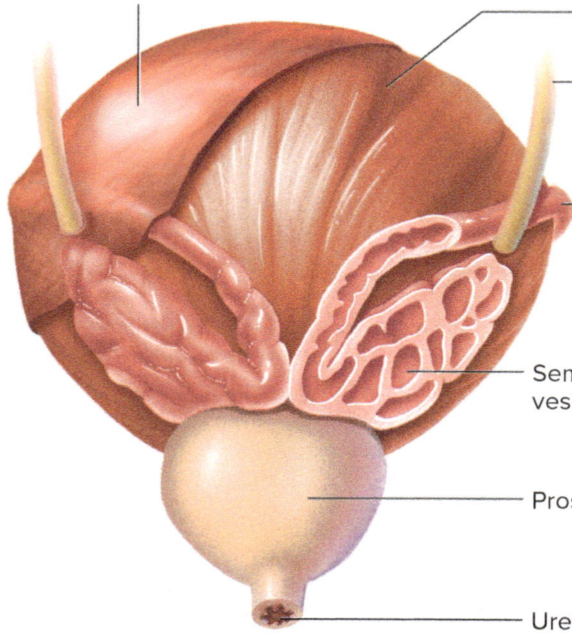

FIGURE 18-2 An illustration identifying the anatomical sites of the prostate

> **Benign Prostatic Hyperplasia (BPH)**
> Enlarged prostate that results in depressing the urethra.

Benign prostatic hyperplasia (BPH), also known as *benign prostatic hypertrophy*, most often diagnosed in men over 50 years of age, is a condition in which the prostate enlarges and results in depressing the urethra. This interferes with the flow of urine from the bladder to the outside. Code category N40 Enlarged prostate with a fourth character would be used to report this condition. BPH also can result in urine retention, severe hematuria (blood in urine), or hydronephrosis.

Hydrocele is a condition that occurs when fluid collects within the tunica vaginalis of the scrotum, the testis, or the spermatic cord. The physician will not only diagnose and treat this condition, but also needs to investigate to determine the underlying cause, especially when associated with pathology that is considered clinically significant. As you abstract the documentation, you will need to identify if the hydrocele is congenital, encysted, infected, or other type, as well as any identified underlying conditions.

N43.0 **Encysted hydrocele**

N43.1 **Infected hydrocele**
Use additional code (B95–B97), to identify infectious agent

N43.2 **Other hydrocele**

P83.5 **Congenital hydrocele**

YOU CODE IT! CASE STUDY

PATIENT NAME: Primiera, Walter

PREOPERATIVE DIAGNOSES:

1. Left hydrocele, possible right.
2. Urethral meatal stenosis.

POSTOPERATIVE DIAGNOSES:

1. Left encysted hydrocele.
2. Urethral meatal stenosis.

OPERATIONS PERFORMED:

1. Left hydrocelectomy.
2. Diagnostic laparoscopy.
3. Urethral meatoplasty.

ANESTHESIA: General and caudal.

DESCRIPTION OF PROCEDURE: After informed consent was acquired, the patient was brought into the surgical suite. The patient was placed on the table in a supine position, and prepped and draped in the usual sterile manner. General anesthesia was accomplished, and a caudal block was administered. A left inguinal skin crease incision was made and the dissection proceeded to expose the external oblique fascia. After placing self-retaining retractors, the external oblique was opened in the direction of its fibers. The external ring was opened. The ilioinguinal nerve was identified and moved away to avoid any injury. The cord was then isolated and a vessel loop placed around it. The fibers of cord were separated and hydrocele sac was identified. This was carefully dissected away from the cord structures, taking care to identify and avoid any injury to the vas or vessels.

Once the sac was completely isolated, bladder was doubly clamped and divided on the proximal aspect as well as up to the internal ring. The sac was then opened, 5-mm laparoscopic trocar sheath was placed under vision into the peritoneum, and a 2-0 silk stitch was secured in order to maintain the pneumoperitoneum. CO_2 was then insufflated to a pressure of 10 mmHg. With the patient in Trendelenburg position, the contralateral internal ring was inspected with a 25-degree lens. The vas and vessels were seen exiting a closed internal ring. Thus, a repair on the right was required. The scope was removed, pneumoperitoneum was released, and the trocar was removed. The hydrocele sac was gathered in the right-angled clamp, twisted, and high ligation was performed with 3-0 Vicryl suture ligature and tied.

Attention was turned to the distal aspect of the sac and the testis was delivered. Tunica vaginalis was opened, redundant tunica was excised, hydrocele fluid drained. A very small testicular appendage was also excised with cautery. The testis was then returned to its normal scrotal location. The floor of the canal was inspected, and there was no evidence of any weakness to suggest a direct hernia. The external oblique was then closed with a running 3-0 Vicryl, taking care to avoid any injury to the nerve. The subcutaneous tissues were closed with interrupted 4-0 chromic, and the skin with running 4-0 Monocryl. Steri-Strip and Tegaderm dressing were placed over the inguinal incision.

Attention was now turned toward the urethral meatus and the tissue in the ventral midline. The meatus was stenotic, so the tissue in the ventral midline was crushed with a mosquito clamp and then opened sharply with Westcott scissors. A 7-0 Vicryl stitch was placed at the apex. Some redundant tissue was crimped and then excised along either the left or right side. To make a normal appearance and help with avoiding interrupting the stream, this tissue was excised. The edge of the urethral mucosa was attached to the glans skin. This was done also with 7-0 Vicryl sutures. Bacitracin ointment was placed over the meatus. The patient was awakened. He was taken to the recovery room in stable condition. All counts were correct. He tolerated the procedure well. There were no complications.

Signed: *Stefan Olsen, MD*

You Code It!

Review Dr. Olsen's operative notes regarding this procedure performed on Walter. Then, determine the accurate ICD-10-CM code or codes that will explain the medical necessity for this encounter.

(continued)

Step #1: Read the case carefully and completely.
Step #2: Abstract the scenario. Which main words or terms describe why the physician cared for the patient during this encounter?
Step #3: Are there any details missing or incomplete for which you would need to query the physician? [If so, ask your instructor.]
Step #4: Check for any relevant guidance, including reading all of the symbols and notations in the Tabular List and the appropriate sections of the Official Guidelines.
Step #5: Determine the correct diagnosis code or codes to explain why this encounter was medically necessary.
Step #6: Double-check your work.

Answer:

Did you determine these to be the correct codes?

N43.0 **Encysted hydrocele**

N35.811 **Other urethral stricture**

Oligospermia is a type of male infertility, commonly known as a low sperm count. ICD-10-CM code options are combination codes that will include the general type of underlying cause, so you will need to be alert for this when you are abstracting the physician's notes. In most cases, you also will need a second code to provide more specifics about that underlying cause.

N46.11 **Organic oligospermia**

N46.121 **Oligospermia due to drug therapy**

N46.122 **Oligospermia due to infection**

N46.123 **Oligospermia due to obstruction of efferent ducts**

N46.124 **Oligospermia due to radiation**

N46.125 **Oligospermia due to systemic disease**

N46.129 **Oligospermia due to other extratesticular causes**

Erectile dysfunction is broadcast in television and Internet ads as easily solved by a little blue pill. However, whether or not it is that simple to cure, the reporting of the diagnosis is complex. As you will discover turning to code category N52 Male erectile dysfunction, you will need to determine, from the documentation, the underlying cause because all of these code options are combination codes.

N52.01 **Erectile dysfunction due to arterial insufficiency**

N52.02 **Corporo-venous occlusive erectile dysfunction**

N52.03 **Combined arterial insufficiency and corporo-venous occlusive erectile dysfunction**

N52.1 **Erectile dysfunction due to diseases classified elsewhere**
Code first **underlying disease**

N52.31 **Erectile dysfunction following radical prostatectomy**

N52.32 **Erectile dysfunction following radical cystectomy**

N52.33 **Erectile dysfunction following urethral surgery**

N52.34 **Erectile dysfunction following simple prostatectomy**

N52.39 **Other and unspecified post-surgical erectile dysfunction**

18.3 Sexually Transmitted Diseases

Age, employment status, income level, gender, number of sexual encounters . . . nothing except taking proper precautions during sex shields someone from getting a sexually transmitted disease (STD). This is true for all types of sexual encounters in which bodily fluids are exchanged–not just intercourse. The paragraphs below present an overview of the STDs considered the most common by the Centers for Disease Control and Prevention (CDC).

Bacterial Vaginosis

Bacterial vaginosis (BV)—the most common vaginal infection in women 16 to 45 years of age, often affecting pregnant women—is caused by an overgrowth of bacteria. Symptoms include odor, itching, burning, pain, and/or a discharge. Code N76.0 Acute vaginitis would be reported, along with a second code to identify the infectious agent.

Chlamydia

Caused by a bacterium *(Chlamydia trachomatis)*, *chlamydia* can result in infertility or other irreversible damage to a woman's reproductive organs. The symptoms are mild or absent, so most women don't know they have a problem unless their partner is diagnosed. Chlamydia can cause a penile discharge in men. It is the most commonly reported bacterial STD in the United States, according to the CDC. In ICD-10-CM, code A55 Chlamydial lymphogranuloma (venereum) is reported for chlamydia that is transmitted by sexual contact. *NOTE:* Do not confuse this with A70 Chlamydia psittaci infections, A74.0 Chlamydial conjunctivitis, A74.81 Chlamydial peritonitis, A74.89 Other chlamydial diseases, or A74.9 Chlamydial infection unspecified, all of which are reported when chlamydia causes another disease.

Genital Herpes

Genital herpes is caused by one of the herpes simplex viruses: type 1 (HSV-1) or type 2 (HSV-2). In this STD, one or more blisters may appear on or in the genital or rectal area. Once the blister bursts, it can take several weeks for the ulcer to heal. The virus will remain in the body indefinitely, even though no more breakouts may be experienced, because there is no cure. Treatment can reduce the number of outbreaks and diminish the opportunity of transmission to a partner. To code from category A60 Anogenital herpesviral [herpes simplex] infections, you must know the specific anatomical site, such as penis or cervix, to determine the additional characters required.

Gonorrhea

Gonorrhea, a bacterial STD, can develop in the reproductive organs of men (urethra) and women (cervix, uterus, fallopian tubes, and urethra), in addition to the mouth, throat, eyes, and anus. Symptoms in men include a burning sensation during urination, a penile discharge (white, yellow, or green), and/or swelling or pain in the testes. Women typically do not experience any symptoms. You will report this diagnosis from ICD-10-CM code category A54 Gonococcal infection, which requires identification of the specific anatomical site of the infection to determine additional characters.

Human Immunodeficiency Virus

Both types of *human immunodeficiency virus (HIV)*—HIV-1 and HIV-2—destroy cells within the body that are responsible for helping fight disease (those that are part of the immune system). Soon after the initial infection, some individuals may suffer flu-like symptoms, while others will have no symptoms at all and feel fine. Current medications can help individuals continue to feel well and decrease their ability to transmit the disease. HIV, especially untreated HIV, has known manifestations, including cardiovascular, renal, and liver disease. In the late stages of the disease, when the patient's immune system is quite damaged, acquired immune deficiency syndrome (AIDS) may develop. Currently, there is no cure for HIV or AIDS. You will report a confirmed diagnosis of HIV with code B20 Human Immunodeficiency Virus [HIV] disease when the patient has, or has had, manifestations or code Z21 Asymptomatic human immunodeficiency virus [HIV] infection status when the patient is asymptomatic.

Human Papillomavirus

There are over 40 different types of *human papillomavirus (HPV)* that can infect the genital regions, mouth, and/or throat of both men and women. This infection will not cause any signs or symptoms; however, it is known to contribute to the development of genital warts as well as cervical cancer (in women). A connection also has been made between HPV and malignancies in the penis, anus, vulva, vagina, and oropharynx. A patient getting a test to screen for HPV will be reported with code Z11.51 Encounter for screening for human papillomavirus (HPV). Reporting for a female patient with a positive test result will come from subcategory R87.8 Other abnormal findings in specimens from female genital organs. Additional characters are required based on the anatomical location (cervix or vagina) and on whether the patient is identified as high risk or low risk. Male and female patients would both be reported with a code from subcategory R85.8 Other abnormal findings in specimens from digestive organs and abdominal cavity for HPV-positive results in the anus. A confirmed diagnosis for either a male or female patient would be reported with A63.0 Anogenital (venereal) warts [due to (human) papillomavirus (HPV)].

Pelvic Inflammatory Disease

Pelvic inflammatory disease (PID) is often a complication of previous chlamydial, gonococcal, or other STD infection, occurring when the bacterium moves from the vagina into a woman's uterus or fallopian tubes. It causes lower abdominal pain. Serious consequences of untreated PID include chronic pelvic pain, formation of abscesses, ectopic pregnancy, and possible infertility. Use code A56.11 Chlamydial female pelvic inflammatory disease or A54.24 Gonococcal female pelvic inflammatory disease, or use a code from category N73 Other female pelvic inflammatory diseases or code N74 Female pelvic inflammatory disorders in diseases classified elsewhere.

Syphilis

In its early stages, *syphilis*, caused by a bacterium *(Treponema pallidum)*, is easy to cure. Signs and symptoms include a rash, particularly on the palmar and plantar surfaces, as well as a small, round, painless sore on the genitals, anus, or mouth. However, these symptoms mimic many other diseases, often resulting in delayed diagnosis. Code category A50 Congenital syphilis, A51 Early syphilis, A52 Late syphilis, or A53 Other and unspecified syphilis would be reported when this condition is sexually transmitted.

Trichomoniasis

Trichomoniasis (trich), a protozoan parasitic *(Trichomonas vaginalis)* STD, is more common in older women than in men. Most individuals do not know they are infected because only approximately 30% develop any symptoms, such as a genital discharge. While the condition is curable, a person who has trich and goes without treatment increases their risk of getting HIV. Trich, when present in a pregnant woman, can cause premature delivery of low-birth-weight neonates. Code category A59 Trichomoniasis requires additional characters to identify the specific anatomical site of the infection.

ICD-10-CM

YOU CODE IT! CASE STUDY

PATIENT: Madison, Amelia

PREOPERATIVE DIAGNOSES:

1. Severe pelvic pain.
2. History of pelvic inflammatory disease and pelvic adhesion.
3. Probable left hydrosalpinx.

POSTOPERATIVE DIAGNOSES:

1. Chronic pelvic inflammatory disease.
2. Extensive pelvic adhesion and left hydrosalpinx.

PROCEDURES PERFORMED:

1. Pelvic examination under anesthesia.
2. Total abdominal hysterectomy.
3. Bilateral salpingo-oophorectomy.
4. Lysis of adhesions.

SURGEON: Gabriel Underwood, MD

ANESTHESIA: General.

ESTIMATED BLOOD LOSS: 100 mL.

COMPLICATIONS: None.

(continued)

DESCRIPTION OF OPERATION: The patient was taken to the operating room, where general anesthesia was administered without complication. The patient was placed in the dorsal lithotomy position, and examination under anesthesia revealed a normal-appearing vagina and cervix. Bimanual exam reveals a normal-sized uterus with no right adnexal pathology noted. There was an adnexal mass in the left adnexa of approximately 4–5 cm. The patient was placed in the supine position. She was prepped and draped in the usual fashion.

A Pfannenstiel skin incision was performed and carried down to the fascial layer. The fascia was transected. The rectus muscles were retracted laterally, and the peritoneum was entered under direct visualization. The pelvic cavity was inspected, and there were extensive pelvic adhesions noted. The bowel was packed into the upper abdomen using moist laps. There was a large left hydrosalpinx present with bilateral tubal-ovarian adhesions. The left hydrosalpinx was first freed up using careful sharp dissection. The tube and ovary on the right side were likewise mobilized with sharp dissection. The right round ligament was doubly clamped, cut, and tied with 0 Vicryl suture. The visceroperitoneum was dissected free to the midline. The left round ligament was likewise doubly clamped, cut, and tied and the visceroperitoneum was dissected free to the midline. The bladder was carefully dissected off the lower uterine segment. The right infundibulopelvic ligament was clamped, cut, and doubly tied with 0 Vicryl suture. The left infundibulopelvic ligament was likewise doubly clamped, cut, and doubly tied with 0 Vicryl suture. The right uterine vessels and cardinal ligament were doubly clamped, cut, and doubly tied with 0 Vicryl suture. The left uterine vessels and cardinal ligament were likewise clamped, cut, and doubly tied with 0 Vicryl suture. The bladder was retracted inferiorly. The right uterosacral ligament was clamped, cut, and tied with 0 Vicryl suture. This step was repeated until the specimen was mobilized on the right side. The left uterosacral ligament was likewise clamped, cut, and tied with 0 Vicryl suture. Again, the step was repeated until the specimen was mobilized on the left side.

The anterior aspect of the vagina was entered with a scalpel and heavy curved scissors were used to remove the uterus, tubes, and ovaries, which were sent to pathology for microscopic examination. Angled sutures were placed on either side of the vaginal cuff using 0 Vicryl suture. The vaginal cuff was closed with interrupted figure-of-eight sutures of 0 Vicryl. A thorough search was made to ensure that there was complete hemostasis. The pelvic peritoneum was reapproximated with 0 Vicryl suture. The instruments were removed from the abdomen. The sponge, needle, and instrument counts were all correct. The parietal peritoneum was reapproximated with 2-0 Vicryl suture. The rectus muscles were reapproximated with interrupted 0 Vicryl suture. The fascia was closed with 0 PDS suture. The subcutaneous tissue was reapproximated with 3-0 Vicryl suture. The skin was closed with staples. A dry sterile dressing was placed over the incision. The patient was then awoken in the operating room and transferred to the recovery room in good condition.

DISPOSITION: The patient was taken to the recovery room in good condition at the end of the procedure.

You Code It!

Read these operative notes, written by Dr. Underwood, about Amelia's procedure, and determine the correct ICD-10-CM code or codes to explain the reason *why* the procedures were medically necessary.

Step #1: Read the case carefully and completely.

Step #2: Abstract the scenario. Which main words or terms describe why the physician cared for the patient during this encounter?

Step #3: Are there any details missing or incomplete for which you would need to query the physician? [If so, ask your instructor.]

Step #4: Check for any relevant guidance, including reading all of the symbols and notations in the Tabular List and the appropriate sections of the Official Guidelines.

Step #5: Determine the correct diagnosis code or codes to explain why this encounter was medically necessary.

Step #6: Double-check your work.

Answer:

Did you determine these to be the codes?

N73.1 Chronic parametritis and pelvic cellulitis

N73.6 Female pelvic peritoneal adhesions (post-infective)

N70.11 Chronic salpingitis

Good job!

18.4 Gynecologic Care

Gynecologist (GYN)
A physician specializing in the care of the female genital tract.

Obstetrics (OB)
A health care specialty focusing on the care of women during pregnancy and the puerperium.

Puerperium
The time period from the end of labor until the uterus returns to normal size, typically 3 to 6 weeks.

Females of all ages may go to the **gynecologist (GYN)** for specialized health care. Sometimes, the physician is referred to as an *OB/GYN*, an abbreviation for the dual specialization of **obstetrics (OB)**, which focuses on care during pregnancy and the **puerperium**, and gynecology. Concerns and disorders relating to other aspects of the female anatomy are not always related to pregnancy. Let's investigate some of the most common reasons a woman would seek the care of a GYN and how to report them.

Routine Encounters

Most women understand the importance of getting their annual well-woman examination. It may take place at the office of a specialized OB/GYN or be performed by a family or general practitioner. Typically, the visit includes a routine physical exam, pelvic exam, and breast exam. Often, the visit also includes a Papanicolaou *cervical* smear, better known as a *Pap smear*. The encounter is coded

Z01.411 Encounter for routine gynecological examination (general) (routine) with abnormal findings

or

Z01.419 Encounter for routine gynecological examination (general) (routine) without abnormal findings

These codes include a *cervical* Pap smear. However, when a *vaginal* Pap smear (which is different from a *cervical* Pap smear and must be specified in the documentation) is included in the visit, add a second code:

Z12.72 Encounter for screening for malignant neoplasm of vagina (vaginal pap smear)

Endometriosis

Endometriosis (code category N80) is an inflammation or swelling of the tissue that lines the uterus. The condition is estimated to affect 2% to 10% of women of childbearing age in the United States. Although the disorder is identified as being within the uterus, endometriosis can be observed in a woman's ovary, cul-de-sac, uterosacral ligaments, broad ligaments, fallopian tube, uterovesical fold, round ligament, vermiform appendix, vagina, and/or rectovaginal septum. This means that a diagnosis of endometriosis is not sufficient to determine the most accurate code. You have to know the specific site of the condition.

Uterine Fibroids

Also known as *uterine leiomyoma* or *uterine fibromyoma*, *uterine fibroids* (code category D25 Leiomyoma of uterus) are tumors located in the female reproductive system. Only about one-third of women with these tumors are actually diagnosed. Uterine fibroids are not related to cancer, do not increase the patient's risk of developing cancer later, and are found to be benign 99% of the time.

Pelvic Pain

Female pelvic and perineal pain (code R10.2) may be related to a specific genital organ or an area around a genital organ or may be psychological in nature. The physician may be able to diagnose a particular cause, such as sexual intercourse or menstruation, or the source of the pain may remain unknown.

ICD-10-CM

YOU CODE IT! CASE STUDY

Clarisse Battle, a 31-year-old female, came to see Dr. Legg with complaints of feeling bloated. She stated that she has felt this way for over a month and cannot connect it to anything she has been eating. After taking a complete history, doing an exam, and performing an ultrasound, Dr. Legg explained that Clarisse had a simple cyst on her right ovary.

(continued)

You Code It!

Go through the steps of coding, and determine the code or codes that should be reported for this encounter between Dr. Legg and Clarisse.

Step #1: Read the case carefully and completely.
Step #2: Abstract the scenario. Which key words or terms describe why the physician cared for the patient during this encounter?
Step #3: Are there any details missing or incomplete for which you would need to query the physician? [If so, ask your instructor.]
Step #4: Check for any relevant guidance, including reading all of the symbols and notations in the Tabular List and the appropriate sections of the Official Guidelines.
Step #5: Determine the correct diagnosis code or codes to explain why this encounter was medically necessary.
Step #6: Double-check your work.

Answer:

Did you determine this to be the correct code?

N83.291 Other ovarian cysts (simple cyst of ovary), right

You are really getting to be a great coder!

Procreative Management

A woman may want to see her physician regarding her desire to have children now or in the future. Code category Z31 Encounter for procreative management is used only for testing conducted with anticipation of procreation (having children). Code subcategory Z31.6 Encounter for general counseling and advice on procreation will provide you with a few fifth-character options to include additional details.

Perhaps a patient comes in for a test to determine whether or not she is a carrier of a genetic disease before getting pregnant. Most often, such a woman wants to be aware of the possibilities of passing inherited diseases, such as sickle cell anemia or Tay-Sachs, to her baby. The code or codes to report her encounter would be code(s):

Z31.430 Encounter of female for testing for genetic diseases carrier status for procreative management

and/or

Z31.438 Encounter for other genetic testing of female for procreative management

Code Z31.5 Encounter for genetic counseling would be used after a genetic test has been done and shown positive results.

With good news so far, our female patient may come in next time for fertility testing or, perhaps, a pregnancy test:

Z31.41 Encounter for fertility testing

Z32.00 Encounter for pregnancy test, result unknown

Z32.01 Encounter for pregnancy test, result positive

Z32.02 Encounter for pregnancy test, result negative

ICD-10-CM

LET'S CODE IT! SCENARIO

Priscilla Sharp, a 25-year-old female, came to see Dr. Trenton to have an intrauterine device (IUD) inserted. She and her husband, Eli, want to wait a while before having children.

(continued)

Let's Code It!

Priscilla came to get an *IUD*. The purpose of this visit is to prevent Priscilla from getting pregnant, also termed *contraception*. Let's go to the Alphabetic Index and look up *contraception*. Look down the list indented under *contraception* and you see *device*. However, none of the terms indented under *device* seems to really match Dr. Trenton's notes. This is the first encounter relating to contraception, so perhaps "initial prescription" would be a place to begin.

Contraception, contraceptive

device (intrauterine) (in situ) Z97.5

initial prescription Z30.014

Turn to the Tabular List and confirm that this is the best, most accurate code:

✓4 **Z30 Encounter for contraceptive management**

There are no notations or directives, so continue reading down the column to determine the most accurate required fourth and fifth characters:

Z30.014 Encounter for initial prescription of intrauterine contraceptive device

Be sure to read further down the column to determine whether any other code descriptions may be more accurate than this description. Sometimes, the Alphabetic Index gets us to only the best subsection of the Tabular List.

Z30.430 Encounter for insertion of intrauterine contraceptive device

There it is! Good job!

18.5 Routine Obstetrics Care

Fertilization and Gestation

Gestation
The length of time for the complete development of a baby from conception to birth; on average, 40 weeks.

When a sperm fertilizes an oocyte, a zygote is created. This will typically occur while the egg is still in the last portion of the fallopian tube. Each oocyte (egg) has 23 chromosomes, and each sperm contains 23 chromosomes (in the nucleus in the head of the sperm). When they combine during fertilization, the zygote then has the complete set of 46 chromosomes. This may be confirmed by a pregnancy test; the medical necessity for this visit is reported with a code such as Z32.01 Encounter for pregnancy tests, result positive.

The *embryonic period*, from weeks 2 through 8 after fertilization, is the time during which external structures and internal organs begin to form. Additionally, the placenta, umbilical cord, amnion, yolk sac, and chorion are established during this time. At week 8, the embryo, about 1 inch in length, is considered a fetus, and all organ systems are in place.

Gestation, the length of the pregnancy, is measured in trimesters, beginning on the first day of the last menstrual period (LMP). For coding purposes, ICD-10-CM provides the following definitions:

- *First trimester:* from the first day of the LMP to less than 14 weeks 0 days.
- *Second trimester:* 14 weeks 0 days to less than 28 weeks 0 days.
- *Third trimester:* 28 weeks 0 days until delivery.
- *Preterm (premature) neonate:* one with a gestation of 28 completed weeks or more but less than 37 completed weeks (between 196 and 258 completed days).
- *Postterm neonate:* one with over 40 completed weeks up to 42 completed weeks of gestation.
- *Prolonged gestation of a neonate:* a gestational period that has lasted over 42 completed weeks (294 days or more).

GUIDANCE CONNECTION

Read the ICD-10-CM Official Guidelines for Coding and Reporting, section **I. Conventions, General Coding Guidelines and Chapter-Specific Guidelines**, subsection **C. Chapter-Specific Coding Guidelines**, chapter **15. Pregnancy, Childbirth, and the Puerperium**, subsections **a.3) Final character for trimester**, **a.4) Selection of trimester for inpatient admissions that encompass more than one trimester**, **a.5) Unspecified trimester**, and **b.3) Episodes when no delivery occurs.**

Weeks of Gestation

Cases in which a complication has been identified require additional specificity, beyond the current trimester of the pregnancy, and you will need to report the specific number of weeks of gestation. Code category Z3A Weeks of gestation provides you with codes that specify the individual week, from 8-week to 42-week gestation. In addition, codes are available for less than 8 weeks and greater than 42 weeks.

When a pregnant patient is admitted and stays in the hospital for more than 1 week, you should use the date of admission to determine the weeks of gestation.

EXAMPLE

Amy went into labor and ultimately delivered the baby. She and her husband were very concerned because the baby was only at 33 weeks:

O60.14X0	Preterm labor third trimester with preterm delivery third trimester, single gestation
Z3A.33	33 weeks gestation of pregnancy

CODING BITES

Code category Z3A codes are not reported in cases of

- Pregnancies with abortive outcomes.
- Elective termination of pregnancy.
- Postpartum conditions.

Prenatal Visits

A woman often has three items noted in her chart: *gravida (G)* reports how many times the woman has been pregnant; *para*, or *parity (P)*, reports how many babies this woman has given birth to (after 20 weeks of gestation); and *abortus (A)* identifies how many pregnancies did not come to term or make it past the 20th week. Gravida and para may be noted using an abbreviation, such as G2 P1.

EXAMPLE

G1 P1	tells you that the woman has been pregnant once and given birth once.
G1 P2	tells you that the woman has been pregnant once and given birth twice—twins!
G2 P1	tells you that the woman has been pregnant twice and given birth once. If she is pregnant now, this is her second pregnancy; if she is not pregnant now, she may have had a miscarriage in the past.

Normal Pregnancy

Routine outpatient **prenatal** checkups are very important to the health and well-being of both the mother and the baby. For a healthy pregnant woman, the visits are typically scheduled at specific points throughout the pregnancy, as determined by the number of weeks of gestation.

Prenatal
Prior to birth; also referred to as *antenatal*.

When coding routine visits, with the patient having no complications, you will choose from the available Z codes. Remember that you will use a Z code when the patient is not encountering the health care provider because of any current illness or injury. A healthy, pregnant woman has neither a current illness nor a current injury.

Z34.01	**Encounter for supervision of normal first pregnancy, first trimester**
Z34.82	**Encounter for supervision of other normal pregnancy, second trimester**

As you can see, you will need to determine which code to use on the basis of the physician's notes on the woman's gravida.

GUIDANCE CONNECTION

Read the ICD-10-CM Official Guidelines for Coding and Reporting, section **I. Conventions, General Coding Guidelines and Chapter-Specific Guidelines**, subsection **C. Chapter-Specific Coding Guidelines**, chapter **15. Pregnancy, Childbirth, and the Puerperium**, subsection **b.1) Routine outpatient prenatal visits**.

High-Risk Pregnancy

In cases where the pregnancy is considered to be medically high risk, you will use a code from category O09 Supervision of high-risk pregnancy for the routine visit.

You will determine the fourth digit for the O09 code according to the reason stated in the physician's notes that the pregnancy is considered high risk. The reason might be a history of infertility (O09.0-), a very young mother (O09.61-), an older mother (O09.51-), or another issue.

The fifth or sixth character is used to report which trimester the patient is in at the encounter.

GUIDANCE CONNECTION

Read the ICD-10-CM Official Guidelines for Coding and Reporting, section **I. Conventions, General Coding Guidelines and Chapter-Specific Guidelines**, subsection **C. Chapter-Specific Coding Guidelines**, chapter **15. Pregnancy, Childbirth, and the Puerperium**, subsection **b.2) Supervision of high-risk pregnancy**.

EXAMPLES

O09.211	Supervision of pregnancy with history of preterm labor, first trimester
O09.32	Supervision of pregnancy with insufficient antenatal care, second trimester

Incidental Pregnant State

You may be in an office when a pregnant woman comes in for services or treatment from a physician for a reason that has nothing to do with her pregnancy at all. Even though the actual treatment or service is not related to her pregnancy, the fact that she is pregnant will affect the way the physician treats her condition. Therefore, you must always include code Z33.1 Pregnant state, incidental, to indicate the pregnancy. It will never be a first-listed code.

EXAMPLE

Wendy Weingarter is 15 weeks pregnant and works at a bank. As she was walking to her car, she slipped and fractured her toe. Dr. Stewart prescribed one pain medication rather than another because Wendy was pregnant. He also took extra precautions while x-raying her foot. You will report these codes:

S92.424A	Nondisplaced fracture of distal phalanx of right great toe, initial encounter
Z33.1	Pregnant state, incidental

YOU CODE IT! CASE STUDY

Genesa Thurston, a 31-year-old female, G1 P0, came to see Dr. Mallard for her routine 20-week prenatal checkup. Dr. Mallard noted that Genesa's blood pressure was elevated and told her to come back in 10 days for a recheck.

You Code It!

Go through the steps of coding, and determine the code or codes that should be reported for this encounter between Dr. Mallard and Genesa.

Step #1: Read the case carefully and completely.

Step #2: Abstract the scenario. Which key words or terms describe why the physician cared for the patient during this encounter?

(continued)

Step #3: Are there any details missing or incomplete for which you would need to query the physician? [If so, ask your instructor.]

Step #4: Check for any relevant guidance, including reading all of the symbols and notations in the Tabular List and the appropriate sections of the Official Guidelines.

Step #5: Determine the correct diagnosis code or codes to explain why this encounter was medically necessary.

Step #6: Double-check your work.

Answer:

Did you determine these to be the correct codes?

Z34.02 **Encounter for supervision of normal first pregnancy, second trimester**

R03.0 **Elevated blood pressure reading, without diagnosis of hypertension**

Good job!

Labor and Delivery

The time has come for the baby to make its way into the world (see **Figure 18-3**). When the event goes picture-perfectly, requiring minimal or very little assistance from the obstetrician, everything is simpler, including the coding. On the mother's chart, every encounter that results in the birth of a baby requires at least two codes:

- The delivery itself.
- The outcome of that delivery–number of babies, alive or not (Z37.-).

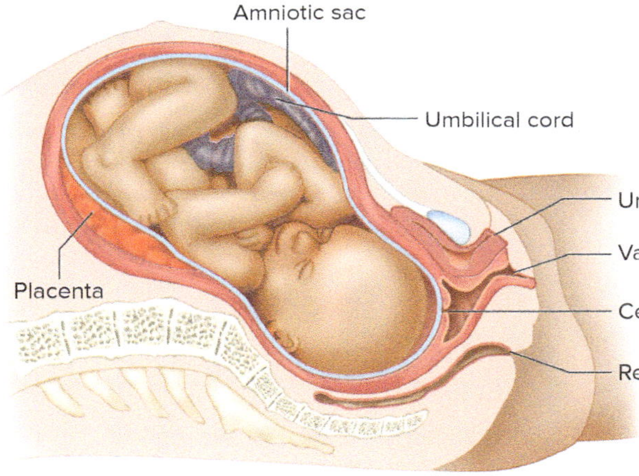

FIGURE 18-3 An illustration identifying the anatomical sites of a pregnant uterus and related parts of the female anatomy

Additional codes may be required if there are any complications.

GUIDANCE CONNECTION

Read the ICD-10-CM Official Guidelines for Coding and Reporting, section **I. Conventions, General Coding Guidelines and Chapter-Specific Guidelines**, subsection **C. Chapter-Specific Coding Guidelines**, chapter **15. Pregnancy, Childbirth, and the Puerperium**, subsections **b.4) When a delivery occurs** and **n. Normal delivery, code O80**.

Normal Delivery

When a baby comes by the old-fashioned route–spontaneous, full-term, vaginal, live-born, single infant–and there are *no current* complications or issues related to the pregnancy, your principal diagnostic code will be

O80 **Encounter for full-term uncomplicated delivery**

Antepartum conditions may have been a concern; however, in order to use code O80, they must have been resolved prior to the big event.

When a pregnant woman is admitted into the hospital and delivers the baby during this admission, the principal diagnosis code should be the reason documented for admitting her, whether or not it is related to the delivery of the baby.

Special Circumstances Related to Delivery

The process of labor and the ultimate delivery of a baby is a natural and joyous occasion. Of course, things don't always happen as they should. There may be an issue that requires ongoing observation, admission into the hospital, or some other factor requiring a change to the original delivery plan (see **Figure 18-4**). For example:

O60.14XX- **Preterm labor third trimester with preterm delivery third trimester**

O64.1XX- **Obstructed labor due to breech presentation**

O69.0XX- **Labor and delivery complicated by prolapse of cord**

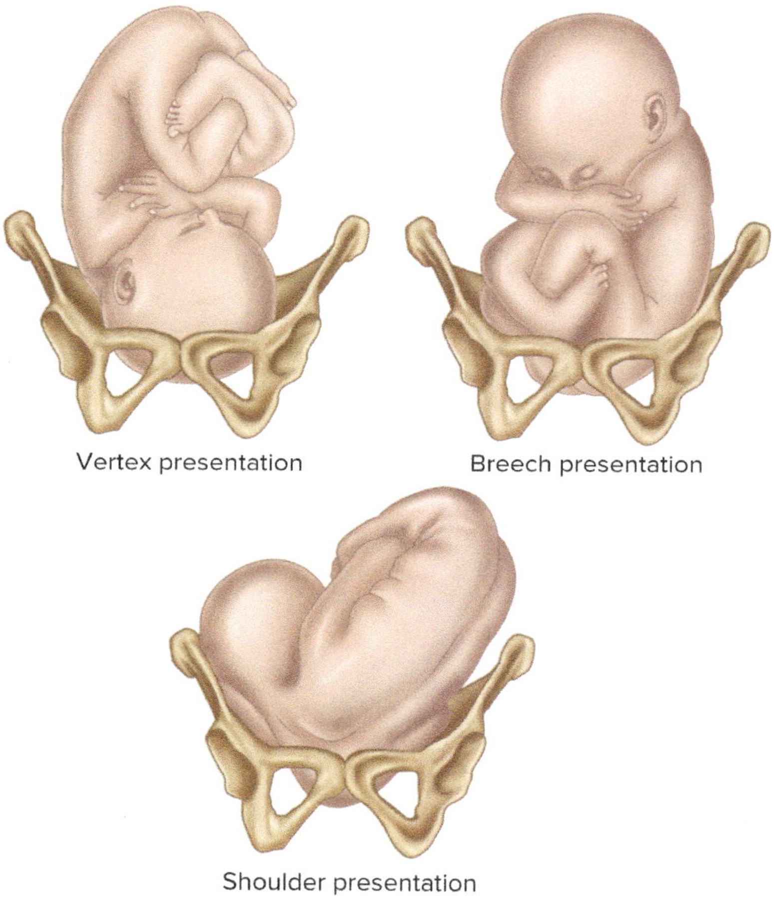

FIGURE 18-4 Illustrations of various birth presentations

GUIDANCE CONNECTION

Read the ICD-10-CM Official Guidelines for Coding and Reporting, section **I. Conventions, General Coding Guidelines and Chapter-Specific Guidelines**, subsection **C. Chapter-Specific Coding Guidelines**, chapter **15. Pregnancy, Childbirth, and the Puerperium**, subsection **a.6) 7th character for fetus identification.**

LET'S CODE IT! SCENARIO

Annette Spearman, a 33-year-old female, G1 P0, is in the birthing room and in full labor, ready to give birth to her baby vaginally. All of a sudden, Dr. Tatum tells her to stop pushing. The umbilical cord has prolapsed, and they cannot seem to move it. Dr. Tatum immediately orders Annette into the OR, where he performs a c-section. Annette's baby girl was born without further incident.

Let's Code It!

Dr. Tatum performed a c-section because the umbilical cord had *prolapsed*, endangering the baby's well-being. This is an example of a complication of childbirth. How should you look it up in the Alphabetic Index? Looking up the word *complication* won't work, so let's take a look at the key diagnostic words, the reason *why* Dr. Tatum performed the c-section (the procedure)—*prolapsed umbilical cord.*

Prolapse, prolapsed

umbilical cord

complicating delivery O69.0

Let's check this out in the Tabular List. You find

✓4 **O69 Labor and delivery complicated by umbilical cord complications**

There is a notation about the seventh character required. First, you must determine the first six characters, so continue reading down. The code suggested by the Alphabetic Index is the first one:

✓7 **O69.0XX Labor and delivery complicated by prolapse of cord**

Notice that the code requires a seventh character. Go back up to the list shown directly below the O69 category. Which is the most accurate seventh character? A single baby was delivered:

O69.0XX0 Labor and delivery complicated by prolapse of cord, single gestation

Good job! You also will need to report an outcome-of-delivery code. Keep reading to learn all about this.

Outcome of Delivery

As stated earlier in this chapter, *every* time a patient gives birth during an encounter, you have to code the birth process (the delivery code) *and* you have to report the result of that birth process (the outcome-of-delivery code).

The very last code on the mother's chart that will have anything to do with the baby is a code chosen from the Z37 Outcome of delivery category. The fourth character for the code is determined by two elements:

1. How many babies were born during this delivery.
2. Live-born, stillborn (dead), or, if a multiple birth, a combination.

GUIDANCE CONNECTION

Read the ICD-10-CM Official Guidelines for Coding and Reporting, section **I. Conventions, General Coding Guidelines and Chapter-Specific Guidelines**, subsection **C. Chapter-Specific Coding Guidelines**, chapter **15. Pregnancy, Childbirth, and the Puerperium**, subsection **b.5) Outcome of delivery**.

CODING BITE

Once a baby is born, the baby gets its own chart. From that point forward, anything having to do with the baby is coded for the baby and stays off the mother's chart.

Remember that the very last code directly relating to the baby that is placed on the mother's chart is a code from category **Z37 Outcome of delivery.** The *very first code on the baby's chart* will be from code category **Z38 Liveborn infants according to place of birth and type of delivery.** This Z code is used to report that a newborn baby has arrived, and it is always the principal (first-listed) code. A code from this category can be used only once, for the date of birth.

LET'S CODE IT! SCENARIO

Shoshanna Betterman, a 29-year-old female, had some third-trimester bleeding, so she went to her physician. Dr. Patterson performed a pelvic examination and was concerned. A transvaginal ultrasound scan confirmed that she was suffering from total placenta previa. Because she is in her 36th week, Dr. Patterson arranged to do a c-section immediately. Shoshanna's baby girl was born without further incident.

Let's Code It!

Dr. Patterson performed a c-section on Shoshanna because she had *total placenta previa with bleeding.* Go to the Alphabetic Index and look up

Placenta, placental — *see* Pregnancy, complicated by (care of) (management affected by), specified condition

So let's turn to

Pregnancy

complicated by (care of) (management affected by)

placenta previa O44.0-

In the Tabular List, you confirm it is an appropriate code. Start reading at

✓4 **O44 Placenta previa**

There are no notations or directives, so keep reading down the column to determine the most accurate fourth character:

✓5 **O44.0- Complete placenta previa NOS or without hemorrhage**

✓5 **O44.1- Complete placenta previa with hemorrhage**

Be certain not to go too fast, or you might miss that the first code, O44.0, states, "without hemorrhage." Shoshanna was hemorrhaging (bleeding). This makes O44.1 more accurate.

Now, you need to determine the required fifth character. As with all codes in this chapter of ICD-1C-CM, you will need to determine, from the documentation, which trimester Paula was in at this encounter. Dr. Patterson stated, "some third-trimester bleeding."

Put it all together and your code for this encounter is

O44.13 Complete placenta previa with hemorrhage, third trimester

That's good. But coding for the encounter with Shoshanna is not complete.

Shoshanna is in only her 36th week of gestation. Therefore, you need to include this detail. Turn to the Alphabetic Index and look up *weeks*—nothing there. Try *gestation*—not there either. Let's turn to

Pregnancy

weeks of gestation

36 weeks Z3A.36

Turn to the Tabular List to confirm, as is required by the Official Guidelines:

✓4 **Z3A Weeks of gestation**

Z3A.36 36 weeks gestation

Terrific! You need one more code, to report the outcome of delivery. Shoshanna had one live-born baby.

✓4 **Z37 Outcome of delivery**

(continued)

There are no notations or directives, so read down the column to determine the required fourth character that will accurately report Shoshanna's outcome of delivery:

Z37.0 **Outcome of delivery, single live birth**

Excellent!

O44.13 **Placenta previa with hemorrhage, third trimester**

Z3A.36 **36 weeks gestation**

Z37.0 **Outcome of delivery, single live birth**

CODING BITES

The last code on the mother's chart regarding the baby is a code from category **Z37 Outcome of delivery**. Once the baby is born, it will get its own chart. The first code on the baby's chart is a code from category **Z38 Liveborn infants according to place of birth and type of delivery**. More information about coding for the baby's medical record is coming up later in this chapter.

CODING BITES

Preterm labor is defined as the spontaneous onset of labor before 37 completed weeks of gestation.

YOU CODE IT! CASE STUDY

Charles Wallace drove his wife, Angela, a 30-year-old female, to the hospital. She had gone into labor, but she was only at 35 weeks gestation. Dr. Callahan assisted in the delivery of her twin girls. However, there was a problem, and one of the twins was stillborn.

You Code It!

Review Dr. Callahan's notes on this encounter with Angela and the birth process, and determine the most accurate codes.

Step #1: Read the case carefully and completely.

Step #2: Abstract the scenario. Which main words or terms describe why the physician cared for the patient during this encounter?

Step #3: Are there any details missing or incomplete for which you would need to query the physician? [If so, ask your instructor.]

Step #4: Check for any relevant guidance, including reading all of the symbols and notations in the Tabular List and the appropriate sections of the Official Guidelines.

Step #5: Determine the correct diagnosis code or codes to explain why this encounter was medically necessary.

Step #6: Double-check your work.

Answer:

Did you determine these to be the correct codes?

O60.14X1 **Preterm labor third trimester with preterm delivery third trimester, fetus 1**

O60.14X2 **Preterm labor third trimester with preterm delivery third trimester, fetus 2**

Z3A.35 **35 weeks gestation**

Z37.3 **Outcome of delivery, twins, one liveborn and one stillborn**

Good job!

18.6 Pregnancies with Complications

A complication of pregnancy is considered to be any condition or illness that may

- Threaten the pregnant state, such as an ectopic pregnancy or an abortion.
- Affect or threaten the health of the woman, such as hemorrhage or vomiting.
- Influence the manner in which the woman will be treated, such as preexisting cardiovascular disease or chromosomal abnormality in the fetus.

A complication may be something as common as mild hyperemesis gravidarum (code O21.0), commonly known as *morning sickness*, or something of concern, such as a kidney infection (e.g., O23.03 Infections of kidney in pregnancy, third trimester).

INFECTIOUS DISEASE: COVID-19

When a pregnant woman is admitted to the hospital with a COVID-19 diagnosis, report the principal diagnosis code as **O98.51- Other viral diseases complicating pregnancy** [sixth character to identify the specific trimester]. This would be followed by code **U07.1 COVID-19**. Any other manifestations or co-morbidities should be reported separately.

YOU CODE IT! CASE STUDY

Vitalita Meadows, a 31-year-old female, G2 P1, is 17 weeks pregnant. Dr. Kramer is meeting with her to discuss her lab test results, which indicate that Vitalita has anemia. Dr. Kramer is concerned about how the anemia will affect her pregnancy.

You Code It!

Go through the steps of coding, and determine the code or codes that should be reported for this encounter between Dr. Kramer and Vitalita.

Step #1: Read the case carefully and completely.
Step #2: Abstract the scenario. Which key words or terms describe why the physician cared for the patient during this encounter?
Step #3: Are there any details missing or incomplete for which you would need to query the physician? [If so, ask your instructor.]
Step #4: Check for any relevant guidance, including reading all of the symbols and notations in the Tabular List and the appropriate sections of the Official Guidelines.
Step #5: Determine the correct diagnosis code or codes to explain why this encounter was medically necessary.
Step #6: Double-check your work.

Answer:

Did you determine this to be the correct code?

O99.012 Anemia complicating pregnancy, second trimester

Good work!

Preexisting Conditions Affecting Pregnancy

Some diseases and illnesses are coded differently when the only thing that has changed is that the woman is now pregnant. Such cases most often involve conditions, such as diabetes mellitus or hypertension, that are systemic (involving the whole body) and, therefore, will complicate the pregnancy, childbirth, or puerperium:

O10.01- **Preexisting essential hypertension complicating pregnancy**

O11- **Preexisting hypertension with pre-eclampsia**

O24.01- **Preexisting diabetes mellitus, type 1, in pregnancy**

O24.11- **Preexisting diabetes mellitus, type 2, in pregnancy**

O24.81- **Other preexisting diabetes mellitus in pregnancy**

O98.7- **HIV complicating pregnancy, childbirth, and the puerperium**

GUIDANCE CONNECTION

Read the ICD-10-CM Official Guidelines for Coding and Reporting, section **I. Conventions, General Coding Guidelines and Chapter-Specific Guidelines**, subsection **C. Chapter-Specific Coding Guidelines**, chapter **15. Pregnancy, Childbirth, and the Puerperium**, subsections **c. Preexisting conditions versus conditions due to the pregnancy**, **d. Preexisting hypertension in pregnancy**, and **g. Diabetes mellitus in pregnancy**.

Gestational Conditions

Other conditions solely related to pregnancy may make caring for a woman and her unborn baby more challenging. Gestational conditions develop as a result of any of the many changes a woman's body goes through and are typically transient, meaning they are expected to go away once the pregnancy is complete.

O13- **Gestational [pregnancy-induced] hypertension without significant proteinuria**

O22.43 **Hemorrhoids in pregnancy, third trimester**

O24.4- **Gestational diabetes mellitus**

Multiple Gestations

Code category O30 provides you with the code options available to report a multiple gestation. In addition to determining the number of fetuses from the documentation, you also will need to determine

- The number of placentae (monochorionic, dichorionic, or more).
- The number of amniotic sacs (monoamniotic, diamniotic, or more).
- The specific trimester the gestation is in during this encounter.

EXAMPLES

O30.032 **Twin pregnancy, monochorionic/diamniotic, second trimester**

O30.111 **Triplet pregnancy with two or more monochorionic fetuses, first trimester**

Fetal Abnormalities

When a woman is pregnant, all care for both her and the baby is provided to the woman herself. Therefore, if there is a change to the treatment or care plan of the mother that is prompted by an issue with the fetus, it must be documented and reported. This may be necessary to support medical necessity for admission to the hospital, for example. Code categories O35 Maternal care for known or suspected fetal abnormality and damage and O36 Maternal care for other fetal problems provide you with the options.

EXAMPLES

O36.593- **Maternal care for other known or suspected poor fetal growth, third trimester**
This diagnosis would explain the medical necessity for the mother being referred to a nutritionist for a special diet.

O35.3XX- **Maternal care for (suspected) damage to fetus from viral disease in mother**
This diagnosis would explain the medical necessity for the mother to have special laboratory tests or an amniocentesis.

NOTE: The seventh character reports which fetus is, or may be, damaged or abnormal. The number 0 (zero) is used for a single gestation, the number 1 for the first of a multiple gestation, the number 2 for the second fetus, and so on.

GUIDANCE CONNECTION

Read the ICD-10-CM Official Guidelines for Coding and Reporting, section **I. Conventions, General Coding Guidelines and Chapter-Specific Guidelines**, subsection **C. Chapter-Specific Coding Guidelines**, chapter **15. Pregnancy, Childbirth, and the Puerperium**, subsection **e. Fetal conditions affecting the management of the mother.**

Seventh Character

You may have noticed that many pregnancy complication codes require a seventh character. If the pregnancy is a single gestation, you will report a zero (0). However, when there is more than one fetus, you will need to determine, from the documentation, which specific fetus is having the problem described by the code. For example:

O64.2XX3 **Obstructed labor due to face presentation, fetus 3**

O69.1XX2 **Labor and delivery complicated by cord around neck, with compression, fetus 2**

Postpartum and Peripartum Conditions

After the birth, the woman's body continues to go through changes. In some cases, treatment of an antepartum condition extends into the postpartum period. On other occasions, health care concerns develop during or after delivery. The *postpartum* period begins at delivery and extends for 6 weeks. The *peripartum* period runs from the beginning of the last month of pregnancy and ends 5 months after delivery.

GUIDANCE CONNECTION

Read the ICD-10-CM Official Guidelines for Coding and Reporting, section **I. Conventions, General Coding Guidelines and Chapter-Specific Guidelines**, subsection **C. Chapter-Specific Coding Guidelines**, chapter **15. Pregnancy, Childbirth, and the Puerperium**, subsection **o. The peripartum and postpartum periods.**

Routine postpartum care, just like routine prenatal care, is reported with a Z code:

Z39.0 **Encounter for care and examination of mother immediately after delivery**

Z39.1 **Encounter for care and examination of lactating mother**

Z39.2 **Encounter for routine postpartum follow-up**

Some postpartum complications may not be routine; for example, if an obstetric surgical wound (cesarean delivery wound or a perineal repair) becomes infected. In addition to the code to identify the infection, you will need an additional code to identify the infectious agent (the pathogen). The notation at the top of the code category O86 reminds you

***Use additional code* (B95–B97), to identify infectious agent**

O86.01 **Infection of obstetric surgical wound, superficial incisional site**

O86.02 **Infection of obstetric surgical wound, deep incisional site**

O86.03 **Infection of obstetric surgical wound, organ and space site**

O86.04 **Sepsis following an obstetrical procedure**
***Use additional code* to identify the sepsis**

Whenever the health care concern arises–even if the diagnosis falls outside the 6-week period–if the physician's notes document that it is a postpartum complication, or pregnancy-related, you are to code it as a postpartum condition.

Sequelae (Late Effects) of Obstetric Complications

Late effects of obstetric complications, as identified by the attending physician in their notes, are coded the same way as all other sequelae. The late effect code–O94 Sequelae of complication of pregnancy, childbirth, and the puerperium–is added when a condition begins during pregnancy but requires continued treatment. The code is placed after the code describing the actual health condition. Notice the notation beneath this code:

***Code first* condition resulting from (sequela) of complication of pregnancy, childbirth, and the puerperium**

ICD-10-CM

YOU CODE IT! CASE STUDY

Marjorie Ableman, a 31-year-old female, gave birth, vaginally, to a beautiful baby girl 3 weeks ago. She comes today to see Dr. Beale because of feelings of fatigue. After exam and blood tests, Dr. Beale diagnoses her with postpartum cervical infection caused by Enterococcus.

You Code It!

Go through the steps of coding, and determine the code or codes that should be reported for this encounter between Dr. Beale and Marjorie.

Step #1: Read the case carefully and completely.

Step #2: Abstract the scenario. Which key words or terms describe why the physician cared for the patient during this encounter?

Step #3: Are there any details missing or incomplete for which you would need to query the physician? [If so, ask your instructor.]

Step #4: Check for any relevant guidance, including reading all of the symbols and notations in the Tabular List and the appropriate sections of the Official Guidelines.

Step #5: Determine the correct diagnosis code or codes to explain why this encounter was medically necessary.

Step #6: Double-check your work.

Answer:

Did you determine these to be the correct codes?

O86.11 **Cervicitis following delivery**

B95.2 **Enterococcus as the cause of diseases classified elsewhere**

O94 **Sequela of complication of pregnancy, childbirth, and the puerperium**

Abortive Outcomes

The term **abortion** should not automatically start a political or religious discussion. Abortions can be spontaneous (caused by a biological or natural trigger) or be induced (initiated by an artificial or therapeutic source). What is commonly known as a *miscarriage* is clinically known as an *abortion*.

Abortion
The end of a pregnancy prior to or subsequent to the death of a fetus.

Many different situations can result in the loss of the fetus:

O00.- **Ectopic pregnancy**

O01.- **Hydatidiform mole**

O02.- **Other abnormal products of conception**

O03.- **Spontaneous abortion**

O04.- **Complications following (induced) termination of pregnancy**

O07.- **Failed attempted termination of pregnancy**

GUIDANCE CONNECTION

Read the ICD-10-CM Official Guidelines for Coding and Reporting, section **I. Conventions, General Coding Guidelines and Chapter-Specific Guidelines**, subsection **C. Chapter-Specific Coding Guidelines**, chapter **15. Pregnancy, Childbirth, and the Puerperium**, subsection **q. Termination of pregnancy and spontaneous abortions**.

EXAMPLE

Nellie, a 22-year-old female who was 10 weeks pregnant, was reading a text message while driving her SUV in slow traffic and didn't notice that the car in front of her had stopped. She hit it. The steering wheel struck and severely bruised her abdomen. This trauma caused her to hemorrhage, resulting in a complete miscarriage. You would report these codes:

O03.6	Delayed or excessive hemorrhage following complete or unspecified spontaneous abortion
V47.5XXA	Car driver injured in collision with fixed or stationary object in traffic accident, initial encounter

18.7 Neonates and Congenital Anomalies

Neonates

Once a baby is born, the baby gets its own chart. From that point forward, anything having to do with the baby is coded for the baby and stays off the mother's chart.

Remember that the very last code directly relating to the baby that is placed on the mother's chart is a code from category Z37 Outcome of delivery. The *very first code on the baby's chart* will be from code category Z38 Liveborn infants according to place of birth and type of delivery. This Z code is used to report that a newborn baby has arrived, and it is always the principal (first-listed) code. A code from this category can be used only once, for the date of birth.

LET'S CODE IT! SCENARIO

Tristan Allen Montegro was born via vaginal delivery in the McGraw Birthing Center at 10:58 a.m. on September 1. He weighed 8 pounds 5 ounces and was 21 inches long, with Apgar scores of 9 and 9. Dr. Grall, a pediatrician, performed a comprehensive examination immediately following Tristan's birth. Baby Tristan was sent home at 6:30 p.m. in the care of his mother, Arashala.

Let's Code It!

Tristan was just born, and this is his first health care chart. As you learned, his very first code must be from the Z38 range. As with all other cases, begin in the Alphabetic Index. What should you look up? *Birth* would be a logical choice. However, when you turn to this term in the Alphabetic Index, you are going to see a long list of adjectives, none of which applies to Tristan, or any other baby being born without a problem. As you look down the list, you may notice this item:

Birth

There is nothing here that fits. Let's go look up the term *newborn.*

Newborn (infant) (liveborn) (singleton) Z38.2

Check Dr. Smith's notes. It is documented that Tristan was a *single, liveborn* baby.

Let's go to the Tabular List and look at our choices. Begin with

✓4 Z38 Liveborn infants according to place of birth and type of delivery

As you read down, you can see that code Z38.2 reports *Single liveborn infant, unspecified as to place of birth.* The documentation clearly indicates where Tristan was born—in the McGraw Birthing Center (not a part of a hospital). So this code is not accurate. Keep reading. The answer from the documentation will bring you to the correct code:

Z38.1 Single liveborn infant, born outside the hospital

Good work!

GUIDANCE CONNECTION

Read the ICD-10-CM Official Guidelines for Coding and Reporting, section **I. Conventions, General Coding Guidelines and Chapter-Specific Guidelines**, subsection **C. Chapter-Specific Coding Guidelines**, chapter **16. Certain Conditions Originating in the Perinatal Period**, subsection **a. General perinatal rules**.

Suspected Conditions Not Found

After a neonate comes into the world, there may be concerns requiring tests to be run or for the baby to stay in the hospital longer. When there is good news, and it turns out the baby is healthy and all the tests are negative, how will you report the medical necessity for the tests and extended stay in the hospital? You will report code Z05 Encounter for Observation and evaluation of newborns for suspected conditions ruled out to explain the circumstances.

For a readmission to the hospital or an outpatient encounter, Z05 may be used as a principal or first-listed diagnosis code.

GUIDANCE CONNECTION

Read the ICD-10-CM Official Guidelines for Coding and Reporting, section **I. Conventions, General Coding Guidelines and Chapter-Specific Guidelines**, subsection **C. Chapter-Specific Coding Guidelines**, chapter **16. Certain Conditions Originating in the Perinatal Period**, subsection **b. Observation and evaluation of newborns for suspected conditions not found**.

Clinically Significant Conditions

The guidelines state that you must code all clinically significant conditions noted on the baby's chart during the standard newborn examination. You may be concerned about how you, as a coder, can determine what is **clinically significant** and what is not. Good news! It is not your decision to make. Only the physician can determine and document this. However, you must ensure that the documentation gives you the diagnostic conditions that support any of the following:

Clinically Significant
Signs, symptoms, and/or conditions present at birth that may impact the child's future health status.

- *Therapeutic treatments performed:* for example, perhaps the baby is placed on a respirator.
- *Diagnostic procedures done:* for example, perhaps additional and specific blood tests are performed on the baby.
- *Keeping the baby in the hospital longer than usual:* perhaps the physician is concerned about an issue so they do not discharge the baby yet.
- *Increased monitoring or nursing care:* perhaps the physician orders 24-hour private-duty nursing care for continuous monitoring.
- *Any implication that the child will need health care services in the future* as a result of a condition, sign, or symptom that can be identified now: perhaps there is evidence that there may be brain damage as a result of the birth process; however, this cannot be confirmed until the child is about 2 years old.

When a congenital or **perinatal** condition has been resolved and no longer has an impact on the child's health and well-being, you will need to assign a code from the range Z85–Z87, Personal history of . . . .

Perinatal
The time period from before birth to the 28th day after birth.

COVID-19 Infection in Newborn

As you have learned, when any patient is confirmed to have COVID-19, you need to report code **U07.1 COVID-19.**

In those cases when the documentation confirms that a neonate was infected, either in utero or during the birth process, you will need to report code **P35.8 Other congenital viral diseases,** followed by **U07.1.**

Of course, if this is documented on the same day as the birth, the principal diagnosis code will still be from code category **Z38**, then followed by the appropriate viral codes.

GUIDANCE CONNECTION

Read the ICD-10-CM Official Guidelines for Coding and Reporting, section **I. Conventions, General Coding Guidelines and Chapter-Specific Guidelines**, subsection **C. Chapter-Specific Coding Guidelines**, chapter **16. Certain Conditions Originating in the Perinatal Period**, subsections **a.6) Code all clinically significant conditions** and **c. Coding additional perinatal diagnoses**.

Maternal Conditions Affecting the Infant

When the physician's notes specify that a mother's illness, injury, or condition had a direct impact on the baby's health, you will include a code on the baby's chart from the subsection code range P00-P04 Newborn affected by maternal factors and by complications of pregnancy, labor, and delivery.

A newborn may be impacted by medication taken by the mother, whether prescribed drugs, such as chemotherapy (P04.11) or anticonvulsants (P04.13), or drugs of addiction, such as cocaine (P04.41) or hallucinogens (P04.42).

Prematurity
Birth occurring prior to the completion of 37 weeks gestation.

Low Birth Weight (LBW)
A baby born weighing less than 5 pounds 8 ounces, or 2,500 grams.

Conditions in the mother, such as nutrition, smoking, high blood pressure, the presence of certain infections, or an abnormal uterus or cervix, can increase the possibilities that the baby might be born **prematurely** and/or with a **low birth weight (LBW)**. A mother's heart, kidney, and/or lung problems also might affect the baby's health.

While the reasons are not completely understood by physicians, a woman may experience spontaneous *p*remature *r*upture *o*f the *m*embranes (PROM), which results in spontaneous preterm labor. There is virtually nothing that can be done to prevent the situation that so often leads to the birth of a premature, LBW baby.

A preterm (premature) neonate is one who has been in gestation for at least 28 completed weeks but less than 37 completed weeks (or between 196 and 258 completed days). While the baby's chart will almost always include a notation of the number of weeks gestation at birth, you are permitted to code "prematurity" only when it is specifically documented by the physician.

A weight of less than 2,500 grams at birth is also an indicator of prematurity. When a fetus has not had the prescribed length of time to grow, the neonate can be susceptible to certain health concerns, realized in the near or distant future.

Premature, LBW babies are more likely to be at risk for developing certain conditions now and later in life. Incomplete growth of the fetus's central nervous system can result in feeding difficulties for the neonate/infant, recurrent apnea, and/or poor vasomotor control. Testing for neonatal hyperbilirubinemia, especially when jaundice is visible, can indicate that the liver did not develop sufficiently to create and excrete bilirubin (a yellowish component of bile that is made by the liver). This is why it is so important that the documentation and the coding accurately report the baby's situation from the beginning. Some of the most common conditions include these:

CODING BITES

Usually, the physician will write the baby's birth weight in grams. However, you should learn how to convert from pounds and ounces to grams:

1 ounce = 28.350 gm
1 pound = 16 oz
1 pound = 453.6 gm

- Breathing problems, including respiratory distress syndrome (RDS).
- Periventricular and/or intraventricular hemorrhage (bleeding in the brain).
- Patent ductus arteriosus (PDA), a dangerous heart problem.
- Necrotizing enterocolitis (NEC), an intestinal problem that leads to difficulties in feeding.
- Retinopathy of prematurity (ROP).
- Low body temperature (caused by a lack of body fat used by newborns to maintain normal body temperature), which promotes slow growth, breathing problems, and other complications.
- Apnea, an interruption in breathing.
- Jaundice, a result of incomplete liver development.
- Anemia.
- Bronchopulmonary dysplasia, also known as *chronic lung disease*.
- Infections, due to the inability of immature immune systems to fight off bacteria and viruses.

Mortality
Death.

Morbidity
Unhealthy.

Respiratory distress syndrome (RDS) is the leading cause of **mortality** and **morbidity** of premature neonates. The immature lungs have an insufficient quantity of surfactant–the secretion within the lungs that supports the alveoli and keeps them from collapsing. Maternal diabetes and neonatal asphyxia are known contributing factors. RDS causes hypoxia, which can then lead to pulmonary ischemia, pulmonary capillary damage, and fluid leaking inappropriately into the alveoli. Cyanosis, increased respiratory effort, anoxia, and acidosis are signs and complications. Report a diagnosis of RDS with code P22.0 Respiratory distress syndrome of newborn.

You will find the codes needed to report an infant's prematurity and/or LBW, as well as long gestation and high birth weight, as documented in the physician's notes, within these code categories:

P05 **Disorders of newborn related to slow fetal growth and fetal malnutrition**

P07 **Disorders of newborn related to short gestation and low birth weight, not elsewhere classified**

P08 **Disorders of newborn related to long gestation and high birth weight**

GUIDANCE CONNECTION

Read the ICD-10-CM Official Guidelines for Coding and Reporting, section **I. Conventions, General Coding Guidelines and Chapter-Specific Guidelines**, subsection **C. Chapter-Specific Coding Guidelines**, chapter **16. Certain Conditions Originating in the Perinatal Period**, subsections **d. Prematurity and fetal growth retardation** and **e. Low birth weight and immaturity status.**

CODING BITES

Codes from category P05 and category P07 may not be reported on the same claim at the same time.

YOU CODE IT! CASE STUDY

Harper Anne Glosick was born today at 27-week, 2-day gestation by cesarean section at Hillside Hospital. She weighed 945 grams at birth, and her lungs are immature. Dr. McArthur admits Harper into the neonatal intensive care unit (NICU) with a diagnosis of extreme immaturity.

You Code It!

Read through Dr. McArthur's notes on Harper, and determine the correct diagnosis code or codes.

Step #1: Read the case carefully and completely.
Step #2: Abstract the scenario. Which key words or terms describe why the physician cared for the patient during this encounter?
Step #3: Are there any details missing or incomplete for which you would need to query the physician? [If so, ask your instructor.]
Step #4: Check for any relevant guidance, including reading all of the symbols and notations in the Tabular List and the appropriate sections of the Official Guidelines.
Step #5: Determine the correct diagnosis code or codes to explain why this encounter was medically necessary.
Step #6: Double-check your work.

Answer:

Did you determine these to be the correct codes?

Z38.01 **Single liveborn infant, delivered by Cesarean**

P07.03 **Extremely low birth weight newborn, 750–999 grams**

P07.26 **Extreme immaturity of newborn, gestational age 27 completed weeks**

CODING BITES

See the notation beneath code category P07:

Note: When both birth weight and gestational age of the newborn are available, both should be coded with birth weight sequenced before gestational age.

Well-Baby Checks

These encounters, just like adult physicals and other checkups, are scheduled by the age of the child: 2 to 4 days, 1 month, 2 months, 4 months, 6 months, 9 months, 1 year, 15 months, 18 months, 2 years, 2.5 years, 3 years, and then annually. The age of the child also influences which codes are reported for the well-baby encounter:

Z00.110 **Health examination for newborn under 8 days old**

Z00.111 **Health examination for newborn 8 to 28 days old**

Z00.121 **Encounter for routine child health examination with abnormal findings**
Use additional code **to identify abnormal findings**

Z00.129 **Encounter for routine child health examination without abnormal findings**

LET'S CODE IT! SCENARIO

Roseanna Glassman brought her 39-day-old daughter, Marisol, to Dr. Granger for her routine health check. During the examination, Roseanna related that Marisol's head accidentally was banged into the table and she was worried about neurologic problems. Dr. Granger checked her head and found no bruise or laceration. To calm Roseanna, he took Marisol down the hall to have a special neurologic screening for traumatic brain injury. Fortunately, the scan was negative.

Let's Code It!

What key words in the notes provide you with the information you need to report this encounter? Why did Dr. Granger care for Marisol? Marisol was brought in for her "*routine health check*"—her regular well-baby visit. What will you look up in the Alphabetic Index? *Routine*? Nothing there. *Well-baby*? Nothing there. Try a term that is not technically a diagnosis: *examination*. Take a look and find

Examination (for) (following) (general) (of) (routine) Z00.00

Read down the long list of additional descriptors and find

child (over 28 days old) Z00.129

That sounds accurate. So let's turn to the Tabular List and check it out:

✓4 **Z00** **Encounter for general examination without complaint, suspected or reported diagnosis**

There are no notations or directives, so read down the column to determine the most accurate fourth and fifth characters:

✓6 **Z00.12** **Encounter for routine child health examination**

Read the notations beneath this code. First, notice that it states "Health check (routine) for child over 28 days old." How old is Marisol? She is 39 days, so this is the correct code. Carefully read the EXCLUDES1 notation, and ask yourself: Does this apply to Dr. Granger's caring for Marisol during this encounter? No, it doesn't. Read down to review the sixth-character choices. The notes state that he did a neurologic screening because of the bang to her head. You will need to check the documentation for the results of this screening so you can report "abnormal findings" or not. The documentation states that "the scan was negative," so you will report this code:

Z00.129 **Encounter for routine child health examination without abnormal findings**

You still need to report the neurologic screening. Go back to the Alphabetic Index and look up

Screening (for) Z13.9

neurological condition Z13.89

That's really the only suggested code, so let's take a look at it in the Tabular List:

✓4 **Z13** **Encounter for screening for other diseases and disorders**

(continued)

Go back to the notes and see that Dr. Granger wrote "neurologic screening for traumatic brain injury." Therefore, you know that **Z13.850 Encounter for screening for traumatic brain injury** is accurate and matches what Dr. Granger wrote in the notes.

One more code—remember, you need to report a code for the bang on the head because this led Dr. Granger to do the screening. Check the notes and see that Dr. Granger found no bruises or lacerations and that Roseanna did not report any other signs or symptoms, such as vomiting or seizure. The bang on the head will have to be reported with an external cause code because it is an external factor that explains why Dr. Granger screened Marisol for a TBI. Check the External Causes Code Alphabetic Index and look up *strike, striking* because Marisol's head struck the table (furniture). Code W22.03 is suggested. Let's check the Tabular List:

✓4 **W22** **Striking against or struck by other objects**

✓7 **W22.03X** **Walked into furniture**

This cannot be accurate because Marisol is only 39 days old and she cannot walk yet. Review all of the other codes in this subsection to determine the code that will report what happened:

W22.8XXA **Striking against or struck by other objects, initial encounter**

So for Marisol's visit to Dr. Granger, you have three codes to report:

Z00.129 **Encounter for routine child health examination without abnormal findings**

Z13.850 **Encounter for screening for traumatic brain injury**

W22.8XXA **Striking against or struck by other objects, initial encounter**

YOU CODE IT! CASE STUDY

Ines Nancy Mulle was born, full term, vaginally at Barton Hospital. Her mother has been an alcoholic for many years and would not stop drinking during the pregnancy. Ines weighed only 1,575 grams, small for a full-term neonate. After testing, she was diagnosed at birth with fetal alcohol syndrome and admitted into the NICU.

You Code It!

Read the notes on Ines, and determine the most accurate diagnosis code(s).

Step #1: Read the case carefully and completely.

Step #2: Abstract the scenario. Which main words or terms describe why the physician cared for the patient during this encounter?

Step #3: Are there any details missing or incomplete for which you would need to query the physician? [If so, ask your instructor.]

Step #4: Check for any relevant guidance, including reading all of the symbols and notations in the Tabular List and the appropriate sections of the Official Guidelines.

Step #5: Determine the correct diagnosis code or codes to explain why this encounter was medically necessary.

Step #6: Double-check your work.

Answer:

Did you determine these to be the correct codes?

Z38.00 **Single liveborn infant, delivered vaginally**

P05.16 **Newborn small for gestational age, 1,500–1,749 grams**

Q86.0 **Fetal alcohol syndrome (dysmorphic)**

Terrific!

Genetics

Genetics is the study of diseases passed from parent to child, a process known as *hereditary transmission*. There are more than 1,000 diseases that might be inherited. A genetic disorder may be *dominant*–the result of one defective gene in a pair–or it may be *recessive*–the result of both alleles being defective. Some examples of dominant genetic disorders are *familial hypercholesterolemia* (code E87.8) and *familial retinoblastoma* (code C69.2-). Examples of recessive genetic disorders include *cystic fibrosis* (code E84.9) and *Gaucher's disease* (code E75.22). Certain diseases that have been correlated to genetics cause accelerated aging, such as *Hutchinson-Guilford progeria* (code E34.8), an inherited endocrine disorder.

If the patient is diagnosed with a specific genetic condition, you will need to report the code for the confirmed diagnosis. However, there are times when the patient does not exhibit any signs or symptoms of the condition. In these cases, it may be important to document the *family history* of the condition to support more frequent screenings or other preventive or early detection services, such as Family history of alcohol abuse and dependence, reported with code Z81.1.

Genetic Conditions versus Congenital Malformations

Congenital
A condition existing at the time of birth.

Anomaly
An abnormal, or unexpected, condition.

Malformation
An irregular structural development.

The term **congenital anomaly** means an abnormality present at birth and therefore refers to any variation from the norm for a neonate. The abnormality may be genetic in nature or may be a malformation that occurred during gestation. A genetic condition may indicate that a chromosomal alteration has been inherited–passed down from parent to child via chromosomal and cell structures. Or the condition may be a congenital malformation, or damage to a chromosome during formation. A congenital **malformation** means that something went awry during the gestational process. Such alterations can occur spontaneously or can be an adverse reaction to a pathogen, drug, radiation, or chemical.

EXAMPLES

Q91.2 Trisomy 18, translocation

Q93.3 Deletion of short arm of chromosome 4

Inherited Conditions

Your blue eyes and brown hair are the products of genetics–qualities in the chromosomes you received from your father and mother. Sadly, a genetic abnormality will negatively affect the health of a child. An inherited mutation in the DNA causes a permanent alteration that will affect each and every cell as it multiplies during the maturation of the zygote to embryo to fetus to neonate. There is also a strong probability that this person will pass this condition along to their children.

Congenital Anomalies

GUIDANCE CONNECTION

Read the ICD-10-CM Official Guidelines for Coding and Reporting, section **I. Conventions, General Coding Guidelines and Chapter-Specific Guidelines**, subsection **C. Chapter-Specific Coding Guidelines**, chapter **17. Congenital Malformations, Deformations, and Chromosomal Abnormalities.**

A congenital malformation, also known as a *birth defect*, is a permanent physical defect–the incomplete development of an anatomical structure–that is identified in a neonate. It may be the effect of a genetic mutation, or it may have been caused by a prenatal event. The fetal development of many organs, including the brain, heart, lungs, liver, bones, and/or intestinal tract, may have been altered by alcohol or drugs used by the mother at a particular point during gestation, by exposure to an environmental factor, or by an injury sustained during delivery.

EXAMPLES

Q14.1 Congenital malformation of retina

Q64.4 Malformation of urachus

Testing

Health care research has found ways to identify the presence or the likelihood of genetic disorders and congenital anomalies.

Genetic testing can be performed prior to fertilization so the potential parents can gain insights on the possibility of passing along certain diseases to their future children. A family tree analysis, called a *pedigree*, is a diagram of the individual's family that includes diseases and causes of death. A geneticist (a physician specializing in the study of genetics) can use this diagram to identify *inheritance patterns* and probabilities. In addition, a blood test known as a *karyotype* can be used. During this test, multiple staining techniques can illuminate each chromosomal band to enable visualization of a mutation.

Prenatal blood and DNA tests can currently detect more than 600 genetic disorders prior to the baby's birth. This information can allow parents to make informed decisions and to become prepared emotionally, intellectually, and financially for the birth of a child with a genetic disorder. In addition, the physician can make certain appropriate arrangements, such as method of delivery and timing of delivery, that may reduce the severity or impact of the condition.

Amniocentesis is the process of collecting a sample of amniotic fluid via needle aspiration from a pregnant uterus. *Chorionic villus sampling* is the process of obtaining tissues from the placenta for prenatal testing by passing a catheter through the vagina and threading it up to the placenta.

Genetic tests are not limited to potential or impending parents. Adults can use this information as well. For example, many women are tested for the BRCA1 or BRCA2 gene that identifies a potential for the development of breast and/or ovarian cancer.

EXAMPLES

Z14.1 Cystic fibrosis carrier

Z15.01 Genetic susceptibility to malignant neoplasm of breast

Gene Therapy

Researchers continue to experiment with gene therapy to prevent or treat these types of diseases. The goal is to find a safe and effective way to correct a malfunctioning gene. Methods currently being investigated include

- Placing a normal gene into the genome in a nonspecific place so it can provide the correct function of the nonfunctional gene.
- Using homologous recombination to remove the abnormal gene and replace it with a normal gene.
- Using selected reverse mutation to actually repair the gene so it will function properly.

In such cases, the term *placed* or *inserted* does not mean the same as it typically does in the context of other health care procedures. One method is to put the therapeutic gene into a carrier molecule, known as a *vector*, which is a genetically altered virus. Nonviral methods include the injection of the therapeutic gene directly into its target cell. However, this can be accomplished only with a limited number of tissue types. Studies are being conducted on the effectiveness of using an artificial liposome and/or certain chemicals to achieve the successful delivery of the therapeutic gene.

Genetic Disorders

Chromosomal Abnormalities

Down syndrome (trisomy 21) is a spontaneous **genetic abnormality** and is not inherited. Manifestations include mental retardation, unusual facial features including slanted eyes and protruding tongue, and congenital heart defects, as well as respiratory and related complications. *Mosaicism* is possible in a child with Down syndrome. This is the occurrence of cells with two different genetic makeups within one person. The possibility of having a child with Down syndrome increases with the age of the mother at the time of delivery. Treatment of manifestations can improve the patient's quality of life and extend the life span. Use code category Q90 Down syndrome (trisomy 21), with an additional character to report nonmosaicism, mosaicism, or translocation. An additional code to identify specific physical and intellectual disabilities is required.

Genetic Abnormality
An error in a gene (chromosome) that affects development during gestation; also known as a *chromosomal abnormality*.

Klinefelter's syndrome is a genetic abnormality that results in the inclusion of an extra X chromosome in a male child. Testicular changes occur at puberty, including eventual infertility due to the deterioration of the testicles. In addition, gynecomastia may develop, learning disabilities may become apparent, facial hair may be sparse, and reduced libido causing impotence will become evident. There is a mosaic form of Klinefelter's. Report this syndrome with a code from category Q98 Other sex chromosome abnormalities, male phenotype, not elsewhere classified.

Autosomal Recessive Inherited Diseases

Cystic fibrosis is seen most often in Caucasian children and rarely seen in black or Asian populations. This disease causes chronic pulmonary disease and deficient exocrine pancreatic function, development of thickened mucus that can block bile flow from the liver, and other manifestations. Use code category E84 Cystic fibrosis, with an additional character to identify manifestations.

Tay-Sachs disease (Tay-Sachs amaurotic familial idiocy) is an inherited disease that results in the child's death before the age of 4. Symptoms include increasing deterioration of motor skills and mental acuity, identifiable in the infant at 6 to 10 months of age. Genetic tests can screen potential parents. Report this disease with code E75.02 Tay-Sachs disease.

Phenylketonuria (PKU) is a genetic disorder that causes a gradual deterioration of the patient's mental faculties, often discernable by 1 year of age. Many hospitals perform a simple blood test for PKU as a part of the birth evaluation. This condition can be treated with a semisynthetic diet. Outcomes improve with early detection. Report PKU with code E70.0 Classical phenylketonuria or E70.1 Other hyperphenylalaninemias (maternal).

Sickle cell anemia is an inherited hemolytic anemia that develops as the result of a defective hemoglobin molecule that causes the red blood cells to be misshapen. This half-moon- (sickle-) shaped cell (instead of the rounded, button shape) interferes with circulation and manifests itself as fatigue, dyspnea, and swollen joints. Pharmaceutical treatments can reduce ill health. Sickle cell disorders are grouped into code category D57 Sickle cell disorders. You will need additional characters to identify the specific type of sickle cell, possibly requiring a pathology report at some point, and to identify whether the patient is having a crisis at this time or not. For example: D57.20 Sickle cell/Hb-C disease without crisis.

Multifactorial Abnormalities

Deformity
A size or shape (structural design) that deviates from that which is considered normal.

Cleft lip and cleft palate are malformations of the upper lip and/or palate that occur during the first 2 months of gestation. This **deformity** may be seen unilaterally or bilaterally (medial is rare) and may extend into the nasal cavity and/or the maxilla (upper jaw). Use code categories Q35 Cleft palate (additional character to identify hard palate, soft palate, etc.), Q36 Cleft lip (additional character to specify laterality), and Q37 Cleft palate with cleft lip (additional character to specify laterality).

X-Linked Inherited Diseases

Hemophilia is an inherited hemostatic disorder that causes difficulty with the occurrence of coagulation. The abnormal bleeding can be problematic, especially after an injury or surgical procedure. On occasion, spontaneous bleeding may occur, causing damage to the brain, nerves, or muscle function, depending upon the location of the hemorrhage. Treatment can extend life expectancy. Report code D66 Hereditary factor VIII deficiency (hemophilia NOS).

Fragile X syndrome is the most frequently diagnosed underlying cause of inherited mental retardation, and it affects both males and females. An accurate pedigree would be important in predicting the likelihood of this condition because probabilities increase with each generation. Males display profound mental retardation, while females may or may not reveal this dysfunction. Use code Q99.2 Fragile X chromosome to report this condition.

Congenital Malformations

Spina bifida is a condition that results from an incomplete closure of the vertebral column, the spinal cord, or both. Presented often by a hole in the skin covering the area of the spine, it is an abnormality in the development of the central nervous system. In the 1990s, researchers discovered that folic acid (a B vitamin), when taken before and during the first trimester of pregnancy, could actually prevent some cerebral and spinal birth defects. In 1996, the U.S. Food and Drug Administration ordered that folic acid be added into breads, cereals, and other grain products. The number of cases of spina bifida dropped from 2,490 in 1995–1996 to 1,640 in 1999–2000. Spina bifida is sometimes accompanied by hydrocephalus. Code category Q05 Spina bifida (aperta) (cystica) requires an additional character to report the location on the spine (cervical, thoracic, lumbar, sacral), as well as to report the presence or absence of hydrocephalus. *Spina bifida occulta* is reported with Q76.0 Spina bifida occulta. This version of spina bifida is evidenced by a tiny gap between vertebrae with no involvement of the nervous system. It can be seen only on an x-ray of the affected area and generally has no signs or symptoms.

Congenital hernia can occur in several locations in the body, just as with adult hernias. The difference with reporting such conditions is the specification in the documentation that the hernia is congenital. Some of the codes include Q40.1 Congenital hiatus hernia, Q79.0 Congenital diaphragmatic hernia, and Q79.51 Congenital hernia of bladder.

Congenital heart defects have been determined by the CDC to affect close to 400,000 babies born in the United States each year. They are the most common type of congenital anomaly and one of the most common causes of death in infants. Research has proved a strong connection between cigarette smoking, especially during the first trimester of gestation, and neonates with pulmonary valve stenosis and type 2 atrial septal defects, among other congenital heart malformations. Code from categories Q20 Congenital malformations of cardiac chambers and connections, Q21 Congenital malformations of cardiac septa, Q23 Congenital malformations of aortic and mitral valves, and Q24 Other congenital malformations of heart. Additional characters are required to provide specific details, such as Q21.1 Atrial septal defect and Q22.1 Congenital pulmonary valve stenosis.

Chapter Summary

The urinary system is designed to remove the urea from the blood, manufacture urine, and perform waste removal by eliminating the urine. It supports many of the other body systems by ensuring fluid balance and eliminating waste products to avoid toxicity. Understanding the components of this system and their functions will help you correctly interpret the documentation to determine the most accurate code or codes. Some conditions affecting organs in the urinary system are the manifestations of other diseases, such as hypertension or diabetes, whereas others may be the result of an infectious organism. Coders must read carefully (as always) to determine the correct coding process.

The anatomical sites included in the female genital system are the definition of the phrase "private places." These organs have important functions and are susceptible to disease and injury, as with other body systems. Female anatomy includes many organs and anatomical sites that can be subject to health concerns. Well-woman exams and preventive tests should be annual events in every woman's life. Each time, a medical necessity for the visit must be documented. Remember that staying healthy or catching illness or disease early is a medical necessity.

Babies are precious and should always be treated with tender loving care. From the moment they are born, babies receive a special version of health care services created especially for them, due to their size and growth patterns. The guidelines for coding the reasons for these services are very specific. Congenital anomalies, whether inherited or caused by an interaction with a chemical, drug, or other environmental factor during gestation, can have a lifelong effect on the child as well as the family. Congenital deficits can cause a minor inconvenience, present a challenge, require years of health care treatments, or result in premature death.

CODING BITES

The *Apgar* test is named for Virginia Apgar, but it also has come to stand for the following:

Activity (muscle tone)
Pulse rate (heart rate)
Grimace (reflex response)
Appearance (skin color)
Respiratory (breathing effort)

Apgar Scoring for Newborns

Score	Interpretation
0–3	Baby needs immediate lifesaving procedures
4–6	Baby needs some assistance; requires careful monitoring
7–10	Normal

CHAPTER 18 REVIEW
Coding Genitourinary, Gynecology, Obstetrics, Congenital, and Pediatrics Conditions

Let's Check It! Terminology

Match each key term to the appropriate definition.

Part I

1. **LO 18.1** The organ system responsible for removing waste products that are left behind by protein, excessive water, disproportionate amounts of electrolytes, and other nitrogenous compounds from the blood and the body.
2. **LO 18.1** Inflammation of any part of the urinary tract: kidney, ureter, bladder, or urethra.
3. **LO 18.7** An error in a gene that affects development during gestation.
4. **LO 18.2** Enlarged prostate that results in depressing the urethra.
5. **LO 18.1** Ongoing malfunction of one or both kidneys.
6. **LO 18.7** A size or shape that deviates from that which is considered normal.
7. **LO 18.1** Glomerular filtration rate, the measurement of kidney function; used to determine the stage of kidney disease.
8. **LO 18.2** Inflammation of the prostate.
9. **LO 18.7** An irregular structural development.
10. **LO 18.1** Malignancy of the urinary bladder.
11. **LO 18.1** A compound that results from the breakdown of proteins and is excreted in urine.
12. **LO 18.1** Suffering from a low red blood cell count.

- **A.** Anemic
- **B.** Benign Prostatic Hyperplasia (BPH)
- **C.** Bladder Cancer
- **D.** Chronic Kidney Disease (CKD)
- **E.** Deformity
- **F.** Genetic Abnormality
- **G.** GFR
- **H.** Malformation
- **I.** Prostatitis
- **J.** Urea
- **K.** Urinary System
- **L.** Urinary Tract Infection (UTI)

Part II

1. **LO 18.4** A health care specialty focusing on the care of women during pregnancy and the puerperium.
2. **LO 18.4** A physician specializing in the care of the female genital tract.
3. **LO 18.5** The length of time for the complete development of a baby from conception to birth; on average, 40 weeks.
4. **LO 18.4** The time period from the end of labor until the uterus returns to normal size, typically 3 to 6 weeks.
5. **LO 18.5** Prior to birth; also referred to as *antenatal*.
6. **LO 18.6** The end of a pregnancy prior to or subsequent to the death of a fetus.

- **A.** Abortion
- **B.** Gestation
- **C.** Gynecologist
- **D.** Obstetrics
- **E.** Prenatal
- **F.** Puerperium

Part III

1. **LO 18.7** An abnormal, or unexpected, condition.
2. **LO 18.7** A condition existing at the time of birth.
3. **LO 18.7** A baby born weighing less than 5 pounds 8 ounces, or 2,500 grams.
4. **LO 18.7** Unhealthy, diseased.
5. **LO 18.5** Prior to birth; also referred to as *antenatal*.

- **A.** Anomaly
- **B.** Clinically Significant
- **C.** Congenital
- **D.** Low Birth Weight (LBW)

6. **LO 18.7** Birth occurring prior to the completion of 37 weeks gestation.
7. **LO 18.7** Signs, symptoms, and/or conditions present at birth that may impact the child's future health status.
8. **LO 18.7** Death.

E. Morbidity
F. Mortality
G. Perinatal
H. Prematurity

Let's Check It! Concepts

Choose the most appropriate answer for each of the following questions.

1. **LO 18.1** GFR below 15 is stage ____ CKD and would be coded ____.
   a. 2, N18.2 b. 3, N18.31 c. 4, N18.4 d. 5, N18.5
2. **LO 18.2** ____ is a condition that occurs when fluid collects within the tunica vaginalis of the scrotum, the testis, or the spermatic cord.
   a. Erectile dysfunction b. Oligospermia
   c. Hydrocele d. Benign prostatic hyperplasia
3. **LO 18.3** The patient is diagnosed with endocarditis. Which ICD-10-CM code should be used?
   a. A51.9 b. A52.06 c. A52.03 d. A51.2
4. **LO 18.4** ____ are tumors located in the female reproductive system.
   a. Uterine leiomyomas b. Uterine fibromyomas c. Uterine fibroids d. All of these
5. **LO 18.5** A woman noted to be G3 P2 has given birth
   a. once. b. never. c. twice. d. four times.
6. **LO 18.5** You would use code Z33.1 for a pregnant woman who came to see the doctor for
   a. a broken leg.
   b. a regular first-pregnancy checkup.
   c. a regular third-pregnancy checkup.
   d. a regular pregnancy checkup for a woman 37 years old.
7. **LO 18.5** The encounter at which a woman gives birth will always have at least
   a. one code. b. four codes. c. two codes. d. three codes.
8. **LO 18.6** All of the following would be considered a complication of a pregnancy except
   a. hyperemesis gravidarum. b. kidney infection.
   c. hemorrhage. d. sprained wrist.
9. **LO 18.7** A congenital malformation is also known as a(n)
   a. inherited condition. b. birth defect. c. breech birth. d. pediatric factor.
10. **LO 18.7** A newborn has been diagnosed with sepsis due to *Staphylococcus aureus*. Which code should be used to report this?
   a. B95.61 b. A41.01 c. P36.8 d. P36.2

Let's Check It! Guidelines

Part I

*Refer to the Official Guidelines and fill in the blanks according to **Chapter 14**, Diseases of Genitourinary System, Chapter-Specific Coding Guidelines.*

mild	2	severe
query	failure or rejection	stage 1-5
based	N18	CKD
sequencing	severity	N18.30-N18.32

3	relationship	I.C.19.g
Z94.0	N18.4	N18.6
diabetes mellitus and hypertension	end-stage-renal disease (ESRD)	chronic kidney disease (CKD)

1. The ICD-10-CM classifies CKD based on ____ .
2. The severity of CKD is designated by ____ .
3. Stage ____ , code N18.2, equates to ____ CKD.
4. Stage ____ , code ____ , equates to moderate CKD.
5. Stage 4, code ____ , equates to ____ CKD.
6. Code N18.6, End stage renal disease (ESRD), is assigned when the provider has documented ____ .
7. If both a stage of CKD and ESRD are documented, assign code ____ only.
8. Patients who have undergone kidney transplant may still have some form of ____ because the kidney transplant may not fully restore kidney function. Therefore, the presence of CKD alone does not constitute a transplant complication. Assign the appropriate ____ code for the patient's stage of CKD and code ____ , Kidney transplant status.
9. If a transplant complication such as ____ or other transplant complication is documented, see section ____ for information on coding complications of a kidney transplant. If the documentation is unclear as to whether the patient has a complication of the transplant, ____ the provider.
10. Patients with ____ may also suffer from other serious conditions, most commonly ____ .
11. The ____ of the CKD code in ____ to codes for other contributing conditions is ____ on the conventions in the Tabular List.

Part II

Refer to the Official Guidelines and fill in the blanks according to ***Chapter 15****, Pregnancy, Childbirth, and the Puerperium, Chapter-Specific Coding Guidelines.*

never	fetus	every	complications
7th	O09	"in childbirth"	"unspecified trimester"
prompted	Z37	priority	Z34
antepartum	trimester	insufficient	maternal
		no	

1. **Chapter 15** codes have sequencing ____ over codes from other chapters.
2. **Chapter 15** codes are to be used only on the ____ record, ____ on the record of the newborn.
3. The majority of codes in **Chapter 15** have a final character indicating the ____ of pregnancy.
4. Whenever delivery occurs during the current admission, and there is an "in childbirth" option for the obstetric complication being coded, the ____ code should be assigned.
5. In instances when a patient is admitted to a hospital for ____ of pregnancy during one trimester and remains in the hospital into a subsequent trimester, the trimester character for the ____ complication code should be assigned on the basis of the trimester when the complication developed, not the trimester of the discharge.
6. The ____ code should rarely be used, such as when the documentation in the record is ____ to determine the trimester and it is not possible to obtain clarification.
7. Where applicable, a ____ character is to be assigned for certain categories to identify the ____ for which the complication code applies.
8. For routine outpatient prenatal visits when no complications are present, a code from category ____ , Encounter for supervision of normal pregnancy, should be used as the first-listed diagnosis.
9. For routine prenatal outpatient visits for patients with high-risk pregnancies, a code from category ____ , Supervision of high-risk pregnancy, should be used as the first-listed diagnosis.
10. In episodes when ____ delivery occurs, the principal diagnosis should correspond to the principal complication of the pregnancy that necessitated the encounter.
11. When an obstetric patient is admitted and delivers during that admission, the condition that ____ the admission should be sequenced as the principal diagnosis.
12. A code from category ____ , Outcome of delivery, should be included on ____ maternal record when a delivery has occurred.

Part III

Refer to the Official Guidelines and fill in the blanks according to ***Chapter 16****, Certain Conditions Originating in the Perinatal Period, Chapter-Specific Coding Guidelines.*

perinatal	condition	type	28th
life	originate	definitive	once
place	before	newborn	first
continue	not	default	Z38
never	clinically	should	

1. For coding and reporting purposes the perinatal period is defined as ____ birth through the ____ day following birth.
2. Codes in this chapter are ____ for use on the maternal record.
3. Codes from Chapter 15, the obstetric chapter, are never permitted on the ____ record.
4. Chapter 16 codes may be used throughout the ____ of the patient if the ____ is still present.
5. When coding the birth episode in a newborn record, assign a code from category ____ , Liveborn infants according to ____ of birth and ____ of delivery, as the principal diagnosis.
6. A code from category Z38 is assigned only ____ , to a newborn at the time of birth.
7. Codes for signs and symptoms may be assigned when a ____ diagnosis has ____ been established.
8. If the reason for the encounter is a ____ condition, the code from Chapter 16 should be sequenced ____ .
9. Should a condition ____ in the perinatal period, and ____ throughout the life of the patient, the perinatal code should continue to be used regardless of the patient's age.
10. If a newborn has a condition that may be either due to the birth process or community acquired and the documentation does not indicate which it is, the ____ is due to the birth process and the code from Chapter 16 should be used.
11. All ____ significant conditions noted on routine newborn examination ____ be coded.

Let's Check It! Rules and Regulations

Please answer the following questions from the knowledge you have gained after reading this chapter.

1. **LO 18.1** Turn to the Official Guidelines for **Chapter 14**, Diseases of Genitourinary System–I.C.14.a.2. Discuss chronic kidney disease and kidney transplant status as outlined in the **Chapter 14** guidelines.
2. **LO 18.3** Discuss how sexually transmitted diseases (STDs) are spread. Include an example of an STD and how it would be coded.
3. **LO 18.5** Explain coding the birth, including what code category goes on the mother's chart (and its sequence) and what code category goes on the newborn's chart, including its sequence and how many times this code can be reported.
4. **LO 18.7** Explain the differences between genetic conditions and congenital malformations.
5. **LO 18.4** Explain what procreative management is. Include the subcategory code for a general counseling and advice encounter.

YOU CODE IT! Basics

First, identify the condition in the following diagnoses, then code the diagnosis.

Example: Glaucoma of newborn:

a. main term: *Glaucoma* **b.** diagnosis: *Q15.0*

1. Acute nephritic syndrome with dense deposit disease:

   a. main term: ______ **b.** diagnosis: ______

2. Recurrent hematuria with membranoproliferative glomeruloephritis:

   a. main term: ______ **b.** diagnosis: ______

3. Chronic interstitial nephritis, reflux associated:

   a. main term: ______ **b.** diagnosis: ______

(continued)

4. Stricture of ureter:
   a. main term: ______ b. diagnosis: ______
5. Left ovarian ectopic pregnancy:
   a. main term: ______ b. diagnosis: ______
6. Cervical shortening, third trimester:
   a. main term: ______ b. diagnosis: ______
7. Spontaneous abortion:
   a. main term: ______ b. diagnosis: ______
8. Embolism following molar pregnancy:
   a. main term: ______ b. diagnosis: ______
9. Respiratory failure of newborn:
   a. main term: ______ b. diagnosis: ______
10. Neonatal tachycardia:
    a. main term: ______ b. diagnosis: ______
11. Dehydration of newborn:
    a. main term: ______ b. diagnosis: ______
12. Neonatal jaundice from breast milk inhibitor:
    a. main term: ______ b. diagnosis: ______
13. Classic hydatidiform mole:
    a. main term: ______ b. diagnosis: ______
14. Hydrocephalus in newborn:
    a. main term: ______ b. diagnosis: ______
15. Thoracic spina bifida:
    a. main term: ______ b. diagnosis: ______

ICD-10-CM

YOU CODE IT! Practice

Using the techniques described in this chapter, carefully read through the case studies and determine the most accurate ICD-10-CM code(s) and external cause code(s), if appropriate, for each case study.

1. Sean Dollarson, an 8-year-old male, is brought in by his parents to see Dr. Greenburg, his pediatrician. Sean has not been feeling well and has had some pinkish-colored urine. Dr. Greenburg completed a physical exam noting elevated blood pressure and periorbital puffiness. Sean is admitted to the hospital. The laboratory tests reveal azotemia, a BUN:Cr ratio of 18, proteinuria of 2.1 g/day, and that RBCs are dysmorphic. After reviewing the results of the tests, Sean is diagnosed with chronic nephritic syndrome with diffused mesangial proliferative glomerulonephritis.
2. Sally Hyman, a 37-year-old female, presents with the complaint of restlessness, nausea, and vomiting. Sally also admits to intermittent abdominal pain. Dr. Moye completes an examination and orders a noncontrast CT scan followed by an intravenous contrast CT scan. The CT results confirmed the diagnosis of a staghorn calculus of kidney.
3. Murphy Jorganson, a 42-year-old male, presents with the complaint of frequent and painful urination. Dr. Reddy completes a physical examination and notes swelling of the testicles. Murphy admits to some soreness and a whitish discharge. Dr. Reddy inserts a cotton swab approximately 3.5 cm into the urethra and rotates it once. Microscopic examination confirmed the diagnosis of non-gonococcal urethritis due to methicillin-resistant *Staphylococcus aureus*.
4. Eugene Applewhite, a 5-year-old male, is brought in by his parents. Eugene is losing weight and his parents are concerned because Eugene prefers drinking water to eating food. Eugene has also been wetting his bed. Dr. Ryant completes a clinical examination and notes mild dehydration and decides to admit Eugene to the hospital. After reviewing the MRI scan and laboratory results, Eugene is diagnosed with nephrogenic diabetes insipidus.
5. Larry Tucker, a 24-year-old male, presents today to see Dr. Dawkins, a urologist, with the complaint of low level of semen with ejaculation. Dr. Dawkins completes a medical history, a physical examination, and the appropriate tests. Larry is diagnosed with azoospermia due to obstruction of efferent ducts.
6. Pamela Cain, a 34-year-old female, presents today 23 weeks pregnant. Pamela has no complaints and states she is feeling well. Pamela was diagnosed with essential hypertension 1 year ago.
7. Gladys Shull, a 17-year-old female, comes in today to see Dr. Henson. Gladys thinks she may be pregnant. Dr. Henson performs a pregnancy test, results positive.
8. Jennifer Addis, a 23-year-old female, presents today with frequent urination and a burning sensation. Jennifer is 25 weeks pregnant. Dr. Pizzuti completes an examination and orders a culture, which reveals *Escherichia coli*. Jennifer is diagnosed with a urinary bladder infection due to *E. coli*.

(continued)

9. Kreshella Goodpaster, a 29-year-old female, 17 weeks pregnant, presents with heavy vaginal bleeding. Dr. Freedenberg admits Kreshella to the hospital with the diagnosis of antepartum hemorrhage.
10. Mazie Iablonovski, a 32-year-old female, 13 weeks pregnant, comes to see Dr. Minick, her OB-GYN. Mazie states she is feeling well and has no complaints. Dr. Minick is concerned because Mazie has a history of miscarriages. Mazie is G3 P0.
11. Judy Sovde, a 28-year-old female, gave birth to a beautiful baby girl today at Weston Hospital. Dr. Kibler assisted in the full-term vaginal delivery. Dr. Kibler diagnoses baby Sovde with congenital entropion, right eye. Code baby Sovde's chart.
12. Jason Eldridge was born today at Weston Hospital. Jason was delivered by cesarean section, full term, by Dr. DeYoung. Jason's laboratory results were positive for metabolic acidemia.
13. Paula Devan, a 2-week-old female, is brought by her parents to see her pediatrician, Dr. Langer, for a checkup. Dr. Langer documents a pansystolic murmur. Paula is diagnosed with a congenital ventricular septal defect (VSD).
14. Dr. Jeffers, a neonatologist, was called in to treat Saddie Hawkins, born in this hospital 2 days ago at 36 completed weeks of gestation. Saddie is showing signs of hypoxia. Dr. Jeffers transferred Saddie to NICU, where the infant pneumogram confirms a diagnosis of apnea of prematurity.
15. Karen Sprague went into labor, and her husband, Allen, was driving her to the hospital when they got caught in a traffic jam. Karen gave birth in the car, and Allen cut the umbilical cord with the utility knife he keeps in the trunk. Upon arrival at the hospital, Dr. Parkerson performed a complete newborn examination and diagnosed the baby with tetanus neonatorum caused by the use of the nonsterile instrument during delivery. Code baby Sprague's chart.

ICD-10-CM YOU CODE IT! Application

The following exercises provide practice in abstracting physicians' notes and learning to work with documentation from our health care facility, Prader, Bracker, & Associates. These case studies are modeled on real patient encounters. Using the techniques described in this chapter, carefully read through the case studies and determine the most accurate ICD-10-CM code(s) and external cause code(s), if appropriate, for each case study.

WESTON HOSPITAL

629 Healthcare Way • SOMEWHERE, FL 32811 • 407-555-6541

PATIENT: OTTMAN, BELINDA

ACCOUNT/EHR #: OTTMBE001

Attending Physician: Renee O. Bracker, MD

S: This 71-year-old female was diagnosed with end-stage renal disease requiring regular dialysis maintenance 6 months ago. She presents today with shortness of breath, nausea, hiccups, and overall weakness. She admits to noncompliance with her dialysis plan.

O: Ht. 5′4″, Wt. 134 lb., P 81, R 28, BP 170/92. HEENT: unremarkable. Serum creatinine of 1.7 mg/dL, GFR 14 mL/min/1.73 m, hemoglobin 6.4, edema pitting 2+.

A: End-stage renal disease with regular dialysis, noncompliance; anemia due to ESRD

P: Admit to inpatient with immediate hemodialysis session and transfusion

Determine the most accurate ICD-10-CM code(s).

(continued)

PRADER, BRACKER, & ASSOCIATES

A Complete Health Care Facility

159 Healthcare Way • SOMEWHERE, FL 32811 • 407-555-6789

PATIENT: BANG, PARC

ACCOUNT/EHR #: BANGPA001

DATE: 10/17/22

Attending Physician: Renee O. Bracker, MD

S: This is a 64-year-old male who comes in today with frequent painful urination and feeling the consistent need to void. He states that he smoked cigarettes for 10+ years but has been smoke-free for 2.5 years.

O: Ht. 6′2″, Wt. 215 lb., P 82, R 18, BP 141/83. HEENT: unremarkable, oxygen saturation 100% in RA. Afebrile. Skin: warm and well perfused with no rash. Back exam: no deformities or defects. Neuro exam: normal tone and strength. Urinalysis is positive for hematuria. Cystoscopy results positive for bladder carcinoma.

A: Bladder cancer, anterior wall, primary

P: Transurethral resection—discussed TUR option with patient. He will think about it and will return in 1 week.

Determine the most accurate ICD-10-CM code(s).

PRADER, BRACKER, & ASSOCIATES

A Complete Health Care Facility

159 Healthcare Way • SOMEWHERE, FL 32811 • 407-555-6789

PATIENT: VANZELL, LEONORE

ACCOUNT/EHR #: VANZLE001

Attending Physician: Oscar R. Prader, MD

S: This is a 58-year-old female who comes in today with concerns about tiredness and urinating during the night. She states that recently she has had interrupted sleep because of being awakened with an urgent need to void. The past 3–4 nights she has gotten up to void at least 4 times during the night. Patient also admits that during the day she has to urinate a good bit and yesterday she counted voiding 9 times within a 24-hour period. She states that her fluid intake has not changed and she is not on any medications. She denies any incontinence at this time.

O: Ht. 5′6″, Wt. 131 lb., P 72, R 16, BP 135/81. HEENT: unremarkable, oxygen saturation 100% in RA. Afebrile. Patient history is noncontributory. Abdomen: flat, soft, nontender. Back exam: no deformities or cutaneous defect. Neuro exam: normal tone, strength, and activity. Finger stick shows glucose levels within normal range. UA is negative for hematuria and infection. Cystourethroscopy ruled out any tumors and kidney stones. Patient denies any pain associated with micturition.

A: Detrusor muscle hyperactivity

P: Rx: Darifenacin

Restrict fluid intake

Determine the most accurate ICD-10-CM code(s).

(continued)

WESTON HOSPITAL

629 Healthcare Way • SOMEWHERE, FL 32811 • 407-555-6541

PATIENT: TERRY, MARIANNA

ACCOUNT/EHR #: TERRMA001

Operative Report

Preoperative DX:	1. First trimester missed abortion; 2. Undesired fertility
Postoperative DX:	Same
Operation:	1. Dilation and curettage with suction; 2. Laparoscopic bilateral tubal ligation using Kleppinger bipolar cautery
Surgeon:	Oscar R. Prader, MD
Assistant:	None
Anesthesia:	General endotracheal anesthesia
Findings:	Pt had products of conception at the time of dilation and curettage. She also had normal-appearing uterus, ovaries, fallopian tubes, and liver edge.
Specimens:	Products of conception to pathology
Disposition:	To PACU in stable condition

Procedure: The patient was taken to the operating room, and she was placed in the dorsal supine position. General endotracheal anesthesia was administered without difficulty. The patient was placed in dorsal lithotomy position. She was prepped and draped in the normal sterile fashion. A red rubber tip catheter was placed gently to drain the patient's bladder. A weighted speculum was placed in the posterior vagina and Deaver retractor anteriorly. A single-tooth tenaculum was placed in the anterior cervix for retraction. The uterus sounded to 9 cm. The cervix was dilated with Hanks dilators to 25 French. This sufficiently passed a #7 suction curet. The suction curet was inserted without incident, and the products of conception were gently suctioned out. Good uterine cry was noted with a serrated curet. No further products were noted on suctioning. At this point, a Hulka tenaculum was placed in the cervix for retraction. The other instruments were removed.

Attention was then turned to the patient's abdomen. A small vertical intraumbilical incision was made with the knife. A Veress needle was placed through that incision. Confirmation of placement into the abdominal cavity was made with instillation of normal saline without return and a positive handing drop test. The abdomen was then insufflated with sufficient carbon dioxide gas to cause abdominal tympany. The Veress needle was removed and a 5-mm trocar was placed in the same incision. Confirmation of placement into the abdominal cavity was made with placement of the laparoscopic camera. Another trocar site was placed two fingerbreadths above the pubic symphysis in the mid-line under direct visualization. The above-noted intrapelvic and intraabdominal findings were seen. The patient was placed in steep Trendelenburg. The fallopian tubes were identified and followed out to the fimbriated ends. They were then cauterized 4 times on either side. At this point, all instruments were removed from the patient's abdomen. This was done under direct visualization during the insufflation. The skin incisions were reapproximated with 4-0 Vicryl suture. The Hulka tenaculum was removed without incident.

The patient was placed back in the dorsal supine position. Anesthesia was withdrawn without difficulty. The patient was taken to the PACU in stable condition. All sponge, instrument, and needle counts were correct in the operating room.

Determine the most accurate ICD-10-CM code(s).

PRADER, BRACKER, & ASSOCIATES

A Complete Health Care Facility

159 Healthcare Way • SOMEWHERE, FL 32811 • 407-555-6789

PATIENT: FAIRBANKS, GREGORY

ACCOUNT/EHR #: FAIRGR001

(continued)

Attending Physician: Renee O. Bracker, MD

Consultant: Vivian D. Pixar, MD

Reason for Consultation: Screening for retinopathy of prematurity

S: The patient was born on 08/19/19, with a birth weight of 2,740 grams, gestational age of 36 weeks; given oxygen in NICU for the first 60 minutes of life. Child discharged third day postpartum with oxygen saturation of 98%.

O: Retinal follow-up examination this date shows normal external exam, well-dilated pupils. Indirect exam shows clear media, normal optic nerves both eyes, with normal right retinal vessel extension to the periphery without evidence of retinopathy. Left retinal vessel extension shows a faint demarcation line at the junction between the vascularized and avascular border.

A: Prematurity retinopathy, stage 1, left eye

P: Follow-up 1 week

Determine the most accurate ICD-10-CM code(s).

19

Factors Influencing Health Status (Z Codes)

Key Terms

Abnormal Findings
Allogeneic
Autologous
Carrier
Isogeneic
Preventive Care
Prosthetic
Screening
Xenogeneic

Learning Outcomes

After completing this chapter, the student should be able to:

LO 19.1 Abstract details about preventive services to report their medical necessity.
LO 19.2 Determine the medical reasons for early detection testing.
LO 19.3 Demonstrate how to report encounters related to genetic susceptibility.
LO 19.4 Identify the reasons for observation services to determine the correct code or codes.
LO 19.5 Apply the Official Guidelines for reporting aftercare and follow-up care.
LO 19.6 Evaluate the specific services provided for organ donation and report the medical necessity.
LO 19.7 Distinguish indications of antimicrobial drug resistance to report this accurately.
LO 19.8 Employ Z codes accurately.
LO 19.9 Social Determinants of Health.

STOP! Remember, you need to follow along in your ICD-10-CM code book for an optimal learning experience.

19.1 Preventive Care

In several chapters throughout this textbook, you got an overview of Z codes, which are codes used to report a reason for a visit to a physician for something other than an illness or injury. As you have learned, there must always be a valid, medical reason for a patient's encounter with a health care professional. And there are occasions for patients to seek attention even when they are not currently ill. These codes give you the opportunity to explain.

Science and research have provided us with a better understanding of disease and disease progression, as well as etiology (underlying cause of disease). This knowledge has resulted in improved **preventive care** services to stop the onset of illness or injury.

Preventive Care
Health-related services designed to stop the development of a disease or injury.

The provision of preventive care services is likely to increase. The enacting of the Affordable Care Act enables more patients to take advantage of more preventive services than ever before. Since September 2010, new health insurance policies must cover preventive services, with no copayment, no coinsurance payments, and no requirement for deductible fulfillment.

Reporting the provision of preventive care will require a Z code to explain the specific reason for the encounter, such as a flu shot or measles vaccination (Z23 Encounter for immunization).

GUIDANCE CONNECTION

Read the ICD-10-CM Official Guidelines for Coding and Reporting, section **I. Conventions, General Coding Guidelines and Chapter-Specific Guidelines**, subsection **C. Chapter-Specific Coding Guidelines**, chapter **21. Factors Influencing Health Status and Contact with Health Services**, subsection **c.2) Inoculations and vaccinations**.

The physician or other health care professional may also be able to provide counseling for the patient and/or family members. This type of counseling is not the same as that provided by a psychiatrist or psychologist; instead, the physician would take the time to discuss options for preventing the development of disease or injury. Perhaps this may include dietary counseling and surveillance (Z71.3) to prevent the onset of hypertension, heart disease, obesity, or other nutrition-related conditions, or a discussion about the patient's tobacco use (Z72.0) could focus on various methodologies available to quit smoking to prevent the patient from developing lung disease. Couples may come in for genetic counseling (Z31.5) to prevent passing chromosomal abnormalities to their future children; for those who do not want to have children yet, general counseling and advice on contraception (Z30.09) may be provided.

LET'S CODE IT! SCENARIO

Bonnie Poggio, a 15-year-old female, came into the clinic with her mother. While searching for seashells at the beach, she went up on the boardwalk barefooted to get ice cream and stepped on a nail, puncturing the sole of her left foot. After checking the puncture wound, cleaning it, and dressing it, Dr. Baldwin gave Bonnie a tetanus shot as a precaution.

Let's Code It!

You are reviewing how to determine Z codes in this chapter, so here's the first code for this encounter: **S91.332A Puncture wound without foreign body, left foot, initial encounter**. Dr. Baldwin's notes state that Bonnie received a preventive tetanus shot. You have learned that, in medical terminology, this is known as an *immunization*. When you turn to the Alphabetic Index, you see

Immunization — *see also* Vaccination

encounter for Z23

When you turn to the Tabular List, you confirm:

Z23 Encounter for immunization

This is great. However, the reason Bonnie went to see Dr. Baldwin was care for the wound. The tetanus shot was secondary. So, you will not report Z23. But you do need an external cause code to explain why Bonnie needed this immunization. Turn to the *Alphabetic Index to External Causes*. Did you find this?

Puncture, puncturing — *see also* Contact, with, by type of object or machine

Let's turn to

Contact (accidental)

with

nail W45.0

Now let's find code category W45 in the Tabular List:

✓4 **W45 Foreign body or object entering through skin**

That sounds right. First, read carefully the EXCLUDES2 notation listing several diagnoses. Take a minute to review them, and determine whether any apply to Bonnie's condition. No, none of them do, so you are in the correct location. Notice the seventh-character options here. You will need them for later. First, you need to determine the first six characters, so continue down and review all of the fourth-, fifth-, and sixth-character choices. Which matches Dr. Baldwin's notes?

✓xx7 **W45.0 Nail entering through skin**

(continued)

Perfect! And the seventh character? The choices are listed at the top of this code category:

W45.0XXA Nail entering through skin, initial encounter

Next, you need the place of occurrence (the beach) and the status code. (Refer to the chapter ***Coding Injury, Poisoning, and External Causes*** to remind yourself about reporting external cause codes whenever you are reporting an injury or poisoning.)

Take a look. Did you find these codes:

Y92.832 Beach as the place of occurrence of the external cause

Y99.8 Other external cause status

Fantastic! You have determined all of the codes required for this encounter:

S91.332A Puncture wound without foreign body, left foot, initial encounter

W45.0XXA Nail entering through skin, initial encounter

Y92.832 Beach as the place of occurrence of the external cause

Y99.8 Other external cause status

You have got this!

19.2 Early Detection

The reason for routine and administrative exams is to ensure continued good health by looking for signs of disease as early as detection may be possible, using a physician's knowledge and technological advancement. Commonly, these health care encounters are known as *annual physicals*, *well-baby checks*, or *well-woman exams*. These routine encounters, most often prompted by the calendar rather than the way the patient feels, are reported with Z codes, such as code Z00.00 Encounter for general adult medical examination without abnormal findings or Z00.129 Encounter for routine child health examination without abnormal findings.

Many schools and organizations require that a physician examine a child before the child joins a sports team (Z02.5), companies may require preemployment exams (Z02.1), and virtually all surgeons will order pre-procedural exams (Z01.81-) for the patient prior to surgery. These are all considered administrative health encounters because they are determined by a specific circumstance, rather than the calendar or the way the patient feels.

Certain conditions, even after being resolved, may continue to identify the patient as being at risk of a recurrence. The patient had a previous condition; however, prudent health care standards require that the physician keep a watchful eye to catch and treat a recurrent episode. Codes such as Z86.11 Personal history of tuberculosis and Z87.11 Personal history of peptic ulcer may provide medical necessity for an extra screening test or encounter.

A **screening** is a test or examination, such as routine lab work or imaging services, administered when there are no current signs, symptoms, or related diagnosis. Report a visit for a screening with a Z code such as code Z13.22 Encounter for screening for metabolic disorder or Z13.820 Encounter for screening for osteoporosis.

Screening
An examination or test of a patient who has no signs or symptoms that is conducted with the intention of finding any evidence of disease as soon as possible, thus enabling better patient outcomes.

The standards of care have established important examinations and tests to detect illnesses at the earliest possible time. However, these tests are typically recommended for specific population subgroups determined to be at the greatest risk, such as mammograms for women over 40 or prostate examinations for men over 50. These encounters would be reported with a Z code such as code Z12.5 Encounter for screening for malignant neoplasm of prostate or Z13.6 Encounter for screening for cardiovascular disorders.

As health care evolves and grows, insights have led to screenings for more conditions not previously identified until signs and symptoms are more obvious. Now, screenings can be used to provide early detection of conditions such as depression, reported with code Z13.31 Encounter for screening for depression, or autism, reported with code Z13.41 Encounter for autism screening.

YOU CODE IT! CASE STUDY

Kathryn Rogers, a 49-year-old female, came in to see Dr. Apter to get a colonoscopy. Dr. Apter explained last week that this was an important screening for malignant neoplasms of the colon and was recommended for all adults aged 50 and over. After the screening, Dr. Apter told Kathryn she was fine and there were no abnormalities.

You Code It!

Go through the steps of coding, and determine the code or codes that should be reported for this encounter between Dr. Apter and Kathryn.

Step #1: Read the case carefully and completely.

Step #2: Abstract the scenario. Which main words or terms describe why the physician cared for the patient during this encounter?

Step #3: Are there any details missing or incomplete for which you would need to query the physician? [If so, ask your instructor.]

Step #4: Check for any relevant guidance, including reading all of the symbols and notations in the Tabular List and the appropriate sections of the Official Guidelines.

Step #5: Determine the correct diagnosis code or codes to explain why this encounter was medically necessary.

Step #6: Double-check your work.

Answer:

Did you determine this to be the correct code?

Z12.11 Encounter for screening for malignant neoplasm of colon

CODING TIP

An encounter for a COVID-19 screening test is reported with code: Z11.52

A patient who has had contact with or suspected exposure to COVID-19 is reported with: Z20.822

Abnormal Findings
Test results that indicate a disease or condition may be present.

Society, especially in the United States, is designed for interaction between individuals. Shopping malls, concert halls and festival venues, public transport sites, classrooms, playgrounds, and other locations draw friends, families, and strangers together in close proximity to one another. Close physical proximity can put someone in contact with a potential health hazard and facilitate (suspected) exposure to a communicable disease. Think of this: two children, Jane and Mary, were playing together, and the next day Jane is diagnosed with rubella. This means that Mary was exposed. When Mary's mom takes her to the physician, this visit will include code Z20.4 Contact with and (suspected) exposure to rubella. Another example: Kenny works for County Animal Control. As he was placing a wild raccoon into his vehicle, the raccoon bit him. Kenny went to the emergency clinic immediately, and code Z20.3 Contact with and (suspected) exposure to rabies was included on the claim.

With all these tests being done to confirm the patient's good health, there are times when the documentation includes **abnormal findings**, meaning the results indicate something is wrong. This is not the same thing as a confirmed diagnosis, necessarily. It may be a signal that a condition is potential or that more extensive and specific examinations must be done.

EXAMPLES

Z00.01 Encounter for general adult medical examination with abnormal findings

Z01.411 Encounter for gynecological examination (general) (routine) with abnormal findings

GUIDANCE CONNECTION

Read the ICD-10-CM Official Guidelines for Coding and Reporting, section **I. Conventions, General Coding Guidelines and Chapter-Specific Guidelines**, subsection **C. Chapter-Specific Coding Guidelines**, chapter **21. Factors Influencing Health Status and Contact with Health Services**, subsections **c.1) Contact/exposure, c.4) History (of), c.5) Screening**, and **c.13) Routine and administrative examinations,** plus section **IV. Diagnostic Coding and Reporting Guidelines for Outpatient Services**, subsection **P. Encounters for general medical examinations with abnormal findings**.

YOU CODE IT! CASE STUDY

Dallas Rossi, a 66-year-old male, came in to see his regular physician, Dr. DeGuisipe, for his annual physical. Dallas said he has been feeling great and working out about twice a week. During the digital rectal exam, Dr. DeGuisipe noted a palpable nodule on the posterior of Dallas's prostate. Dr. DeGuisipe told Dallas that he appears in good health except for the nodule. They discussed this and scheduled an appointment for a biopsy.

You Code It!

Go through the steps of coding, and determine the code or codes that should be reported for this encounter between Dr. DeGuisipe and Dallas.

Step #1: Read the case carefully and completely.
Step #2: Abstract the scenario. Which main words or terms describe why the physician cared for the patient during this encounter?
Step #3: Are there any details missing or incomplete for which you would need to query the physician? [If so, ask your instructor.]
Step #4: Check for any relevant guidance, including reading all of the symbols and notations in the Tabular List and the appropriate sections of the Official Guidelines.
Step #5: Determine the correct diagnosis code or codes to explain why this encounter was medically necessary.
Step #6: Double-check your work.

Answer:

Did you determine these to be the correct codes?

Z00.01 Encounter for general adult medical examination with abnormal findings

N40.2 Nodular prostate without lower urinary tract symptoms

You did great!

19.3 Genetic Susceptibility

A patient might be a **carrier** or suspected carrier of a disease. They need to know this so the condition is not unintentionally passed on. Or the patient may have an abnormal gene that may increase a patient's chances of developing a disease. This is of particular concern when there is a known family history for conditions that are, or may be, inherited.

> **Carrier**
> An individual infected with a disease who is not ill but can still pass it to another person; an individual with an abnormal gene that can be passed to a child, making the child susceptible to disease.

In most cases, the documentation will note that the patient has a family history of a condition, such as code Z80.6 Family history of leukemia or Z83.3 Family history of diabetes mellitus. In these cases, no additional genetic testing may be done. However, the knowledge of family members with a particular condition could support more frequent screenings, such as a patient getting a mammogram every 6 months instead of the standard annual test.

A patient may have reason to believe they are the carrier of a disease, such as diphtheria (Z22.2) or viral hepatitis B (Z55.51). A carrier is an individual who has been infected with a pathogen yet has no signs or symptoms of the disease. Carriers, while not ill themselves, are still able to pass the condition to another person.

EXAMPLE

Cystic fibrosis, the result of mutations in the CFTR gene, is a common genetic disease. Due to its nature, both parents must each carry a copy of the mutated gene in order for the child to inherit and develop the disease. However, the parents may not show any signs or symptoms.

Risk is measured by family history and ethnic background. If the patient has a family history of CF, then the probability of being a carrier is increased above the risk based on ethnicity alone. The probability increases if the patient is a close relative of an individual with CF, such as a parent, sibling, or child.

To report medical necessity to perform the genetic testing:

Z84.81 **Family history of carrier of genetic disease**

Z13.71 **Encounter for nonprocreative screening for genetic disease carrier status**

or

Z31.430 **Encounter of female for testing for genetic disease carrier status for procreative management**

or

Z31.440 **Encounter of male for testing for genetic disease carrier status for procreative management**

If the woman is currently pregnant and needs to be screened, use this code:

Z36.- **Encounter for antenatal screening of mother**

If the test is positive, report

Z14.1 **Cystic fibrosis carrier**

You may have heard about genetic susceptibility to malignant neoplasm of the breast (Z15.01) and genetic susceptibility to malignant neoplasm of the ovary (Z15.02), identified by the BRCA1 and BRCA2 tests. These tests may be used to confirm, or deny, the presence of an abnormality in a gene that may have been inherited, which can serve as a prediction of the potential for developing a disease–in these cases, cancer. Some patients have opted for prophylactic (preventive) surgery after a positive finding of an abnormal gene. If a patient had this procedure, you would report it with code Z40.01 Encounter for prophylactic removal of breast.

GUIDANCE CONNECTION

Read the ICD-10-CM Official Guidelines for Coding and Reporting, section **I. Conventions, General Coding Guidelines and Chapter-Specific Guidelines**, subsection **C. Chapter-Specific Coding Guidelines**, chapter **21. Factors Influencing Health Status and Contact with Health Services**, subsections **c.3) Status** and **c.14) Miscellaneous Z codes–Prophylactic organ removal.**

19.4 Observation

There might be a reason that a physician suspects a patient may be ill despite the absence of signs and symptoms. Code categories Z03 and Z04 enable you to report the reason these types of encounters are medically necessary.

✓4 **Z03** **Encounter for medical observation for suspected diseases and conditions ruled out**

✓4 **Z04** **Encounter for examination and observation for other reasons**

Imagine that a mother brings her 2-year-old son into the emergency department because she found him in her bathroom with her allergy pill bottle tipped over and pills strewn about the floor. She does not know whether he ingested any of the pills and, if he did, how many. After an examination showing no signs or symptoms of overdose or poisoning, the physician decides to keep the boy in the hospital for observation, just in case. The next day, the boy appears to be fine, and his blood tests show no signs of the allergy medication at all. He is discharged with a clean bill of health. You would report this with code Z03.6 Encounter for observation for suspected toxic effect from ingested substance, ruled out.

CODING BITES

Notice that these codes are used when the physician determines observation is required "to be sure" and the result is nothing is wrong [ruled out]. If the determination is that there *is* a problem, you would then report the code for the problem, not the observation.

GUIDANCE CONNECTION

Read the ICD-10-CM Official Guidelines for Coding and Reporting, section **I. Conventions, General Coding Guidelines and Chapter-Specific Guidelines**, subsection **C. Chapter-Specific Coding Guidelines**, chapter **21. Factors Influencing Health Status and Contact with Health Services**, subsection **c.6) Observation**.

YOU CODE IT! CASE STUDY

Tracey Morales, a 33-year-old male, was brought into the ED after an accident on his construction job site. He tripped and hit his head against a pile of bricks. There was a 3-cm laceration on his temporal lobe scalp, but he did not lose consciousness. CT scan of his head was inconclusive. After the laceration was stitched up with a simple repair, Dr. Tribow placed Tracey into observation status so they could watch for signs of a concussion. After 20 hours with normal vital signs and a normal neurologic exam, he was determined to not have suffered a concussion and released.

You Code It!

Review Dr. Tribow's documentation about Tracey's stay in observation. Then, determine the correct ICD-10-CM code or codes to report the reasons why Tracey needed care.

Step #1: Read the case carefully and completely.
Step #2: Abstract the scenario. Which main words or terms describe why the physician cared for the patient during this encounter?
Step #3: Are there any details missing or incomplete for which you would need to query the physician? [If so, ask your instructor.]
Step #4: Check for any relevant guidance, including reading all of the symbols and notations in the Tabular List and the appropriate sections of the Official Guidelines.
Step #5: Determine the correct diagnosis code or codes to explain why this encounter was medically necessary.
Step #6: Double-check your work.

Answer:

Did you determine these to be the codes?

Z04.2	**Encounter for examination and observation following work accident**
S01.01XA	**Laceration without foreign body of scalp, initial encounter**
W01.198A	**Fall on same level from slipping, tripping, and stumbling with subsequent striking against other object, initial encounter**
Y92.61	**Building [any] under construction as the place of occurrence of the external cause**
Y99.0	**Civilian activity done for income or pay**

19.5 Continuing Care and Aftercare

GUIDANCE CONNECTION

Read the ICD-10-CM Official Guidelines for Coding and Reporting, section **I. Conventions, General Coding Guidelines and Chapter-Specific Guidelines**, subsection **C. Chapter-Specific Coding Guidelines**, chapter **21. Factors Influencing Health Status and Contact with Health Services**, subsections **c.7) Aftercare**.

Chronic illness may require long-term use of medication, known as *drug therapy*. When a patient is taking any type of pharmaceutical on an ongoing basis, regular monitoring can identify potential concerns, such as side effects or loss of potency. Some individuals' body chemistry can get used to certain drugs, making them less effective. When coding an encounter for such monitoring, you may begin with Z51.81 Encounter for therapeutic drug level monitoring, along with a code to identify the type of therapeutic drug, such as Z79.01 Long-term (current) use of anticoagulants or Z79.811 Long-term (current) use of aromatase inhibitors.

Of course, the physician-patient relationship in treating a specific illness or injury does not end at the end of a surgical procedure or other type of therapeutic service. A healing illness or injury may require aftercare, reported with a code such as Z47.1 Aftercare following joint replacement surgery, Z48.00 Encounter for change or removal of nonsurgical wound dressing, or Z45.24 Encounter for aftercare following lung transplant.

Patients with implanted medical devices may need more frequent encounters to check the device to ensure it is working properly, as is the case with a patient with a cardiac pacemaker (Z45.01) or a patient with a cochlear implant (Z45.321).

Follow-up examinations may be necessary for a condition that has already been treated or no longer exists. Examples of such follow-ups include an encounter for the removal of sutures (stitches), reported with code Z48.02, or an encounter after the patient has completed treatment for a malignant neoplasm (Z08), once the patient has finished the chemotherapy or radiation treatment plan.

GUIDANCE CONNECTION

Read the ICD-10-CM Official Guidelines for Coding and Reporting, section **I. Conventions, General Coding Guidelines and Chapter-Specific Guidelines**, subsection **C. Chapter-Specific Coding Guidelines**, chapter **21. Factors Influencing Health Status and Contact with Health Services**, subsection **c.8) Follow-up.**

LET'S CODE IT! SCENARIO

Adelina Plenner, a 43-year-old female, came in to see Dr. Buldar, her gastroenterologist. She had a colostomy 6 weeks ago, and this is a standard postprocedural follow-up. He noted that there was some irritation and he applied some ointment and gave Adelina a prescription for more ointment. Dr. Buldar examined the area and told Adelina to return prn.

Let's Code It!

This encounter is a standard follow-up post-surgically to ensure all is well with the patient. Dr. Buldar was checking Adelina's condition post-colostomy.

In the ICD-10-CM Alphabetic Index, find

Aftercare (*see also* Care) Z51.89

Read all of the indented items. Hmm, there doesn't seem to be anything that matches this encounter. Let's try this:

Care (of) (for) (following)

Wow, nothing here seems to fit, either. What about . . .

Encounter (with health service) (for) Z76.89

(continued)

Not here, either! One more idea. . . . Dr. Buldar paid attention to Adelina's stoma. Take a look at this:

Attention (to)

artificial

opening (of) Z43.9

digestive tract NEC Z43.4

colon Z43.3

Finally!!! Success!! This proves that you cannot give up. You must keep thinking and looking because it will always be there . . . somewhere.

Turn in the ICD-10-CM Tabular List and find

✓4 **Z43 Encounter for attention to artificial openings**

Read carefully the diagnoses listed next to the INCLUDES, EXCLUDES1, and EXCLUDES2 notations. Did you check the *artificial opening status only, without need for care (Z93.-)*? Was there a need for care? The ointment could support this. Did you check to see if this qualifies as a *complication of external stoma* . . . particularly K94.-? When on the job, you could query the physician for confirmation. This documentation does not really describe a complication, so let's continue on to confirm this code:

Z43.3 Encounter for attention to colostomy

Good job!

19.6 Organ Donation

The number of organs and tissues that can be successfully transplanted has dramatically increased over the years, and many can be provided by a living donor. Code category Z52 Donors of organs and tissues includes various types of blood donors (Z52.0-), skin donors (Z52.1-), and bone donors (Z52.2-). You will notice that all three of these code subcategories require you, as the professional coder, to determine from the documentation whether the donor is **autologous** or is providing another type of graft or donation (see **Table 19-1**). It is not unusual for a patient to donate their own blood prior to having a surgical procedure so that in the event the patient needs a transfusion, their own blood will be used. When an injury to the skin is so severe that a graft is needed, there are times when the surgeon will take the graft from another part of the patient's own body and transfer it to the injured site.

Autologous
The donor tissue is taken from a different site on the same individual's body (also known as an *autograft*).

TABLE 19-1 Types of Grafts

Autologous	**The donor tissue is taken from a different site on the same individual's body (also known as an *autograft*).**
Isogeneic	The donor and recipient individuals are genetically identical (i.e., monozygotic twins).
Allogeneic	**The donor and recipient are of the same species, e.g., human → human, dog → dog (also known as an *allograft*).**
Xenogeneic	The donor and recipient are of different species, e.g., bovine cartilage → human (also known as a *xenograft* or *heterograft*).
Prosthetic	**Lost tissue is replaced with synthetic material such as metal, plastic, or ceramic.**

Allogeneic
The donor and recipient are of the same species, e.g., human → human, dog → dog (also known as an *allograft*).

Isogeneic
The donor and recipient individuals are genetically identical (i.e., monozygotic twins).

Xenogeneic
The donor and recipient are of different species, e.g., bovine cartilage → human (also known as a *xenograft* or *heterograft*).

Prosthetic
Fabricated artificial replacement for a damaged or missing part of the body.

A kidney (Z52.4) and cornea (Z52.5) as well as a part of the liver (Z52.6) may come from a living donor. Fertility issues occur and some women donate their oocytes (eggs) for in vitro fertilization for themselves or someone else (Z52.81-). The donation of any of these organs would almost always be used as an **allogeneic** donation to another individual.

A donation from the recipient's monozygotic twin is called **isogeneic**, while a **xenogeneic** donation involves a donor and recipient who are of different species. Synthetic organ and tissue replacements are referred to as **prosthetics**.

YOU CODE IT! CASE STUDY

Ilani Marhefka, a 31-year-old female, came in to donate her eggs. Her sister, Serita, had lesions on her ovaries and had to have them removed many years ago. Dr. Stark is going to harvest eggs from Ilani to implant in Serita so she and her husband, Jude, can have children. Ilani wanted to help her sister and brother-in-law by donating her eggs.

You Code It!

Go through the steps of coding, and determine the code or codes that should be reported for this encounter between Dr. Stark and Ilani.

Step #1: Read the case carefully and completely.
Step #2: Abstract the scenario. Which main words or terms describe why the physician cared for the patient during this encounter?
Step #3: Are there any details missing or incomplete for which you would need to query the physician? [If so, ask your instructor.]
Step #4: Check for any relevant guidance, including reading all of the symbols and notations in the Tabular List and the appropriate sections of the Official Guidelines.
Step #5: Determine the correct diagnosis code or codes to explain why this encounter was medically necessary.
Step #6: Double-check your work.

Answer:

Did you determine this to be the correct code?

Z52.811 Egg (oocyte) donor under age 35, designated recipient

Very good!

Of course, prior to the actual procedure to harvest the organ or tissue, an examination will need to be done, reported with code Z00.5 Encounter for examination for potential donor of organ or tissue.

19.7 Resistance to Antimicrobial Drugs

You learned about antimicrobial resistance (AMR) in the chapter about coding infectious diseases. Let's review these codes again, just to reinforce how to report these situations using Z codes.

Take a look at code category Z16 Resistance to antimicrobial drugs. You can see that ICD-10-CM provides a note with some direction about the proper use of these Z codes:

> ***NOTE:*** **The codes in this category are provided for use as additional codes to identify the resistance and non-responsiveness of a condition to antimicrobial drugs.**

And you can see the ***Code first*** **the infection** notation that provides sequencing direction.

Z16.10 Resistance to unspecified beta lactam antibiotics

Z16.11 Resistance to penicillins (amoxicillin) (ampicillin)

Z16.12 Extended spectrum beta lactamase (ESBL) resistance

Z16.19 Resistance to other specified beta lactam antibiotics (cephalosporins)

Z16.20 Resistance to unspecified antibiotic (antibiotics NOS)

Z16.21 Resistance to vancomycin

Z16.22 Resistance to vancomycin related antibiotics

Z16.23 **Resistance to quinolones and fluoroquinolones**

Z16.24 **Resistance to multiple antibiotics**

Z16.29 **Resistance to other single specified antibiotic (aminoglycosides) (macrolides) (sulfonamides) (tetracylines)**

Z16.342 **Resistance to multiple antimycobacterial drugs**

Z16.35 **Resistance to multiple antimicrobial drugs** EXCLUDES1 **resistance to multiple antibiotics only (Z16.24)**

Reporting these conditions is not exclusive to the Z code chapter. When a patient is confirmed to have an infection that is resistant, you might report one of these codes instead:

A41.02 **Sepsis due to methicillin resistant Staphylococcus aureus**

A49.02 **Methicillin resistant Staphylococcus aureus infection, unspecified site**

J15.212 **Pneumonia due to methicillin resistant Staphylococcus aureus**

And remember, back in the ***Coding Infectious Diseases*** chapter, you learned about using the additional codes to identify the bacterial or viral pathogen in a specific other infection, such as a urinary tract infection or infected laceration, by using an additional code from B95–B97, including these:

B95.61 **Methicillin susceptible Staphylococcus aureus infection as the cause of diseases classified elsewhere**

B95.62 **Methicillin resistant Staphylococcus aureus infection as the cause of diseases classified elsewhere**

These code descriptions change the language a bit, so you will need to know the difference between "resistant" and "susceptible." In this context:

- *Resistant* means that those certain antibiotics will not be effective in combating this pathogen.
- *Susceptible* (also referred to as *sensitive*) means that the named antibiotic is expected to be successful in killing off the infection.

YOU CODE IT! CASE STUDY

PATIENT: Paulina Stohl

PHYSICIAN REQUESTING THE CONSULT: Ada Carole, MD

REASON FOR CONSULTATION: Resistant infection.

CHIEF COMPLAINT: Fatigue.

HISTORY OF PRESENT ILLNESS: The patient is a 57-year-old female with a history of type 2 diabetes mellitus, pancreatitis, and chronic hepatitis C who presented with complaints of fever and generalized malaise. She was seen and evaluated by Dr. Koehler in the ED and subsequently admitted. Vital signs identified a low grade fever [99.8 F] and blood cultures taken in ED were positive for gram-positive cocci. In addition, urinalysis was positive for MRSA. Patient was given Zosyn, 3.375g q6h. Infectious disease was requested in for a consultation.

At bedside, the patient stated a cystoscopy was performed by her urologist for chronic obstructive uropathy. The following biopsy was negative for malignancy. A few days later, the patient began to experience generalized malaise and then experienced fever and chills. The urine culture taken in ED was noted to be positive for MRSA and one of two blood cultures was positive. Since admission 1 day ago, blood cultures were repeated, with positive results in both tests for gram-positive cocci in clusters.

FAMILY HISTORY: No immune dysfunction other than diabetes.

ALLERGIES: No known drug allergies.

REVIEW OF SYSTEMS: A 14-system review is as per history of present illness, otherwise negative.

CURRENT MEDICATIONS: List is reviewed.

PHYSICAL EXAMINATION:

(continued)

VITAL SIGNS: Upon my initial evaluation, patient has T 100.2 degrees Fahrenheit, pulse 104, respirations 20, and blood pressure 120/70.

GENERAL: Patient is alert and oriented x3, in no apparent distress at rest.

HEENT: Head is normocephalic and atraumatic. Extraocular muscle movements are intact. No scleral icterus. Oropharynx is clear.

NECK: Free of palpable adenopathy.

HEART: Regular at 100. No auscultated rub.

LUNGS: Clear to auscultation and percussion bilaterally. No rhonchi and no wheezing.

ABDOMEN: Positive bowel sounds, soft, nontender, and nondistended. No rebound, rigidity, or guarding.

EXTREMITIES: Lower extremities are without clubbing or cyanosis.

NEUROMUSCULAR: Neurologically, patient is nonfocal with normal cranial nerves. Muscle strength is normal in the upper extremities.

LABORATORY STUDIES: A complete blood count, basic metabolic profile, full microbiologic database, all of which have been reviewed.

IMPRESSION:

1. Methicillin-resistant *Staphylococcus aureus* urinary tract infection in a patient who has recently undergone a genitourinary procedure for outlet obstruction.
2. Type 2 diabetes mellitus with poor control.
3. Fever.

RECOMMENDATIONS:

1. Place the patient in contact isolation.
2. Repeat blood cultures x2.
3. Start vancomycin.
4. Discontinue Zosyn [the extended-spectrum penicillin that has proved ineffective to patient's MRSA].

Thank you for this interesting consult and allowing us to participate in this patient's care.

Allen B. Dechante, MD

You Code It!

Read Dr. Dechante's notes regarding his evaluation of Paulina Stohl and determine the accurate ICD-10-CM diagnosis code or codes for this encounter.

Step #1: Read the case carefully and completely.
Step #2: Abstract the scenario. Which main words or terms describe why the physician cared for the patient during this encounter?
Step #3: Are there any details missing or incomplete for which you would need to query the physician? [If so, ask your instructor.]
Step #4: Check for any relevant guidance, including reading all of the symbols and notations in the Tabular List and the appropriate sections of the Official Guidelines.
Step #5: Determine the correct diagnosis code or codes to explain why this encounter was medically necessary.
Step #6: Double-check your work.

Answer:

Did you determine these to be the codes?

N39.0 **Urinary tract infection, site not specified**

B95.62 **Methicillin resistant Staphylococcus aureus infection as the cause of diseases classified elsewhere**

E11.9 **Type 2 diabetes mellitus without complication**

19.8 Z Codes as First-Listed/Principal Diagnosis

During most encounters, a Z code may be the only code you report, or it may be reported along with others, determined by the specific circumstances. Except for 20 of the Z codes, sequencing is determined by the facts of the encounter and the Official Guidelines, as explained in Sections II and III. The other 20 Z codes are permitted to be *only* first-listed or principal diagnosis codes:

Z00	**Encounter for general examination without complaint, suspected or reported diagnosis**
Z01	**Encounter for other special examination without complaint, suspected or reported diagnosis**
Z02	**Encounter for administrative examination**
Z03	**Encounter for medical observation for suspected diseases and conditions ruled out**
Z04	**Encounter for examination and observation for other reasons**
Z31.81	**Encounter for male factor infertility in female patient**
Z31.83	**Encounter for assisted reproductive fertility procedure cycle**
Z31.84	**Encounter for fertility preservation procedure**
Z33.2	**Encounter for elective termination of pregnancy**
Z34	**Encounter for supervision of normal pregnancy**
Z38	**Liveborn infants according to place of birth and type of delivery**
Z39	**Encounter for maternal postpartum care and examination**
Z40	**Encounter for prophylactic surgery**
Z42	**Encounter for plastic and reconstructive surgery following medical procedure or healed injury**
Z51.0	**Encounter for antineoplastic radiation therapy**
Z51.1-	**Encounter for antineoplastic chemotherapy and immunotherapy**
Z52	**Donors of organs and tissues *Except:* Z52.9, Donor of unspecified organ or tissue**
Z76.1	**Encounter for health supervision and care of foundling**
Z76.2	**Encounter for health supervision and care of other healthy infant and child**
Z99.12	**Encounter for respirator [ventilator] dependence during power failure**

GUIDANCE CONNECTION

Read the ICD-10-CM Official Guidelines for Coding and Reporting, section **I. Conventions, General Coding Guidelines and Chapter-Specific Guidelines**, subsection **C. Chapter-Specific Coding Guidelines**, chapter **21. Factors Influencing Health Status and Contact with Health Services**, subsection **c.16) Z codes that may only be principal/first-listed diagnosis**.

LET'S CODE IT! SCENARIO

Alfredo "Al" Martinelli, a 43-year-old male, was admitted to the hospital today because he is donating one of his kidneys to his son Anthony. The surgery is scheduled for this afternoon.

Let's Code It!

Even though he is perfectly healthy, Alfredo Martinelli is admitted into the hospital. Why? Because he is an organ donor. You don't have too much information here, so how will you look this up? Turn in the ICD-10-CM Alphabetic Index to

Donor (organ or tissue) Z52.9

(continued)

Read down the indented list beneath and find:

kidney Z52.4

This appears to be very straightforward, so go to the code category in the Tabular List:

✓4 **Z52 Donors of organs and tissues**

Directly below this you will see INCLUDES and EXCLUDES1 notations. Good that you saw these. Read them carefully. Alfredo is definitely a living donor. Is this "autologous"? In transplantation, the term "autologous" means that the donor and the recipient are the same person. This is not the case here because Alfredo is donating to his son. Does this mean you cannot use a code from this code category? Remember that the term "and" also means "and/or," so because Alfredo is a living donor, this situation is included here. What about the EXCLUDES1 notation? Is Alfredo here to be examined as a "potential" donor? No, it is evident that this has been done previously because Alfredo is here to donate, and the surgery is scheduled. Good! So, you can now read all of the fourth-character options and determine which is accurate for this encounter. . . .

Now you can report, with confidence, this code to specify the medical necessity for Alfredo's admission into the hospital.

Z52.4 Kidney donor

Good job!

19.9 Social Determinants of Health

There are circumstances found in patients' everyday lives that will directly affect their health and their ability to get healthy and stay healthy. These factors can range from an individual's education and literacy level to their housing and other economic considerations, and so much more. The path to health equity begins with knowing what these factors are, so we can then, as a society, address them. To this end, these Z code categories have been created, so when the physician or provider has documented these details, we can code/report them. Only then, can the data be analyzed and used to make the healthcare system work with greater consistency. For these purposes, medical coding professionals can collect these details from the physician's notes as well as patient self-reported influences, and notes from social workers, community healthcare workers, case managers, and nurses, as long as they are documented in the patient's official medical record. Include as many SDOH codes as necessary to represent all social problems, conditions, and/or risk factors the provider has documented.

GUIDANCE CONNECTION

Read the ICD-10-CM Official Guidelines for Coding and Reporting, section **I. Conventions, General Coding Guidelines and Chapter-Specific Guidelines**, subsection **C. Chapter-Specific Coding Guidelines**, chapter **21. Factors Influencing Health Status and Contact with Health Services**, subsection **17) Social Determinants of Health.**

Social determinants of health codes are located primarily in these ten Z code categories:

Z55 Problems related to education and literacy

Z56 Problems related to employment and unemployment

Z57 Occupational exposure to risk factors

Z58 Problems related to physical environment

Z59 Problems related to housing and economic circumstances

Z60 Problems related to social environment

Z62 Problems related to upbringing

Z63 Other problems related to primary support group, including family circumstances

Z64 Problems related to certain psychosocial circumstances

Z65 Problems related to other psychosocial circumstances

Chapter Summary

As a professional coder, you are responsible to ensure that every physician-patient encounter is supported as medically necessary. You probably know from your own personal experience that there are legitimate reasons for a healthy person to seek the attention of a physician or other health care professional. In ICD-10-CM, virtually all of the codes used to explain these valid reasons are found in the Z code chapter. Here, you will find codes to report the medical necessity for providing preventive care services, performing a screening, observing a patient, and checking for the viability of a potential organ donor.

CODING BITES

Free Preventive Services under Affordable Care Act

All marketplace plans and many other plans must cover the following list of preventive services without charging you a copayment or coinsurance. This is true even if you haven't met your yearly deductible. This applies only when these services are delivered by a network provider.

1. *Abdominal aortic aneurysm one-time screening* for men of specified ages who have ever smoked.
2. *Alcohol misuse screening and counseling.*
3. *Aspirin use* to prevent cardiovascular disease for men and women of certain ages.
4. *Blood pressure screening* for all adults.
5. *Cholesterol screening* for adults of certain ages or at higher risk.
6. *Colorectal cancer screening* for adults over 45–75.
7. *Depression screening* for adults.
8. *Diabetes (type 2) screening* for adults 40 to 70 years who are overweight or obese.
9. *Diet counseling* for adults at higher risk for chronic disease.
10. Fall prevention for adults 65 years and over.
11. Hepatitis B screening for people high risk.
12. Hepatitis C screening aged 15–65 years.
13. *HIV screening* for everyone ages 15 to 65, and other ages at increased risk.
14. PrEP (pre-exposure prophylaxis) HIV prevention medication
15. *Immunization vaccines* for adults—doses, recommended ages, and recommended populations vary:
    - Diphtheria
    - Hepatitis A
    - Hepatitis B
    - Herpes zoster
    - Human papillomavirus
    - Influenza (flu shot)
    - Measles
    - Meningococcal
    - Mumps
    - Pertussis
    - Pneumococcal
    - Rubella
    - Shingles
    - Tetanus
    - Varicella
16. Lung cancer screening for adults 50–80 years at high risk.
17. Obesity screening and counseling.
18. Sexually transmitted infection (STI) prevention counseling.
19. Statin preventive medication for adults 40 to 75 years.
20. Syphilis screening for adults at higher risk.
21. Tobacco use screening and cessation interventions for tobacco users.
22. Tuberculosis screening.

Source: "Preventive Health Benefits," https://www.healthcare.gov/what-are-my-preventive-care-benefits/

CHAPTER 19 REVIEW
Factors Influencing Health Status (Z Codes)

Let's Check It! Terminology

Match each key term to the appropriate definition.

1. **LO 19.6** The donor and recipient individuals are genetically identical.
2. **LO 19.3** An individual infected with a disease who is not ill but can still pass it to another person; an individual with an abnormal gene that can be passed to a child, making the child susceptible to disease.
3. **LO 19.2** Test results that indicate a disease or condition may be present.
4. **LO 19.6** The donor and recipient are of different species.
5. **LO 19.2** An examination or test of a patient who has no signs or symptoms that is conducted with the intention of finding any evidence of disease as soon as possible, thus enabling better patient outcomes.
6. **LO 19.6** Lost tissue that is replaced with synthetic materials such as metal, plastic, or ceramic.
7. **LO 19.6** The donor tissue is taken from a different site on the same individual's body.
8. **LO 19.1** Health-related services designed to stop the development of a disease or injury.
9. **LO 19.6** The donor and recipient are of the same species.

A. Abnormal Findings
B. Allogeneic
C. Autologous
D. Carrier
E. Isogeneic
F. Preventive Care
G. Prosthetic
H. Screening
I. Xenogeneic

Let's Check It! Concepts

Choose the most appropriate answer for each of the following questions.

1. **LO 19.2** The patient, a 38-year-old adult, presents for an annual physical examination, without abnormal findings. You would use code _____.
   a. Z00.00 **b.** Z01.00 **c.** Z00.2 **d.** Z00.70
2. **LO 19.1** When the patient has a preventive care encounter, you will use a _____ code.
   a. W **b.** Z **c.** X **d.** Y
3. **LO 19.6** If the donor and recipient are of different species, the graft is
   a. isogeneic. **b.** allogeneic. **c.** xenogeneic. **d.** autologous.
4. **LO 19.2** Abnormal findings are
   a. test results that indicate a disease or condition may be present.
   b. test results that are negative.
   c. test results showing that the donor and recipient are of the same species.
   d. test results that are inconclusive.
5. **LO 19.8** All of the following "Z" codes can be reported as the principal diagnosis except _____.
   a. Z00 **b.** Z33.2 **c.** Z76.2 **d.** Z46.0
6. **LO 19.6** James Davis presents today to donate his bone marrow. How would you code this?
   a. Z52.3 **b.** Z52.21 **c.** Z52.29 **d.** Z52.20
7. **LO 19.3** An individual has been found to be a typhoid carrier. How would you code this?
   a. Z22.1 **b.** A01.00 **c.** A01.03 **d.** Z22.0
8. **LO 19.5** The patient presents today to have his surgical wound dressing changed. What code would you use?
   a. Z48.00 **b.** Z48.01 **c.** Z48.02 **d.** Z48.03

9. **LO 19.4** If a patient is without signs or symptoms and is being watched for a suspected illness, then the patient is under

   a. preventive care. **b.** observation. **c.** continuous care. **d.** aftercare.

10. **LO 19.7** Ben Harris, an 8-year-old male, has an ear infection. Dr. Whitman prescribed a round of penicillin, but Ben's condition has not improved. Ben's infection is resistant to penicillin. You would first code the infection and then code _____.

   a. Z16.10 **b.** Z16.11 **c.** Z16.21 **d.** Z16.22

Let's Check It! Guidelines

Part I

Refer to the Official Guidelines and fill in the blanks according to ***Chapter 21****, Factors Influencing Health Status and Contact with Health Services, Chapter-Specific Coding Guidelines.*

first-listed	secondary	any
screening	present	past
potential	Z	carrier
procedure	specifically	higher
depending	Family	no
sequelae	not	

1. _____ codes are for use in _____ health care setting.
2. Z codes may be used as either a _____ (principal diagnosis code in the inpatient setting) or secondary code, _____ on the circumstances of the encounter.
3. Z codes are _____ procedure codes.
4. A corresponding _____ code must accompany a Z code to describe any procedure performed.
5. Contact/exposure codes may be used as a first-listed code to explain an encounter for testing, or, more commonly, as a _____ code to identify a potential risk.
6. Status codes indicate that a patient is either a _____ of a disease or has the _____ or residual of a past disease or condition.
7. Personal history codes explain a patient's _____ medical condition that _____ longer exists and is not receiving any treatment, but that has the _____ for recurrence, and therefore may require continued monitoring.
8. _____history codes are for use when a patient has a family member(s) who has had a particular disease that causes the patient to be at _____ risk of also contracting the disease.
9. A _____ code may be a first-listed code if the reason for the visit is _____ the screening exam.
10. The observation codes are not for use if an injury or illness or any signs or symptoms related to the suspected condition are _____.

Part II

Z40	routine	support
surveillance	continued	living
multiple	prophylactic	initial
aftermath	Z52	risk

1. Aftercare visit codes cover situations when the _____ treatment of a disease has been performed and the patient requires _____ care during the healing or recovery phase, or for the long-term consequences of the disease.
2. The follow-up codes are used to explain continuing _____ following completed treatment of a disease, condition, or injury.
3. A follow-up code may be used to explain _____ visits.
4. Codes in category _____, Donors of organs and tissues, are used for _____ individuals who are donating blood or other body tissue.

5. Counseling Z codes are used when a patient or family member receives assistance in the ____ of an illness or injury, or when ____ is required in coping with family or social problems.
6. The Z codes allow for the description of encounters for ____ examinations, such as, a general checkup, or, examinations for administrative purposes, such as, a preemployment physical.
7. For encounters specifically for ____ removal of an organ (such as prophylactic removal of breasts due to a genetic susceptibility to cancer or a family history of cancer), the principal or first-listed code should be a code from category ____, Encounter for prophylactic surgery, followed by the appropriate codes to identify the associated ____ factor (such as genetic susceptibility or family history).

Let's Check It! Rules and Regulations

Please answer the following questions from the knowledge you have gained after reading this chapter.

1. **LO 19.2** Why is early detection important? Include examples of early detection encounters.
2. **LO 19.3** Why is it important for a patient to know if they have a genetic susceptibility?
3. **LO 19.5** Why would a patient need continuing care or aftercare?
4. **LO 19.6** Explain the difference between *autologous*, *allogeneic*, and *xenogeneic*.
5. **LO 19.8** List 10 of the Z codes, including descriptions, that are permitted to be only first-listed or principal codes.

YOU CODE IT! Basics

First, identify the condition in the following diagnoses; then code the diagnosis.

Example: Awaiting organ transplant status:

a. main term: *Status* **b.** diagnosis: *Z76.82*

1. Encounter for disability limiting activities:
   a. main term:______ **b.** diagnosis:______
2. Encounter for screening for human papillomavirus:
   a. main term:______ **b.** diagnosis:______
3. Personal history of leukemia:
   a. main term:______ **b.** diagnosis:______
4. Genetic susceptibility to malignant neoplasm:
   a. main term:______ **b.** diagnosis:______
5. Contact with and suspected exposure to rubella:
   a. main term:______ **b.** diagnosis:______
6. Carrier of diphtheria:
   a. main term:______ **b.** diagnosis:______
7. Encounter for surveillance of injectable contraceptive:
   a. main term:______ **b.** diagnosis:______
8. Encounter for procreative management:
   a. main term:______ **b.** diagnosis:______
9. Encounter for fitting and adjustment of external right breast prosthesis:
   a. main term:______ **b.** diagnosis:______
10. Aftercare following explantation of knee joint:
    a. main term:______ **b.** diagnosis:______
11. Cornea donor:
    a. main term:______ **b.** diagnosis:______
12. High-risk bisexual behavior:
    a. main term:______ **b.** diagnosis:______
13. Acquired absence of left upper limb below elbow:
    a. main term:______ **b.** diagnosis:______
14. Encounter for examination of blood pressure without abnormal findings:
    a. main term:______ **b.** diagnosis:______
15. Presence of heart assist device:
    a. main term:______ **b.** diagnosis:______

YOU CODE IT! Practice

Using the techniques described in this chapter, carefully read through the case studies and determine the most accurate ICD-10-CM code(s) and external cause code(s), if appropriate, for each case study.

1. Donald DuFour, an 8-month-old male, is brought in by his mother and Kent Fuller to determine if Kent is the biological father. Don's mother is applying for child support and social welfare benefits and needs proof of the biological father before she can proceed. Dr. Sanderson completes a paternity test; results 99.99% that Kent is the biological father.
2. Jane Ellerbe, a 36-year-old female, presents today to see Dr. Molly, her dentist. Dr. Molly's dental hygienist cleans Jane's teeth and Dr. Molly completes a dental examination. Dr. Molly notes no abnormalities.
3. Charles Copeland, a 48-year-old male, presents today to see Dr. McElmurray. Charles is scheduled to have a cardiac pacemaker implanted. Dr. McElmurray completes the pre-procedural cardiovascular examination and clears Charles for the implant.
4. Betty Junketer, a 32-year-old female, was plugging in a light fixture at work when it shocked her badly. She was taken to the ER by the office manager. After the appropriate tests were completed, Dr. Peterson, the ER physician, put Betty under observation.
5. Tammy Coco, a 33-year-old female, went on a tour of 19th-century buildings last week. The company that conducted the tour just announced asbestos was found in some of these buildings. Tammy comes to see Dr. Kiefer today because she is concerned she might have been exposed to asbestos. Dr. Kiefer completes the appropriate tests, which return a negative result for asbestos exposure.
6. Kelly Richardson, a 46-year-old female, comes in today with the complaints of painful and burning urination. Dr. Keyton completes the appropriate tests and diagnoses Kelly with a UTI due to *Staphylococcus aureus;* the culture shows the UTI is resistant tovancomycin.
7. Connie Burton, a 63-year-old female, presents today for a screening for malignant neoplasm of the ovaries. Connie's mother died at age 58 of ovarian cancer. Dr. Bales performs the screening; results were negative.
8. Bennie Cantrell, a 45-day-old male, is brought in by his parents for a well-baby check. Dr. Davis notes that Bennie's heel prick is slow to coagulate and stop bleeding. After the appropriate tests, Dr. Davis diagnoses Bennie with hemophilia A, symptomatic carrier.
9. Ross Risinger, a 47-year-old male, presents today for screening of a malignant neoplasm of the prostate. Ross's grandfather died of prostate cancer. Dr. Richardson completes the appropriate test; results were negative.
10. Nellie Preacher, a 27-year-old female, is in her second trimester of pregnancy, G2 P1. Nellie presents today for her regular checkup. Dr. Williams notes no abnormalities and tells Nellie she is doing fine.
11. Alexandra Smith, a 31-year-old female, presents today to donate blood platelets for her child, who has been diagnosed with thrombocytopenia.
12. Martha Henry, a 38-year-old female, was diagnosed with breast cancer. Martha had a mastectomy 1 month ago, and Dr. Martin chose to delay the breast reconstruction. Martha presents today for the breast reconstruction procedure.
13. Van Poteat, a 59-year-old male, was diagnosed with colon cancer and now has an end colostomy. Van comes to see Dr. Holland, who inspects and cleans the colostomy opening. Dr. Holland tells Van he is doing well.
14. Edwina Henning, a 61-year-old female, was diagnosed with atrial fibrillation and her cardiologist, Dr. Balestrero, prescribed heparin, an anticoagulant. Edwina is taking the heparin as prescribed and presents today for therapeutic drug monitoring.
15. Andrew Medders, a 12-year-old male, is brought in by his parents to see Dr. Hearn, his pediatrician. Andrew has been cross and having some temper tantrums. Dr. Hearn notes Andrew has yawned three times since he has been in the examination room. Dr. Hearn also notes minor periorbital dark circles and slight periorbital puffiness. Andrew admits he has not been sleeping well. Andrew is diagnosed with sleep deprivation.

(continued)

YOU CODE IT! Application

The following exercises provide practice in abstracting physicians' notes and learning to work with documentation from our health care facility, Prader, Bracker, & Associates. These case studies are modeled on real patient encounters. Using the techniques described in this chapter, carefully read through the case studies and determine the most accurate ICD-10-CM code(s) and external cause code(s), if appropriate, for each case study.

PRADER, BRACKER, & ASSOCIATES

A Complete Health Care Facility

159 Healthcare Way • SOMEWHERE, FL 32811 • 407-555-6789

PATIENT: ELLIOTT, ELLYN

ACCOUNT/EHR #: ELLIEL001

Attending Physician: Oscar R. Prader, MD

S: Patient is a 27-year-old female who came in for a physical. I last saw this patient approximately 1 month ago when she received her annual flu shot. She is starting a new job on the first of next month and is required by her employment contract to get a complete physical including blood pressure check, cholesterol screening, blood glucose levels, tetanus-diphtheria and acellular pertussis (TdAP), and flu vaccine.

O: Vital signs charted by the nurse, including BMI. Finger stick glucose test was normal, showing there were no indications of patient being prediabetic. Cholesterol screening is within normal limits. The TdAP immunization was administered on 5/24/2019. The flu vaccine was administered on 09/14/2023.

A: Preemployment examination.

P: Form completed, and attached the documentation showing the TdAP and flu administration dates, and signed it.

Determine the most accurate ICD-10-CM code(s).

WESTON HOSPITAL

629 Healthcare Way • SOMEWHERE, FL 32811 • 407-555-6541

PATIENT: GALLOP, MICHAEL

ACCOUNT/EHR #: GALLMI001

Attending Physician: Renee O. Bracker, MD

S: Neonate was born 8 hours ago via spontaneous vaginal delivery, full-term, this hospital.

O: Newborn screening exam performed in the well-baby nursery included pulse oximetry showing normal percentage of hemoglobin in his blood that is saturated with oxygen. However, the test for hypothyroidism was positive. Prior to discharge, I met with the parents and explained this condition and discussed thyroxine, the medication required so the baby can avoid problems such as slowed growth and brain damage.

A: Congenital hypothyroidism without goiter

P: Rx: Thyroxine

Follow-up in office in 2 days

Determine the most accurate ICD-10-CM code(s).

(continued)

PRADER, BRACKER, & ASSOCIATES

A Complete Health Care Facility

159 Healthcare Way • SOMEWHERE, FL 32811 • 407-555-6789

PATIENT: BELLOW, SANDRA

ACCOUNT/EHR #: BELLSA001

Attending Physician: Oscar R. Prader, MD

Patient and her husband, Wayne, are thinking about starting a family, so they came in to learn about genetic screenings. They wanted to get all the information possible before Sandra gets pregnant so preparations can be employed to have a healthy child. I counseled them and discussed many options. Both Sandra and Wayne decided to complete a preconception genetic test, and family histories were reviewed.

Determine the most accurate ICD-10-CM code(s).

PRADER, BRACKER, & ASSOCIATES

A Complete Health Care Facility

159 Healthcare Way • SOMEWHERE, FL 32811 • 407-555-6789

PATIENT: LESZEK, OGLEV

ACCOUNT/EHR #: LESZOG001

Attending Physician: Renee O. Bracker, MD

S: This 13-year-old male was last seen in this office for his back-to-school annual exam 3 months ago. This exam revealed a healthy young man without any significant medical history.

Today Oglev presents complaining of a cough and a sore throat, of approximately 1-week duration. He is accompanied by his mother. He and his mother deny fever, nasal congestion, or runny nose. He says he feels more tired than usual, and his mom states that she can't get him out of bed to go to school. Oglev has been truant from school over the last 6 weeks. Patient states that his "mom won't get off my back." He admits that his grades have been dropping and he quit the baseball team. Mom leaves the room, and patient admits to smoking pot every day, sometimes several times a day, for the last month or so. He denies any other drug use and states smoking pot is "no big deal."

O: Physical examination is remarkable only for a mildly erythematous throat without petechiae. Lungs are clear, and the rest of his exam is normal. Vital signs are also unremarkable.

COUNSELING: Patient is assured that physician-patient confidentiality is secure. We discussed side effects and risks of abusing pot. He states he has tried to quit but can't make it through an entire day without smoking. It is pointed out to him that his pot use is already having a negative impact on his life. He understands that his parents need to know about this but that he must tell them himself. We discussed options and methodologies for his quitting with reduced effects. He agrees to regular surveillance.

A: Marijuana abuse counseling

P: Refer to drug counselor

Determine the most accurate ICD-10-CM code(s).

(continued)

PRADER, BRACKER, & ASSOCIATES

A Complete Health Care Facility

159 Healthcare Way • SOMEWHERE, FL 32811 • 407-555-6789

PATIENT: MONETS, ARNOLD

ACCOUNT/EHR #: MONEAR001

Attending Physician: Oscar R. Prader, MD

S: Patient is a 37-year-old male who came to our office for his annual physical exam. Blood was taken and processed in our in-house lab while the rest of the exam was completed. The results of his blood work revealed a random elevated transferrin saturation of 82%.

O: Past Medical History: Noncontributory

Family History: Noncontributory

Social History: Active; states he works out in the gym three times a week; apparently healthy; married for 4 years to Valerie, no children. He states that his wife gives him a multivitamin daily, but he is not certain which one or its exact contents. His diet includes raw oysters on the half shell and sushi about once a week; denies eating red meat or organ meat; drinks coffee, about three cups a day, but denies drinking teas or caffeinated beverages.

Physical Exam: Unremarkable; Height: 6′1″; Weight: 215 lb.; Vital signs: within normal limits.

A: Hemochromatosis

P: Quantitative phlebotomy of 500 mL of whole blood per week for an estimated 5 months.

Regular monitoring via blood tests every month: serum ferritin, hemoglobin, and hematocrit over the course of the phlebotomy treatments.

Dietary modifications, including elimination of all iron supplements and multivitamins containing iron, as well as no more consumption of raw shellfish.

Determine the most accurate ICD-10-CM code(s).

20

Inpatient (Hospital) Diagnosis Coding

Key Terms

Co-morbidity
Complication
Concurrent Coding
Diagnosis-Related Group (DRG)
Hospital-Acquired Condition (HAC)
Major Complication and Co-morbidity (MCC)
Present-On-Admission (POA)
Uniform Hospital Discharge Data Set (UHDDS)

Learning Outcomes

After completing this chapter, the student should be able to:

LO 20.1 Evaluate concurrent and discharge coding methodologies.
LO 20.2 Utilize the Official Guidelines specific for inpatient reporting.
LO 20.3 Apply the Present-On-Admission (POA) indicators properly.
LO 20.4 Determine the impact of diagnosis-related groups (DRGs) on the coding process.
LO 20.5 Recognize the importance of the Uniform Hospital Discharge Data Set (UHDDS).

STOP! Remember, you need to follow along in your ICD-10-CM code book for an optimal learning experience.

20.1 Concurrent and Discharge Coding

Concurrent Coding
System in which coding processes are performed while a patient is still in the hospital receiving care.

Some acute care facilities have patients who may spend weeks or months in the hospital. In these cases, professional coding specialists may do what is called **concurrent coding**. This means that coders actually go up to the nurse's station on the floor of the hospital and code from the patient's chart while the patient is still in the hospital. Concurrent coding enables the hospital to gain reimbursement to date without having to wait until the patient is discharged, improving cash flow for the facility. **Figure 20-1** shows you an example of progress notes that might be found in a patient's chart. A coder performing concurrent coding would read these, as well as other documentation, to determine what diagnoses to report.

Once a patient is discharged, you will go through the complete patient record. The most important documentations to look for include:

- *Discharge summary or discharge progress notes*, signed by the attending physician.
- *Hospital course*, which is a summary of the patient's hospital stay.
- *Discharge instructions*, a copy of which is given to the patient.
- *Discharge disposition*, which contains orders for the patient to be transferred home with special services, transferred to another facility, etc.
- *The death/discharge summary*, which is used if the patient expired prior to discharge.

All of these documents should be reviewed to provide you with a complete picture of what procedures, services, and treatments were provided to the patient, along with signs, symptoms, and diagnoses to support medical necessity.

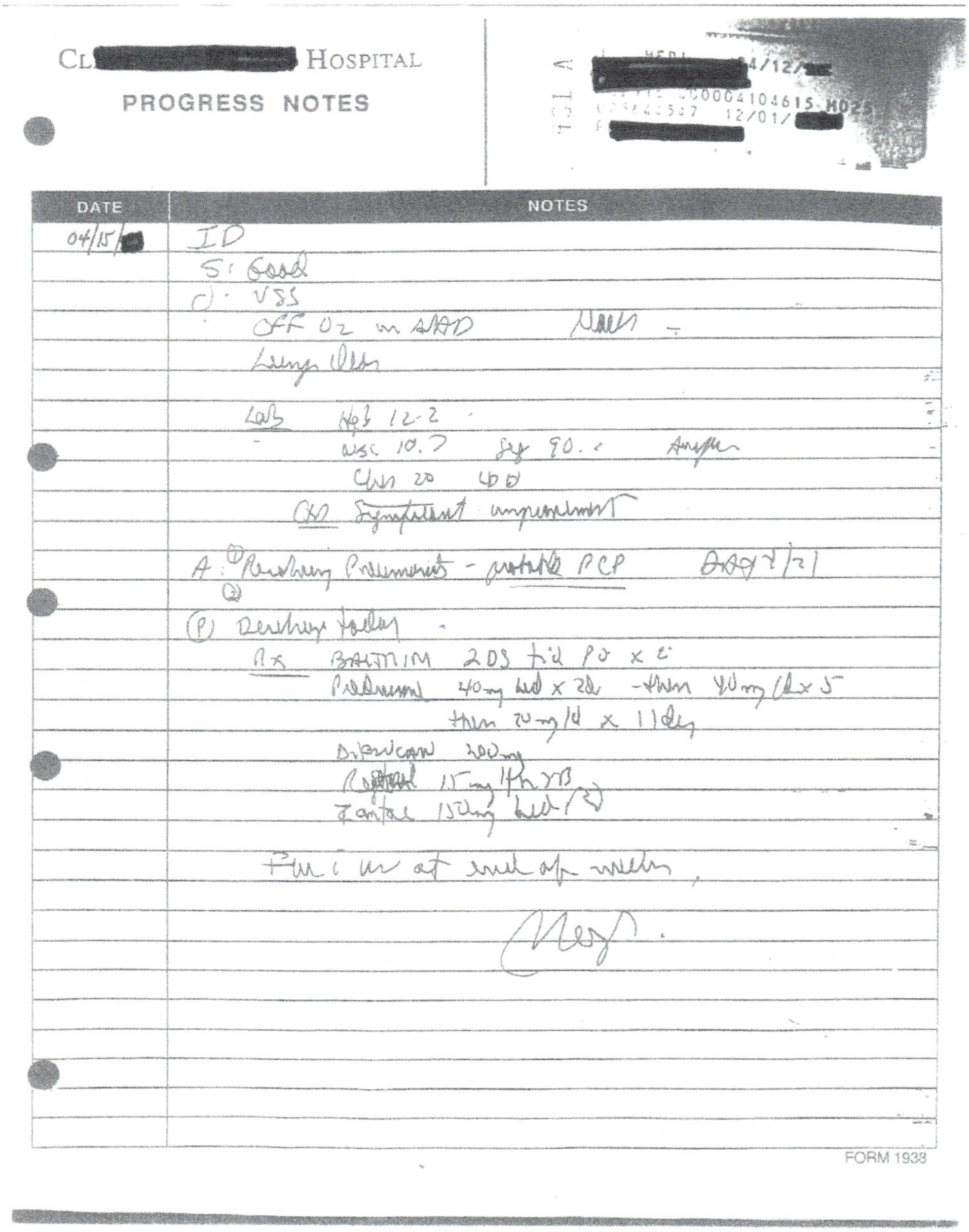

FIGURE 20-1 An example of a handwritten physician's progress note

LET'S CODE IT! SCENARIO

The attending physician, Raymond Morrison, MD, included this in the discharge summary:

Admission Diagnosis: Abdominal pain, status post appendectomy

Final Diagnosis: Abdominal pain, unknown etiology, status post appendectomy

Brief History: Patient underwent an appendectomy for perforated appendicitis 6 weeks ago. . . . Three days prior to admission, she had a recurrent bout of diffuse, dull abdominal pain in the right upper quadrant with associated nausea and anorexia. She was admitted to the hospital at the time for workup of this pain.

At this time, the patient has just had a regular meal without difficulty and feels like returning home. She will be discharged home at this time and can follow up with her primary MD. We will see her on an as-needed basis.

(continued)

Let's Code It!

This discharge documentation provides you the information you need to code the diagnosis supporting this patient's stay in the hospital. (To code the procedures, you would have to review the complete record.)

You have the admitting diagnosis and the final diagnosis. Remember, the Official Guidelines state that the principal diagnosis is "that condition established after study." This tells you that the final diagnosis would be used. You have two conditions to report: *abdominal pain, unknown etiology*, and *status post appendectomy*.

As always, begin in the Alphabetic Index, and find

Pain(s) – *see also* Painful R52

abdominal R10.9

Turn to the Tabular List to review the complete code description:

✓4 **R10 Abdomen and pelvis pain**

The EXCLUDES1 and EXCLUDES2 notations do not appear to include any diagnosis documented in these notes, so continue reading down the column to determine the most accurate fourth character:

✓5 **R10.1 Pain localized to upper abdomen**

Virtually all of the choices you have for the fifth character are specific to the location of the pain in the abdomen. Dr. Morrison did state that when the patient was admitted, she had "abdominal pain in the right upper quadrant," leading you to the fifth character 1. So, here is how this diagnosis code will be reported:

R10.11 Right upper quadrant pain

Are you done? Do you need to report that the patient was status post appendectomy? Yes, you do. It is not known if the pain is related to the surgical procedure or the condition for which it was performed. So let's turn back to the Alphabetic Index and look up

Status (post) – *see also* Presence (of)

Appendectomy is not listed. What can you look up? Think about the patient status post: What exactly is an appendectomy? Surgery. No, *surgery* is not listed in this index either. Hmmmm. Try looking at *postsurgical*. Aha!

Status (post) – *see also* Presence (of)

postsurgical (postprocedural) NEC Z98.890

(*Postoperative NEC* is also shown, leading to the same code.)

Let's turn to the Z code section and check this code out:

✓4 **Z98 Other postprocedural states**

The EXCLUDES2 notes don't relate to this discharge summary, so continue reading down the column to find the correct fourth character. No other fourth character is accurate to report postappendectomy, so let's take a look at what the Alphabetic Index suggested:

✓5 **Z98.8 Other specified postprocedural status**

✓6 **Z98.89 Other specified postprocedural states**

Z98.890 Other specified postprocedural states

When you review the other procedures included in this classification, none seem to relate to an appendectomy. This code description is the most accurate of those available. Therefore, these are the diagnosis codes you will report for this case:

R10.11 Right upper quadrant pain

Z98.890 Other specified postprocedural states

Good job!

> **CODING BITES**
>
> What about the part of the diagnosis where Dr. Morrison wrote "Abdominal pain, *unknown etiology*"? How is that reported? Notice that the code R10.11 for the abdominal pain is located in the ICD-10-CM code book's ***Chapter 18: Symptoms, Signs, and Abnormal Clinical and Laboratory Conditions, Not Elsewhere Classified***. This is the part that reports the physician could not determine the cause (etiology) of the pain. Had the cause of the pain been identified, you would be reporting that with a different code.

20.2 Official Coding Guidelines

In the front of your ICD-10-CM code book are the Official Coding Guidelines. Included are some specific directions that focus on inpatient coding, rather than on outpatient coding or both. They are always at your fingertips, right there in your code book, but please become familiar with them, so you can gain confidence to use them correctly.

Uncertain Diagnosis

Remember, you learned for *out*patient coding (as shown in *Section IV, subsection H. Uncertain diagnosis*) that you are *not permitted* to ever code something identified by the physician in their documentation as "rule out," "probable," "possible," "suspected," or other similar terms of an unconfirmed nature.

For *in*patient coding, this guidance (as shown in *Section II, subsection H. Uncertain diagnosis*) is different.

> **GUIDANCE CONNECTION**
>
> Read the ICD-10-CM Official Guidelines for Coding and Reporting, section **II. Selection of Principal Diagnosis**, subsection **H. Uncertain diagnosis**.

The guidance for inpatient coders is that you *are permitted* to "code the condition as if it existed or was established." This is done so that medical necessity can be reported for tests, observation, or other services and resources used to care for the patient whether or not these efforts resulted in a confirmed diagnosis.

Patient Receiving Diagnostic Services Only

> **GUIDANCE CONNECTION**
>
> Read the ICD-10-CM Official Guidelines for Coding and Reporting, section **III. Reporting Additional Diagnoses**, subsection **B. Abnormal findings**.

In the outpatient world, the guidelines instruct you to wait until the test results have been determined and interpreted by the physician as documented in the final report before coding. At that time, confirmed diagnoses, or the signs and symptoms that were documented as the reason for ordering the test, are reported.

When you are coding for inpatient services, abnormal test results are not reported unless the physician has documented the clinical significance of those results. Interestingly, in this section of the guidelines, it is reiterated that if the coding professional notices abnormal test results and documentation is unclear from the physician, it is "appropriate to ask the provider whether the abnormal finding should be added."

YOU CODE IT! CASE STUDY

The attending physician, Thomas Talbott, MD, included this in the discharge summary:

Admission Diagnosis: Acute cervical pain, admitted through ED after MVA

Final Diagnosis: Acute cervical pain and radiculitis secondary to degenerative disc disease with post-traumatic activation of pain

Brief History: Patient is a 41-year-old male who was involved in a motor vehicle accident, admitted after being brought to the ED by the ambulance that responded to the accident scene. Patient showed signs of neck and arm pain associated with cervical radiculopathy, radiating into the shoulders along with constant headaches. He has numbness and tingling into the hands and fingers.

(continued)

Radiology: X-rays AP and lateral cervical spinal x-rays demonstrate evidence of significant degenerative disc disease at C5–6 and C6–7 levels. MRI of cervical spine demonstrates evidence of significant degenerative disc disease at the C5–6 and C6–7 levels with osteophyte formation and canal compromise with the spinal canal diameter reduced to approximately 9 mm. Lumbar spine MRI demonstrates mild degenerative disc disease; otherwise normal.

Recommendation to patient is to undergo an anterior cervical diskectomy and fusion utilizing an autologous iliac bone grafting and placement of anterior titanium plate. After reviewing with patient regarding risks and benefits of surgery, the patient refused and requested to be discharged immediately.

You Code It!

In this case, the patient received only diagnostic services. Determine the most accurate diagnosis code or codes for this inpatient encounter.

Step #1: Read the case carefully and completely.
Step #2: Abstract the scenario. Which main words or terms describe why the physician cared for the patient during this encounter?
Step #3: Are there any details missing or incomplete for which you would need to query the physician? [If so, ask your instructor.]
Step #4: Check for any relevant guidance, including reading all of the symbols and notations in the Tabular List and the appropriate sections of the Official Guidelines.
Step #5: Determine the correct diagnosis code or codes to explain why this encounter was medically necessary.
Step #6: Double-check your work.

Answer:

Did you determine the accurate codes?

M50.122 **Cervical disc disorder at C5–C6 level with radiculopathy**

M50.123 **Cervical disc disorder at C6–C7 level with radiculopathy**

G89.11 **Acute pain due to trauma**

V43.92XA **Unspecified car occupant injured in collision with other type car in traffic accident, initial encounter**

Good job!

20.3 Present-On-Admission Indicators

Present-On-Admission (POA) indicators are required for each diagnosis code reported on UB-04 and 837 institutional claim forms. They are used to report additional detail about the patient's condition.

Centers for Medicare and Medicaid Services (CMS), in CR5499, requires a POA indicator for every diagnosis appearing on a claim from an acute care facility. Claims are returned stamped "unpaid" to the facility if POA indicators are not included. Hospitals are permitted to enter the POA indicators and refile the claim; however, think about all the time and work wasted by having to do this.

Present-On-Admission (POA)
A one-character indicator reporting the status of the diagnosis at the time the patient was admitted to the acute care facility.

GUIDANCE CONNECTION

Read the ICD-10-CM Official Guidelines for Coding and Reporting, **Appendix I. Present on Admission Reporting Guidelines**.

General Reporting Guidelines

According to CMS Publication 100-04, "*Present on admission is defined as present at the time the order for inpatient admission occurs—conditions that develop during an outpatient encounter, including emergency department, observation, or outpatient surgery, are considered as present on admission.*"

CODING BITES

A POA indicator is required to be assigned to the principal diagnosis codes as well as all secondary diagnoses, including external cause of injury codes.

What does this mean? This means professional coders must carefully review the admitting physician's history and physical (H&P)–the documentation that supports the order to admit the patient into the hospital (see **Figure 20-2** for an example)–to determine whether or not the condition was identified at that time. Then you will assign the POA indicator to report this fact: Yes–this diagnosis was present when the patient was admitted; No–it was not present; and so on.

Rm: PIC

STEPHEN

MR#

Date of Admission: 03/15/

ADMITTING DIAGNOSIS:
Chest pain.

HISTORY OF PRESENT ILLNESS: This 80-year-old black male presented to the emergency room with chest pain radiating to the back and shoulders. He was here at the emergency room within the past week with similar complaints.

PAST MEDICAL HISTORY: Coronary artery disease, noninsulin-dependent diabetes mellitus, hypertension, TURP.

SOCIAL HISTORY: Not available.

FAMILY HISTORY: Not available.

MEDICATIONS: Nitroglycerin, Naprosyn.

ALLERGIES: No known allergies.

REVIEW OF SYSTEMS: Not available.

PHYSICAL EXAMINATION

VITAL SIGNS: This 80-year-old black male admitted with temperature 96.8°, pulse 67, respirations 20, blood pressure 160/94.

SKIN: Skin turgor good.

EYES: Pupils react equally to light and distance.

ENT: No lesions noted.

NECK: Supple.

CHEST: Clear.

HEART: Regular rate and rhythm. No murmurs.

ABDOMEN: Soft and nontender.

History and Physical
1 of 2

ORIGINAL CHART COPY

FIGURE 20-2 An example of an admitting history and physical (H&P) (Page 1 of 2)

(continued)

Rm: PIC

STEPHEN

MR#

GENITALIA: Not done.

RECTAL: Not done.

EXTREMITIES: No edema.

NEUROLOGIC: Intact.

ADMISSION IMPRESSION:
1. Chest pain.
2. Noninsulin-dependent diabetes mellitus.
3. Hypertension.

TREATMENT PLAN: The patient went to the telemetry floor. He was seen in consultation by Dr. Dennis, cardiologist. CPK, LDH, troponin, q.8h. x 3, EKG daily x 3. He was given an inch of nitro paste q.6h. Further recommendations to follow.

PROGNOSIS: Guarded.

STEPHEN

SMS:rd 3847
d: 03/15/ 5:29 P
t: 03/16/ 7:09 A
cc: STEPHEN

History and Physical
2 of 2

ORIGINAL CHART COPY

FIGURE 20-2 An example of an admitting history and physical (H&P) (Page 2 of 2)

One reason for the importance of gathering POA data is to identify **hospital-acquired conditions (HACs)**. A hospital-acquired condition (HAC) is exactly what it sounds like: an illness or injury that the patient contracted solely due to the fact that they were in the hospital at the time. HAC data are used for many different purposes, including evaluating patient safety directives and limiting payment to a facility for errors it may have made that caused the problem.

Hospital-Acquired Condition (HAC)
A condition, illness, or injury contracted by the patient during their stay in an acute care facility; also known as *nosocomial condition.*

GUIDANCE CONNECTION

Go to:

www.cms.gov

> Medicare

. . . scroll down to . . .

> Hospital-Acquired Conditions (Present on Admission Indicator)

On the next screen, on the left side, click on the link ***Hospital-Acquired Conditions*** and then click on ***ICD-10 HAC LIST*** for a current list of the conditions included in this program.

https://www.cms.gov/medicare/payment/fee-for-service-providers/hospital-aquired-conditions-hac/icd-10

The ICD-10 HAC LIST actually shows you the diagnosis and then the procedures, with ICD-10-PCS codes included. Very interesting!

CODING BITES

POA indicators are not required for external cause codes unless the code is being reported as an "other diagnosis."

POA Indicators

The POA indicators are used to clearly identify whether or not the signs, symptoms, and diagnoses reported on the claim form were documented by the admitting physician at the time the patient was admitted into the hospital.

The indicators are Y, N, U, W, and 1:

- **Y** **Yes** This condition was documented by the admitting physician as present at the time of inpatient admission.

EXAMPLE

POA—"Y" Indicator

Felicia was admitted to the hospital from the emergency department with severe angina (chest pains), dyspnea (shortness of breath), and paresthesia (tingling) in her left arm. After all the tests were run, Dr. Gordon diagnosed her with an ST elevation, acute myocardial infarction (AMI) of the anterior wall, left main coronary artery; discussed diet, exercise, and medications; and discharged her. Reported with **I21.01 ST elevation (STEMI) myocardial infarction involving left main coronary artery** would be POA indicator Y because the signs and symptoms that caused her admission to the hospital were those of an AMI. Her heart attack was present on admission.

- **N** **No** This condition was *not* present at the time of inpatient admission.

CODING BITES

If any part of the diagnosis code description was NOT present at the time of admission, report this with an N.

EXAMPLE

POA—"N" Indicator

Porter was admitted with an esophageal ulcer that did not begin bleeding until after admission. Reported with code **K22.11 Ulcer of esophagus with bleeding** is POA indicator N because the entire description of this code was not present at admission.

- **U** **Unknown** Documentation from the admitting physician is insufficient to determine if the condition is present on admission.

EXAMPLE

POA—"U" Indicator

David was admitted to the hospital to have his tonsils removed due to his chronic tonsillitis. The second day, the physician noted a diagnosis of urinary tract infection (UTI) and ordered antibiotics. Upon discharge, code **J35.01 Chronic tonsillitis** will get POA indicator Y; however, code **N39.0 Urinary tract infection, site not specified**, would receive a U because the documentation is not clear whether the UTI was not present and developed while he was in the hospital or was present and not diagnosed when David was admitted.

CODING BITES

It is the responsibility of the physician or health care provider admitting the patient into the hospital to clearly document which conditions are POA. However, it is the professional coder's responsibility to query the physician if the documentation is incomplete with regard to this issue.

- **W** **Clinically Undetermined** Provider is unable to clinically determine whether the condition was present on admission or not.

EXAMPLE

POA—"W" Indicator

Torrie was admitted with diabetic gangrene. After a blood workup early on her third day in the hospital, the physician documented an additional diagnosis of septicemia. Upon discharge, the code for the diabetic gangrene (E11.52) would be reported with a POA of Y; however, the septicemia (A41.9) would receive POA indicator W because the physician documented that there is no way to be certain clinically whether the septicemia was not present and developed while she was in the hospital or present and not diagnosed when Torrie was admitted.

- **1** **Exempt**

You can find a list of the conditions, and their diagnosis codes, that are exempt from POA reporting in the Official Coding Guidelines in your ICD-10-CM book or on the CMS website. (*NOTE:* Some third-party payers prefer this box remain blank instead of using the numeral 1.)

EXAMPLE

POA—"Exempt" Diagnoses

Belinda was admitted to the hospital in full labor and delivered a beautiful baby boy the next morning. Upon discharge, both codes **O80 Normal delivery** and **Z37.0 Outcome of delivery, single liveborn**, are reported with POA indicator 1. You will notice that both of these codes are on the ***Categories and Codes Exempt from Diagnosis Present on Admission Requirement*** list shown on the CMS website at:

FY 2024 Present On Admission (POA) Exempt List (ZIP) . . . The website of the Centers for Medicare & Medicaid Services (CMS). The landing page outlines the coding guidelines and policies related to hospital-acquired conditions (HACs) for providers participating in Medicare.

GUIDANCE CONNECTION

Read the ICD-10-CM Official Guidelines for Coding and Reporting, **Appendix I, Present on Admission Reporting Guidelines**, subsection **Condition is on the "Exempt from Reporting" list**.

CODING BITES

The CDC website has the detailed list of ICD-10-CM codes that are exempt from (do not require) the use of a POA indicator:

The website of the Centers for Medicare & Medicaid Services (CMS). The landing page outlines the coding guidelines and policies related to hospital-acquired conditions (HACs) for providers participating in Medicare.

.. scroll to the bottom of the screen to find the Exempt List.

The conditions on this exempt list represent categories and/or codes for circumstances regarding the health care encounter or factors influencing health status that do not represent a current disease or injury or are always present on admission.

LET'S CODE IT! SCENARIO

Kimberly Byner was admitted into the hospital because she was suffering acute exacerbation of her obstructive chronic bronchitis. After 2 days of treatment, while still in the hospital, she tried to get out of bed without help, fell, and broke her left wrist.

Let's Code It!

The reason Kimberly was admitted into the hospital was because she was having exacerbation of her bronchitis. Therefore, the documentation (the physician's H&P) identifies this as being present when she was admitted:

J44.1 **Chronic obstructive pulmonary disease with (acute) exacerbation**
POA: Y

When she was discharged, Kimberly also had her wrist in a cast, due to the break suffered from her fall. This is very clearly a condition she did not have when she was admitted:

S62.102A **Fracture of unspecified carpal bone, left wrist, initial encounter**
POA: N

20.4 Diagnosis-Related Groups

Diagnosis-Related Group (DRG)
An episodic care payment system basing reimbursement to hospitals for inpatient services upon standards of care for specific diagnoses grouped by their similar usage of resources for procedures, services, and treatments.

In addition to dealing with diagnosis and procedure codes, hospitals must work with **diagnosis-related groups (DRGs)** for Medicare reimbursement, under Medicare Part A–Hospital Insurance. To determine how much an acute care facility will be paid, the Inpatient Prospective Payment System (IPPS) was developed. Within IPPS, each and every patient case is sorted into a DRG.

Each DRG has a payment weight assigned to it determined by the typical resources used to care for the patient in that case. This calculation includes the labor costs, such as nurses and technicians, as well as nonlabor costs, such as maintenance for equipment and supplies.

GUIDANCE CONNECTION

Go to:

www.cms.gov

> Medicare

. . . *scroll down to* . . .

> Acute Inpatient PPS

Here, along with the links on the left side, you will find up-to-date information on the Inpatient Prospective Payment System.

Typically, professional coding specialists do not have to worry about assigning the DRG for a patient's case. This is determined, most often, by a special software program known as a "DRG grouper."

Medicare-Severity Diagnosis-Related Groups (MS-DRGs) are a subset of 745 subclassifications used in the IPPS (Inpatient Prospective Payment System) that Medicare uses to determine reimbursement for services provided to Medicare beneficiaries by acute care health care facilities (hospitals). MS-DRGs are subdivided into three payment tiers based on the presence (or lack) of major complications and co-morbidities (MCC) and/or complications and co-morbidities (CC).

EXAMPLE

There are several other versions of DRG systems that focus on different details:

APR-DRG = All-Patient Refined Diagnosis-Related Group

APS-DRG = All-Patient Severity-Adjusted DRG

MS-LTC-DRG = Medicare-Severity—Long-Term Care DRG

R-DRG = Refined DRG

AP-DRG = All Patient DRG

S-DRG = Severity DRG

IR-DRG = International-Refined DRG

Principal Diagnosis

So why do you need to know all this? The *principal* diagnosis assigned is one of the factors used to determine which DRG is most accurate. Particularly when it comes to coding for reporting inpatient services to a Medicare beneficiary, the sequence in which you place the diagnosis codes can make a big difference in how accurately the hospital will be reimbursed.

GUIDANCE CONNECTION

Read the ICD-10-CM Official Guidelines for Coding and Reporting, section **II. Selection of Principal Diagnosis.**

Remember that the principal, or first-listed, diagnosis as defined by the guidelines is "that condition established after study to be chiefly responsible for occasioning the admission of the patient to the hospital for care." This is the diagnosis that explains the most serious reason for the patient to be in the hospital. This might be the reason for admission, it might be the most serious condition, or it might be the condition that required the greatest number of services, treatments, or procedures during the patient's stay in the hospital.

Complications and Co-morbidities

Complication
An unexpected illness or other condition that develops as a result of a procedure, service, or treatment provided during the patient's hospital stay.

As each diagnosis is evaluated for its standard of care, CMS understands that a patient in a hospital may have multiple conditions or concerns (signs, symptoms, diagnoses) that are interrelated and create a more complex need for care. These may be *complications and/or co-morbidities (CCs).*

In some cases, regardless of the precautions that may be taken, **complications** of a procedure or treatment may arise during the patient's stay. Such a condition must be coded and reported to support the medical necessity for the treatment provided to resolve the concern.

EXAMPLE

Lori had surgery this morning and is now having a bronchospasm, a reaction to the general anesthesia. This bronchospasm is a complication of the administration of general anesthesia and must be coded and reported to identify the medical necessity for the treatments to help alleviate this condition.

You have learned that a patient may have, or end up with, several different conditions treated during a stay in the hospital. The individual also may have preexisting conditions that have nothing to do with the reason for admission but still need attention by hospital personnel.

Co-morbidity
A separate diagnosis existing in the same patient at the same time as an unrelated diagnosis.

EXAMPLE

Henry was admitted into the hospital with appendicitis. During his stay, the physician had to order and the nurses had to continue to give Henry his Lipitor, prescribed for his preexisting hypercholesterolemia (high cholesterol). Even though this condition has nothing to do with the appendicitis or the appendectomy (surgery to remove the infected appendix), this **co-morbidity** must be coded and reported to support the medical necessity for the hospital supplying the medication.

Major Complication and Co-morbidity (MCC)
A complication or co-morbidity that has an impact on the treatment of the patient and makes care for that patient more complex.

Major Complications and Co-morbidities

Conditions, illnesses, and injuries come in all shapes and sizes, as well as severities, and so do complications and co-morbidities. Typically, a **major complication and co-morbidity (MCC)** is a condition that is systemic, making treatment for the principal diagnosis more complex and/or making the health concern life-threatening.

EXAMPLES

MS-DRG 799	Splenectomy with MCC	Weight: 4.7488
MS-DRG 800	Splenectomy with CC	Weight: 2.7250
MS-DRG 801	Splenectomy without CC or MCC	Weight: 1.7473

You can see how the presence, or absence, of MCC and/or CC alters the weight applied to the reimbursement for this procedure.

GUIDANCE CONNECTION

Read the ICD-10-CM Official Guidelines for Coding and Reporting, section **III. Reporting Additional Diagnoses**.

20.5 Uniform Hospital Discharge Data Set

Uniform Hospital Discharge Data Set (UHDDS)
A compilation of data collected by acute care facilities and other designated health care facilities.

The **Uniform Hospital Discharge Data Set (UHDDS)** is a collection of specific data gathered about hospital patients at discharge. No, this is not an invasion of privacy, nor is it a collection of personal data. The information pulled from hospital claim forms is related to demographic and clinical details.

Demographic data include

- *Gender.*
- *Age.*
- *Race and ethnicity.*
- *Geographic location.*
- *Provider information*, such as the hospital facility National Provider Identifier (NPI) as well as attending and operating physician(s).
- *Expected sources of payment*, including primary and other sources of payment for this care.
- *Length of stay (LOS)*, determined by date of admission and date of discharge.
- *Total charges billed by the hospital* for this admission (this will not include physician and other professional services billed).

Clinical data collected evaluate

- *Type of admission*, described as *scheduled* (planned in advance with preregistration at least 24 hours prior) or *unscheduled*.
- *Diagnoses*, including principal and additional diagnoses.
- *Procedures, services, and treatments provided* during this admission period.
- *External causes of injury*, determined by the reporting of external cause codes.

Definitions of these, and other, categories as determined by the UHDDS are used by ICD-10-CM in the Official Coding Guidelines. Over the years that the UHDDS has been in place, these definitions have been used to assist the reporting of patient data not only in acute care facilities (hospitals) but also for inpatient short-term care, long-term care, and psychiatric hospitals. Outpatient providers including home health agencies, nursing homes, and rehabilitation facilities also use these definitions for their data.

Chapter Summary

The coding process remains the same for inpatient and outpatient services for which coders are determining and reporting accurate diagnosis codes. The same code set, ICD-10-CM, is used; the same guidelines are used (with the exception of the two specific guidelines). Therefore, with the additional knowledge provided in this chapter, a professional coder can be successful in any type of facility.

CODING BITES

POA Reporting Options

Y = Yes
N = No
U = Unknown
W = Clinically undetermined
Unreported/Not used = Exempt from POA reporting

POA Reporting Definitions

Y = Present at the time of inpatient admission
N = Not present at the time of inpatient admission
U = Documentation is insufficient to determine if condition is present on admission
W = Provider is unable to clinically determine whether condition was present on admission or not

CHAPTER 20 REVIEW
Inpatient (Hospital) Diagnosis Coding

Let's Check It! Terminology

Match each key term to the appropriate definition.

1. **LO 20.4** A complication or co-morbidity that has an impact on the treatment of the patient and makes care for that patient more complex.
2. **LO 20.4** A separate condition or illness present in the same patient at the same time as another, unrelated condition or illness.
3. **LO 20.5** A compilation of data collected by acute care facilities and other designated health care facilities.

A. Co-morbidity
B. Complication
C. Concurrent Coding
D. Diagnosis-Related Group (DRG)

4. **LO 20.1** System in which coding processes are performed while a patient is still in the hospital receiving care.
5. **LO 20.3** A condition, illness, or injury contracted by the patient during their stay in an acute care facility; also known as a *nosocomial condition*.
6. **LO 20.4** An unexpected illness or other condition that develops as a result of a procedure, service, or treatment provided during the patient's hospital stay.
7. **LO 20.4** An episodic-care payment system basing reimbursement to hospitals for inpatient services upon standards of care for specific diagnoses grouped by their similar usage of resources for procedures, services, and treatments.
8. **LO 20.3** A one-character indicator reporting the status of the diagnosis at the time the patient was admitted to the acute care facility.

E. Hospital-Acquired Condition (HAC)
F. Major Complication and Co-morbidity (MCC)
G. Present-On-Admission (POA)
H. Uniform Hospital Discharge Data Set (UHDDS)

Let's Check It! Concepts

Choose the most appropriate answer for each of the following questions.

1. **LO 20.1** Which of the following is signed by the attending physician?
   a. Hospital course **b.** Discharge instructions **c.** Discharge summary **d.** Discharge disposition
2. **LO 20.2** Martha Jameson was found to have a breast lump during a mammogram last month. She is admitted today for a breast biopsy of her left breast. The pathology report returns with lower-inner quadrant breast carcinoma of the left breast. Martha's mother had breast cancer in her fifties. What is the correct code assignment?
   a. D05.12 **b.** D05.12, Z80.3 **c.** C50.312 **d.** C50.912, Z80.3
3. **LO 20.3** All of the following are POA indicators except
   a. X. **b.** Y. **c.** W. **d.** 1.
4. **LO 20.5** The UHDDS is a new code set that will replace ICD-10-CM in 2025.
   a. True **b.** False
5. **LO 20.3** Bobby was admitted into the hospital with a compound fracture of the left femur head. Three days later, during his stay, he developed pneumonia. The POA indicator for the pneumonia is
   a. Y. **b.** 1. **c.** W. **d.** N.
6. **LO 20.4** An example of a complication is a
   a. known allergy to penicillin. **b.** family history of breast cancer.
   c. high-risk pregnancy. **d.** postoperative wound infection.
7. **LO 20.2** Inpatient coders are not permitted to ever code something identified in the physician's notes as "suspected" or "probable."
   a. True **b.** False
8. **LO 20.5** The UHDDS collects all of these data elements except
   a. gender. **b.** credit card number. **c.** geographic location. **d.** age.
9. **LO 20.1** Once a patient is discharged, the coder will go through the complete patient record. The most important documentation to look for includes all of the following except
   a. the discharge summary. **b.** the hospital course.
   c. the discharge disposition. **d.** all of these documentations are important.
10. **LO 20.4** DRGs are used for reimbursement from Medicare to
    a. physician offices. **b.** acute care facilities.
    c. ambulatory surgical centers. **d.** walk-in clinics.

Let's Check It! Guidelines

Part I

Refer to the Official ICD-10-CM Guidelines and fill in the blanks according to Sections II and III.

inpatient	diagnostic	Abnormal
outside	one	principal
admitted	complete	discharge
not	unusual	worsens
ask	existed	established
equally	overemphasized	led

1. The circumstances of _____ admission always govern the selection of principal diagnosis.
2. The principal diagnosis is defined in the Uniform Hospital Discharge Data Set (UHDDS) as "that condition _____ after study to be chiefly responsible for occasioning the admission of the patient to the hospital for care."
3. The importance of consistent, _____ documentation in the medical record cannot be _____ .
4. Codes for symptoms, signs, and ill-defined conditions from Chapter 18 are _____ to be used as _____ diagnosis when a related definitive diagnosis has been established.
5. In the _____ instance when two or more diagnoses _____ meet the criteria for principal diagnosis as determined by the circumstances of admission, diagnostic workup and/or therapy provided, and the Alphabetic Index, Tabular List, or another coding guidelines does not provide sequencing direction, any _____ of the diagnoses may be sequenced first.
6. If the diagnosis documented at the time of _____ is qualified as "probable," "suspected," "likely," "questionable," "possible," or "still to be ruled out," or other similar terms indicating uncertainty, code the condition as if it _____ or was established.
7. When a patient is _____ to an observation unit for a medical condition, which either _____ or does not improve, and is subsequently admitted as an inpatient of the same hospital for this same medical condition, the principal diagnosis would be the medical condition which _____ to the hospital admission.
8. If the provider has included a diagnosis in the final _____ statement, such as the discharge summary or the face sheet, it should ordinarily be coded.
9. _____ findings (laboratory, x-ray, pathologic, and other diagnostic results) are not coded and reported unless the provider indicates their clinical significance.
10. If the findings are _____ the normal range and the attending provider has ordered other tests to evaluate the condition or prescribed treatment, it is appropriate to _____ the provider whether the abnormal finding should be added.

Part II

Go to www.cms.gov and click on the Medicare tab in the upper navigation bar. In the left column, select Payment. On the right side select Prospective Payment System. Scroll down to the related links and click on Acute Inpatient PPS. Fill in the blanks accordingly.

(IPPS)	add-on	approved	prospectively
census	diagnosis-related group	unusually	outlier
multiplied	added	divided	low-income
inpatient	qualify	wage	ratio
disproportionate	prospective	cost of living	average

1. Section 1886(d) of the Social Security Act (the Act) sets forth a system of payment for the operating costs of acute care hospital _____ stays under Medicare Part A (Hospital Insurance) based on _____ set rates.
2. This payment system is referred to as the inpatient _____ payment system _____ .
3. Under the IPPS, each case is categorized into a _____ (DRG). Each DRG has a payment weight assigned to it, based on the _____ resources used to treat Medicare patients in that DRG.
4. The base payment rate is _____ into a labor-related and nonlabor share.

5. The labor-related share is adjusted by the ____ index applicable to the area where the hospital is located, and if the hospital is located in Alaska or Hawaii, the nonlabor share is adjusted by a ____ adjustment factor.
6. This base payment rate is ____ by the DRG relative weight.
7. If the hospital treats a high percentage of ____ patients, it receives a percentage ____ payment applied to the DRG-adjusted base payment rate.
8. This add-on, known as the ____ share hospital (DSH) adjustment, provides for a percentage ____ in Medicare payment for hospitals that _____ under either of two statutory formulas designed to identify hospitals that serve a disproportionate share of low-income patients.
9. Also if the hospital is an ____ teaching hospital it receives a percentage add-on payment for each case paid through IPPS.
10. This add-on known as the indirect medical education (IME) adjustment, varies depending on the ____ of residents-to-beds under the IPPS for operating costs, and according to the ratio of residents-to-average daily ____ under the IPPS for capital costs.
11. Finally, for particular cases that are ____ costly, known as ____ cases, the IPPS payment is increased.
12. Any outlier payment due is ____ to the DRG-adjusted base payment rate, plus any DSH or IME adjustments.

Let's Check It! Rules and Regulations

Please answer the following questions from the knowledge you have gained after reading this chapter.

1. **LO 20.3** Define "Present-On-Admission" according to CMS Publication 100-04.
2. **LO 20.2** What are the two instances in which the ICD-10-CM guidelines direct inpatient coders differently than outpatient?
3. **LO 20.4** Explain what DRG stands for and what it is.
4. **LO 20.4** Differentiate between a co-morbidity and a complication.
5. **LO 20.5** What does UHDDS stand for, and what is its function? Include the type of data UHDDS collects.

ICD-10-CM

YOU CODE IT! Application

The following exercises provide practice in abstracting physicians' notes and learning to work with documentation from our health care facility, Westward Hospital. These case studies are modeled on real patient encounters. Using the techniques described in this chapter, carefully read through the case studies and determine the most accurate ICD-10-CM code(s) and external cause code(s), if appropriate, for each case study.

WESTWARD HOSPITAL

591 Chester Road

Masters, FL 33955

DISCHARGE SUMMARY

PATIENT: FALSONE, LEWIS

ADMITTING DIAGNOSIS: Right breast mass

DISCHARGE DIAGNOSIS: Malignant neoplasm of areola, right breast, estrogen receptor status negative; postsurgical respiratory congestion

This 52-year-old African American male was admitted to the hospital with a palpable 2.25-cm nodule in the right breast in the superficial aspect of the right breast in the 4 o'clock axis near the periphery.

(continued)

Excision of the right breast mass with an intermediate wound closure of 3 cm was accomplished. Patient tolerated the procedure well; however, some respiratory complications were realized as a result of the general anesthesia so the patient was kept in the facility for an extra day.

Patient is discharged home with his wife. Discharge orders instruct him to make a follow-up appointment with Dr. Facci, the oncologist, to discuss treatment.

Benjamin Johnston, MD

Determine the most accurate ICD-10-CM code(s).

WESTWARD HOSPITAL

591 Chester Road

Masters, FL 33955

DISCHARGE SUMMARY

PATIENT: FRIZZELLI, ALLISON

ADMITTING DIAGNOSIS: Schizoaffective disorder

DISCHARGE DIAGNOSIS: Schizoaffective disorder; hypothyroidism; hypercholesterolemia; borderline hypertension

The patient is a 34-year-old white female with a long history of schizoaffective disorder with numerous hospitalizations, brought in by ambulance for increasing paranoia; increasing arguments with other people; and, in general, an exacerbation of her psychotic symptoms, which had been worsening over the previous 2 weeks.

She is now discharged to return to her home at the YMCA and also to return to her weekly psychiatric appointments with Dr. Mulford. The patient also is advised to follow up with her primary care physician for her hypertension.

The patient was advised during this admission to start on hydrochlorothiazide 12.5 mg daily, but she refused.

She has been compliant with her medication until the recently refused hydrochlorothiazide. She is irritable at times, but overall she is redirectable and is considered to be at or close to her best baseline. She is considered in no imminent danger to herself or to others at this time.

Roxan Kernan, MD

Determine the most accurate ICD-10-CM code(s).

WESTWARD HOSPITAL

591 Chester Road

Masters, FL 33955

DISCHARGE SUMMARY

PATIENT: TAPPEN, KENNETH

ADMITTING DIAGNOSIS: Major depressive disorder

DISCHARGE DIAGNOSIS: Alcohol dependence; cocaine dependence; major depressive disorder, recurrent; HIV positive (previous HIV infection resolved); hepatitis C; and history of asthma

This 39-year-old single male was referred for this admission, his second lifetime rehabilitation. The patient has a history of alcohol and cocaine dependence since age 17.

During the course of admission, the patient was placed on hydrochlorothiazide 25 milligrams for hypertension, to which he responded well. He participated in this rehabilitation program and worked rigorously throughout.

(continued)

On discharge, the patient is alert and oriented x3. Mood is euthymic. Affect is full range. The patient denies SI, HI, denies AH, VH. Thought process is organized. Thought content—no delusions elicited. There is no evidence of psychosis. There is no imminent risk of suicide or homicide.

Benjamin Johnston, MD

Determine the most accurate ICD-10-CM code(s).

WESTWARD HOSPITAL

591 Chester Road

Masters, FL 33955

DISCHARGE SUMMARY

PATIENT: ENGELS, WARREN

ADMITTING DIAGNOSIS: Mass in bladder

DISCHARGE DIAGNOSIS: High-grade transitional cell carcinoma of the left bladder wall; low-grade transitional cell carcinoma in situ, bladder; underlying mild chronic inflammation, bladder

This 59-year-old male was admitted with a suspicious mass identified in the lateral bladder wall. Biopsy was performed, and upon pathology report of malignancy, a transurethral resection of the bladder tumors was performed. Patient was kept overnight. Foley catheter removed second day, and discharged with orders to make appointment to be seen in the office in about 2 weeks to start weekly BCG bladder installation treatments for recurrent bladder tumors.

Kenzi Bloomington, MD

Determine the most accurate ICD-10-CM code(s).

WESTWARD HOSPITAL

591 Chester Road

Masters, FL 33955

DISCHARGE SUMMARY

PATIENT: BROCKTON, BRIAN

ADMITTING DIAGNOSIS: Hematuria

DISCHARGE DIAGNOSIS: Benign prostatic hypertrophy; hematuria

This 51-year-old male had a transurethral resection of prostate 10 years ago, complicated by a postoperative bleed as well as evaluation with an attempted ureteroscopy. This hematuria is secondary to prostatic varices.

Flexible cystoscopy demonstrated a normal urethra and obstructed bladder outlet secondary to a very large nodular regrowth of the prostate at the medium lobe.

A transurethral resection of prostate was performed with success.

Phillip Carlsson, MD

Determine the most accurate ICD-10-CM code(s).

(continued)

WESTWARD HOSPITAL

591 Chester Road

Masters, FL 33955

DISCHARGE CLINICAL RESUME

PATIENT: LOGAN, PETER

ADMITTING DIAGNOSES:

1. Dyspnea
2. Congestive heart failure (CHR) exacerbation
3. Hypertension
4. Heart murmur
5. Inferior vena cava filter placed July 2021 secondary to lower extremity deep venous thrombosis (DVT)
6. Hypothyroidism with TSH 9.1
7. Peripheral vascular disease—peripheral arterial disease

DISCHARGE DIAGNOSES:

1. Dyspnea, resolved
2. Diastolic CHR, ejection fraction 70%
3. Hypertension, controlled
4. Aortic stenosis with insufficiency
5. Catheter placed secondary to deep venous thrombosis, on Coumadin, INR in 2 on discharge
6. Hypothyroidism
7. Peripheral vascular disease
8. Renal ultrasound with medical disease

HISTORY: A 76-year-old male was admitted with dyspnea. He was found with diastolic CHF exacerbation. The patient was seen by Dr. Shah, vascular surgeon, who believed that he had some mild arterial insufficiency and continued anticoagulation. He wants to see him in his office as an outpatient. During admission, on and off he was having numbness in bilateral feet and hands and cyanosis that resolved by themselves with no problems. Probably Raynaud phenomenon. During the admission he also was seen by cardiologist, who diuresed the patient with no complications. He believes that the patient needs to be started on 1 mg po Bumex. Weigh every day. If the weight gain is more than 3 pounds, Bumex is to be increased by 1 mg po. The patient also was seen by Dr. Almeada, who believed that the patient can go home and continue follow-up as an outpatient. Pulmonology saw the patient as well and believed the same thing. The patient has been stable. Vital signs stable, afebrile, 98% O_2 stat on room air. He was complaining of some biting itching. The daughter had taken him to the dermatologist and wants to continue follow-up with the dermatologist as an outpatient.

RECOMMENDATIONS: Discharge patient home. Follow up with Dr. Yablakoff in the nursing home.

DISCHARGE MEDICATIONS

1. The patient is going with alendronate 70 mg every week, bumetanide 1 mg twice a day if the weight gain is more than 3 pounds
2. Diovan 80 mg once a day
3. Levothyroxine was increased to 200 mcg every day, and check TSH in 4 weeks with Dr. Yablakoff
4. Metolazone 2.5 mg once a day
5. Potassium 20 mEq prn every day
6. Warfarin 5 mg every day. Check INR every day and let Dr. Yablakoff know if the INR is more than 2.5
7. Medrol Dosepak as directed

The outpatient care plan was discussed with the patient and his daughter. They understood, had no questions, and agreed with the plan.

Keith Kappinski, MD

cc. Carole Yablakoff, MD

Determine the most accurate ICD-10-CM code(s).

(continued)

WESTWARD HOSPITAL

591 Chester Road

Masters, FL 33955

DISCHARGE CLINICAL RESUME

PATIENT: DRYLER, ARTHUR

DATE OF ADMISSION: 06/03/26

DATE OF DISCHARGE: 06/06/26

ADMITTING DIAGNOSIS: Ischemia, transient ischemic attack, rule out myocardial infarction, arrhythmia

DISCHARGE DIAGNOSES: Transient ischemic attack (TIA)
Hyperlipidemia
Coronary artery disease, status post coronary artery bypass graft and cardioversion
Urinary tract infection

CONSULTATIONS: Dr. Jenson for neurology and Dr. Balmer for cardiology

PROCEDURES: Echocardiogram, TEE, Thallium stress test

COMPLICATIONS: None

INFECTIONS: None

HISTORY: Eighty-one-year-old white male with significant history of coronary artery disease, status post coronary artery bypass graft 3 years ago and cardioversion in February 2016, who presented with difficulty speaking. He stated that he had difficulty obtaining the right words when he spoke. This lasted about 15 minutes; however, when the patient came to the emergency room he was completely okay. He did not have any deficits. The patient was admitted and consultants were called in to provide evaluation of possible TIA with rule out cardiac source. Carotid Doppler was done. Echocardiogram was done. This showed dilated left ventricle, severe global left ventricular dysfunction, estimated ejection fraction 20% and left atrial enlargement, mitral annular calcification with severe mitral regurgitation, aortic sclerosis with moderate aortic insufficiency, and severe tricuspid regurgitation with estimated pulmonary study pressure of 70 mm. Thallium stress test was uneventful. Persantine infusion protocol and no clinical EKG changes of ischemia and radionuclide showed fixed defect anteroseptal, anteroapical, and adjacent inferior wall with hypokinesis; no ischemia seen. The ejection fraction was calculated 40%. CT of the brain showed white matter ischemic changes and atrophy, no acute intracranial abnormalities. MRI showed extensive periventricular white matter ischemia changes. MRA was normal. EKG was within normal limits, showing sinus bradycardia with average of 50 to 56.

The patient went to TEE to rule out cardiac source. The TEE was not conclusive and there was no hypokinesis, as described in the previous echocardiogram, and it was considered the patient needs to have lifetime Coumadin because of previous events.

The hospital course was uneventful. He never presented with any other new deficit or any new symptoms.

Today, the patient is asymptomatic; vital signs are stable. Monitor shows sinus rhythm, and he is discharged in stable condition to be followed by Dr. Curran in 1 week, by Dr. Jenson in 2 weeks, and by Dr. Balmer in 2 weeks. He will have home health nurse to inject him Lovenox until PT and INR reach therapeutic levels of 2/3. He will be on Coumadin 5 mg po qd, and home health nurse will draw PT and INR daily until Dr. Roman thoroughly assesses the patient. He will receive the last dose of Bactrim today for urine; however, urine culture has been negative.

Rudolph Langer, MD

cc. Karyn Curran, MD

Determine the most accurate ICD-10-CM code(s).

(continued)

WESTWARD HOSPITAL

591 Chester Road

Masters, FL 33955

DISCHARGE DOCUMENT SUMMARY

PATIENT: WESTCOTT, ROSEANNE

DATE OF ADMISSION: 02/09/26

DATE OF DISCHARGE: 02/10/26

ADMISSION DIAGNOSIS: Abdominal pain, status postappendectomy

DISCHARGE DIAGNOSIS: Abdominal pain, unknown etiology, status postappendectomy

BRIEF HISTORY: The patient is a 21-year-old female who, 6 weeks ago, underwent an appendectomy for perforated appendicitis. About 3 weeks following that, she had episodes of nausea and vomiting and diffuse abdominal pain. This was worked up at Kinsey Urgent Care Center, including CT scan, Meckel scan, and laboratory, which were unremarkable. It resolved spontaneously over a 3-day period. Three days prior to admission, she had a recurrent bout of diffuse, dull, abdominal pain with associated nausea and anorexia. She was admitted to our hospital at the time for workup of this pain.

CLINICAL COURSE: On examination, the patient was found to have a diffuse, mild tenderness without any rebound or peritoneal signs. Plain radiographs of the abdomen were obtained, which were within normal limits. A CT scan of the abdomen and pelvis was also obtained, which was unremarkable. She was without leukocytosis. Dr. Pointer of GI saw the patient in consultation, and an upper GI with small bowel follow-through was obtained. This was performed today and was found to be normal.

At this time, the patient has just had a regular meal without difficulty and feels like returning home. She will be discharged home at this time and can follow up with her primary MD. We will see her on an as-needed basis.

Robyn Charne, MD

Determine the most accurate ICD-10-CM code(s).

WESTWARD HOSPITAL

591 Chester Road

Masters, FL 33955

DISCHARGE DOCUMENT SUMMARY

PATIENT: ROMANSKI, CESAR

DATE OF ADMISSION: 08/01/26

DATE OF DISCHARGE: 08/22/26

FINAL DIAGNOSES:

1. Alcohol dependence, methamphetamine dependence
2. Major depressive disorder, recurrent, current episode severe
3. HIV
4. Tuberculosis of the lung, primary
5. Hepatitis C, chronic

DISCHARGE MEDICATIONS:

1. Zoloft 100 mg po qam
2. Seroquel 50 mg po qhs
3. Truvade 1 tab qam

(continued)

4. Regataz 300 mg po qam
5. Norvir 100 mg po qam with breakfast
6. Dapsone 100 mg po qam
7. Hydrochlorothiazide 25 mg po qam

DISPOSITION: The patient will return to his residence at the Daylight Hotel. He will attend the hospital continuing day treatment program.

PROGNOSIS: Guarded

HISTORY: He is noted to have significant immunosuppression related to his HIV. Currently there is no stigmata of opportunistic infection.

During the course of admission, the patient was placed on hydrochlorothiazide 25 mg for hypertension, which he responded well to.

CONDITION ON DISCHARGE: The patient is a 43-year-old single black male referred for his first BRU admission, his second lifetime rehabilitation. The patient has a history of alcohol and methamphetamine dependence since age 21. Prior to this admission, he had attained no significant period of sobriety other than time spent incarcerated.

The patient participated in a 21-day MICA rehabilitation program. He worked rigorously throughout the entire program. He had perfect attendance and participated well as a peer support provider. The patient attended eight groups daily. He worked well in individual therapy with his nurse practitioner and social worker.

On discharge, the patient is alert and oriented x3. Mood is euthymic. Affect is full range. The patient denies SI, HI, denies AH, VH. Thought process is organized. Thought content—no delusions elicited. There is no evidence of psychosis. There is no imminent risk of suicide or homicide.

Kelsey Berge, MD

Determine the most accurate ICD-10-CM code(s).

WESTWARD HOSPITAL

591 Chester Road

Masters, FL 33955

DISCHARGE CLINICAL RESUME

PATIENT: MORETTA, TERACIA

DATE OF ADMISSION: 11/05/26

DATE OF DISCHARGE: 11/28/26

This is a 36–37-week-old female neonate delivered to a 25-year-old, gravida 2, para 1, who was a known breech presentation. Mother presented with complaint of vaginal bleeding, rupture of membranes, and abdominal pain and cramping. On exam found to be complete with large fecal impaction. Fetal heart rate 120 by monitor. To c-section room for disimpaction and cesarean section for breech. Delivered precipitously immediately after impaction was removed, breech presentation. OB moved baby to warmer. She was pale with no respiratory effort or heart rate. Ambu bagged with mask for 30 seconds. Intubation attempted. Code called. UAC was placed. ENT in place and bagged. No heart rate, no breath sounds, pale, cyanotic. Reintubated with chest rise, heart rate about 60. Chest compression stopped when heart rate above 120, color improved. Apgar 0 at 1 minute, 1 at 5 minutes, and 4 at 10 minutes. No spontaneous respiratory effort. Received sodium bicarbonate, epinephrine, and calcium. No grimace, no spontaneous movements. Pupils midpoint, nonreactive to light. NG placed for distended abdomen. Cord pH 7.33. Mother noted to have 50% abruptio placenta. Transferred to Neo. UAC was removed and replaced. UVC also placed.

Physical exam on admission: weight 2,620 grams, pink, fontanelle soft, significant clonus of extremities, tone decreased. Pupils 2 cm and round, nonreactive to light. No movement, no grimace, no suck, good chest rise. Equal breath sounds, no murmur. Pulses 2+. Perfusion good. Abdomen soft and full. No masses. Normal female genitalia externally. Anus patent. Extremities no edema. Skin—Mongolian spot sacrum and both arms, single café-au-lait spot left flank 1.5 cm × 0.5 cm. Palate intact.

(continued)

IMPRESSION:

1. 36–37 week AGA female
2. Status postcardiopulmonary arrest
3. Rule out sepsis
4. At risk for hypoxic ischemic encephalopathy

Physical exam on discharge: 23 days of age, weight 2,520 grams, head circumference 35, pink. Anterior fontanelle soft. Heart—II/VI murmur radiating to the axilla. Chest clear. Abdomen soft, positive bowel sounds, gastrostomy tube intact, wound is okay. Neuro—irritable. The infant has an anal fissure at 12 o'clock that has caused some blood streaks in the stool.

FINAL DIAGNOSES:

1. 36–37 week appropriate for gestational age female
2. History post cardiac arrest
3. Respiratory arrest
4. Rule out sepsis
5. Hypoxic ischemic encephalopathy, mild
6. Gastroesophageal reflux and feeding problems

Nancy Odom, MD

Determine the most accurate ICD-10-CM code(s).

21

Diagnostic Coding Capstone

Learning Outcomes

After completing this chapter, the student should be able to:

LO 21.1 Apply the techniques learned, carefully read through the case studies, and determine the accurate ICD-10-CM code(s) and the external cause code(s), as required.

As you worked your way through the last 20 chapters, you have learned how to abstract documentation and interpret the reasons *WHY* a physician needed to care for a patient–known as the diagnosis–into ICD-10-CM codes. You also learned to distinguish signs and symptoms, and other conditions, and when to code those–or not. Now, this chapter provides you with case studies so you can get some hands-on practice.

For each of the following case studies, read through the documentation and:

- Determine what code or codes report these reasons, to their most specific level.
- Determine how many ICD-10-CM codes you will need to tell the whole story as to WHY the patient required care.
- Identify external cause codes in cases of injury or poisoning.
- If more than one code is required, determine the sequence in which to report the codes.

Remember, the notations, symbols, and Official Guidelines are there to help you get it correct.

You Code It! Diagnosis Capstone

CASE STUDY 1: JELYSA HANSON

JeLysa Hanson, a 41-year-old female, presents to the ED complaining of shortness of breath and tightness in her chest. Following examination, she is discharged with a diagnosis of musculoskeletal pain due to overexertion while practicing her new hobby, boxing, in her backyard.

CASE STUDY 2: HARRIS TEAL

Harris Teal, a 19-year-old male, reports to the hospital-based urgent care clinic for headache and wheezing. Following examination, he is discharged with an acute frontal sinus infection, recurrent, and exacerbated asthma due to environmental dust allergies.

CASE STUDY 3: ROGER GILL

Roger Gill, a 39-year-old retired professional athlete, comes in with complaints of intermittent joint pain, particularly in his left shoulder. He was a pitcher on a AA league baseball team. He also states he feels tenderness at the outer aspect of the left shoulder, most often when he raises his arm. He states that simply putting on his shirt is very painful. Dr. Jeneau asks Roger if he suffered any shoulder injuries while playing baseball. Roger admitted that his left proximal humerus was fractured when hit by a thrown ball during a game. Roger quickly added that it healed OK. Dr. Jeneau confirms a diagnosis of abscess of the bursa of his shoulder.

CASE STUDY 4: ANGEL DUNBAR

Angel Dunbar, a 27-year-old male, presents to see his physician, Dr. Davison, with the complaints of difficulty breathing, muscle weakness, and fatigue. Following a complete examination, Dr. Davison notes ataxia and sudden muscle spasms in Angel's legs. The lab results are positive for lactic acidosis. CSF results show elevated protein, and the muscle biopsy is positive for ragged red fiber. Angel is diagnosed with MERRF syndrome.

CASE STUDY 5: RENAY GRIFFITH

Renay Griffith, a 25-year-old female, recently returned from working for the Red Cross overseas. She presents to the clinic for an evaluation of a rash. Dr. Leisom evaluates the patient and diagnoses her with cutaneous leishmaniasis related to her recent deployment to Iraq.

CASE STUDY 6: MARYBELLE OSTENKOWSKY

Patient: Marybelle Ostenkowsky

Physician: Fiona McNally, MD

History

This 87-year-old female has been a patient of the McGraw Health Center and Clinic since 2009. Chronic conditions: pernicious anemia, osteoarthritis, and urinary incontinency. She is fully functional and fully independent. She provides care for her homebound husband, who has severe COPD. They live in a home chosen because it was "close to the hospital" to ensure access to house calls for her husband.

In September 2015, the husband died as a result of respiratory arrest. Her only relative is a niece who talks with her about once a month. In October 2020, her home was broken into and our patient was raped and robbed. She was taken to a local hospital specializing in rape. Here, she was distressed, delusional, and reported to be very emotionally distraught.

Examination

I saw the patient about 3 weeks after the rape in a community nursing home, where she was moved after a 4-day stay at the hospital. She was very distressed, delusional, and confused. She slowly improved over 2 months and was discharged to a senior living center.

In March 2022, the patient was seen in the office. She is still very emotionally unstable. She is crying, depressed (not suicidal), and stressed about her new home. She wants to move to a different Senior Housing unit because it would be on the bus route, making it easier to get around. She has also hired a middle-aged woman as a caregiver.

In November 2022, 9 months after moving to the new facility, she becomes acutely ill with psychotic symptoms and severe paranoia. She hallucinates that men and women are in her bed and calls others all hours of the day. I admitted her into a hospitalized psychiatric unit and she shows improvement over about 14 days without antipsychotic medication.

Today, 1 week following discharge from the hospital, symptoms rapidly recurred when she returned to the senior apartment. She was disruptive and threatened with eviction unless something was done rapidly. An emergency petition was prepared because she refused medical care. With the help of her companion, we were finally able to persuade her to take a neuroleptic drug (Haloperidol 0.025–1.0 mg/day) for her recurrent incapacitating hallucinations. Initial injection was administered IM 5 mg. Our office nurse and staff called her later in the day to guide her through the process of taking her medicines. She slowly but steadily improved and became stabilized.

Diagnosis: Chronic Post Traumatic Stress Disorder

Rx: Haloperidol 0.025–1.0 mg/day

CASE STUDY 7: RAYONNETTA CALHOUN

Patient: Rayonnetta Calhoun

Physician: Robert Morgan, MD

ADMISSION to McGraw Hill Hospital

History

A fully functional, independent female who is nearly 89 years old; lives with her two sons. A history finds that she has

- high blood pressure
- CAD
- congestive heart failure
- cataracts
- hearing impairments
- knee osteoarthritis

Current Medications: lisinopril, furosemide, ASA, and metoprolol

Examination

Patient develops abdominal pain increasing over 4 days; obstipation for 1 day. She is acutely ill and appears uncomfortable and volume depleted. On exam, she has abdominal distention, she has hypoactive bowel sounds, and no mass is found. Her heart is enlarged and no S3.

Laboratory findings:

- WBC . . . 13290
- HCT . . . 42
- Na . . . 128
- K . . . 2.6
- Bun/creatinine . . . normal

An abdominal CT scan shows the cecum is very dilated to 13 cm and the left image shows a possible mass in the descending colon.

Recognizing the seriousness of her illness, she was quickly stabilized with volume repletion due to her dehydration. She was in the emergency department 2 hours, then admitted to a nonintensive care surgical unit and cared for by a general surgeon, Herman Canton, MD, and a geriatrician, Kyla Mondolano, MD.

Upon Admission

Protocol calls for endoscopy, but to do so would require a delay before surgery that is clearly needed. There was an urgency to get her to surgery as delays would likely lead to complications. Accordingly, no colonoscopy was performed. Prior to surgery, careful anesthesia planning and intra-operative management were designed. A shortened bowel prep was initiated.

A left hemicolectomy was performed on day 2 with pathology confirmation of malignant neoplasm of the sigmoid colon. Pain was controlled with low doses of morphine and fluid management was tightly managed. She was provided a single, quiet room and a family member stayed with her continuously. The patient was discharged to subacute rehabilitation on day 5, and then to home on day 10.

CASE STUDY 8: WINSTON WALLER

Patient: Winston Waller

Physician: Morris Johnston, MD

History:

This patient is a 73-year-old male nonsmoker with type 2 diabetes mellitus and hypertension. He presented to this ED with shortness of breath and was found to have had an acute myocardial infarction of the anterior wall of his heart showing an ST elevation that had previously been left untreated. He developed several complications, including renal failure from a combination of cardiogenic shock and toxicity from the dye used for emergency catheterization of his heart.

(continued)

Hemodialysis was started during this hospitalization because of his renal failure. After spending almost a month in the hospital and developing severe deconditioning, he was discharged to a subacute rehabilitation facility.

Examination

While he was there he was noted to have symptoms consistent with mild depression, as well as a prior history of a major depressive episode in 2024. Mirtazapine (Remeron) 25 mg/day was started.

He was transferred to a skilled nursing unit for another month of rehabilitation management of his medical conditions and then discharged home to the care of his wife.

CASE STUDY 9: GERALD YOUNG

Patient: Gerald Young

Physician: Hannah Cohen, MD

This 37-year-old man presents to the psychiatry emergency room for inappropriate behavior and confusion. He works as a janitor and has had reasonably good work attendance. His coworkers say that he has appeared "fidgety" for several years. They specifically mention jerky movements that seem to affect his entire body more recently. His mother is alive and well, although his father died at age 28 in an auto accident.

On examination, he is alert but easily distracted. His speech is fluent without paraphasias but is noted to be tangential. He has trouble with spelling the word "world" backwards and serial seven's, but recalls three objects at 3 minutes. His constructions are good. When he walks, there is a lot of distal hand movement, and his balance is precarious, although he can stand with both feet together. His reflexes are increased bilaterally, and there is bilateral ankle clonus. A urine drug screen is negative.

Most likely diagnosis: Huntington disease.

Next diagnostic step: Genetic counseling and genetic testing for Huntington disease. Review the history very carefully with patient and his relatives and assess medications—either illicit or licit that could be responsible.

Molecular or genetic basis: Repeat CAG triplets present in a gene called huntingtin located on chromosome 4p16.3. Repeat lengths greater than 40 are nearly always associated with clinical Huntington's disease. Confirmed Huntington's disease.

CASE STUDY 10: MARLENE SMITHSON

Patient: Marlene Smithson

Marlene Smithson, a 31-year-old pregnant female, G1 P0, at 29 weeks, 5 days gestation, developed a cough with expectoration on March 26, 2025. On March 27, she developed a fever, with her body temperature fluctuating between 99F and 101 F. She was admitted to the hospital with common pneumonia and treated with oral cephalosporin for 3 days. Her pulmonary computed tomography (CT) scan on March 30, 2025 (30 weeks, 2 days gestation) showed scattered consolidation and ground-glass shadow of both lungs. In addition, the routine blood test results showed that her white blood cell count was extraordinarily high. She tested negative for influenza A and B virus antigens, Mycoplasma pneumoniae, and Chlamydia pneumoniae.

Based on the criteria of COVID-19 pneumonia in the New Coronavirus Prevention and Control Program (5th edition) dated February 3, 2022, she was diagnosed as a clinically confirmed case, so quarantine treatment including nebulized inhalation and oral cephalosporin could begin. Five days later (30-week gestation), patient's body temperature returned to normal and the symptoms, including cough and expectoration, disappeared. Subsequently, the pharyngeal swab test of SARS-CoV-2 revealed twice negative on April 5 and April 7, 2025.

CASE STUDY 11: BLAIZE MASTERS

PATIENT: Blaize Masters

IMPRESSION: This is a 49-year-old male who has significant multivessel coronary artery disease. He has atypical anginal symptoms, suspected to be secondary to his type 1 diabetes mellitus. Still it is believed that he is at risk for ischemia. To reduce this risk, surgical myocardial revascularization is recommended.

The patient is given complete details about the procedure, the risks, and the benefits. We also discuss alternative treatments that may be viable. The patient signs the informed consent and the surgery is scheduled.

PLAN: Proceed with coronary artery bypass graft operation utilizing the left internal mammary artery as conduit to the left anterior descending. The remaining conduit will come from the greater saphenous veins.

CASE STUDY 12: CAROLINA SPENCER

PATIENT: Carolina Spencer

REASON FOR ENCOUNTER: Assistance with tracheostomy management.

HISTORY OF PRESENT ILLNESS: The patient is a 73-year-old female admitted to McGraw Hospital on July 17th with acute ischemic CVA and DKA. The patient has a very complicated medical history, including respiratory failure, on prolonged mechanical ventilation. She underwent tracheostomy placement on July 19 and was weaned from mechanical ventilation within 12 hours. She was also diagnosed with hospital-acquired pneumonia, multi-organism, and pulmonary embolism by CTPA. She is currently on heparin drip, while started on Warfarin. She also has end-stage renal disease and is on hemodialysis.

PAST MEDICAL HISTORY: In addition to the above, the patient was found to have some type of intracardiac shunt per echocardiogram, not otherwise defined; atherosclerosis of the internal carotid arteries; positive lupus anticoagulants; and long-standing history of diabetes mellitus, type II.

SOCIAL HISTORY: Tobacco and alcohol use are unknown.

MEDICATIONS: Sliding scale insulin, Reglan, Lantus insulin, diltiazem, Timentin, heparin drip, Warfarin, Bactrim, Pepcid, and iron sulfate.

ALLERGIES: No known allergies.

REVIEW OF SYSTEMS: Not available.

FAMILY HISTORY: Not available.

PHYSICAL EXAMINATION: GENERAL: She is an unresponsive female, in no acute distress.

VITAL SIGNS: Temperature is 98.6 degrees; respiratory rate is 21 to 25, somewhat irregular; pulse is 102; blood pressure is 122/80; and pulse oximetry is 97% on 50% cuffless tracheostomy.

HEENT: Unable to visualize posterior pharynx secondary to the patient's resistance to mouth opening. The patient does have some natural dentition anteriorly. No coating of the tongue is appreciated. The patient has an eschar on the left upper lip, presumably secondary to ET tube. Conjunctivae are clear. Gaze is conjugate. The patient has a size 8 Portex cuffless tracheostomy tube in the midline.

CHEST: The patient has a few crackles at the right base, few anterior coarse rhonchi. No wheeze or stridor with the tracheostomy tube, patent. With finger occlusion of the cuffless #8 Portex, the patient does have stridor and increased respiratory rate. Unable to adequately percuss the chest.

CARDIOVASCULAR: The patient has regular rate and rhythm. No murmur or gallop is appreciated. No heaves or thrills.

ABDOMEN: Soft and obese. The patient has G-tube in position and normoactive bowel sounds. No guarding.

EXTREMITIES: She has decreased pulse in lower extremities bilaterally. No discrepancy in calf size is appreciated. No clubbing, cyanosis, or edema.

NEUROLOGIC: The patient does withdraw, on the left side; grimaces to pain. She is not cooperative with exam at this time.

LABORATORY DATA: BUN 16 and creatinine 3.3 on July 18 with venous CO_2 of 24, calcium 9.1, white count 9200, hemoglobin 9.2, and platelets 515,000. Chest x-ray is not available for review.

(continued)

IMPRESSION: The patient is a 73-year-old female, status post respiratory failure, prolonged mechanical ventilation, necessitating tracheostomy tube placement. She has had multiple complications including pulmonary embolism, for which she is now anticoagulated with heparin and reportedly intracardiac shunt, which would help explain her Aa gradient. She also reported she had a right-sided cavitary lesion and had negative AFB on bronchoalveolar lavage.

RECOMMENDATIONS:

1. Change to #8 Portex cuffless tracheostomy tube. Would not plan on downsizing, capping tracheostomy at this time secondary to poor patient cough, decreased mental status, and inability to protect airway. She does have some evidence with occlusion of the tracheostomy of possible upper airway obstruction, and so, if her ability to protect her airway improves, she may need evaluation of the upper airway before considering progressing toward decannulation as well.
2. Repeat chest x-ray to evaluate right cavitary lesion and obtain films from the primary care physician for comparison.

CASE STUDY 13: LINDA BROTHERS

This is a 33-year-old female, primigravida, who came in experiencing early labor. Patient is at 40 weeks gestation. The patient had been scheduled for a cesarean section due to breech presentation.

This patient has had no significant problems during first, second, or third trimester. The patient's past medical history is noncontributory. The patient's LMP was 06/22/2026, placing her EDC at 04/05/2026. Ultrasounds were performed throughout the pregnancy and revealed adequate growth during the pregnancy and EDC remained technically the same.

The patient's initial blood work showed blood type to be A positive, VDRL was nonreactive, rubella titer indicated immunity, hepatitis B surface antigen (HbsAg) was negative, HIV screen was negative, GC and *Chlamydia* cultures were negative. Pap smear was normal. Her 1-hour glucose tolerance test was within normal parameters. The patient's blood count also remained well within normal parameters. Her quad screen for maternal serum alpha-fetoprotein (MSAFP) was normal. Strep culture was likewise negative at 34–35 weeks.

The patient, upon admission, was having contractions approximately every 4–5 minutes, moderate in intensity. The patient had no dilation; presenting part was still in a breech presentation, per bedside ultrasound; and the patient was therefore made ready for primary cesarean section.

The patient was taken to surgery, where primary classical cesarean section was performed with delivery of a breech infant from left sacral anterior positioning, male weighing 6 pounds 10 ounces with Apgars 8 and 8 at 1 and 5 minutes. Placenta delivered intact. Membranes were removed. The patient tolerated the procedure quite well. Estimated blood loss was less than 600 mL.

The patient has had an uneventful postoperative period. She is ambulating well and moving well at this time. The patient is passing gas, moving her bowels, and urinating well; moderate lochia is present; uterus is firm. The patient is discharged from the hospital, being given careful instructions to avoid douching, intercourse, strenuous activity, going up and down stairs, and traveling by car. She is to keep her incision clean with peroxide. She was discharged with Darvocet-N 100 as needed for pain. She will be followed up in 1 week for staple removal. The patient was given information and instructions. Should she experience unusual bleeding; difficulty urinating, voiding, or having a bowel movement; or temperature elevation, she is to contact this physician. The patient's baby is showing some jaundice and may be kept for another 24–48 hours to evaluate bilirubin levels.

CASE STUDY 14: STEWART ALLEN

DISCHARGE DIAGNOSES:

AXIS I:

1. Bipolar disorder, depressed, with psychotic features, symptoms in remission.
2. Attention deficit hyperactivity disorder, symptoms in remission.

AXIS II: Deferred.

AXIS III: None.

AXIS IV: Moderate.

(continued)

AXIS V: Global assessment of functioning 65 on discharge.

REASON FOR ADMISSION: The patient was admitted with a chief complaint of suicidal ideation. The patient was brought to the hospital after his guidance counselor found a note the patient wrote, which detailed to whom he was giving away his possessions when he dies. The patient told the counselor that he hears voices telling him to hurt himself and others. The patient reports over the last month these symptoms have exacerbated. The patient had a fight in school recently, which the patient blames on the voices. Three weeks ago, he got pushed into a corner at school and threatened to shoot himself and others with a gun. The patient was suspended for that remark.

PROCEDURES AND TREATMENT:

1. Individual and group psychotherapy.
2. Psychopharmacologic management.
3. Family therapy with the patient and the patient's family for the purpose of education and discharge planning.

HOSPITAL COURSE: The patient responded well to individual and group psychotherapy, milieu therapy, and medication management. As stated, family therapy was conducted.

DISCHARGE ASSESSMENT: At the time of discharge, the patient is alert and fully oriented. Mood euthymic. Affect broad range. He denies any suicidal or homicidal ideation. IQ is at baseline. Memory intact. Insight and judgment good.

PLAN: The patient may be discharged as he no longer poses a risk of harm toward himself or others.

The patient will continue on the following medications: Ritalin LA 60 mg q.a.m., Depakote 500 mg q.a.m. and 750 mg q.h.s., Abilify 20 mg q.h.s. Depakote level on date of discharge was 110. Liver enzymes drawn were within normal limits.

The patient will follow up with Dr. Wallace for medication management and Dr. Deiter for psychotherapy. All other discharge orders per the psychiatrist, as arranged by social work.

CASE STUDY 15: NOAH LOGAN

PATIENT: Noah Logan

PREOPERATIVE DIAGNOSIS: Midface deficiency.

POSTOPERATIVE DIAGNOSIS: Cleft hard palate with cleft soft palate.

OPERATIVE PROCEDURE: LeFort I osteotomy with advancement.

ANESTHESIA: General via nasal intubation.

BLOOD LOSS: 200.

FLUIDS: 600.

URINE OUTPUT: 125.

DRAINS: No drains.

COMPLICATIONS: No complications.

BRIEF HISTORY: The patient is an 8-month-old male who has been under the care of Dr. Grayson for his pre-surgical orthodontics in order to address a midface deficiency. He was also found to have a maxillary midline deficit of approximately 3 mm to his left side. It was determined that he would benefit from a maxillary advancement of approximately 6 mm with rotation in order to set the midline straight.

OPERATIVE PROCEDURE: He was seen in the preop area, brought to the operating room, placed in supine position. General anesthesia was induced. Head and neck were prepped and draped in normal fashion. Time-out was performed. An NG was placed. The external reference marks were made using the right and left medial canthal tendon areas. The nasal width was also measured.

Next, a vestibular incision was made between the right and left first molars in the maxilla. Subperiosteal dissection was performed, as well as dissection around the piriform rim into the nasal fossa. Next, using a reciprocating saw, a standard LeFort 1 osteotomy was made. The osteotomy was taken posteriorly into the pterygomaxillary junction. Next, using a series of guarded chisels, the osteotomies were completed. The nasal septum was disarticulated as were the lateral nasal walls and finally pterygomaxillary disjunction was completed with chisels. The maxilla was brought down quite easily without any bleeding. All bony interferences were removed. The maxilla was then mobilized appropriately.

(continued)

Next, the maxilla was placed into intermaxillary fixation, and four 1.5-mm KLS plates were placed across the right and left piriform rims as well as the zygomaticomaxillary buttresses in order to plate the LeFort 1 osteotomy. Once this was done, the intermaxillary fixation was released and the occlusion was found to be stable and repeatable. This was approximately a 6-mm advancement move with about a 2-mm rotation to the left. At this point, a V-Y closure of the upper lip was performed. An alar cinch suture was also used to reestablish the alar width. The vestibular incision was then irrigated and closed. The throat pack was removed. NG was maintained. The patient was extubated and taken to the recovery room.

PART III

REPORTING PHYSICIAN SERVICES AND OUTPATIENT PROCEDURES

INTRODUCTION

Now that you have learned to better understand the reasons why *a patient may need the attention and care from a physician or other health care provider, the next phase–layer 2–of your learning will be about reporting* what *is done for this patient.*

Procedures, services, and treatments are essentially all-inclusive to cover anything and everything a health care provider can do to, or for, someone. These actions may be preventive in nature, such as a vaccination; diagnostic such as an x-ray; or therapeutic–something done to fix or repair an existing problem.

While you think of all the actions a physician may perform in care of the patient, keep in mind that this includes advice and recommendations. Most of us rely on our health care providers for guidance related to improving our health. As the professional coder, a "service" might be conversation with the patient. This counts, too!

22

Introduction to CPT

Key Terms

- Category I Codes
- Category II Codes
- Category III Codes
- Experimental
- Outpatient
- Outpatient Facility
- Procedure
- Service
- Treatment
- Unlisted Codes

Learning Outcomes

After completing this chapter, the student should be able to:

LO 22.1	Recognize the main terms for procedure codes.
LO 22.2	Distinguish the various sections of CPT and how to use them.
LO 22.3	Analyze complete code descriptions.
LO 22.4	Recall the meanings of notations and symbols within CPT.
LO 22.5	Interpret accurately the Official Guidelines, shown before sections and in-section.
LO 22.6	Utilize Category II and Category III codes, as required.

STOP! **Remember, you need to follow along in your CPT code book for an optimal learning experience.**

22.1 Abstracting for Procedure Coding

Procedures, **services**, and **treatments** are the terms used for anything and everything that occurs between a health care professional and a patient. Remember, you learned about distinguishing *what* the provider did for the patient and reporting them in the chapter ***Introduction to the Languages of Coding***. CPT is one of the languages—the terminologies—we use to communicate these details.

CPT stands for Current Procedural Terminology and lists services, procedures, and treatments provided by all types of health care professionals. Services such as counseling, treatments such as the application of a cast, and procedures such as the surgical removal of a mole are each assigned a special code to simplify reporting for purposes of reimbursement and statistical analysis. In addition, ancillary services, such as imaging (x-rays, CT scans, magnetic resonance imaging), pathology, and laboratory (biopsy analysis, blood tests, cultures), also are reported using CPT codes. These services may range from intense surgical procedures, such as a heart transplant, to everyday treatments or services, such as removing a splinter or providing professional advice regarding a treatment plan or preventive service.

When you are coding for a physician or other health care professional, or on behalf of an **outpatient** facility, you will use CPT codes to report the actions taken for the health and well-being of a patient.

An **outpatient facility** may be in the same building as a hospital, for example, an emergency room, ambulatory care center, or same-day surgery center, or it may be a free-standing facility, such as a physician's office, a walk-in clinic, or an independent same-day surgery center.

Procedure
Action taken, in accordance with the standards of care, by the physician to accomplish a predetermined objective (result); a surgical operation.

Services
Spending time with a patient and/or family about health care situations.

Treatment
The provision of medical care for a disorder or disease.

Outpatient
A patient who receives services for a short amount of time (less than 24 hours) in a physician's office or clinic, without being kept overnight.

Outpatient facility
An **outpatient facility** includes a hospital emergency room, ambulatory care center, same-day surgery center, or walk-in clinic.

CODING BITES

CPT codes explain *what* the physician or health care professional did to or for the patient.

EXAMPLES

Outpatient Facilities

- Physicians' offices
- Urgent care and walk-in clinics
- Ambulatory care centers
- Same-day surgery centers
- Emergency departments

When you are abstracting the physician's documentation to collect the details, you need to determine the codes that report what actions the physician accomplished for the patient during this encounter. This is a different perspective from when you are abstracting for diagnosis coding. As you read through the case, look for action verbs: inserted; excised; administered; discussed; dilated; and many, many more. Then, you will be able to identify which terms to interpret into CPT codes.

CODING BITES

IMPORTANT: You are only permitted to report codes for procedures, services, and treatments provided to the patient during the encounter. If the physician "*orders*" something to be done at a later date or at a different location, you are not permitted to report it.

YOU INTERPRET IT!

Identify the term in the sentence that describes WHY the physician treated the patient and the term that describes WHAT the physician did for the patient.

1. Liam O'Connor fractured his thumb when building a bookshelf in his house. Dr. Brazinski placed a cast on Liam's hand.
2. Emma Burgeron has been using tobacco for 20 years, and she wants to quit, once and for all. Dr. Spencer discussed with her several ways to help her.
3. Jacob Treviani was found to have cholelithiasis (gallstones), so Dr. Myverson performed a cholecystectomy.

GUIDANCE CONNECTION

Read the CPT **Introduction**, subsection **Instructions for Use of the CPT Codebook**.

CODING BITES

Not all publishers of CPT books present the sections in this order. This is an excellent time to become familiar with the layout of *your* CPT book and know where you can find all of this key information.

22.2 CPT Code Book

The Organization of the CPT Book

The CPT book has two parts, each of which has many sections.

1. The main body of the CPT book has six sections, presented in numeric order (generally speaking) by code number:
   - Evaluation and Management: 98000-98016, 99202-99499
   - Anesthesia: 00100-01999 and 99100-99140
   - Surgery: 10004-69990
   - Radiology: 70010-79999
   - Pathology and Laboratory: 80047-89398, 0001U-0599U
   - Medicine: 90281-99199, 99500-99607

   You may notice that, while each section within itself is in numeric order (for the most part), the sections are also in numeric order, for the most part. Bottom line . . . *read carefully*.
2. The second part of the CPT book contains several sections, including:
   - *Category II codes*: for supplemental tracking of performance measurement.
   - *Category III codes*: temporary codes for emerging technological procedures.
   - *Appendixes A-P*: modifiers and other relevant additional information.
   - *Alphabetic Index*: all the CPT codes in alphabetical order by short code description, presented in four classes of entries:
     a. Procedures or services, such as removal, implantation, or debridement.
     b. Anatomical site or organ, such as heart, mouth, or pharynx.

c. Condition, such as miscarriage, cystitis, or abscess.
d. Eponyms, synonyms, or abbreviations, such as Baker's cyst or EKG.

As you prepare to learn and improve your knowledge about medical procedures, and build your skills for interpreting the documentation into CPT codes, you will find that your education in medical terminology will be very useful. A medical dictionary may be very helpful.

YOU INTERPRET IT!

Identify the term that explains WHAT the physician did for the patient and from which SECTION that would be reported.

4. Dr. Harper excised a mole from Katrina's arm.
5. Dr. Aubrey administered general anesthesia prior to the beginning of the surgery.
6. Dr. Davine took and evaluated the MRI images of Lawrence's head after the car accident.

CPT Resequencing Initiative

The American Medical Association (AMA) was faced with the challenge of fitting new codes for evolving health care innovation and technology into a preexisting set of numbers. So, the AMA determined that resequencing codes would be easier, and less confusing, than renumbering the entire code set. (That certainly would have caused havoc!)

Therefore, when new codes needed to be added to CPT and there were no more available numbers in the correct sequence, the next available code number was assigned. Different publishers of CPT books present this new information in various ways.

In the AMA-published CPT book, the new code is listed in two places:

1. In its correct numeric sequence. The code is shown in the correct numeric sequence with a notation that informs you where to find the code in its topic-related location.

EXAMPLE

Directly after code 46200 is code

46220 **Code is out of numerical sequence. See 46200–46255**

You can actually find code 46220 with its description between codes 46948 and 46230.

2. In its correct topic-related location. The code is placed with the other codes that report the same procedure or service based on the specific code description. This is highlighted by a symbol to the left of the code number–# (the hashtag sign)–to bring your attention to the fact that this code is not in numeric order.

EXAMPLES

The codes in the subsection for Anus, Excision are listed:

46221	Hemorrhoidectomy, internal, by rubber band ligation(s)
# 46945	Hemorrhoidectomy, internal, by ligation other than rubber band; single hemorrhoid column/group
# 46946	2 or more hemorrhoid columns/groups

As you can see, it makes much more sense for all of the hemorrhoidectomy codes to be in the same place so that you can read through all of the code descriptions and choose the one that most accurately matches the physician's notes. If the new codes were just placed in numeric order, you would need to keep flipping back and forth.

GUIDANCE CONNECTION

Read the CPT **Introduction**, subsection **Instructions for Use of the CPT Codebook–Code Symbols**, last paragraph.

22.3 Understanding Code Descriptions

As you look through the CPT book, both the numeric listings and the Alphabetic Index show their data in columns. Notice that some information is indented under other descriptions or terms. An indented description or term attaches to the description or term that appears at the margin of the column above, or before, the indented words.

In the Alphabetic Index

The Alphabetic Index uses a *list with an indented list* as a space-saving format. Take a look at this example:

EXAMPLE

Find "excision" in the Alphabetic Index:

Excision

Abdomen

    Tumor 49203-49205

Look at the words at the margin and those indented.

The term *Excision*, a type of procedure, is the heading of this part of the index. This heading is at the margin of the column, in bold. Beneath this, also at the margin of the column, is the word *Abdomen*, to indicate the anatomical site where the excision was performed. Underneath this, indented, is the word *Tumor*, to report what specifically was being excised, followed by a short range of suggested codes. Read backward and you have *Tumor, Abdomen, Excision*. The physician's notes are more likely to read:

Excision of a tumor in the abdomen

Just as with the descriptions in the numeric listing, you must be careful as you read and connect the indented words and phrases. Using a ruler or other straight edge may make it easier to see which words are indented and which are at the margins.

Notice that the CPT Alphabetic Index will not necessarily direct you toward one code. Very often, there will be multiple or a range of codes suggested. Take a look at the example for the *Excision* of an abdominal tumor; the Index suggests the range of codes 49203-49205. This means that you are required to investigate ALL of these codes before making a decision as to which code will accurately report *what* the physician did.

As you compare these three code descriptions in the *Main Section* of CPT, you can identify which additional specific detail or details you will need to abstract from the documentation. Continue to the *Main Section* as you learn the steps to determine an accurate CPT code.

In the Main Section (Numeric Listing)

Turn to the *Main Section* of CPT and find the first code suggested by the Alphabetic Index:

49203 Excision or destruction, open, intra-abdominal tumors, cysts, or endometriomas, 1 or more peritoneal, mesenteric, or retroperitoneal primary or secondary tumors; largest tumor 5 cm diameter or less

Look carefully. Do you see that this description is set at the inner margin of the column? The positioning indicates that it is the complete description of this code. Now, let's look right below this code, at the next two codes listed, which were included in the Alphabetic Index's suggested range.

49203 **Excision or destruction, open, intra-abdominal tumors, cysts, or endometriomas, 1 or more peritoneal, mesenteric, or retroperitoneal primary or secondary tumors; largest tumor 5 cm diameter or less**

49204 **largest tumor 5.1–10.0 cm diameter**

49205 **largest tumor greater than 10.0 cm diameter**

CODING BITES

Remember, the rule is to read the part of the code *up to the semicolon* and then attach the indented description to it. The CPT book does this to save space.

You can see that the descriptions next to codes 49204 and 49205 are both indented, not in line at the inner margin of the column. This means you must not only read 49204 or 49205's description but also attach it to the description above. How do you know what parts or how much? Look at the punctuation of the first code:

49203 **Excision or destruction, open, intra-abdominal tumors, cysts, or endometriomas, 1 or more peritoneal, mesenteric, or retroperitoneal primary or secondary tumors; largest tumor 5 cm diameter or less**

Notice the *semicolon (the dot over the comma)* after the word *tumors*. The semicolon is very important. When you read the description for a code that has an indented term or phrase, attach it to the description of the code above, but only the part of the description *up to the semicolon*. Read it as shown by the colored text:

49203 **Excision or destruction, open, intra-abdominal tumors, cysts, or endometriomas, 1 or more peritoneal, mesenteric, or retroperitoneal primary or secondary tumors; largest tumor 5 cm diameter or less**

49204 **largest tumor 5.1–10.0 cm diameter**

Putting both lines together means that the actual complete description of code 49204 is

49204 **Excision or destruction, open, intra-abdominal tumors, cysts, or endometriomas, 1 or more peritoneal, mesenteric, or retroperitoneal primary or secondary tumors; largest tumor 5.1–10.0 cm diameter**

Now that you know the trick to reading these code descriptions, you can understand the precise details reported by each of these three codes, and how they differ:

49203 **Excision or destruction, open, intra-abdominal tumors, cysts, or endometriomas, 1 or more peritoneal, mesenteric, or retroperitoneal primary or secondary tumors; largest tumor 5 cm diameter**

49204 **Excision or destruction, open, intra-abdominal tumors, cysts, or endometriomas, 1 or more peritoneal, mesenteric, or retroperitoneal primary or secondary tumors; largest tumor 5.1–10.0 cm diameter**

49205 **Excision or destruction, open, intra-abdominal tumors, cysts, or endometriomas, 1 or more peritoneal, mesenteric, or retroperitoneal primary or secondary tumors; largest tumor greater than 10.0 cm diameter**

GUIDANCE CONNECTION

Read the CPT **Introduction**, subsection **Instructions for Use of the CPT Codebook–Format of the Terminology**.

LET'S CODE IT! SCENARIO

Dr. Cragen performed a subtotal pericardiectomy using cardiopulmonary bypass on Lucy Brockton.

Let's Code It!

The procedure performed by Dr. Cragen was a pericardiectomy. Let's begin in the CPT Alphabetic Index, and read

Pericardiectomy, Subtotal 33030, 33031

Turn in the *Main Section* of CPT, and find these codes:

(continued)

33030 **Pericardiectomy, subtotal or complete; without cardiopulmonary bypass**

33031 **with cardiopulmonary bypass**

To determine the complete description for 33031, put it together, as you learned earlier. Remember, use the part of the first code description ***up to the semicolon*** plus the indented information:

33030 **Pericardiectomy, subtotal or complete; without cardiopulmonary bypass**

33031 **Pericardiectomy, subtotal or complete; with cardiopulmonary bypass**

Dr. Cragen documented that this pericardiectomy was performed with a cardiopulmonary bypass. Now, you know exactly which code to report!

33031 **Pericardiectomy, subtotal or complete; with cardiopulmonary bypass**

Good job!

Unlisted Codes
Codes shown at the end of each subsection of the CPT used as a catch-all for any procedure not represented by an existing code.

Unlisted Procedure or Service

On rare occasions, the physician for whom you are coding may perform a service or procedure that does not yet have a designated CPT Category I or CPT Category III code. When this is the case, you may find it necessary to report an **unlisted code**. There is one of these codes at the end of almost every section or subsection.

EXAMPLES

You will typically find an unlisted procedure code at the end of each section or subsection.

01999 **Unlisted anesthesia procedure(s)**

19499 **Unlisted procedure, breast**

78699 **Unlisted nervous system procedure, diagnostic nuclear medicine**

In these situations, report the unlisted code and attach a special report to the claim that includes the specific details of the procedure or service. Make certain you, as the professional coder, have done everything possible, including querying the physician, to confirm there are no other codes that will sufficiently or accurately report what was done.

22.4 Notations and Symbols

Throughout the CPT book, you will see notations and symbols. Let's review them together.

See

A "*see*" reference is found under a heading in the Alphabetic Index. Let's review an example to better understand this reference.

EXAMPLE

Leukocyte

See White Blood Cell

In this example, under the heading "Leukocyte," the notation "*See* White Blood Cell" provides an alternate term that the physician may have used in his or her notes. The CPT book is suggesting that, if you cannot find a match to the documentation under "Leukocyte," you might find it under the heading "White Blood Cell."

+ Plus Sign

The plus symbol (+) identifies an *add-on code*. An add-on procedure is most often performed with a main procedure. These services or treatments are in addition to, and associated with, the main procedure and are never performed or reported alone (without the main procedure). Due to this relationship with the main procedure, add-on codes *never* use the modifier 51 Multiple Procedures. (You will learn all about modifiers later in this book.) All the add-on codes are grouped and listed in the CPT code book's Appendix D for additional reference.

GUIDANCE CONNECTION

Read the CPT **Introduction**, subsection **Instructions for Use of the CPT Codebook–Add-on Codes**.

EXAMPLE

Add-On Code Listing—the Plus Symbol

+22328 each additional fractured vertebra or dislocated segment (List separately in addition to code for primary procedure)

(List Separately in Addition to Code for Primary Procedure)

This notation can be seen at the end of the description of an add-on code and reminds you that the code represents a procedure that is done as a part of another procedure, reported separately. Again, this should also remind you that this code cannot be used by itself.

EXAMPLE

Add-On Code Listing—the Parenthetical Notations

22630 Arthrodesis, posterior interbody technique, including laminectomy and/or discectomy to prepare interspace (other than for decompression), single interspace; lumbar

+22632 each additional interspace (List separately in addition to code for primary procedure)

(Use 22632 in conjunction with 22612, 22630, or 22633 when performed at a different interspace.)

(Use . . . in Conjunction with . . .)

The notation "*Use . . . in conjunction with . . .*" is found below the description of an add-on code. Here, the CPT book is going one step further. In addition to the + symbol and the notation "List separately," the book states the primary procedure code or codes with which the add-on code may be reported.

● Bullet Symbol

The bullet symbol (●) identifies a new code, one that is in the CPT book for the first time. During the annual update of the CPT book, various codes and guidelines are added, deleted, or revised. The new, updated, printed version of CPT is effective every January 1.

GUIDANCE CONNECTION

Read the CPT **Introduction**, subsection **Instructions for Use of the CPT Codebook–Code Symbols**. Also, be certain to check across the bottom of each page throughout the book. A legend will help remind you about the meaning for the symbols.

CODING BITES

If a claim form is received listing codes that have been deleted or changed, the claim will be rejected for the use of invalid codes.

▲ Triangle Symbol

The triangle symbol (▲) distinguishes a code whose description has been changed, or revised, since the last edition of CPT.

EXAMPLE

An Example of the ▲ (Triangle) Symbol

In the 2023 Code book, see

96446 Chemotherapy administration into the peritoneal cavity via indwelling port or catheter

In the 2024 Code book, see

96446 Chemotherapy administration into the peritoneal cavity via implanted port or catheter

The ▲ alerts you to the change, so you can make the appropriate adjustments to your coding process. From January 1, 2024, going forward, you will need to check the physician's notes for the new required details.

The double sideways triangles (▶ ◀) mark the beginning and end of text that has been revised or is being shown for the first time in this year's CPT book. This symbol may highlight code descriptions, guidelines, and/or instructional paragraphs throughout the CPT book.

EXAMPLE

76984 Ultrasound, intraoperative thoracic aorta (eg epiaortic)
▶ (For diagnostic intraoperative epicardial cardiac ultrasound (ie, echocardiography), see 76987, 76988, 76989)

You can see that it is helpful to have this new notation here, so you do not make the mistake of coding the wrong approach for the procedure.

★ Star Symbol

The star symbol (★), is placed to the left of those procedure codes that are permitted to be reported when the service has been provided using synchronous telemedicine services, and appended with modifier 95. These synchronous (real-time) telemedicine services engage physician and patient by use of equipment with functioning audio and video. These codes are listed in the CPT code book's Appendix P.

EXAMPLE

★ 90832 Psychotherapy, 30 minutes with patient

The star lets you know that if this physician and patient met in person, you can report this code. And if this physician and patient met via telemedicine (such as FaceTime or other telehealth technology), you can report this same code, appended with modifier 95.

There will be more about modifiers in the chapter ***CPT and HCPCS Level II Modifiers***.

⦸ Open Circle with Slash

The symbol of a circle with a slash through it (⦸), also called the Forbidden Symbol, identifies codes that are *not* permitted to be appended with modifier 51 Multiple Procedures. These codes are procedures that are sometimes done at the same time as another procedure (like an add-on code) but also can be performed alone (unlike an add-on code). Consequently, when such a procedure is performed along with other procedures, you are not allowed to attach the multiple procedure modifier. All codes that are modifier 51 exempt are grouped and listed in the CPT code book's Appendix E. There will be a lot more about modifiers as you go through this text.

EXAMPLE

⊘44500 Introduction of long gastrointestinal tube (e.g., Miller-Abbott) (separate procedure)

Hashtag

When you see this symbol, a hashtag (#), to the left of a CPT code, this identifies a code that has been added and placed into the code set out of numeric order. For more on this, see the section on the *CPT Resequencing Initiative* in the section ***CPT Code Book*** of this chapter.

♓ Duplicate PLA Test

Proprietary laboratory analyses (PLA) tests are represented by U codes, found in the Pathology and Laboratory section of CPT. Occasionally, the same description of a test may be connected by two different codes, and only differentiated by the proprietary name. When this has happened, this symbol ♓ will appear to the left of the code number, and a notation beneath will identify the matching code. Appendix O will provide additional details to enable you to identify which code you should report.

EXAMPLE

♓ 0202U Infectious disease (bacterial or viral respiratory tract infection), pathogen-specific nucleic acid (DNA or RNA), 22 targets including severe acute respiratory syndrome coronavirus 2 (SARSOCoV-2), qualitative RT-PCR, nasopharyngeal swab, each pathogen reported as detected or not detected.

(For additional PLA code with identical clinical descriptor, see 0223U. See Appendix O or the most current listing on the AMC CPT website to determine appropriate code assignment)

○ Open Circle

An open circle (○) identifies a recycled or reinstated code, which is a code that was previously deleted and now is found to be necessary, so it has been reactivated.

CODING BITES

There is a legend across the bottom of the pages throughout the CPT code book to remind you what each symbol represents, so you don't have to worry about memorizing all of these notations and symbols.

➲ Arrow in a Circle

Some versions of the CPT book may also include a circle with an arrow symbol (➲). This symbol (➲) points you toward an AMA-published reference that may be of additional guidance. The notation may direct you toward a particular edition of either the *CPT Assistant* newsletter or the book *CPT Changes: An Insider's View*. The AMA describes this subscription-only publication, *CPT Assistant*, as "*instrumental to many in their appeal of insurance denials, validating coding to auditors, training their staff and simply making answering day-to-day coding questions second nature.*"

LET'S CODE IT! SCENARIO

Kevin Kewly was in a fight with a member of his rival company's softball team. The other player took out a knife and stabbed him. When he arrived at the Emergency Department, Dr. Jarrenson repaired his 12 cm laceration, including debridement and retention sutures, on his lower right arm.

(continued)

Let's Code It!

Dr. Jarrenson stitched a 12 cm laceration on Kevin's arm. You learned in medical terminology class that this is known in health care services as a wound repair. Turn to the Alphabetic Index in your CPT code book and find

Wound

Read down the list to find Repair, and indented beneath this, Arms.

Wound

Repair

Arms

Complex 13120–13122

Intermediate . . . 12031, 12032, 12034–12037

Simple 12001, 12002, 12004–12007

Do you know whether Kevin's wound required a simple repair, intermediate repair, or complex repair? Not yet (you will learn), so for now, let's turn to the first code—12001—and see what we can find out.

Look at the in-section guidelines that are here, in the Repair (Closure) subsection, above code 12001. As you read the descriptions of the three types of repairs, notice that debridement and retention sutures are mentioned in both the case scenario and the description of Complex Repair.

Turn to the subsection Repair—Complex and find

13120 Repair, complex, scalp, arms and/or legs; 1.1 cm to 2.5 cm

13121 2.6 cm to 7.5 cm

+ 13122 each additional 5 cm or less (List separately in addition to code for primary procedure)

Look back at the case scenario. It states the wound was 12 cm. You learned earlier in this chapter that the plus sign (**+**) means you will need two codes because code 13122 cannot be reported alone. So, you will have to do some addition.

Code 13121 reports the first 7.5 cm, and you also will need to report 13122 for the additional 4.5 cm to total 12 cm.

That completes the story. Now, you can report Dr. Jarrenson's procedure performed on Kevin with confidence . . .

13121 Repair, complex, scalp, arms and/or legs; 2.6 cm to 7.5 cm

13122 each additional 5 cm or less (List separately in addition to code for primary procedure)

Good job!

22.5 Official Guidelines

Section Guidelines

The Official Guidelines you will use to ensure that you are coding procedures correctly are presented right in your CPT code book. Notice the pages in front of each of the six sections of the main part of the book.

- Evaluation and Management Guidelines
- Evaluation and Management Numerical Listings
- Anesthesia Guidelines
- Anesthesia Numerical Listings
- Surgery Guidelines
- Surgery Numerical Listings
- Radiology Guidelines
- Radiology Numerical Listings

- Pathology and Laboratory Guidelines
- Pathology and Laboratory Numerical Listings
- Medicine Guidelines
- Medicine Numerical Listings

The guidelines identify important rules and directives that coders must follow when assigning codes from each section–for example:

- Evaluation and management services guidelines include the definitions of commonly used terms.
- Surgery guidelines include a listing of services that are bundled into the surgical package definition (see **Figure 22-1**).
- Medicine guidelines include instructions on how to code multiple procedures and the proper use of add-on codes.

Surgery Guidelines

Guidelines to direct general reporting of services are presented in the **Introduction.** Some of the commonalities are repeated here for the convenience of those referring to this section on **Surgery.** Other definitions and items unique to Surgery are also listed.

Services

Services rendered in the office, home, or hospital, consultations, and other medical services are listed in the **Evaluation and Management Services** section (99201-99499) beginning on page 11. "Special Services and Reports" (99000-99091) are listed in the **Medicine** section.

CPT Surgical Package Definition

By their very nature, the services to any patient are variable. The CPT codes that represent a readily identifiable surgical procedure thereby include, on a procedure-by-procedure basis, a variety of services. In defining the specific services "included" in a given CPT surgical code, the following services related to the surgery when furnished by the physician or other qualified health care professional who performs the surgery are included in addition to the operation per se:

- Evaluation and Management (E/M) service(s) subsequent to the decision for surgery on the day before and/or day of surgery (including history and physical)
- Local infiltration, metacarpal/metatarsal/digital block or topical anesthesia
- Immediate postoperative care, including dictating operative notes, talking with the family and other physicians or other qualified health care professionals
- Writing orders
- Evaluating the patient in the postanesthesia recovery area
- Typical postoperative follow-up care other concomitant conditions is not included and may be listed separately.

Follow-Up Care for Therapeutic Surgical Procedures

Follow-up care for therapeutic surgical procedures includes only that care which is usually a part of the surgical service. Complications, exacerbations, recurrence, or the presence of other diseases or injuries requiring additional services should be separately reported.

Supplied Materials

Supplies and materials (eg, sterile trays/drugs), over and above those usually included with the procedure(s) rendered are reported separately. List drugs, trays, supplies, and materials provided. Identify as 99070 or specific supply code.

Reporting More Than One Procedure/Service

When more than one procedure/service is performed on the same date, same session or during a post-operative period (subject to the "surgical package" concept), several CPT modifiers may apply (see Appendix A for definition).

Separate Procedure

Some of the procedures or services listed in the CPT codebook that are commonly carried out as an integral component of a total service or procedure have been identified by the inclusion of the term "separate procedure." The codes designated as "separate procedure" should not be reported in addition so the code for the

FIGURE 22-1 A portion of the Surgery Guidelines in the CPT code book, including the CPT Surgical Package Definition

Source: *CPT Professional Manual*, American Medical Association

In-Section Guidelines

There are additional guidelines and instructions throughout each section, shown in paragraphs under various subheadings. These instructional notations, ranging from a short sentence to several paragraphs, provide specific information regarding the proper coding appropriate to that anatomical site or type of procedure (see **Figure 22-2**).

EXAMPLES

Instructional Notations in a Subsection

Biopsy

Directly above code 11102 is more than a page of guidance containing important details for coders preparing to report a code from this subsection.

Cardiography

Above code 93000, critical coding guidelines in addition to important definitions and descriptions are provided at the beginning of this subsection.

Stereotactic Radiation Therapy

Thoracic stereotactic body radiation therapy (SRS/SBRT) is a distinct procedure which may involve collaboration between a surgeon and radiation oncologist. The surgeon identifies and delineates the target for therapy. The radiation oncologist reports the appropriate code(s) for clinical treatment planning, physics and dosimetry, treatment delivery, and management from the Radiation Oncology section (see 77295, 77331, 77370, 77373, 77435). The same physician should not report target delineation services with radiation treatment management codes (77427–77499).

Target delineation involves specific determination of tumor borders to identify tumor volume and relationship with adjacent structures (e.g., chest wall, intraparenchymal vasculature and atelectatic lung) and previously placed fiducial markers, when present. Target delineation also includes availability to identify and validate the thoracic target prior to treatment delivery when a fiducial-less tracking system is utilized.

Do not report target delineation more than once per entire course of treatment when the treatment requires greater than one session.

32701 Thoracic target(s) delineation for stereotactic body radiation therapy (SRS/SBRT), (photon or particle beam), entire course of treatment

CPT Changes: An Insider's View 2013

(Do not report 32701 in conjunction with 77261–77799)

(For placement of fiducial markers, see 31626, 32553)

FIGURE 22-2 In-section guidelines from the Surgery section of the CPT code book related to reporting Stereotactic Radiation Therapy

Source: *CPT Professional Manual*, American Medical Association

Remember, the CPT code book will actually support your efforts to code accurately. The Official Guidelines are right there at your fingertips, and it is your obligation to read them before you confirm a code is ready to be reported. This is to your benefit . . . as you will improve your accuracy!

YOU INTERPRET IT!

Identify the pre-section or in-section guideline that you need to report the procedure accurately.

7. Dr. Singer documented that he debrided Jesse's abdominal wall. What specific details do you need to know to determine this code?
8. Dr. Trenton documented performing a sleep study with simultaneous recording of vital signs for Kent Burlington. The CPT code description is

   95807 Sleep study, simultaneous recording of ventilation, respiratory effort, ECG or heart rate, and oxygen saturation, attended by a technologist

   What does "attended by" mean?
9. Dr. Obatunda completed his documentation on his evaluation of Adam. To determine the correct Evaluation and Management code, you must determine the level of history documented in the notes. What exactly is included in a problem-focused history?

22.6 Category II and Category III Coding

In the chapter ***Introduction to the Languages of Coding***, you learned about the three categories of codes located in the CPT code book: **Category I codes** in the main text of the CPT book, **Category II codes**, and **Category III codes**. Let's briefly review how Category II and Category III codes are used.

Category I Codes
The codes listed in the main text of the CPT book, also known as CPT codes.

Category II Codes
Codes for performance measurement and tracking.

Category III Codes
Codes for emerging technology.

Category II Codes

Category II codes are used for statistical purposes–to track and measure performance and the quality of care provided in a health care facility.

While the number of Category II codes is small, these codes identify specific services that have been proven to be connected to quality patient care. Category II codes have five characters: four numbers followed by the letter *F*.

EXAMPLES

0015F Melanoma follow-up completed (includes assessment of all of the following components): history obtained regarding new or changing moles, complete physical skin exam performed, and patient counseled to perform a monthly self-skin examination.

1220F Patient screened for depression

As you can see from these examples, Category II codes provide detailed information about the encounter between physician and patient . . . details that are important to research.

Each code's description explains clinical fundamentals (such as vital signs), lab test results, patient education, or other facets that might be provided within a typical office visit. However, individually, these component services do not have any billable value and, therefore, are not assigned a code from Category I CPT codes. Assigning Category II codes simply is a way for the health care researchers to specifically calculate how often these services are being provided.

Merit-Based Incentive Payment System (MIPS)

Beginning in 2017, the Merit-Based Incentive Payment System (MIPS) was launched by the Centers for Medicare and Medicaid Services (CMS) to provide a way to reward participating providers with a performance-based payment adjustment to their earned Medicare reimbursements. This program replaces the Physician Quality Reporting System (PQRS) program. Coders are instructed to report when designated sets of quality measures are provided by an eligible professional (EP), using CPT Category II codes on a standard claim form, with a charged amount of $0.00 (zero) or $0.01 (zero dollars and one cent).

LET'S CODE IT! SCENARIO

Michael Catapano, a 71-year-old male, comes to see Dr. Sheridan, his primary care physician for the last 5 years, for his annual checkup. Michael has a family history of cardiac disease, so Dr. Sheridan takes extra care to examine Michael and speak with him about angina (severe acute chest pain caused by inadequate supply of oxygen to part of the heart). Dr. Sheridan documents that angina is absent.

Let's Code It!

As the coder for Dr. Sheridan, you will report a preventive medicine evaluation and management (E/M) code for the annual physical, along with codes for any specific tests or exams that she ordered to make certain Dr. Sheridan is properly reimbursed for her work. Dr. Sheridan was a good health care professional taking the time to discuss angina with Michael, and to carefully confirm that angina is not present. How can you, as the coder, report this service to Medicare?

Turn to the Category II code section in your CPT book.

Under the heading *Patient History*, find the code that identifies this patient does not have angina. You will see this code:

1012F Angina absent

So your report for this encounter will include two codes to tell the whole story about this encounter:

99397 Periodic comprehensive preventive medicine reevaluation and management of an individual including an age and gender appropriate history, examination, counseling/participatory guidance/risk factor reduction interventions, and the ordering of laboratory/diagnostic procedures; 65 years and older

1012F Angina absent

NOTE: You will learn more about annual physical exam coding in the chapter ***CPT Evaluation and Management Coding***, section on ***Preventive Medicine Services***.

Category III Codes

Category III codes offer the opportunity to collect detailed information on the use of new technological advancements, services, and procedures at their entry point into the practice of health care throughout the United States. Each code identifies an innovative procedure that is at the forefront of the health care industry but not yet widely used or accepted as a standard of care. It is why the codes in this section of the CPT book are considered temporary.

Category III codes may eventually become Category I codes (the codes in the main text of the CPT book). New procedures and services are assigned a Category III code so that actual usage can be accurately measured. They are placed in this section of the CPT book and assigned a code that has five characters: four numbers followed by the letter *T* (for *temporary*) in the fifth position.

EXAMPLES

0184T Excision of rectal tumor, transanal endoscopic microsurgical approach (i.e., TEMS), including muscularis propria (i.e., full thickness)

0509T Electroretinography (ERG) with interpretation and report, pattern (PERG)

The use of Category III codes is mandatory, as appropriate, according to the physician's notes. If there aren't any accurate Category I codes in the CPT book to report the physician's services, you must check the Category III section for an appropriate code *before* you are permitted to use a Category I **unlisted code**. The good news is that the CPT book will continue to help you. Category III codes *are* included in the Alphabetic Index. In addition, there are notations throughout the main sections that will direct you to a Category III code, if applicable.

It is important that you are aware of the fact that Category III codes represent up-and-coming technology. Because of this, the third-party payers from whom you seek reimbursement may consider some services **experimental**. When you work in a health care facility that uses any procedures or services reported with a Category III code, it is critical that you determine the carrier's rules and coverage with regard to the treatment or test. Should the carrier exclude it and refuse to pay, both the patient and your facility are better off knowing this as soon as possible.

GUIDANCE CONNECTION

Read the additional explanation in the guidelines directly under the section heading **Category III Codes** in your CPT book.

Experimental
A procedure or treatment that has not yet been accepted by the health care industry as the standard of care.

Keep good communication open with the physicians for whom you code. There are multiple benefits for this, including you finding out about a new technique or procedure before it is provided to any patient. Then, you can determine if this procedure will require a Category III code. Knowing this before a patient is involved will give you time. You may be able to petition the payer to convince it of the medical necessity and the cost efficiency of the new technology, and you may receive an approval after all. Waiting for a denial notice is not an efficient way to handle the situation. That is also not respectful to the patient.

A particular Category III code, once assigned, is reserved for 5 years, whether the code is upgraded to a Category I code or deleted altogether. It allows for the fact that certain technologies or procedures may take time to find acceptance.

YOU CODE IT! CASE STUDY

Dr. Rasmussen performed an automated eye-movement analysis without spatial calibration on Grave Emerson. He documented his interpretations in a report to her internist.

You Code It!

Go through the steps of coding, and determine the code(s) that should be reported for this test provided by Dr. Rasmussen to Grace Emerson.

Step #1: Read the case carefully and completely.
Step #2: Abstract the scenario. Which key words or terms describe what service the physician provided to the patient during this encounter?
Step #3: Are there any details missing or incomplete for which you would need to query the physician? [If so, ask your instructor.]
Step #4: Determine the correct CPT procedure code or codes to explain the details about what was provided to the patient during this encounter.
Step #5: Check for any relevant guidance, including reading all of the symbols and notations.
Step #6: Do you need to append any modifiers to ensure complete and accurate information is provided?
Step #7: Double-check your work.

Answer:

Did you determine this to be the code?

0615T **Automated analysis of binocular eye movements without spatial calibration, including disconjugacy, saccades, and papilary dynamics for the assessment of concussion, with interpretation and report**

Good job!

Chapter Summary

In this chapter, you learned about the important role that coding plays in our health care system, with specific focus on procedure codes used to report physician services and outpatient facility services. As an up-and-coming professional coding specialist, you must strive to accurately report the procedure, services, and treatments provided to every patient using CPT codes. Health care professionals are responsible for ensuring that the supporting documentation is complete so that you have the information necessary to find the most accurate code or codes.

CODING BITES

Steps to Coding Procedures

Step #1: Read the case carefully and completely.
Step #2: Abstract the scenario. Which key words or terms describe what service the physician provided to the patient during this encounter?
Step #3: Are there any details missing or incomplete for which you would need to query the physician? [If so, ask your instructor.]
Step #4: Determine the correct CPT procedure code or codes to explain the details about what was provided to the patient during this encounter.
Step #5: Check for any relevant guidance, including reading all of the symbols and notations.
Step #6: Do you need to append any modifiers to ensure complete and accurate information is provided?
Step #7: Double-check your work.

You Interpret It! Answers

1. Fracture = diagnosis code reported to explain why; Cast = CPT code reported to explain what Dr. Brazinski did for Liam.
2. Tobacco use = diagnosis code reported to explain why; Discuss = CPT code reported to explain what Dr. Spencer did for Emma.
3. Cholelithiasis = diagnosis code reported to explain why; Cholecystectomy = CPT code reported to explain what Dr. Myverson did for Jacob.
4. Excision = surgical removal . . . report a code from the Surgery section.
5. Anesthesia . . . report a code from the Anesthesia section.
6. MRI (Magnetic Resonance Imaging) = imaging . . . report a code from the Radiology section.
7. Inside the Surgery section of CPT, above the many codes available to report debridement, are in-section guidelines that include *Debridement*. Wound debridements (11042-11047) are reported by depth of tissue that is removed and by surface area of the wound.
8. 95807 Sleep study, simultaneous recording of ventilation, respiratory effort, ECG or heart rate, and oxygen saturation, attended by a technologist. What does "attended by" mean? The CPT book includes this definition right there, along with in-section guidelines for Sleep Medicine Testing: "*Attended: a technologist or qualified health care professional is physically present*.
9. Turn to the Evaluation and Management (E/M) Services Guidelines directly in front of the E/M code section in the CPT book and find this subsection: "**Determine the Extent of History Obtained** . . . ***Problem focused:*** Chief complaint; brief history of present illness or problem."

CHAPTER 22 REVIEW
Introduction to CPT

Let's Check It! Terminology

Match each term to the appropriate definition.

1. **LO 22.1** The provision of care for a patient using advice, recommendations, or discussion.
2. **LO 22.1** A treatment or service provided by a health care professional.
3. **LO 22.1** A patient who receives services for a short term (less than 1 day) in a physicians office or clinic, without being kept overnight.
4. **LO 22.1** The provision of medical care for a disorder or disease.
5. **LO 22.6** Codes for performance measurement and tracking.
6. **LO 22.6** The codes listed in the main text of the CPT book, also known as CPT codes.

A. Category I
B. Category II
C. Category III
D. Experimental
E. Outpatient
F. Procedure
G. Service

7. **LO 22.6** Codes for emerging technology.	**H.** Treatments
8. **LO 22.6** A procedure or treatment that has not yet been accepted by the health care industry as the standard of care.	**I.** Unlisted Code
9. **LO 22.3** Codes shown at the end of each subsection of the CPT used as a catch-all for any procedure not represented by an existing code.	

Let's Check It! Concepts

Choose the most appropriate answer for each of the following questions.

1. **LO 22.1** CPT stands for
   - **a.** Current Procedural Trailers.
   - **b.** Classification of Procedural Techniques.
   - **c.** Current Procedural Terminology.
   - **d.** Classification of Procedural Terms.
2. **LO 22.2** The main body of the CPT book has ___ sections, presented in numeric order (for the most part) by code number.
   - **a.** 2
   - **b.** 4
   - **c.** 6
   - **d.** 8
3. **LO 22.3** When reading a code description, the rule is to read the part of the code ___ and then attach the indented description to it.
   - **a.** up to the comma
   - **b.** up to the semicolon
   - **c.** up to the period
   - **d.** up to the hyphen
4. **LO 22.5** CPT guidelines
   - **a.** must be memorized by professional coders.
   - **b.** can be found in the front of every CPT section.
   - **c.** can be found in a separate guidelines book.
   - **d.** change every 2 months.
5. **LO 22.4** The **+** plus symbol identifies
   - **a.** a new code.
   - **b.** a revised code.
   - **c.** an add-on code.
   - **d.** a code that includes conscious sedation.
6. **LO 22.4** The ★ star symbol identifies
   - **a.** a new code.
   - **b.** an add-on code.
   - **c.** a revised code.
   - **d.** a telemedicine encounter.
7. **LO 22.4** The ● bullet symbol identifies
   - **a.** a new code.
   - **b.** an add-on code.
   - **c.** a revised code.
   - **d.** a code that includes conscious sedation.
8. **LO 22.4** The # hashtag symbol identifies
   - **a.** a reinstated or recycled code.
   - **b.** a product pending FDA approval.
   - **c.** an out-of-numeric-sequence code.
   - **d.** an exemption from modifier 51.
9. **LO 22.3** An unlisted code should only be used when
   - **a.** an accurate Category I code is not available.
   - **b.** an accurate Category I code is not available *and* an accurate Category III code is not available.
   - **c.** an accurate Category III code is not available.
   - **d.** an accurate Category I code is not available *or* an accurate Category III code is not available.
10. **LO 22.6** The ___ program provides for a bonus payment to those eligible professionals who meet the criteria for successful reporting, and a negative payment adjustment is applied when reporting is not submitted as required.
    - **a.** MIPS
    - **b.** AMA
    - **c.** RVU
    - **d.** PQRS

Let's Check It! Symbols and Sections

Part I

Match each symbol to the appropriate definition.

1.	**LO 22.4** Add-on code	A.	▲
2.	**LO 22.4** New or revised text	B.	○
3.	**LO 22.4** Telemedicine	C.	●
4.	**LO 22.4** Out-of-numeric-sequence code	D.	★
5.	**LO 22.4** New code	E.	⊘
6.	**LO 22.4** Revised code	F.	✚
7.	**LO 22.4** Exempt from modifier 51	G.	▶◀
8.	**LO 22.4** Reinstated or recycled code	H.	#
9.	**LO 22.4** Duplicate PLA Test	I.	♓
10.	**LO 22.4** Audio-only	J.	🔈

Part II

The main body of the CPT book has six sections. Match the code range to the correct section name.

1.	**LO 22.2** Surgery	A.	98000-98016, 99202-99499
2.	**LO 22.2** Pathology and Laboratory	B.	00100-01999 and 99100-99140
3.	**LO 22.2** Evaluation and Management	C.	10004-69990
4.	**LO 22.2** Medicine	D.	70010-79999
5.	**LO 22.2** Anesthesia	E.	80047-89398, 0001U-0559U
6.	**LO 22.2** Radiology	F.	90281-99199, 99500-99607

Let's Check It! Rules and Regulations

Please answer the following questions from the knowledge you have gained after reading this chapter.

1. **LO 22.1** Explain what is meant by *outpatient*. Include three examples of an outpatient facility.
2. **LO 22.2** Explain the CPT Resequencing Initiative.
3. **LO 22.3** Discuss unlisted procedure or service codes, when it is appropriate to use them, and any attachment that should be included.
4. **LO 22.4** What does the arrow in a circle symbol identify?
5. **LO 22.6** Differentiate between a CPT Category I code, Category II code, and Category III code, including any special characteristics of how they are identified.

YOU CODE IT! Basics

First, identify the procedural main term in the following statements; then code the procedure or service.

Example: Drainage of eyelid abscess

a. main term: *Drainage* **b.** procedure: *67700*

1. Ligation salivary ducts, intraoral:

   a. main term:______ **b.** procedure:______

2. Carpal scaphoid fracture manipulation:

   a. main term:______ **b.** procedure:______

3. Thoracotomy with cardiac massage:

   a. main term:______ **b.** procedure:______

(continued)

4. Ureter meatotomy:
   a. main term:______ b. procedure:______
5. Intraocular pressure monitoring for 36 hours:
   a. main term: ______ b. procedure:______
6. Tendon sheath incision, finger:
   a. main term: ______ b. procedure:______
7. Immunoassay antigen detection influenza B:
   a. main term:______ b. procedure:______
8. Anesthesia for ear biopsy:
   a. main term:______ b. procedure:______
9. Data analysis of implantable defibrillation, wearable device:
   a. main term:______ b. procedure:______
10. Keratoplasty, anterior lamellar:
   a. main term: ______ b. procedure:______
11. Lower arm x-ray:
   a. main term: ______ b. procedure:______
12. Kidney cyst injection:
   a. main term: ______ b. procedure:______
13. Lithotripsy with cystourethroscopy:
   a. main term:______ b. procedure:______
14. Percutaneous spinal cord biopsy:
   a. main term:______ b. procedure:______
15. Pediatric gastroenteritis education, individual:
   a. main term:______ b. procedure:______

YOU CODE IT! Practice

Using the techniques described in this chapter, carefully read through the case studies and determine the most accurate CPT code(s) for each case study.

1. Kelley Gaylord, a 7-year-old female, saw Dr. Roberts for a screening audiologic function test, pure tone, air only, to check her hearing.
2. Marlene Carrington, a healthy 42-year-old female, was taken to the operating room (OR) for an anterior cervical discectomy with decompression of a single interspace of the spinal cord and nerve roots and including osteophytectomy.
3. Rosa Phillips, a 34-year-old female, presents today for a percutaneous breast biopsy, needle core.
4. Sandra Lewis, a 55-year-old female, has been experiencing pain in her lower left back that wraps around to her inner thigh. Dr. Janson does a renal ultrasound, limited, real time with image documentation.
5. Hoyt Markum, a 78-year-old male, was taken to the OR for a single lung transplant with a cardiopulmonary bypass. Dr. Cannelloni was concerned because Hoyt was not expected to survive without the transplant.
6. Sunshine Thomas, an otherwise healthy 24-year-old female, was taken to the OR for a total thyroidectomy to remove a left thyroid mass.
7. Elaine Coker, an otherwise healthy 41-year-old female, was admitted to the same-day surgery center after having an abnormal shoulder x-ray in the clinic the week before. Dr. Logan decided to do a diagnostic arthroscopy.
8. Dr. Unentl inserted a nontunneled centrally inserted central venous catheter into Kevin Lorenzi, a 4-year-old male.
9. Anna Mourning, a 24-year-old female who is an amateur gymnast, was brought to the OR for the insertion of a plate with screws to assist the healing of the malunion of a humeral shaft fracture, open treatment.
10. Viviana Shank, a 5-month-old female, was taken to the OR for an excision, radical resection, of a 1.3-cm malignant neoplasm on the soft tissue of her left cheek right below her eye. It is expected that the carcinoma was caught before any spread. The patient is in otherwise healthy condition.
11. Nancy Hansen, an 18-year-old female, was brought to the OR for a c-section. Anesthesia was administered. She has type 1 diabetes that is currently under control. Dr. Klackson came to perform the cesarean delivery only. Code Dr. Klackson's procedure.
12. Ted Garrison, a 37-year-old male, was rushed to the hospital by ambulance and taken directly to the OR for an appendectomy for a ruptured appendix and generalized peritonitis. The patient is otherwise healthy.

(continued)

13. Dr. Simmons performed a 2.67 cm spigelian hernia repair in the lower abdomen on Drew Avalino, a 7-month-old male.
14. Barbara Cannin, an 18-year-old female, came to see her physician, Dr. Cordoba. She had something in her eye, and it was irritating her. Nothing she did could get it out. Dr. Cordoba took a problem-focused history and examined the area. He then applied a topical anesthetic and removed the foreign body from the superficial conjunctiva of her eye. Code the removal of the foreign body only.
15. Michael Munsey, an 84-year-old male, was seen by his physician at an ambulatory surgical center for the insertion of a temporary transvenous single-chamber cardiac electrode. The patient tolerated the procedure well.

YOU CODE IT! Application

The following exercises provide practice in the application of abstracting the physicians' notes and learning to work with SOAP notes from our textbook's health care facility, Prader, Bracker, & Associates. These case studies (SOAP notes) are modeled on real patient encounters. Using the techniques described in this chapter, carefully read through the case studies and find the most accurate CPT code(s) for each case study.

SOAP notes are a standardized documentation method used by health care providers to build a patient's chart. The SOAP note has four parts and each part will vary in length depending on the patient's encounter for that day.

So, what does the acronym SOAP stand for?

S = subjective
O = objective
A = assessment
P = plan

What does the **subjective** portion of the SOAP note include?

The chief complaint, a short statement in the patient's own words as to the reason for the encounter.

What does the **objective** portion of the SOAP note include?

The results of the physical examination and any measurable result; a few examples are vital signs, height, weight, and lab and diagnostic results.

What does the **assessment** portion of the SOAP note include?

A brief summation of the physician's diagnosis.

What does the **plan** portion of the SOAP note include?

The physician's plan of care (treatment) for the patient's encounter.

PRADER, BRACKER, & ASSOCIATES

A Complete Health Care Facility

159 Healthcare Way • SOMEWHERE, FL 32811 • 407-555-6789

PATIENT: MURRAY, CARMEL

ACCOUNT/EHR #: MURRCA001

Attending Physician: Oscar R. Prader, MD

S: This new patient is a 32-year-old female who comes in with a complaint of severe neck pain and difficulty turning her head. She states she was in a car accident 2 days ago; her car was struck from behind when she was driving home from work.

O: PE reveals tightness upon palpitation of ligaments in neck and shoulders, most pronounced C3 to C5. X-rays are taken of the cervical vertebrae, three views (AP, Lat, and PA). Radiologic review denies any fracture.

(continued)

A: Anterior longitudinal cervical sprain

P: 1. Prescribed cervical collar to be worn during all waking

2. Rx Vicodin (hydrocodone) 500 mg po prn
3. 1,000 mg aspirin
4. Pt to return in 2 weeks for follow-up

Determine the most accurate CPT code(s) for the x-ray(s).

PRADER, BRACKER, & ASSOCIATES

A Complete Health Care Facility

159 Healthcare Way • SOMEWHERE, FL 32811 • 407-555-6789

PATIENT: AUSTIN, BRUCE

ACCOUNT/EHR #: AUSTBR001

Attending Physician: Renee O. Bracker, MD

Preoperative Dx: Orbital mass, OD

Postoperative Dx: Herniated orbital fat pad, OD

Procedure: Excision of lesion and repair, right superior conjunctiva

Surgeon: Marc Zammarrelli, MD

Anesthesia: Local

PROCEDURE: After proparacaine was instilled in the eye, it was prepped and draped in the usual sterile manner and 2 percent lidocaine with 1:200,000 epinephrine was injected into the superior aspect of the right orbit. A corneal protective shield was placed in the eye. The eye was placed in down-gaze.

The upper lid was everted and the fornix examined. The herniating mass was viewed and measured at 0.75 cm in diameter. Westcott scissors were used to incise the fornix conjunctivae. The herniating mass was then clamped, excised, and cauterized. It appeared to contain mostly fat tissue, which was sent to pathology.

The superior fornix was repaired using running suture of 6-0 plain gut. Bacitracin ointment was applied to the eye followed by an eye pad. The patient tolerated the procedure well and left the OR in good condition.

Determine the most accurate CPT code(s) for the excision of the lesion.

WESTON HOSPITAL

629 Healthcare Way • SOMEWHERE, FL 32811 • 407-555-6541

PATIENT: WOODARD, HOPE

ACCOUNT/EHR #: WOODHO001

Attending Physician: Oscar R. Prader, MD

The patient is a 54-year-old female with a very long history of schizoaffective disorder with numerous hospitalizations who was brought in by ambulance due to increasing paranoia; increasing arguments with other people; and, in general, an exacerbation of her psychotic symptoms, 14-day duration.

I am here to provide psychoanalysis.

Initially, the patient was very agitated and uncooperative. She refused medications. A 2PC* was done and the patient had a court hearing that results in retention. Eventually, the patient agreed to a trial of Risperdal; she fairly rapidly improved once she was started on Risperdal 2 mg twice daily. At the time of discharge compared with admission, the patient is much improved. She is usually pleasant and cooperative, with occasional difficult moments and some continuing mild paranoia. She has no hallucinations. She has no thoughts of harming herself or anyone else. She has been compliant with her medication until she recently refused hydrochlorothiazide. She is irritable at times, but overall she is redirectable and is considered to be at or close to her best baseline. She is considered no imminent danger to herself or to others at this time.

(continued)

FINAL DX: Schizoaffective disorder; hypothyroidism; hypercholesterolemia; borderline hypertension.

Prescriptions for 30-day supplies were given:

Ativan 2 mg po tid; Celexa 40 mg po daily; Risperdal 2 mg po bid; Synthroid 0.088 mg po qam; Zocor 40 mg po qhs

**2PC* stands for "two physicians certify"—a medical certification testifying that an individual requires involuntary treatment at a psychiatric facility.

Determine the most accurate CPT code(s) for the psychoanalysis.

PRADER, BRACKER, & ASSOCIATES

A Complete Health Care Facility

159 Healthcare Way • SOMEWHERE, FL 32811 • 407-555-6789

PATIENT: JOHNS, CHARLENE

ACCOUNT/EHR #: JOHNCH001

Attending Physician: Renee O. Bracker, MD

S: This patient is a 34-year-old female who I have not seen in 6 months. She has a history of recurrent sinus infections. She has been well until 6 days ago. She presents with fever, severe frontal headache, facial pain, and runny nose. Patient states she has been having difficulty concentrating.

O: PE reveals: T 101.5°. HEENT: Tenderness over frontal and left maxillary sinuses. Nasal congestion visible. CT scan of the maxillofacial area, without contrast, reveals opacification of both frontal, left maxillary, and sphenoid sinuses and a possible large nonenhanced lesion in the brain.

A: Epidural abscess with frontal lobe lesions caused by significant compression on frontal lobe.

P: Recommendation for surgery to evacuate the abscess. Patient will think about it and call in a day or two.

Rx: Amoxil 875 mg q12h

Sudafed 120 mg q12h

Determine the most accurate CPT code(s) for the CT scan.

PRADER, BRACKER, & ASSOCIATES

A Complete Health Care Facility

159 Healthcare Way • SOMEWHERE, FL 32811 • 407-555-6789

PATIENT: PYKE, JOEL

ACCOUNT/EHR #: PYKEJO001

Diagnosis: Primary cardiomyopathy with chest pain

Procedure: Arterial catheterization

Physician: Oscar R. Prader, MD

Anesthesia: Local

Procedure: The patient was placed on the table in supine position. Local anesthesia was administered. Once we were assured that the patient had achieved no nervous stimuli, the incision was made and the catheter was introduced percutaneously. The incision was sutured with a simple repair. The patient tolerated the procedure well and was transferred to the recovery room.

Determine the most accurate CPT code(s) for the catheterization.

23

CPT and HCPCS Level II Modifiers

Key Terms

Alphanumeric
Ambulatory Surgery Center (ASC)
AMCC
Category II Modifiers
Class A Finding
Class B Finding
Class C Finding
Clinical Laboratory Improvement Amendment (CLIA)
CPT Code Modifier
Early and Periodic Screening, Diagnostic, and Treatment (EPSDT)
End-Stage Renal Disease (ESRD)
HCPCS Level II Modifier
Liters per Minute (LPM)
Locum Tenens Physician
Modifier
Nonphysician
Parenteral Enteral Nutrition (PEN)
Personnel Modifier
Physical Status Modifier
Service-Related Modifier
Supplemental Report
Urea Reduction Ratio (URR)

Learning Outcomes

After completing this chapter, the student should be able to:

LO 23.1 Recognize the purpose of procedure code modifiers.
LO 23.2 Apply personnel modifiers per the guidelines.
LO 23.3 Correctly use anesthesia Physical Status Modifiers.
LO 23.4 Implement ambulatory surgery center modifiers.
LO 23.5 Append anatomical site modifiers, as required.
LO 23.6 Identify circumstances that require a service-related modifier.
LO 23.7 Analyze the guidelines to correctly sequence multiple modifiers.
LO 23.8 Determine when a supplemental report is necessary.

STOP! Remember, you need to follow along in your CPT and HCPCS Level II code books for an optimal learning experience.

23.1 Modifiers Overview

In addition to the code for the specific procedure or service provided to the patient, there may be times when you will have to append a **modifier**. Modifiers are two-character codes that add clarification and additional details to the procedure code's original description, as written in the main portion of the *Current Procedural Terminology* (CPT) book.

Sometimes, the modifier provides necessary explanation to the third-party payer that directly relates to the reimbursement that the facility or physician should receive. It might explain that

- A service or procedure had both a professional component and a technical component.
- A service or procedure was performed by more than one physician.
- A service or procedure was performed in more than one location.
- A service or procedure was not performed in total (only part of it was done).
- The provider has special qualifications or training.
- An optional extra service was performed.
- A bilateral procedure was performed.
- A service or procedure was performed more than once.
- Unusual events arose.

Modifier
A two-character code that affects the meaning of another code; a code addendum that provides more meaning to the original code.

One of the most important reasons to properly report a procedure code with a modifier is to provide more information about that procedure–additional details that need to be added to the code description to make certain you are completely and accurately reporting what was *actually* provided to the patient during the encounter. Some modifiers will result in the physician or facility getting paid more money because the circumstances resulted in their having to do more work than usual. For example, modifier 22 Increased Procedural Service reports that the procedure was more complex than usual.

GUIDANCE CONNECTION

Read the CPT **Introduction**, subsection **Instructions for Use of the CPT Codebook–Modifiers** on how to properly use modifiers.

CODING BITES

Bookmark ***Appendix A*** in your CPT code book. This is the section containing the CPT modifiers and their full descriptions. It is important that you reference these prior to using any modifier. Your HCPCS Level II book has its own section that lists those modifiers with their complete descriptions.

CPT Code Modifier
A two-character code that may be appended to a code from the main portion of the CPT book to provide additional information.

Some modifiers will result in the physician or facility getting paid less money for the typical procedure but truthfully and accurately report that less work than usual was provided. For example, modifier 52 Reduced Services reports fewer services were provided.

Other modifiers will prevent a claim for reimbursement from being denied because it brings attention to the fact that unusual circumstances required unusual work. For example, modifier 23 Unusual Anesthesia alerts that a procedure that typically only uses a local anesthetic, for example, required general anesthesia. In these cases, you also will need to provide a supplemental report to explain what those circumstances were so that they will understand because you are telling the *whole* story.

As you go through the lists, you will find there are modifiers that have no effect at all on reimbursement but provide specific details about the procedure that will be important for continuity of care, as well as for research and statistics. An example is modifier RC Right Coronary Artery to identify the specific anatomical site upon which the procedure was completed.

You will find many modifiers listed in their own section of the CPT code book's ***Appendix A***. Listed in numeric order, each modifier is shown by category, accompanied by an explanation of when and how you should use that modifier. The rest can be found in the separate HCPCS Level II code book.

Types of Modifiers

There are five categories of modifiers:

- **CPT code modifiers** are two characters that can be attached to regular codes from the main portion of the CPT book and to HCPCS Level II codes.

EXAMPLE

CPT Modifiers

23 Unusual Anesthesia

66 Surgical Team

Physical Status Modifier
A two-character alphanumeric code used to describe the condition of the patient at the time anesthesia services are administered.

Alphanumeric
Containing both letters and numbers.

- Anesthesia **Physical Status Modifiers** consist of two characters and are **alphanumeric**. They are used only with CPT codes reporting anesthesia services.

EXAMPLE

Physical Status Modifiers

P1 A normal healthy patient

P3 A patient with severe systemic disease

Ambulatory Surgery Center (ASC)
A facility specially designed to provide surgical treatments without an overnight stay; also known as a *same-day surgery center.*

- **Ambulatory surgery center (ASC)** hospital outpatient modifiers are two digits and are used only when reporting services provided at this type of outpatient facility.

EXAMPLE

ASC Modifiers

27 Multiple outpatient hospital E/M encounters on the same date

73 Discontinued outpatient procedure prior to anesthesia administration

- **HCPCS Level II modifiers** are two characters and alphabetic or alphanumeric. They are used to provide additional information about services when appended to CPT and HCPCS Level II codes.

HCPCS Level II Modifier
A two-character alphabetic or alphanumeric code that may be appended to a code from the main portion of the CPT book or a code from the HCPCS Level II book.

EXAMPLE

HCPCS Level II Modifiers

E1	Upper left eyelid
RT	Right side (of body)

- **Category II modifiers** are two characters: a number followed by the letter P. Only appended to Category II codes, these modifiers provide explanations as to why a particular service should not be included in the qualifications for a specific performance measure.

Category II Modifiers
Modifiers provided for use with Category II CPT codes to indicate a valid reason for a portion of a performance measure to be deleted from qualification.

EXAMPLES

1P	Performance Measure Exclusion Modifier due to Medical Reasons
2P	Performance Measure Exclusion Modifier due to Patient Reasons

CODING BITES

HCPCS Level II modifiers can be appended to either CPT codes or HCPCS Level II codes.

Using Modifiers

Using modifiers is, most often, a judgment that you, the coding specialist, will have to make as you review the details of each case. As you analyze the descriptions of the procedures performed, as documented by the physician, and compare them with the descriptions of the codes in the CPT book, you may find that there is more to the story than the code description provides. This is important because it is a coding professional's job to relate the *whole story* of the encounter.

EXAMPLE

Dr. Kennedy determined that Patricia's tear ducts were blocked. He dilated and irrigated both the right and left eyes.

[Remember from medical terminology class, the medical term for the tear duct = lacrimal punctum (plural = puncta). If you don't remember, it is important to use your medical dictionary to ensure you can determine the accurate code or codes.]

CPT Modifier Notation

68801 Dilation of lacrimal punctum, with or without irrigation

(To report a bilateral procedure, use 68801 with modifier 50)

Modifier 50 is used to identify that a service or procedure was performed bilaterally (both sides). If the physician's documentation states that this procedure was done on both sides, you can see that the code description does not include this detail. Therefore, you must add a modifier . . . to tell the whole story.

CODING BITES

On occasion, the CPT book will remind you of a special circumstance that requires a modifier. However, most of the time, it is *you* who must determine when to use a modifier and which modifier or modifiers to append to the code.

EXAMPLE

Jason has been deaf in his left ear since he was 16. Today, Dr. Sangar is performing a speech audiometry threshold test on his right ear.

92555 Speech audiometry threshold

Does this code report the test on one ear or two ears? It doesn't specifically state this important detail. How do you know how to report this accurately? The CPT in-section guidelines give you the answer.

CPT Instructional Paragraph

Paragraph above code 92550:

Audiologic Function Tests

". . . All services include testing of both ears. Use modifier 52 if a test is applied to one ear instead of two ears."

Modifier 52 indicates that the service or procedure, as described, was not completed in full. If both ears are included in the code, but only one ear was tested, then a reduced service was provided. This is why it is so very important to read all of these in-section guidelines, in addition to the those in the front of the section, to help you code accurately. Therefore, if the physician's documentation states that only one ear was examined during this encounter, you must append modifier 52 to tell the whole *story.*

LET'S CODE IT! SCENARIO

Dinah Chen, a 21-year-old female, came into the emergency clinic with two lacerations: one on her right hand and the second on her right arm. Dr. Padmore debrided and provided a complicated repair of the 3.1-cm laceration on her upper right arm and a layered closure of a 2.5-cm laceration on her right hand, proximal to the second digit.

Let's Code It!

What exactly did Dr. Padmore do for Dinah Chen? *A complicated repair of a laceration on her upper arm + a layered repair on her hand.* Begin in the CPT Alphabetic Index, and look up

Repair . . . Arm, Upper would make sense, but wait a minute. Dr. Padmore did not actually repair Dinah's arm, with regard to its muscles or tendons, etc. He repaired the laceration. Check this out . . .

Repair . . . Laceration does not work either. None of the anatomical sites listed beneath match arm or hand. Pull out your medical dictionary and check the meaning of laceration: a wound or cut in the tissue. Let's try . . .

Repair . . . Wound—this has possibilities. The three terms showing—Complex, Intermediate, Simple—make sense, and Dr. Padmore did provide a "complicated repair," which could translate to Complex. The Alphabetic Index suggests codes in the range 12001–13160. Turn in the CPT *Main Section* to find code **12001 Simple repair**. How do you know what actually constitutes a complex, intermediate, or simple repair?

Directly above this first code [12001] are Official Guidelines under the subheading **Repair (Closure)**. These in-section guidelines explain the definitions of **Simple Repair**, **Intermediate Repair**, and **Complex Repair**, along with other important details that you need to report these repairs accurately.

The chapter ***CPT Surgery Section*** will provide you with more in-depth instruction about this.

For this chapter, on Modifiers, you want to focus on paragraph 2 of these *in-section guidelines*. It tells you that, when multiple wounds are repaired, reported with different levels of repair, you will need to append modifier **59 Distinct Procedural Service** to the second code and all thereafter. This will help you understand that, to report Dr. Padmore's services to Dinah Chen, you will submit these codes:

13121 **Repair, complex, scalp, arms, and/or legs; 2.6 cm to 7.5 cm**

12041-59 **Repair, intermediate, wounds of neck, hands, feet and/or external genitalia; 2.5 cm or less, distinct procedural service**

GUIDANCE CONNECTION

Read the **in-section** Official Guidelines, in the subsection **Repair (Closure)**, including paragraph **2. When multiple wounds are repaired**.

23.2 Personnel Modifiers

As you read through the descriptions of the modifiers, most of them will seem very straightforward. **Personnel modifiers** explain special circumstances relating to the health care professionals involved in the treatment of the patient. These modifiers specifically identify the qualifications of the health care professional who provided the service reported by the code to which this modifier is being attached, while other modifiers identify the provider's special training. You will note that some of the modifier descriptions also include a location as a part of their meaning.

Personnel Modifier
A modifier adding information about the professional(s) attending to the provision of this procedure or treatment to the patient during this encounter.

Nonphysician
A nonphysician can be a nurse practitioner, certified registered nurse anesthetist, certified registered nurse, clinical nurse specialist, or physician assistant.

EXAMPLES

Personnel Modifier

62	Two Surgeons
66	Surgical Team
80	Assistant Surgeon
GF	**Nonphysician** services in a critical access hospital
AQ	Physician providing a service in an unlisted health professional shortage area (HPSA)

Modifier 62 Two Surgeons clearly is used when the operative notes indicate that two surgeons worked side by side, both as primary surgeons, during a procedure. If the modifier is not there to explain that there *were* two primary surgeons involved, how else could the insurance carrier know that receiving two separate claim forms for the same patient on the same day is legitimate? The insurance carrier would certainly think that one of the physicians is fraudulently billing for work done by another. The second claim filed, and possibly even the first one, might be denied or set aside for further determination to find out why the second claim was submitted, and/or the carrier may even initiate a fraud investigation. This little two-digit modifier tells the insurance carrier that no one is cheating and both surgeons actually did provide for the patient.

The same scenario works for other CPT personnel modifiers:

- 66 Surgical Team
- 80 Assistant Surgeon
- 81 Minimum Assistant Surgeon
- 82 Assistant Surgeon (when qualified resident surgeon not available)

Using any of these modifiers, or any of the HCPCS Level II modifiers (see **Table 23-1**), provides an explanation, very directly and simply, why more than one health care professional is claiming reimbursement for providing service to the same patient on the same date, or the specific qualifications of that professional.

Locum Tenens Physician
A physician who fills in, temporarily, for another physician.

TABLE 23-1 HCPCS Level II Personnel Modifiers

AE	Registered dietitian
AF	Specialty physician
AG	Primary physician
AH	Clinical psychologist
AI	Principal physician of record

(continued)

AJ	Clinical social worker
AK	Nonparticipating physician
AM	Physician, team member service
AQ	Physician providing service in unlisted HPSA
AR	Physician provider services in a physician scarcity area
AS	Physician assistant, nurse practitioner, or clinical nurse specialist services for assistant at surgery
DA	Oral health assessment by professional other than a dentist
GC	Service performed in part by a resident under the direction of a teaching physician
GE	Service performed by a resident without the presence of a teaching physician under the primary care exception
GF	**Nonphysician** services in a critical access hospital
GJ	"Opt out" physician or practitioner emergency or urgent service
GV	Attending physician not employed or paid under arrangement by the patient's hospice provider
HL	Intern
HM	Less than bachelor degree level
HN	Bachelor's degree level
HO	Master's degree level
HP	Doctoral level
HT	Multidisciplinary team
Q4	Service for ordering/referring physician that qualifies as a service exemption
Q5	Service furnished by a substitute physician under a reciprocal billing arrangement
Q6	Service furnished by a **locum tenens physician**
SA	Nurse practitioner rendering service in collaboration with a physician
SB	Nurse midwife
SD	Services provided by registered nurse with specialized, highly technical home infusion training
SW	Services provided by a certified diabetic educator
TD	Registered nurse (RN)
TE	Licensed practical nurse (LPN) or LVN

CPT

LET'S CODE IT! SCENARIO

Valerie Ferguson, a 43-year-old female, has been diagnosed with endometriosis and is admitted to Midtown Hospital to have Dr. Lissard perform a vaginal, radical hysterectomy. While Valerie is in the operating room (OR) and under anesthesia, Dr. Rasmussen is going to perform an open sling operation for stress incontinence on her bladder, and Dr. Barlow is an assistant surgeon who is there to assist Dr. Lissard. She tolerates both procedures well and is taken back to her room.

Let's Code It!

The codes for these procedures are 58285 and 57288. You will learn more about how to determine these codes in the following chapters. For now, let's focus on the modifiers.

(continued)

The CPT procedure codes explain what was done for Valerie during this procedure. Afterwards, Dr. Lissard's coder will submit a claim and send it to Valerie's health insurance company, including the services provided for both Dr. Lissard and Dr. Barlow. The coder forgets to append any modifiers.

Dr. Rasmussen's coder sent the claim for her work performed for Valerie 2 days later. This claim also fails to include any modifiers.

Now, Bernice Cannelloni, claims adjuster for Valerie's health insurance company, looks at Dr. Rasmussen's claim. Wait a minute. We just paid a claim for two other physicians who stated a totally different surgical procedure was provided to the same patient on the same date! Perhaps someone is trying to defraud this company! An investigation begins, delaying payment by several months until it is all straightened out.

If there were modifiers that could explain what role each of these surgeons played, working side-by-side to care for this patient, the entire fraud investigation and delay in payment could be prevented.

Open your CPT code book to ***Appendix A*** and read through the list of modifiers to see if any might enable Dr. Lissard's coder and Dr. Rasmussen's coder to more clearly explain the whole story. Take a look at

62 **Two Surgeons:** When 2 surgeons work together as primary surgeons performing distinct part(s) of a procedure, each surgeon should report his/her distinct operative work by adding modifier 62 to the procedure code . . .

This looks perfect to explain this unusual situation, doesn't it?

Now what about Dr. Barlow? How do we explain his role during this procedure? Review the modifiers in ***Appendix A*** to determine if there are any that will help explain. Take a look at

80 **Assistant Surgeon:** Surgical assistant services may be identified by adding modifier 80 to the usual procedure number(s).

So, Dr. Lissard's coder would report this code:

58285-62 **Vaginal hysterectomy, radical (Schauta type operation); two surgeons**

And Dr. Rasmussen's coder would report this code:

57288-62 **Sling operation for stress incontinence; two surgeons**

And Dr. Barlow's coder would report this:

58285-80 **Vaginal hysterectomy, radical (Schauta type operation); assistant surgeon**

Good job!

Anesthesia Personnel Modifiers

The following modifiers (see **Table 23-2**), used only with anesthesia codes, are actually HCPCS Level II modifiers. You can see that they provide specific details about the personnel administering the anesthetic to the patient. These details are important for reimbursement as well as responsibility.

TABLE 23-2 Anesthesia Personnel Modifiers

AA	Anesthesia services that are performed personally by anesthesiologist
AD	Medical supervision by a physician: more than four concurrent anesthesia procedures
G8	Monitored anesthesia care (MAC) for deep complex, complicated, or markedly invasive surgical procedure
G9	Monitored anesthesia care for patient who has history of severe cardiopulmonary condition
QK	Medical direction of two, three, or four concurrent anesthesia procedures involving qualified individuals
QS	Monitored anesthesia care (MAC) service
QX	Qualified nonphysician anesthetist with medical direction by a physician
QY	Medical direction of one qualified nonphysician anesthetist by an anesthesiologist
QZ	CRNA service without medical direction by a physician

YOU CODE IT! CASE STUDY

CPT HCPCS Level II

Dr. Charleston, an anesthesiologist, was asked to provide anesthesia care while Dr. Ablione performed a needle biopsy of the pleura of Rosalind Bowman's left lung. Gerald Mathinson, a CRNA, will administer the anesthesia for this procedure, with Dr. Charleston's supervision.

You Code It!

Gerald Mathinson is administering this anesthesia, but he is not an anesthesiologist. Dr. Charleston is not administering the anesthesia for this procedure; however, his presence and expertise are still needed. The procedure code for this anesthesia service is this:

00522 Anesthesia for closed chest procedures; needle biopsy of pleura

Good. Now, you must find a way to explain that this was not an anesthesiologist who provided the service, but a CRNA (Certified Registered Nurse Anesthetist), with direction by Dr. Charleston. The code description is correct. You just need to clearly communicate what health care professionals were actually involved in this procedure. A modifier can provide this additional explanation.

Answer:

Did you determine this to be the correct modifier?

00522-QX Anesthesia for closed chest procedures; needle biopsy of pleura, CRNA service: with medical direction by a physician

Good job!!

23.3 Anesthesia Physical Status Modifiers

Anesthesia Physical Status Modifiers are two-character alphanumeric codes: the letter *P* followed by a number. These modifiers identify the condition of the patient at the time anesthesia services were provided and highlight health circumstances that might dramatically affect the anesthesiologist's ability to successfully care for the patient. An explanation of the patient's health level at the time the anesthesiologist administers the service helps the third-party payer get a better understanding of how hard this physician (anesthesiologist) had to work.

For example, if a patient has uncontrolled hypertension at the time anesthesia is administered, the anesthesiologist must monitor the patient more carefully, must perhaps use a different type of anesthetic, and must watch for possible complications that would not be an issue with an otherwise healthy patient. This status modifier, for the most part, does not relate to the reason the patient is having the anesthesia administered but is indicative of the patient's overall health. You can see that, without understanding the difference between treatment issue and overall health, it might be hard for you to identify a patient as "P1 A normal healthy patient" when the person is in your facility to have a diseased gallbladder removed. However, if the patient is *otherwise healthy*, P1 is the correct status modifier.

The Physical Status Modifiers, P1–P6, may be appended *only* to codes from the Anesthesia section of the CPT book, codes 00100–01999.

GUIDANCE CONNECTION

Read the anesthesia Physical Status Modifiers and their descriptions in the **Official Guidelines** located immediately prior to the **Anesthesia** code section in the main part of CPT and/or in **Appendix A**.

All anesthesia codes and *only* anesthesia codes are appended with a Physical Status Modifier, immediately following the anesthesia code.

EXAMPLE

Use of a Physical Status Modifier

Anesthesia for a diagnostic arthroscopy of the knee on a 67-year-old male with diabetes mellitus, controlled well with medication.

01382-P2

There may be a case when a CPT modifier must also be used with an anesthesia code. When this is done, the Physical Status Modifier is to be placed closest to the anesthesia code.

EXAMPLE

Using a Physical Status Modifier with a CPT Modifier

Anesthesia for a third-degree burn excision, 5% of total body surface area, for a patient with uncontrolled diabetes. The procedure was discontinued due to sudden onset of arrhythmia.

01952-P3-53

Modifier **P3** reports that this patient has a severe systemic disease [the uncontrolled diabetes mellitus].

Modifier **53** reports a Discontinued Procedure.

You will read more about the anesthesia Physical Status Modifiers in the chapter ***CPT Anesthesia Section***.

LET'S CODE IT! SCENARIO

Carson Crosby, a healthy and fit 18-year-old male, fell from a girder on a construction site, fracturing three ribs and two vertebrae, and sustaining a hairline fracture of his pelvis. Dr. Pollack, an anesthesiologist, was brought in to administer general anesthesia so the body cast could be applied by Dr. Abrams, an orthopedist.

Let's Code It!

You are the professional coding specialist for Dr. Pollack, the anesthesiologist. Our focus in this case is the application of anesthesia modifiers; however, you will need a code to which to append that Physical Status Modifier. So, let's begin with the Alphabetic Index:

Anesthesia

The long list beneath includes mostly anatomical sites. Hmmm. You have two terms: body + cast, so try these.

There is listing for *Body*; however, there are two listings for *Cast*:

Cast
- Knee 01420

Cast Application
- Forearm, Wrist, and Hand . . 01860
- Leg 01490
- Pelvis 01130
- Shoulder 01680

Cast Application matches the documentation; however, none of these anatomical areas match. The scenario did mention Carson's pelvis being fractured, so let's start with that code.

01130 Anesthesia for body cast application or revision

(continued)

This is perfect! Now, you learned that all codes from the Anesthesia section require a Physical Status Modifier. So, turn to ***Appendix A*** and find the heading **Anesthesia Physical Status Modifiers** [it is after modifier **99 Multiple Modifiers**]. Go back to the documentation and look for a description of Carson's current health. This is in regard to his overall health, not in relation to this specific issue. Did you read that the scenario states, "*Carson Crosby, a healthy and fit 18-year-old male*"? Healthy and fit! Review all of the Physical Status Modifier descriptions and determine which is most accurate about Carson's condition during this encounter.

P1 A normal healthy patient

Good job! Now put them together and you can report this, with confidence, to communicate what Dr. Pollack did for Carson during this session:

01130-P1 Anesthesia for body cast application or revision; a normal healthy patient

23.4 Ambulatory Surgery Center Hospital Outpatient Use Modifiers

When you are reporting the code or codes for procedures provided to a patient in a same-day surgery center or outpatient surgery center, you might determine that a modifier may be necessary. In these cases, you will append modifiers from those provided specifically for these locations. The ASC Hospital Outpatient Use Modifiers are shown in ***Appendix A*** of your CPT book, in their own subsection. Some of the modifiers in this subheading are the same as the CPT modifiers. However, there are three additional modifiers specifically for ASC coders. Open your CPT book to ***Appendix A*** and read along as we review some of these modifiers.

Modifier 27

27 Multiple Outpatient Hospital E/M Encounters on the Same Date: For hospital outpatient reporting purposes, utilization of hospital resources related to separate and distinct E/M encounters performed in multiple outpatient hospital settings on the same date may be reported by adding modifier 27 to each appropriate level outpatient and/or emergency department E/M code(s). This modifier provides a means of reporting circumstances involving evaluation and management services provided by physician(s) in more than one (multiple) outpatient hospital setting(s) (e.g., hospital emergency department, clinic).

Using modifier 27 will not be a common occurrence, but still, it can be complex. So, let's use an example scenario to work through together:

CODING BITES

Many hospitals have outpatient departments providing same-day or outpatient surgical procedures. If the patient is "admitted" and "discharged" the same day, this is coded as an outpatient procedure, using CPT and, when necessary, this group of modifiers.

EXAMPLE

Alexandra Benson, a 41-year-old female, cut her hand and went to the Mulford General Hospital clinic. After Dr. Williams evaluated her hand, he sent her to the emergency department (ED) because the cut was so deep it needed more intense care. Dr. Kinsey evaluated the injury and repaired Alexandra's laceration in the ED.

As the coding specialist for the hospital, you would be responsible for coding the services provided in all your facilities, including the clinic as well as the ED. Alexandra Benson was seen in two different facilities on the same day for the same injury. First, you would code the services that Dr. Williams did—the E/M of Alexandra's injury and his decision to send her to the ED for a higher level of care. Second, you would report the services that Alexandra received in the ED, which certainly included additional evaluation and then the repair of her wound.

For Dr. Williams, report: 99201-27

For Dr. Kinsey, report: 99281-27

Without the use of modifier 27, you would have difficulty in getting the claim paid because the third-party payer may think that this is a case of duplicate billing, an error, or fraud.

Modifiers 73 and 74

Occasionally, a planned surgical event is not performed due to circumstances that might put the patient in jeopardy. In such cases, all the preparation was done, the team was ready, and your facility needs to be reimbursed, even though you have not performed the service or treatment. Modifiers 73 and 74 will identify these unusual circumstances.

73 **Discontinued Outpatient Hospital/Ambulatory Surgery Center (ASC) Procedure Prior to the Administration of Anesthesia:** Due to extenuating circumstances or those that threaten the well-being of the patient, the physician may cancel a surgical or diagnostic procedure subsequent to the patient's surgical preparation (including sedation when provided, and being taken to the room where the procedure is to be performed), but prior to the administration of anesthesia (local, regional block(s) or general). Under these circumstances, the intended service that is prepared for but canceled can be reported by its usual procedure number and the addition of modifier 73.

74 **Discontinued Outpatient Hospital/Ambulatory Surgery Center (ASC) Procedure After Administration of Anesthesia:** Due to extenuating circumstances or those that threaten the well-being of the patient, the physician may terminate a surgical or diagnostic procedure after the administration of anesthesia (local, regional block(s) or general), or after the procedure was started (incision made, intubation started, scope inserted, etc.). Under these circumstances, the procedure started, but terminated can be reported by its usual procedure number and the addition of modifier 74.

The extenuating circumstances mentioned are generally accepted situations that would be reasonable to stop a procedure at this late point in time. Prior to the administration of anesthesia, it might be that the nurse, while taking the patient's vital signs, documents that the patient has a fever. It is the standard of care to avoid surgical procedures on a patient with a fever, so the proper thing to do would be to postpone. Once the patient is in the procedure room, and anesthesia has been administered, there may be a need to stop the procedure, such as the patient experiencing a seizure or dramatic drop in blood pressure. Make certain that you not only append one of these modifiers, when appropriate, but also include a special report to explain exactly what happened to make cancelling the procedure the right action to take.

LET'S CODE IT! SCENARIO

Cole Dennali, a 59-year-old male, was brought into Room 5 to be prepared for a bunionectomy. He changed into a gown, he got into bed, and the nurse took his vital signs. Cole's breathing was labored—it appeared he was having an asthma attack. Dr. Fraumann ordered respiratory therapy to come in and provide a nebulizer treatment. Because general anesthesia could not be administered, the bunionectomy was canceled.

Let's Code It!

Dr. Fraumann and her team were prepared and ready to perform a bunionectomy. However, it is not wise to administer general anesthesia to a patient having difficulty breathing, so the procedure had to be canceled in the best interest of the patient. The facility still deserves to be reimbursed for its time, materials and supplies, and efforts. Therefore, the facility will submit a claim form to Cole's insurance carrier with the code for the bunionectomy and the modifier 73 to indicate that the procedure was canceled *prior to the administration of anesthesia*:

28292-73 **Correction, hallux valgus (bunionectomy), with sesamoidectomy, when performed; with resection of proximal phalanx base, when performed, any method, Discontinued Out-Patient Hospital/Ambulatory Surgery Center (ASC) Procedure Prior to the Administration of Anesthesia**

23.5 Anatomical Site Modifiers

Anatomical site modifiers (see **Table 23-3**) provide additional specific detail about the target of the service or procedure not provided by the code. These pieces of information are important to include for those providing continuity of care as well as for reimbursement purposes.

- E1–E4 identify right/left/upper/lower eyelids
- F1–FA identify each of the 10 fingers
- T1–TA identify each of the 10 toes
- LC–LD identify portions of the left coronary artery

- RC identifies the right coronary artery
- LT = left
- RT = right

EXAMPLE

28008 Fasciotomy, foot and/or toe

Adding a modifier such as T7 would include very important information for the claim, especially if the patient had a preexisting condition involving a different toe.

T7 Right foot, third digit

Therefore, you would report: **28008-T7 Fasciotomy, right foot, third digit.**

TABLE 23-3 Anatomical Site Modifiers

E1	Upper left eyelid
E2	Lower left eyelid
E3	Upper right eyelid
E4	Lower right eyelid
FA	Left hand, thumb
F1	Left hand, second digit
F2	Left hand, third digit
F3	Left hand, fourth digit
F4	Left hand, fifth digit
F5	Right hand, thumb
F6	Right hand, second digit
F7	Right hand, third digit
F8	Right hand, fourth digit
F9	Right hand, fifth digit
LC	Left circumflex coronary artery
LD	Left anterior descending coronary artery
LT	Left side (i.e., left side of the body)
RC	Right coronary artery
RT	Right side (i.e., right side of the body)
TA	Left foot, great toe
T1	Left foot, second digit
T2	Left foot, third digit
T3	Left foot, fourth digit
T4	Left foot, fifth digit
T5	Right foot, great toe
T6	Right foot, second digit
T7	Right foot, third digit
T8	Right foot, fourth digit
T9	Right foot, fifth digit

YOU CODE IT! CASE STUDY

Beatrice Burmuda, a 37-year-old female, came to the Upton Ambulatory Surgery Center so that Dr. Thomas could excise a benign tumor from her left foot's big toe (known medically as the great toe). She tolerated the procedure well and was discharged.

You Code It!

Go through the steps to determine the procedure code(s) that should be reported for this encounter between Dr. Thomas and Beatrice Burmuda.

Step #1: Read the case carefully and completely.
Step #2: Abstract the scenario. Which key words or terms describe what service the physician provided to the patient during this encounter?
Step #3: Are there any details missing or incomplete for which you would need to query the physician? [If so, ask your instructor.]
Step #4: Determine the correct CPT procedure code or codes to explain the details about what was provided to the patient during this encounter.
Step #5: Check for any relevant guidance, including reading all of the symbols and notations.
Step #6: Do you need to append any modifiers to ensure complete and accurate information is provided?
Step #7: Double-check your work.

Answer:

The procedure code is 28108. Did you determine the correct modifier?

28108-TA **Excision or curettage of bone cyst or benign tumor, phalanges of foot, left foot, great toe**

Terrific!

23.6 Service-Related Modifiers

As you learn and expand your abilities to accurately report procedures, services, and treatments provided to the patients of your facility, you will discover that to tell the complete story about what was done, you may need to add a detail or two to the existing code description. Modifiers are created to enable this.

Preventive Services

The Affordable Care Act mandates most health plans to cover preventive services and early detection screening services, with no cost to the patient. When this service is ordered by the physician, the reason would be based on the patient's age and include documentation that there are no signs or symptoms apparent. In these cases, modifier 33 should be appended to the procedure code.

33 **Preventive Services:** When the primary purpose of the service is the delivery of an evidence-based service in accordance with a US Preventive Services Task Force A or B rating in effect or is another preventive service identified in preventive services mandates (legislative or regulatory), the service may be identified by adding modifier 33 to the procedure. For separately reported services specifically identified as preventive, the modifier should not be used.

Telemedicine Synchronous Services

We live in a world integrated with technology, enabling us to improve patient care. Now, encrypted versions of Facetime and other synchronous, interactive, audio-only or audiovisual software programs permit an encounter between physician and patient who are not in the same room– sometimes not even in the same city. In the CPT code book's *Appendix T*, you will find a list of 58 CPT codes permitted to be appended with modifier 93 when the service is performed using audio-only synchronous electronic communications equipment. These codes are primarily located in the E/M and Medicine sections of CPT, marked with a little audio speaker (🔈) symbol to the left of the code.

In *Appendix P*, you will find a list of 79 CPT codes permitted to be appended with modifier **95** when the service is performed using synchronous electronic communications equipment. These codes are primarily located in the E/M and Medicine sections of CPT, marked with a star (★) symbol to the left of the code.

The documentation for these encounters must confirm that the content of the physician/patient meeting is sufficient to meet the requirements for the code to be reported whether the service was provided face-to-face, real time audio-only, or with the use of audiovisual telemedicine services, (as indicated by the appending of either modifier 93 or 95.

93 **Synchronous Telemedicine Service Rendered Via Telephone or Other Real-Time Interactive Audio-Only Telecommunications System:** Synchronous telemedicine service is defined as a real-time interaction between a physician or other qualified health care professional and a patient who is located away at a distant site from the physician or other qualified health care professional. The totality of the communication of information exchanged between the physician or other qualified health care professional and the patient during the course of the synchronous telemedicine service must be of an amount and nature that is sufficient to meet the key components and/or requirements of the same service when rendered via a face-to-face interaction.

95 **Synchronous Telemedicine Service Rendered Via a Real-Time Interactive Audio and Video Telecommunications System:** Synchronous telemedicine service is defined as a real-time interaction between a physician or other qualified health care professional and a patient who is located at a distant site from the physician or other qualified health care professional. The totality of the communication of information exchanged between the physician or other qualified health care professional and the patient during the course of the synchronous telemedicine service must be of an amount and nature that would be sufficient to meet the key components and/or other requirements of the same service when rendered via a face-to-face interaction. Modifier 95 may only be appended to the services listed in Appendix P. Appendix P is the list of CPT codes for services that are typically performed face-to-face, but may be rendered via a real-time (synchronous) interactive audio and video telecommunications system.

EXAMPLES

Dr. Lappin has been working with Louisa providing psychotherapy to help her deal with panic attacks. Today, they had a good, 30-minute session in the office.

90832 **Psychotherapy, 30 minutes with patient**

Dr. Lappin has been working with Louisa providing psychotherapy to help her deal with panic attacks. Today, Louisa is on a plane, traveling to visit her parents in another state. As she feels a panic attack coming on, she uses the airplane's WiFi system to Skype with Dr. Lappin. They spend 30 minutes talking things through and helping Louisa get through.

90832-95 **Psychotherapy, 30 minutes with patient, synchronous telemedicine service rendered via a real-time interactive audio and video telecommunications system**

By appending modifier 95, you are clearly communicating the difference in Dr. Lappin's service to her patient.

Wound Care

Typically, a dressing change is required for a wound many times throughout the healing process. In addition, it is not unusual that a patient might have more than one wound that needs care at the same time. Therefore, to make the coding process easier and more efficient, one modifier can explain the extent of such care so that listing the same code multiple times is not necessary. The list in **Table 23-4** contains the modifiers for multiple wounds.

TABLE 23-4 Modifiers for Multiple Wounds

A1	Dressing for one wound
A2	Dressing for two wounds
A3	Dressing for three wounds
A4	Dressing for four wounds
A5	Dressing for five wounds
A6	Dressing for six wounds
A7	Dressing for seven wounds
A8	Dressing for eight wounds
A9	Dressing for nine or more wounds

LET'S CODE IT! SCENARIO

Ted Kercher, a 33-year-old male, is a firefighter who sustained partial-thickness burns the entire length of his right arm when something exploded. He comes in to see Dr. Taggert to have the dressings changed on four wounds.

Let's Code It!

Ted comes in to have his *dressings changed* on *four* burn wounds. First, you must find the CPT code for the procedure; second, you can address the modifier. Let's go to the Alphabetic Index and look up *dressings*. You find

Dressings

Burns 16020–16030

Change

    Anesthesia 15852

You know that Dr. Taggert is changing Ted's dressings; however, there is nothing in the notes that states anesthesia was involved. In addition, Ted's wounds are burns, so let's turn to the numeric listing and carefully read the descriptions for the codes shown next to *burns*. Do you agree that this is the best code?

16025 **Dressings and/or debridement of partial-thickness burns, initial or subsequent; medium (e.g., whole face or whole extremity, or 5% to 10% total body surface area)**

The notes indicate that Dr. Taggert changed the dressings for *four wounds*. So rather than just list this code four times, we can use a modifier to communicate this fact: 16025-A4 tells the whole story clearly.

16025-A4 **Dressings and/or debridement of partial-thickness burns, initial or subsequent; medium (e.g., whole face or whole extremity, or 5% to 10% total body surface area); four wounds dressed**

Good work!

Ophthalmology/Optometry

Sometimes, when ophthalmic or optometric services are provided, more detail is necessary to ensure proper reimbursement. Following are the HCPCS Level II modifiers used with these services:

AP	Determination of refractive state was not performed in the course of diagnostic ophthalmologic examination
LS	FDA-monitored intraocular lens implant
PL	Progressive addition lenses
VP	Aphakic patient

ESRD/Dialysis

Dialysis and other services for a patient with renal conditions, including those with **end-stage renal disease (ESRD)**, may involve extenuating circumstances requiring further explanation. The dialysis modifiers in **Table 23-5** provide that information.

End-Stage Renal Disease (ESRD)
Chronic, irreversible kidney disease requiring regular treatments.

AMCC
Automated Multi-Channel Chemistry–Automated organ disease panel tests performed on the same patient, by the same provider, on the same day.

Urea Reduction Ratio (URR)
A formula to determine the effectiveness of hemodialysis treatment.

TABLE 23-5 ESRD/Dialysis Modifiers

CB	Service ordered by a renal dialysis facility (RDF) physician as part of the beneficiary's benefit is not part of the composite rate and is separately reimbursable
CD	**AMCC** test has been ordered by an ESRD facility or MCP physician that is part of the composite rate and is not separately billable
CE	AMCC test has been ordered by an ESRD facility or MCP physician that is a composite rate test but is beyond the normal frequency covered under the rate and is separately reimbursable based on medical necessity
CF	AMCC test has been ordered by an ESRD facility or MCP physician that is not part of the composite rate and is separately billable
EM	Emergency reserve supply (for ESRD benefit only)
G1	Most recent **urea reduction ratio (URR)** reading of less than 60
G2	Most recent URR reading of 60 to 64.9
G3	Most recent URR reading of 65 to 69.9
G4	Most recent URR reading of 70 to 74.9
G5	Most recent URR reading of 75 or greater
G6	ESRD patient for whom less than six dialysis sessions have been provided in a month

LET'S CODE IT! SCENARIO

Amie Gander, a 39-year-old female, was diagnosed with ESRD. Dr. Linnger prescribed her treatments to begin on May 29 at the Southside Dialysis Center (SDC). Code for the services provided at SDC for the month of May.

Let's Code It!

End-stage renal disease (ESRD) services are billed on a monthly basis. However, Amie only received 3 days of services during the month of May (May 29, May 30, and May 31) from Southside Dialysis Center. In the Alphabetic Index, you will find:

End-Stage Renal Disease Services

Dialysis 90951-90970

Home 90963-90966

Inpatient 90935, 90937, 90945, 90947

Outpatient 90951-90962

Less Than a Full Month 90967-90970

After reading the complete code descriptions in the suggested range, you find the best procedure code to be this:

90970 End-stage renal disease (ESRD) related services (less than full month), per day; for patients twenty years of age and over

This means you will have to list the code three times because the code description says per day. Are there any modifiers than can help you communicate this situation?

G6 ESRD patient for whom less than six dialysis sessions have been provided in a month

The modifier that will complete this report is G6 because she has had fewer than six sessions in 1 month: **90970-G6; 90970-G6; 90970-G6** *or* **90970-G6 × 3**.

Good job!

Habilitative and Rehabilitative Services

In the 2018 CPT code set, two modifiers were added:

96 Habilitative Services

97 Rehabilitative Services

These modifiers would most often be appended to codes from the *Physical Medicine and Rehabilitation* subsection of the Medicine section. More about this in the chapter ***CPT Medicine Section***.

Pharmaceuticals

Pharmaceuticals, the industry term for medications, are items that must be monitored very carefully: the purchase, the storage, and the dispensing. The modifiers in **Table 23-6** provide important information that must be tracked.

TABLE 23-6 Pharmaceutical Modifiers

JW	Drug amount discarded/not administered to any patient
KD	Drug or biological infused through DME
KO	Single drug unit dose formulation
KP	First drug of a multiple drug unit dose formulation
KQ	Second or subsequent drug of a multiple drug unit dose formulation
QE	Prescribed amount of oxygen is less than 1 **liter per minute (LPM)**
QF	Prescribed amount of oxygen exceeds 4 LPM and portable oxygen is prescribed
QG	Prescribed amount of oxygen is greater than 4 LPM
QH	Oxygen-conserving device is being used with an oxygen delivery system
RD	Drug provided to beneficiary, but not administered "incident to"
SL	State-supplied vaccine
SV	Pharmaceuticals delivered to patient's home but not utilized

Liters per Minute (LPM)
The measurement of how many liters of a drug or chemical are provided to the patient in 60 seconds.

Modifier RD Drug provided to beneficiary, but not administered "incident to" indicates that a particular pharmaceutical was provided to the patient but not administered. For example, the nurse brings the patient's pills into his room to administer them when she notices he has a rash. She notifies the physician on call and he orders the medication stopped to investigate if the patient is allergic. Once the pills have been taken out of the pharmacy, they cannot be returned. If the patient does not take them, they must be discarded but still accounted for in the system and billing.

Modifier SV Pharmaceuticals delivered to patient's home but not utilized might be used by a mail-order pharmaceutical service to show that the medications were shipped and delivered to the patient's house but have nothing to do with how, when, or if the patient uses those drugs.

EXAMPLES

RD Drug provided to beneficiary, but not administered "incident to"

SV Pharmaceuticals delivered to patient's home but not utilized

Parenteral Enteral Nutrition (PEN)
Nourishment delivered using a combination of means other than the gastrointestinal tract (such as IV) in addition to via the gastrointestinal tract.

Clinical Laboratory Improvement Amendment (CLIA)
Federal legislation created for the monitoring and regulation of clinical laboratory procedures.

Items/Services

The modifiers in **Table 23-7** cover a variety of circumstances relating to the provision of an item or a service.

TABLE 23-7 Items/Services Modifiers

AU	Item furnished in conjunction with a urologic, ostomy, or tracheostomy supply
AV	Item furnished in conjunction with a prosthetic device, prosthetic, or orthotic
BA	Item furnished in conjunction with **parenteral enteral nutrition (PEN)** services
BL	Special acquisition of blood and blood products
BO	Orally administered nutrition, not by feeding tube
EY	No physician or other licensed health care provider order for this item or service
FX	X-ray taken using film
GK	Reasonable and necessary item/item associated with GA or GZ modifier
GL	Medically unnecessary upgrade provided instead of standard item, no charge, no advance beneficiary notice (ABN)
GY	Item or service statutorily excluded or does not meet the definition of any Medicare benefit, not a contract benefit
GZ	Item or service expected to be denied as not reasonable and necessary
KS	Glucose monitor supply for diabetic beneficiary not treated with insulin
KZ	New coverage not implemented by managed care
Q1	Routine clinical service provided in a clinical research study that is in an approved clinical research study
QW	**Clinical Laboratory Improvement Amendment (CLIA)** waived test
SC	Medically necessary service or supply
SF	Second opinion ordered by a professional review organization (PRO)
SM	Second surgical opinion
SN	Third surgical opinion
SQ	Item ordered by home health

LET'S CODE IT! SCENARIO

Oscar Barkley, a 57-year-old male, was diagnosed with type 2 diabetes mellitus. Dr. Habersham wants to try a new medication to control Oscar's blood glucose levels and delay, or avoid, putting him on insulin. Dr. Habersham gives Oscar the prescription for the medication and a second prescription for a home blood glucose monitor.

Let's Code It!

The code you will report for the provision of the home glucose monitor is this:

E0607 Home blood glucose monitor

Now, you need a way to explain that this monitor is for a patient who is a non-insulin-dependent diabetic. Sounds like the perfect job for a modifier!

Did you determine this to be the correct modifier?

E0607-KS Home blood glucose monitor; Glucose monitor supply for diabetic beneficiary not treated with insulin

Purchase/Rental Items

Often, when durable medical equipment (DME) is supplied, the patient has a choice to rent the equipment or purchase it outright. This will depend upon the patient's personal situation. A modifier (see **Table 23-8**) provides important details, especially to the payor.

TABLE 23-8 Purchase/Rental Items Modifiers

BP	The beneficiary has been informed of the purchase and rental options and has elected to purchase the item
BR	The beneficiary has been informed of the purchase and rental options and has elected to rent the item
BU	The beneficiary has been informed of the purchase and rental options and after 30 days has not informed the supplier of his/her decision
KH	DMEPOS item, initial claim, purchase or first month rental
KI	DMEPOS item, second or third month rental
KJ	DMEPOS item, parenteral enteral nutrition (PEN) pump or capped rental, months four to fifteen
KR	Rental item, billing for partial month
LL	Lease/rental (use when DME rental payments are to be applied against the purchase price)
MS	Six-month maintenance and servicing fee for reasonable and necessary parts and labor not covered under any manufacturer or supplier warranty
NR	New when rented
RR	Rental DME

YOU CODE IT! CASE STUDY

Darryl Rosen, an 81-year-old male, fell and broke his hip last winter. Even though it healed, Darryl is still experiencing difficulty walking long distances. Dr. Sorrel prescribed a power wheelchair for him. Darryl decided to purchase a lightweight, portable, motorized/power wheelchair from Hammermill Medical Supply Systems.

You Code It!

Go through the steps of coding, and determine the code or codes that should be reported for the supply of Darryl Rosen's new equipment. [*NOTE:* The wheelchair is reported with an HCPCS Level II code.]

Step #1: Read the case carefully and completely.
Step #2: Abstract the scenario. Which key words or terms describe what service the physician provided to the patient during this encounter?
Step #3: Are there any details missing or incomplete for which you would need to query the physician? [If so, ask your instructor.]
Step #4: Determine the correct CPT procedure code or codes to explain the details about what was provided to the patient during this encounter.
Step #5: Check for any relevant guidance, including reading all of the symbols and notations.
Step #6: Do you need to append any modifiers to ensure complete and accurate information is provided?
Step #7: Double-check your work.

Answer:

The code for the provision of the wheelchair is K0012. Did you determine this to be the correct modifier?

K0012-KH **Lightweight portable motorized/power wheelchair; DMEPOS item, initial claim, purchase or first month rental**

Good work!

Deceased Patient

Should a patient expire (die) while services are in the process of being rendered, certainly the situation changes and there must be some indication of the death. The following modifiers are used in such circumstances:

- CA Procedure payable only in the inpatient setting when performed emergently on an outpatient who expires prior to admission
- QL Patient pronounced dead after ambulance called

Claims and Documentation

The modifiers shown in **Table 23-9** directly provide additional information relating to the claims and documentation involved in certain health care encounters.

TABLE 23-9 Claims and Documentation Modifiers

CC	Procedure code change (used to indicate that a procedure code previously submitted was changed either for an administrative reason or because an incorrect code was filed)
GA	Waiver of liability statement issued, individual case
GB	Claim being resubmitted for payment because it is no longer covered under a global payment
KB	Beneficiary requested upgrade for ABN, more than four modifiers identified on claim
KX	Requirements specified in the medical policy have been met
QP	Documentation is on file showing that the laboratory test(s) was ordered individually or ordered as a CPT-recognized panel other than automated profile codes 80002-80019, G0058, G0059, and G0060

YOU CODE IT! CASE STUDY

CPT HCPCS Level II

Jonny Craig, a 45-year-old male, had a mass on his left upper eyelid. Dr. Neilsen performed a biopsy on the eyelid. The pathology report determined it was a benign neoplasm. Gwen Sanders, the professional coding specialist, mistakenly put code 68710-E1 on the claim form instead of 67810-E1. She didn't realize this until the claim came back denied.

You Code It!

What additional modifier should Gwen append to code 67810-E1 on the second claim form, which she needs to submit as a corrected claim?

Answer:

Did you determine this to be the correct code?

67810-E1-CC **Incisional biopsy of eyelid skin including lid margin; upper left, eyelid, Procedure code change because an incorrect code was filed**

Good job!!

Family Services

Services provided under Medicaid's **Early and Periodic Screening, Diagnostic, and Treatment (EPSDT)** program must be identified with the EP modifier, shown in **Table 23-10**. In addition, other family services may benefit from further explanation by the use of one of the modifiers found in that list.

Early and Periodic Screening, Diagnostic, and Treatment (EPSDT)
A Medicaid preventive health program for children under 21.

TABLE 23-10 Family Services Modifiers

EP	Service provided as part of Medicaid early periodic screening diagnosis and treatment (EPSDT) program
FP	Service provided as part of family planning program
G7	Pregnancy resulted from rape or incest or pregnancy certified by physician as life threatening
TL	Early intervention/individualized family service plan (IFSP)
TM	Individualized education plan (IEP)
TR	School-based individualized education program (IEP) services provided outside the public school district responsible for the student

Treatments/Screenings

The modifiers shown in **Table 23-11** are directly related to the provision of mammography and infusion therapeutic services.

TABLE 23-11 Treatments/Screenings Modifiers

GG	Performance and payment of a screening mammogram and diagnostic mammogram on the same patient, same day
GH	Diagnostic mammogram converted from screening mammogram on same day
SH	Second concurrently administered infusion therapy
SJ	Third, or more, concurrently administered infusion therapy

LET'S CODE IT! SCENARIO

Cheryl Baxett, a 41-year-old female, came into the hospital for her annual screening mammogram. Dr. Ogden ordered the screening to be completed with computer-aided detection, due to a prior history of breast cancer. Later that day, after the images were analyzed, Dr. Ogden diagnosed her with a considerable mass in her left breast.

Let's Code It!

Cheryl came in for a screening mammogram with computer-aided detection on her left breast. Let's go to the Alphabetic Index of the CPT book and find the best, most appropriate procedure code:

77067 Screening mammography, bilateral (two view film study of each breast), including computer-aided detection (CAD) when performed

Once the results of the mammogram became the basis for a decision to have surgery, the screening mammogram became a diagnostic mammogram. Cheryl's insurance carrier accepts HCPCS Level II codes and modifiers, so you must adapt the definition of the mammogram from screening to diagnostic by appending a modifier: 77065-GH. The **GH** modifier means that a **diagnostic mammogram was converted from a screening mammogram on the same day**.

77065-GH-LT Diagnostic mammography, including computer-aided detection (CAD) when performed; unilateral, diagnostic mammogram converted from screening mammogram on same day, left side

77067-52-RT Screening mammography, bilateral (two view film study of each breast), including computer-aided detection (CAD) when performed, reduced services, right side

Great job!

Transportation

Table 23-12 has the modifiers that provide additional details with relation to transportation services provided to patients.

TABLE 23-12 Transportation Modifiers

GM	Multiple patients on one ambulance trip
LR	Laboratory round trip
QM	Ambulance service provided under arrangement by a provider of services
QN	Ambulance service furnished directly by a provider of services
TK	Extra patient or passenger, non-ambulance
TP	Medical transport, unloaded vehicle
TQ	Basic life support transport by a volunteer ambulance provider

Funded Programs

When a service or treatment is provided under the terms or conditions of a formalized program or plan, the services must be identified so that statistical tracking can be accomplished accurately and reimbursement is not received from two sources. The modifiers shown in **Table 23-13** enable such tracking.

TABLE 23-13 Funding Modifiers

GN	Services delivered under an outpatient speech language pathology plan of care
GO	Services delivered under an outpatient occupational therapy plan of care
GP	Services delivered under an outpatient physical therapy plan of care
H9	Court-ordered
HA	Child/adolescent program
HB	Adult program, nongeriatric
HC	Adult program, geriatric
HE	Mental health program
HF	Substance abuse program
HG	Opioid addiction treatment program
HH	Integrated mental health/substance abuse program
HI	Integrated mental health and mental retardation/developmental disabilities program
HJ	Employee assistance program
HK	Specialized mental health programs for high-risk populations
HU	Funded by child welfare agency
HV	Funded by state addictions agency
HW	Funded by state mental health agency
HX	Funded by county/local agency
HY	Funded by juvenile justice agency
HZ	Funded by criminal justice agency
SE	State and/or federally funded programs/services

Individual/Group

Most often, modifiers for individuals or groups are going to be used in conjunction with psychiatric and psychotherapeutic codes to clarify how many patients were involved in the session. The modifiers shown in **Table 23-14** relate to the number, and sometimes the type, of patient(s) being helped at one time.

TABLE 23-14 Individual/Group Modifiers

HQ	Group setting
HR	Family/couple with client present
HS	Family/couple without client present
TJ	Program group, child and/or adolescent
TT	Individualized service provided to more than one patient in same setting
UN	Two patients served
UP	Three patients served
UQ	Four patients served
UR	Five patients served
US	Six or more patients served

Prosthetics

When services are provided relating to the supply or adjustment of a prosthetic device, you might have to include additional information by using one of the modifiers shown in **Table 23-15**.

TABLE 23-15 Prosthetics Modifiers

K0	Lower extremity prosthesis functional level 0–does not have the ability or potential to ambulate or transfer safely with or without assistance and prosthesis does not enhance his or her quality of life or mobility
K1	Lower extremity prosthesis functional level 1–has the ability or potential to use a prosthesis for transfers or ambulation on level surfaces at fixed cadence, typical of the limited and unlimited household ambulatory
K2	Lower extremity prosthesis functional level 2–has the ability or potential for ambulation with the ability to traverse low-level environmental barriers such as curbs, stairs, uneven surfaces, typical of limited community ambulatory
K3	Lower extremity prosthesis functional level 3–has the ability or potential for ambulation with variable cadence. Typical of the community ambulatory who has the ability to traverse most environmental barriers and may have vocational, therapeutic, or exercise activity that demands prosthetic utilization beyond simple locomotion
K4	Lower extremity prosthesis functional level 4–has the ability or potential for prosthetic ambulation that exceeds the basic ambulation skills, exhibiting high impact, stress, or energy levels, typical of the prosthetic demands of the child, active adult, or athlete
KM	Replacement of facial prosthesis including new impression/moulage
KN	Replacement of facial prosthesis using previous master model

LET'S CODE IT! SCENARIO

Sam Tanner, a 29-year-old male, returned home after being in a rehabilitation center for 3 months. He had a below-knee amputation (BKA) after he was hurt in a rescue mission following a major hurricane. Alice Conner fitted him for an initial, below-knee patellar tendon bearing (PTB) type socket prosthesis because he has the ability to walk on and even maneuver over such low obstacles as sidewalk curbs and stairs.

Let's Code It!

Alice Conner ordered and supplied an *initial, below-knee PTB type socket prosthesis*. In the HCPCS Level II Alphabetic Index, you find

Prosthesis

Fitting, L5400–L5460, L6380–L6388

(continued)

The notes did say that Alice fitted him, so this should provide a good lead. When you get to this section, beginning with L5400, you find a code whose description matches the notes very well:

L5500 **Initial, below knee PTB type socket, non-alignable system, pylon, no cover, SACH foot, plaster socket, direct formed**

(*NOTE:* SACH stands for solid ankle, cushioned heel.)

You also have to support the service with a modifier to explain Sam's abilities:

K2 **Lower extremity prosthesis functional level 2—has the ability or potential for ambulation with the ability to traverse low-level environmental barriers such as curbs, stairs, or uneven surfaces. Typical of the limited community ambulator**

And report this as

L5500-K2 **Initial, below knee PTB type socket, non-alignable system, pylon, no cover, SACH foot, plaster socket, direct formed, lower extremity prosthesis functional level 2**

Durable Medical Equipment

When the services relate to the provision of or adjustments to a piece of durable medical equipment (DME), a modifier from **Table 23-16** may be needed to clarify a certain condition or circumstance.

TABLE 23-16 DME Modifiers

KA	Add on option/accessory for wheelchair
KC	Replacement of special power wheelchair interface
KF	Item designated by FDA as Class III device
NB	Nebulizer system, any type, FDA-cleared for use with specific drug
NR	New when rented
NU	New equipment
RA	Replacement of a DME, orthotic, or prosthetic item
RB	Replacement of a part of a DME, orthotic, or prosthetic item furnished as part of a repair
TW	Backup equipment
UE	Used durable medical equipment (DME)

HCPCS Level II

YOU CODE IT! CASE STUDY

On January 5, a respiratory suction pump was provided to Teresa Christley, who was diagnosed with emphysema. On January 6, another suction pump was delivered to Teresa. The first unit had to be replaced because of a defective piece.

You Code It!

Go through the steps, and determine the HCPCS Level II code or codes that should be reported for these services for Teresa Christley.

Step #1: Read the case carefully and completely.

Step #2: Abstract the scenario. Which key words or terms describe what service the physician provided to the patient during this encounter?

(continued)

Step #3: Are there any details missing or incomplete for which you would need to query the physician? [If so, ask your instructor.]
Step #4: Determine the correct CPT procedure code or codes to explain the details about what was provided to the patient during this encounter.
Step #5: Check for any relevant guidance, including reading all of the symbols and notations.
Step #6: Do you need to append any modifiers to ensure complete and accurate information is provided?
Step #7: Double-check your work.

Answer:

The code for the provision of the pump is E0600. Did you determine the correct modifier for the second claim?

Jan 5: E0600 Respiratory suction pump, home model, portable or stationary, electric

Jan 6: E0600-RA Respiratory suction pump, home model, portable or stationary, electric; replacement of DME, orthotic, or prosthetic item

Location

The following modifiers describe situations when you will need to clarify the location at which services were provided:

PN Non-excepted service provided at an off-campus, outpatient, provider-based department of a hospital

PO Expected services provided at off-campus, outpatient, provider-based department of a hospital

SG Ambulatory surgical center (ASC) facility service

SU Procedure performed in physician's office (i.e., to denote use of facility and equipment)

TN Rural/outside providers' customary service area

Podiatric Care

There are times when particular services are recategorized, determined by certain signs and/or symptoms that the patient may be exhibiting. The following list identifies modifiers used to indicate some of these circumstances when a podiatrist provides treatment to a patient:

Q7 One **class A finding**

Q8 Two **class B findings**

Q9 One class B and two **class C findings**

Class A Finding
Nontraumatic amputation of a foot or an integral skeletal portion.

Class B Finding
Absence of a posterior tibial pulse; absence or decrease of hair growth; thickening of the nail, discoloration of the skin, and/or thinning of the skin texture; and/or absence of a posterior pedal pulse.

Class C Finding
Edema, burning sensation, temperature change (cold feet), abnormal spontaneous sensations in the feet, and/or limping.

Recording

The following modifiers indicate the use of recording equipment as a part of the service, treatment, or procedure provided to the patient:

QC Single-channel monitoring

QD Recording and storage in solid-state memory by a digital recorder

QT Recording and storage on tape by an analog tape recorder

Other Services

The modifiers shown in **Table 23-17** do not seem to fit into any of the other categories we have established. Review all the modifiers in the list, and see if you can come up with examples of how and when they would be used.

Medicaid Services

Each state administers its own version of the federal Medicaid program and determines its own specific descriptions of the different levels of care. To maintain consistency, HCPCS Level II has the modifiers shown in **Table 23-18** that can be used nationwide—even though the description of each modifier will change, as defined by each state.

TABLE 23-17 Other Services Modifiers

AT	Acute treatment (to be used only with 98940, 98941, 98942)
EJ	Subsequent claims for a defined course of therapy
ET	Emergency services
GQ	Via asynchronous telecommunications system
GT	Via interactive audio and video telecommunication systems
GW	Service not related to the hospice patient's terminal condition
Q2	HCFA/ORD demonstration project procedure/service
Q3	Live kidney donor surgery and related services
QJ	Services/items provided to a prisoner or patient in state or local custody, however the state or local government, as applicable, meets the requirements in 42 CFR 411.4(b)
SK	Member of high-risk population (use only with immunization codes)
ST	Related to trauma or injury
SY	Persons who are in close contact with member of high-risk population (use with immunization codes only)
TC	Technical component
TG	Complex/high-tech level of care
TH	Obstetrical treatment/services, prenatal or postpartum
TS	Follow-up service
UF	Services provided in the morning
UG	Services provided in the afternoon
UH	Services provided in the evening
UJ	Services provided at night
UK	Services provided on behalf of the client to someone other than the client (collateral relationship)

TABLE 23-18 Medicaid Services Modifiers

U1	Medicaid level of care 1, as defined by each state
U2	Medicaid level of care 2, as defined by each state
U3	Medicaid level of care 3, as defined by each state
U4	Medicaid level of care 4, as defined by each state
U5	Medicaid level of care 5, as defined by each state
U6	Medicaid level of care 6, as defined by each state
U7	Medicaid level of care 7, as defined by each state
U8	Medicaid level of care 8, as defined by each state
U9	Medicaid level of care 9, as defined by each state
UA	Medicaid level of care 10, as defined by each state
UB	Medicaid level of care 11, as defined by each state
UC	Medicaid level of care 12, as defined by each state
UD	Medicaid level of care 13, as defined by each state

Special Rates

The following two modifiers are used to indicate that a service or procedure was provided to a patient during an unusual time frame, that is, not during regular working hours:

TU Special payment rate, overtime

TV Special payment rates, holidays/weekends

Use of CDSS

There are eight (8) modifiers available to explain if the health care professional ordering a service, test, medication, or procedure has consulted the Clinical Decision Support System (CDSS) prior to making the decision to document the order. CDSS is an add-on to Electronic Health Records (EHR) systems that enable the professional to access state-of-the-art evidence-based research at the click of a mouse.

The descriptions of these modifiers report circumstances why the ordering professional may or may not have checked CDSS prior to writing the order. The reasons may include: loss of Internet, access or lack of access to EHR, emergency situations, and there is one modifier to express "unknown." Be sure you do not append the "unknown" modifier as a default. Instead, educate your physician to document these details, so you can append an accurate modifier. Check your HCPCS Level II modifiers: MA, MB, MC, MD, ME, MF, MG, and MH.

23.7 Sequencing Multiple Modifiers

There may be circumstances where one case is so complex, unusual, or special that you need more than one modifier to explain the whole scenario.

Two or Three Modifiers Needed

There are occasions when a particular procedure code will require the amendment of more than one modifier. In these cases, you must place the modifiers in a particular order depending upon what each modifier represents. Let's review a few different situations.

Generally, the CPT modifier that most directly changes, or modifies, the specific code description will be placed closest to the procedure code. These are called **service-related modifiers** because they change, or alter, the description of the service (such as 23 Unusual Anesthesia or 32 Mandated services), rather than those modifiers that explain personnel in attendance (such as 62 Two Surgeons) or an event (such as 57 Decision for Surgery).

Service-Related Modifier
A modifier relating to a change or adjustment of a procedure or service provided.

EXAMPLE

Dr. Weaver, and his surgical team, began the pancreatic transplantation procedure on Kenneth. Once the incision had been made, the patient's heartbeat became erratic and could not be brought back under control, so the procedure was discontinued. The procedure code reported requires two modifiers: 48554-53-66.

Modifier 53 explains that the procedure was discontinued. This modifier relates the fact that everyone involved, including the facility, prepared for the surgery and began the procedure but had to stop. This will explain why, sometime down the road, this same patient may again go through a pancreatic transplantation. In addition, this modifier will enable the health care professionals and the facility to get some reimbursement to cover the cost of the services they did provide.

Modifier 66, on the other hand, explains that a surgical team was participating in the surgery. This does not affect the specific code description of the procedure. It explains why the third-party payer will need to reimburse more than one surgeon. This modifier also may help to prevent the claim for each of those additional team members from being denied, or placed into determination, slowing the reimbursement process and avoiding an audit.

When an HCPCS Level II modifier is used in addition to a CPT modifier, the CPT modifier is placed closest to the procedure code, and the HCPCS Level II modifier follows.

EXAMPLE

24201-76-LT Removal of foreign body, upper arm or elbow area; deep, repeat procedure by same physician, left side

There is an exception to this rule when reporting anesthesia services. The Physical Status Modifier always is reported closest to the anesthesia procedure code.

EXAMPLE

Dr. Cowles administered the general anesthesia when Dr. Dean had to take the patient back into the surgery unexpectedly to attend to a problem with the replantation procedure for the patient's index finger of his right hand. For Dr. Cowles, the code is 01810-P1-76.

LET'S CODE IT! SCENARIO

Dr. Tuders performed a bilateral osteotomy on the shaft of Arlis Richardson's femur. Another surgeon performed the same procedure on Arlis 2 weeks ago but was unsuccessful, so Dr. Tuders repeated the procedure. As an expert in this procedure, he was brought in to perform the surgery only and will not be involved in any preoperative or postoperative care of the patient.

Let's Code It!

To accurately report Dr. Tuders's surgical services to Arlis Richardson, you would need the following:

27448 **Osteotomy, femur, shaft, or supracondylar; without fixation**

-50 **Modifier to report that it was a bilateral procedure**

-54 **Modifier to report Dr. Tuders was providing surgical care only**

-77 **Modifier to report that this is a repeat procedure by another physician**

Therefore, the code you report will look like this:

27448-50-54-77

More Than Three Modifiers Needed

The outpatient claim form, upon which you will record your chosen codes and other information to request reimbursement from a third-party payer, has a limited amount of space in which to place the necessary information, particularly when it comes to including modifiers. Some third-party payers do not permit multiple modifiers to be listed on the same line as the CPT code. Therefore, should your case require three or more modifiers to completely explain all of the circumstances involved, you can use modifier 99.

99 **Multiple Modifiers:** Under certain circumstances two or more modifiers may be necessary to completely delineate a service. In such situations modifier 99 should be added to the basic procedure, and other applicable modifiers may be listed as part of the description of the service.

Sequencing Multiple Modifiers

When you need more than one modifier with a procedure or service code, you must place the modifiers in order of specificity, with the most important, most precise modifier closest to the main code.

YOU CODE IT! CASE STUDY

Dr. Cabbot drained an abscess on Mark Swanson's left thumb and another on his second finger. Both were simple procedures.

(continued)

You Code It!

Go through the steps of coding, and determine the code or codes that should be reported for this encounter between Dr. Cabbot and Mark Swanson.

Step #1: Read the case carefully and completely.
Step #2: Abstract the scenario. Which key words or terms describe what service the physician provided to the patient during this encounter?
Step #3: Are there any details missing or incomplete for which you would need to query the physician? [If so, ask your instructor.]
Step #4: Determine the correct CPT procedure code or codes to explain the details about what was provided to the patient during this encounter.
Step #5: Check for any relevant guidance, including reading all of the symbols and notations.
Step #6: Do you need to append any modifiers to ensure complete and accurate information is provided?
Step #7: Double-check your work.

Answer:

The correct procedure code for the I&D of the abscess is 10060. Did you determine the correct modifiers?

10060-FA **Incision and drainage of abscess, simple or single; left hand, thumb**

10060-F1-59 **Incision and drainage of abscess, simple or single; left hand, second digit; separate procedure**

Without the modifiers *FA* for left hand, thumb; *F1* for left hand, second digit; and *59* for distinct procedural service, the claim form could not clearly communicate that Dr. Cabbot did work on two different fingers.

23.8 Supplemental Reports

Remember, *documentation* is your watchword. It is the backbone of the health information management industry. In many situations when a modifier is used, a **supplemental report** is needed for additional clarification.

Supplemental Report
A letter or report written by the attending physician or other health care professional to provide additional clarification or explanation.

Generally, the modifier itself provides a certain amount of explanation; however, the insurance carrier wants more details. You can be efficient and send the specific information along with the claim, or you can wait until the carrier requests additional information. Either way, you will have to supply all the facts. However, if you wait to be asked, you will be delaying payment to your facility.

You will need to use your judgment, so as you look at the modifiers you include to tell the whole story, review the codes and modifiers to evaluate if there are any unanswered questions so you can use a supplemental report to answer them.

EXAMPLES

Here a just a few of the modifiers that might need a supplemental report to ensure complete communications.

22 **Increased Procedural Services** . . . *what was it that required the additional time and effort?*

23 **Unusual Anesthesia** . . . *why was this necessary?*

52 **Reduced Services** . . . *why couldn't the physician complete the planned procedure in full?*

53 **Discontinued Procedure** . . . *why did the physician have to stop?*

LET'S CODE IT! SCENARIO

Aden Carrington, a 9-year-old boy, had a superficial cut, about 3.3 cm, on his left cheek, after being in a car accident and hit by broken glass. Dr. Kern is ready to perform a simple repair of the wound, but she is very concerned. Aden has Tourette's syndrome, which causes him to jerk or move abruptly, especially when nervous. Although anesthesia is not typically used for a simple repair of a superficial wound, Dr. Kern administers general anesthesia. Sharon Haverty, a CRNA, assists Dr. Kern with monitoring Aden during the procedure.

Let's Code It!

Dr. Kern performed a *simple repair* of Aden's *superficial wound* on his *face.* Go to the Alphabetic Index in your CPT code book and look up *Repair.* As you look down the list of anatomical sites, you do not see face or cheek listed. You know that the repair was simple, and when you look at that listing, you note the direction "*See* Integumentary System, Repair, Simple." Once you go to that listing, you find the suggested codes 12001–12021. Let's take a look at the complete description in the numeric listing.

12011 Simple repair of superficial wounds of face, ears, eyelids, nose, lips and/or mucous membranes; 2.5 cm or less

The basic description matches the notes exactly. However, several choices are determined by the size of the wound. The notes state that Aden's wound was 3.3 cm. This brings you to the correct code:

12013 Simple repair of superficial wounds of face, ears, eyelids, nose, lips and/or mucous membranes; 2.6 cm to 5.0 cm

Great! Now, you have to address the fact that Dr. Kern gave Aden *general anesthesia.* This was done for a very valid medical reason, and Dr. Kern (and her facility) should be properly reimbursed for the service. Anesthesia is not included with code 12013 because it is not normally required. Aden's case is unusual. Unusual circumstances often require modifiers, so let's look at the CPT code book's ***Appendix A*** to see if there is an applicable modifier. Modifier 23 seems to fit.

23 Unusual Anesthesia: *Occasionally, a procedure, which usually requires either no anesthesia or local anesthesia, because of unusual circumstances must be done under general anesthesia. This circumstance may be reported by adding modifier 23 to the procedure code of the basic service.*

So modifier 23 should be appended, or attached, to the procedure code.

12013-23

You know that you have to code the anesthesia service as well.

00300 Anesthesia for all procedures on the integumentary system, muscles and nerves of head, neck, and posterior trunk, not otherwise specified

Let's look to see if there is an applicable CPT modifier to explain that an anesthesiologist was not involved. Modifier 47 seems to fit.

47 Anesthesia by Surgeon: *Regional or general anesthesia provided by the surgeon may be reported by adding modifier 47 to the basic service. (This does not include local anesthesia.) Note: Modifier 47 would not be used as a modifier for the anesthesia procedures.*

Well, the note within the description of modifier 47 tells you that this modifier is necessary but that it cannot be used with code 00300. You have to attach the modifier to the procedure code. Therefore, you submit the claim with one CPT code and two modifiers: 12013-23-47. In addition, it is smart to include a supplemental report with the claim to explain the use of general anesthesia. You are aware that the insurance company needs to know the details before paying the claim.

Chapter Summary

Modifiers provide additional explanation to the third-party payer so that it can fully appreciate any special circumstances that affected the procedures and services provided to the patient. In health care, as well as in so many other instances of our lives, most things do not fit neatly into predetermined descriptions. By using modifiers correctly, you provide an additional explanation and promote the efficient and more accurate reimbursement of your facility.

CODING BITES

CPT MODIFIER REFERENCES:

Inside the front cover of your CPT code book: CPT modifiers and short descriptions

Appendix A: CPT modifiers, some Level II (HCPCS/National) Modifiers, and full descriptions

HCPCS LEVEL II MODIFIER REFERENCE:

Appendix 2: Modifiers

[*NOTE:* Different publishers may place the Modifier listing in different locations of the HCPCS Level II code book.]

CHAPTER 23 REVIEW
CPT and HCPCS Level II Modifiers

connect

Enhance your learning by completing these exercises and more at mcgrawhillconnect.com!

Let's Check It! Terminology

Match each key term to the appropriate definition.

Part I

1. **LO 23.1** Containing both letters and numbers.
2. **LO 23.1** A two-character alphabetic or alphanumeric code that may be appended to a code from the main portion of the CPT book or a code from the HCPCS Level II book.
3. **LO 23.8** A letter or report written by the attending physician or other health care professional to provide additional clarification or explanation.
4. **LO 23.1** A modifier relating to a change or adjustment of a procedure or service provided.
5. **LO 23.2** A nurse practitioner, certified registered nurse anesthetist, certified registered nurse, clinical nurse specialist, or physician assistant.
6. **LO 23.1** A two-character code that affects the meaning of another code; a code addendum that provides more meaning to the original code.
7. **LO 23.1** A facility specially designed to provide surgical treatments without an overnight stay; also known as a same-day surgery center.
8. **LO 23.2** A modifier adding information about the professional(s) attending to the provision of this procedure or treatment to the patient during this encounter.
9. **LO 23.1** A two-character code that may be appended to a code from the main portion of the CPT book to provide additional information.
10. **LO 23.1** A two-character alphanumeric code used to describe the condition of the patient at the time anesthesia services are administered.

A. Alphanumeric
B. Ambulatory Surgery Center (ASC)
C. CPT Code Modifier
D. HCPCS Level II Modifier
E. Modifier
F. Nonphysician
G. Personnel Modifier
H. Physical Status Modifier
I. Service-Related Modifier
J. Supplemental Report

Part II

1. **LO 23.6** Nontraumatic amputation of a foot or an integral skeletal portion.
2. **LO 23.6** A Medicaid preventive health program for children under 21.
3. **LO 23.6** Nourishment delivered using a combination of means other than the gastrointestinal tract (such as IV) in addition to via the gastrointestinal tract.
4. **LO 23.6** Edema, burning sensation, temperature change (cold feet), abnormal spontaneous sensations in the feet, and/or limping.
5. **LO 23.6** Chronic, irreversible kidney disease requiring regular treatments.
6. **LO 23.6** Absence of a posterior tibial pulse; absence or decrease of hair growth; thickening of the nail, discoloration of the skin, and/or thinning of the skin texture; and/or absence of a posterior pedal pulse.
7. **LO 23.6** The measurement of how many liters of a drug or chemical are provided to the patient in 60 seconds.
8. **LO 23.2** A physician who fills in, temporarily, for another physician.
9. **LO 23.6** Federal legislation created for the monitoring and regulation of clinical laboratory procedures.
10. **LO 23.6** A formula to determine the effectiveness of hemodialysis treatment.
11. **LO 23.6** Automated organ disease panel tests performed on the same patient, by the same provider, on the same day.

A. Automated Multi-Channel Chemistry (AMCC)
B. Class A Finding
C. Class B Finding
D. Class C Finding
E. Clinical Laboratory Improvement Amendment (CLIA)
F. Early and Periodic Screening, Diagnostic, and Treatment (EPSDT)
G. End-stage renal disease (ESRD)
H. Locum Tenens Physician
I. Liters per Minute (LPM)
J. Parenteral Enteral Nutrition (PEN)
K. Urea Reduction Ratio (URR)

Let's Check It! Concepts

Choose the most appropriate answer for each of the following questions.

Part I

1. **LO 23.1** A modifier explains
   a. the reason a procedure was performed. **b.** an unusual circumstance.
   c. the date of service. **d.** the level of education of the physician.
2. **LO 23.1** CPT code modifiers are appended to
   a. policy numbers. **b.** diagnosis codes. **c.** procedure codes. **d.** pharmaceutical codes.
3. **LO 23.2** Service performed by a resident without the presence of a teaching physician under the primary care exception is identified with modifier
   a. AG **b.** AK **c.** GC **d.** GE
4. **LO 23.3** A Physical Status Modifier may only be appended to
   a. surgical codes. **b.** radiology codes.
   c. anesthesia codes. **d.** evaluation and management codes.
5. **LO 23.1** An example of an HCPCS Level II modifier is
   a. 23 **b.** LT **c.** P4 **d.** 99
6. **LO 23.2** An example of a personnel modifier is
   a. 81 **b.** 47 **c.** LC **d.** 57
7. **LO 23.7** If a third-party payer limits your use of multiple modifiers, you should use
   a. no modifiers **b.** 91 **c.** 51 **d.** 99

8. **LO 23.3** P5 is an example of a(n)
   a. HCPCS Level II modifier.
   b. CPT modifier.
   c. Physical Status Modifier.
   d. personnel modifier.
9. **LO 23.7** When appending both a CPT modifier and an HCPCS Level II modifier to a procedure code,
   a. the HCPCS Level II modifier comes first.
   b. the CPT modifier comes first.
   c. it doesn't matter which comes first.
   d. use neither—they cancel each other out.
10. **LO 23.8** A(n) ___ is a letter or report written by the attending physician or other health care professional to provide additional clarification or explanation.
   a. supplemental report
   b. service-related report
   c. ambulatory surgery report
   d. personnel report

Part II

1. **LO 23.6** Appending modifier A7 identifies a(n)
   a. aphakic patient.
   b. most recent URR reading of 65 to 69.9
   c. state-supplied vaccine.
   d. dressing for seven wounds.
2. **LO 23.4** Discontinued outpatient hospital/ambulatory surgery center (ASC) procedure prior to the administration of anesthesia is identified with modifier
   a. 27 b. 73 c. 74 d. AJ
3. **LO 23.6** LPM stands for
   a. local procedure modality.
   b. licensed practical medicine.
   c. local patient median.
   d. liters per minute.
4. **LO 23.4** Multiple outpatient hospital E/M encounters on the same date are identified by modifier
   a. 27 b. 73 c. 74 d. 82
5. **LO 23.6** An example of DME is
   a. an aspirin.
   b. the administration of a vaccination.
   c. a wheelchair.
   d. the removal of a cyst.
6. **LO 23.6** CLIA is identified with modifier
   a. BL b. QW c. SQ d. AV
7. **LO 23.6** EPSDT for school-based individualized education program (IEP) services provided outside the public school district responsible for the student is identified by
   a. TR b. EP c. G7 d. TM
8. **LO 23.5** Dr. Fullmark repairs a laceration on Johnny's left lower eyelid. What modifier would be appended?
   a. E4 b. E3 c. E2 d. E1
9. **LO 23.5** Which of the following modifiers identifies the right foot, third digit?
   a. T2 b. T7 c. T8 d. T9
10. **LO 23.8** Which of the following modifiers may need a supplemental report?
   a. 50 b. 57 c. 66 d. 53

Let's Check It! Rules and Regulations

Please answer the following questions from the knowledge you have gained after reading this chapter.

1. **LO 23.1** Why are modifiers used?
2. **LO 23.3** Explain what an anesthesia Physical Status Modifier is and why it is used.
3. **LO 23.2** Explain what an anesthesia personnel modifier is and why it is important to use them. Include an example.

4. **LO 23.8** What is a supplemental report? Why would a supplemental report be needed, and when do you submit it?
5. **LO 23.6** Explain the difference between a Class A finding, a Class B finding, and a Class C finding.

YOU CODE IT! Practice

Using the techniques described in this chapter, carefully read through the case studies and determine the most accurate modifier(s) for each case study. NOTE: All insurance carriers and third-party payers for the patients accept HCPCS Level II codes and modifiers.

Part I

1. Dr. Clayton removed Ricky Pujara's gallbladder 10 days ago. Today, he comes to see Dr. Clayton because of a problem with his knee. Which modifier should be appended to the encounter's E/M code?
2. Dr. Smyth performed an appendectomy on Lynda Lyman. However, the operation took twice as long as usual because Lynda weighs 356 pounds.
3. Dr. Julienne performed a biopsy on the left external ear of Ben Maas, a 69-year-old male.
4. Christopher Slice, a 17-year-old male, was brought into the OR in the Bracker ASC to have a programmable pump inserted into his spine for pain control. After the anesthesia was administered and Chris was fully unconscious, Dr. Sutton made the first incision. Chris began to hemorrhage. The bleeding was stopped, the incision was closed, and the procedure was discontinued. The coder is coding for the ASC facility.
5. Glenda Roberts, a 61-year-old female, goes to see Dr. Zentz at the referral of her family physician, Dr. Younts, for his opinion as to whether or not she should have surgery. After the evaluation and Glenda's agreement, Dr. Zentz schedules surgery for Thursday. Which modifier should be appended to Dr. Zentz's consultation code for today's evaluation?
6. Patricia Harris, an 82-year-old female, is having Dr. Harmon remove a cyst from her left ring finger.
7. Charles McBroom, a 4-week-old male, was rushed into surgery for repair of a septal defect. If the repair is not completed successfully, he may not survive. What is the correct anesthesia Physical Status Modifier?
8. Dr. Shull is preparing to perform open-heart surgery on Fred Faulkner. Dr. Lowell is asked to assist because a surgical resident is not available. Which modifier should be appended to the procedure code on Dr. Lowell's claim for services?
9. Carolyn Lovett, a 37-year-old female, comes to see Dr. Richardson for a complete physical examination, required by her insurance carrier.
10. George Carlos, a 9-week-old male, was born prematurely and weighs 3.8 kg. Dr. Wilson performs a cardiac catheterization on George.
11. Dr. Kelley excised an abscess on Clyde Hawken's great toe, right foot.
12. Annie Mathewson, a 12-year-old female, has been complaining of hearing a constant ringing in her right ear. Dr. Burwell performs an assessment for tinnitus in the right ear only.
13. Dr. Maxwell performed a percutaneous transluminal coronary atherectomy, by mechanical method, on Ronald Yates's left circumflex artery.
14. John Davis, a 25-year-old male, came to Dr. Browne to have corrective surgery on both of his eyes.
15. Tamara Connelly, a 16-year-old female, hurt her shoulder while camping. The clinic in the area took an x-ray but did not have a radiologist, so Tamara took the films to Dr. Evely, a radiologist, for interpretation and evaluation. Which modifier should Dr. Evely's coder append to the code for the x-rays?

Part II

1. Dr. White performed a blepharotomy on Vanetta Regis, draining the abscess on her upper left eyelid.
2. Stacey Maxell, a nurse midwife, helped Janise Edge deliver her first baby, a girl.

(continued)

3. Wilfred Edmonds, a 67-year-old male diagnosed with terminal bone cancer, has been in the hospice facility for 3 weeks and is showing signs of an ear infection. Dr. Johns was called in to attend Wilfred's ear problem.
4. Blake Gamble, an EMT, answered a call, with his partner, to Bracker Nursing Home. There was a small fire in the laundry room, and two patients were overcome by smoke enough to require hospitalization. Blake transported both patients at the same time in his ambulance and made one trip to the hospital.
5. Donnie Hentschell, a licensed psychotherapist, began the first of a series of court-ordered therapy sessions with Sonia Jacobs.
6. Dr. Rodriguez was called in to provide monitored anesthesia care for a procedure that will be performed on Malaka Kinlaw. Malaka has a history of acute cardiopulmonary problems.
7. Doon Jung, a registered nurse, works at the Bracker Nursing Facility. He changed the dressing on three wounds that Sang Killingsworth had on her leg.
8. Frank Wenami is the coding specialist for Bracker Dialysis Center. He is preparing the claim for services provided to Jenny Fortner, a patient with ESRD, who moved to the area just last week. Bracker Dialysis provided four dialysis treatments for Jenny during the month.
9. Cindy Kidman, one of the coding specialists at Weston Hospital, discovered that a claim had been submitted with an incorrect code. She has corrected the procedure code and is resubmitting the claim.
10. Nancy Nemeir works at Bracker Medical Equipment Inc. She meets with Earl Hillier, who was recently prescribed an electric wheelchair by Dr. Franks. Nancy explains the options of purchasing and renting the chair, and Earl decides to purchase the wheelchair.
11. Dr. Ott excised a lesion from Oliver Olden's right thumb.
12. Gwen Osby gave Frances Volkesberg, a 72-year-old female, a flu shot.
13. Dr. Parker saw Barbara Gillins and provided service defined as level 3 by Medicaid in her state.
14. Keren Haynes is a certified diabetic educator. She met with Bonnie Haversat to provide services.
15. The peer review organization (PRO) ordered Dr. Dumont to provide a second opinion on the surgical options for Maxine Nevradi.

YOU CODE IT! Application

The following exercises provide practice in abstracting the physician's notes and learning to work with physician documentation for various types of situations that might require a modifier. These case studies are modeled on real patient encounters. Using the techniques described in this chapter, carefully read through the case studies and determine the most accurate CPT code(s) and modifiers, if appropriate, to report the physician's services for each case study. NOTE: All insurance carriers and third-party payers for the patients accept HCPCS Level II codes and modifiers.

GREGORY SAME DAY SURGERY

955 East Healthcare Boulevard • SOMEWHERE, FL 32811 • 407-555-1597

PATIENT: RISHER, BELVA

ACCOUNT/EHR #: RISHBE001

Diagnosis: Fecal incontinence, diarrhea, constipation

Procedure: Total colonoscopy with hot biopsy destruction of sessile 3-mm mid-sigmoid colon polyp and multiple cold biopsies taken randomly throughout the colon

Physician: Marion M. March, MD

Anesthesia: Demerol 50 mg and Versed 3 mg, both given IV

PROCEDURE: Pt is a 43-year-old female. Patient was placed into position. Digital examination revealed no masses. The pediatric variable flexion Olympus colonoscope was introduced into the rectum and advanced to the cecum. A picture was taken of the appendiceal orifice and the ileocecal valve.

(continued)

The scope was then carefully extubated. The mucosa looked normal. Random biopsies were taken from the ascending colon, the transverse colon, the descending colon, the sigmoid colon, and the rectum. There was a 3-mm sessile polyp in the mid-sigmoid colon that a hot biopsy destroyed.

IMPRESSION: Sigmoid colon polyp destroyed by hot biopsy

RECOMMENDATIONS: Follow-up in 7 days for biopsy results.

Determine the most accurate CPT code(s) and necessary modifier(s) for the colonoscopy.

GREGORY SAME DAY SURGERY

955 East Healthcare Boulevard • SOMEWHERE, FL 32811 • 407-555-1597

PATIENT: GILMORE, STEVEN

ACCOUNT/EHR #: GILMST001

Diagnosis: Family history of colon cancer

Procedure: Colonoscopy

Physician: Marion M. March, MD

Anesthesia: Versed 4 mg, Demerol 75 mg

PROCEDURE: Pt is a 59-year-old male presenting for a colonoscopy. Pt receives educational material and is informed of the risks. He acknowledges he understands the nature of the procedure, the risks, and the consequences, and consents to the procedure.

The patient is placed in the left lateral decubitus position. The rectal exam reveals normal sphincter tone and no masses. A colonoscope is introduced into the rectum and advanced to the distal sigmoid colon. Further advancement is impossible due to the marked fixation and severe angulation of the rectosigmoid colon. Procedure is discontinued.

On withdrawal, no masses or polyps are noted, and the mucosa is normal throughout. Rectal vault is unremarkable. The patient tolerates the procedure without difficulty.

IMPRESSION: Normal colonoscopy, only to the distal sigmoid colon

PLAN: Strong recommendation for a barium enema

Determine the most accurate CPT code(s) and necessary modifier(s) for the colonoscopy.

WESTON HOSPITAL

591 Chester Road • Masters, FL 33955

PATIENT: SCHERINI, STEPHANIE

ACCOUNT/EHR #: SCHEST001

Diagnosis: Chronic obstructive lung disease

Procedure: Lung transplant, single, with cardiopulmonary bypass

Surgical Team: Marion M. March, MD, primary; Fredrick Avatar, MD; Gene Lavelle, MD

Anesthesia: General

PROCEDURE: Pt is a 37-year-old female brought into the OR, placed on the table, and draped in sterile fashion. Anesthesia was administered. At thoracotomy, the left lung was removed by dividing the left main stem bronchus at the level of the left upper lobe. The two pulmonary veins and single pulmonary artery were divided distally. An allograft left lung was inserted. The recipient left main stem bronchus and pulmonary artery were re-resected to accommodate the transplant. The recipient pulmonary veins were opened into the left atrium. An end-to-end anastomosis

(continued)

of the recipient's respective structures (pulmonary artery, main stem bronchus, and left atrial cuffs) was made to the similar donor structures. Two chest tubes were inserted. Bronchoscopy was performed in the OR. Cardiopulmonary bypass was successfully completed.

Patient tolerated the procedure well and was taken to the recovery room.

Determine the most accurate CPT code(s) and necessary modifier(s) for the transplantation. TIP: Don't forget your Anesthesia code with modifier.

PRADER, BRACKER, & ASSOCIATES

A Complete Health Care Facility

159 Healthcare Way • SOMEWHERE, FL 32811 • 407-555-6789

PATIENT: WILBORN, AMANDA

ACCOUNT/EHR #: WILBAM001

Attending Physician: Renee O. Bracker, MD

Referring Physician: Valerie R. Reymond, MD

S: Pt is a 41-year-old female who was injured in a car accident. She presents today at the recommendation of Dr. Reymond for a fitting for a prosthetic spectacle.

O: HEENT is unremarkable. Monofocal measurements are taken, and data for the creation of an appropriate prosthesis are recorded.

A: Aphakia, left eye

P: Return in 2 weeks for final fitting

Determine the most accurate CPT code(s) and necessary modifier(s) for the fitting of the prosthetic spectacle.

PRADER, BRACKER, & ASSOCIATES

A Complete Health Care Facility

159 Healthcare Way • SOMEWHERE, FL 32811 • 407-555-6789

PATIENT: HOLDER, ANDREW

ACCOUNT/EHR #: HOLDAN001

Procedure Performed: CT brain w/o contrast

Radiologist: Michael B. Hawkins, MD

Clinical Information: Evaluation for VP shunt, postsurgical

Attending Physician: Renee O. Bracker, MD

TECHNICAL INFORMATION: Contiguous 3-mm-thick axial images were obtained through the skull base and posterior fossa structures followed by 7-mm-thick axial images through the remainder of the brain. The examination was performed without the use of intravenous contrast material. The scan was performed at an independent imaging center and sent to me via secured PACS system, so I could interpret.

INTERPRETATION: Evaluation of the posterior fossa demonstrates bilateral vertebral artery calcification. No abnormal intra- or extra-axial collections are noted. There is no evidence of midline shift.

Analysis of the region of the sella turcica demonstrates calcification, likely atherosclerotic involving the cavernous carotid arteries bilaterally seen on series 2 image 7.

(continued)

Supratentorially, the lateral ventricles are prominent in size. A ventriculostomy catheter is seen coursing from the region of the postcentral sulcus with its distal tip terminating within the frontal horn of the right lateral ventricle abutting the septum pellucidum. Hypodensity is seen within the periventricular white matter particularly abutting the frontal horns of the lateral ventricles bilaterally. There is a mild degree of cerebral volume loss. No abnormal intra- or extra-axial collections are noted.

Evaluation of the visualized skull and paranasal sinuses demonstrates a right parietal burr hole defect for placement of the patient's ventriculostomy catheter. A subcutaneous ventriculostomy valve is seen on series 3 image 26.

RECOMMENDATIONS: There is mild prominence of the lateral ventricles bilaterally without evidence of dilation of the cerebral aqueduct or fourth ventricle.

Determine the most accurate CPT code(s) and necessary modifier(s) for the CT scan.

24

CPT Evaluation and Management Coding

Key Terms

- Anticipatory Guidance
- Basic Personal Services
- Care Plan Oversight Services
- Consultation
- Critical Care Services
- End-Stage Renal Disease (ESRD)
- Established Patient
- Evaluation and Management (E/M)
- Global Surgical Package
- Hospice
- Level of Patient History
- Level of Physical Examination
- Medical Decision Making (MDM)
- New Patient
- Nursing Facility
- Past, Family, and Social History (PFSH)
- Preventive
- Problem-Pertinent System Review
- Relationship
- Risk Factor Reduction Intervention
- Transfer of Care

Learning Outcomes

After completing this chapter, the student should be able to:

LO 24.1 Explain the purpose of E/M codes.
LO 24.2 Abstract the details for determining the location of the encounter.
LO 24.3 Interpret the relationship between physician and patient.
LO 24.4 Analyze the documentation to accurately determine the type of E/M service provided.
LO 24.5 Ascertain the correct code for preventive care (annual physicals).
LO 24.6 Cull the appropriate information from the documentation related to E/M services.
LO 24.7 Apply the rules of the global surgical package.
LO 24.8 Assign E/M modifiers and add-on codes accurately.
LO 24.9 Determine the most accurate way to report special evaluation services.
LO 24.10 Validate and report the provision of coordination and management services.

STOP! Remember, you need to follow along in your CPT code book for an optimal learning experience.

24.1 What Are E/M Codes?

Evaluation and Management (E/M) is the first section in the CPT book and lists codes numbered 99202–99499. These codes are used to report and reimburse physicians for their expertise and thought processes involved in diagnosing and treating patients, such as

- Talking with the patient and his or her family.
- Reviewing data such as complaints, signs, symptoms, and examination results.
- Doing research in medical books and journals.
- Consulting with other health care professionals.

All these elements, including the training and education that this health care professional has had, go into the decision of what to do next for the patient—what advice, what prescription, what test, what treatment, what procedure. E/M codes provide a way to reimburse the health care professional for his or her assessment and supervision of the patient and the determination of the best course for his or her care.

E/M services go beyond those included in the typical office or hospital visit. **Preventive** medicine assessments—more commonly called annual physicals or wellness visits, evaluations of patients in short-term and long-term care facilities, counseling, and critical care—are just some of the areas of focus that might be required of the attending physician. This chapter reviews these subcategories of E/M codes.

> **Preventive**
> A type of action or service that stops something from happening or from getting worse.

As you just read, E/M codes are used to describe specifically the physician's expertise and assessment that was provided during an encounter between him or her and a patient. There are many different types of E/M codes, as you will learn throughout this and the next chapter. Let's begin by reviewing the pieces of information you will need to abstract from the physician's documentation to code the E/M portion of the encounter properly.

Face-to-Face (Office and Other Outpatient Visits)

You may have noticed the phrase *face-to-face* in the code description qualification about time. CPT is very specific about what is included in this element of E/M services provided by a physician to a patient, such as the time it takes to collect health care-related history, perform the physical examination, and counsel the patient (as discussed previously).

Everyone understands that most physicians will spend time, before and after their encounters with patients, reviewing records, going over test results, conferencing with other professionals and the patients by writing letters and reports, making phone calls, and performing other non-face-to-face tasks. Officially, these are included in the time component of the E/M codes.

GUIDANCE CONNECTION

When a specific code is approved for use in reporting services provided using synchronous, audiovisual, telecommunications equipment [indicated by a star (★) symbol to the left of the code], face-to-face may also occur electronically. Refer to the chapter ***CPT and HCPCS Level II Modifiers***, where you will find a section on ***Service-Related Modifiers***, specifically modifier 95.

GUIDANCE CONNECTION

Read the additional explanations in the **Evaluation and Management (E/M) Services Guidelines**, subhead **Time**, paragraphs **Face-to-face . . .** and **Unit/floor time . . .**, in your CPT book directly in front of the E/M section that lists all the codes.

Unit/Floor Time (Hospital and Other Inpatient Visits)

When a physician attends to a patient in a facility, such as a hospital or nursing home, the measure of time, for purposes of E/M coding, is described a bit differently than for outpatient encounters.

In outpatient encounters, time is measured by face-to-face—the number of minutes spent with the patient. With inpatient services, in addition to the face-to-face time that the physician may spend at bedside examining the patient, there are additional components included in the measure of time. These additional components are known as *unit/floor time*, which include

- Meeting with nursing staff and other health care professionals.
- Speaking with family members.
- Time the physician spends going over the patient's chart and reviewing notes by other professionals caring for the patient while the physician is still physically present in the hospital unit.

24.2 Location Where the E/M Services Were Provided

The first element you must identify when coding E/M services is the location of the encounter between the health care professional (physician) and the patient. Exactly where did the provider see the patient: in an outpatient location (such as a physician's office), in the hospital, in a skilled nursing facility? Did they just speak on the phone, or did the provider see the patient somewhere else?

Unlike when you are coding other procedures, it can be more efficient to go directly to the E/M section of CPT rather than beginning with the Alphabetic Index. Knowing where this encounter took place between the provider and the patient will enable you to narrow down the range of possible codes and get to the accurate one more effectively. In addition, going to the location subsection of the E/M section will let you know what additional information you need to determine the right code.

For example, when the encounter occurs at the physician's office, you will need to know the level of history taken, the level of examination performed, and the complexity of medical decision making (MDM). However, when the encounter occurs on the telephone, you will need to know how long the physician was on the phone and the date of the most recent face-to-face E/M service. You will learn more about non-face-to-face encounters, such as telephone calls, later in this chapter and in the next chapter.

Evaluation and Management (E/M) The codes that describe the specific components of a meeting between a health care professional and a patient.

Take out your copy of the *Current Procedural Terminology* (CPT) code book so we can go through this together. Go to the ***Evaluation and Management (E/M)*** section of the CPT book. Look at the first subheading on the first page: **Office or Other Outpatient Services**.

This header, like many others throughout the section, identifies the location of the encounter—where the physician met with the patient.

Once you are in the subsection that identifies where the encounter happened, you can see what additional information you will need to gather from the physician's notes to determine the correct code. For example, in the **Office or Other Outpatient Services** subsection, you can see that the next piece of data you need to know is the relationship between this provider and this patient—whether this patient is a *new patient* or an *established patient*. However, under the **Hospital Inpatient Services** subsection, the next piece of information you will need to cull from the documentation is whether this is the *initial* hospital care visit or a *subsequent* hospital care visit.

CODING BITES

When a physician sees a patient in the office and then, that same physician admits that patient to the hospital on the same day, the entire encounter for that day would be reported with an E/M code from ***Initial Hospital Inpatient or Observation Care***.

EXAMPLES

Nicholas Marrin, a 59-year-old male, was brought into the emergency department (ED) with sharp pain in his chest radiating downward into his left arm. The best, most appropriate E/M code will be found in the 99281–99288 range of codes, under **Emergency Department Services**.

Dr. Harman goes to the Sother Nursing Home to see his patient Robin Farber, a 93-year-old female. The best, most appropriate E/M code will be found in the 99304–99318 range of codes, under **Nursing Facility Services**.

Armani Belez, a 35-year-old female, comes to see Dr. Abrahams at his office. The best, most appropriate E/M code will be found in the 99201–99215 range of codes, under **Office or Other Outpatient Services.**

Location-Specific Headings in the E/M Section

The location-specific headings in the E/M section:

- **Office or Other Outpatient Services**
- **Hospital Inpatient and Observation Care Services**
- **Consultations**
- **Emergency Department Services**
- **Critical Care Services**
- **Nursing Facility Services**
- **Home or Residence Services**
- **Non-Face-to-Face Services**
- **Delivery/Birthing Room Attendance and Resuscitation Services**
- **Inpatient Neonatal Intensive Care Services and Pediatric and Neonatal Critical Care Services**

Nursing Facility
A facility that provides skilled nursing treatment and attention along with limited medical care for its (usually long-term) residents, who do not require acute care services (hospitalization).

LET'S CODE IT! SCENARIO

Suzette Kabole, an 87-year-old female, broke her hip 1 month ago. She has been a patient of Dr. Okine for several years. Since her release from the hospital, Suzette has been homebound until her hip completely heals. Therefore, Dr. Okine went to her home to check on her progress.

(continued)

Let's Code It!

Read the notes again, and look for the key words that tell you the location of the encounter and the relationship between patient and physician.

The notes state that the doctor went to "*her home*." That phrase tells us the location of the encounter. Look through the E/M section of the CPT book, and find the group of E/M codes that report this location: **Home or Resident Services . . .** codes 99341–99350.

YOU INTERPRET IT!

Match the E/M subsection code range for each of these locations:

1. Preventive medicine services **a.** 99202-99205

2. Telephone with patient **b.** 99252-99255

3. Emergency Department **c.** 99381-99429

4. Inpatient Consultations **d.** 99441-99443

5. Walk-in clinic **e.** 99281-99288

24.3 Relationship between Provider and Patient

Throughout the E/M section of the CPT book, subheadings identify the **relationship** between the provider and the individual. E/M codes use different types of relationship for determining the best, most appropriate code. You may have to identify, from the documentation, if the relationship between the physician and patient is as a **new patient** or **established patient**; if this is initial care or subsequent care; or if this qualifies as a temporary relationship—a **consultation**.

Relationship
The level of familiarity between provider and patient.

New Patient
A person who has not received any professional services within the past 3 years from either the provider or another provider of the same specialty and the same subspecialty who belongs to the same group practice.

Established Patient
A person who has received professional services from the physician/qualified health care professional or another physician/qualified health care professional of the exact same specialty and subspecialty who belongs to the same group practice, within the past three years.

Consultation
An encounter for purposes of a second physician's opinion or advice, requested by another physician, regarding the management of a patient's specific health concern. A consultation is planned to be a short-term relationship between a health care professional and a patient.

New or Established Patient

In many cases, you must know the relationship between the patient and the provider so that you can communicate an understanding of how familiar the physician is with the patient; the patient's personal history, social history, and family history; and other elements that may affect the physician's decisions regarding the patient's health. Certainly you can understand that the first time they meet, the physician knows absolutely nothing about the patient. He or she must spend time asking questions to help collect the information that will be critical to determining the correct diagnosis and course of treatment. When the physician sees the patient again, however, all the doctor will need to do is quickly read through the patient's file to refresh his or her memory of past conditions and issues.

New Patient

The CPT code set defines a new patient as "*one who has not received any professional services from the physician within the past three years.*" This includes not only this specific physician but also any other group practice member who belongs to the exact same specialty or subspecialty, whether they are a physician or another health care professional.

Established Patient

It is logical, then, to understand that an established patient is one who *has* received professional services from this physician *or* another physician or health care professional in this same group practice who has the exact same specialty and subspecialty credentials, within the last 3 years.

Some location subsections have different codes for a new patient and an established patient, and others do not. You must read the descriptions at the beginning of each subsection to be certain whether this is a criterion for a particular E/M code. For example, the subheading **Emergency Department Services** offers the same codes whether the individual is a new or an established patient.

EXAMPLE

Leonora Lopez, a 25-year-old female, comes to see Dr. Poker at his office and complains of severe pain in her right wrist and forearm. She just moved to the area, and this is the first time Dr. Poker has seen her.

"*. . . at his office . . .*" identifies the LOCATION of the encounter.

"*. . . this is the first time Dr. Poker has seen her*" identifies the RELATIONSHIP for this professional and this patient.

Therefore, the E/M codes applicable for this encounter are now in the smaller range of 99202–99205, **Office or Other Outpatient Services, New Patient**.

GUIDANCE CONNECTION

Read the additional explanations in the **Evaluation and Management (E/M) Services Guidelines**, subhead **Definitions of Commonly Used Terms–New and Established Patient**, in your CPT book directly in front of the E/M section that lists all the codes.

Initial or Subsequent Care

For services located in hospitals, nursing facilities, intensive neonatal and pediatric critical care departments, and intensive care locations, you will need to identify whether the encounter is the initial or a subsequent visit rather than if the relationship is new or established. This distinction is similar to the *new* or *established* concept, as these two terms describe how up-to-date the physician is on the current condition of this patient.

Initial care visits are reported for the first time a physician, the one for whom you are coding, sees a patient *at a location* for a specific course of treatment or care.

Subsequent care visits are reported for the second time and all visits thereafter that a physician sees a patient *at a location* during the course of the same treatment or care.

EXAMPLE

Barry Balmer is admitted to the hospital on Saturday after having a myocardial infarction (MI) while playing tennis. His regular cardiologist, Dr. Hamilton, is out of town for the weekend, so Dr. Zenbar admits Barry to the hospital on Saturday and checks in on his care on Sunday. Monday, when Dr. Hamilton returns, she goes to see Barry in the hospital and takes charge of his care.

- On Saturday, an *initial* hospital care visit is reported for Dr. Zenbar because this is his first time seeing Barry during this course of treatment at the hospital.
- On Sunday, a *subsequent* hospital care visit is reported for Dr. Zenbar because this is his second time seeing Barry during this course of treatment at the hospital.
- On Monday, an *initial* hospital care visit is reported for Dr. Hamilton because this is her first time seeing Barry during this course of treatment at the hospital, even though it is Barry's third day in the hospital.
- On Tuesday, a *subsequent* hospital care visit is reported for Dr. Hamilton because this is her second time seeing Barry during this course of treatment at the hospital.

Consultations

There are times when the relationship between a patient and a health care provider is expected to be temporary, typically lasting only one visit. In such cases, one physician or health care professional will ask another physician to meet with a patient and evaluate a patient's condition only to offer his or her own professional opinion about the patient's diagnosis and/or treatment options. This temporary relationship is known as a consultation.

When a patient goes to a physician for a *consultation* because the first physician is merely seeking a *second opinion* from the consulting physician regarding diagnosis and/or treatment of the patient, it will be reported from the **Consultations** subsection of E/M. Different from other subsections, the consultation codes 99242-99255 are separated into two parts on the basis of the location of where the consultation took place: **Office and Other Outpatient Consultations** and **Inpatient or Observation Care Consultations**.

EXAMPLE

Dr. Gail reviews Derita Beck's lab tests and notices that her lipase level is very high. This may indicate a problem with the patient's pancreas. While Derita is healthy overall, Dr. Gail does not want to take any chances, so he refers Derita to Dr. Keith, a gastroenterologist, for a second opinion. Derita goes to see Dr. Keith, who examines her, reviews the test results, and writes a letter to Dr. Gail agreeing with his assessment. Derita goes back to Dr. Gail and does not see Dr. Keith again.

The relationship between Dr. Keith and Derita Beck is not defined as new or established but as a consultation–a second opinion requested by another physician. Therefore, Dr. Keith's coder will report this one encounter from the **Consultations** subsection, codes 99242-99255.

GUIDANCE CONNECTION

Read the additional explanations in the in-section guidelines located within the **Evaluation and Management (E/M)** section, subhead **Consultations**, directly above code 99242 in your CPT book.

If the second opinion is requested by the patient or a family member instead of another health care professional, this is *not* reported as a Consultation. It would be reported as a New Patient encounter.

LET'S CODE IT! SCENARIO

ICD-10-PCS

Denny Rossman, a 49-year-old male, was having pain in his lower abdomen, especially when going to the bathroom. His primary care physician, Dr. Lein, did a PSA and was not very concerned, so he told Denny to come back in 6–8 months for a follow-up. Denny did not feel comfortable about Dr. Lein's decision and made an appointment for a second opinion with Dr. Ellis, a urologist.

Let's Code It!

The notes indicate that it was Denny, "the patient," who "requested the consultation" with Dr. Ellis. Therefore, it is coded as a new patient office visit, and you will find the correct code in the 99202–99205 range.

Referral or Consultation?

Referral and consultation are two terms that are commonly used and confused. When one physician *transfers* the care and treatment for a patient (in total or for one particular issue) to another physician, this is a *referral*. The patient is merely being recommended to see another physician and is expected to become a patient of the other physician. These visits are reported using the regular E/M codes, based on the location of the encounter between the new physician (the specialist) and the patient–for example, physician's office 99202-99205, etc.

Transfer of Care
When a physician gives up responsibility for caring for a patient, in whole or with regard to one specific condition, and another physician accepts responsibility for the care of that patient.

If the patient goes back to see the "consultant" again, this second E/M encounter will be reported as an established patient encounter because this means that the "consultant" has accepted this individual as a patient for continued care. This is the same as when the first physician may refer the patient to another physician for continuing care and not just a second opinion. More commonly known as a referral, the industry term for this is **transfer of care**. Transfer of the care of a patient can be complete, such as when a physician is retiring, or just for one particular portion of a patient's care, such as a primary care physician sending a patient to a specialist for care of just the one issue.

EXAMPLE

Dr. Sanger has been Penny Condrel's primary care physician for many years. Today, Penny comes in complaining of a rash all over her legs. Dr. Sanger refers Penny to Dr. Arias, a dermatologist, so that he can take over the diagnosis and treatment of this skin condition. Dr. Arias agrees to take Penny on as his patient to treat this rash. In this case, there has been a transfer of care for Penny's rash from Dr. Sanger to Dr. Arias.

For that first visit, the relationship between Dr. Arias and Penny is one of a new patient, not a consultation, because Dr. Arias has accepted Penny as a patient and the relationship is not a temporary one. This relationship will be ongoing until Penny's problem is resolved. However, Dr. Sanger will remain Penny's primary care physician.

24.4 Types of E/M Services

As you read through the documentation, you also will need to identify the specific *type of service* provided by the physician. This detail will contribute to your ability to determine which subsection of the E/M codes will provide you with accurate code descriptions related to this specific encounter.

- Active Care
- Critical Care
- Case Management
- Care Plan Oversight
- Preventive Medicine
- Non-Face-to-Face
- Special Services
- Newborn Care
- Delivery/Birthing Room
- Care Management Services

Level of Service

While accurately reporting the level of expertise and knowledge used by the physician during a visit may seem intangible, the ***Evaluation and Management (E/M) Services Guidelines*** provide you with the criteria–very specific and tangible measurements to help you determine the appropriate level of service based on the documentation for the encounter. Let's begin this step of E/M by discussing what you need to determine which level has been provided:

- MDM required to determine a diagnosis, or possible diagnoses, and a treatment plan or next step.

Level of Patient History and Level of Physical Examination

Physicians need to document the **level of patient history** and observations noted during a documentation of the **level of physical examination** for the purposes of continuity of care. These are key details that health care professionals should track over time to support early diagnoses and predictive indicators, which may support more effective treatment plans. While important components of a physician's evaluation of the patient's condition, the measure of history and physical examination is not a component in the determination of which E/M code to report.

Level of Patient History
The amount of detail involved in the documentation of patient history.

Level of Physical Examination
The extent of a physician's clinical assessment and inspection of a patient.

CODING BITES

A **PFSH** has three key components that you should be watching for while abstracting that will help you differentiate a detailed history: **P**ast history, **F**amily history, and **S**ocial **H**istory.

(continued)

Past History [Patient's Medical History (PMH)]

- Prior major illnesses and injuries
- Prior operations
- Prior hospitalizations
- Current medications
- Allergies (e.g., drug, food)
- Age-appropriate immunization status
- Age-appropriate feeding/dietary status

Family History

- The health status or cause of death of parents, siblings, and children
- Specific diseases related to problems identified in the chief complaint, history of present illness, and/or system review
- Diseases of family members that may be hereditary or place the patient at risk

Social History

- Marital status and/or living arrangements
- Current employment
- Occupational history
- Use of drugs, alcohol, and tobacco
- Level of education
- Sexual history
- Other relevant social factors

Level of Medical Decision Making

Beginning January 1, 2023, the level of **medical decision making (MDM)** provided by the physician during this encounter is the determining factor when identifying the appropriate E/M code. This can be the most challenging component because, in essence, you need to determine from the documentation how hard the physician had to think to determine what to do next to help this patient with this concern. It may be that the physician writes a prescription, recommends a treatment or surgery, or orders some diagnostic tests to provide further information. Your understanding of anatomy and physiology will help you with this portion of determining the most accurate code. There are four levels of MDM.

CODING BITES

A *complete* PFSH would cover details about the patient's health that covers all or most body systems and health-related behaviors.

Medical Decision Making (MDM) The level of knowledge and experience needed by the provider to determine the diagnosis and/or what to do next.

Straightforward MDM

a. A small number of possible diagnoses.
b. A small number of treatment or management options.
c. A low to no risk for complications.
d. Little to no data or research to be reviewed.

EXAMPLE

Antonio

If when Dr. Grace looked down Antonio's throat he observed inflammation of his tonsils, and if Antonio has no problematic history, then Dr. Grace's decision making may be very straightforward. Dr. Grace was trained to recognize tonsillitis and knows exactly what to prescribe to help Antonio heal.

Low-Level MDM

a. A limited number of possible diagnoses.
b. A limited number of treatment or management options.
c. A limited amount of data to be reviewed.
d. A low risk for complications.

EXAMPLE

Antonio

If Dr. Grace observed Antonio had a different type of inflammation (other than tonsillitis), such as some indication that his condition might be strep throat or pharyngitis, the process of determining what is best to do is slightly more complex. If so, then a culture would need to be taken for a lab test.

Moderate-Level MDM

a. A multiple number of possible diagnoses.

b. A multiple number of treatment or management options.

c. A moderate amount of data to be reviewed.

d. A moderate level of risk for complications, possibly due to other existing diagnoses or medications currently being taken.

EXAMPLE

Antonio

In addition to the inflammation Dr. Grace observed, he also noted worrisome sounds in Antonio's lungs. This complicates matters because the diagnosis possibilities now extend from tonsillitis to strep throat to asthma, bronchitis, or pneumonia. Or perhaps Antonio has a history of asthma or previous bouts with pneumonia. Or perhaps Antonio has other known current illnesses, such as hypertension or diabetes, which may make diagnosing and treating this condition much more complicated.

CODING BITES

Certain terms in the physician's notes may indicate a more complex process of MDM on the physician's part. Orders for several tests with terms such as *rule out*, *possible*, and *likely* might indicate the physician is looking for evidence of several possible diagnoses.

High-Level MDM

a. A large number of possible diagnoses.

b. A large number of treatment or management options.

c. A large amount of data and/or research to be reviewed.

d. A high level of risk for complications, possibly due to other existing diagnoses and/or medications currently being taken.

EXAMPLE

Antonio

In highly complex cases, the documentation will show issues such as multiple co-morbidities (other conditions or diseases), current multiple medications that may make determining the best treatment for a problem more dangerous for fear of adverse interactions, perhaps allergies to medications under consideration, or other factors that make the determination of the best course of treatment for the patient incredibly complicated.

Table 24-1 may provide you with help to determine what level of MDM is documented.

TABLE 24-1 Determine Level of Medical Decision Making Documented

	Straightforward	Low Level	Moderate Level	High Level
Number of possible diagnoses	1 or 2	Few	Several	Many
Number of management options	1 or 2	Few	Several	Many
Quantity of information to be obtained, reviewed, analyzed (test results, records, etc.)	None, 1, or 2	Few	Several	Many
Risk of significant complications (morbidity, mortality, interactions, allergies, co-morbidities, systemic underlying conditions, etc.)	None, 1, or 2	Few	Several	Many

EXAMPLE

Bernard Clinton comes in to the Emergency Department with a large shard of glass in his hand. You can see that the number of potential diagnoses is very small: a foreign body in his hand. There are a small number of treatment options: remove the shard. There are no real health complications, and the physician should not have to research Bernard's condition before deciding what to do. This is a straightforward level of MDM.

EXAMPLE

Karen Potts lives in a domiciliary and is seen by Dr. Seridan. She complains of malaise and fatigue. She denies any major changes in her diet or lifestyle prior to the onset of her symptoms. This is a complex situation that will take a lot of investigation and knowledge on the part of the physician to determine Karen's underlying condition. There are numerous possible diagnoses and, therefore, a large number of management options. Dr. Seridan may have to perform several diagnostic tests to help him determine the problem. This is a highly complex case.

GUIDANCE CONNECTION

Read the additional explanations in the **Evaluation and Management (E/M) Services Guidelines**, subhead **Determine the Complexity of Medical Decision Making**, in your CPT book directly in front of the E/M section that lists all the codes.

YOU CODE IT! CASE STUDY

Dr. Sternan was asked by Dr. MacAndrews to provide a second opinion on Arthur Jankowski, a 17-year-old male. Arthur's pulmonary specialist, Dr. MacAndrews, wants to perform a lung transplant because of his diagnosis of cystic fibrosis. Dr. Sternan examined Arthur's respiratory system in his hospital room, reviewed the x-rays ordered by Dr. MacAndrews, and wrote a report agreeing that Dr. MacAndrews should perform the surgery.

You Code It!

Go through the steps of E/M coding, and determine the E/M code that should be reported for this encounter between Dr. Sternan and Arthur Jankowski.

Step #1: Read the case completely.
Step #2: Abstract the notes: Which key words can you identify relating to the E/M service performed?
Step #3: What is the location?
Step #4: What is the relationship?
Step #5: What level of MDM was required?
Step #6: What is the most accurate E/M code for this encounter?
Step #7: Double-check your work.

Answer:

Did you determine this to be the correct code?

99252 Inpatient or observation consultation, straightforward medical decision making

Good work!

GUIDANCE CONNECTION

Read the additional explanations in the **Evaluation and Management (E/M) Services Guidelines**, subhead **Instructions for Selecting a Level of E/M Service**, in your CPT book directly in front of the E/M section that lists all the codes.

LET'S CODE IT! SCENARIO

Sadie Adanson, an 89-year-old female, was admitted today into McGraw Skilled Nursing Facility (SNF) by Dr. Domino for rehabilitation and care. She suffered a stroke 2 weeks ago and was just discharged from the hospital. Dr. Domino documented a comprehensive level of history. She performed a detailed level of physical exam. Due to the patient's advanced age, co-morbidities, and long list of current medications, as well as the late effects of the stroke, Dr. Domino's MDM was of high level.

Let's Code It!

First, identify the location where the encounter between Dr. Domino and Sadie Adanson occurred. The notes state, "*admitted into McGraw Skilled Nursing Facility.*" Turn in the CPT book, E/M section, to **Nursing Facility Services**. This subsection of E/M is divided into two parts: **Initial Nursing Facility Care** and **Subsequent Nursing Facility Care**.

The documentation states that Sadie was admitted today, so this must be the first time Dr. Domino is caring for Sadie at this nursing home. Now you know that the correct code for Dr. Domino's evaluation of Sadie for this visit must be within the **Initial Nursing Facility Care 99304–99306** range.

This scenario is provided with a shortcut, indicating the level for you: *MDM high level.*"

MDM *high* level meets the description of 99306.

LET'S CODE IT! SCENARIO

Patrick Chapman, a 77-year-old male, has been living at Northside Assisted Living Facility for 6 months. Dr. Colon, his primary physician since he moved in, comes in today to see Patrick because of a complaint of leg pain. Dr. Colon documents a problem-focused interval history, an expanded problem-focused exam, and MDM of moderate level.

Let's Code It!

Read through the scenario, and identify the location where Dr. Colon provided his evaluation and management services: "*assisted living facility.*"

Let's turn to the **Home or Residence Services** subsection of E/M. Why? In the first paragraph under this heading, you will see that CPT directs you to use this category of E/M codes "to report evaluation and management services in an assisted living facility."

This subsection is divided into **New Patient** and **Established Patient**, so go back to the scenario. It states, "*Dr. Colon, his primary physician since he moved in,*" meaning that Patrick qualifies as an established patient. This narrows down the choices to **Established Patient 99347-99350**.

As we did before, this scenario is provided with a shortcut, indicating the level for you:

MDM moderate level meets the requirement for 99349.

YOU CODE IT! CASE STUDY

Daman Cordero, a 81-year-old male, was seen at his home by Dr. Decklin for the first time because of a cough, fever, excessive sputum production, and difficulty in breathing. He had been reasonably well until now. Dr. Decklin did a physical exam of the patient's respiratory system and took Daman's personal, family, and social history in detail. After a chest x-ray was taken to rule out pneumonia, Dr. Decklin's straightforward MDM led her to diagnose him with bronchitis and prescribe an antibiotic and a steroid.

You Code It!

Go through the steps of E/M coding, and determine the E/M code that should be reported for this encounter between Dr. Decklin and Daman Cordero.

Step #1: Read the case completely.
Step #2: Abstract the notes: Which key words can you identify relating to the E/M service performed?
Step #3: What is the location?
Step #4: What is the relationship?
Step #5: What level of MDM was required?
Step #6: What is the most accurate E/M code for this encounter?
Step #7: Double-check your work.

Answer:

Did you determine the correct code to be **99341**? Good work!

You know, from the notes, that Daman saw the doctor "at his home." This tells you the location. You also can detect that Daman is a new patient because Dr. Decklin is seeing him "for the first time."

Code 99341 is supported by the "straightforward medical decision making."

The correct E/M code for this scenario is **99341**.

Telemedicine Services

Synchronous Communication Technology E/M

By now, most people are familiar with telemedicine services where technology enables a provider and patient to meet, in real time, synchronously, via an encrypted software program. We now have specific codes to report evaluation and management (E/M) services conducted using this technology. As professional coding specialists, we must determine, from the physician's documentation, details to further clarify which code to report:

First, was the encounter...

Synchronous Audio-Video

Synchronous Audio-Only

You are looking for the clarification of whether or not video was involved [e.g., similar to Zoom or FaceTime], or did they communicate with audio only [e.g., a phone call].

Second, was this encounter with a new patient or an established patient. You learned about this earlier in this chapter (**24.3 Relationship between Provider and Patient**).

Once you have determined whether or not video was used, and the patient's relationship during the encounter, you can next determine which subsection from which to choose the code to report.

Synchronous Audio-Video E/M New Patient: 98000-98003

Synchronous Audio-Video E/M Established Patient: 98004-98007

Synchronous Audio-Only E/M New Patient: 98008-98011

Synchronous Audio-Only E/M Established Patient: 98012-98015

To further narrow down to the most accurate code, you will need to identify the level of medical decision-making from the documentation, just as you would do to choose a code from 99202-99215 for other E/M office services. The same choices are present here: straightforward MDM, low MDM, moderate MDM, or high MDM. Each code description includes approximate time measures, again, just as you see under the other Office or Other Outpatient Services codes.

Brief Synchronous Communication Technology Service (e.g., Virtual Check-In)

Code 98016, new for 2025, is used for a quick conversation, between 5 and 7 minutes in length, initiated by an established patient, to discuss if there is a need for another, longer E/M visit. This succinct exchange may be conducted with or without video.

EXAMPLE

Fiona Friedlander called to speak with her physician. Dr. Ellynton prescribed a new medication for Fiona at their last appointment, 2 weeks ago. She has been experiencing itching on her arms and legs and wanted to ask the physician about this concern. She asked if she needs to make an appointment to come in again or just stop taking the medication. Dr. Ellynton recommends that she come in so he can examine her and determine a solution. This phone call was documented at five minutes in length and Fiona was scheduled to come into the office the day after tomorrow. This would be reported with code 98016.

Critical Care Services

Critical care services include the management and care of severely ill patients, and this takes a great deal of skill, knowledge, and time. Critically ill or injured patients have a high likelihood of developing a deteriorating life-threatening condition. E/M services reported include

Critical Care Services
Care services for an acutely ill or injured patient with a high risk for life-threatening developments.

- Highly complex decision-making to assess, manipulate, and support vital system function.
- Treatment of single or multiple vital organ system failure.
- Efforts to avoid additional life-threatening decline of the patient's condition.
- Interpretation of various vital function factors.
- Evaluation of advantages and disadvantages of using advanced technology.

The health care provider must document the amount of time spent so that you will know how to code the encounter. The physician may spend his or her time

- Reviewing test results and films at the nurses' station.
- Discussing the patient's treatment and care with the other members of the medical team.
- Charting (writing in the patient's chart).
- Attending to the patient at bedside.

All such activities are a part of the time spent providing critical care.

Critical care services can be, but do not have to be, provided in a coronary care unit (CCU), an intensive care unit (ICU), a respiratory care unit (RCU), or an emergency care facility.

The codes you choose to report critical care services are determined by the services provided for the critically ill or injured patient and the total length of unit/floor time of the encounter. Use the following for coding physician services for the critically ill or injured patient:

99291 **Critical care, evaluation and management of a critically ill or critically injured patient; first 30–74 minutes**

+99292 **each additional 30 minutes**

(*NOTE:* If the physician spends *less than 30 minutes* of unit/floor E/M time with a critically ill or critically injured patient, regular E/M inpatient codes should be reported. Critical care codes do not become applicable until the 30th minute.)

CODING BITES

If a physician goes to see a patient who is currently in the hospital and given a bed in the CCU but who is not critically ill, you are not permitted to use the critical care codes 99291-99292. You have to code it as a regular hospital visit.

GUIDANCE CONNECTION

Read the additional explanations in the in-section guidelines located within the **Evaluation and Management (E/M)** section, subhead **Critical Care Services**, directly above code 99291 in your CPT book.

LET'S CODE IT! SCENARIO

Rafael Soriano, a 17-year-old male, was brought into the ED by ambulance after being involved in a motorcycle accident. He was not wearing a helmet, and his head hit a brick wall. After initial evaluation and testing by the ED physician, Rafael was sent to the CCU and Dr. Haung spent 2 hours reviewing test results, performing a complete physical exam of Rafael, and discussing a care management plan with the rest of the medical team.

Let's Code It!

Dr. Haung spent "*2 hours*" managing the care of Rafael Soriano in the "*critical care unit.*" Turn to the Critical Care codes, and let's look at the chart. Two hours *equals* 2 *times* 60 minutes, or 120 minutes. When you look at the chart, you will see that 105–134 minutes (120 minutes is right in the middle of this range) is coded with 99291 × 1 and 99292 × 2 (read ×2 as reported twice). Look at the following complete description:

99291 **Critical care, evaluation and management of the critically ill or critically injured patient; first 30–74 minutes**

+99292 **each additional 30 minutes**

You know that Dr. Haung spent 120 minutes and that 120 minutes *minus* 74 minutes (which is represented by code 99291) leaves 46 minutes unreported. Therefore, you must add 99292 to report an additional 30 minutes. However, 16 minutes still remains. So you must include 99292 again to account for the leftover minutes. The claim form that you complete will show **99291, 99292, 99292** *or* **99291, 99292 × 2.** Great job!

CODING BITES

If the same physician provides critical care services to the same patient on the same date as other E/M services, codes from both subheadings may be reported.

Inpatient Neonatal and Pediatric Critical Care

These services will most often be provided in sections of a hospital known as a neonatal intensive care unit (NICU) or pediatric intensive care unit (PICU), but these codes are not exclusive to those designated areas. The guidelines included in the CPT directly above code 99468 contain a great deal of detail on the specific services that are included in these codes and not reported separately.

Determining the most accurate code in this subsection will require you to have two essential pieces of information:

- Age: Is the patient 28 days or younger, 29 days to 24 months, or 2–5 years of age?
- Initial or subsequent: Was this the first day of care for this baby or second/additional day of care by this physician for this newborn?

Note that these code descriptions report a day of E/M service, not just history/exam/MDM or even time spent.

Intensive Care Services—Child

There is a difference between a patient who is critically ill and one who requires intensive care services, such as intensive observation, cardiac and respiratory monitoring, vital sign monitoring, and other services detailed in the guidelines for this subsection (shown above code 99477).

Determining the most accurate code in this subsection will require you to have two essential pieces of information:

- 99477 reports the initial hospital care for a neonate, 28 days of age or younger, who requires intensive care, as per those services identified in the guidelines.
- Subsequent intensive care codes 99478-99480 are distinguished by the present weight of the neonate.

Note that these code descriptions report a day of E/M service, not just history/exam/MDM or even time spent.

GUIDANCE CONNECTION

Read the additional explanations in the in-section guidelines located within the **Evaluation and Management (E/M)** section, subhead **Initial and Continuing Intensive Care Services**, directly above code 99477 in your CPT book.

Time

Under certain circumstances, the correct E/M code is not determined by the key components of history, physical exam, and MDM but is based on the amount of time the physician spent evaluating the patient's condition and managing his or her care. In these cases, the time shown in the last paragraph of the E/M code description is used as a guide. This detail can be found following the three bullets for the key components. You will see that the last sentence reads something like *When using time for code selection, 15–29 minutes of total time is spent on the date of the encounter* (found in the last portion of the code 99202 description). This gives you an approximate time frame that may be used instead of the other key components to determine the appropriate level. In order to use this guideline to choose a code, the documentation must contain the appropriate specific information.

GUIDANCE CONNECTION

Read the additional explanations of these elements used to determine the most accurate E/M code involving the measurement of time spent with the patient in the **Evaluation and Management (E/M) Services Guidelines**, subhead **Time**, in your CPT book directly in front of the E/M section that lists all the codes.

Counseling between Physician and Patient

If the physician spends more than half (51% or more) of the total time *counseling* the patient, then time spent shall be used as the key element in determining the best, most appropriate E/M code. This is not psychological counseling with a therapist (reported with codes 90785-90899) but the physician's discussing diagnosis and treatment with the patient. It might be to review test results or to go over care options with a family member. The CPT guidelines specify the following:

- The results of recommendations for diagnostic tests and/or the review of the results of tests and impressions already gathered.

EXAMPLE

The doctor writes, "*I discussed with the patient that the MRI shows an area of concern. . . .*"

- The options of multiple treatments, including risks and benefits.

EXAMPLE

The doctor writes, "*I explained to the patient that his condition can be treated with medication or surgery. The research shows that this new drug has been quite effective; however, there are some side effects. . . .*"

- Directions to the patient for treatment and/or follow-up.

> **EXAMPLE**
>
> The doctor writes, "*Prescription provided with instructions to take one tablet three times a day. I want to see you in 1 week.*"

- Emphasis on the importance of compliance with the agreed-upon treatment plan.

> **EXAMPLE**
>
> The doctor writes, "*I informed the patient that she needs to take all of the pills in this pack. Even if she is feeling better, I instructed her to keep taking them until they are all gone.*"

- Risk factor reduction.

> **EXAMPLE**
>
> The doctor writes, "*The test was negative this time. However, I discussed with the patient how to prevent possible exposure in the future.*"

- Patient and family education.

> **EXAMPLE**
>
> The doctor writes, "*I explained to the daughter that her mother is going to need oxygen to treat her respiratory insufficiency. What this means is. . . .*"

> **GUIDANCE CONNECTION**
>
> Read the additional explanations in the **Evaluation and Management (E/M) Services Guidelines**, subhead **Counseling**, in your CPT book directly in front of the E/M section that lists all the codes.

Counseling and/or Risk Factor Reduction Intervention

A physician may see a patient at a visit, separate from the annual preventive medicine evaluation, for the purposes of helping the patient learn about, understand, and/or adopt better health practices, including

- Preventing injury or illness, such as the proper way to lift or the importance of testing one's blood glucose levels regularly.
- Encouraging good health, such as nutritional counseling or a new exercise regime.

Services such as these are reported with codes from

99401–99404	**Preventive medicine, individual counseling**
99406–99409	**Behavior Change Interventions, Individual**
99411–99412	**Preventive medicine, group counseling**
99429	**Unlisted preventive medicine services**

EXAMPLE

Dr. DeSalva meets a group of students from the local university to counsel them on preventing sexually transmitted diseases. He speaks with them for an hour. It should be reported with code **99412 Preventive Medicine Counseling and/or risk factor reduction intervention(s) provided to individuals in a group setting; approximately 60 minutes**.

GUIDANCE CONNECTION

Read the additional explanations in the in-section guidelines located within the **Evaluation and Management (E/M)** section, subhead **Counseling Risk Factor Reduction and Behavior Change Intervention**, directly above code 99401 in your CPT book.

Long-Term Care Services

Specific codes are used to report E/M services provided to patients in residential care facilities.

Use 99304–99316 for reporting services to patients in the following places:

- Skilled nursing facilities (SNF).
- Intermediate care facilities (ICF).
- Long-term care facilities (LTCF).
- Psychiatric residential treatment centers.

Home or Residence Services

Use 99341–99350 for reporting services to patients in locations where room, meals, and **basic personal services** are provided, but medical services are not included:

- Assisted living facilities
- Domiciliaries
- Rest homes
- Custodial care settings
- Alzheimer's facilities

Basic Personal Services
Services that include washing/bathing, dressing and undressing, assistance in taking medications, and assistance getting in and out of bed.

GUIDANCE CONNECTION

Read the additional explanations in the in-section guidelines located within the **Evaluation and Management (E/M)** section, subhead **Nursing Facility Services**, directly above code 99304 in your CPT book.

EXAMPLE

Dr. Banks goes to see Peter Lister at the halfway house where he resides. Peter is autistic, and Dr. Banks wants to examine him and adjust his medication for asthma. You should report Dr. Banks's visit to Peter with code 99347.

Care Plan Oversight Services

When a physician provides **care plan oversight services**, you have to use the appropriate code determined by the length of time involved and the type of facility in which the patient is located.

99374–99375 **for home health care patients in assisted living or domiciliary facility**

99377–99378 **for hospice patients**

99379–99380 **for residents in a nursing facility—but only if the management of the patient involves repeated direction of therapy by the attending physician**

Care Plan Oversight Services
E/M of a patient, reported in 30-day periods, including infrequent supervision along with preencounter and postencounter work, such as reading test results and assessment of notes.

Hospice
Care that is provided to all patients with a terminal illness with a prognosis of 6 months or less to live.

Admission to a Nursing Facility

When a patient is admitted into a nursing facility as a continued part of an encounter at the physician's office or the emergency department (ED) (on the same day by the same physician), you report only one code (from the **Nursing Facility** section of the E/M codes) that will include all the services provided from all the locations on that day. The admission to the hospital from the physician's office or ED is reported all in the one hospital admission E/M code. The same rule also applies to admission to a nursing facility.

However, if the patient has been discharged from inpatient status on the same day as being admitted to a nursing facility, you code the physician's discharge services separately from the admission.

Three key components, similar to other E/M codes, are used to determine the appropriate level of E/M service provided by the attending physician to a patient on the first day at a nursing facility. There is no differentiation made in this section of codes between a new patient and an established patient.

Physicians use different methods and tools to assess a patient's status and to create and/or update an appropriate treatment plan for the ongoing care of the individual. Such methods and tools include

- Resident assessment instrument (RAI)
- Minimum data set (MDS)
- Resident assessment protocols (RAP)

Subsequent Nursing Facility Care

> **Interval**
> The time measured between one point and another, such as between physician visits.

Once the patient is in the facility, it is expected that the physician will continue to review the patient's chart, as well as assess test results and changes in the patient's health status. Notice that the code description for the history key component includes the term **interval**. The physician needs to evaluate the patient's history only back to the last visit to gain a complete, up-to-date picture of the individual's health. The continuing care type of assessment is reported with the most appropriate code from the 99307–99310 range.

LET'S CODE IT! SCENARIO

Mara Morietty, a 55-year-old female, was diagnosed with advanced pancreatic cancer and is being cared for at her home by her family, with the help of a home health agency. Dr. Clarke is providing care plan oversight services for the first month of care. The plan includes home oxygen, IV medications for pain control management, and diuretics for edema and ascites control. Dr. Clarke also discusses end-of-life issues, living will directive, and other concerns with the family, the nurse, and the social worker. Dr. Clarke includes documentation of his 45-minute assessment, as well as notes on modifications to the care plan. Certifications of care from the nursing staff, the social worker, the pharmacy, and the company supplying the durable medical equipment for support are also in the record.

Let's Code It!

Dr. Clarke documented that he provided "*care plan oversight services*" for Mara Morietty. Turn to the Alphabetic Index, and look up *Care Plan Oversight Services*. The index instructs you to see *Physician Services*. Turn to *Physician Services*, and you will see *Care Plan Oversight Services*.

As you look at the indented list below that phrase, note that you have to identify the location at which the patient is being cared for. Mara is being cared for at home by a home health agency. This index entry suggests codes 99374 and 99375.

Physician services

Care Plan Oversight Services

Home Health Agency Care. 99374, 99375

(continued)

Now, let's turn to code 99374 to read the entire code description:

99374 **Physician supervision of a patient under care of home health agency (patient not present) in home, domiciliary or equivalent environment requiring complex and multidisciplinary care modalities involving regular physician development and/or revision of care plans; 15–29 minutes**

99375 **30 minutes or more**

Dr. Clarke's notes report that he spent 45 minutes. Therefore, the correct code is **99375**.

Case Management Services

If a patient has several or complex health issues or diagnoses, a team of health care professionals may have to work together to provide proper management and treatment. The team may involve several physicians or the attending physician and a physical therapist, for example, conferencing together. To properly reimburse the health care professional for the time and expertise spent on the patient's behalf with other professionals, you report such services using codes from ranges

99366–99368	**Medical Team Conferences**
99441–99443	**Telephone Services**
99421–99423	**Online Digital Evaluation and Management Services**
99446–99452	**Interprofessional Telephone/Internet/Electronic Health Record Consultations**
99453–99454, 99091	**Digitally Stored Data Services/Remote Physiologic Monitoring**
99457–99458	**Remote Physiologic Monitoring Treatment Management Services**

GUIDANCE CONNECTION

Read the additional explanations in the in-section guidelines located within the **Evaluation and Management (E/M)** section, subhead **Care Management Services**, including **Medical Team Conferences.**

YOU CODE IT! CASE STUDY

Scott Germain, an 81-year-old male, is still having pain and swelling in his hands. Dr. Daniels, an orthopedist, came in to evaluate Scott 2 weeks ago, and Ira Hansrani's last physical therapy session with Scott was yesterday.

Dr. Rubine, the gerontologist and primary care physician for Scott, reads the up-to-date notes and test results, and sets up a meeting in the conference room with Ira Hansrani, the physical therapist, and Dr. Daniels to discuss adjusting Scott's therapy plan, based on current test results. The meeting lasts 45 minutes.

You Code It!

Go through the steps of coding, and determine the E/M code that should be reported for the encounter between Dr. Rubine, Dr. Daniels, and Ira Hansrani.

Step #1: Read the case completely.
Step #2: Abstract the notes: Which key words can you identify relating to the E/M service performed?
Step #3: What is the location?
Step #4: Is this an "interdisciplinary team"?
Step #5: Is the patient or patient's family present (in the meeting)?
Step #6: How long did the meeting last?
Step #7: Double-check your work.

(continued)

Answer:

Did you determine these to be the correct codes?

Reported for Dr. Rubine:

99367 **Medical team conference with interdisciplinary team, 30 minutes or more; participation by physician**

Reported for Dr. Daniels:

99367 **Medical team conference with interdisciplinary team, 30 minutes or more; participation by physician**

Reported for Ira Hansrani, PT:

99368 **Medical team conference with interdisciplinary team, 30 minutes or more; participation by nonphysician qualified health care professional**

Great work!

Newborn and Pediatric E/M Care

The E/M for a newborn or child may be performed by a neonatologist, pediatrician, or other physician. This portion of the E/M section is divided into several parts:

Newborn Care

CODING BITES

A newborn is described as a baby aged 28 days old or younger.

Determining the most accurate code in this subsection will require you to have two essential pieces of information:

- Location: Hospital or birthing center, or other location.
- Initial or subsequent: Was this the first day of care for this newborn or the second/additional day of care by this physician for this newborn?

Note that these code descriptions report a day of E/M service, not just history/exam/MDM or even time spent.

Delivery/Birthing Room Attendance and Resuscitation

CODING BITES

When a physician sees a newborn at an office visit after seeing the baby initially at the hospital or other birth location, the visit is coded as an established patient visit (as long as it is within 3 years, of course).

When requested by the delivering physician (most often the obstetrician), a neonatologist or pediatrician may need to be there in the delivery room to resuscitate and/or stabilize a baby immediately upon his or her birth.

EXAMPLE

Dr. Baldwin is a neonatologist. Dr. Matthews, an obstetrician, asked Dr. Baldwin to be in attendance during the delivery of Anita Mescale's baby because of a concern over her excessive alcohol consumption during pregnancy. Dr. Baldwin was there and stabilized the baby after birth. You would report Dr. Baldwin's service with code 99464.

Home or Residence Services

If a physician provides E/M services to a patient at his or her private residence, use codes 99341-99350. Determine the most appropriate code by determining the level of MDM.

Some home health agencies employ physicians, some physicians may volunteer to see homebound patients, while others visit only established patients who are homebound.

When a health care professional other than the physician—such as a nurse or respiratory therapist—cares for a patient at the patient's home, report these services with a code from the range 99500-99602 in the ***Medicine*** section of CPT.

LET'S CODE IT! SCENARIO

Jules Paganto, a 39-year-old male, suffers from agoraphobia and cannot leave his home. Dr. Volente went to the house to examine Jules because he was complaining of chest congestion. Dr. Volente took a problem-focused history, as this was the first time he had seen Jules. The doctor examined Jules's HEENT and chest and concluded that Jules had a chest cold. He told Jules to get some over-the-counter cold medicine and to call if the symptoms did not go away within a week.

Let's Code It!

You need to find the appropriate code to reimburse Dr. Volente for his E/M services to Jules Paganto. You know that "*Dr. Volente went to the house*," so the location section is titled **Home Services**. The notes say that "*this was the first time he had seen Jules*," meaning that Jules is a new patient, narrowing the choices to codes 99341–99345. According to the notes, Dr. Volente

Concluded, without tests or additional resources: *straightforward*.

When you assess the levels and use the meet or exceed rule, the most accurate code for the visit is **99341**. Good job!

Non-Face-to-Face: Telephone Services and Online Medical Evaluation

Everyone is trying to work more efficiently by using the telephone or the Internet to communicate with an established patient and/or the patient's family, coordinate care, discuss test results, or answer a question. This makes good sense.

To report E/M services provided by the physician over the telephone, a code from the range 99441-99443 should be used. The different codes are distinguished by the length of time of the call. However, before you report one of these codes, there are restrictions. If the phone call is a follow-up to an E/M service provided for a related problem or concern that occurred within the previous 7 days, none of these codes can be reported because the phone call is considered part of that service. In the same light, if the phone call results in the decision for the patient to come in to see the physician as soon as possible, this phone call is considered a part of that future E/M service, so one of these codes would not be used, either.

Codes 99421-99423 are used to report an online E/M service to an established patient, a guardian, or a health care provider as a response to a patient's question. Similar to the restriction on the reporting of a telephone call, code 99444 should not be reported when this e-mail or Internet communication is connected to an E/M service provided for a related concern that occurred within the previous 7 days or within a surgical procedure's postoperative period.

GUIDANCE CONNECTION

Read additional explanations in the in-section guidelines within the **Evaluation and Management (E/M) Services** section, subhead **Non-Face-to-Face Services**, related to codes 99441-99457 in your CPT book.

YOU CODE IT! CASE STUDY

Renay Miller, a 47-year-old female, had just seen the doctor during her annual physical 2 weeks earlier. Today she phoned Dr. Reese to ask if she could travel out of the country, due to her condition. They spoke for about 12 minutes reviewing her history and discussing details regarding his recommended precautions.

(continued)

You Code It!

Go through the steps of coding, and determine the E/M code that should be reported for the encounter between Dr. Reese and Renay Miller.

Step #1: Read the case completely.
Step #2: Abstract the notes: Which key words can you identify relating to the E/M service performed?
Step #3: Is this a "face-to-face" or "non-face-to-face" call?
Step #4: Is this synchronous audio-video or audio only?
Step #5: Is Renay Miller a new patient or an established patient?
Step #6: How long did the call last?
Step #7: Double-check your work.

Answer:

Did you determine this to be the correct code?

98012 Synchronous audio-only visit for the evaluation and management of an established patient, which requires a medically appropriate history and/or examination, straightforward medical decision making, and more than 10 minutes of medical discussion

24.5 Preventive Medicine Services

CODING BITES

Online Digital Evaluation and Management Services codes: 99421-99423 Check your CPT coding manual for details.

Anticipatory Guidance
Recommendations for behavior modification and/or other preventive measures.

Risk Factor Reduction Intervention
Action taken by the attending physician to stop or reduce a behavior or lifestyle that is predicted to have a negative effect on the individual's health.

There may be times when the physician's notes do not clearly identify all the individual components (for instance, history, exam, and MDM) of an encounter, such as when a patient comes in for an annual physical. In these cases, you should be careful not to force the components or make them up. Instead, you should look at other areas of the E/M section. For example, the ***Preventive Medicine*** section, codes 99381-99429, may be more appropriate.

When provided at the same time as a comprehensive preventive medical examination, preventive medicine service codes 99381-99397 include

- Counseling
- **Anticipatory guidance**
- **Risk factor reduction interventions**

In regard to these preventive evaluations, the term *counseling* does not refer to a formalized relationship between a mental health counselor, psychologist, or psychiatrist but to the advice and guidance provided by a health care professional to his or her patient. From your own personal experience, you may be familiar with discussions with your physician during your annual physical. The talks cover everything from quitting smoking to exercising more and perhaps having a better diet. These are all examples of counseling.

Anticipatory guidance refers to the physician's offering suggestions for behavior modification or other preventive measures related to a patient's high risk for a condition. The concern may be based on specifics in a patient's condition or history (or perhaps a family history or an occupational hazard).

EXAMPLE

Dr. Herbert provides anticipatory guidance to Kenneth Simons with regard to being careful about protecting his respiratory health. Kenneth works at an automobile paint shop, and the fumes are very dangerous if a breathing mask is not worn.

A physician prescribing a patch to help a patient quit smoking or referring a patient to a registered dietitian to help him or her with a new diet—each of these is considered a risk factor reduction intervention. It means the physician is taking action to intervene with, or help stop, patient behaviors that put the patient at a higher risk for certain illnesses or conditions.

Specific **Preventive Medicine** codes are determined first by New Patient or Established Patient, and second by the patient's age:

- Infant (age younger than 1 year).
- Early childhood (age 1 through 4 years).

- Late childhood (age 5 through 11 years).
- Adolescent (age 12 through 17 years).
- 18-39 years.
- 40-64 years.
- 65 years and older.

You may be familiar with the standards of care that have physicians check different parts of the body in different ways, determined by the patient's age, such as:

- Behavioral assessments for children ages 0-11 months, 1-4 years, 5-10 years, 11-14 years, and 15-17 years.
- Hearing screening for all newborns.
- Diabetes (type 2) screening for adults with high blood pressure.

If elements such as risk factor reduction intervention or counseling occur during a separate visit (not at the same time as the physical examination), you have to code them separately with a code from the 99401-99412 range.

> **CODING BITES**
>
> Vaccination administration and sera, screening tests, and other ancillary studies which have a specific CPT code are reported separately from these Preventive Medicine Services.

If, during the course of the preventive medicine examination, the physician finds something of concern that warrants special and extra attention involving the key components of a problem-oriented E/M service, the extra work should be coded with a separate E/M code appended with modifier 25. It is applicable only when the same physician does the extra service on the same date.

LET'S CODE IT! SCENARIO

Kensie Hamilton, a 47-year-old female, comes to see her regular physician, Dr. Granger, for her annual physical. During the examination, Dr. Granger finds a mass in her abdomen that concerns him. After the exam, he sits and talks with Kensie about past or current problems with her abdomen, including pain, discomfort, and other details regarding her abdominal issue. He asks whether any family members have had problems in that area, as well as about her alcohol consumption and sexual history as they relate to this concern. Dr. Granger then goes into his office to analyze the multiple possibilities of diagnoses, evaluates the information in Kensie's chart, and reviews the moderate risk of complications that might occur due to her current list of medications. He orders an abdominal CT scan, blood work, and a UA for further input.

Let's Code It!

According to the notes, *Dr. Granger* performed an "*annual physical exam,*" also known as a preventive medicine exam, on Kensie, a "*47-year-old.*" Go to the Alphabetic Index and look up *Evaluation and Management, Preventive Services*, or go directly to the E/M section and look for the **Preventive Medicine Services** subheading. The phrase "*her regular physician*" reveals that Kensie is an established patient, helping you to determine to report code

99396 Periodic comprehensive preventive medicine, established patient, 40–64 years

Dr. Granger's notes also reveal that during the exam he found a mass in Kensie's abdomen that he felt needed further investigation. He spent additional time getting details about her personal, family, and social history regarding abdominal problems; he reviewed concerns about multiple possible diagnoses, complications, and treatments. As per the guidelines, this is extra work done on Dr. Granger's part, and, therefore, he is entitled to additional reimbursement, reported with a separate E/M code. As you review the notes, you should be able to determine the best, most appropriate E/M code for the additional service. Dr. Granger did a comprehensive examination, and his MDM was certainly at a high level of complexity, leading you to the code

99215 Office or other outpatient visit with comprehensive exam and medical decision making of high complexity

plus this modifier:

-25 Significant, separately identifiable evaluation and management service

(continued)

The claim form for Dr. Granger's encounter with Kensie will show **99396** and **99215-25**. Good job!

Code 99396 will reimburse Dr. Granger for his time and services for the annual physical, and code 99215 will reimburse him for the extra work he did regarding the abdominal mass. The modifier −25 explains that, while unusual, Dr. Granger did both of these services at the same encounter.

(*NOTE:* More information on E/M modifiers is provided later in this chapter.)

GUIDANCE CONNECTION

Read additional explanations in the in-section guidelines located within the **Evaluation and Management (E/M)** section, subhead **Preventive Medicine Services**, directly above code 99381 in your CPT book.

24.6 Abstracting the Physician's Notes

You learned about abstracting clinical documentation in the chapter ***Abstracting Clinical Documentation***. Abstracting for details regarding E/M is a bit different because you have to cull out details about the physician's thought processes, in addition to specifically *what* was done and *why*. Very rarely will physicians actually identify the level of MDM in their notes with a statement such as "MDM was low complexity." So, you really need to hone your interpretative skills.

YOU CODE IT! CASE STUDY

Gloria Merro, a 33-year-old female, comes to see Dr. Feldner at his office with complaints of severe pain in her right wrist and forearm. She just moved to the area, and this is the first time Dr. Feldner has seen her. Gloria sees Dr. Feldner for a very specific concern. The doctor asks Gloria about any medical history she may have related to her arm (diagnosed osteoporosis, previous broken bones, etc.). Next, Dr. Feldner examines Gloria's arm. He suspects that the arm is broken and orders an x-ray to be taken.

You Code It!

Go through the steps to determine the E/M code that should be reported for this encounter between Dr. Feldner and Gloria Merro.

Step #1: Read the case completely.
Step #2: Abstract the notes: Which key words can you identify relating to the E/M service performed?
Step #3: What is the location?
Step #4: What is the relationship?
Step #5: What level of MDM was required?
Step #6: What is the most accurate E/M code for this encounter?
Step #7: Double-check your work.

Answer:

Did you determine this to be the correct code?

99202 Office or other outpatient visit, new patient

Let's carefully review the physician's notes.

- Where did the encounter occur? Gloria went "*to see Dr. Feldner at his office.*" This will lead us to the first subheading in the E/M section, **Office or Other Outpatient Services.**

(continued)

- What is the relationship? The notes state, *"She just moved to the area, and this is the first time Dr. Feldner has seen her."* This brings us to the category of **New Patient,** and the code range 99202–99205.
- What is the level of MDM? In this case, did you analyze the situation and determine that the MDM was *straightforward*? However, you can see that the documentation supports the definition of this level: there is only one diagnosis, the management options are limited (put a cast on it), there are very few complications, and Dr. Feldner didn't really have to do any research to recommend a course of treatment.

This brings you to the best, most appropriate E/M code: **99202.**

Please understand that the physicians will not come right out and use the same words as the code descriptions to describe what occurred during the encounter. Let's inspect various statements from patients' charts and identify the key words that lead to the correct E/M code.

1. George Semple, a 57-year-old male, was seen for the first time by Dr. Brieo in the office for a contusion of his hand. Dr. Brieo asked questions about the bruise on George's hand and examined his hand thoroughly.
   a. Location: *Office* tells us where the encounter took place.
   b. Relationship: *First time* tells us this is a new patient.
   c. Key components: *medical decision making–straightforward*. Therefore, the correct code is **99202**.
2. Dr. Fein performed an initial observation at the hospital of Lois Martin, a 31-year-old female. After asking about her personal medical history, including pertinent history of stomach problems, digestive problems, and pertinent family and social history directly relating to her complaints, he examined Lois's abdomen, chest, neck, and back, which revealed lower right quadrant pain accompanied by nausea, vomiting, and a low-grade fever. Dr. Fein made the straightforward decision to admit Lois overnight to the hospital to rule out appendicitis.
   a. Location: *Initial observation at the hospital* tells us this code is in the **Hospital Inpatient and Observation Care Services** section.
   b. Relationship: Initial Hospital inpatient care because the patient was just admitted.
   c. Key components: *medical decision making–straightforward*, and *overnight admission to the hospital* all lead us to the correct code of **99221**.
3. Dr. Murphy, a general surgeon, saw Teena Harrison, a 46-year-old female, in her office for a second opinion requested by Teena's gynecologist, Dr. Enterez, regarding a lump in her right breast. Dr. Murphy took a brief history of Teena's present illness and a personal and family medical history relating to her hematologic and lymphatic system, which was positive for breast cancer on her maternal side. After reviewing the mammogram and performing a limited physical exam of her breasts and chest area, the physician made the straightforward decision to advise a lumpectomy.
   a. Location: *In her office* tells us where the encounter took place.
   b. Relationship: *Second opinion requested by a physician* tells us this is a consultation.
   c. Key components: *medical decision making–straightforward* lead us directly to the correct code of **99242**.
4. David Emerson, a 17-year-old male, presented at the ED with a painful, swollen wrist. The patient stated he had been hurt at a softball game. Dr. Lubner took a brief history and asked some key questions about David's arm/hand. He then examined David's wrist and arm, checked his musculoskeletal system, and ordered x-rays to be taken. It was rather simple to determine that David's diagnosis was a sprained wrist.
   a. Location: *ED* tells you the location.
   b. Relationship: Codes in the **Emergency Department Services** section do not differentiate between new and established patients.
   c. Key components: *medical decision making–low level* tell us the extent of the encounter. The correct code is **99282**.

24.7 E/M in the Global Surgical Package

As a part of the standard of care, there are certain E/M encounters that are already included in the code for a surgical procedure. This is called the **global surgical package**. Specific details about this will be included in the ***CPT Surgery Section*** chapter. For now, let's skip to the time frame, after the procedure is over and the patient is discharged.

Global Surgical Package
A group of services already included in the code for the operation and not reported separately.

You are probably familiar with this: a patient is being discharged after a procedure, and the physician says, "I want to see you in my office in a week." A physician gets paid for performing surgery *and* for the time spent checking on the patient after the surgery to make certain the body is healing correctly. When the follow-up visit in the office (or wherever) occurs, you will not report this by using a regular E/M code because the physician will not be paid separately. However, you do need to report that this encounter occurred. Therefore, you will report a *special services* code from the **Medicine** section of the CPT book. Take a look at this code:

99024 Postoperative follow-up visit, normally included in the surgical package to indicate that an evaluation and management service was performed during a postoperative period for a reason(s) related to the original procedure

YOU CODE IT! CASE STUDY

Ten days after Dr. Rollins performed a carpal tunnel revision on Nicole Letchin's left hand, Nicole, a 23-year-old female, came to see him in his office, as instructed when he discharged her. He asked how she was feeling, checked the flexibility of the wrist, removed the stitches, and checked the healing of the incision. She was doing fine, so Dr. Rollins told her to come in only if she needed anything.

You Code It!

Go through the steps of coding, and determine the E/M code that should be reported for the encounter between Dr. Rollins and Nicole Letchin.

Step #1: Read the case completely.
Step #2: Abstract the notes: Which key words can you identify relating to the E/M service performed?
Step #3: What is the location?
Step #4: What is the relationship?
Step #5: Is this E/M service already included in the global surgical package?
Step #6: What is the most accurate E/M code for this encounter?
Step #7: Double-check your work.

Answer:

Did you determine this to be the correct code?

99024 Postoperative follow-up visit, normally included in the surgical package . . .

I knew you could do it!

24.8 E/M Modifiers and Add-On Codes

Several modifiers may be used in conjunction with an E/M code to provide additional information about an encounter. Each modifier specifically explains an unusual circumstance that may justify the payment to the provider and helps you avoid having to appeal a denied claim later on. CPT Level I modifiers are two-digit codes that are listed in ***Appendix A*** of the CPT book. You first learned about these modifiers in the chapter ***CPT and HCPCS Level II Modifiers*** in this textbook.

Open your CPT book to ***Appendix A*** and read along as we review some of these modifiers.

24 Unrelated Evaluation and Management Service by the Same Physician or Other Qualified Health Care Professional During a Postoperative Period: The physician or other qualified health care professional may need to indicate that an E/M service was performed during a postoperative period for a reason(s) unrelated to the original procedure. This circumstance may be reported by adding modifier 24 to the appropriate level of E/M service.

As a part of the standard of care and the global surgical package, a physician gets paid for performing surgery and for the time spent checking on the patient after the surgery to make certain the body is healing correctly. Modifier 24 would explain that the physician had to see the patient about a *totally different concern* during this time period.

YOU CODE IT! CASE STUDY

Dr. Marple removed Christen Ellison's gallbladder (cholecystectomy) on February 27. The global period for this surgical procedure is 90 days. On March 15, Christen came to see Dr. Marple because he had been out in his garden and developed a rash on his arms. The physician examined Christen's arms and gave him an ointment for the rash.

You Code It!

Go through the steps of coding, and determine the E/M code that should be reported for the encounter between Dr. Marple and Christen Ellison.

Step #1: Read the case completely.
Step #2: Abstract the notes: Which key words can you identify relating to the E/M service performed?
Step #3: What is the location?
Step #4: What is the relationship?
Step #5: What level of MDM was required?
Step #6: What is the most accurate E/M code for this encounter?
Step #7: Do you need to clarify any detail or explain something with a modifier?
Step #8: Double-check your work.

Answer:

Did you determine the correct code to be **99212-24**? Good for you!

Christen came to see Dr. Marple, meaning the encounter happened at the doctor's office. Considering that *Dr. Marple just performed surgery on Christen* 2 weeks ago, it is very reasonable to consider Christen an established patient. Dr. Marple did an *appropriate examination* (limited exam of the problem area), and his *decision making was straightforward.* This directs us to code 99212.

Ninety days from February 27 goes all the way to May 27. That means the visit for the rash, which is a concern totally unrelated to the gallbladder surgery, occurred within the 90-day period. We must explain that Dr. Marple should be compensated separately for the encounter because it has nothing to do with the surgery. So our code will be 99212-24.

25 **Significant, Separately Identifiable E/M Service by the Same Physician or Other Qualified Health Care Professional on the Same Day of the Procedure or Other Service:** It may be necessary to indicate that on the day a procedure or service identified by a CPT code was performed, the patient's condition required a significant, separately identifiable E/M service above and beyond the other service provided or beyond the usual preoperative and postoperative care associated with the procedure that was performed. A significant, separately identifiable E/M service is defined or substantiated by documentation that satisfies the relevant criteria for the respective E/M service to be reported. The E/M service may be prompted by the symptom or condition for which the procedure and/or service was provided. As such, different diagnoses are not required for reporting of the E/M services on the same date. This circumstance may be reported by adding modifier 25 to the appropriate level of E/M service.
Note: This modifier is not used to report an E/M service that resulted in a decision to perform surgery. See modifier 57. For significant, separately identifiable non-E/M services, see modifier 59.

Certainly this happens quite frequently: A patient goes to see the doctor for a minor procedure in the office. Then the patient says, "*Oh, Doc, while I'm here, I want to talk to you about. . . .*" Should that happen, you have to append the E/M code with modifier 25 to explain that there were two visits in one at this encounter.

CODING BITES

In order for modifier 25 to be used correctly, it is best if the E/M code links or relates to a different diagnosis from the procedure performed that day. So there would be at least two diagnosis codes on the same claim form before you consider using this modifier. Although different diagnoses are not required, there is concern in the industry about overuse of modifier 25, so this may trigger an audit without a separately identifiable diagnosis.

LET'S CODE IT! SCENARIO

Gladys Topfer goes to see her dermatologist for a scheduled appointment to have a 1.5-cm mole removed from her cheek. Once Dr. Assanti completes the procedure, Gladys asks the doctor to look at a cyst that has developed under her arm. Dr. Assanti discusses the presence of the cyst with her (How long has it been there? Does it hurt? etc.), and then he examines her underarm area and determines that the best course of action is to wait and see what happens with the cyst. He advises Gladys to keep the area clean and to come back in 3 weeks if the cyst has not gone away.

Let's Code It!

Gladys met with *her dermatologist* (documenting that she is an established patient), Dr. Assanti, at his office (identifying an outpatient location). The notes document that Dr. Assanti did an *appropriate history* (because they discussed nothing else other than the cyst) and an *appropriate examination* (because Dr. Assanti examined only the area where the cyst is located), and his *decision making was straightforward* (because he is very knowledgeable about cysts and Gladys has no other conditions or medications that would cause more evaluation). This directs you to code 99212.

But wait! The claim for this encounter is going to include the code for the surgical removal of the mole—a totally different concern from the reason prompting the E/M of the patient. In essence, there were two encounters in one: the first for the removal of the mole and the second for the concern about the cyst. Therefore, the correct code would be **99212-25** (plus the procedure code for the excision of the mole: CPT code 11312).

32 **Mandated Services:** Services related to *mandated* consultation and/or related services (e.g., third-party payer, governmental, legislative, or regulatory requirement) may be identified by adding modifier 32 to the basic procedure.

Modifier 32 indicates that a third-party payer, a governmental agency, or other regulatory or legislative action required the encounter, consultation, and/or procedure(s).

LET'S CODE IT! SCENARIO

Alene Morgen, a 49-year-old female, went to see Dr. Blume for a comprehensive physical assessment, as a requirement for her special coverage application. The insurance carrier would not consider the policy without the examination. She had never seen Dr. Blume before today's visit.

Let's Code It!

Alene met with the physician at his office and had never seen Dr. Blume before, meaning that she is a new patient. According to the notes, Dr. Blume did an initial comprehensive preventive medicine E/M of a 49-year-old female. That directs you to code 99386.

Notice that the insurance carrier, a third-party payer, mandated the evaluation. Therefore, you must add the modifier to the E/M code to get **99386-32** to explain this fact.

CODING BITES

Modifier 32 can be used with both E/M codes and procedure or treatment codes.

57 **Decision for Surgery:** An E/M service that resulted in the initial decision to perform the surgery may be identified by adding modifier 57 to the appropriate level of E/M service.

Documentation of an encounter may start off with the discussion between physician and patient about test results and treatment options. If the two (physician and patient) agree that a surgical procedure should be scheduled, then the E/M code should be appended with modifier 57.

LET'S CODE IT! SCENARIO

Dr. Richards referred Timothy Dunne, a 67-year-old male, to Dr. Eliot for a consultation to determine whether he needs a prostatectomy. After taking a comprehensive history, performing a comprehensive examination, and reviewing all the previous test results, Dr. Eliot informs Timothy that he recommends the procedure. Timothy agrees, and they select a date the following week for the surgery to be performed.

Let's Code It!

Timothy met with Dr. Eliot at his office at the request of *Dr. Richards* for a *consultation*. According to the documentation, Dr. Eliot did a *comprehensive history* and a *comprehensive examination*. His medical decision making was of moderate complexity. This directs you to code 99244. BUT this encounter ended in Timothy's decision to have Dr. Eliot perform the surgery. As you learned earlier in this chapter, this means there has been a transfer of care in addition to the decision for surgery. Therefore, you must add the modifier 57 to the E/M code for a new patient office visit: **99244-57**.

Prolonged Services: 99358-99359, 99415-99416, 99417-99418

In some cases, patients require more than the usual amount of attention from a physician, more time than would regularly be spent—either face-to-face or without direct contact.

Prolonged service codes report E/M services that are at least 15-30 minutes longer than the amount of time represented by standard E/M codes. These codes may be reported in addition to standard E/M codes, as appropriate. Time spent while providing other services, procedures, or treatments which are reported by codes other than E/M is not included in the calculation for prolonged service.

To determine the most accurate code from this subcategory, you need to identify the situation for the Prolonged services. There are three categories:

- Prolonged Service on Date Other Than the Face-to-Face Evaluation and Management Services Without Direct Patient Contact - these codes are used when a prolonged service is provided *on a date other than the date of a face-to-face E/M encounter.* Note: the topic of what was discussed must be related to the same patient or an E/M service that has occurred or will occur. Prolonged service of less than 30 minutes above the time allotted for the standard E/M code is not separately reported.
  - 99358 Prolonged evaluation and management service before and/or after direct patient care, first hour
  - +99359 . . . each additional 30 minutes
- Prolonged Clinical Staff Services with Physician or Other Qualified Health Care Professional Supervision - used to report overtime in which clinical staff face-to-face E/M services are provided in a physician's office or other outpatient location. A physician must be present to supervise the staff member during the service. Time total for this prolonged E/M begins counting at 30 minutes beyond the allotted amount of time for the standard E/M being reported.
  - +99415 Prolonged clinical staff service (beyond the highest time in the range of total time) in the office or outpatient setting, direct patient contact with physician supervision, first hour
  - +99416 . . . each additional 30 minutes
- Prolonged Service With or Without Direct Patient Contract on the Date of an Evaluation and Management Service - used to report total time of the E/M service, with and without direct patient contact, on the same date, by a physician or other qualified healthcare professional. These codes are only reported when a) only time is used to determine the original E/M code, and b) when the highest level of the time for that code is exceeded by at least 15 minutes.
  - +99417 Prolonged outpatient E/M services, each 15 minutes
  - +99418 Prolonged inpatient or observation E/M, each 15 minutes

This may all sound like a lot to digest however, your CPT coding manual has some tables, within the in-text guidelines, that may help you figure it out.

CODING BITES

When the health care provider has spent more than the standard time but less than 15-30 minutes with the patient, it is not reported separately.

EXAMPLE

Dr. Alfredo spent a total of 75 minutes, in his office, with Mona Catzer working with her to stabilize her diabetes mellitus. The codes used to report this E/M encounter are

99215	Office visit, established patient, moderate MDM*	55 min.
+99417	Prolonged physician service in the office; first hour	15 min.
+99417	additional 15 minutes	15 min.
	TOTAL	**75 min.**

*While 99214 reports a moderate level of MDM, when using time to determine the code for prolonged services, you must report the code with the highest amount of time

GUIDANCE CONNECTION

Read the additional explanations in the in-section guidelines located within the **Evaluation and Management (E/M)** section, subhead **Prolonged Services**, directly above code 99358 in your CPT book.

24.9 Special Evaluation Services

In cases when a patient is about to have a life insurance or disability certificate issued, the insurer often requires the attending physician to provide an evaluation to establish a baseline of data. The visit does not involve any actual treatment or management of the patient's condition–it accounts for the time to create the appropriate documentation. The codes in range 99450-99456 apply to both new and established patients.

The three codes within this subsection are very specific as to which services are included:

99450 **Basic life and/or disability examination that** includes:

- Measurement of height, weight, and blood pressure;
- Completion of a medical history following a life insurance pro forma;
- Collection of blood sample and/or urinalysis complying with "chain of custody" protocols; and
- Completion of necessary documentation/certificates.

99455 **Work related or medical disability examination** by the treating physician that includes:

- Completion of a medical history commensurate with the patient's condition;
- Performance of an examination commensurate with the patient's condition;
- Formulation of a diagnosis, assessment of capabilities and stability, and calculation of impairment;
- Development of future medical treatment plan; and
- Completion of necessary documentation/certificate and report.

CODING BITES

Be aware of codes 99000-99091 in the **Special Services, Procedures and Reports** subsection of the **Medicine** section of CPT–most specifically 99080. Read the notes carefully, as well as the descriptions of the codes, to choose the most accurate.

99456 **Work related or medical disability examination** by other than the treating physician that includes:

- Completion of a medical history commensurate with the patient's condition;
- Performance of an examination commensurate with the patient's condition;
- Formulation of a diagnosis, assessment of capabilities and stability, and calculation of impairment;
- Development of future medical treatment plan; and
- Completion of necessary documentation/certificate and report.

Be aware of the notation beneath code 99456:

(Do not report 99455, 99456 in conjunction with 99080 for the completion of Workman's Compensation forms)

99080 **Special reports such as insurance forms, more than the information conveyed in the usual medical communications or standard reporting form**

24.10 Coordination and Management Services

Complex Chronic Care Coordination Services

Patients with chronic illnesses, such as diabetes mellitus or hypertension, need more attention from their health care team. Code 99487 represents the first hour of clinical staff time for complex chronic care coordination directed by a physician or other qualified health care professional with no face-to-face time. Code 99487 is used for a face-to-face visit, and code 99489 is an add-on code for each additional 30 minutes of complex chronic care coordination.

Numerous studies have proven that patients with chronic illnesses and conditions benefit from coordinated care across the many disciplines of physicians and other members of the clinical staff in addition to community service agencies. This specific subset of E/M codes focuses on support services and management of care provided to patients who are living in their own homes, domiciliaries, rest homes, or assisted living facilities.

These services are provided to patients who

- Require repeated hospital admissions or ED visits.
- Are diagnosed with one or more chronic continuous or episodic medical and/or psychiatric conditions lasting at least 1 year (12 months).
- Are at significant risk of death, acute exacerbation, decompensation, and/or functional decline.
- Require continuing care from multiple health care specialties that need to be coordinated for efficacy and efficiency of medical conditions, psychosocial conditions, and activities of daily living (ADLs).
- Require moderate or highly complex MDM during treatment.

Physicians and other qualified health care professionals must implement a documented care plan to coordinate multiple disciplines and agencies, which is shared with the patient and/or family or caregiver.

With all of the services and activities involved with the care of a chronically ill patient, CPT has specifically identified those services characteristically reported by these codes, including

- Developing and maintaining a comprehensive care plan.
- Facilitating access to care and services needed by the patient and/or family.
- Assessing and supporting patient compliance with the treatment plan, including schedule of medication.
- Educating the patient, family, and/or caregiver to enable and support self-management, independent living, and ADLs.
- Identifying community and health care resources available to the patient and/or family.
- Communicating with home health agencies and other community services available and used by the patient.
- Communicating aspects of care to the patient, family, and/or caregiver.
- Collecting health outcomes data and registry documentation.

Services identified by code 99487 overlap long-standing E/M codes. Therefore, when reporting 99487 (to set off clause), do not separately report the following:

- Care plan oversight services (CPT codes 99339, 99340, 99374–99378).
- Prolonged services without direct patient contact (99358, 99359).
- Anticoagulant management (99363, 99364).
- Medical team conferences (99366–99368).
- Education and training (98966–98968, 99441–99443).
- Online medical evaluation (98969, 99444).
- Preparation of special reports (99080).
- Analysis of data (99090, 99091).
- Transitional care management services (99495, 99496).
- Medication therapy management services (99605–99607).

Codes 99487 and 99489 should not be reported separately, nor should they include the time spent when reporting the following:

- End-stage renal disease services (ESRD) (90951–90970) during the same month.
- Postoperative care services during the global period.
- E/M services (99211–99215, 99334–99337, 99347–99350).

- E/M services while patient is an inpatient or in observation (99217-99239, 99241-99255, 99291-99318).
- Transitional care management services (99495, 99496).

GUIDANCE CONNECTION

Read the additional explanations in the in-section guidelines located within the **Evaluation and Management (E/M)** section, subhead **Complex Chronic Care Management Services**, directly above code 99487 in your CPT book.

As you can see, 99487 would be reported only once per month by the physician or health care professional who has taken on the role of coordinator for this patient for the first 60–89 minutes of services.

Add-on code 99489 can be reported in conjunction with 99487 to represent time greater than 89 minutes during the month.

Transitional Care Management Services

It can be a complex event to transfer the care and management of a patient's ongoing condition from one facility to another, especially when the new location will involve a new care team. Code 99495 (transitional care management services) requires the physician to document the following elements:

- Communication (direct contact, telephone, electronic) with the patient and/or caregiver within 2 business days of discharge.
- MDM of at least moderate complexity during the service period.
- Face-to-face visit within 14 calendar days of discharge.

Code 99496 (transitional care management services) requires the following elements:

- Communication (direct contact, telephone, electronic) with the patient and/or caregiver within 2 business days of discharge.
- MDM of high complexity during the service period.
- Face-to-face visit within 7 calendar days of discharge.

Providers are often concerned that patients with multiple medical and/or psychosocial issues may "slip through the cracks" when transferred from inpatient status to the care of an assisted living facility, a domiciliary, or the patient's own home. These two codes provide an effective way to report the provision of these services to an established patient by the physician or other qualified health care professional or licensed clinical staff member under direction of the physician.

Transitional care management (TCM) includes one episode of face-to-face contact along with non-face-to-face services provided by the physician and clinical staff. The period of TCM service begins on the date of discharge and runs for 29 consecutive days.

Within 48 hours (2 days) after discharge, the first TCM interactive contact between the reporting physician and the patient must occur. This contact may be face-to-face, over the telephone, or by use of electronic communication. The contact must encompass the professional's ability to promptly act upon patient needs and go beyond simply scheduling follow-up care.

When the provider documents two or more attempted contacts within the prescribed time period and is unable to connect with the patient, family, and/or caregiver, the provider may still report TCM services as long as the other transitional care management criteria have been met.

Reporting either of the two TCM codes requires at least one face-to-face visit, as well as reconciliation of prescribed medication, with the patient. For patients requiring highly complex MDM services, the provider must meet with the patient face-to-face within the first 7 calendar days after the patient is discharged from inpatient status.

For patients requiring a moderate level of MDM, the first face-to-face visit must occur during the first 14 calendar days of discharge. This first patient contact is included in the TCM code and not reported separately. However, any additional E/M services provided afterwards may be reported with a separate E/M code accordingly.

The CPT guidelines include specific services by the physician or other health care professional included in TCM, as well as services provided by clinical staff under the direction of that physician.

Services provided by the physician or other qualified health care professional include

- Obtaining and reviewing the discharge information.
- Reviewing the need for or follow-up on pending diagnostic tests and treatments.
- Educating the patient, family, and/or caregiver.
- Establishing (or reestablishing) referrals.
- Arranging for required community resources.

- Assisting in scheduling any required follow-up with community providers and services.
- Interacting with other qualified health care professionals who will assume (or reassume) care of the patient's system-specific problems.

Services provided by clinical staff under the direction of the physician include

- Communicating about various aspects of care with the patient, family, caregiver, and/or other professionals.
- Identifying available community and health resources.
- Assessing and supporting compliance with the treatment plan, including medication management.
- Communicating with home health agencies and other community services used by the patient.
- Educating the patient, family, and/or caregiver to support self-management, independent living, and ADL.
- Facilitating access to care and services required by the patient, family, and/or caregiver.

When reporting 99495 or 99496, do *not* separately report the following:

- Care plan oversight services (CPT codes 99339, 99340, 99374-99380)
- Prolonged services without direct patient contact (99358, 99359)
- Medical team conferences (99366-99368)
- Education and training (98960-98962, 99071, 99078)
- Telephone services (98966-98968, 99441-99443)
- **ESRD** services (90951-90970)
- Online medical evaluation (98969, 99444)
- Preparation of special reports (99080)
- Analysis of data (99090, 99091)
- Complex chronic care coordination services (99487-99489)
- Medication therapy management services (99605-99607)

End-Stage Renal Disease (ESRD) Chronic, irreversible kidney disease requiring regular treatments.

GUIDANCE CONNECTION

Read the additional explanations in the in-section guidelines located within the **Evaluation and Management (E/M)** section, subhead **Transitional Care Management Services**, directly above code 99495 in your CPT book.

TCM may be reported only once within 30 days of discharge by only one health care professional, even if there is a subsequent discharge within that time. This professional is permitted to report hospital or observation discharge services concurrently with TCM services, but not within the global period of postoperative care.

Cognitive Assessment, Psychiatric Collaborative, and General Behavioral Health Integration Care Management Services

Health care professionals have gained greater understanding about those who may benefit from cognitive, mental, or behavioral support. These are some of the codes available for reporting these services from the appropriate professionals:

99483	**Assessment of and care planning for a patient with cognitive impairment**
99484	**Care management services for behavioral health conditions**
99492	**Initial psychiatric collaborative care management**
99493	**Subsequent psychiatric collaborative care management**
+99494	**Initial or subsequent psychiatric collaborative care management, each add'l 30 mins**

Chapter Summary

E/M codes report the energy and knowledge a health care professional puts into gathering information, reviewing data, and determining the best course of treatment for the patient's current condition. Many health information management professionals find these difficult to correctly determine due to the complex formula of such codes. Don't become overwhelmed. Once you get a job, you will find that a particular portion of this section will become your main focus.

EXAMPLE

- If you work for a provider in a private medical office, most of your E/M codes will be found under the **Office** heading on the first two pages of the section.
- If you work for a physician who cares for patients at a skilled nursing facility, you will use codes from under the **Nursing Facility Services** heading.

So in the real world, most of the time, you will be using the same small set of codes over and over again. But because you don't know where you will be working in the future, you should learn the entire section.

In this chapter you learned that, for the key components of coding for services rendered in a nursing home, a long-term care facility, or the patient's home, you use a different set of codes from those reporting physician services in an office or a hospital.

Understand that the elements of the distinct types of encounters, such as annual physicals (preventive medical assessments) and case management services, also use varying sets of parameters.

Your job as a professional coding specialist is to understand the variety of essentials involved in coding E/M services properly and to report those services accurately.

CODING BITES

The steps to determine some E/M codes:

Step #1: Read the case completely.
Step #2: Abstract the notes: Which key words can you identify relating to the E/M service performed?
Step #3: What is the location?
Step #4: What is the relationship?
Step #5: What level of MDM was required?
Step #6: What is the most accurate E/M code for this encounter?
Step #7: Double-check your work.

You Interpret It! Answers

1. c (99381–99429), **2.** d (99441–99443), **3.** e (99281–99288), **4.** b (99252–99255), **5.** a (99202–99205)

CHAPTER 24 REVIEW CPT Evaluation and Management Coding

connect

Enhance your learning by completing these exercises and more at mcgrawhillconnect.com!

Let's Check It! Terminology

Match each key term to the appropriate definition.

Part I

1. **LO 24.3** The level of familiarity between provider and patient.
2. **LO 24.3** An encounter for purposes of a second physician's opinion or advice, requested by another physician, regarding the management of a patient's specific health concern.
3. **LO 24.4** The extent of a physician's clinical assessment and inspection of a patient.
4. **LO 24.4** The collection of details about the patient's chief complaint, the current issue that prompted this encounter: duration, specific signs and symptoms, etc.
5. **LO 24.4** The level of knowledge and experience needed by the provider to determine the diagnosis and/or what to do next.

A. Consultation
B. Established Patient
C. Evaluation and Management (E/M)
D. History of Present Illness

6. **LO 24.4** The amount of detail involved in the documentation of patient history.
7. **LO 24.4** Collection of details, related to the chief complaint, regarding possible signs, symptoms, behaviors, genetic connection, etc.
8. **LO 24.3** A person who has received professional services from the physician/qualified health care professional or another physician/qualified health care professional of the exact same specialty and subspecialty who belongs to the same group practice, within the past three years.
9. **LO 24.3** A person who has not received any professional services within the past 3 years from either the provider or another provider of the same specialty and the same subspecialty who belongs to the same group practice.
10. **LO 24.2** The codes that describe the specific components of a meeting between a health care professional and a patient.
11. **LO 24.4** The physician's collection of details of signs and symptoms, as per the patient, affecting only those body systems connected to the chief complaint.

E. Level of Patient History
F. Level of Physical Examination
G. Medical Decision Making (MDM)
H. New Patient
I. PFSH
J. Problem-Pertinent System Review
K. Relationship

Part II

1. **LO 24.7** A group of services already included in the code for the operation and not reported separately.
2. **LO 24.5** Action taken by the attending physician to stop or reduce a behavior or lifestyle that is predicted to have a negative effect on the individual's health.
3. **LO 24.4** Care that is provided to all patients with a terminal illness with a prognosis of 6 months or less to live.
4. **LO 24.4** Services that include washing/bathing, dressing and undressing, assistance in taking medications, and getting in and out of bed.
5. **LO 24.1** A type of action or service that stops something from happening or from getting worse.
6. **LO 24.2** A facility that provides skilled nursing treatment and attention along with limited medical care for its (usually long-term) residents, who do not require acute care services (hospitalization).
7. **LO 24.4** The time measured between one point and another, such as between physician visits.
8. **LO 24.4** Services for a patient who has a life-threatening condition expected to worsen.
9. **LO 24.10** Chronic, irreversible kidney disease requiring regular treatments.
10. **LO 24.4** E/M of a patient, reported in 30-day periods, including infrequent supervision along with pre-encounter and post-encounter work, such as reading test results and assessment of notes.
11. **LO 24.5** Recommendations for behavior modification and/or other preventive measures.
12. **LO 24.3** When a physician gives up responsibility for caring for a patient, in whole or with regard to one specific condition, and another physician accepts responsibility for the care of that patient.

A. Anticipatory Guidance
B. Basic Personal Services
C. Care Plan Oversight Services
D. Critical Care Services
E. ESRD
F. Global Surgical Package
G. Hospice
H. Interval
I. Nursing Facility
J. Preventive
K. Risk Factor Reduction Intervention
L. Transfer of Care

Let's Check It! Concepts

Choose the most appropriate answer for each of the following questions.

Part I

1. **LO 24.1** E/M codes enable the physician to be reimbursed for all of these services except
   a. talking with the patient and his or her family.
   b. taking continuing education classes.
   c. consulting with other health care professionals.
   d. reviewing data such as test results.

2. **LO 24.2** Often, finding the correct E/M code begins with knowing
   - **a.** where the patient met with the physician.
   - **b.** which credential is held by the provider.
   - **c.** what type of insurance policy is held by the patient.
   - **d.** what the patient does for an occupation.
3. **LO 24.3** A patient who has not seen a particular physician in the last 3 years is categorized as
   - **a.** an established patient. **b.** a referral. **c.** a consultation. **d.** a new patient.
4. **LO 24.3** A ___ is when one physician transfers the care and treatment for a patient to another physician.
   - **a.** consultation **b.** PMH **c.** referral **d.** PFSH
5. **LO 24.4** The key details health care professionals track over time to support early diagnoses and predictive indictors is known as the
   - **a.** Level of History.
   - **b.** Level of Exam.
   - **c.** Level of Chief Complaint.
   - **d.** Level of History and Level of Physical Examination.
6. **LO 24.4** Which of the following is the determining factor when identifying the appropriate E/M code.
   - **a.** Medical Decision Making **b.** History
   - **c.** Exam **d.** Chief Complaint
7. **LO 24.4** According to the E/M section guidelines Number and Complexity of Problems Addressed at the Encounter A problem that runs a definite and prescribed course, is transient in nature, and is not likely to permanently alter health status is a:
   - **a.** minimal problem **b.** acute problem
   - **c.** self-limited or minor problem **d.** chronic problem
8. **LO 24.4** Physician or other qualified health care professional time includes the following activities, when performed except
   - **a.** Preparing to see the patient. **b.** Obtaining and/or reviewing separately obtains history.
   - **c.** Travel. **d.** Counseling and educating the patient/family/caregiver.
9. **LO 24.3** A consultation is expected to be a(n) ___ relationship with the patient.
   - **a.** extended **b.** transferred **c.** temporary **d.** continuing
10. **LO 24.3** A patient seen in the office and then admitted to the hospital by the same physician on the same day should be coded with E/M codes from subsection(s)
    - **a.** Office Visit only. **b.** Office Visit and Initial Hospital Care.
    - **c.** Initial Hospital Care only. **d.** Emergency Department.

Part II

1. **LO 24.5** A preventive medical E/M encounter may include any of these services *except*
   - **a.** counseling. **b.** admission into the hospital.
   - **c.** anticipatory guidance. **d.** risk factor reduction intervention.
2. **LO 24.8** If the physician finds a health concern during a preventive medicine examination requiring additional E/M services and the extra service is performed by the same physician on the same day, then the extra service should be coded with
   - **a.** the preventive medicine code only. **b.** the additional E/M code.
   - **c.** whichever code is reimbursable at a higher rate. **d.** a separate E/M code appended with modifier 25.

3. **LO 24.8** Prolonged service codes report E/M services that are at least ___ minutes longer than the amount of time represented by standard E/M codes.

 a. 5-15 **b.** 15-30 **c.** 30-45 **d.** 45-60

4. **LO 24.4** If a patient is discharged from the hospital and admitted into a skilled nursing facility (SNF) on the same day by the same physician, report the E/M services with

 a. an admission to the nursing facility E/M code only.
 b. a hospital discharge code and an admission to the nursing facility code.
 c. one outpatient E/M services code.
 d. a subsequent nursing facility E/M code.

5. **LO 24.4** Care plan oversight services provided for a patient in a hospice setting are coded from the

 a. 99315-99316 range. **b.** 99374-99375 range. **c.** 99377-99378 range. **d.** 99379-99380 range.

6. **LO 24.4** Frank Brookshire goes to Dr. Corriher's office for an appointment. After a full history, an exam, and comprehensive MDM, Dr. Corriher recommends that Frank be admitted into a psychiatric residential treatment center. He takes him over and admits him into the facility that afternoon. You will code the E/M services with

 a. one office visit code.
 b. an admission to nursing facility code.
 c. both an office visit code and an admission to nursing facility code.
 d. a domiciliary, rest home, custodial care center code only.

7. **LO 24.4** Arlen Flowers, a 5-day-old male, was admitted into the NICU for complications of his low birthweight status. Dr. Hohman saw him yesterday and is in again today. You will code today's E/M services from the

 a. 99468-99469 range. **b.** 99478-99479 range. **c.** 99307-99310 range. **d.** 99211-99215 range.

8. **LO 24.4** Critical care codes are determined by

 a. length of time. **b.** inpatient or outpatient status.
 c. MDM. **d.** new or established patient.

9. **LO 24.4** Conferencing with other health care professionals regarding management and/or treatment of a patient is

 a. included in all E/M codes. **b.** coded as a consultation E/M code.
 c. coded from 99366-99368. **d.** coded from 99202-99205.

10. **LO 24.8** A modifier

 a. explains an unusual circumstance. **b.** has five digits.
 c. begins with the letter *M*. **d.** explains how a patient became injured.

Let's Check It! Guidelines

Refer to the Official Evaluation and Management (E/M) Services Guidelines and fill in the blanks accordingly.

not	history	management
counseling	Medical decision making	separate
face-to-face	exact	examination
discussion	E/M	Stable
four	emergency department	time
personally	subspecialty	problem

1. Solely for the purposes of distinguishing between new and established patients, professional services are those___ services rendered by physicians and other qualified health care professionals who may report evaluation and management services reported by a specific CPT code(s).
2. An established patient is one who has received professional services from the physician/qualified health care professional or another physician/qualified health care professional of the ___ same specialty and ___ who belongs to the same group practice, within the past 3 years.

3. A ___ is a disease, condition, illness, injury, symptom, sign, finding, complaint, or other matter addressed at the encounter, with or without a diagnosis being established at the time of the encounter.
4. ___ for the purposes of categorizing MDM is defined by the specific treatment goals for an individual patient.
5. Levels of E/M services are ___ interchangeable among the different categories or subcategories of service.
6. There are ___ recognized types of MDM.
7. Time is not a descriptive component for the ___ levels of E/M services because emergency department services are typically provided on a variable intensity basis, often involving multiple encounters with several patients over an extended period of time. Therefore, it is often difficult to provide accurate estimates of the time spent face-to-face with the patient.
8. When the physician or other qualified health care professional is reporting a ___ service for ___ of ___ with a physician or another qualified health care professional, the discussion is not counted toward the MDM when selecting a level of ___ services.
9. The nature and extent of the ___ and/or physical examination are determined by the treating physician or other qualified health care professional reporting the service.
10. The extent of history and physical ___ is not an element in the selection of the level of E/M service codes.
11. The basic format of codes with levels of E/M services based on ___ or time is the same.
12. When ___ is being used to select the appropriate level of services for which time-based reporting is allowed, the time ___ spent by the physician(s) and other qualified health care professional(s) assessing and managing the patient and/or ___, educating, communicating results to the patient/family/caregiver on the date of the encounter is summed to define total time.

Let's Check It! Rules and Regulations

Please answer the following questions from the knowledge you have gained after reading this chapter.

1. **LO 24.2** List the location-specific headings in the E/M section.
2. **LO 24.9** Explain *Special Evaluation Services*, include the three codes within this subsection.
3. **LO 24.5** Explain anticipatory guidelines.
4. **LO 24.7** Explain a global surgical package.
5. **LO 24.10** When transferring care and management of a patient to another facility, code 99495 requires the physician to document what elements?

YOU CODE IT! Basics

Using the techniques described in this chapter, carefully read through the case studies and determine the most accurate E/M code(s) for each case study.

1. Makayla Sorensen, a 4-year-old female, sees Dr. Pitassin, a pediatrician, for the first time with itchy spots all over her body. After a medically appropriate history and examination, his MDM is of a low level. Dr. Pitassin diagnoses her with chickenpox.
2. Loretta Stabler, an 81-year-old female, comes to see Dr. Gilman for her semi-annual check-up Dr. Gilman notes he last saw the patient 6 months ago for a regular checkup. Dr. Gilman completes a medically appropriate history and examination. He reviews and affirms the present medical plan of care. Loretta's condition is stable, her hypertension and diabetes (type 2) are in good control, and she has no new problems. There are minimal data for Dr. Gilman to review and several diagnoses to consider. The MDM is moderate.
3. George Terazzo, an 81-year-old male, collapsed at church during services and was brought to the ED. Dr. Horatio took a comprehensive history, performed a comprehensive examination, and made the decision to admit George into the observation unit of the hospital due to an irregular heartbeat with an unknown cause. MDM is of moderate level.
4. Sue Appleton, a 46-year-old female, was admitted this morning for observation after an MVA. Dr. Rhodes documents a detailed history and a comprehensive exam with a straightforward MDM. Sue is doing fine; all test results are within normal range. Dr. Rhodes discharges Sue the same afternoon.

(continued)

5. Reisa Haven, a 39-year-old female, was sent by Dr. Alfaya to Dr. Avery, an OB-GYN, for an office consultation. She had been suffering with moderate pelvic pain, a heavy sensation in her lower pelvis, and marked discomfort during sexual intercourse. In a detailed history, Dr. Avery noted the location, severity, and duration of her pelvic pain and related symptoms. In the review of systems, Reisa had positive findings related to her gastrointestinal, genitourinary, and endocrine body systems. Dr. Avery noted that her past medical history was noncontributory to the present problem. The detailed physical examination centered on her gastrointestinal and genitourinary systems with a complete pelvic exam. Dr. Avery ordered lab tests and a pelvic ultrasound in order to consider uterine fibroids, endometritis, or other internal gynecologic pathology. MDM level was moderate.
6. Catalina King came into the ED with what appeared to be a wrist sprain that she sustained during a baseball game when she slid into home base. She was in obvious pain, and the wrist was swollen and too painful upon attempts to flex. Dr. Ervin performed a medically appropriate and exam before he ordered x-rays. Reports confirmed a simple fracture of the distal radius. MDM was low.
7. George Carter was discharged today from the Bracker Nursing Center after Dr. Mintz spent 25 minutes performing a final examination, discussing George's stay, and providing instructions to George's wife for continuing care.
8. Heather Swann, a 68-year-old female, in good health, is a new patient at Victors Boarding Home. Dr. Cannon comes by to complete Heather's evaluation and documents a medically appropriate history and exam with an MDM of low level.
9. Marla Olden, a 38-year-old female, G2 P1, was admitted to Weston Hospital to deliver. Marla is considered a high-risk delivery. Dr. Kucherin was on standby for 30 minutes in the event a c-section was necessary. Marla delivered vaginally. Marla and baby are doing well. Code Dr. Kucherin's services.
10. Loretta Reubens, an 18-month-old female, is admitted today by Dr. Smallerman into the pediatric critical care unit because of severe respiratory distress.

YOU CODE IT! Practice

Using the techniques described in this chapter, carefully read through the case studies and determine the most accurate E/M code(s) and modifier(s), if appropriate, for each case study.

1. Zena Awtrey, a 58-year-old female, sees Dr. Lunden for the first time for a variety of medical problems. She was diagnosed 5 years ago with insulin-dependent diabetes mellitus with complicating eye and renal problems. In addition, she suffers from hypertensive heart disease with episodes of congestive heart failure. Her peripheral vascular disease has worsened, and she can walk only a block before being crippled with extreme leg pain. The patient reports that a new problem has surfaced: throbbing headaches with radiating neck pain. Dr. Lunden and Zena thoroughly discuss her health concerns and issues. In order to manage and investigate the multiplicity of problems, Dr. Lunden takes a complete PFSH. A complete review of systems (ROS) is performed and a medically appropriate examination is completed. Dr. Lunden has to take a multitude of factors into consideration, as the patient's problems are highly complex. MDM was high.
2. Jamie Farmer, a 32-year-old male, goes to his family physician, Dr. Mitchell, for a tetanus shot after stepping on a rusty nail at the beach. While there, he asks Dr. Mitchell to look at a cut on his left hand. Dr. Mitchell examines the wound and tells him to keep the wound clean and bandaged. Dr. Mitchell documents a medically appropriate history and exam of the left hand, MDM straightforward. Code only the E/M.
3. Owen Unger, a 19-month-old male, is admitted to the hospital by his pediatrician, Dr. Curtis, after a chest x-ray confirmed the child has pneumonia. Dr. Curtis and Mrs. Unger, Owen's mother, discuss the child's fever, cough, and diarrhea. Mrs. Unger provides a pertinent PFSH. An extended problem-focused ROS is completed and an extended examination of the cardiovascular and respiratory systems is performed. The course of treatment planned by Dr. Curtis is straightforward as the child's condition is of low severity.
4. Raymond Johnston, a 3-year-old male, showed no sign of improvement after 5 days of antibiotic therapy, so Dr. Servina admits Raymond into the hospital with a diagnosis of bacterial pneumonia. At Raymond's admittance, his vitals showed a temperature of 38.3°C (101°F), with a mild rash on his torso. The following day, Dr. Servina performed a problem-focused history and examination with MDM of low level. Code Dr. Servina's visit on the second day.

(continued)

5. Tom Seihill, a 23-year-old male, was admitted into the hospital 2 days ago for bronchitis. While in the hospital, Tom requested that his family physician, Dr. Selbiger, perform a circumcision, so Dr. Selbiger called in Dr. Wacker, a urologist, for a consultation. Dr. Wacker discussed the request with Tom and took a brief history and performed a limited genitalia examination. Afterward, Dr. Wacker made a straightforward decision and recommended that Tom have the surgical procedure done at a later date as an outpatient procedure. Code for Dr. Wacker's services.
6. Dr. Modesta spent 2½ hours administering critical care services and evaluating Carolina Tanner upon her admission into the ICU.
7. Howard Shires, a 78-year-old male, was diagnosed with advanced Alzheimer's disease about 1 year ago and has been in this facility for approximately 10 months. He was seen today by the nursing facility's physician, Dr. Bowyer, over concern of the development of urinary and fecal incontinence, as well as a number of other medical problems that have appeared to increase in severity. In addition to the detailed interval history, the physician spoke with family members and the nursing staff. Then, Dr. Bowyer reviewed the patient's record to create an extended history necessary for an extended review of systems (ROS). Dr. Bowyer performed a comprehensive physical exam to assess all body systems. Afterward, he wrote all new orders due to the dramatic change in the patient's physical and mental condition. A new complex treatment plan was created.
8. Royce Onoton's legs have finally healed to the point that he can be discharged from the nursing facility, where he has been for the last 6 weeks. Before he can go home, Dr. Zandi comes in for the final examination and to provide continuing care instructions to Royce's wife, who will be caring for Royce at home. Dr. Zandi prepares the discharge records and writes a prescription for Royce for pain. This whole process takes Dr. Zani about 45 minutes to complete.
9. Bernard Kristenson moved into the Prader Assisted Living Center today. Dr. Ramada, the center's resident physician, introduced himself to Bernard and then took an extended HPI and pertinent PFSH. Dr. Ramada performed a comprehensive examination. After reviewing the results of the examination, Dr. Ramada found management of Barnard's case to be moderate level.
10. Dr. Harrington provided care plan oversight services for Verniece Dantini, one of her patients at the Bracker Assisted Living Center. It took her 20 minutes with no direct patient contact.
11. Dr. Kaminsky spends approximately 1 hour in a meeting with an oncologist in Texas and a reconstructive surgeon in California. The three professionals discussed treatments and options for Karyn Cassey, a 41-year-old female, who was recently diagnosed with parosteal osteogenic sarcoma. Code the conference.
12. Raymond Catertell, a 23-year-old male, is the son of two alcoholics. Dr. Lowen spends 40 minutes with him providing risk factor reduction behavior modification techniques to help him avoid becoming an alcoholic himself.
13. Premier Life & Health Insurance Company required David Harrison, a 39-year-old male, to get Dr. Dijohn, his regular physician, to complete a certificate confirming that David's current disability prevents him from working at his regular job and makes him eligible for disability insurance.
14. Dr. Anderson works in a very small town in Ohio and travels up to 200 miles to see his patients in the surrounding rural areas. His patient Brenda Viard gave birth at her home the previous day to a 6-lb 3-oz baby girl, Alice Rose. Dr. Anderson sees Alice Rose for the first time today, does a complete history and exam, and prepares her medical chart. Alice Rose is a healthy newborn.
15. Petula Carter, a 4-day-old female, currently weighs 2,000 grams and requires intensive cardiac and respiratory monitoring. This is her third day in the NICU, and Dr. Wadhwa comes in to do his E/M of her condition.

YOU CODE IT! Application

The following exercises provide practice in the application of abstracting the physicians' notes and learning to work with documentation from our health care facility, Prader, Bracker, & Associates. These case studies are modeled on real patient encounters. Using the techniques described in this chapter, carefully read through the case studies and determine the most accurate E/M code(s) and modifier(s), if appropriate, for each case study.

(continued)

WESTON HOSPITAL

629 Healthcare Way • SOMEWHERE, FL 32811 • 407-555-6541

PATIENT: TURNER, CHARLES

ACCOUNT/EHR #: TURNCH001

Attending Physician: Renee O. Bracker, MD

S: This 27-year-old male was brought to the ED by ambulance after he was found unconscious on the living room floor. He regained consciousness within several minutes but complained of a severe headache and nausea. Pt states that the last thing he remembers he was on a ladder, changing a light bulb. He believes he lost his balance trying to reach too far and fell, hitting his head on the end-table.

O: Ht 5′10″, Wt 195 lb., R 16. Head: Scalp laceration on the right posterior parietal bone. Bruise indicates trauma to this area. Eyes: PERRLA. Neck: Neck muscles are tense; there is minor pain upon rotation of the head. Musculoskeletal: All other aspects of the shoulders, arms, and legs are unremarkable. X-rays of skull, two views, and soft tissue of the neck are all benign.

A: Concussion

P: 1. MRI to rule out subdural hematoma

2. Repair laceration and bandage

Determine the most accurate E/M code(s) and modifier(s), if appropriate.

PRADER, BRACKER, & ASSOCIATES

A Complete Health Care Facility

159 Healthcare Way • SOMEWHERE, FL 32811 • 407-555-6789

PATIENT: BROMWELL, BRANDON

ACCOUNT/EHR #: BROMBR001

Attending Physician: Oscar R. Prader, MD

S: Brandon is a 9-month-old male brought in today by his mother. I last saw this patient at his regular 6-month checkup. He has been irritable lately and is tugging at his right ear. Brandon has been running a low-grade fever since yesterday. There has been no cough. Pt has a history of problems with his ears and sinuses.

O: Ht 25″, Wt 26 lb., R 20, T 101.3. HEENT: Purulent nasal discharge, yellow-green in color, is noted. Right TM is erythematous unilaterally, bulging, and with purulent effusions. Oropharynx is nonerythematous without lesions. One tooth on the bottom. Tonsils are unremarkable. Neck: Neck is supple with good range of motion (ROM). Positive cervical adenopathy. Lungs: Clear. Heart: Regular rate and rhythm without murmurs.

A: Acute suppurative otitis media, right side

P: 1. Rx Augmentin 40 mg/kg divided tid 10 days

2. Bed rest, lots of fluids

3. Follow-up prn or if no improvement in 10 days

Determine the most accurate E/M code(s) and modifier(s), if appropriate.

PRADER, BRACKER, & ASSOCIATES

A Complete Health Care Facility

159 Healthcare Way • SOMEWHERE, FL 32811 • 407-555-6789

PATIENT: HENSLEY, ERNEST

ACCOUNT/EHR #: HENSER001

(continued)

Attending Physician: Benjamin L. Johnston, MD

Referring Physician: Oscar R. Prader, MD

S: Pt is a 35-year-old male, referred by Dr. Prader for a consultation regarding a sore on his left temple, at the hairline. Pt states he is very involved in water sports. He knows the importance of sunscreen; however, he does not always remember to put it on. He has not had any dermatologic concerns prior to this. Patient states that his skin is occasionally dry and that he has adult onset acne.

O: Ht 6′1″, Wt 225 lb., R 17, T 98.6. After an examination of the skin along the hairline, as well as the rest of the face and neck, a culture is taken of the lesion. The pathology report confirms a malignant melanoma of the skin of the scalp.

A: Malignant melanoma, scalp

P: 1. Discuss surgical and pharmaceutical options for treatment

2. Report sent to Dr. Prader

Determine the most accurate E/M code(s) and modifier(s), if appropriate.

PRADER, BRACKER, & ASSOCIATES

A Complete Health Care Facility

159 Healthcare Way • SOMEWHERE, FL 32811 • 407-555-6789

PATIENT: SARGENT, ALEXANDER

ACCOUNT/EHR #: SARGAL001

Attending Physician: Renee O. Bracker, MD

S: This 85-year-old male is seen today at Northside Assisted Living Center, where he has been living for the last 6 months. The last time I saw this patient was right before he moved into the center. Nurse Thomas states that he has been complaining of mild abdominal pain and some discomfort upon urination. Other than this issue, he has been well and stable.

O: Ht 5′6.5″, Wt 145 lb., R 18, P 73, BP 137/81. Abdomen is unremarkable. No masses or rigidity noted.

A: Suspected bladder infection

P: Order written for UA to rule out bladder infection.

Determine the most accurate E/M code(s) and modifier(s), if appropriate.

WESTON HOSPITAL

629 Healthcare Way • SOMEWHERE, FL 32811 • 407-555-6541

PATIENT: LEAMAN, HESTER

ACCOUNT/EHR #: LEAMHE001

Attending Physician: Renee O. Bracker, MD

This 18-month-old female is being admitted to the pediatric critical care. Mother claims onset of symptoms was sudden. She states that she rushed the child to the ED immediately.

Child is unresponsive. Respiration is shallow. B/P 85/60 mmHg, T 102.

Complete blood workup ordered: CBC with diff, tox screen, bilirubin, and basic metabolic panel. IV fluids to keep hydrated.

Await test results.

Determine the most accurate E/M code(s) and modifier(s), if appropriate.

25

CPT Anesthesia Section

Key Terms

Anesthesia
Anesthesiologists
Certified Registered Nurse Anesthetist (CRNA)
Conscious Sedation
General Anesthesia
Local Anesthesia
Monitored Anesthesia Care (MAC)
Regional Anesthesia
Topical Anesthesia

Learning Outcomes

After completing this chapter, the student should be able to:

LO 25.1 Interpret the types of anesthesia provided.
LO 25.2 Determine the accurate code and physical status modifier for the administration of anesthesia.
LO 25.3 Incorporate the Official Guidelines for reporting.
LO 25.4 Apply the formula for using time to report anesthesia services.
LO 25.5 Select the accurate qualifying circumstances add-on codes.
LO 25.6 Identify special circumstances requiring a CPT modifier.
LO 25.7 Abstract the notes to append HCPCS Level II modifiers.

STOP! Remember, you need to follow along in your CPT and HCPCS Level II code books for an optimal learning experience.

25.1 Types of Anesthesia

Anesthesia is defined as the suppression of nerve sensations to relieve or prevent the feeling of pain, usually by the use of pharmaceuticals. Essentially, it is more commonly described as the administration of drugs to enable a patient to avoid the feeling of pain. While there are many types of anesthesia, they are all primarily divided into three preliminary categories: topical/local, regional, and general.

Anesthesia
The loss of sensation, with or without consciousness, generally induced by the administration of a particular drug.

Topical Anesthesia
The application of a drug to the skin to reduce or prevent sensation in a specific area temporarily.

Local Anesthesia
The injection of a drug to prevent sensation in a specific portion of the body; includes local infiltration anesthesia, digital blocks, and pudendal blocks.

Topical and/or Local Anesthesia

Topical anesthesia refers to the numbing of surface nerves, whereas **local anesthesia** refers to the dulling of feeling in a limited area of the body.

Topical anesthesia is applied directly to the skin or mucous membranes, using a liquid or gel form. Typically, this is administered prior to very minor procedures on the epidural layer of the skin, or the eye, anus, vagina, mouth, gums, eardrum, or nose. Local anesthetics are most often administered by injection, directly into the anatomical site that is the object or target of the procedure. Lidocaine is one of the frequently used anesthetics.

EXAMPLE

Dr. Victors, a general dentist, rubbed a *topical anesthetic* onto Walter's gum to prevent him from feeling any pain from the injection of the *local anesthetic*. The local anesthetic will prevent him from feeling pain while the doctor drills the cavity that Walter has in his left, lower molar.

CODING BITES

Topical: Think top, for the top layer of skin

Local: The effect of the anesthesia stays close to the injection site

Neither of these types of anesthesia is separately reported. They are already included in the procedure code.

Regional Anesthesia

> **Regional Anesthesia**
> The administration of a drug in order to interrupt the nerve impulses without loss of consciousness.

Regional anesthesia prevents a section of the body from transmitting pain and includes epidural, caudal, spinal, axillary, stellate ganglion blocks, regional blocks, and brachial anesthesia.

Regional anesthesia is most often used when the procedure

- Is focused on a specific region of the body.
- Involves a larger area of the body than could be treated with a local injection.
- Does not require general anesthesia.

In these cases, the chosen anesthetic is injected directly into a nerve, nerve plexus, or the spinal cord. There are two types of regional anesthesia:

- Peripheral nerve blocks, which are typically used for procedures performed on the extremities: arms or legs, or the groin, or the face.
- Epidural and spinal anesthesia, which employs an anesthetic injected into the spinal cord, most often to numb the lower abdomen, pelvic area, or the lower extremities.

EXAMPLE

Dr. Carloni, an anesthesiologist, was paged to come to the maternity ward to administer *epidural anesthesia* for Kimberly Saunders. After the epidural was given, Kimberly was able to proceed with the birth of her baby without the pain of childbirth. The loss of sensation was only from the waist down. She was otherwise awake and alert.

General Anesthesia

> **General Anesthesia**
> The administration of a drug in order to induce a loss of consciousness in the patient, who is unable to be aroused even by painful stimulation.

General anesthesia, also called *surgical anesthesia*, creates a total loss of consciousness and sensation. General anesthesia is given to the patient by inhalation, intravenous (IV) injection, or, on rare occasions, intramuscular (IM) injection.

Propofol is the drug most commonly used, administered by slow intravenous infusion. In some cases, a slow inhalation of anesthetic vapors is administered using a face mask.

EXAMPLE

Dr. Carver, an anesthesiologist, administered general anesthesia to Darnell Liberty after he was brought into the operating room (OR) and positioned on the table. Dr. Mendosa was preparing to remove Darnell's gallbladder because of the collection of stones in that organ, and everyone wanted to be certain that Darnell would not feel anything during the surgical procedure.

Moderate (Conscious) Sedation

> **Conscious Sedation**
> The use of a drug to reduce stress and/or anxiety.

One additional type of anesthesia that you should know about when coding anesthetic and surgical services is called **conscious sedation**. It is a form of ultralight general anesthesia that affects the entire body.

With conscious sedation, the physician gives the patient medication to reduce anxiety and stress. A short-acting benzodiazepine, such as midazolam (Versed), either alone or in combination with an opioid analgesic, such as fentanyl, is most often used for this purpose. The patient remains awake and aware of his or her surroundings and what is going on. He or she can answer questions and respond to verbal commands.

Most often, conscious sedation is used for procedures that will not typically cause pain but may be worrisome to patients, causing them to be nervous and frightened. The services of an anesthesiologist are not required for the provision of conscious sedation, so the physician performing the procedure, or a member of the nursing staff, may administer this before the patient goes into the procedure room. This is one of the reasons the codes for this service are not found in the ***Anesthesia*** section of CPT, but in the ***Medicine*** section.

Codes 99151-99157 report the administration of moderate (conscious) sedation and include

- Assessing the patient.
- Establishing IV access and fluids to maintain patency, when performed.
- Administering the drug.
- Maintaining the sedated level.
- Monitoring oxygen saturation, heart rate, and blood pressure.
- Observing and assessing the patient during recovery.

Coding for the administration of conscious sedation also has a few guidelines to help you determine the best, most appropriate code:

Anesthesiologists
Physicians specializing in the administration of anesthesia.

Monitored Anesthesia Care (MAC)
The administration of sedatives, anesthetic agents, or other medications to relax but not render the patient unconscious while under the constant observation of a trained anesthesiologist; also known as "twilight" sedation.

1. Who is administering the sedation?
   a. If the physician performing the procedure also administers the conscious sedation, use a code from the 99151-99153 range (located in the ***Medicine*** section of the CPT book).
   b. If a different physician or other health care professional, other than the professional performing the procedure, administers the conscious sedation, use a code from the 99155-99157 range (located in the ***Medicine*** section of the CPT book).
   c. If an **anesthesiologist** administers the moderate sedation, this is known as **Monitored Anesthesia Care (MAC)**, which is reported from the ***Anesthesia*** section of CPT (codes 00100-01999).
2. The time spent with the patient under conscious sedation helps to determine the correct code or codes. Intraservice work is measured in an initial 15-minute segment, followed by 15-minute segments. The clock starts when the physician administers the sedative and stops when the patient is discharged and the physician is no longer required to supervise the patient. Total time is calculated only for the minutes the physician continuously spends face-to-face with the patient.
3. The patient's age is the other factor that will lead you to the correct code.
4. Codes 99151-99153 require the presence of an independent qualified observer to monitor the patient's conscious status during the procedure. This is the sole responsibility for this individual.

EXAMPLES

99151	Moderate sedation services provided by the same physician or other qualified health care professional performing the diagnostic or therapeutic service that the sedation supports, requiring the presence of an independent trained observer to assist in the monitoring of the patient's level of consciousness and physiological status; initial 15 minutes of intraservice time, patient younger than 5 years of age
99152	initial 15 minutes of intraservice time, patient age 5 years or older
+99153	each additional 15 minutes intraservice time (List separately in addition to code for primary service)

GUIDANCE CONNECTION

Read the additional explanations in the in-section guidelines located within the **Medicine** section, subhead **Moderate (Conscious) Sedation**, directly above code 99151 in your CPT book.

Certified Registered Nurse Anesthetist (CRNA)
A registered nurse (RN) who has taken additional, specialized training in the administration of anesthesia.

LET'S CODE IT! SCENARIO

Caterina Zingler, a 41-year-old female, came into the same day surgery center to have Dr. Freeman perform a hemorrhoidopexy by stapling. She was very nervous because she had never had this procedure before. Raymond Elvers, a ***certified registered nurse anesthetist (CRNA)****, administered Versed, IV, a sedative to relieve her anxiety. The procedure is not*

(continued)

really painful, so there was no need for a full anesthetic or painkiller. Raymond sat with Caterina throughout the procedure to ensure her safety and comfort level. Dr. Freeman accomplished the procedure in one stage, taking 30 minutes.

Let's Code It!

Raymond Elvers, a CRNA, administered Versed, a mild "sedative," to Caterina before Dr. Freeman performed the procedure. Read the complete description for the procedure code used to report the performing of a "*hemorrhoidopexy by stapling*" (46947). This includes all of the details about the procedure, except the administration of the moderate sedation. Let's go to the Alphabetic Index and find *moderate sedation.*

Moderate Sedation

See Sedation

Turn to *Sedation,* where you find:

Sedation

Moderate 99151–99153, 99155–99157

with independent observation 99151–99153

Read, carefully, the complete descriptions of all of these codes in the *Main Section* of the CPT book and analyze the details within each.

Code 99151 requires the physician who performed the procedure to administer the moderate sedation, whereas 99155 requires another physician or health care professional. Which is correct? Go back to the documentation, which states, "*Raymond Elvers, a certified registered nurse anesthetist (CRNA), administered Versed, IV, a sedative to relieve her anxiety.*" This would lead you to 99155.

You will see that code 99155 is the more accurate. This identifies **moderate sedation,** administered by a **different health care professional** [Raymond Elvers, CRNA] **than the professional who performed the procedure** [Dr. Freeman]**, initial 15 minutes intraservice, patient younger than 5 years of age**.

Wait a minute; the documentation states the patient is "*a 41-year-old female.*" Take a look at code **99156 initial 15 minutes intraservice time, patient age 5 years or older**. That's more accurate.

Are you done? Not yet. Code 99156 only reports 15 minutes. The documentation states, "*taking 30 minutes.*" You will need to also report code 99157 for the next 15 minutes, so Dr. Freeman and Raymond Elvers can be accurately reimbursed for all of the time they spent.

So, in addition to the code for the *hemorrhoidopexy* (46947), you need to include two additional codes for the *moderate sedation* (99156 and 99157) on the report and claim form.

Good job!

25.2 Coding Anesthesia Services

When coding anesthesia services, you should follow these steps to find the best, most appropriate code.

1. *Confirm* that the physician who performed the procedure for which the anesthesia was required is a different professional from the person who administered the anesthesia.

   On those occasions when the same physician who performs the procedure also administers regional or general anesthesia, you must append modifier 47 Anesthesia by Surgeon to the appropriate procedure code. The modifier is <u>not</u> attached to an anesthesia procedure code; it is added to the basic procedure code. No additional code from the **Anesthesia** section will be used. See the subsection ***Special Circumstances*** later in this chapter to learn more about using modifier 47.
2. *Identify* the anatomical site of the patient's body upon which the surgical procedure was performed.
3. *Confirm* the exact surgical procedure performed, as documented in the physician's notes (also known as the *operative report*).
4. *Consult* the Alphabetic Index of the CPT book, look under the heading of **Anesthesia**, and read down the list to find the anatomical site shown below that heading. Identify the suggested code or codes for this site.

EXAMPLE

Anesthesia
Skull 00190

5. *Turn* to the *Main Section* of the CPT book, ***Anesthesia*** section, and find the subsection identifying that anatomical site.

EXAMPLES

00212 Anesthesia for intracranial procedures; subdural taps

00216 vascular procedures

6. *Read* the descriptions written next to each code option suggested in the Alphabetic Index carefully. Then compare them with the terms used by the physician in his or her notes documenting the procedure. This will lead you to the best, most appropriate code available.

LET'S CODE IT! SCENARIO

Dr. Fonda is called in to administer general anesthesia to Morgan Saffire, a 6-month-old female, diagnosed with congenital tracheal stenosis. Dr. Caudwell performs a surgical repair of her trachea.

Let's Code It!

The notes indicate that Dr. Fonda administered the anesthesia and Dr. Caudwell performed a "*surgical repair of her trachea.*" Remember, this means that an anesthesia code will be used, not a modifier appended to the procedure code. So let's go ahead and find the best code for the anesthesia service.

Turn to the Alphabetic Index and look up *anesthesia.* Going down the alphabetic listing of the sites beneath this heading, look for more than a page until you get to the correct anatomical site: *Trachea.*

Trachea 00320, 00326, 00542

Reconstruction 00539

The physician's notes state that Dr. Caudwell performed a "*repair,*" not a reconstruction, so focus on the codes shown next to *Trachea.* Turn to the *Main Section* of the CPT book to find the codes 00320, 00326, and 00542. Read the descriptions written next to each code, as well as the others found in the subsection, in order to determine the best, most appropriate code available.

Neck

00320 Anesthesia for all procedures on esophagus, thyroid, larynx, trachea and lymphatic system of neck; not otherwise specified, age 1 year or older

00322 Anesthesia for all procedures on esophagus, thyroid, larynx, trachea and lymphatic system of neck; needle biopsy of thyroid

00326 Anesthesia for all procedures on the larynx and trachea in children less than 1 year of age

00542 Anesthesia for thoracotomy procedures involving lungs, pleura, diaphragm, and mediastinum (including surgical thoracoscopy); decortication

As you review the code descriptions, you can identify which terms or words are most important in matching the code to the physician's documentation of the procedure. Look at the physician's notes one more time and identify the key terms.

(continued)

Dr. Fonda is called in to administer general anesthesia to Morgan Saffire, a 6-month-old female, diagnosed with congenital tracheal stenosis. Dr. Caudwell performs a surgical repair of her trachea.

The combination of all these terms matches only one of our available code descriptions, doesn't it?

00326 Anesthesia for all procedures on the larynx and trachea in children younger than 1 year of age

You found the best, most appropriate code for the administration of general anesthesia for Morgan's surgery.

GUIDANCE CONNECTION

Read the additional explanations in the **Anesthesia Guidelines** in your CPT book directly before the **Anesthesia** section that lists all the codes.

Physical Status Modifiers

The American Society of Anesthesiologists (ASA) established six levels of measuring the physical condition of a patient with regard to the administration of anesthesia. Each level, identified by the letter *P* and a number from 1 to 6, denotes issues that may increase the complexity of delivering anesthetic services and is measured at the time the anesthetic is about to be administered. The anesthesiologist is the professional who determines the correct Physical Status Modifier. However, you, as the coding specialist, must be certain to look for the information and include it on the claim form.

Physical Status Modifiers are mandatory with every code from the ***Anesthesia*** section of the CPT book and are placed directly after the five-digit CPT code (with a hyphen between the two). For example: 00000-P1. (*NOTE:* Physical Status Modifiers are different from the regular CPT and HCPCS modifiers.)

Following are the Physical Status Modifiers that are to be used only with anesthesia codes:

P1 (*a normal healthy patient*). Modifier P1 indicates that the patient to whom the anesthetic was given had no medical concerns that would interfere with the anesthesiologist's responsibilities for keeping the patient sedated and safe.

EXAMPLE

Dr. Tristan administered general anesthesia to Austin Berger, a 15-year-old otherwise healthy female gymnast, before Dr. Armaden performed an arthroscopic extensive debridement of her shoulder joint. The correct code is 01630-P1.

P2 (*a patient with mild systemic disease*). When a patient has a disease that may affect the general workings of his or her body, it must be taken into consideration with regard to administering anesthesia. However, if the disease is under control, then its involvement is less of a concern.

EXAMPLE

Dr. Steiner administered general anesthesia to Venice Binle, a 41-year-old female with controlled type 1 diabetes mellitus, for her radical mastectomy with internal mammary node dissection, to be performed by Dr. Cabara. The correct code is 00406-P2.

P3 (*a patient with severe systemic disease*). In this case, the patient's disease is serious throughout his or her body and is an important factor for the anesthesiologist to contend with, in addition to the reason for the procedure.

EXAMPLE

Dr. Jeffries administered general anesthesia to Wilson Meyers, a 62-year-old male with benign hypertension due to Cushing's disease. Wilson came today for Dr. Ephron to perform a laparoscopic cholecystectomy with cholangiography for acute cholecystitis. The correct code is 00790-P3.

P4 (*a patient with severe systemic disease that is a constant threat to life*). Modifier P4 describes any patient having medical problems that have invaded or affected multiple systems of the body. The large number of issues regarding the effects of the disease, along with existing medications and treatments that have been ongoing in the patient's system, and the potential interactions with the anesthetic make it a very complex case.

EXAMPLE

Dr. Rockenbach administers general anesthesia to Ethan Vox, a 71-year-old male. Ethan has advanced esophageal cancer that has metastasized throughout his body. Dr. Glasser will be performing a partial esophagectomy. The correct code is 00500-P4.

P5 (*a moribund patient who is not expected to survive without the operation*). This is a life or death situation, but not necessarily an emergency. In such cases, the patient is in critical condition, and there are serious medical complications that make administering anesthesia more challenging.

EXAMPLE

Dr. Jeppapi administered general anesthesia to Zena Afronski, a 31-year-old female with acute arteriosclerosis. Dr. Able was called back in from vacation to perform a heart/lung transplant this morning. The correct code is 00580-P5.

P6 (*a declared brain-dead patient whose organs are being removed for donor purposes*). This modifier is provided by the ASA for use with brain-dead patients. Individuals in this condition need to have anesthesia administered to slow bodily functions and give the transplant team time to harvest the viable organs.

YOU INTERPRET IT!

Determine which Physical Status Modifier is most accurate from the descriptions below of the patients' conditions.

1. Uma Koslozki, a 53-year-old female, with controlled hypertension. __________
2. Zachery Gregson is brought into the OR to have knee replacement surgery. He has acute COPD. __________
3. Tyler Madison is brought in to have his tonsils out. He is a healthy 12-year-old male. __________

GUIDANCE CONNECTION

Read the additional explanations in the **Anesthesia Guidelines**, subsection **Anesthesia Modifiers**, in your CPT book directly in front of the **Anesthesia** section that lists all the codes, and read the entire descriptions in **Appendix A**, subsection **Anesthesia Physical Status Modifiers**, in your CPT book.

25.3 Anesthesia Guidelines

Anesthesia Guidelines

The Official Guidelines specifically intended for coding anesthesia services (general and regional anesthesia) are shown at length on the pages at the beginning of the *Anesthesia* section of the CPT book. Go through these guidelines and review how they might help you determine the best, most appropriate anesthesia code.

- *Time Reporting:* You will learn more about this method sometimes used to report anesthesia services provided. Guidelines for this are included in this front part of the section.
- *Supplied Materials:* You might have questions if the anesthesiologist's documentation includes the use of special drugs or equipment such as a surgical tray. These guidelines include some direction.
- *Separate or Multiple Procedures:* When multiple procedures are performed during the same operative session, but the anesthesia is continuous, the anesthesia should be coded for the most complicated procedure only. These guidelines will provide you with the correct way to report these situations on behalf of the anesthesiologist.
- *Special Report:* There are times when something unusual occurs, or a situation where a less-than-common procedure is performed. How will this affect your reporting for the anesthesiologist? Check these guidelines.
- *Anesthesia Modifiers:* You learned about these in the previous chapter on ***CPT and HCPCS Level II Modifiers***. They are repeated here for your convenience.
- *Qualifying Circumstances:* Later in this chapter, you will learn about these add-on codes that are used to explain when an anesthesiologist has an additional challenge keeping the patient sedated and safe. These are listed here, for your ease of reference.

CPT HCPCS Level II

YOU CODE IT! CASE STUDY

Gerald Chang, a healthy 19-year-old male, was in a motorcycle accident. Today, Dr. Oliver, an anesthesiologist, was called in to administer general anesthesia so Dr. Joshua could insert internal fixation on Gerald's compound fracture of the right distal ulna and radius, as well as complete an arthroscopic repair of the right rotator cuff.

You Code It!

You need to determine the correct code or codes to report Dr. Oliver's work during this surgical event. He administered general anesthesia while Dr. Joshua performed two procedures: insertion of internal fixation on a compound fracture (01830) + repair of a rotator cuff injury (01630). Identify which Official Guideline will guide you in how to accurately code Dr. Oliver's work in this case.

Step #1: Read the case carefully and completely.
Step #2: Abstract the scenario. Which key words or terms describe what service the physician provided to the patient during this encounter?
Step #3: Are there any details missing or incomplete for which you would need to query the physician? [If so, ask your instructor.]
Step #4: Determine the correct CPT procedure code or codes to explain the details about what was provided to the patient during this encounter.
Step #5: Check for any relevant guidance, including reading all of the symbols and notations.
Step #6: Do you need to append any modifiers to ensure complete and accurate information is provided?
Step #7: Double-check your work.

Answer:

Did you determine this to be the correct code to report, and which Official Guideline did you use?

01830-P1-AA **Anesthesia for open or surgical arthroscopic/endoscopic procedures on distal radius, distal ulna, wrist, or hand joints; not otherwise specified, healthy patient, anesthesia administered by anesthesiologist**

Two procedures were performed during this one anesthetic administration: the compound fracture is more complex and severe than a rotator cuff injury. Therefore, in accordance with the Official Guidelines titled *Separate or Multiple Procedures*, you will only report the one code for the "most complex procedure."

Good work!

Anesthesia Code Package

All the codes within the ***Anesthesia*** section of the CPT book include activities that are most often performed by **anesthesiologists** when they are preparing to administer anesthesia to a patient. The following services are included in the *anesthesia code package* and are not coded separately.

> **Anesthesiologists**
> Physicians specializing in the administration of anesthesia.

1. *Usual preoperative visits.* Most of the time, the anesthesiologist will stop in to interview the patient, in addition to taking the time to thoroughly read the chart and patient history, before administering the anesthesia. It gives the physician the opportunity to discuss any potential reactions or other considerations with the patient.
2. *Anesthesia care during the procedure.* The time and expertise the anesthesiologist spends in addition to administering the actual anesthetic, including observing the patient throughout the procedure, are very important parts of his or her job responsibilities.
3. *Administration of fluids.* The anesthesiologist gives the patient fluids as well as analgesics (liquid form) as needed during the procedure.
4. *Usual monitoring services* (such as ECG [electrocardiogram], temperature, BP [blood pressure]). As a part of the natural course of the anesthesiologist's duties, he or she must monitor the patient's vital signs throughout the procedure and make certain that there are no unexpected effects from the anesthesia.
5. *Usual postoperative visits.* The anesthesiologist normally visits the patient while he or she is in recovery to ensure that there are no lingering effects of the anesthesia and there are no other concerns as a result of the anesthesia.

YOU CODE IT! CASE STUDY

PATIENT: Darlena Eskine

PREOPERATIVE DIAGNOSIS: Avascular necrosis, right hip.

POSTOPERATIVE DIAGNOSIS: Avascular necrosis, right hip.

OPERATION PERFORMED: Right total hip arthroplasty.

SURGEON: Arthur Hunter, MD

ANESTHESIOLOGIST: Samuel Samahdi, MD

INDICATIONS FOR OPERATION: The patient is an overall healthy 39-year-old former athlete who presents for hip arthroplasty having failed nonoperative treatment options. The risks, benefits, and treatment alternatives were discussed including, but not limited to, infection, bleeding, blood clots, nerve injury, dislocation, leg length inequality, prosthetic wear, loosening, need for further surgery, failure to relieve pain, etc. The patient's questions were answered, and the surgical plan was approved.

DESCRIPTION OF OPERATION: The patient was taken into the operating room, the appropriate extremity was identified, and the patient was positioned with appropriate padding to all pressure areas. After sterile skin preparation and draping, a posterior incision was performed. The skin and subcutaneous tissues were divided to the level of the fascia, which was then incised along the course of its fibers for a posterior approach. Leg lengths were measured prior to dislocation and then the hip capsule was excised, and a femoral neck cut was made. The acetabulum was then exposed and examined. No significant osteophytes were found. No significant acetabular defect was found.

The acetabulum was prepared. The last reamer used was 51 mm. No bone graft was used to reconstruct the acetabular defect. The acetabular component, 52 mm Pinnacle, was positioned appropriately and impacted into position, and mechanical stability was achieved. Supplemental screw fixation was not used. A neutral 36 liner was then appropriately chosen and positioned and the device assembled. Femoral exposure was obtained and the femoral canal was prepared. A trial reduction was performed and hip stability was assessed.

After the appropriate component position was determined, final canal preparation was completed. The component was then impacted into position, and mechanical stability was achieved. A trial reduction was performed, leg length and hip stability were assessed, the appropriate neck length was chosen, and a +8.5 ceramic head was impacted into position. The final reduction was performed, and hip stability was assessed. The hip was stable to 90 degrees of internal rotation, 20 degrees of abduction, 20 degrees of extension, 20 degrees of adduction, and 60 degrees of external rotation really with no tendency to dislocate.

(continued)

The wound was irrigated profusely, a final inspection was performed, and bleeding was controlled and the wound was closed in layers. The hip capsule was not sutured. A drain was not placed. Sterile dressings were applied, and a radiograph was ordered. The components were found to be in appropriate alignment. The plan is for a routine postoperative course with weight bearing as tolerated and ambulation. Sciatic nerve was explored at the end of the procedure and found to be intact.

You Code It!

Read this operative report and determine what code or codes should be reported for Dr. Samadhi's services.

Step #1: Read the case carefully and completely.
Step #2: Abstract the scenario. Which key words or terms describe what service the physician provided to the patient during this encounter?
Step #3: Are there any details missing or incomplete for which you would need to query the physician? [If so, ask your instructor.]
Step #4: Determine the correct CPT procedure code or codes to explain the details about what was provided to the patient during this encounter.
Step #5: Check for any relevant guidance, including reading all of the symbols and notations.
Step #6: Do you need to append any modifiers to ensure complete and accurate information is provided?
Step #7: Double-check your work.

Answer:

Did you determine this to be the correct code to report?

01214-P1-AA **Anesthesia for open procedures involving hip joint; total hip arthroplasty, healthy patient, anesthesia administered by anesthesiologist**

25.4 Time Reporting

Time reporting may be used for billing general anesthesia services in certain areas or by certain third-party payers instead of CPT codes. If this is the custom in your local area, the clock begins when the anesthesiologist starts to prepare the patient for the administration of the anesthetic drug in the OR and is typically measured in 15-minute increments. The time ends when the anesthesiologist is no longer required to be present, once the patient has been safely transferred to postoperative supervision. When multiple procedures are completed during the same operative session, the time calculated should be the total time for all the procedures performed. A formula is used to calculate the amount of compensation the anesthesiologist will receive. The formula is

$$\textbf{Compensation} = (B + T + M) \times CF$$

where

B = base unit

T = time spent by the anesthesiologist with the patient

M = modifying factors

CF = conversion factor

The base unit is assigned by the American Society of Anesthesiologists (ASA), as published in the annual *Relative Value Guide*. The unit includes reimbursement for the usual time and services performed by the anesthesiologist preoperatively and postoperatively. Modifying factors are any adjustments made to allow for the additional challenges presented by the physical status of the patient at the time anesthesia is administered. The conversion factor is the number used to translate units into dollars.

Figure 25-1 is an example of an anesthesiologist's sedation record showing the time log of service.

GUIDANCE CONNECTION

Read the additional explanations in the **Anesthesia Guidelines**, subhead **Time Reporting**, in your CPT book directly before the **Anesthesia** section that lists all the codes.

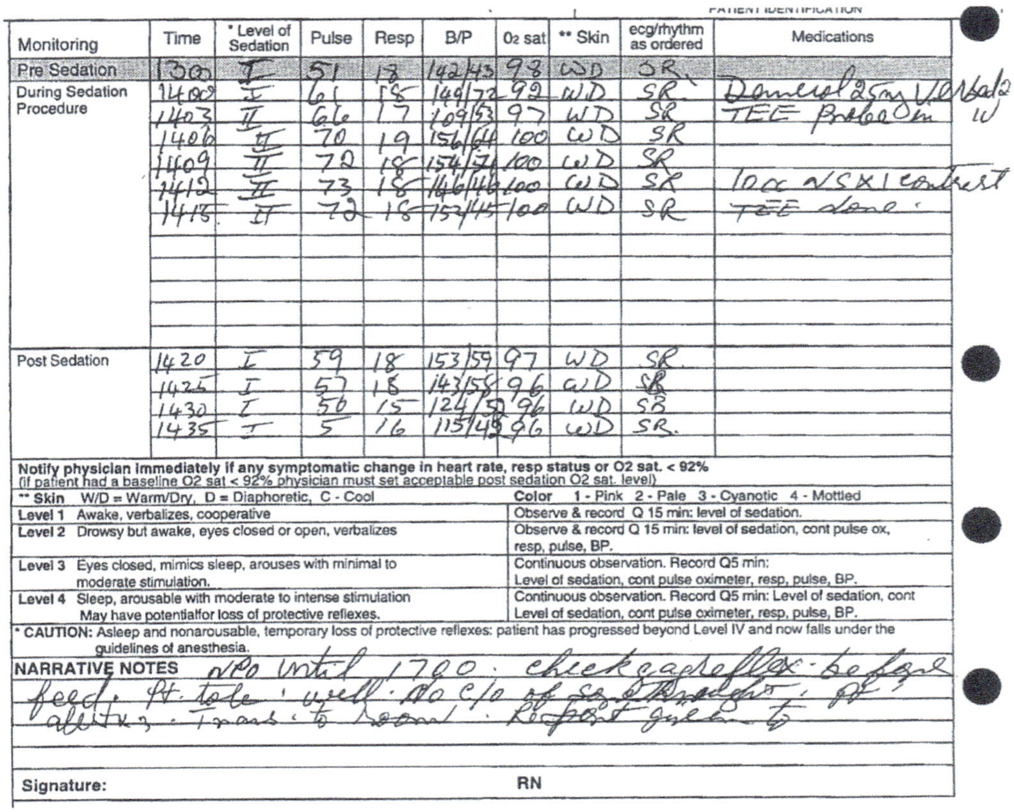

PATIENT IDENTIFICATION

Monitoring	Time	* Level of Sedation	Pulse	Resp	B/P	O2 sat	** Skin	ecg/rhythm as ordered	Medications
Pre Sedation	1300	I	51	18	142/43	98	WD	SR	
During Sedation Procedure	1400	I	61	18	149/72	92	WD	SR	Demerol 25mg Versed 2
	1403	II	66	17	109/53	97	WD	SR	TEE probe in
	1406	II	70	19	156/64	100	WD	SR	
	1409	II	72	18	154/74	100	WD	SR	
	1412	II	73	18	146/46	100	WD	SR	10cc NS x1 contrast
	1415	II	72	18	153/45	100	WD	SR	TEE done
Post Sedation	1420	I	59	18	153/59	97	WD	SR	
	1425	I	57	18	143/55	96	WD	SR	
	1430	I	56	15	124/52	96	WD	SR	
	1435	I	5	16	115/49	96	WD	SR	

Notify physician immediately if any symptomatic change in heart rate, resp status or O2 sat. < 92%
(If patient had a baseline O2 sat < 92% physician must set acceptable post sedation O2 sat. level)

** Skin W/D = Warm/Dry, D = Diaphoretic, C - Cool	Color 1 - Pink 2 - Pale 3 - Cyanotic 4 - Mottled
Level 1 Awake, verbalizes, cooperative	Observe & record Q 15 min: level of sedation.
Level 2 Drowsy but awake, eyes closed or open, verbalizes	Observe & record Q 15 min: level of sedation, cont pulse ox, resp, pulse, BP.
Level 3 Eyes closed, mimics sleep, arouses with minimal to moderate stimulation.	Continuous observation. Record Q5 min: Level of sedation, cont pulse oximeter, resp, pulse, BP.
Level 4 Sleep, arousable with moderate to intense stimulation May have potentialfor loss of protective reflexes.	Continuous observation. Record Q5 min: Level of sedation, cont Level of sedation, cont pulse oximeter, resp, pulse, BP.

* CAUTION: Asleep and nonarousable, temporary loss of protective reflexes: patient has progressed beyond Level IV and now falls under the guidelines of anesthesia.

NARRATIVE NOTES NPO until 1700. check gag reflex before feed. Pt. tol. well. No c/o of [illegible]. Pt. alert. Trans. to room. Report given to

Signature: RN

FIGURE 25-1 Anesthesiologist's sedation record

YOU INTERPRET IT!

Here are the facts as reported by Dr. Haverall's sedation record of general anesthesia administered to Allen Dagmar for his perineal prostatectomy, performed by Dr. Kessler.

Base unit(s): 6

Time: 60 minutes [15 minutes × 4]

Modifying factors: None

Conversion factor: 21.9935

4. Determine the compensation the anesthesiologist should receive.

Remember . . . $(B + T + M) \times CF$ = Compensation

25.5 Qualifying Circumstances

Sometimes special circumstances, also called qualifying circumstances, cause the anesthetic process to be more complicated than usual. In these cases, a second–or add-on–code is used to identify that circumstance.

The available add-on codes for qualifying circumstances are

+99100 *Patient of extreme age . . . younger than 1 year or older than 70 years*
—This add-on code is not to be used when the code description already includes an age definition, such as code 00326, 00834, or 00836.

+99116 *Anesthesia complicated by total body hypothermia*
—Hypothermia is defined as *extremely low body temperature*, below 36.1°C (97°F). Because monitoring vital signs, including body temperature, is an important part of the anesthesia process, a very low body temperature would make the safe administration of anesthesia more complex.

+99135 *Anesthesia complicated by controlled hypotension*
—Hypotension is defined as *abnormally low BP*. The critical connection between BP and heart rate makes this situation very intricate for the anesthesiologist. Controlled hypotension is utilized during surgical procedures to reduce bleeding and the need for blood transfusions. This has become more popular, as it contributes to a satisfactory bloodless surgical field.

+99140 *Anesthesia complicated by emergency conditions*
—An emergency is characterized as a situation in which the patient's life, or an individual body part, would be threatened if there were any delay in providing treatment. In such a case, the anesthesiologist may not have the time to get the patient history or other information necessary to do his or her job most efficiently or effectively.

GUIDANCE CONNECTION

Read the additional explanations in the **Anesthesia Guidelines**, subsection **Qualifying Circumstances**, in your CPT book directly in front of the **Anesthesia** section that lists all the codes.

YOU CODE IT! CASE STUDY

Arlena Smithson, a 77-year-old female, comes to see Dr. Beele for a total knee arthroplasty due to acute arthritis. Dr. Knight is called in to administer the general anesthesia for the procedure. Arlena is in otherwise good health.

You Code It!

Go through the steps, and determine the code(s) that should be reported for the anesthesia provided by Dr. Knight to Arlena.

Step #1: Read the case carefully and completely.
Step #2: Abstract the scenario. Which key words or terms describe what service the physician provided to the patient during this encounter?
Step #3: Are there any details missing or incomplete for which you would need to query the physician? [If so, ask your instructor.]
Step #4: Determine the correct CPT procedure code or codes to explain the details about what was provided to the patient during this encounter.
Step #5: Check for any relevant guidance, including reading all of the symbols and notations.
Step #6: Do you need to append any modifiers to ensure complete and accurate information is provided?
Step #7: Double-check your work.

Answer:

Did you determine these to be the correct codes?

01402-P1 **Anesthesia for open or surgical arthroscopic procedures on knee joint; total knee arthroplasty; a normal healthy patient**

99100 **Anesthesia for patient of extreme age, younger than 1 year and older than 70**

25.6 Special Circumstances

Unusual Anesthesia

Unusual circumstances might require the administration of general anesthesia for a procedure that typically requires either local anesthesia or no anesthesia. In these cases, the modifier 23 Unusual Anesthesia must be appended to the procedure code for that basic service (not to the anesthesia code); you will not assign a code from the *Anesthesia* section of CPT.

Turn to the CPT code book's ***Appendix A*** and read the CPT modifier description:

23 **Unusual Anesthesia:** Occasionally, a procedure, which usually requires either no anesthesia or local anesthesia, because of unusual circumstances must be done under general anesthesia. This circumstance may be reported by adding modifier 23 to the procedure code of the basic service.

LET'S CODE IT! SCENARIO

Louisa Cabaña, a 61-year-old female, arrived for the excision of the cataract in her right eye. Dr. Snyder, knowing that Louisa has been diagnosed with Parkinson's disease, causing her to have uncontrollable tremors, decided that conscious sedation (which is the standard of care) was insufficient to ensure the patient's safety. He called Dr. Corman to administer general anesthesia.

Let's Code It!

Dr. Snyder decided that Louisa needed general anesthesia for this procedure, even though it is not the standard, because her Parkinson's disease made the procedure unsafe without it. The procedure notes state that a secondary membranous cataract was removed. Dr. Corman, an anesthesiologist, administered the anesthesia.

The Alphabetic Index shows

Cataract

Excision 66830

Dilated Fundus Evaluation 2020F

Review the full description of code 66830 to see if it matches the physician's documentation.

66830 **Removal of secondary membranous cataract (opacified posterior lens capsule and/or anterior hyaloid) with corneo-scleral section, with or without iridectomy (iridocapsulotomy, iridocapsulectomy)**

Before you move on to the next section, remember that Dr. Snyder administered general anesthesia. Remember that conscious sedation is the standard of care for this procedure. Generally, there is no need for general anesthesia—the cost or the risk. General anesthesia is unusual. How will you ensure Dr. Snyder and Dr. Corman get properly reimbursed for the administration of the anesthesia? This is what modifiers do—identify unusual circumstances. Modifier 23 is specifically for a case when unusual anesthesia is used.

In this case, the correct code is **66830-23**.

You also would include a Supplemental Report to explain the medical necessity for providing this patient with general anesthesia, so the third-party payer and anyone else will understand this was the right thing to do for this patient.

Same Physician Administering Anesthesia and Performing the Procedure

If the physician performing the procedure also administers either regional or general anesthesia, the modifier 47 Anesthesia by Surgeon must be appended to the procedure code for that basic service (not to the anesthesia code). In such cases, an anesthesia code would *not* be reported. However, it is permissible to report a code for the injection of the anesthetic drug.

Turn to the CPT code book's ***Appendix A*** and read the CPT modifier description:

47 **Anesthesia by Surgeon:** Regional or general anesthesia provided by the surgeon may be reported by adding modifier 47 to the basic service. (This does not include local anesthesia.) *NOTE:* Modifier 47 would not be used as a modifier for the anesthesia procedures.

GUIDANCE CONNECTION

Read the additional explanations in the **Anesthesia Guidelines**, first column, last paragraph, in your CPT book directly before the **Anesthesia** section that lists all the codes, and read the entire description of modifier 47 in **Appendix A**, subsection **Modifiers**, in your CPT book.

YOU CODE IT! CASE STUDY

Hallie Van Masters, a 27-year-old female, came to see Dr. Knowles for a repair of her extensor tendon in her right wrist. Dr. Knowles administered a regional nerve block and then performed the repair.

You Code It!

Go through the steps, and determine the procedure code(s) that should be reported for this encounter between Dr. Knowles and Hallie Van Masters.

Step #1: Read the case carefully and completely.
Step #2: Abstract the scenario. Which key words or terms describe what service the physician provided to the patient during this encounter?
Step #3: Are there any details missing or incomplete for which you would need to query the physician? [If so, ask your instructor.]
Step #4: Determine the correct CPT procedure code or codes to explain the details about what was provided to the patient during this encounter.
Step #5: Check for any relevant guidance, including reading all of the symbols and notations.
Step #6: Do you need to append any modifiers to ensure complete and accurate information is provided?
Step #7: Double-check your work.

Answer:

Did you determine these to be the correct codes?

25270-47 **Repair, tendon or muscle, extensor, forearm and/or wrist; primary, single, each tendon or muscle, regional anesthesia administered by surgeon**

64450 **Injection, anesthetic agent; other peripheral nerve or branch**

Excellent!

25.7 HCPCS Level II Modifiers

Specific HCPCS Level II modifiers are designated for use with anesthesia service codes (see **Table 25-1**). These modifiers are used only if the insurance carrier, such as Medicare, accepts HCPCS Level II codes and modifiers. It is your responsibility, as a professional coder, to know the rules for the different third-party payers with which you will work.

TABLE 25-1 HCPCS Level II Anesthesia-Related Modifiers

AA	Anesthesia services performed personally by the anesthesiologist
AD	Medical supervision by a physician: *more than 4 concurrent anesthesia procedures*
G8	Monitored anesthesia care (MAC) for deep complex, complicated, or markedly invasive surgical procedure
G9	Monitored anesthesia care (MAC) for a patient who has a history of a severe cardiopulmonary condition
QK	Medical direction of *2, 3, or 4 concurrent anesthesia procedures involving qualified individuals*
QS	Monitored anesthesiology care services (can be billed by a qualified nonphysician anesthetist or a physician)
QX	Qualified nonphysician anesthetist with medical direction by a physician
QY	Medical direction of one qualified nonphysician anesthetist by an anesthesiologist
QZ	CRNA without medical direction by a physician

The QY modifier would be used to indicate that an anesthesiologist was available and oversaw the administration of anesthesia services provided by someone else, such as a CRNA. The QY modifier is for the supervision of one case at a time. QK is used for two to four cases at one time, and AD is for more than four cases at one time.

GUIDANCE CONNECTION

Read the HCPCS Level II code book, subsection **Level II National Modifiers**.

LET'S CODE IT! SCENARIO

PATIENT: Randolph Butterman

PREOPERATIVE DIAGNOSIS: Caries and tooth eruption disturbance.

POSTOPERATIVE DIAGNOSIS: Caries and tooth eruption disturbance.

SURGICAL PROCEDURE: Extraction of tooth and alveoplasty

#6, 7, 8, 9, 10, 11, 14, 18, 19, 20, 21, 22, 23, 24, 25, 26, 27, 28, 29, 30, 31, 32

IV FLUIDS: 1,200 mL of normal saline.

ESTIMATED BLOOD LOSS: 20 cc.

INDICATIONS FOR PROCEDURE: Extractions of remaining teeth under general anesthesia due to severe periodontal disease.

PROCEDURE IN DETAIL: The patient was identified in the preoperative holding area, at which time informed consent was given by the patient after addressing risks, benefits, and alternatives, and answering all questions. The patient was then transferred to the operating room. The patient was prepped and draped in a normal fashion.

The patient was anesthetized using general anesthesia due to the extensive nature of the procedure. Dr. Kendale, an anesthesiologist, personally cared for this patient due to the patient's uncontrolled type 2 diabetes mellitus.

A bite block was placed, a throat pack was placed, and attention was addressed to teeth #6, 7, 8, 9, 10, 11, 14, 18, 19, 20, 21, 22, 23, 24, 25, 26, 27, 28, 29, 30, 31, 32. These teeth were extracted using elevators and forceps. A mucoperiosteal buccal flap was elevated along the maxilla and mandibular alveolus. The alveolus of the maxilla and mandible (upper left, right, lower left, right) was trimmed and carved using rongeur forceps and bone files to appropriately remove undercuts and sharp points. Specimens were sent to pathology. The surgical sites were irrigated thoroughly with normal saline. Gel foam was packed into the extraction sockets for hemostasis. The tissue was closed with 3-0 chromic gut sutures.

Dentures were fitted and found to have adequate retention and occlusion. Gauze was then packed over dentures for pressure hemostasis.

Let's Code It!

You are going to report Dr. Kendale's services as the anesthesiologist during this surgery. First, the anesthesia code. Turn to the Alphabetic Index in your CPT book, and find:

Anesthesia

There is a very long list beneath this main term. Look for teeth—no listing, extraction—no listing, . . . try . . .

Mouth 00170, 00172

Turn to the ***Anesthesia*** section in the *Main Part* of CPT, and take a look:

00170 Anesthesia for intraoral procedures, including biopsy; not otherwise specified

00172 Anesthesia for intraoral procedures, including biopsy; repair of cleft palate

There is no documentation that Randolph had a cleft palate, so 00172 cannot be reported. What about 00170? Intraoral means within the oral cavity. That's accurate. But what about the biopsy? There is no indication a biopsy was performed during these extractions, or was it. Read again, the sentence "*Specimens were sent to pathology.*" That supports the biopsy, so you now can confirm 00170 as the correct code.

(continued)

Do you need any modifiers? You have already learned that every anesthesia code requires a Physical Status Modifier. Is there anything in the documentation that will help you? Look at "*the patient's uncontrolled type 2 diabetes mellitus.*" This sentence will lead you to Physical Status Modifier P3.

Do you need to report any other modifiers? Dr. Kendale is an anesthesiologist, and he personally administered the anesthesia for this procedure. Is there a modifier that can report this? Check the list. Modifier AA explains this perfectly.

Now, you can report this code with these modifiers to clearly communicate Dr. Kendale's work during this procedure.

00170-P3-AA **Anesthesia for intraoral procedures, including biopsy; not otherwise specified, patient with severe systemic disease, anesthesia services performed personally by the anesthesiologist**

Good work!

Chapter Summary

For the most part, anesthesia coding is for the purposes of submitting health insurance claim forms on behalf of the anesthesiologist or a member of his or her staff, such as a CRNA.

To find the best, most appropriate code that accurately represents the anesthesia services administered, you first must know which type of anesthesia was used. Then you must determine the anatomical site upon which the procedure was performed and exactly which procedure was provided to the patient. In addition, you must know who administered the anesthesia to the patient: Was it the physician who also performed that procedure, or was it a different health care professional? When using HCPCS Level II modifiers, you also need to know whether the physician who administered the anesthetic was an anesthesiologist.

Once you determine the best, most appropriate code for the dispensation of the anesthesia, you also have to append the correct modifiers, when applicable.

CODING BITES

Physical Status Modifiers

P1 *A normal healthy patient*
P2 *A patient with mild systemic disease*
P3 *A patient with severe systemic disease*
P4 *A patient with severe systemic disease that is a constant threat to life*
P5 *A moribund patient who is not expected to survive without the operation*
P6 *A declared brain-dead patient whose organs are being removed for donor purposes*

Qualifying Circumstances Add-On Codes

+99100 Patient of extreme age
+99116 Anesthesia complicated by total body hypothermia
+99135 Anesthesia complicated by controlled hypotension
+99140 Anesthesia complicated by emergency conditions

You Interpret It! Answers

1. P2, **2.** P4, **3.** P1, **4.** $219.94

CHAPTER 25 REVIEW
CPT Anesthesia Section

Enhance your learning by completing these exercises and more at mcgrawhillconnect.com!

Let's Check It! Terminology

Match each key term to the appropriate definition.

1. **LO 25.1** The administration of sedatives, anesthetic agents, or other medications to relax but not render the patient unconscious while under the constant observation of a trained anesthesiologist; also known as "twilight" sedation.
2. **LO 25.1** The loss of sensation, with or without consciousness, generally induced by the administration of a particular drug.
3. **LO 25.1** The application of a drug to the skin to reduce or prevent sensation in a specific area temporarily.
4. **LO 25.1** The administration of a drug in order to interrupt the nerve impulses without loss of consciousness.
5. **LO 25.1** The administration of a drug in order to induce a loss of consciousness in the patient, who is unable to be aroused even by painful stimulation.
6. **LO 25.1** The use of a drug to reduce stress and/or anxiety.
7. **LO 25.3** Physicians specializing in the administration of anesthesia.
8. **LO 25.1** A registered nurse (RN) who has taken additional, specialized training in the administration of anesthesia.
9. **LO 25.1** The injection of a drug to prevent sensation in a specific portion of the body; includes local infiltration anesthesia, digital blocks, and pudendal blocks.

A. Anesthesia
B. Anesthesiologists
C. Certified Registered Nurse Anesthetist (CRNA)
D. Conscious Sedation
E. General Anesthesia
F. Local Anesthesia
G. Monitored Anesthesia Care (MAC)
H. Regional Anesthesia
I. Topical Anesthesia

Let's Check It! Concepts

Choose the most appropriate answer for each of the following questions.

1. **LO 25.1** The categories of anesthesia include all *except*
   a. topical/local. **b.** moderate sedation. **c.** regional. **d.** general.
2. **LO 25.2** A normally healthy patient presents today for lens surgery. What would be the correct anesthesia code for this procedure?
   a. 00140-P1 **b.** 00142-P2 **c.** 00142-P1 **d.** 00144-P3
3. **LO 25.6** Unusual circumstances might require the administration of general anesthesia for a procedure that typically requires either local anesthesia or no anesthesia. What modifier would be appended to the procedure code in these circumstances?
   a. 23 **b.** QZ **c.** 47 **d.** G9
4. **LO 25.1** MAC is an acronym that stands for
   a. medically administered care. **b.** mutually accessible care.
   c. monitored anesthesia care. **d.** medical anesthetic characters.
5. **LO 25.7** All of the following are HCPCS Level II modifiers *except*
   a. AD **b.** G8 **c.** 57 **d.** QX

6. **LO 25.2** When the physician performing the procedure also administers regional or general anesthesia, modifier 47 should
   - **a.** be appended to the correct anesthesia code.
   - **b.** be appended to the correct procedure code.
   - **c.** be appended to either the correct anesthesia code or the correct procedure code.
   - **d.** not be used in this circumstance.
7. **LO 25.3** The anesthesia code package includes all *except*
   - **a.** preoperative visits.
   - **b.** postoperative visits.
   - **c.** usual monitoring services.
   - **d.** home health follow-up.
8. **LO 25.4** When reporting anesthesia services using time reporting, the formula used is
   - **a.** $(B + T + M) \times CF$
   - **b.** $(B + Q + CF) \times T$
   - **c.** $(Q + T + CF) \times B$
   - **d.** $(CF + B + T) \times M$
9. **LO 25.5** Qualifying circumstances are conditions that might require more work on the part of the anesthesiologist, including all *except*
   - **a.** extreme age.
   - **b.** emergency conditions.
   - **c.** severe systemic disease.
   - **d.** total body hypothermia.
10. **LO 25.2** A Physical Status Modifier describes issues that may increase the complexity of delivering anesthetic services, including
    - **a.** emergency situations.
    - **b.** mild systemic disease.
    - **c.** extreme age.
    - **d.** controlled hypotension.

Let's Check It! Guidelines

Refer to the Anesthesia Guidelines and fill in the blanks accordingly.

five-digit	over	99155, 99156, 99157	safely	Medicine
minimal	second	All	complex	moderate
multiple	ends	anesthesia	99070	physical status modifier
plus	total	not	facility	deep
99151, 99152, 99153	nonfacility	single	above	"P"
time	separately	monitored	1 to 6	

1. Services involving administration of ___ are reported by the use of the anesthesia ___ procedure code plus modifier codes.
2. To report ___ (conscious) sedation provided by a physician also performing the service for which conscious sedation is being provided, see codes ___.
3. When a second physician other than the health care professional performing the diagnostic or therapeutic services provides moderate (conscious) sedation in the ___ setting, the second physician reports the associated moderate sedation procedure/service ___; when these services are performed by the second physician in the ___ setting, codes 99155, 99156, 99157 would ___ be reported.
4. Moderate sedation does not include ___ sedation (anxiolysis), ___ sedation, or ___ anesthesia care.
5. Anesthesia ___ begins when the anesthesiologist begins to prepare the patient for the induction of anesthesia in the operating room and ___ when the anesthesiologist is no longer in personal attendance, that is, when the patient may be ___ placed under postoperative supervision.
6. "Special Services and Reporting" are listed in the ___ section.
7. Supplies and materials provided ___ and ___ those usually included in the office visit or other services rendered may be listed ___. Drugs, tray supplies, and materials provided should be listed and identified with ___ or the appropriate supply code.
8. When ___ surgical procedures are performed during a ___ anesthetic administration, the anesthesia code representing the most ___ procedure is reported. The time reported is the combined ___ for all procedures.
9. ___ anesthesia services are reported by use of the anesthesia five-digit procedure code ___ the addition of a ___.
10. Physical Status Modifiers are represented by the initial letter ___ followed by a single digit from ___.

HCPCS Level II

Let's Check It! Rules and Regulations

Please answer the following questions from the knowledge you have gained after reading this chapter.

1. **LO 25.2** List the six steps to coding anesthesia.
2. **LO 25.3** What is included in the anesthesia code package?
3. **LO 25.4** Why is time important to coding anesthesia? When does the clock start and stop?
4. **LO 25.5** List the qualifying circumstance add-on codes with their description.
5. **LO 25.7** Explain the difference between HCPCS Level II modifiers QX, QY, and QZ.

CPT HCPCS Level II

YOU CODE IT! Basics

Using the techniques described in this chapter, carefully read through the case studies and determine the most accurate anesthesia code(s) and modifier(s), if appropriate, for each case study.

1. Dr. Carey administers general anesthesia so Dr. Tucker can perform a transconjunctival blepharoplasty. Patient has a diagnosis of controlled hypertension.
2. Dr. Tumbokon administers general anesthesia and performs an incisional biopsy to rule out salivary duct carcinoma. Patient is otherwise healthy.
3. Dr. Lynn administers anesthesia so Dr. Buckner can perform a bone marrow aspiration on Mayra Magazine's posterior iliac crest. Mayra is a 36-year-old female who has been diagnosed with anemia and congestive heart failure.
4. Tierra, a healthy 29-year-old female, is taken to the OR, where Dr. Denmark administers spinal anesthesia so Dr. Martin can perform a tubal ligation by bipolar coagulation method.
5. Geoffrey Foulks, an otherwise healthy 11-week-old male, is taken to the OR to repair his congenital cleft lip. Geoffrey weighs 12 lbs. and has a 10 g/dL hemoglobin. Dr. Fairbanks administers general anesthesia, and Dr. Olafson successfully performs the Millar procedure.
6. Paulette Milling, a 51-year-old female, has been diagnosed with a thyroid cyst. She presents today for a needle biopsy of the thyroid cyst which is performed by Dr. Harvard. Dr. Singletary, anesthesiologist, administers general anesthesia. Otherwise, she is healthy.
7. Brian, a healthy 13-month-old male, is brought to the OR, where Dr. Thomas administers general anesthesia so Dr. Richardson, a pediatric urologist, can perform a laparoscopic orchiopexy.
8. Jessica Hamilton, an otherwise healthy 12-year-old female, was playing in a treehouse when she fell approximately 6 feet, causing a tracheobronchial injury (TBI). Jessica was taken to the OR on an emergency basis, where Dr. Mortimer administers general anesthesia so Dr. Skipper can perform the tracheobronchial reconstruction.
9. The patient is taken to the OR, where Dr. Sidney administers the general anesthesia so Dr. Weigle, an orthopedic surgeon, can perform an ankle arthroplasty. Patient has an implanted pacemaker.
10. Dr. Benefield administers anesthesia and performs a vasectomy. Patient is otherwise healthy.
11. Dr. Simmons administers anesthesia and performs a thoracentesis, no imaging guidance.
12. Dr. Coleman administers anesthesia for Dr. Cho to harvest a liver from a brain-dead patient for transplantation.
13. Dr. Caulkins administers anesthesia so Dr. Murphy can perform a pelvic body cast application revision. The patient is otherwise healthy.
14. Dr. Jones administers anesthesia so Dr. Britten can perform an osteotomy of the humerus. Patient has been diagnosed with ongoing cardiac ischemia
15. Dr. Payne administers anesthesia so Dr. Almond can perform a third-degree burn debridement; total body surface 5%. Patient has been diagnosed with well-controlled DM/HTN.

CPT HCPCS Level II

YOU CODE IT! Practice

Using the techniques described in this chapter, carefully read through the case studies and determine the most accurate anesthesia code(s) and modifier(s), if appropriate, for each case study.

1. Connie Huffman, a healthy 28-year-old female, received anesthesia before delivering her son at the hospital. It was a vaginal delivery. Patient is otherwise healthy.
2. Dr. Masters administered general anesthesia to Ashton Hopkins, an otherwise healthy 32-year-old firefighter. Dr. Woody performed a third-degree burn excision, followed by a skin grafting on Ashton's chest, where 9% of his body surface was burned while he was rescuing a little girl from a house fire.
3. David Wolff, a 53-year-old male, was previously diagnosed with benign hypertension due to morbid obesity. Dr. Adams administers general anesthesia so that Dr. McKnight can perform a direct venous thrombectomy on his lower left leg.
4. Dr. Carroll administered anesthesia to Margaret Lindler, a 41-year-old female, diagnosed with a malignant neoplasm of the uterus. Her gynecologist, Dr. Ramage, performed a vaginal hysterectomy.
5. Dr. Billingsworth administered anesthesia to Ralph Skipper, a 7-month-old male requiring a hernia repair in the lower abdomen. Dr. Sims, the neonatologist, noted that, without the surgery, Ralph was not expected to survive.
6. Martha Gantt, a 76-year-old female with a history of hypertension and diabetes mellitus, is brought into the OR for Dr. Brunson to perform a corneal transplant. Dr. Williams, the anesthesiologist, administers the anesthesia.
7. Dr. Elliston is preparing to perform a ventriculography with burr holes on Daniel Ewing, a 12-year-old male, who fell off the monkey bars onto a cement floor yesterday. Dr. Hallbeck administers the anesthesia. Daniel is otherwise healthy.
8. Dr. Hanh administers anesthesia so that Dr. Lindholm can perform a diagnostic lumbar puncture on Keith Franklin, a 56-year-old male. Over the course of the last year, Keith, a construction worker, has developed essential hypertension, which is currently controlled by diet. This lumbar puncture is to confirm the suspected diagnosis of bacterial meningitis.
9. Gerry Sherman, a healthy 28-year-old male, plays professional basketball and is given anesthesia by Dr. Wallace before having a diagnostic arthroscopy of his right knee by Dr. Hook.
10. Carlton Dazquez, a 17-year-old male, was in a go-kart accident and fractured his upper arm 3 months ago. Today, Dr. Hytower operated on him to repair the malunion of his humerus. Dr. Murphy, the anesthesiologist, administered the anesthesia. Carl is otherwise healthy.
11. Trisha Moultrie brought her 3-year-old daughter, Tamara, into the emergency room with a deep laceration of her scalp above her right ear, measuring 2.25 cm. Tamara was distraught, crying, and combative, kicking at the physician and the nurse as they attempted to clean the wound. At the recommendation of Dr. White, Trisha held Tamara in her lap, while the physician administered 1 mg of Versed, IM. Once the sedation took effect, Dr. White was able to perform a layered repair of the laceration while the nurse monitored Tamara's vital signs. The entire procedure took 25 minutes. Code the moderate sedation only.
12. Regina Weyeneth, a healthy 23-year-old female, was given an epidural during labor, with the expectations of a vaginal delivery. After a time, Dr. Bedenbaugh, her obstetrician, determined that the labor was obstructed and notified the hospital staff that they would have to do a cesarean (c-section).
13. Dr. Anderson administered anesthesia to Barbara Brooks, a 52-year-old female, in preparation of the breast reconstruction with TRAM flap to be performed by Dr. Mocase. Barbara has a history of breast cancer and is postmastectomy; she is otherwise healthy.
14. Dr. Solington brought Howard Chen, a 10-month-old male, into the OR for repair of his complete transposition of the great arteries under cardiopulmonary bypass. Pump oxygenation was used. Howard was not expected to survive without the surgery. Dr. Misher, the anesthesiologist, administered the anesthesia.
15. Meredith Susswell, a 79-year-old female, was given anesthesia by Dr. Yabsley, the anesthesiologist, in preparation for the repair of her ventral hernia in her lower abdomen, to be performed by Dr. Carrouth. Meredith has uncontrolled diabetes mellitus and essential hypertension.

(continued)

YOU CODE IT! Application

The following exercises provide practice in the application of abstracting the physicians' notes and learning to work with documentation from our health care facility, Anytown Anesthesiology Associates. These case studies are modeled on real patient encounters. Using the techniques described in this chapter, carefully read through the case studies and determine the most accurate anesthesia code(s) and modifier(s), if appropriate, for each case study.

ANYTOWN ANESTHESIOLOGY ASSOCIATES

241 MAIN STREET • ANYTOWN, FL 32711 • 407-555-1234

PATIENT: PERSILE, LORRAINE

ACCOUNT/EHR #: PERSLO001

Preoperative DX: Locked right knee, rule out medial meniscus tear

Postoperative DX: 1. Grade 2 tear, anterior, cruciate ligament

2. Medial meniscus tear, anterior, horn

3. Grade 2 chondrosis, medial femoral condyle

Procedure: 1. Arthroscopy

2. Partial anterior cruciate ligament debridement

3. Partial medial meniscectomy

Attending Physician: Renee O. Bracker, MD

Anesthesia: General

Anesthesiologist: Lawrence Miller, MD

INDICATIONS: The patient is a 33-year-old female who was in her usual state of good health until about 10 days ago when she sustained a twisting injury to the right knee with inability to fully extend the knee, with pain and swelling.

PROCEDURE: Estimated blood loss: None. Complications: None. Tourniquet time: See anesthesia notes. Specimens: None. Drains: None. Disposition: To the recovery room in stable condition.

Pt was taken to surgery and placed on the OR table in the supine position. After adequate general anesthesia was administered, she received a gram of intravenous Kefzol preoperatively. A proximal thigh tourniquet was applied. Examination revealed no significant Lachman or drawer and a moderate effusion. No varus or valgus instability. Distal pulses intact. The right lower extremity was placed in the arthroscopic leg holder; shaved, prepped, and draped in the usual meticulously sterile fashion for lower extremity surgery. Esmarch exsanguinations of the limb were performed, and the tourniquet was inflated. Proximal medial, anteromedial, and anterolateral portals were fashioned. A systematic evaluation of the knee was performed. The undersurface of the patella demonstrated normal tracking with no chondrosis.

The suprapatellar pouch, medial, and lateral gutters were well within normal limits, and in the notch a grade 2 tear of the anterior cruciate ligament was identified. There were some bloody fragments of the ACL that seemed to be impinging in the medial compartment. This was meticulously debrided. Approximately 50% of the ACL appeared to be intact. Attention was turned to the lateral compartment. The articular surface of the meniscus was normal. On the medial side, a grade 2 lesion in medial femoral condyle, lateral side, was noted. This was not debrided. Also, an anterior tear of the medial meniscus, which was frayed and torn, was another potential source of impingement. This was meticulously debrided to a smooth, stable mechanical limb, and the wound was irrigated and closed with 4-0 nylon simple interrupted sutures. Xeroform, 4 × 4s, Webril and Ace bandage from the tips of the toes to the groin completed the sterile dressing. There were no intraoperative or immediate postoperative complications. The prognosis is good, although it may be limited by potential for arthritis and instability in the future.

Determine the most accurate anesthesia code(s) and modifier(s), if appropriate.

(continued)

ANYTOWN ANESTHESIOLOGY ASSOCIATES

241 MAIN STREET • ANYTOWN, FL 32711 • 407-555-1234

PATIENT: HAMMOND, NEIL

ACCOUNT/EHR #: HAMMNE001

Preoperative DX: C5–C6 and C6–C7 herniated nucleus pulposus

Postoperative DX: Same

Procedure: C5–C6 and C6–C7 anterior cervical diskectomy and fusion with cadaver bone and plate

Attending Physician: Oscar R. Prader, MD

Anesthesia: General endotracheal

Anesthesiologist: Eric Keist, MD

INDICATIONS: The patient is a 35-year-old male with a history of neck and arm pain. MRI scan showed disk herniation at C5–C6 and C6–C7. The patient failed conservative measures and was subsequently set up for surgery. Patient has been diagnosed with DM/HTN, which is well under control.

PROCEDURE: The patient was taken to the OR. The patient was induced, and an endotracheal tube was placed. A Foley catheter was placed. The patient was given preoperative antibiotics. The patient was placed in slight extension. The left neck was prepped and draped in the usual manner. A linear incision was made above the C6 vertebral body. The platysma was divided. Dissection was continued medial to the sternocleidomastoid to the prevertebral fascia. The longus colli were cauterized and elevated. The C5–C6 disk space was addressed first. A retractor was placed. A large anterior osteophyte was removed with a large Leksell and drill. Distraction pins were then placed. The disk space was drilled out. Large bone spurs were drilled posteriorly. The posterior longitudinal ligament was removed. A free fragment was removed from beneath the ligament. The dura was visualized. A piece of bank bone was measured and slightly countersunk. The C6–C7 disk space was then addressed. Distraction pins were placed. A large anterior osteophyte was removed with a large Leksell and drill. The disk space was drilled out. Large bone spurs were drilled posteriorly. The Kerrison punch was used to remove the posterior longitudinal ligament. The dura was visualized. One piece of bank bone was in the C5, one in the C6, and two in the C7 vertebral bodies. The locking screws were tightened. The wound was irrigated. A drain was placed. The platysma was approximated with simple interrupted Vicryl. The dressing was applied. The patient was placed in a soft collar. The patient tolerated the procedure without difficulty. All counts were correct at the end of the case. The patient was extubated and transferred to recovery.

Determine the most accurate anesthesia code(s) and modifier(s), if appropriate.

ANYTOWN ANESTHESIOLOGY ASSOCIATES

241 MAIN STREET • ANYTOWN, FL 32711 • 407-555-1234

PATIENT: WAYMEN, MARK

ACCOUNT/EHR #: WAYMMA001

Preoperative DX: Inguinal hernia, right

Postoperative DX: Inguinal hernia, right, direct and indirect

Procedure: Repair of right inguinal hernia with mesh

Attending Physician: Oscar R. Prader, MD

Anesthesia: General

Anesthesiologist: Lawrence Miller, MD

PROCEDURE: The patient is a 41-year-old male who was taken to the OR and prepped in the usual sterile fashion. After Dr. Miller, the anesthesiologist, administered anesthesia and a satisfactory state was achieved, a transverse incision was made above the inguinal ligament and carried down to the fascia of the external oblique, which was

(continued)

then opened, and the cord was mobilized. The ilioinguinal nerve was identified and protected. A relatively large indirect hernia was found. However, there was an extension of the hernia, such that one could definitely tell there had been a long-standing hernia here that probably had enlarged fairly recently. The posterior wall, however, was quite dilated and without a great deal of tone and bulging as well, and probably fit the criteria for a hernia by itself. Nonetheless, the hernia sac was separated from the cord structures, and a high ligation was done with a purse string suture of 2-0 silk and a suture ligature of the same material prior to amputating the sac. The posterior wall was repaired with Marlex mesh, which was sewn in place in the usual manner, anchoring two sutures at the pubic tubercle tissue, taking one lateral up the rectus sheath and one lateral along the shelving border of Poupart's ligament past the internal ring. The mesh had been incised laterally to accommodate the internal ring. Several sutures were used to tack the mesh down superiorly and laterally to the transversalis fascia. Then the two limbs of the mesh were brought together lateral to the internal ring and secured to the shelving border of Poupart's ligament. The mesh was irrigated with Gentamicin solution. The subcutaneous tissue was closed with fine Vicryl, as was the internal oblique. Marcaine was infiltrated in the subcutaneous tissue and skin. The wound was closed with fine nylon. The patient tolerated the procedure well.

Determine the most accurate anesthesia code(s) and modifier(s), if appropriate.

ANYTOWN ANESTHESIOLOGY ASSOCIATES

241 MAIN STREET • ANYTOWN, FL 32711 • 407-555-1234

PATIENT: DRESSLER, SIMONE

ACCOUNT/EHR #: DRESSI001

Preoperative DX: Chronic cholelithiasis

Postoperative DX: Chronic cholelithiasis; subacute cholecystitis

Procedure: Laparoscopic cholecystectomy; intraoperative cholangiogram

Attending Physician: Renee O. Bracker, MD

Anesthesia: General endotracheal

Anesthesiologist: Melinda Abruzzo, MD

PROCEDURE: The patient, a 57-year-old female, was taken to the OR. The patient was induced and an endotracheal tube was placed. The patient was then placed in the supine position. The abdomen was prepped and draped in the usual fashion. The patient had several previous lower midline incisions and right flank incision; therefore, the pneumoperitoneum was created via epigastric incision to the left of the midline with a Verres needle. After adequate pneumoperitoneum, the 11-mm trocar was placed through the extended incision in the left epigastrium just to the left of the midline, and the laparoscope and camera were in place. Inspection of the peritoneal cavity revealed it to be free of adhesions, and another 11-mm trocar was then placed under direct vision through a small infraumbilical incision. The scope and camera were then moved to this position, and the gallbladder was easily visualized. The gallbladder was elevated, and Hartmann's pouch was grasped. Using a combination of sharp and blunt dissection, the cystic artery was identified. The gallbladder was somewhat tense and subacutely inflamed. Therefore, a needle was passed through the abdominal wall into the gallbladder, and the gallbladder was aspirated free until it collapsed. One of the graspers was held over this region to prevent any further leakage of bile. Again, direction was turned to the area of the triangle of Calot. The cystic duct was dissected free with sharp and blunt dissection. A small opening was made in the duct, and the cholangiogram catheter was passed. The cholangiogram revealed no stones or filling defects in the bile duct system. The biliary tree was normal. There was good flow into the duodenum, and the catheter was definitely in the cystic duct. The catheter was removed, and the cystic duct was ligated between clips, as was the cystic artery. The gallbladder was then dissected free from the hepatic bed using electrocautery dissection, and it was removed from the abdomen through the umbilical port. Inspection of the hepatic bed noted that hemostasis was meticulous. The region of dissection was irrigated and aspirated dry. The trocars were removed, and the pneumoperitoneum was released. The incisions were closed with Steri-Strips, and the umbilical fascial incision was closed with 2-0 Maxon. The patient tolerated the procedure well; there were no complications. She was returned to the recovery room awake and alert.

Determine the most accurate anesthesia code(s) and modifier(s), if appropriate.

(continued)

ANYTOWN ANESTHESIOLOGY ASSOCIATES

241 MAIN STREET • ANYTOWN, FL 32711 • 407-555-1234

PATIENT: LYNDON, JAMES

ACCOUNT/EHR #: LYNDJA001

Preoperative DX: Sensory deficit of common digital nerve; tendon laceration

Postoperative DX: Same

Procedure: Repair of digital nerve, right hand; repair of tendon laceration

Attending Physician: Renee O. Bracker, MD

Anesthesia: General

Anesthesiologist: Eric Keist, MD

INDICATIONS: The patient is a 23-year-old male who was stabbed in the right hand during a street fight. Examination showed a sensory deficit of the thumb and index finger due to an injury to the common digital nerve and a tendon laceration involving the abductor pollicis and first dorsal interosseous. He was taken immediately to the OR for repair.

PROCEDURE: The patient was taken to the OR. General anesthesia was administered personally by Dr. Eric Keist, a tourniquet was applied, and the wound was explored. The common digital nerve to the thumb was identified and found to be divided at the level just proximal to the first metacarpal. The digital nerve to the radial aspect of the index finger was also divided. The abductor pollicis and the first dorsal interosseous tendons were then repaired with 3-0 Vicryl to the fascia.

Following this, both digital nerves were repaired by using interrupted 9-0 Nylon, suturing epineurium to epineurium. When completed, the wound was thoroughly irrigated with saline solution and the skin was closed with interrupted Ethilon. A dorsal splint was applied to the thumb and remains in IP flexion at about 30 degrees and slight adduction. Tourniquet time totaled 190 minutes.

Determine the most accurate anesthesia code(s) and modifier(s), if appropriate.

26

CPT Surgery Section

Key Terms

Allotransplantation
Arthrodesis
Closed Treatment
Complex Closure
Donor Area (Site)
Excision
Fornix
Full-Thickness
Global Period
Harvesting
Intermediate Closure
Laminectomy
Manipulation
Open Treatment
Percutaneous Skeletal Fixation
Recipient Area
Saphenous Vein
Simple Closure
Standard of Care
Surgical Approach
Transplantation

Learning Outcomes

After completing this chapter, the student should be able to:

LO 26.1 Distinguish among the types of surgical procedures.
LO 26.2 Determine which services are included in the global surgical package.
LO 26.3 Interpret the impact on coding of the global time frames.
LO 26.4 Identify unusual services and treatments and report them accurately.
LO 26.5 Abstract physician documentation of procedures on the integumentary system.
LO 26.6 Apply the guidelines, accurately, for coding procedures on the musculoskeletal system.
LO 26.7 Recognize the details required to accurately report procedures on the respiratory system.
LO 26.8 Identify guidelines to correctly report services to the cardiovascular system.
LO 26.9 Distinguish the various procedures on the digestive system.
LO 26.10 Ascertain the elements of coding services to the urinary system.
LO 26.11 Determine how to accurately report procedures on the genital systems: male and female.
LO 26.12 Interpret documentation to accurately report procedures on the nervous system.
LO 26.13 Recognize the necessary details to report procedures on the eye, ocular adnexa, and auditory system.
LO 26.14 Report accurately the different services provided during an organ transplant.
LO 26.15 Demonstrate the proper way to report the use of an operating microscope with a CPT code.

STOP! **Remember, you need to follow along in your CPT code book for an optimal learning experience.**

26.1 Types of Surgical Procedures

Typically, a surgical procedure can be performed in any one of several locations: the physician's office, an ambulatory care center, or a hospital. Of course, the location will most often be determined by the intensity or complexity of the procedure. You certainly would not expect an entire operating room (OR) at the hospital to be used for a physician repairing a simple laceration (cut), and no one could imagine agreeing to have a heart transplant performed in a physician's office. As a coding specialist, your responsibilities will vary, depending upon where you work, when it comes to coding surgical procedures. In addition, there may be more than one coding specialist involved with reporting one procedure.

EXAMPLE

For a surgical procedure performed in a hospital operating room (OR), there may be as many as three coders involved:

1. The hospital's coder codes for the support personnel, facilities, and supplies.
2. The surgeon's coder codes for his or her professional services.
3. The anesthesiologist's coder codes for his or her professional services.

Coding operative reports and procedure notes becomes easier with experience because the longer you work for a physician or facility, the more you will learn about the procedures and services he or she performs. Experience will train you to decipher which services are included in procedures and which are not. Throughout this chapter and the next, the guidelines and specifications for coding the various types of surgical and nonsurgical procedures are reviewed.

In CPT, the term *surgery* is not limited to only those services and treatments performed in an OR or even in a hospital. Within this section of the CPT book, codes are listed that report

- Incision and drainage (I&D) of a cyst.
- Debridement.
- Simple repair of a superficial wound.

All these services can easily be performed in a physician's office. In addition, many procedures are now performed at an ambulatory surgical center or outpatient department.

When hearing the word *surgery*, most people picture an all-white room with health care professionals dressed in masks, gowns, and gloves and a patient under general anesthesia. However, this is a very narrow perspective on surgical procedures. You, as a professional coding specialist, need to understand the various types of surgical processes because this detail may be important for determining the most accurate code.

Prophylactic, Diagnostic, and Therapeutic Procedures

Under certain circumstances, the purpose of a procedure will affect the code you use to report the service. Three key terms to watch for are *prophylactic*, *diagnostic*, and *therapeutic*.

- A *prophylactic* treatment is one that is performed to prevent a condition from developing. This may be a surgical procedure, a series of injections, or a prescription.
- A *diagnostic* procedure or test is performed so that the physician can gather more details about a condition or concern at issue. In other words, the reason for performing the test or procedure is to get closer to an accurate diagnosis.
- A *therapeutic* procedure is provided, most often, to correct or fix a problem.

EXAMPLES

27187	Prophylactic treatment (nailing, pinning, plating or wiring) with or without methylmethacrylate, femoral neck and proximal femur
49320	Laparoscopy, abdomen, peritoneum and omentum, diagnostic, with or without collection of specimen(s) by brushing or washing (separate procedure).
50541	Laparoscopy, surgical; ablation of renal cysts

There are times when, for the safety of the patient, a procedure begins as a diagnostic examination and turns into a therapeutic procedure. Generally, a therapeutic or surgical procedure will include the diagnostic portion, thereby requiring only one code when both are done during the same encounter.

Above, in both of the two laparoscopic codes (49320 and 50541), CPT includes the guideline "*Surgical laparoscopy always includes diagnostic laparoscopy*." Therefore, if the physician performed a diagnostic laparoscopy solely to determine what was wrong with the patient, the correct code might be 49320. However, if while the physician was performing the diagnostic laparoscopy, he observed a renal cyst and decided to ablate the cyst at the same time, this would mean that a diagnostic procedure (to discover the cyst) and a therapeutic procedure (ablation of the cyst) were done at the same time. In that case, only 50541 might be reported, as it is one code that includes both the diagnostic and therapeutic portions of the procedure.

GUIDANCE CONNECTION

Read additional explanations in the **Surgery Guidelines**, subheads **Follow-Up Care for Diagnostic Procedures** and **Follow-Up Care for Therapeutic Surgical Procedures**, in your CPT book directly in front of the Surgery section that lists all the codes.

Follow-Up Care for Diagnostic Procedures

When a diagnostic procedure is performed, the code includes only that care related to the recovery from this procedure, not any treatment for the condition identified. Care for the condition (therapeutic services) is not included.

Follow-Up Care for Therapeutic Surgical Procedures

The code reporting the provision of a therapeutic procedure only includes the care related to that procedure. Complications, exacerbations, recurrence, or the presence of other diseases or injuries requiring additional services should be reported separately.

Surgical Approaches

Procedure coding requires that you understand the various **surgical approaches** a physician can take to provide care for a patient:

Surgical Approach
The methodology or technique used by the physician to perform the procedure, service, or treatment.

- A *noninvasive*, or *external*, procedure is one that does not enter the patient's body; these are procedures that are applied or performed directly to the skin without physical entry into the visceral (internal) part of the body. An example of a noninvasive procedure is a shave biopsy, a technique to acquire pathology specimens of an elevated growth on the skin by razor.
- *Minimally invasive* procedures are becoming more and more available as health care researchers continue to find methods to diagnose and correct problems with the least amount of trauma to the patient. Although there is a big difference in our perception between a patient being stabbed by a mugger and a patient being cut open by a physician during a surgical procedure, the human body knows only that it is being invaded by a sharp piece of metal. It is traumatic, and healing must occur at the point of the incision as well as to whatever was done to internal organs.
- The *percutaneous approach* uses instruments inserted into the body by way of a puncture or small incision to access the intended anatomical site. Example: needle biopsy.
- The *percutaneous endoscopic approach* uses instruments inserted into the body by way of a puncture or small incision to access and visualize the intended anatomical site. Example: diagnostic anoscopy.
- The *via natural or artificial opening approach* involves instrumentation entered into the body through a natural opening (such as the vagina) or an artificial opening (such as a stoma) to visualize the intended anatomical site. Example: flexible esophagoscopy.
- The *via natural or artificial opening endoscopic approach* involves insertion of a scope through a natural opening (such as the mouth) or an artificial opening (such as a stoma) to visualize and aid in the performance of a procedure on the intended anatomical site. Example: colonoscopy with polyp removal.
- *Open approach* procedures are fully invasive, as the surgeon cuts the body open to enable access to internal tissues and organs. These procedures involve using a scalpel or laser to cut through the skin, membranes, and body layers to access the intended anatomical site.

EXAMPLES

Surgical procedures on a woman's uterus can be performed using

- The vaginal canal as the entry point (endoscopic using a natural opening) to avoid surgical entry through the abdomen, reported with

  58262 Vaginal hysterectomy, for uterus 250 g or less; with removal of tube(s) and/or ovary(s)

- Laparoscopy (a minimally invasive procedure through the abdominal cavity) via small incisions into the patient's skin and muscle, reported with

  58542 Laparoscopy, surgical, supracervical hysterectomy, for uterus 250 g or less; with removal of tube(s) and/or ovary(s)

- Open procedure with a longer incision through the abdominal wall, reported with

  58150 Total abdominal hysterectomy (corpus and cervix), with or without removal of tube(s), with or without removal of ovary(s)

You can see that all three of these codes accurately report a hysterectomy (the surgical removal of the uterus) with the removal of the fallopian tubes and ovaries. The difference between these codes is the surgical technique reported: 58150 reports an open abdominal procedure using an incision through the patient's abdominal wall, 58262 reports a procedure using a natural orifice (the vagina) so that no surgical incision was required, and 58542 reports a laparoscopic procedure that uses three tiny incisions in the patient's abdomen. The information provided by the reporting of these different versions of this procedure includes not only the level of work required by the physician to perform the procedure but also the level of postoperative care that the patient will require.

YOU INTERPRET IT!

Interpret each of these procedural statements to determine the type of procedure being documented: Diagnostic, Prophylactic, or Therapeutic.

1. Biopsy was performed to determine if mass is benign or malignant. ____________

2. Lithotripsy to destroy kidney stones. ____________

3. Cholecystectomy. ____________

4. Pneumonia vaccine administered. ____________

Interpret each of these procedural statements to determine the type of surgical approach being documented: Open, Percutaneous, or Endoscopic/Laparoscopic.

5. A 7-cm incision was made. ____________

6. A needle-biopsy was performed. ____________

7. The scope was passed through the patient's mouth into the stomach. ____________

GUIDANCE CONNECTION

Read additional explanations in the **Surgery Guidelines**, subhead **CPT Surgical Package Definition**, in your CPT book directly in front of the Surgery section that lists all the codes.

Standard of Care
The accepted principles of conduct, services, or treatments that are established as the expected behavior.

Global Period
The length of time allotted for postoperative care included in the surgical package, which is generally accepted to be 90 days for major surgical procedures and up to 10 days for minor procedures.

CODING BITES

Remember that an encounter that ends with an agreement to have surgery is reported with an E/M code appended with modifier **57 Decision for Surgery**. This is a notification of a surgical package that will soon begin.

26.2 The Surgical Package

One of the trickiest portions of coding surgical events is distinguishing between which services and procedures are included in the code and which services and procedures might need to be coded separately for additional reimbursement. Whereas the services included in each surgical protocol may vary with the procedure itself, some elements are already integrated in most CPT codes.

Services Always Included

Let's begin by reviewing services that are *always included* in CPT surgical procedure codes.

Once the physician and patient agree to move forward with the operation or procedure, the surgical package includes the following elements:

1. *Evaluation and management (E/M) encounters provided after the decision to have surgery.* These visits may begin the day before the surgical procedure (for more complex procedures) or the day of the procedure (for minor procedures), as needed.
2. *Local infiltration, metacarpal/metatarsal/digital block, or topical anesthesia.* You learned about the different types of anesthesia in the chapter ***CPT Anesthesia Section***. The surgical package includes specific types of local and regional anesthesia services only when they are provided by the surgeon (the same professional who will be performing the procedure).
3. *The operation itself, along with any services normally considered a part of the procedure being performed.* This would include supplies, as well as applying sutures, bandages, casts, and so on to enable the patient to leave the OR safely after the procedure.
4. *Immediate postoperative care.* This includes assessing the patient in the recovery area; attending to any complications exhibited by the patient (not including any additional trips to the OR); dictating or writing the operative notes; talking with the patient, the patient's family, and other health care professionals; and writing orders.
5. *Follow-up care.* This care includes postoperative visits; care for typical complications following surgery; pain management; dressing changes; removal of sutures, staples, tubes, casts, and so on; and any other services considered to be the **standard of care** during the **global period** for the specific surgical procedure. However, be careful. Some procedures may require a longer period of postoperative care by the surgeon. The period is determined by the accepted standard of care guidelines for each specific procedure and the details regarding the particular patient's health. More about this in the section ***Global Period Time Frames***.

6. *Supplies provided in a physician's office.* With a few specific exceptions, included supplies are determined by the insurance carrier.
7. *Graft procurement.* When a physician is performing a procedure involving the use of a graft, the codes that include obtaining or harvesting a graft already include procuring the autograft (from the patient) during the same operative session. Therefore, this would not be reported separately.

Services Not Included

Some functions that are commonly performed when a patient is going to have, or has had, surgery are *not included* in the surgical package. When such services and/or procedures are performed, you must code them separately.

1. *Diagnostic tests and procedures.* Tests or procedures that the physician needs to confirm the medical necessity for the surgery or investigate other issues related to the surgery are coded separately.

EXAMPLE

Diagnostic tests and procedures, such as biopsies, blood tests, and x-rays.

2. *Postoperative therapies.* Examples of postoperative therapies include immunosuppressive therapy after an organ transplant and chemotherapy after surgery to remove a malignancy.
3. *A more comprehensive version of the original procedure.* If the physician attempted to use a less extensive procedure first that was not sufficient to treat the patient, the second, more extensive procedure would be coded separately, with its own surgical package; it is not an extension of the first procedure. Also, the CPT code for the second event would be appended with modifier 58.

EXAMPLE

Dr. Keystone performed a lumpectomy on Joan Calcanne's left breast. The biopsy of the tissue removed during the lumpectomy showed that the malignancy had spread farther through the breast. Dr. Keystone had to take Joan back into the OR 1 week later for a simple, complete mastectomy. The code for the mastectomy is appended with modifier 58.

19301	Mastectomy, partial (e.g., lumpectomy, tylectomy, quadrantectomy, segmentectomy)
19303-58	Mastectomy, simple, complete, more extensive procedure

CODING BITES

For a surgical biopsy followed by a surgical procedure in response to the results of that biopsy, the surgical procedure (not the biopsy) code would be appended with modifier **58 Staged or related procedure or service by the same physician during the postoperative period**.

4. *Staged or multipart procedures.* Each stage or operation has its own surgical package and global period for aftercare. You must add modifier 58 to the second procedure code and all additional procedure codes reported for the same encounter.

58 **Staged or Related Procedure or Service by the Same Physician During the Postoperative Period.** It may be necessary to indicate that the performance of a procedure or service during the postoperative period was: (a) planned or anticipated (staged); (b) more extensive than the original procedure; or (c) for therapy following a surgical procedure. This circumstance may be reported by adding modifier 58 to the staged or related procedure.

CODING BITES

There are some codes that are *exempt* from using modifier 58. Take a look at codes 67141-67229 for some examples. Notice that each code's description includes the phrase "one or more sessions."

EXAMPLE

Albert Rodgers, a 31-year-old male, suffered a fracture to his upper arm that severely damaged the shaft of his right humerus. Dr. Curran decides to first do a bone graft to support the healing process of the fracture and to follow that with a second surgical procedure—an osteotomy—in about 4 weeks. This is a staged, or multipart, surgical procedure.

24516	Treatment of humeral shaft fracture, with insertion of intramedullary implant, with or without cerclage and/or locking screws
24400-58	Osteotomy, humerus, with or without internal fixation, staged procedure by the same physician during the postoperative period

5. *Management of postoperative complications that require additional surgery.* As you may remember about the surgical package from *Services Always Included* (earlier in this section), the physician's attention to any postoperative complications is included in the original package *unless* those complications require the patient to return to the OR. In such cases, you must use a modifier with the CPT code for the procedure performed.

76 **Repeat Procedure by the Same Physician.** It may be necessary to indicate that a procedure or service was repeated subsequent to the original procedure or service. This circumstance may be reported by adding modifier 76 to the repeated procedure or service.

78 **Unplanned Return to the Operating/Procedure Room by the Same Physician Following Initial Procedure for a Related Procedure During the Postoperative Period.** It may be necessary to indicate that another procedure was performed during the postoperative period of the initial procedure (unplanned procedure following initial procedure). When this procedure is related to the first, and requires the use of an operating/procedure room, it may be reported by adding modifier 78 to the related procedure.

EXAMPLE

Lilly Drummond, a 14-year-old female, was burned on her left forearm when she missed catching a flaming baton during cheerleading practice. Five days ago, Dr. Cheng applied a skin allograft to the burned area. Lilly is admitted today because the graft is not healing properly, and Dr. Cheng is going to apply a new allograft of 20 sq. cm.

15271-76	Application of skin substitute graft to trunk, arms, legs, total wound surface area up to 100 sq. cm; first 25 sq. cm or less wound surface area; repeat procedures by the same physician

77 **Repeat Procedure by Another Physician.** The physician may need to indicate that a basic procedure or service performed by another physician had to be repeated. This situation may be reported by adding modifier 77 to the repeated procedure/service.

EXAMPLE

Ray DeVilldus, an 18-year-old male, was stabbed in the chest during a fight. Dr. Swartz performed a complex repair of a 6-cm laceration of the chest. The next day, Dr. Swartz left for a medical conference. The guy who stabbed Ray showed up at the hospital, and Ray got out of bed, against doctor's orders, and engaged in another fight, ripping open his stitches. Dr. Tyson, filling in for Dr. Swartz, had to take Ray back into the OR and redo the repair. Dr. Tyson will send the claim with the following code:

13101-77	Repair, complex, trunk; 2.6 cm to 7.5 cm; repeat procedure by another physician

6. *Unrelated surgical procedure during the postoperative period.* If the same physician must perform an unrelated surgical procedure during the postoperative period, you have to include a modifier to explain that this procedure has nothing to do with the first.

79 **Unrelated Procedure or Service by the Same Physician During the Postoperative Period.** The physician may need to indicate that the performance of a procedure or service during the postoperative period was unrelated to the original procedure. This circumstance may be reported by using modifier 79.

EXAMPLE

Judith Conchran, a 41-year-old female, had a gastric bypass performed by Dr. Fellowes 10 days ago. She comes to see him today because she has a fever and pain radiating across her abdomen. Dr. Fellowes examines her, calls an ambulance, and takes her to the hospital and up to the operating room, where he performs an appendectomy to remove her ruptured appendix. The global postoperative period for a gastric bypass is 90 days. Dr. Fellowes performed Judith's appendectomy during the postoperative period for the bypass, and it had nothing to do with the first procedure. Therefore, our correct code would be

44960-79 Appendectomy; for ruptured appendix with abscess or generalized peritonitis; unrelated procedure or service by the same physician during the postoperative period

7. *Supplies.* In certain cases, for certain procedures performed in a physician's office, a separate code is permitted for supplies, such as a surgical tray, casting supplies, splints, and drugs. You have to check the reimbursement rules for the specific third-party payer.

CODING BITES

Code 99072 was added in 2022 to report the use of additional supplies, materials, and clinical staff, only during a Public Health Emergency (as defined by law). For example, during the COVID-19 pandemic, personal protective equipment (PPE) had to be used and changed for each individual patient seen in person.

EXAMPLE

Illea Beurus was prepped and ready for the procedure to begin. Dr. Hernandez performed the closed manipulation of the fracture. Instead of the usual plaster cast, fiberglass was used.

99070 Supplies and materials (except spectacles), provided by the physician or other qualified health care professional over and above those usually included with the office visit or other services rendered (list drugs, trays, supplies, or materials provided)

YOU INTERPRET IT!

Determine if the service or procedure provided in these statements is Included in the Surgical code (package) *or* Reported with a separate code.

8. Jeanine came to see Dr. Kidmon in his office 1 week after he performed her hysterectomy, as he instructed her to do. He wanted to check her sutures and healing progress. ____________________
9. While at Dr. Kidmon's office, Jeanine asked him to check her left breast because she felt a lump. He was concerned and performed a biopsy on the lump. ____________________
10. After Dr. Kidmon performed a mastectomy on Jeanine's left breast, he explained to her that they would need to complete a series of skin grafts. One graft would be done each month for 3 months. All are part of the postoperative care for mastectomy patients. Jeanine agreed. ____________________

26.3 Global Period Time Frames

Essentially, all procedures have assigned global period time frames based on the standard of care for a treatment or service. These range from 0 (zero) for a very simple procedure to 10 days for a minor procedure to 90 days for major surgery.

Zero-Day Postoperative Period

For procedures such as endoscopies and some minor procedures:

- No preoperative period.
- No postoperative days.
- Visit on day of procedure is generally not payable as a separate service.

10-Day Postoperative Period

For other minor procedures, 10 days following the day of the surgery:

- No preoperative period.
- Visit on day of the procedure is generally not payable as a separate service.

EXAMPLE

Dr. Bartlett performed a diagnostic flexible esophagoscopy with a biopsy on Wendy Crosek on April 5. The last day of the global period for this procedure will be April 15.

90-Day Postoperative Period

For major procedures, the total global period is actually 92 days: 1 day before the day of the surgery plus the day of surgery plus 90 days immediately following the day of surgery.

- One day preoperative included.
- Day of the procedure is generally not payable as a separate service.

EXAMPLE

Dr. Brennan saw Mira Sisto in his office on February 4 to confirm the arrangements and answer any last-minute questions for her intestinal allotransplantation surgery the next day.

On February 5, Dr. Brennan performed the intestinal allotransplantation from a cadaver donor to Mrs. Sisto.

The last day of the postoperative period is May 5.

GUIDANCE CONNECTION

Refer to the *Global Surgery Booklet* from CMS:

https://www.cms.gov/files/document/mln907166-global-surgery-booklet.pdf

To find the official Global Surgery Period for each CPT code, use the Physician Fee Schedule Look-Up Tool:

https://www.cms.gov/Medicare/Medicare-Fee-for-Service-Payment/PFSlookup/index.html

Scroll all the way down the page to ACCEPT. This will bring you to the next screen, where you will specify the parameters about the code for which you are seeking information. Remember, CPT is also known as HCPCS Level I, so in that field, you can enter the CPT code. Click SUBMIT.

On the next screen, be certain to click "Show All Columns."

YOU INTERPRET IT!

Use your resources and good critical thinking to determine the global surgery period for these procedures.

11. Metacarpal osteotomy [CPT code 26565] ________________

12. Initial pericardiocentesis [CPT code 33010] ________________

13. Cervical lymphadenectomy [CPT code 38724] ________________

14. Placement of seton [CPT code 46020] ________________

15. Cystourethroscopy, with biopsy [CPT code 52204] ________________

26.4 Unusual Services and Treatments

Treatment Plan Provided by More Than One Physician

It is expected that the same physician will provide all of the surgical package's elements. This is an umbrella that covers only one health care professional.

Occasionally, however, more than one physician will be involved in providing all the necessary services for one patient having one operation. In such cases, modifiers explain to the third-party payer who did what and when.

54 **Surgical Care Only.** You must add this modifier to the correct CPT surgical procedure code when your physician is only going to perform the procedure itself, and not provide or be involved in any preoperative or postoperative care of the patient.

55 **Postoperative Management Only.** This modifier is added to the CPT code for the surgical procedure included on a claim from the physician who only cares for the patient after the operation.

56 **Preoperative Management Only.** When a physician, other than the surgeon who performed the procedure, cares for the patient from the decision to have surgery up to but not including the operation itself, modifier 56 is appended to the CPT code for the procedure.

ICD-10-PCS

LET'S CODE IT! SCENARIO

Nadia Forrester, a 37-year-old female, was on vacation, hiking through the mountains, when she fell over a log and wrenched her knee very badly. She was flown to the nearest hospital and placed under the care of Dr. Petrone. After the diagnostic tests were completed, Dr. Petrone recommended arthroscopic surgery to treat the knee. Dr. Petrone called in Dr. Wellington, an orthopedic surgeon, to perform the procedure. Dr. Wellington performed a surgical arthroscopy and repaired the medial meniscus. Immediately after the surgery, Nadia flew home, and she went to her family physician, Dr. Shields, for the follow-up appointments.

Let's Code It!

The notes indicate that Dr. Petrone, Dr. Wellington, and Dr. Shields were all involved, to some extent, in caring for Nadia during the procedure—*surgical arthroscopy* and *repair of the medial meniscus*. Let's go to the Alphabetic Index and look up the procedure.

Find *arthroscopy*. As you go down the list, you will see the subcategories *Diagnostic* and *Surgical*. You know from the notes that this was surgical. Continue down and find the anatomical site for this procedure: **Knee . . . 29871–29889**. Indented under knee, you will find additional listings that don't really match, so let's look at the suggested codes:

29871 Arthroscopy, knee, surgical; for infection, lavage and drainage

The description is correct, up to the semicolon. So continue down the page to find any additional information that might be applicable to the case, according to our documentation. (Remember: Read up to the semicolon on the code because it is at the margin, and then finish the description with each indented description.)

Continue reading until you see

29882 with meniscus repair (medial OR lateral)

The complete description of this code is

29882 Arthroscopy, knee, surgical; with meniscus repair (medial OR lateral)

This matches the notes exactly, doesn't it? It does! Good job!

As you have learned, the surgical package for this procedure includes all the services and treatments that Nadia received. However, instead of just one physician, Nadia actually had three doctors caring for her throughout. Each physician will send his or her own claim form in an effort to get paid for the services he or she provided. You need to supply some explanation to the third-party payer so that it can understand receiving three claim forms for one procedure provided to the one patient.

(continued)

Dr. Petrone will have the 29882-56 code with modifier to indicate he only provided the preoperative care.

Dr. Wellington will have the 29882-54 code with modifier to indicate he only performed the surgery.

Dr. Shields will have the 29882-55 code with modifier to indicate she only provided the postoperative care.

Increased Procedural Services

Every service and treatment or procedure has an industry standard of care. Included in the assessment of each service is a calculation of how much work is involved and how long it will take to complete the procedure. It is all part of the formula used by third-party payers to determine how much to pay the health care professional. As you might expect, though, particularly in health care, things do not always go exactly as planned. There may be an issue with a patient that requires more work on the physician's part. When this happens, the physician should receive additional compensation. Therefore, you have to attach the modifier 22 to the procedure code to identify an unusual circumstance. You also have to attach documentation that fully explains the circumstances.

22 **Increased Procedural Services.** When the work required to provide a service is substantially greater than typically required, it may be identified by adding modifier 22 to the usual procedure code. Documentation must support the substantial additional work and the reason for the additional work (i.e., increased intensity, time, technical difficulty of procedure, severity of patient's condition, physical and mental effort required). *Note:* The modifier should not be appended to an E/M service.

ICD-10-PCS

YOU CODE IT! CASE STUDY

Frederick Stiner, a 15-year-old male, is 5 ft. 6 in., 365 lb. Dr. Girst performs a partial colectomy with anastomosis. The procedure, however, takes several hours longer than usual due to the fact that Frederick is morbidly obese.

You Code It!

Go through the steps, and determine the procedure code(s) that should be reported for this encounter between Dr. Girst and Frederick Stiner.

Step #1: Read the case carefully and completely.
Step #2: Abstract the scenario. Which key words or terms describe what service the physician provided to the patient during this encounter?
Step #3: Are there any details missing or incomplete for which you would need to query the physician? [If so, ask your instructor.]
Step #4: Determine the correct CPT procedure code or codes to explain the details about what was provided to the patient during this encounter.
Step #5: Check for any relevant guidance, including reading all of the symbols and notations.
Step #6: Do you need to append any modifiers to ensure complete and accurate information is provided?
Step #7: Double-check your work.

Answer:

Did you determine this to be the correct code?

44140-22 **Colectomy, partial; with anastomosis, increased procedural service**

In addition to the code, you should attach a letter with the claim to explain the circumstance that complicated the procedure.

CODING BITES

Read the entire description of these modifiers, and all others, in your **CPT book, Appendix A.**

Separate Procedure

Throughout the CPT book, you will see code descriptions that include the notation "separate procedure." Such services and treatments are generally performed along with a group of other procedures. When this happens, you will be able to find a combination, or bundled, code that includes all the treatments together. However, this particular procedure also can be performed alone. If so, you would use the code for the "separate procedure."

GUIDANCE CONNECTION

Read the additional explanations in the **Surgery Guidelines**, subhead **Separate Procedure**, in your CPT book directly in front of the Surgery section that lists all the codes.

LET'S CODE IT! SCENARIO

Dr. Capella performed a repair of the secondary tendon flexor in Bruce Roden's right foot. He first performed an open tenotomy and then did the repair with a free graft.

Let's Code It!

The *repair* that Dr. Capella performed on Bruce Roden actually includes the *tenotomy*. Therefore, we will use the one combination code for the entire procedure.

Go to the Alphabetic Index, and look up the procedure: *repair.* Under *Repair*, let's find the anatomical site: *foot.* Under *foot*, let's find the part of the foot that was treated: *tendon*. The Alphabetic Index suggests the code range 28200–28226, 28238. Let's go to the first one.

28200 Repair, tendon, flexor, foot; primary or secondary, without free graft, each tendon

28202 secondary with free graft, each tendon (includes obtaining graft)

It seems we have found the code description that matches the physician's notes.

28202 Repair, tendon, flexor, foot; secondary with free graft, each tendon (includes obtaining graft)

Great job!

Had Dr. Capella performed the tenotomy only, the correct code would be

28230 Tenotomy, open, tendon flexor; foot, single or multiple tendon(s) (separate procedure)

On occasion, you may find that the "separate procedure" is performed along with other procedures, not those in the bundle. Should this be the situation, you have to add the modifier 59 to the "separate procedure" code. Documentation must support these facts, as always.

59 Distinct Procedural Service. When the physician performs a procedure or service that is not normally performed with the other procedures or services, modifier 59 should be added to the second procedure.

26.5 Integumentary System

The largest organ of the human body, the skin, is the main component of the integumentary system, along with the hair and nails. Most people take this for granted. Yet this is the body's protective layer, the first line of defense for the anatomical organs and systems within.

Incision and Drainage (I&D)

A cyst, an abscess, a furuncle (boil), or a paronychia (infected skin around a fingernail or toenail) can harbor infection. When this happens, most often a physician will perform an incision (cut into the tissue) and drainage (I&D) to extract the infectious material.

CODING BITES

Remember: There is a difference between *incision* and *excision*.

Incision means *cut into*, while excision means *cut out*.

Debridement

The process of carefully cleaning out a wound to encourage the healing process is called *debridement*. The basis of this term comes from the word *debris*, meaning wreckage or rubble, and relates to the process of taking away necrotic (dead or dying) tissue that can impede the creation of new, healthy tissue. This may be necessary for burn patients, for victims of penetrating wounds, and sometimes for patients with complex wounds such as an open, penetrating fracture.

EXAMPLE

11000 Debridement of extensive eczematous or infected skin; up to 10% of body surface

+11001 each additional 10% of the body surface, or part thereof

You can see, from the descriptions of the codes in this subsection, that you will need to identify the total body surface area (TBSA) that was debrided, in order to determine an accurate code.

Biopsies

Biopsies are performed, most often, for diagnostic purposes. These procedures are done to obtain a sampling of cells or piece of tissue from the body that can then be pathologically analyzed. Although a specimen of tissue may be excised, shave removed, or lased and then sent to pathology for testing, this does not automatically indicate the need for a separate biopsy code. The guidelines state that you should use a biopsy procedure code only when the procedure is conducted individually, or distinctly separate, from any other procedure or service performed at the same time.

EXAMPLE

Paula had a rash that would not go away. So, she went to see Dr. Denardo, a dermatologist, who took a biopsy of one of the pustules, using a curette, in an effort to diagnose the cause of her rash. Dr. Denardo closed the small defect with one stitch. Dr. Denardo's coder would report

11102 Tangential biopsy of skin (e.g., shave, scoop, saucerize, curette); single lesion

There are many different types of biopsies, and you will need to know the details (from the documentation) to help you determine the correct code:

GUIDANCE CONNECTION

Read the additional explanations in the in-section guidelines located within the **Surgery** section, subhead **Biopsy**, directly above code 11102 in your CPT book.

- ***Fine-needle aspiration biopsy:*** The physician uses a thin needle to draw out—or drain—a specimen (some fluid or gas) to be used for pathology testing.
- ***Core-needle biopsy:*** The physician uses a hollow needle, a bit larger than the needle used during a fine-needle biopsy, to extract a cylindrical section of tissue to be analyzed. This category includes a punch biopsy.
- ***Excisional biopsies** and **incisional biopsies:*** A sampling of tissue of the abnormal area; an entire organ or tumor is taken during the procedure and sent to the pathology lab. These can include tangential biopsy, punch biopsy, and incisional biopsy.
- ***Endoscopic biopsy:*** During a percutaneous endoscopy or via a natural or artificial opening endoscopic procedure, a specimen of an abnormal or suspicious tissue is obtained and sent to the lab.

LET'S CODE IT! SCENARIO

Seth Berensen, a 69-year-old male, came to see Dr. Tyner to get rid of some skin tags on his left cheek. After applying a local anesthetic, Dr. Tyner removed nine tags and sent them to the lab.

(continued)

Let's Code It!

Let's go to the Alphabetic Index and find the key term for the procedure: *removal.* Now, what did the physician remove? *Skin tags.* Find the term "skin tags" indented under *Removal . . . skin tags . . .* : The codes suggested are 11200–11201. Turn to the numeric listing of the book, in the ***Surgery*** section, and look for those codes. You will see

11200 Removal of skin tags, multiple fibrocutaneous tags, any area; up to and including 15 lesions

+11201 each additional 10 lesions or part thereof (list separately in addition to code for primary procedure)

(Use 11201 in conjunction with 11200)

The next question is . . . How many skin tags (lesions) did the physician remove from Seth's face? When you reread the notes, you will see that he removed *nine tags.* This confirms the correct code is 11200.

The notes also indicate that the lesions were sent to pathology, meaning a biopsy. Should we add another code for the biopsy? Remember that the guidelines state that a separate code for the biopsy is used only when the biopsy is a procedure distinctly separate from other procedures and not a part of another service. In this case, the biopsy is a part of the removal of the skin tags and does not require a second code.

Excisions

When the physician removes a lesion from a patient, you must code the **excision** of each lesion separately. Codes for the excision, or **full-thickness** removal (**Figure 26-1**), of a lesion are determined first by the anatomical site from where the lesion was removed and then by the size of the lesion removed. The code for the excision includes the administration of a local anesthetic and a **simple closure** of the excision site, as mentioned in the definition.

Excision
The full-thickness removal of a lesion, including margins; includes (for coding purposes) a simple closure.

Full-Thickness
A measure that extends from the epidermis to the connective tissue layer of the skin.

Simple Closure
A method of sealing an opening in the skin (epidermis or dermis), involving only one layer. It includes the administration of local anesthesia and/or chemical or electrocauterization of a wound not closed.

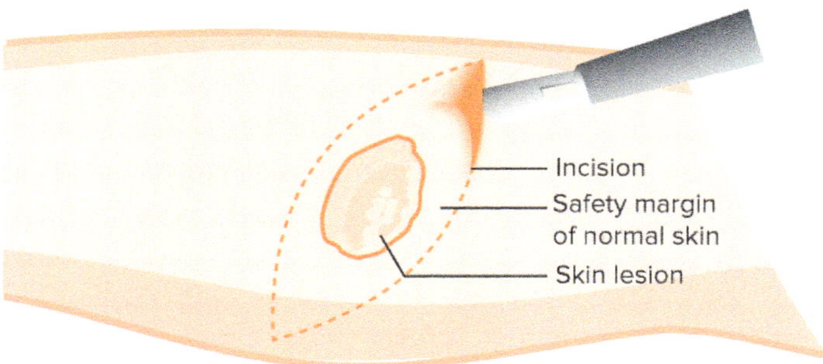

FIGURE 26-1 This illustration shows how you will determine the size of the lesion for coding

To correctly measure what was excised, you must look at the dimensions of the lesion itself *plus* a proper margin around the lesion. That will give you the total amount actually excised by the physician and lead you to the correct code. In order to find the correct size of the lesion excised, we must do the following: add the size of the lesion to the size of the margin doubled (margins *all around* means that the diameter will have a margin on each side).

The formula is

Coded size of lesion = size of lesion + (size of margins × 2)

As always, you must read carefully. Some surgeons include the measurement of the margins in their operative notes. In other cases, you may need to review the pathologist's report to determine an accurate measurement. And, typically, the measurements will be presented in centimeters (cm). Just in case:

1 centimeter (cm) = 10 millimeters (mm) = 0.4 inch (in.)

1 millimeter (mm) = 0.1 centimeter (cm) = 0.04 inch (in.)

1 inch (in.) = 2.54 cm

ICD-10-PCS

LET'S CODE IT! SCENARIO

Dr. Lanahan excised a lesion that measured 2.0 cm by 1.0 cm, with 0.2-cm margins all around, from Anson Hillam's neck. The pathology report confirmed that the lesion was benign.

Let's Code It!

Let's go to the Alphabetic Index and find the suggested code or codes. Look up *excision* for the procedure and then *neck* for the anatomical site, right? Well, you will see that there is no listing for *neck* under *excision*. What should you do now? Analyze what you see in the physician's notes. Where exactly is the lesion? It isn't really on his *neck*; it is on his *skin*. So look at *excision, skin*. Aha! Under *skin*, you will see *lesion*. Good. And now, look for *benign*, as per the notes, to find suggested codes 11400–11471.

When you go to the numeric listing, you will see the description for the first code in our range:

11400 Excision, benign lesion including margins, except skin tag (unless listed elsewhere), trunk, arms or legs; excised diameter 0.5 cm or less

The description for code 11400 matches our physician's notes except for the mention of the anatomical sites: trunk, arms, or legs. Our patient had the lesion on her neck. Continue looking down the listings, and take a look at the description for code 11420.

11420 Excision, benign lesion including margins, except skin tag (unless listed elsewhere), scalp, neck, hands, feet, genitalia; excised diameter 0.5 cm or less

This matches our physician's notes! Next, you must determine the size of the lesion. Remember the formula:

Coded size of lesion = size of lesion + (size of margins × 2)

To the size of the lesion (2.0 cm, which is its largest measurement), we add the size of the margin (0.2 cm) times 2 (margins *all around* mean that the diameter will have a margin on each side). With the figures in place, our formula becomes

Coded size of lesion = 2.0 cm + (0.2 cm × 2) = 2.4 cm

Therefore, the total size of the lesion excised is 2.4 cm. Now find the descriptions indented underneath 11420.

11423 Excision, benign lesion including margins, except skin tag (unless listed elsewhere), scalp, neck, hands, feet, genitalia; excised diameter 2.1 to 3.0 cm

This matches exactly. You have found the code: 11423. Good work!

GUIDANCE CONNECTION

Read the additional explanations in the in-section guidelines within the **Surgery** section, subheads **Excision–Benign Lesions**, directly above code 11400; **Excision–Malignant Lesions**, directly above code 11600; and **Excision**, directly above code 19081, in your CPT book.

You may find that the physician's notes indicate that the excision of the lesion was complicated or unusual in some way. Should this be the situation, remember to add modifier 22 Increased Procedural Services to the procedure code. The difficulty is related to the process of excising the lesion, not the closure.

CPT

LET'S CODE IT! SCENARIO

Dr. Samsune excised a lesion that measured 2.1 by 3.0 cm, with 0.5-cm margins on each side, from Sally Hardy's abdomen. Sally is diagnosed clinically obese and the excess fatty tissue around the lesion required a complex closure of the excision site. The pathology report confirmed that the lesion was malignant.

(continued)

Let's Code It!

The Alphabetic Index will direct you to a slightly different group of codes—*excision, skin, lesion, malignant*—suggesting a code within the range of 11600–11646. Just as before, you will need to find the code in this range that identifies the correct anatomical location of the lesion:

11600 Excision, malignant lesion including margins, trunk, arms or legs; excised diameter 0.5 cm or less

The abdomen is a part of the trunk, so this code is OK. Next, you will need to add up the size of the lesion.

Coded size of lesion = 3.0 cm + (0.5 cm × 2) = 4.0 cm

The answer 4.0 cm leads to the code

11604 Excision, malignant lesion including margins, trunk, arms or legs; excised diameter 3.1 to 4.0 cm

Excellent! Sally's case was not as complicated as Anson's, so modifier 22 will not be required. However, Dr. Samsune did note that Sally's procedure "required a complex closure of the excision site." The guidelines tell you that only a simple closure is included in the excision code. A complex closure, just like an intermediate closure, is coded in addition to the code for the excision. So let's code it!

Let's go back to the Alphabetic Index and find the key term *closure*. None of the indented descriptors seem to match, so you should investigate the code range shown next to the word *closure*: 12001–13160.

You will notice the heading immediately above the first code in the range: 12001. It reads "Repair—Simple." But you are looking for a complex closure, so continue down the page. The next section, above code 12031, is "Repair—Intermediate." This is closer to what you need, but not exactly. Above code 13100 you find the heading you have been looking for: "Repair—Complex."

Remember that Sally's lesion was located on her abdomen (trunk). Look at the codes in this section, and find the best code for the *complex closure* of her excision site.

13100 Repair, complex, trunk; 1.1 cm to 2.5 cm

Excellent! You have found the correct level of closure (repair) for the correct anatomical site (trunk). Now, you must find the correct size of the excision site. Your calculation totaled 4.0 cm, which brings you to the correct code:

13101 Repair, complex, trunk; 2.6 cm to 7.5 cm

Excellent! You now know that, for this one procedure on Sally, the claim form will include these codes:

11604 Excision, malignant lesion including margins, trunk, arms or legs; excised diameter 3.1 to 4.0 cm

13101 Repair, complex, trunk; 2.6 cm to 7.5 cm

Good job!

Reexcision

When the pathology report indicates that the physician did not excise around the lesion (the margins) widely enough to get all the malignancy, an additional excision procedure may be needed.

If the reexcision is performed during the same operative session, adjust the total size of the lesion being coded to include the new total measurement. Report just the one code, with the largest measurement shown in the operative or procedure notes.

If the reexcision is performed during a subsequent encounter during the postoperative period, you should attach modifier 58 Staged Procedure to the procedure code for that second excision. The reexcision to remove additional tissue around the original site during the postoperative period would directly apply to modifier 58's description: (b) more extensive than the original procedure.

Repair (Closures)

Simple closure is included in the excision code. However, if the closure of the excision site becomes more involved and is described as an **intermediate closure** or a **complex closure**, the repair is no longer included in the code for the excision procedure. You need to report an additional code.

As you read the procedure notes or operative report, pay close attention to the description documented as to how deep into the skin the physician worked. When you see a layered closure that involves the deeper layers of the subcutaneous tissue, the superficial fascia, and the epidermal and dermal layers of the skin, you will report an intermediate repair. Also reported as an intermediate repair is a single-layer closure that first requires extensive cleaning or particulate matter removal before closing.

When a complex repair has been performed, the documentation will include more than just a layered enclosure: scar revision, traumatic laceration debridement, avulsions, extensive undermining, stent insertion, or retention suture(s) all describe this more involved level of repair.

When multiple wounds are repaired with the same complexity on the same anatomical site(s) as indicated by the code descriptor, add all the lengths together to use one code for the total repair. You may sometimes have more than one code to report repairs performed at this encounter. In these cases, the codes should be listed in order from the most complex to the simplest, then from head to toe. All procedure codes, after the first, should have the modifier 59 Distinct Procedural Service appended.

Intermediate Closure
A multilevel method of sealing an opening in the skin involving one or more of the deeper layers of the skin. Single-layer closure of heavily contaminated wounds that required extensive cleaning or removal of particulate matter also constitutes intermediate closure.

Complex Closure
A method of sealing an opening in the skin involving a multilayered closure and a reconstructive procedure such as scar revision, debridement, or retention sutures.

GUIDANCE CONNECTION

Read the additional explanations in the in-section guidelines located within the **Surgery** section, subhead **Repair (Closure)**, directly above code 12001 in your CPT book.

CODING BITES

Modifier 59 is used to report multiple procedures that are performed at the same encounter by the same provider. This modifier is appended to the codes reporting the second and additional services, not the primary procedure code.

GUIDANCE CONNECTION

In-Section Guidelines (above code 12001 in the Surgery section)

The multiple wound repair guideline is different from the guideline for multiple lesions. Remember that, with lesions, each lesion is coded separately. With wounds, you will *report one code for the total length of all wounds being repaired on the same anatomical site with the same level of repair (simple, intermediate, complex).*

When more than one level of wound repair is used during the same encounter for the same patient, list the more complicated as the primary procedure and the less complicated as the secondary procedures, using modifier 59.

Debridement or decontamination of a wound is included in the code for the repair of that wound. However, if the contamination is so extensive that it requires extra time and effort, it should be coded separately. Also, if the debridement is performed and the wound is not closed or repaired during the same session, code the debridement separately.

LET'S CODE IT! SCENARIO

Fiona Curtis, a 27-year-old female, got into a bar fight and sustained multiple wounds to her hand and arm. Dr. Rockville performed intermediate repair of a 5- by 2-cm wound and a 3.1- by 1-cm wound on Fiona's right hand and a simple repair to a 3.2- by 1-cm wound to her right forearm.

Let's Code It!

You can see by Dr. Rockville's notes that Fiona had two wounds treated with intermediate closures, both on her right hand, and one wound with a simple repair, on her right forearm. Let's go to the Alphabetic Index and find *repair, wound, intermediate* (suggesting code range 12031–12057) and *repair, wound, simple* (suggesting code range 12001–12021).

(continued)

The intermediate repairs were done to the right *hand*, so let's turn to the numeric listing for the code range 12031–12057 and find the best code for this anatomical site.

12041 Repair, intermediate, wounds of neck, hands, feet and/or external genitalia; 2.5 cm or less

There were two wounds on Fiona's right hand (the first is 5 × 2 cm and the second 3.1 × 1 cm). The guidelines state that, because the wounds are on the same anatomical site as per the code description (*hands*) and received the same level of repair (*intermediate*), you must add them together. Let's add the two longest measurements together (5 cm + 3.1 cm) for a total of 8.1 cm. This brings us to the correct code:

12044 Repair, intermediate, wounds of neck, hands, feet and/or external genitalia; 7.6 cm to 12.5 cm

Good job! Now, the last wound on Fiona's forearm is different. It is a simple repair rather than an intermediate repair, and the wound is on her arm, not her hand. Therefore, this wound repair will have its own code. Follow the code descriptions and see if you can come up with the most accurate code. Did you determine this to be the correct code?

12002 Simple repair of superficial wounds of scalp, neck, axillae, external genitalia, trunk and/or extremities (including hands and feet); 2.6 cm to 7.5 cm

Now that you know the guideline regarding multiple wound repairs, do you think any adjustments should be made to the claim form you are preparing for Dr. Rockville to be reimbursed for his work on Fiona? You need to report them in the correct sequence and append a modifier:

12044 (The intermediate repair tells us this was the more severe or complicated procedure. Therefore, this code is reported first.)

12002-59 (This was the simple repair of a smaller wound. This was less complicated and, therefore, the code is listed second and appended with the modifier 59.)

That's great! You did excellent work!

YOU CODE IT! CASE STUDY

A woman was screaming in a parking lot and calling for help. She had accidentally locked her keys in the car, along with her infant son. It was a hot day, and she was quite concerned about her child. Alex Franklin came along and used a rock to break a window on the other side of the car, reached in through the broken glass, and unlocked the door. Without question, Alex is a hero, but he also cut his wrist on the broken glass. At the ED, Dr. Zander discovered that the subcutaneous tissue at the laceration site was littered with tiny shards of glass. Dr. Zander administered a local anesthetic. It took Dr. Zander quite a long time to debride the 5.3- by 1.6-cm wound of all the glass before he was able to suture it.

You Code It!

Go through the steps, and determine the procedure code(s) that should be reported for this encounter between Dr. Zander and Alex Franklin.

Step #1: Read the case carefully and completely.
Step #2: Abstract the scenario. Which key words or terms describe what service the physician provided to the patient during this encounter?
Step #3: Are there any details missing or incomplete for which you would need to query the physician? [If so, ask your instructor.]
Step #4: Determine the correct CPT procedure code or codes to explain the details about what was provided to the patient during this encounter.
Step #5: Check for any relevant guidance, including reading all of the symbols and notations.
Step #6: Do you need to append any modifiers to ensure complete and accurate information is provided?
Step #7: Double-check your work.

(continued)

Answer:

Did you determine these to be the correct codes?

11042	**Debridement, subcutaneous tissue (includes, epidermis and dermis, if performed); first 20 sq. cm or less**
12002-51	**Simple repair of superficial wounds of scalp, neck, axillae, external genitalia, trunk and/or extremities (including hands and feet); 2.6 cm to 7.5 cm; multiple procedures**

Excellent! You are really learning how to code!

Adjacent Tissue Transfer and/or Rearrangement

When an excision is repaired with an adjacent tissue transfer or rearrangement, you will see several terms in the procedure notes that are included in this code subcategory.

- Z-plasty is a double transposition flap, most often used to correct a skin web or perform a scar revision.
- W-plasty uses several small, triangular-shaped flaps, alternating inversion, just like the letter "W," to break up a long scar.
- V-Y plasty uses a V-shaped flap that is next to the defect with surrounding skin raised up and brought into the wound.
- Rotation flap is a raised subdermal plane, semicircular in shape, pivoted around into the defect.
- Random island flap is a section of skin moved into the defect with its blood supply.
- Advancement flap involves a subdermal place of skin, longitudinally moved to the defect.

GUIDANCE CONNECTION

Read additional explanations in the in-section guidelines located within the **Surgery** section, subhead **Adjacent Tissue Transfer or Rearrangement**, directly above code 14000 in your CPT book.

The correct code to report a tissue transfer or rearrangement requires two elements from the physician's notes:

- Anatomical site: The anatomical location of the primary defect–the skin opening that needs to be repaired–as well as the location of the secondary defect–the skin area from where the surgeon took the skin being transferred.
- Size of the defect: Add together the sizes of the primary defect and the secondary defect.
- For all defects over 30 sq. cm, all anatomical sites are reported with the same codes–code 14301 with code 14302, depending upon the total size.

LET'S CODE IT! SCENARIO

Larissa Cheek had a 2.5 cm × 1 cm contracted scar on the back of her hand, making it difficult to use her fingers completely. Dr. Villa performed a Z-plasty tissue transfer to disrupt the scar tissue and elongate the transferred tissues. He notes that the secondary defect was 3 sq. cm.

Let's Code It!

Dr. Villa did a "*Z-plasty tissue transfer*" on Larissa. However, when you look in the CPT Alphabetic Index for *Z-plasty*, you will find nothing. Take a look at the Alphabetic Index for *transfer*. There are a few items listed below, but none of these seem to relate to the procedure on Larissa. So let's take a look at the CPT Alphabetic Index listings for *tissue*. Below this you will see:

(continued)

Tissue

Transfer

Adjacent

Skin 14000–14350

As you review the guidelines in this subsection, shown above code 14000, you can see that Z-plasty is included in this section, confirming that you are in the right area. Next, you can see that the code descriptions require you to know the anatomical location of the procedure.

14000 **Adjacent tissue transfer or rearrangement, trunk**

14020 **Adjacent tissue transfer or rearrangement, scalp, arms, and/or legs**

14040 **Adjacent tissue transfer or rearrangement, forehead, cheeks, chin, mouth, neck, axillae, genitalia, hands and/or feet**

14060 **Adjacent tissue transfer or rearrangement, eyelids, nose, ears, and/or lips**

Go back to the scenario and identify the anatomical site: "*on the back of her hand.*" This leads you to code 14040. You must now choose between the following two codes, determined by the size of the defects:

14040 **Adjacent tissue transfer or rearrangement, forehead, cheeks, chin, mouth, neck, axillae, genitalia, hands and/or feet; defect 10 sq. cm or less**

14041 **defect 10.1 sq. cm to 30.0 sq. cm**

How big was the defect? In the guidelines above code 14000, it says, "*The primary defect resulting from the excision and the secondary defect resulting from flap design to perform the reconstruction are measured together to determine the code.*"

Larissa's original scar—the primary defect—is noted to be 2.5 cm × 1. Multiply these two numbers to get 2.5 sq. cm. The secondary defect, the source of the tissue transfer, is noted to be 3 sq. cm. Add 2.5 sq. cm to 3 sq. cm and get a total of 5.5 sq. cm. Compare this measurement to the measurements included in the code descriptions for tissue transfers done on the hands. This confirms the correct code for the procedure Dr. Villa did for Larissa:

14040 **Adjacent tissue transfer or rearrangement, forehead, cheeks, chin, mouth, neck, axillae, genitalia, hands and/or feet; defect 10 sq. cm or less**

Good job!

Skin Replacement Surgery and Flaps

The codes for skin grafts are determined by three things:

1. The size of the **recipient area** (the size of the wound to be grafted).
2. The location of the recipient area (the anatomical site).
3. The type of graft (pinch graft, split graft, full-thickness graft, and so on).

> **Recipient Area**
> The area, or site, of the body receiving a graft of skin or tissue.

> **Harvesting**
> The process of taking skin or tissue (on the same body or another).

The codes include a simple debridement, or avulsion, of the recipient site. Through **harvesting**, grafts can be taken from another part of the patient's body, another body (a live donor), a cadaver (a deceased person), skin substitutes (such as neodermis, synthetic skin), or another species (for instance, a porcine graft). You have to know where the graft came from in order to determine the best, most appropriate code.

It is not uncommon for skin grafts to be planned, from the beginning, to be done in stages. When this is the case, the second and subsequent portions of the staged procedure should be appended with modifier 58. This is directly described in CPT's modifier 58 description: (a) planned or anticipated (staged).

If the **donor area (site)** requires a skin graft or a local flap to repair it, it should be coded as an additional procedure. When evaluating the size of the wound that has been grafted, the measurement of *100 sq. cm* is used with patients aged 10 and older. The code descriptor referring to a *percentage of the body area* applies only to patients under the age of 10.

> **Donor Area (Site)**
> The area or part of the body from which skin or tissue is removed with the intention of placing that skin or tissue in another area or body.

EXAMPLE

15002 Surgical preparation or creation of recipient site by excision of open wounds, burn eschar, or scar (including subcutaneous tissues), or incisional release of scar contracture, trunk, arms, legs; first *100 sq. cm* or *1% of body area of infants and children*

GUIDANCE CONNECTION

Read additional explanations in the in-section guidelines located within the **Surgery** section, subhead **Skin Replacement Surgery**, directly above code 15002 in your CPT book.

In the subheading relating to flaps and grafts, when the physician attaches a flap, either in transfer or to the final site, the anatomical site identified in the code's description is the *recipient* site, not the donor site.

EXAMPLE

15733 Muscle, myocutaneous, or fasciocutaneous flap; head and neck with named vascular pedicle (ie, buccinators, genioglossus, temporalis)

When a tube is formed to be used later, or when "delay" of flap is done before the transfer, the anatomical sites indicated in the code description refer to the *donor* site, not the recipient site.

GUIDANCE CONNECTION

Read the additional explanations in the in-section guidelines located within the **Surgery** section, subhead **Flaps (Skin and/or Deep Tissues)**, directly above code 15570 in your CPT book.

EXAMPLE

15620 Delay of flap or sectioning of flap (division and inset); at forehead, cheeks, chin, mouth, neck, axillae, genitalia, hands or feet

When extensive immobilization is performed, such as large plaster casts or traction, the application of the immobilization device should be coded as a separate procedure. However, make note that the procedure codes in the range 15570–15738 already include small or standard immobilization, such as a sling or splint.

YOU CODE IT! CASE STUDY

Evan Riggs, an 11-year-old male, had burn eschar on his face from an accident. Dr. Charne performed a surgical preparation of the area. Two days later, Dr. Charne applied a dermal autograft to the 30-sq.-cm area.

(continued)

You Code It!

Based on the notes, find the best, most appropriate procedure code(s) to report all of Dr. Charne's work for Evan's injury.

Step #1: Read the case carefully and completely.
Step #2: Abstract the scenario. Which key words or terms describe what service the physician provided to the patient during this encounter?
Step #3: Are there any details missing or incomplete for which you would need to query the physician? [If so, ask your instructor.]
Step #4: Determine the correct CPT procedure code or codes to explain the details about what was provided to the patient during this encounter.
Step #5: Check for any relevant guidance, including reading all of the symbols and notations.
Step #6: Do you need to append any modifiers to ensure complete and accurate information is provided?
Step #7: Double-check your work.

Answer:

Did you determine the following codes?

15004 **Surgical preparation or creation of recipient site by excision of open wounds, burn eschar, or scar (including subcutaneous tissues), or incisional release of scar contracture, face, scalp, eyelids, mouth, neck, ears, orbits, genitalia, hands, feet, and/or multiple digits; first 100 sq. cm or 1% of body area of infants and children**

15135-58 **Dermal autograft, face, scalp, eyelids, mouth, neck, ears, orbits, genitalia, hands, feet, and/or multiple digits; first 100 sq. cm or less, or 1% of body area of infants and children; staged procedure**

Great work!

Destruction

Destruction is the term used for the removal of diseased or unwanted tissue from the body by surgical or other means, such as surgical curettement (also known as curettage), laser treatment, electrosurgery, chemical treatment, or cryosurgery. Ablation is the surgical destruction of tissue or a body part. When the tissue is destroyed rather than excised, there is nothing left. Therefore, there will be no specimens sent to pathology for analysis. The codes in the destruction subheading of the surgical section include the administration of local anesthesia.

There are several methods that a physician can use to destroy tissue.

- *Cauterization* is the process of destroying tissue with the use of a chemical or electricity to seal a wound and stop bleeding. Some cauterizations can be accomplished with extreme heat or cold. For example, you might see physician's notes document the removal of an internal polyp with the use of hot forceps.
- *Cryosurgical* or *cryotherapy* techniques use liquid nitrogen or freezing carbon dioxide to destroy the tissue of concern.
- *Curettage* is the method of using a special surgical tool, called a curette, to scrape an organ, a muscle, or other anatomical site.
- *Electrosurgical* methods use high-frequency electrical current instead of a scalpel to separate and destroy tissue. One example of this is electrolysis, which removes hair by using electricity to destroy the hair follicle.
- *Laser* surgery uses light to cut, separate, or destroy tissue. The term *laser* is actually an acronym for "light amplification by stimulated emission of radiation."

GUIDANCE CONNECTION

Read additional explanations in the in-section guidelines located within the **Surgery** section, subhead **Destruction**, directly above code 17000 in your CPT book.

LET'S CODE IT! SCENARIO

Derrick Franks, a 54-year-old male, came to see Dr. Johnston, his podiatrist, for the removal of a benign plantar wart from the sole of his left foot. Dr. Johnston administered a local anesthetic and then destroyed the wart using a chemosurgical technique. A protective bandage was applied to the foot, and Frank was sent home with an appointment to return in 1 week for a follow-up check.

Let's Code It!

The notes indicate that Derrick had a *benign plantar wart* that Dr. Johnston *destroyed* using *chemosurgery*.

Let's go to the Alphabetic Index and look up *destruction*.

Under *destruction*, you will see an alphabetical list that includes both anatomical sites as well as skin conditions, such as cysts and lesions. You know from the notes that Dr. Johnston destroyed a wart on Derrick's foot. There are no listings for foot or sole of foot. However, there is a listing for *Warts, flat . . . 17110–17111*. Do you know if a plantar wart is a flat wart? Because this is the only choice here, let's go to the codes suggested and see if the numeric listing can provide more information.

The code descriptions read

17110 **Destruction (e.g., laser surgery, electrosurgery, cryosurgery, chemosurgery, surgical curettement), of benign lesions other than skin tags or cutaneous vascular proliferative lesions; up to 14 lesions**

17111 **15 or more lesions**

These descriptions do not really answer our question about whether a plantar wart is a flat wart or a benign lesion. But before you query the doctor, go to the beginning of this subsection and read down.

Directly below the description for code 17111 is a notation:

(For destruction of extensive cutaneous neurofibroma over 50–100 lesions, see 0419T, 0420T)

Directly below the description for code 17003 is a notation:

(For destruction of common or plantar warts, see 17110, 17111.)

This is an excellent example of how you must investigate all possibilities and really give the CPT book a chance to point you toward the correct code.

Dr. Johnston destroyed with chemosurgery Derrick's benign lesion that was not a skin tag or a cutaneous vascular proliferative lesion, and he only had one. Code 17110 is perfect!

Mohs Micrographic Surgery

The group of codes for Mohs micrographic surgery (17311–17315) will be used only when you are coding for a physician who is specially trained in this type of procedure because it requires one doctor to act as *both* surgeon and pathologist. If two different professionals perform these functions, these codes cannot be used.

If a repair is performed during the same session, the repair, flap, or graft procedures should be coded separately.

If a biopsy is performed on the same day as the Mohs surgery because the physician suspects that the patient has skin cancer, it should be reported separately as well, appended with modifier 59 Distinct Procedural Service.

GUIDANCE CONNECTION

Read the additional explanations in the in-section guidelines located within the **Surgery** section, subhead **Mohs Micrographic Surgery**, directly above code 17311 in your CPT book.

26.6 Musculoskeletal System

The musculoskeletal system subsection of codes reports procedures and treatments performed on the bones, ligaments, cartilage, muscles, and tendons in the human body (**Figure 26-2**).

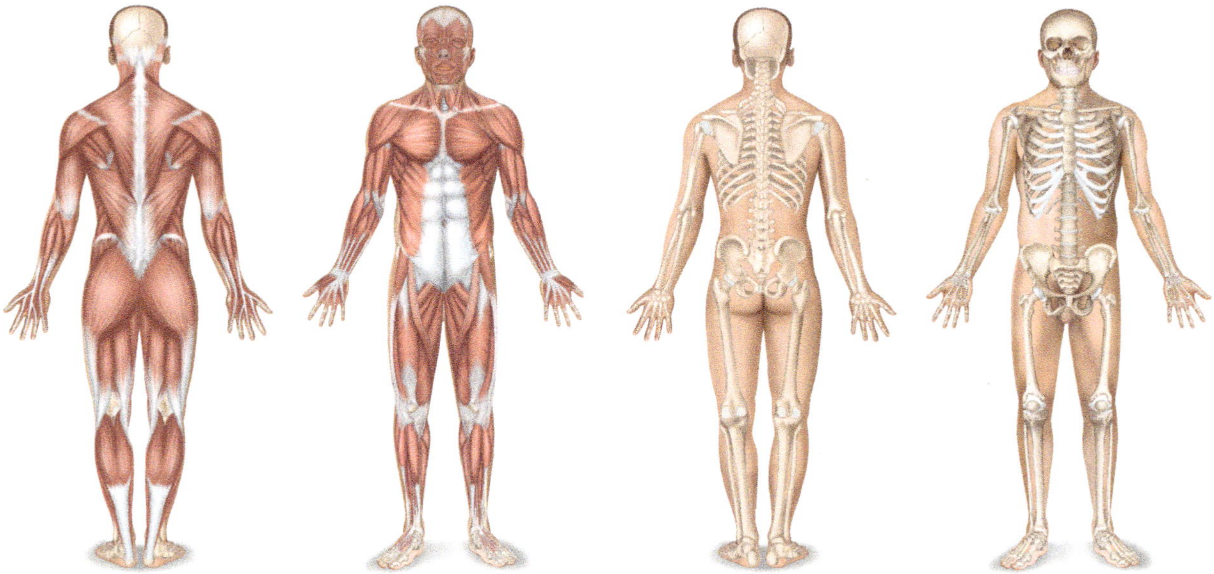

FIGURE 26-2 These illustrations show some of the over 600 muscles and 206 bones in the human body

Cast Application

Earlier in this chapter, you learned about the surgical package, and all of the services it includes. In addition, codes in this subsection already include the application and removal of a cast or traction device as a part of the procedure performed.

So, when would you report a code from the subsection **Application of Casts and Strapping**, codes 29000 through 29799? There are times when no other procedure is performed. When the only service provided is the cast application, this will be reported from here.

GUIDANCE CONNECTION

Read additional explanations in the in-section guidelines located within the **Surgery** section, subhead **Application of Casts and Strapping**, directly above code 29000 in your CPT book.

EXAMPLES

Dr. Philphot performed a closed realignment, manipulating the fractured calcaneal bone back together, and applied a foot-to-knee plaster cast.

- The application of this cast would be included in the code for the treatment of the fracture:

  28405 Closed treatment of calcaneal fracture; with manipulation

Justine had fractured her ulna and radius after falling off her skateboard. She got caught in an unexpected rainstorm that drenched her, and her cast. Dr. Keller replaced the long-arm cast.

- The application of this cast was the only service provided for the treatment of Justine's fracture; therefore, it would be reported separately.

  29065 Application, cast; shoulder to hand (long arm)

Fracture Reduction

> **Manipulation**
> The attempted return of a fracture or dislocation to its normal alignment manually by the physician.

A fracture reduction is the process of returning the bone fragments back to their original and correct location and configuration. The type of fracture will determine the specific components of this procedure. For example, a simple fracture might possibly be reduced with a closed treatment, while a multifragmentary fracture or one with bone loss may require an open treatment with additional work, such as a bone graft or internal fixation, to restore the bone to its previous length, alignment, and ability to rotate (such as with an articulation). Reduction or **manipulation** may be necessary to realign the bone pieces so that union can occur properly. This may be done externally (closed reduction, known as manipulation) or surgically (open reduction).

Details from the CPT Coding Guidelines, found at the beginning of the **Musculoskeletal System** section of the ***Surgery*** section of CPT, remind you that

> *Manipulation is used throughout the musculoskeletal fracture and dislocation subsections to specifically mean the attempted reduction or restoration of a fracture or joint dislocation to its normal anatomic alignment by the application of manually applied forces.*

This will support your determination for the correct code as you see that the codes for treatment of either an open fracture or a closed fracture are categorized by the method of reduction (manipulation) and fixation/immobilization used to stabilize the realigned bone.

Certainly, you already know that the CPT procedure code will be determined, in part, by which specific bone is fractured and therefore needs treatment.

EXAMPLES

23525 Closed treatment of sternoclavicular dislocation; with manipulation

27178 Open treatment of slipped femoral epiphysis; closed manipulation with single or multiple pinning

The key terms you will need to identify from the documentation also will vary depending upon the particular fractured bone that is being treated. For example:

Open treatment and/or reduction of vertebral fracture(s) and/or dislocation(s), posterior approach, 1 fractured vertebra or dislocated segment;

Lumbar 22325

Cervical 22326

Thoracic 22327

Additional fractured vertebra . . . . . +22328

When the fractured bone is a segment of the spinal column, you will need to abstract three key important pieces of information: the location of the bone on the vertebral column (i.e., cervical, thoracic, lumbar), the number of fractured vertebrae reduced, and the approach–posterior or anterior. The codes shown above (22325-22328) are only to be reported when the physician used a posterior, or back, approach. When the approach used to visualize and reduce the fracture was from the front–an anterior approach–codes 63081-63091 are used instead.

Open or Closed Treatment

Procedures and services can be provided for various sites of the musculoskeletal system as an open treatment or a closed treatment. These two words, *open* and *closed*, are used for both the description of the fracture itself (in the diagnostic statement) and the description of the procedure. Be careful not to confuse these identifiers because they are NOT interrelated–that is, a compound (open) fracture is not automatically treated with an open procedure. Be certain to differentiate the description of the fracture from the description of the procedure. Let's begin with understanding what CPT means by open treatment or closed treatment.

Open Treatment

CPT defines **open treatment** as a procedure provided to treat a fractured bone that is either

> Surgically opened, so that the fracture can be visualized and internal fixation may be applied.

or

> Not opened surgically, but the fractured bone is opened remotely from the site to enable the surgeon to insert an intramedullary nail.

Open Treatment
Surgically opening the fracture site, or another site in the body nearby, in order to treat the fractured bone.

Closed Treatment

According to CPT, the **closed treatment** of a fracture is performed

- With or without manipulation.
- With or without traction.
- Without the fracture being opened and visualized.

Closed Treatment
The treatment of a fracture without surgically opening the affected area.

Penetrating Trauma Wounds

The CPT book distinguishes between wounds and penetrating trauma wounds. A penetrating trauma wound requires

1. Surgery to explore the wound.
2. Determination of the depth and complexity of the wound.
3. Identification of any damage created by the penetrating object (such as the stabbing from a knife or the wound from a bullet).
4. Debridement of the wound to remove any particles, dirt, and foreign fragments.
5. Ligation or coagulation of minor subcutaneous tissue, muscle fascia, and/or muscle (not severe enough to require a thoracotomy or laparotomy).

You will use codes 20100–20103 to report the exploration of such wounds. Then, code whichever repair the physician actually performs, as documented in the notes.

GUIDANCE CONNECTION

Read the additional explanations in the in-section guidelines located within the **Surgery** section, subhead **Musculoskeletal System**, subsection **Wound Exploration–Trauma (e.g., Penetrating Gunshot, Stab Wound)**, directly above code 20100 in your CPT book.

Bone Grafts and Implants

Medical science and technology have progressed amazingly. Be certain to differentiate between skin grafts (reported from the **Integumentary System** subsection of CPT) and bone, cartilage, tendon, and fascia lata grafts that are coded from the **Musculoskeletal System** subsection.

If the code description does not specifically reference the harvesting of the graft or implant (e.g., code 20936 "includes harvesting the graft"), then the procedure for obtaining autogenous bone, cartilage, tendon, fascia lata grafts, or other tissues should be reported separately.

Spine

As you may remember from anatomy class, the human spine is referred to in sections: cervical (at or near the neck), thoracic (the chest area), lumbar (at the waist and lower back), and sacral. References to the individual vertebrae are most often identified by their alphanumeric identifiers, such as C1 (cervical vertebra number 1), L5 (lumbar vertebra number 5), or S3 (sacral vertebra number 3), as you can see in **Figure 26-3**.

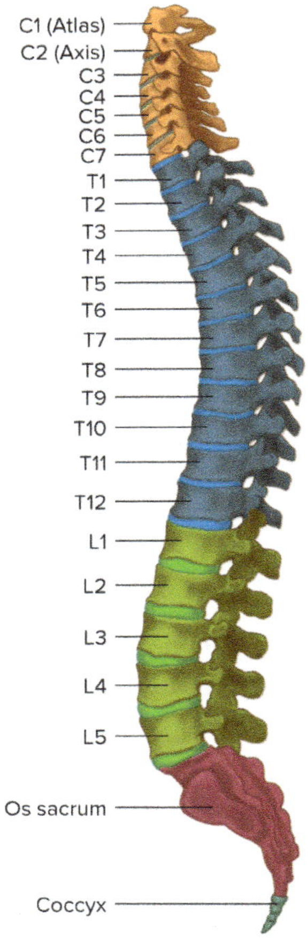

FIGURE 26-3 The vertebrae of the spinal column are numbered from the head to the coccyx

Source: www.boundless.com

GUIDANCE CONNECTION

Read the additional explanations in the in-section guidelines within the **Surgery** section, subhead **Spine (Vertebral Column)**, directly above code 22010 in your CPT book.

Laminotomy

A laminotomy is a partial laminectomy used to treat lumbar disc herniation. Removing a portion of the lamina is often sufficient to access the affected nerve root. Then, the disc herniation can be visualized and accessed from beneath the nerve root. This procedure should be reported with the most accurate code, based on the details in the documentation:

63020 **Laminotomy (hemilaminectomy), with decompression of nerve root(s), including partial facetectomy, foraminotomy and/or excision of herniated intervertebral disc, including open or endoscopically-assisted approach; one interspace, cervical**

63030 **Laminotomy (hemilaminectomy), with decompression of nerve root(s), including partial facetectomy, foraminotomy and/or excision of herniated intervertebral disc, including open or endoscopically-assisted approach; one interspace, lumbar**

+63035 **each additional interspace, cervical or lumbar (List separately in additional to code for primary procedure.)**

Compare these two different codes. What's the difference?

63020	63030
Laminotomy (hemilaminectomy)	Laminotomy (hemilaminectomy)
With decompression of nerve root(s)	With decompression of nerve root(s)
Including partial facetectomy, foraminotomy and/or excision of herniated intervertebral disc	Including partial facetectomy, foraminotomy and/or excision of herniated intervertebral disc
Including open or endoscopically-assisted approach	Including open or endoscopically-assisted approach
One interspace, cervical	One interspace, lumbar

You can see that the only difference between the two code descriptions is the location of the vertebra being treated. This is a piece of information you will need to determine the correct code.

Then, depending upon how many discs were involved, you might add

+63035 **each additional interspace, cervical or lumbar**

CODING BITES

CPT describes a vertebral interspace as the nonbony compartment between two adjacent vertebral bodies. This space houses the intervertebral disc and includes the nucleus pulposus, the annulus fibrosus, and two cartilaginous endplates.

Arthrodesis

Arthrodesis The immobilization of a joint using a surgical technique.

Arthrodesis is the surgical immobilization of a joint so that the bones can heal, or grow solidly, together. While this is most often performed on the spine, it also can be done on any joint in the body, including ankle, elbow, shoulder, etc.

When coding arthrodesis, you will need to identify the approach technique used by the physician, such as

- Lateral extracavitary technique.
- Anterior transoral or extraoral technique.
- Anterior interbody technique.
- Posterior technique: craniocervical or atlas-axis.
- Posterior or posterolateral technique.
- Posterior interbody technique with number of interspaces treated.

Arthrodesis can be performed alone or in combination with other procedures such as bone grafting, osteotomy, fracture care, vertebral corpectomy, or **laminectomy**. When arthrodesis is done at the same time as another procedure, modifier 51 Multiple Procedures should be appended to the code for the arthrodesis. This applies to almost all procedures, with the exception of bone grafting and instrumentation. Modifier 51 Multiple Procedures is not used in those cases because bone grafts and instrumentation are never performed without arthrodesis.

Laminectomy
The surgical removal of a vertebral posterior arch.

LET'S CODE IT! SCENARIO

Caryn Philips, a 51-year-old female, was diagnosed with degenerative disc disease 3 months ago. She is admitted today for Dr. Cheffer to perform a posterior arthrodesis of L5–S1 (transverse process), utilizing a morselized autogenous iliac bone graft harvested through a separate fascial incision. Caryn tolerates the procedure well and is returned to her hospital room after 2 hours in recovery.

Let's Code It!

Pull out the description of the procedures that Dr. Cheffer performed. First, note the "*posterior arthrodesis of L5–S1*" and then the "*morselized autogenous iliac bone graft harvested through a separate fascial incision.*"

Let's begin in the Alphabetic Index with the listing for *arthrodesis*. The designation of L5–S1 tells you this was done to Caryn's spine. However, *spine* isn't listed under arthrodesis. Keep reading and you will see *vertebra* listed, *lumbar* underneath that, and *posterior* beneath that. However, the physician noted "transverse process," which is listed here as well. Let's investigate code 22612, as suggested by the Alphabetic Index.

22612 Arthrodesis, posterior or posterolateral technique, single level; lumbar (with or without lateral transverse technique)

This matches the physician's notes.

Now, let's move to the next procedure performed. Look in the Alphabetic Index under *bone graft*. Read through the list until you reach the item that reflects what was done for Caryn: *spine surgery*. Indented below that you will see *autograft* (the same as *autogenous*) and then *morselized*. The index suggests code 20937. Turn to the numeric list and take a look at the code's description:

+20937 Autograft for spine surgery only (includes harvesting the graft); morselized (through separate skin or fascial incision)

Notice the symbol to the left of code 20937: **+**. The plus sign means this is an add-on code and it cannot be used alone. However, the notation below 20937 indicates that you are permitted to use this code along with 22612.

In addition, the guidelines state that when arthrodesis is performed with another procedure, you need to add modifier 51 to the arthrodesis code *except* when the other procedure is a bone graft. This is the case in Caryn's record, so the claim form for Caryn Phillip's surgery will show procedure codes 22612 and 20937—with no modifiers. Great job!

GUIDANCE CONNECTION

Read the additional explanations in the in-section guidelines within the **Surgery** section, subhead **Spine**, subsection **Arthrodesis**, directly above code 22532 in your CPT book.

Skeletal Fixation

Whether the fracture is open or closed, it may require fixation. *Internal fixation* is the process of placing plates and screws, or pins, or other devices directly onto or around the bone, inside of the patient. When *external fixation* is used, a device–such as a brace, cast, or halo–prevents motion in a certain area of the body. The care for a fracture also may include the external application of traction.

Percutaneous Skeletal Fixation
The insertion of fixation instruments (such as pins) placed across the fracture site. It may be done under x-ray imaging for guidance purposes.

It is not always necessary for the physician to visualize the specific fracture directly, yet some type of immobilization is required to ensure proper healing. X-ray imaging is used to provide guidance so pins or other fixation can be accurately applied. This is known as **percutaneous skeletal fixation** because the procedure is not an open procedure, yet it is not completely closed either.

EXAMPLE

25606 Percutaneous skeletal fixation of distal radial fracture or epiphyseal separation

External fixation, as the name implies, is the attachment of skeletal pins along with a device to provide stability and corrective action on either a permanent or temporary basis. This is only reported separately when this portion of the process is not already part of the procedure.

EXAMPLE

21454 Open treatment of mandibular fracture with external fixation

Internal fixation is, most often, applied directly to the bone during an open procedure or treatment.

EXAMPLE

29855 Arthroscopically aided treatment of tibial fracture, proximal (plateau); unicondylar, includes internal fixation, when performed (includes arthroscopy)

GUIDANCE CONNECTION

Read the additional explanations in the in-section guidelines located within the **Surgery** section, subhead **Spine (Vertebral Column)**, subsection **Fracture and/or Dislocation**, directly above code 22310 in your CPT book.

LET'S CODE IT! CASE SCENARIO

Peter Kessler, a 17-year-old male, plays basketball on his high school team. While practicing in his driveway, he fell and fractured the shaft of his tibia. Dr. Warden, the orthopedist on duty at the emergency room, is able to use a percutaneous fixation using pins.

Let's Code It!

Let's turn to the Alphabetic Index. This time, we won't look up the procedure by the type of treatment (*percutaneous*), but we will look at the condition that was treated: *fracture*. Under *fracture*, find the anatomical site of the fracture—*tibia*—and then the *percutaneous fixation*. The index suggests code 27756. Let's check the description in the numeric listing:

27756 Percutaneous skeletal fixation of tibial shaft fracture (with or without fibular fracture) (e.g., pins or screws)

That's exactly what Dr. Warden did. Great job!

Spinal Procedures

There are several procedures often performed on patients with spinal concerns:

- *Arthrodesis* is the surgical immobilization of a joint.
- *Arthroplasty* is the insertion of an artificial disc.
- *Discectomy* is the surgical removal of an intervertebral disc, either a portion of the disc or the entire component.
- *Laminectomy* is the surgical removal of the lamina (posterior arch) of the vertebra.
- *Osteotomy* is performed to remove, or cut out, a portion of a bone.
- *Vertebroplasty* and *kyphoplasty* may be performed surgically or percutaneously for the purpose of repairing a vertebra that has been compromised by a compression fracture.

Spinal Fusion

Spinal fusion permanently locks two or more spinal vertebrae together so that they move as a single unit utilizing bone grafts, with or without screws, plates, cages, or other devices. The bone grafts are placed around the problem area of the spine during surgery. As the body heals itself, the graft helps join the bones together.

Performed under general anesthesia, fusion of lumbar vertebrae is generally done using a posterior lumbar approach, whereas cervical vertebrae are accessed using an anterior cervical approach. An anterior thoracic approach is normally used for fusion of thoracic vertebrae.

Spinal fusion is known to diminish mobility because of the connections made between the individual vertebrae involved in the procedure. This is one of the primary reasons health care technology has been working diligently on an artificial intervertebral disc that can continue to permit individual vertebral motion. Artificial discs have been evidenced to allow for six degrees of freedom.

GUIDANCE CONNECTION

Read the additional explanations in the in-section guidelines located within the **Surgery** section, subhead **Spine (Vertebral Column)**, subsection **Spinal Instrumentation**, directly above code 22840 in your CPT book.

After removing the ineffective or damaged disc, two metal plates are pressed into the bony endplates above and below the interspace and held into place by metal spikes. A plastic spacer, usually made of a polyethylene core, is inserted between the plates. The patient's own body weight compresses the spacer after the surgery is complete.

YOU CODE IT! CASE STUDY

Allyssa Erickson, an 83-year-old female, fell and sustained a fracture to the C4 vertebral body. Due to the position of the fracture, Dr. Rubbine was able to use a closed treatment without having to put her through a surgical procedure. Dr. Rubbine then put Allyssa into a brace.

You Code It!

Go through the steps, and determine what procedure code(s) should be reported for this encounter between Dr. Rubbine and Allyssa Erickson.

Step #1: Read the case carefully and completely.
Step #2: Abstract the scenario. Which key words or terms describe what service the physician provided to the patient during this encounter?
Step #3: Are there any details missing or incomplete for which you would need to query the physician? [If so, ask your instructor.]
Step #4: Determine the correct CPT procedure code or codes to explain the details about what was provided to the patient during this encounter.
Step #5: Check for any relevant guidance, including reading all of the symbols and notations.
Step #6: Do you need to append any modifiers to ensure complete and accurate information is provided?
Step #7: Double-check your work.

(continued)

Answer:

Did you find this to be the correct code?

22310 **Closed treatment of vertebral body fracture(s), without manipulation, requiring and including casting or bracing**

Great job!

Lumbar Puncture (Spinal Tap)

When a patient exhibits certain signs and symptoms, the physician may decide to perform a lumbar puncture, commonly known as a spinal tap. In this procedure, a needle is inserted into the spinal canal between two lumbar vertebrae to collect cerebrospinal fluid (CSF).

The two key procedure codes are differentiated by the reason the procedure is performed—diagnostic or therapeutic.

62270 **Spinal puncture, lumbar, diagnostic;**

62272 **Spinal puncture, therapeutic, for drainage of cerebrospinal fluid (by needle or catheter);**

26.7 Respiratory System

The organs and tissues involved with bringing oxygen into the body and discharging gases make up the respiratory system. Procedures and treatments affecting this sector are coded from the **Respiratory System** subsection.

GUIDANCE CONNECTION

Read the additional explanations in the in-section guidelines located within the **Surgery** section, subhead **Respiratory System**, subsection **Endoscopy**, directly above code 31231 in your CPT book.

Sinus Endoscopy

The upper respiratory system includes the nasal passages and sinus cavities. The standard for a nasal/sinus endoscopic procedure, performed for diagnostic purposes, includes assessment of the interior nasal cavity, the middle and superior meatus, the turbinates, and the sphenoethmoid recess. Therefore, the inspection of all of these areas is included in the diagnostic sinus endoscopy procedure code.

When a surgical sinus endoscopy is provided, the code descriptions include both the sinusotomy and a diagnostic endoscopy.

LET'S CODE IT! SCENARIO

Epharim Habbati, a 41-year-old male, had been diagnosed with chronic sinusitis many years ago and has tried everything. He told Dr. Tolber that no medication has worked and the inflammation just won't go away. Dr. Tolber performed a nasal/sinus diagnostic endoscopy via the inferior meatus, with a maxillary sinusoscopy.

Let's Code It!

The documentation explains that Dr. Tolber performed a "*diagnostic endoscopy via the inferior meatus, with a maxillary sinusoscopy,*" so let's turn to the CPT Alphabetic Index and find *endoscopy*. You can see a long list of anatomical sites beneath. On what anatomical site did Dr. Tolber perform this endoscopy? The notes state "*nasal/sinus.*" Find the term *nose* under *endoscopy* and you will see there are three choices: *Diagnostic*, *Surgical*, and *Unlisted Services and Procedures*. Let's go back to the notes and find out which of these is most appropriate. The notes state specifically "*diagnostic endoscopy.*" The Alphabetic Index suggests a range of codes: 31231–31235. Let's turn to the *Main Portion* of CPT to read the complete code descriptions.

(continued)

31231 **Nasal endoscopy, diagnostic; unilateral or bilateral (separate procedure)**

31233 **Nasal/sinus endoscopy, diagnostic; with maxillary sinusoscopy (via inferior meatus or canine fossa puncture)**

31235 **Nasal/sinus endoscopy, diagnostic; with sphenoid sinusoscopy (via puncture of sphenoidal face or cannulation of ostium)**

Let's go back to the physician's notes to confirm exactly what was done for Mr. Habbati.

diagnostic endoscopy . . . all three code choices include this term

via the inferior meatus . . . only code 31233 mentions the inferior meatus specifically

with a maxillary sinusoscopy . . . only code 31233 mentions the maxillary sinusoscopy

The code description for 31233 matches the notes and is our most accurate code to report.

Pleural and Lung Biopsies

A biopsy of the pleural tissue or lung tissue may be accomplished in one of several different ways.

Percutaneous Needle

When a percutaneous needle biopsy is performed, a hollow needle is inserted through a tiny incision and directed toward the internal area, typically with the support of imaging guidance. Only local anesthesia is used, and with only tiny incisions to mend, getting back to normal daily activities is quick.

32400 **Biopsy, pleura, percutaneous needle**

32405 **Biopsy, lung or mediastinum, percutaneous needle**

Thoracotomy with Biopsy

When a thoracotomy is performed, along with a lung or pleural biopsy, the patient's chest is surgically opened (an open procedure rather than a percutaneous approach). You will need to abstract, from the documentation, if the biopsy is performed to establish a diagnosis (diagnostic biopsy) or for therapeutic purposes (to surgically remove the abnormal tissues).

32096 **Thoracotomy, with diagnostic biopsy of lung infiltrate (e.g., wedge, incisional), unilateral**

32097 **Thoracotomy, with diagnostic biopsy of lung nodule or masses (e.g., wedge, incisional), unilateral**

32098 **Thoracotomy, with biopsy(ies) of pleura**

NOTE: Other thoracotomy procedures can be reported with a code from the range of 32100–32160.

CPT

YOU CODE IT! CASE STUDY

Harrison Matthews, a 37-year-old male, was having frequent nosebleeds. Finally, after all other methods failed to provide relief, Dr. French performed an endoscopic surgical procedure to control his nasal hemorrhages.

You Code It!

Review the details of what Dr. French did for Harrison Matthews, and determine the CPT code or codes.

Step #1: Read the case carefully and completely.

Step #2: Abstract the scenario. Which key words or terms describe what service the physician provided to the patient during this encounter?

(continued)

Step #3: Are there any details missing or incomplete for which you would need to query the physician? [If so, ask your instructor.]
Step #4: Determine the correct CPT procedure code or codes to explain the details about what was provided to the patient during this encounter.
Step #5: Check for any relevant guidance, including reading all of the symbols and notations.
Step #6: Do you need to append any modifiers to ensure complete and accurate information is provided?
Step #7: Double-check your work.

Answer:

Did you determine this to be the procedure code?

31238 Nasal/sinus endoscopy, surgical; with control of nasal hemorrhage

26.8 Cardiovascular System

Treatments and procedures on the heart as well as the entire network of veins, arteries, and capillaries are coded from the **Cardiovascular System** subsection.

Pacemakers

When a physician inserts a standard pacemaker system (CPT codes 33202–33275), the procedure includes the placement of a pulse generator into a subcutaneous envelope that has been created beneath the abdominal muscles distally to the ribs or placement in a subclavicular site. The generator itself contains a battery and one or more leads (electrodes) that are inserted transvenously (through a vein) or epicardially (on the surface of the heart) (see **Figure 26-4**).

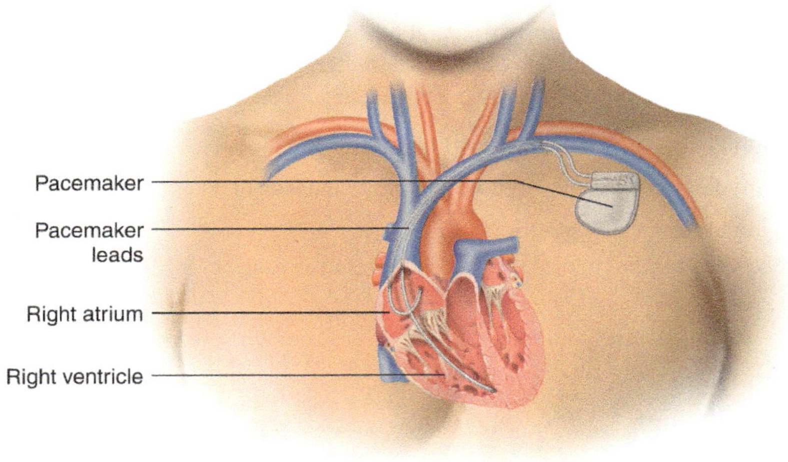

FIGURE 26-4 An illustration showing the location of all of the components of an implanted dual-lead pacemaker

When the epicardial placement is used, a thoracotomy or thoracoscopy is necessary to insert the electrodes accurately.

33202 Insertion of epicardial electrode(s); open incision (e.g., thoracotomy, median sternotomy, subxiphoid approach)

33203 Insertion of epicardial electrode(s); endoscopic approach (e.g., thoracoscopy, pericardioscopy)

When a physician inserts a single-chamber pacemaker system into a patient, it includes the pulse generator and one electrode inserted into *either* the atrium or the ventricle.

When a dual-chamber pacemaker system is placed, the system includes the pulse generator and one electrode into *both* the right atrium and the right ventricle.

When the pulse generator is inserted at the same encounter, report 33202 or 33203 in addition to

33212 Insertion of pacemaker pulse generator only; with existing single lead

33213 Insertion of pacemaker pulse generator only; with existing dual leads

33221 Insertion of pacemaker pulse generator only; with existing multiple leads

In addition to the insertion method (epicardial or transvenous), coders must abstract from the physician's documentation the specific chamber or chambers of the heart affected. These codes include the insertion of the pulse generator subcutaneously, the transvenous placement of the electrode or electrodes, and moderate (conscious) sedation. If, during the insertion process, the skin pocket requires revision, this is also included in these codes (and all others from 33206 through 33249).

33206 Insertion of new or replacement of permanent pacemaker with transvenous electrode(s); atrial

33207 Insertion of new or replacement of permanent pacemaker with transvenous electrode(s); ventricular

33208 Insertion of new or replacement of permanent pacemaker with transvenous electrode(s); atrial and ventricular

You may notice that these code descriptions include the term *replacement*, insinuating that the patient already had a pacemaker in place. It is important to note that these codes do not include the work to remove a previous system, only the insertion of a new one. To report the physician's services to remove a previous system and insert a replacement system (pulse generator and transvenous electrode(s)) during the same encounter, you will report

33233 Removal of permanent pacemaker pulse generator only

+

33234 Removal of transvenous pacemaker electrode(s); single lead system, atrial or ventricular

or

33235 Removal of transvenous pacemaker electrode(s); dual lead system + *One of these codes: 33206 or 33207 or 33208*

When the physician documents that the patient has been upgraded from a single-chamber system to a dual-chamber system, the removal of the existing pulse generator and the insertion of the new dual-chamber system are reported with one code:

33214 Upgrade of implanted pacemaker system, conversion of single chamber system to dual chamber system (includes removal of previously placed pulse generator, testing of existing lead, insertion of new lead, insertion of new pulse generator)

For some patients, the physician determines that an additional lead (electrode) inserted into the left ventricle would be beneficial. This is known as *biventricular pacing*. When this additional electrode is inserted, it is separately reported:

33224 Insertion of pacing electrode, cardiac venous system, for left ventricular pacing, with attachment to previously placed pacemaker or pacing cardioverter-defibrillator pulse generator (including revision of pocket, removal, insertion, and/or replacement of existing generator)

or

+33225 Insertion of pacing electrode, cardiac venous system, for left ventricular pacing, at time of insertion of pacing cardioverter-defibrillator or pacemaker pulse generator (e.g., for upgrade to dual chamber system) (List separately in addition to code for primary procedure)

Commonly referred to as replacing the battery in the pacemaker or cardioverter-defibrillator, this procedure involves the removal of the old pulse generator and the insertion of a new pulse generator. These two actions should be coded individually–one code for the removal of the old and another code for the insertion of the new. When this is documented, report the code determined by the number of leads (electrodes) already in place:

33227 Removal of permanent pacemaker pulse generator with replacement of pacemaker pulse generator; single lead system

33228 Removal of permanent pacemaker pulse generator with replacement of pacemaker pulse generator; dual lead system

33229 Removal of permanent pacemaker pulse generator with replacement of pacemaker pulse generator; multiple lead system

After a length of time, some patients may develop an erosion of the dermal and subcutaneous tissues, or an infection, at the location of the pulse generator. A situation of this nature may require the physician to relocate the "pocket." When this is documented, report the physician's services with this:

33222 **Relocation of skin pocket for pacemaker**

Reporting the insertion and replacement of a pacing cardioverter-defibrillator (ICD) system is very similar, but often does require different codes from within this subsection of CPT.

33249 **Insertion or replacement of permanent implantable defibrillator system, with transvenous lead(s), single or dual chamber**

33270 **Insertion or replacement of permanent subcutaneous implantable defibrillator system, with subcutaneous electrode, including defibrillation threshold evaluation, induction of arrhythmia, evaluation of sensing for arrhythmia termination, and programming or reprogramming of sensing or therapeutic parameters, when performed**

33271 **Insertion of subcutaneous implantable defibrillator electrode**

GUIDANCE CONNECTION

Read the additional explanations in the in-section guidelines located within the **Surgery** section, subhead **Cardiovascular System**, subsection **Pacemaker or Implantable Defibrillator**, directly above code 33202 in your CPT book.

Implantable Defibrillators

Pacing cardioverter-defibrillator systems are similar to pacemaker systems. While they also consist of a pulse generator and electrodes, the units may use several leads inserted into a single chamber (ventricle) or into dual chambers (atrium and ventricle) (**Figure 26-4**). The system is actually a combination of antitachycardia pacing, low-energy cardioversion, and/or defibrillating shocks to address a patient's ventricular tachycardia or ventricular fibrillation.

In some cases, an additional electrode may be needed to regulate the pacing of the left ventricle, called *biventricular pacing*. When this occurs, the placement of the electrode transvenously should be coded separately, just as the pacemaker is coded, with either 33224 or 33225.

Leadless Pacemakers

An intracardiac pacemaker functions in much the same way as other pacemakers to regulate heart rate. However, these newly FDA-approved units are self-contained, one-inch-long devices that are implanted directly into the right ventricle chamber of the heart, and have _no_ leads and _no_ pockets. This pulse generator has an internal battery and electrode and is inserted into a cardiac chamber by transfemoral catheter (through an artery in the thigh). No incision or creation of a pocket reduces the opportunity for infection and eliminates unsightly scars. No leads avoid the repercussions of lead failure and result in no possible discomfort when moving, increasing mobility for the patient.

33274 **Transcatheter insertion or replacement of permanent leadless pacemaker, right ventricular, including imaging guidance (e.g., fluoroscopy, venous ultrasound, ventriculography, femoral venography) and device evaluation (e.g., interrogation or programming), when performed**

33275 **Transcatheter removal of permanent leadless pacemaker, right ventricular, including imaging guidance (e.g., fluoroscopy, venous ultrasound, ventriculography, femoral venography), when performed**

Bypass Grafting

Venous Grafts

Saphenous Vein
Either of the two major veins in the leg that run from the foot to the thigh near the surface of the skin.

When a venous graft is performed, use codes from the range 33510–33516. All these codes include a **saphenous vein** graft.

However, if the graft is harvested from an upper extremity (arm) vein, you need to code this separately, using code 35500, in addition to the code for the bypass procedure itself.

+35500 **Harvest of upper extremity vein, 1 segment, for lower extremity or coronary artery bypass procedure (List separately in addition to code for primary procedure.)**

+35572 **Harvest of femoropopliteal vein, one segment, for vascular reconstruction procedure (e.g., aortic, vena caval, coronary, peripheral artery) (List separately in addition to code for primary procedure.)**

> **CODING BITES**
>
> The same exceptions apply as before: if the graft is harvested from an upper extremity artery, code it separately from the bypass procedure, using code 35600. And if the graft is obtained from the femoropopliteal vein, code it with 35572 in addition to the code for the bypass procedure.

Combined Arterial-Venous Grafts

When both venous grafts and arterial grafts are used during the same procedure, you will use two codes. First, code the combined arterial-venous graft from the range 33517-33523. Just like the codes for the venous grafts, these include getting the graft from the saphenous vein. Second, code the appropriate arterial graft from the range 33533-33536. Harvesting the arterial vein section is included in those codes.

GUIDANCE CONNECTION

Read the additional explanations in the in-section guidelines within the **Surgery** section, subhead **Cardiovascular System**, subsection **Venous Grafting Only for Coronary Artery Bypass**, directly above code 33510 in your CPT book.

Arterial Grafts

When an arterial graft is performed, use codes from the range 33533-33536. All these codes include the use of grafts from the internal mammary artery, gastroepiploic artery, epigastric artery, radial artery, and arterial conduits harvested from other sites. For example, examine the following code descriptions:

33533 **Coronary artery bypass, using arterial graft(s); single arterial graft**

33534 **Coronary artery bypass, using arterial graft(s); 2 coronary arterial grafts**

33535 **Coronary artery bypass, using arterial graft(s); 3 coronary arterial grafts**

33536 **Coronary artery bypass, using arterial graft(s); 4 or more coronary arterial grafts**

Use one of the following codes (in addition to the code for the bypass procedure) if the graft is harvested from another site:

- From an upper extremity artery, add code 35600.
- From an upper extremity vein, add code 35500.
- From the femoropopliteal vein, use code 35572.

GUIDANCE CONNECTION

Read the additional explanations in the in-section guidelines within the **Surgery** section, subhead **Cardiovascular System**, subsection **Combined Arterial-Venous Grafting for Coronary Bypass**, directly above code 33517 in your CPT book.

Composite Grafts

When two or more vein segments are harvested from a limb other than that part of the body undergoing the bypass, you must use the best, most appropriate code from the range 35681-35683 to report the harvesting and anastomosis of the multiple vein segments.

+35681 **Bypass graft; composite, prosthetic and vein (List separately in addition to code for primary procedure.)**

+35682 **Bypass graft; autogenous composite, two segments of veins from two locations (List separately in addition to code for primary procedure.)**

+35683 **Bypass graft; autogenous composite, three or more segments of vein from two or more locations (List separately in addition to code for primary procedure.)**

A little confusing? Hopefully, **Table 26-1** will help you organize all the rules for coding bypass grafts.

TABLE 26-1 Bypass Grafts

Graft	Harvested from	Use Code(s)
Venous graft	Saphenous vein	Choose from 33510 to 33516
Venous graft	Upper extremity vein	Choose from 33510 to 33516; + 35500
Venous graft	Femoropopliteal vein	Choose from 33510 to 33516; + 35572
Arterial-venous	Saphenous vein	Choose from 33517 to 33523; + choose from 33533 to 33536
Arterial-venous	Upper extremity vein	Choose from 33510 to 33516; + choose from 33533 to 33536; + 35500
Arterial-venous	Upper extremity artery	Choose from 33510 to 33516; + choose from 33533 to 33536; + 35600
Arterial-venous	Femoropopliteal vein	Choose from 33510 to 33516; + choose from 33533 to 33536; + 35572
Arterial graft	Internal mammary artery Gastroepiploic artery Epigastric artery Radial artery Arterial conduits from other sites	Choose from 33533 to 33545
Arterial graft	Upper extremity vein	Choose from 33533 to 33545; + 35500
Arterial graft	Upper extremity artery	Choose from 33533 to 33545; + 35600
Arterial graft	Femoropopliteal vein	Choose from 33533 to 33545; + 35572
Composite graft	Two or more segments from another part of body	+ 35682 or 35683

Arteries and Veins

The primary vascular procedure codes 34001-37799 include

1. Ensuring both the inflow and the outflow of the arteries and/or veins involved (**Figure 26-5**).
2. The operative arteriogram that is performed by the surgeon during the procedure.
3. Sympathectomy for aortic procedures.

GUIDANCE CONNECTION

Read the additional explanations in the in-section guidelines within the **Surgery** section, subhead **Cardiovascular System**, subsection **Arterial Grafting for Coronary Artery Bypass**, directly above code 33533 in your CPT book.

Endovascular Repair of Abdominal Aorta and/or Iliac Arteries

There are many therapeutic procedures available to treat conditions affecting the abdominal aorta and/or iliac arteries. Often, this involves the insertion, positioning, or deployment of a device known as a covered stent (see **Figure 26-6**). You may find the physician documentation may specify an endograft, endovascular graft, stentgraft, tube endograft, or endoprosthesis–all of which are variations of a stent.

CPT codes 34701 through 34834 provide the details of these various procedures from which you can determine the code that best reports where [which artery] as well as what specifically was done for this patient.

GUIDANCE CONNECTION

Read the additional information in the in-section guidelines within the **Surgery** section, subhead **Cardiovascular System**, subsection **Endovascular Repair of Abdominal Aortic and/or Iliac Arteries,** directly above code 34701 in your CPT book.

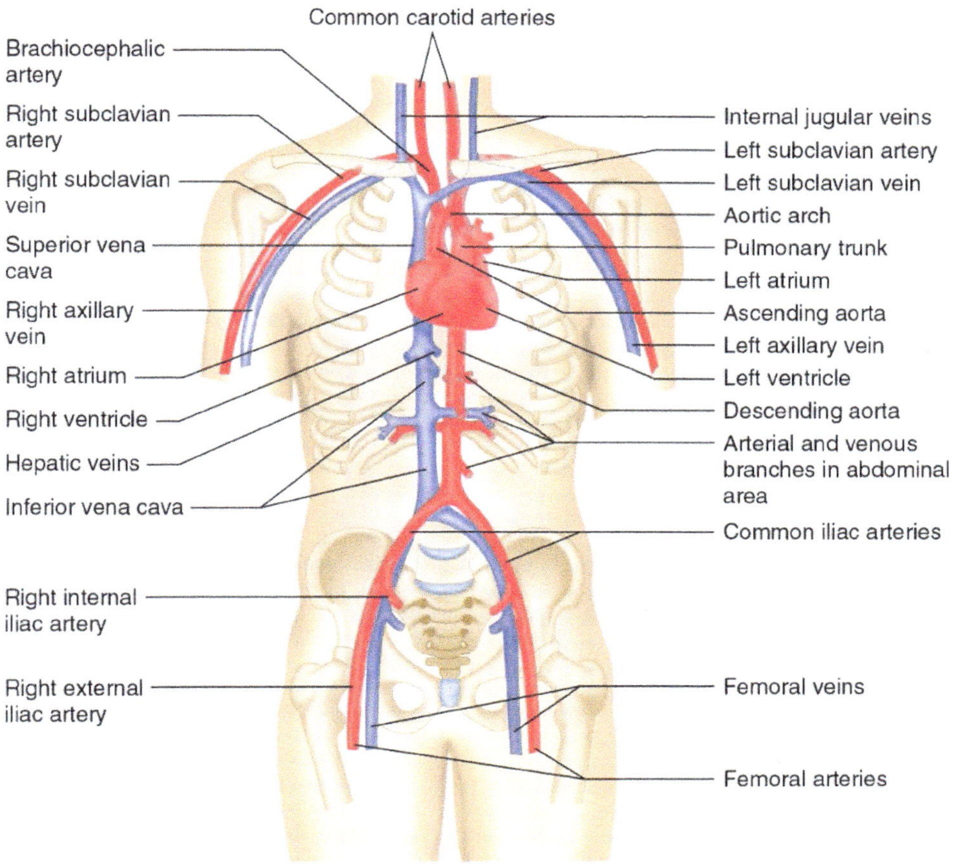

FIGURE 26-5 An illustration showing some of the arteries and veins of the body

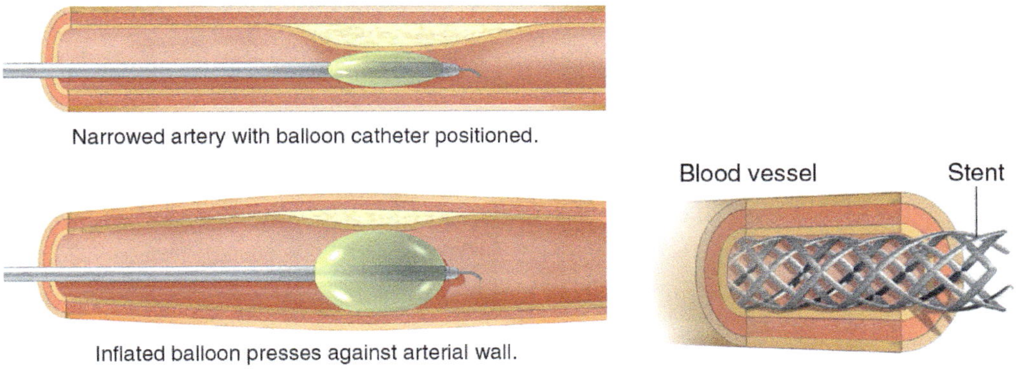

FIGURE 26-6 Illustrations of a balloon catheterization and the placement of a stent

YOU CODE IT! CASE STUDY

Jason Antone, a 54-year-old, was admitted to the hospital by Dr. Sabrina Jordan, for treatment of a chronic, contained rupture of an aneurysm of the infrarenal aorta. Jason was prepped and draped in the usual manner, and the procedure to deploy an aorto-bi-iliac endograft was performed.

(continued)

You Code It!

Go through the steps, and determine the procedure code(s) that should be reported for this encounter between Dr. Jordan and Jason Antone.

Step #1: Read the case carefully and completely.
Step #2: Abstract the scenario. Which key words or terms describe what service the physician provided to the patient during this encounter?
Step #3: Are there any details missing or incomplete for which you would need to query the physician? [If so, ask your instructor.]
Step #4: Determine the correct CPT procedure code or codes to explain the details about what was provided to the patient during this encounter.
Step #5: Check for any relevant guidance, including reading all of the symbols and notations.
Step #6: Do you need to append any modifiers to ensure complete and accurate information is provided?
Step #7: Double-check your work.

Answer:

Did you determine this to be the correct code?

34705 Endovascular repair of infrarenal aorta and/or iliac artery(ies) by deployment of an aorto-bi-iliac endograft . . .

Good job!

Catheterizations and Vascular Families

Understanding the vascular families can be useful to coders when reporting the provision of a catheterization. **Table 26-2**, **Table 26-3**, and **Table 26-4** show some examples of the vascular orders when reporting the catheterization of the aorta. The catheterization of the femoral or carotid arteries would each have their own families, of course. A full listing can be found in your CPT code book, ***Appendix L, Vascular Families***.

TABLE 26-2 Vascular Families: Superior Mesenteric

First Order	Second Order Branch	Third Order Branch
Superior mesenteric	Middle colic	
	Inferior pancreaticoduodenal	Posterior inferior pancreaticoduodenal
		Anterior inferior pancreaticoduodenal
	Jejunal	
	Ileocolic	
	Appendicular	
	Posterior cecal	
	Anterior cecal	
	Marginal	
	Right colic	

A vascular family begins with the vessel that branches off from the aorta, femoral artery, or carotid artery and continues to track all vessels that branch from that. For example, in **Table 26-2**, in the first order (first column), you see the superior mesenteric, which is one of the arteries that branch off the aorta. The middle colic, interior pancreaticoduodenal, jejunal, ileocolic, appendicular, posterior cecal, anterior cecal, marginal, and right colic arteries all branch off the superior mesenteric. From this point, only the interior pancreaticoduodenal has additional vessels branching off it—the posterior inferior pancreaticoduodenal and the anterior inferior pancreaticoduodenal.

TABLE 26-3 Vascular Families: Left Common Carotid

First Order	Second Order Branch	Third Order Branch
Left common carotid	Left internal carotid	Left ophthalmic
		Left posterior communicating
		Left middle cerebral
		Left anterior cerebral
	Left external carotid	Left superior thyroid
		Left ascending pharyngeal
		Left facial
		Left lingual
		Left occipital
		Left posterior auricular
		Left superficial temporal
		Left internal maxillary

LET'S CODE IT! SCENARIO

Lisa Westerly, an 11-week-old female, was diagnosed with ventricular septal defect (VSD) after her pediatrician, Dr. Harris, ordered an echocardiography. A large VSD was identified in the septum. Due to the size of the defect, Dr. Harris admitted Lisa into the hospital today to close the defect with a patch graft.

Let's Code It!

Review the notes and abstract the key terms. Let's go to the Alphabetic Index and look up *closure*, the procedure being performed. Under the word *closure*, you will find *septal defect*, ventricular which suggests three codes: 33776, 33780, 93581.

While we are in the Alphabetic Index, let's try one other way to look up the code. Let's go to *heart*, the anatomical site where the procedure is being performed. When you read the column below *heart*, you will see *septal defect*, which directs you to *See* Septal Defect. You also can look in the Alphabetic Index under the term *repair* (another word for the procedure being done). Under *repair*, find the anatomical site *heart*, then below that *septal defect*, which suggests 33545, 33608–33610, 33681–33688, 33692–33697, 33782, 33783. Indented below this adds *atrial and ventricular* with only one code suggestion—33647. *Ventricular septal defect septum* is a more specific match to the physician's notes than *septal defect*, but not exactly? Not certain? That's great because you need to let the actual code descriptions in the numeric listing give you more details before you make a decision. Therefore, you need to check them all.

This is where time and patience are important to the coding process. Read carefully through the description of each code suggested by the Alphabetic Index. You will probably agree that the best, most appropriate code is

33681 Closure of single ventricular septal defect, with or without patch

Great job!

Central Venous Access Procedures

Venous access devices (VADs) can be challenging to report because of the various types of procedures involved with their insertion as well as the multitude of purposes for the procedure itself. According to the CPT guidelines, the tip of the VAD or catheter must come to an end in the subclavian vein, brachiocephalic (innominate) vein, iliac vein, superior or inferior vena cava, or right atrium of the heart to be considered a *central* VAD or catheter.

TABLE 26-4 Vascular Families: Common Iliac

First Order	Second Order Branch	Third Order Branch	Beyond Third Order Branches
Common iliac	Internal iliac	Iliolumbar	
		Lateral sacral	
		Superior gluteal	
		Umbilical	
		Superior vesical	
		Obturator	
		Inferior vesical	
		Middle rectal	
		Inferior rectal	
		Internal pudendal	
		Inferior gluteal	
	External iliac	Inferior epigastric	Cremasteric
			Pubic
		Deep circumflex iliac	Ascending deep circumflex iliac
	Common femoral	Profunda femoris	Medial descending
			Perforating branches
			Lateral descending
			Lateral circumflex
		Deep external pudendal	
		Superficial external pudendal	
		Ascending lateral circumflex femoral	
		Descending lateral circumflex femoral	
		Transverse lateral circumflex femoral	
		Superficial femoral	Geniculate
			Popliteal
			Anterior tibial
			Peroneal
			Posterior tibial

Catheter or Device

A catheter is a tube that is used for various medical reasons. It may be inserted to withdraw bodily fluids, as a urinary catheter collects urine from the bladder. Catheters also can be used to deliver medications, such as an intravenous (IV) injection of drugs directly into the patient's veins. In addition, catheters can be used as a vehicle to enable the insertion of a device such as a stent.

In this usage, a device is most often a subcutaneous pump or a subcutaneous port designed to achieve ongoing access internally without the need to repeatedly obtain a new entry site.

Entry Site: Centrally Inserted or Peripherally Inserted

For these procedures, it is important to the coding process that you read the physician's notes carefully to determine exactly where on the patient's body the VAD or catheter was inserted. A centrally inserted device enters the body at the jugular, subclavian, or femoral vein or the inferior vena cava. A VAD or catheter that enters the body at either the basilic vein or the cephalic vein is called a peripherally inserted central catheter, often referred to by its initials–a PICC line.

Nontunneled or Tunneled

A tunneled catheter does exactly as its name describes–it tunnels under the skin. These tubes are more flexible; they are inserted into a vein at one location, such as the neck, chest, or groin, and wended through beneath the skin to emerge at a separate site in the body. A nontunneled catheter is inserted directly into the vein by venipuncture.

GUIDANCE CONNECTION

Read the additional explanations in the in-section guidelines within the **Surgery** section, subhead **Cardiovascular System**, subsection **Central Venous Access Procedures**, directly above code 36555 in your CPT book.

YOU CODE IT! CASE STUDY

Elias McGynty is a 54-year-old male who has significant multivessel coronary artery disease. He has atypical anginal symptoms, which are probably secondary to his insulin-dependent (type 1) diabetes mellitus. Nonetheless, he is at risk for ischemia, and in order to reduce this risk, surgical myocardial revascularization is recommended.

PROCEDURE: A coronary artery bypass graft operation utilizing the left internal mammary artery as conduit to the left anterior descending. The remaining conduit will come from the greater saphenous veins. The risks and benefits of this procedure were explained to the patient. He signed the informed consent. The patient tolerated the procedure well and was brought into recovery conscious and aware.

Francis Lamiere, MD

You Code It!

Dr. Lamiere performed a coronary artery bypass graft on Elias McGynty. Determine the code or codes to report this work.

Step #1: Read the case carefully and completely.
Step #2: Abstract the scenario. Which key words or terms describe what service the physician provided to the patient during this encounter?
Step #3: Are there any details missing or incomplete for which you would need to query the physician? [If so, ask your instructor.]
Step #4: Determine the correct CPT procedure code or codes to explain the details about what was provided to the patient during this encounter.
Step #5: Check for any relevant guidance, including reading all of the symbols and notations.
Step #6: Do you need to append any modifiers to ensure complete and accurate information is provided?
Step #7: Double-check your work.

Answer:

Did you determine these to be the correct codes?

33533 **Coronary artery bypass, using arterial graft(s); single coronary arterial grafts**

+33517 **Coronary artery bypass, using venous graft(s) and arterial graft(s); single venous graft**

26.9 Digestive System

The digestive tract begins at the mouth and travels through the body all the way to the anus. The organs along the pathway process food and nourishment so cells can absorb nutrients and eliminate waste. The digestive tract also is referred to as the alimentary canal or the gastrointestinal (GI) tract.

Endoscopic Procedures

There are times when a physician needs to visually examine and/or obtain a specimen for pathological testing of the interior of an organ, such as the throat, stomach, or bladder, in order to make a more accurate diagnosis. In these cases, an endoscope may be used.

An esophagogastroduodenoscopy (EGD), more commonly known as an upper endoscopy, enables the physician to view the patient's esophagus, stomach, and duodenum without a surgical invasion of the body.

Endoscopic retrograde cholangiopancreatography (ERCP) uses a combination of x-rays and the endoscope to enable visualization of the patient's stomach, the duodenum, and the bile ducts in the biliary tree and pancreas.

Sigmoidoscopy and colonoscopy are endoscopic procedures used to examine the internal aspects of the lower digestive system. A sigmoidoscopy permits the physician to visually investigate a patient's anus, rectum, and sigmoid colon. A colonoscopy permits the physician to look at the entire large intestine: the anus, the rectum, the descending (sigmoid) colon, the transverse colon, the ascending colon, and the cecum.

Endoscopy can be used for therapeutic procedures as well, as when Dr. Sanger had to remove a penny (foreign body) from little Billy's esophagus after he tried to swallow the coin, code 43247 Esophagogastroduodenoscopy, flexible, transoral; with removal of foreign body(s).

Gastric Intubation

The insertion of a nasogastric (NG) tube may be done for many reasons. The stomach contents may need to be removed, presurgery, postsurgery, or to remove ingested substances (commonly known as "pumping the stomach"). In other cases, the tube may be required to deliver nutrition directly into the stomach. This may be done for a patient after a surgical procedure on the esophagus or the esophogastric junction. Alternately, the tube may be inserted through the mouth instead of the nose, known as oro-gastric tube placement, or percutaneously through the abdominal wall, known as a gastrostomy tube.

EXAMPLES

43752 Naso- or oro-gastric tube placement, requiring physician's skill and fluoroscopic guidance (includes fluoroscopy, image documentation, and report)

43753 Gastric intubation and aspiration(s), therapeutic, necessitating physician's skill (e.g., for gastrointestinal hemorrhage), including lavage if performed

Hernia Repair

A hernia is a situation where an organ pushes through an abnormal opening within a muscle or other structure that contains it. A hernia may occur in the inner groin (inguinal hernia), in the outer groin (femoral hernia), in the umbilicus (umbilical hernia), between the esophagus and stomach (hiatal hernia), and as the result of an incision (an incisional hernia).

Of course, the procedure will be different to repair a hernia, as determined by the anatomical location. As you can see by looking in the CPT Alphabetic Index, just knowing the physician performed a hernia repair is not enough detail to determine the code. You must identify, from the documentation, the specific anatomical site.

As with many other procedures, hernia repair can be done as an open procedure or laparoscopically. With some types of hernias, you also may need to know the patient's age. Diaphragmatic, inguinal, and umbilicus hernias are known to occur in neonates and children. And more specifics are needed about the hernia itself: initial or recurrent; incarcerated or strangulated. All of these details also will impact the determination of the code to report.

YOU CODE IT! CASE STUDY

Thomas Mouldare, a 47-year-old male, was diagnosed with a diaphragmatic (hiatal) hernia that required surgery. Dr. Wallabee performed a Nissen fundoplication, laparoscopically. The upper area of the stomach (gastric fundus) is plicated (wrapped) around the distal portion of the esophagus. This is done to support and reinforce the effectiveness of the lower esophageal sphincter. Then, the esophageal hiatus is sutured to narrow the opening back to the correct width.

(continued)

You Code It!

Review the details in this case study, and determine the code or codes required to accurately report Dr. Wallabee's surgical procedure on Thomas Mouldare.

Step #1: Read the case carefully and completely.
Step #2: Abstract the scenario. Which key words or terms describe what service the physician provided to the patient during this encounter?
Step #3: Are there any details missing or incomplete for which you would need to query the physician? [If so, ask your instructor.]
Step #4: Determine the correct CPT procedure code or codes to explain the details about what was provided to the patient during this encounter.
Step #5: Check for any relevant guidance, including reading all of the symbols and notations.
Step #6: Do you need to append any modifiers to ensure complete and accurate information is provided?
Step #7: Double-check your work.

Answer:

Did you determine this to be the correct code?

43280 Laparoscopy, surgical, esophagogastric fundoplasty (e.g., Nissen, Toupet procedures)

Bariatric Surgery

Bariatric surgical procedures may be performed on the stomach, the duodenum, the jejunum, and/or the ileum and are most often provided to patients who have been diagnosed as morbidly obese. Consideration for performing this surgery may include the physician's evaluation of the candidate's eating behaviors as well as the patient's predisposition for serious obesity-related co-morbidities such as coronary heart disease, type 2 diabetes mellitus, and/or acute sleep apnea.

These surgeries may be performed as an open procedure or laparoscopically, and this detail will affect the determination of the correct code. The four most common versions of this surgery are

- *Adjustable gastric band (AGB).* See codes 43770–43774. AGB is a procedure that places a small, adjustable band to create a proximal pouch, thereby limiting the passage of food. The attending physician can increase or decrease the size of the passage using saline solution to inflate or deflate as needed for the patient's situation.
- *Roux-en-Y gastric bypass (RYGB).* See codes 43846, 43847, 43644. RYGB limits food intake by use of a small pouch that is similar in size to that created by the adjustable gastric band. In addition, absorption of food in the digestive tract is reduced by excluding most of the stomach, duodenum, and upper intestine from contact with food by routing food directly from the pouch into the small intestine.
- *Biliopancreatic diversion with a duodenal switch (BPD-DS).* See code 43845. BPD-DS, most often referred to as a "duodenal switch," includes transection of the stomach, a bypass to route digested material away from the small intestine, as well as re-routing bile and other digestive juices that impair digestion.
- *Vertical sleeve gastrectomy (VSG).* See code 43775. A VSG is performed and connected to a very short segment of the duodenum, which is then directly connected to a lower part of the small intestine. A small portion of the duodenum is untouched to provide passage for food and absorption of some vitamins and minerals. The distance between the stomach and colon is made much shorter after this operation, resulting in malabsorption.

A VSG procedure includes the resectioning of the stomach and is most often performed solely as the first stage of the multistaged BPD-DS on those patients determined to be unable to go through such a long procedure at one encounter. VSG is not without benefits, as research has shown that some VSG patients report significant weight loss. Should a second-stage procedure be performed, that second procedure and any others in the sequence would be reported with the appropriate procedure code appended by modifier 58 Staged Procedure.

During the postoperative period, adjustments of an adjustable gastric restrictive device are included in the global surgical package and therefore not coded separately.

GUIDANCE CONNECTION

Read the additional explanations in the in-section guidelines located within the **Surgery** section, subhead **Digestive System**, subsection **Bariatric Surgery**, directly above code 43770 in your CPT book.

LET'S CODE IT! SCENARIO

Justin Abernathy, a 61-year-old male, was suffering from fecal incontinence, diarrhea, and constipation. He came to the Ambulatory Care Center so that his gastroenterologist, Dr. Minton, could perform a colonoscopy. First, Ellen Brennon, RN, administered Demerol and Versed by IV, and the patient was brought into the examination room. The variable flexion Olympus colonoscope was introduced into the rectum and advanced to the cecum. In the midsigmoid colon, a 3-mm sessile polyp was destroyed. The procedure took about 30 minutes, and Justin tolerated the procedure well.

Let's Code It!

We know that the main procedure was a *colonoscopy*, so let's look that up in the Alphabetic Index. When you refer to the notes, what else was done for Justin in conjunction with the colonoscopy? *A polyp was destroyed.*

Find *destruction* beneath *colonoscopy*. Do you know whether a polyp is a lesion or a tumor? It happens to be a lesion; however, you don't have to know this because the index suggests the same code for both: 45388. Let's look at the complete description in the numeric listing.

45388 Colonoscopy, flexible; with ablation of tumor(s), polyp(s), or other lesion(s) (includes pre- and post-dilation and guide wire passage, when performed)

You also will need to code the administration of the moderate sedation that was given to Justin (the Demerol and Versed).

99156 Moderate sedation services provided by a physician or other qualified health care professional other than the physician or other qualified health care professional performing the diagnostic or therapeutic service that the sedation supports; initial 15 minutes of intraservice time, patient age 5 years or older

+99157 each additional 15 minutes of intraservice time (List separately in addition to code for primary service.)

You have three codes to report the whole story as to what Dr. Minton did for Justin during this encounter: **45388, 99156, 99157**.
Great job!

26.10 Urinary System

The urinary system is responsible for maintaining the proper level and composition of fluids in the body.

Urinary Catheterization

There are many reasons why a urinary catheter might need to be inserted: patients with incontinence, especially those who are chronically bedridden or those with lower paralysis; those about to go through a surgical procedure, especially when general anesthesia is administered; as well as patients who suffer from reduced or blocked urine flow, such as male patients with enlarged prostates or female patients with uterine fibroid tumors. A patient with reduced renal function may require a catheterization so health care professionals can accurately monitor their urinary output.

GUIDANCE CONNECTION

Read the additional explanations in the in-section guidelines within the **Surgery** section, subhead **Urinary System**, subsection **Urodynamics**, directly above code 51725 in your CPT book.

The documentation may include details, such as the type of catheter used, including a Foley, a Robinson, a Carson, or a Tieman catheter. Each type performs differently with various features, determined by the specific issue being addressed.

Urodynamics

The codes listed for the procedures in the **Urodynamics** section, 51725–51798, include the services of the physician to perform the procedure (or directly supervise the performance of the procedure), as well as the use of all instruments, equipment, fluids, gases, probes, catheters, technician's fees, medications, gloves, trays, tubing, and other sterile supplies.

If the physician for whom you are coding did not actually perform the procedure but only interpreted the results, then the appropriate procedure code from this section should be appended with modifier 26 Professional Component.

YOU CODE IT! CASE STUDY

Rachel Naviga, a 39-year-old female, G3 P3, states she has been dealing with stress incontinence increasingly over the last several years. She had three vaginal deliveries, with the largest infant weighing 7.5 lb. Rachel states that her leakage frequency, volume, timing, and associated symptoms (urgency, stress, urinary frequency, nocturia, enuresis, incomplete emptying, straining to empty, leakage without warning) have become bothersome and she wants to do something about it.

Today she presents for a complex cystometrogram with voiding pressure study to confirm or deny the diagnosis of stress urinary incontinence prior to the scheduling of surgery.

You Code It!

Go through the steps, and determine what procedure code(s) should be reported for the encounter with Rachel.

Step #1: Read the case carefully and completely.
Step #2: Abstract the scenario. Which key words or terms describe what service the physician provided to the patient during this encounter?
Step #3: Are there any details missing or incomplete for which you would need to query the physician? [If so, ask your instructor.]
Step #4: Determine the correct CPT procedure code or codes to explain the details about what was provided to the patient during this encounter.
Step #5: Check for any relevant guidance, including reading all of the symbols and notations.
Step #6: Do you need to append any modifiers to ensure complete and accurate information is provided?
Step #7: Double-check your work.

Answer:

Did you determine this to be the correct code?

51728 Complex cystometrogram (ie. calibrated electronic equipment); with voiding pressure studies (ie., bladder voiding pressure), any technique

Transurethral Surgery

When a diagnostic or therapeutic cystourethroscopic intervention is performed, the appropriate codes, 52204–52356, include the insertion and removal of a temporary stent. Therefore, those services are not reported separately—when done at the same time as the cystourethroscopy (**Figure 26-7**).

If the physician, however, inserts a self-retaining, indwelling stent during the diagnostic or therapeutic cystourethroscopic intervention, use one of the following:

1. Code 52332 with the modifier 51, along with the code for the cystourethroscopy for a unilateral procedure.
2. Code 52332 with modifier 50 for a bilateral insertion of self-retaining, indwelling ureteral stents.

Note that when the physician removes the self-retaining, indwelling ureteral stent, use either 52310 or 52315 with modifier 58.

LET'S CODE IT! SCENARIO

Ena Colby, a 41-year-old female, is admitted today for the surgical removal of a kidney stone. The stone was too big for her to pass, so Dr. Olympia decided to remove it surgically. The nephrolithotomy, with complete removal of the calculus, went as planned, and Ena tolerated the entire procedure well.

(continued)

Let's Code It!

Dr. Olympia performed a *nephrolithotomy*, involving the *removal of a kidney stone*, also known as *calculus*. Let's try something direct and look up *nephrolithotomy* in the Alphabetic Index.

The Alphabetic Index suggests the code range 50060–50075. Let's go to the numeric listing and read the different code descriptions.

Do you agree that, according to the physician's notes, the best, most appropriate code available is the following?

50060 Nephrolithotomy; removal of calculus

You are getting very good at this.

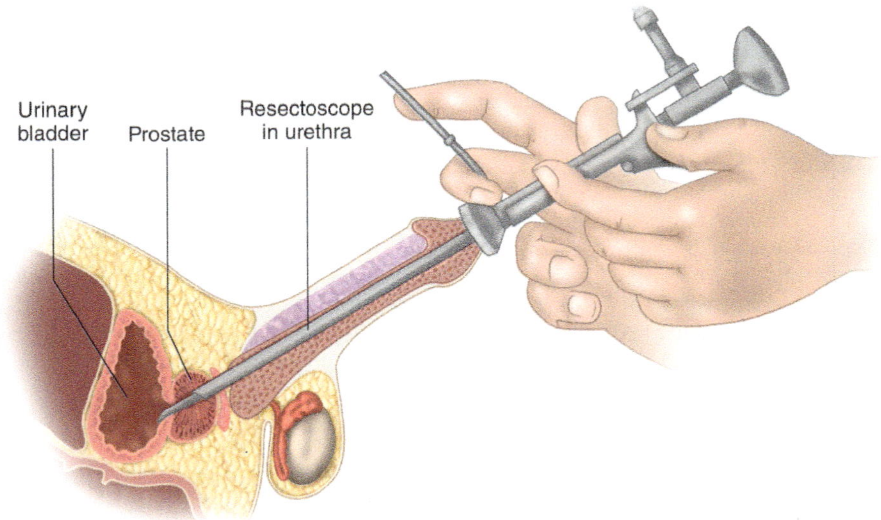

FIGURE 26-7 An illustration of a resectoscope inserted through the urethra of a male patient

Percutaneous Genitourinary Procedures

Diagnostic procedures, such as a nephrostogram or a ureterogram, are most often performed percutaneously, using some type of imaging to guide them. The most common are ultrasound and fluoroscopy.

A patient may have a nephrostomy catheter inserted due to ureter stenosis or obstruction preventing the flow of urine from the kidney to the bladder. A nephrostogram is done to confirm that the tube is positioned and working properly.

50432 Placement of nephrostomy catheter, percutaneous, including diagnostic nephrostogram and/or ureterogram when performed, imaging guidance (e.g., ultrasound and/or fluoroscopy) and all associated radiological supervision and interpretation

> **GUIDANCE CONNECTION**
>
> Read the additional explanations in the in-section guidelines within the **Surgery** section, subhead **Urinary System**, and throughout this subsection in your CPT book.

Wondering if you should also report a second code for the injection of the contrast material, such as code 50430 or 50431? No worries, just read the guidelines beneath 50432 and you will know exactly how to report this:

(Do not report 50432 in conjunction with 50430, 50431, 50432, 50694, 50695, 74425 for the same renal collecting system and/or associated ureter)

This informs you that you cannot report 50430 or 50431 at the same time with 50432. The guidelines are there to help you do this all correctly!

26.11 The Genital Systems: Male and Female

The Male Genital System

The male genital system is closely situated with the urinary bladder, so a urologist may be the specialist most often performing procedures on this area of the male anatomy.

Penile Plaque

This type of plaque is a flat layer of scar tissue that can form on the inside of a thick membrane called the tunica albuginea, which envelops the erectile tissues, and is known as Peyronie disease. This is believed to begin as an inflammation, and the plaque is benign, not contagious, and not sexually transmitted. However, it can cause discomfort and pain in men with this condition. There are several ways to treat the problem.

Injections of steroids and chemotherapy agents, such as interferon, can be directly delivered to the site of the plaque to work to reduce the effect. These procedures may be reported with

54200 Injection procedure for Peyronie disease

54205 Injection procedure for Peyronie disease; with surgical exposure of plaque

The plaque can be surgically removed. This procedure may be performed just to excise the plaque, or it may include the grafting of material to replace tissue that was excised.

54110 Excision of penile plaque (Peyronie disease)

54111 Excision of penile plaque (Peyronie disease); with graft to 5 cm in length

54112 Excision of penile plaque (Peyronie disease); with graft greater than 5 cm in length

Severe cases may require more extensive reconstruction and will be reported with code

54360 Plastic operation on penis to correct angulation

CPT

YOU CODE IT! CASE STUDY

Glenn Hagger, a 15-year-old male, came to see his regular physician, Dr. Carboni, for help. Glenn and his friends were fooling around at his father's construction company, and a staple gun went off, projecting a staple into his scrotum. Dr. Carboni carefully removed the staple and applied some antibiotic ointment to prevent infection until the two small wounds healed.

You Code It!

Go through the steps, and determine the procedure code(s) that should be reported for this encounter between Dr. Carboni and Glenn Hagger.

Step #1: Read the case carefully and completely.
Step #2: Abstract the scenario. Which key words or terms describe what service the physician provided to the patient during this encounter?
Step #3: Are there any details missing or incomplete for which you would need to query the physician? [If so, ask your instructor.]
Step #4: Determine the correct CPT procedure code or codes to explain the details about what was provided to the patient during this encounter.
Step #5: Check for any relevant guidance, including reading all of the symbols and notations.
Step #6: Do you need to append any modifiers to ensure complete and accurate information is provided?
Step #7: Double-check your work.

(continued)

Answer:

Did you determine this to be the correct code?

55120 Removal of foreign body in scrotum

This matches the physician's description perfectly!

The Female Genital System

Vulvectomy

Sometimes physicians use direct terms in their notes, such as *simple*, *partial*, *radical*, or *complete*, when describing vulvectomies. Such terms make finding the best code easier. However, other physicians may be more descriptive in their notes regarding the procedure. Therefore, you have to know what these terms mean. The CPT book defines them as follows:

- *Simple:* The removal of skin and *superficial* subcutaneous tissues.
- *Radical:* The removal of skin and *deep* subcutaneous tissues.
- *Partial:* The removal of *less than* 80% of the vulvar area.
- *Complete:* The removal of *more than* 80% of the vulvar area.

EXAMPLES

56620 Vulvectomy, simple; partial

The description of this code represents a physician's statement that he or she removed less than 80% of the skin and superficial subcutaneous tissues of the vulvar area.

56633 Vulvectomy, radical; complete

The description of this code represents a physician's statement that he or she removed more than 80% of the skin and deep subcutaneous tissues of the vulvar area.

GUIDANCE CONNECTION

Read the additional explanations in the in-section guidelines within the **Surgery** section, subhead **Female Genital System**, subsection **Vulva, Perineum, and Introitus**, directly above code 56405 in your CPT book.

Maternity Care and Delivery

The complete package of services provided to a woman for uncomplicated maternity care includes the antepartum (prenatal) care, the delivery of the baby, and the postpartum care of the mother. Similar to working with the services already provided in the global surgical package, you must know the components of the maternity care package. This is the only way you can determine what is already included and what services should be reported separately.

Antepartum Care

- Initial patient history.
- Subsequent patient history.
- Physical examinations.
- Documentation of weight, blood pressure, fetal heart tones, routine chemical urinalysis.
- Monthly visits from conception up to 28 weeks gestation.
- Biweekly visits from 28 weeks to 36 weeks gestation.
- Weekly visits from 36 weeks gestation to delivery.

Delivery Services

- Admission to the hospital.
- Admission history and physical examination (H&P).
- Management of uncomplicated labor.
- Delivery: vaginal (with or without episiotomy, with or without forceps) or cesarean section.

Postpartum Care

- Hospital and office visits following the delivery.

Should a physician provide one portion of the services, but not all, this will affect the determination of the correct code.

EXAMPLE

Dr. Barber provided antepartum care for Nancy Trainer. While on vacation in Europe, Nancy suffered a miscarriage (spontaneous abortion) and lost the baby. Dr. Barber provided postpartum care for Nancy when she returned home. Therefore, instead of reporting

59400 Routine obstetric care including antepartum care, vaginal delivery (with or without episiotomy, and/or forceps) and postpartum care

or

59510 Routine obstetric care including antepartum care, cesarean delivery, and postpartum care

Dr. Barber's complete care for Nancy will be reported with two codes:

59425 Antepartum care only; 4–6 visits

59430 Postpartum care only (separate procedure)

GUIDANCE CONNECTION

Read the additional explanations in the in-section guidelines within the **Surgery** section, subhead **Maternity Care and Delivery**, directly above code 59000 in your CPT book.

LET'S CODE IT! SCENARIO

PATIENT: Gloria Valdez

ADMITTING DIAGNOSIS: Intrauterine pregnancy at 36 weeks and 5 days estimated gestational age. Presented with contractions and in latent labor.

DISCHARGE DIAGNOSIS: Status post normal spontaneous vaginal delivery at 36 weeks and 5 days estimated gestational age.

HISTORY OF PRESENT ILLNESS/HOSPITAL COURSE: This patient is a 31-year-old G4, P1-0-2-1 female for whom I have been attending through all prenatal care. She is at 36 weeks and 5 days estimated gestational age who presented with contractions and in latent labor. On vaginal examination, the patient was found to be 3 cm dilated, 70% effaced and −3 station. The fetal heart tracing at the time was in the 140s and reactive. The patient was admitted to Labor and Delivery for antibiotics and epidural. The patient continued to have a good labor pattern and proceeded to deliver a viable female infant weighing 5 pounds 7 ounces over an intact perineum with Apgars of 9 and 9 at 1 and 5 minutes. There were no nuchal cords, no true knots, and the number of vessels in the cord were three. Her postpartum course was uncomplicated and the patient was discharged to home in stable and satisfactory condition on postpartum day #2.

(continued)

PROCEDURES PERFORMED: Normal spontaneous delivery and repair of midline episiotomy in the usual fashion.

COMPLICATIONS: None.

FINAL DIAGNOSIS: Status post normal spontaneous vaginal delivery at 36 weeks and 5 days estimated gestational age.

DISCHARGE INSTRUCTIONS: Call for increased pain, fever, or increased bleeding.

DIET: Advance as tolerated.

ACTIVITY: Pelvic rest for 6 weeks and nothing inserted into the vagina for 6 weeks, i.e., no tampons, douche, or sex.

MEDICATIONS AND FOLLOW-UP: Instructed patient to call me in the morning, or prn with any concerns. Then, I will see her in the office in 1 week.

Felicia Washington, MD

Let's Code It!

Dr. Washington has been caring for Gloria throughout this pregnancy and delivery. This is the big event, so turn to the CPT Alphabetic Index to

Table Cell

See Cesarean Delivery; Vaginal Delivery

Gloria has a vaginal delivery, so turn to

Vaginal Delivery. 59400, 59610-59614

Are there any items listed below this that match what Dr. Washington did for Gloria? Not exactly. So, turn to review the full descriptions of these codes.

59400 **Routine obstetric care including antepartum care, vaginal delivery (with or without episiotomy, and/or forceps) and postpartum care**

59610 **Routine obstetric care including antepartum care, vaginal delivery (with or without episiotomy, and/or forceps) and postpartum care, after previous cesarean delivery**

59612 **Vaginal delivery only after previous cesarean delivery (with or without episiotomy and/or forceps);**

59614 **Vaginal delivery only after previous cesarean delivery (with or without episiotomy and/or forceps); including postpartum care**

Do any of these codes accurately and completely report what Dr. Washington provided to Gloria for this pregnancy and delivery?

59400 **Routine obstetric care including antepartum care, vaginal delivery (with or without episiotomy, and/or forceps) and postpartum care**

Good work!

26.12 Nervous System

Procedures performed on the nervous system organs (the brain, spinal cord, nerves, and ganglia) and connective tissues are coded from the **Nervous System** subsection. These components of the human body are responsible for sensory, integrative, and motor activities.

Skull Surgery

The skull is, technically, the bone-shell that covers and protects the brain and organs within. To cushion the tissues, blood vessels, and nerves, the dura mater, arachnoid mater, and pia mater lie between the skull and these components (**Figure 26-8**).

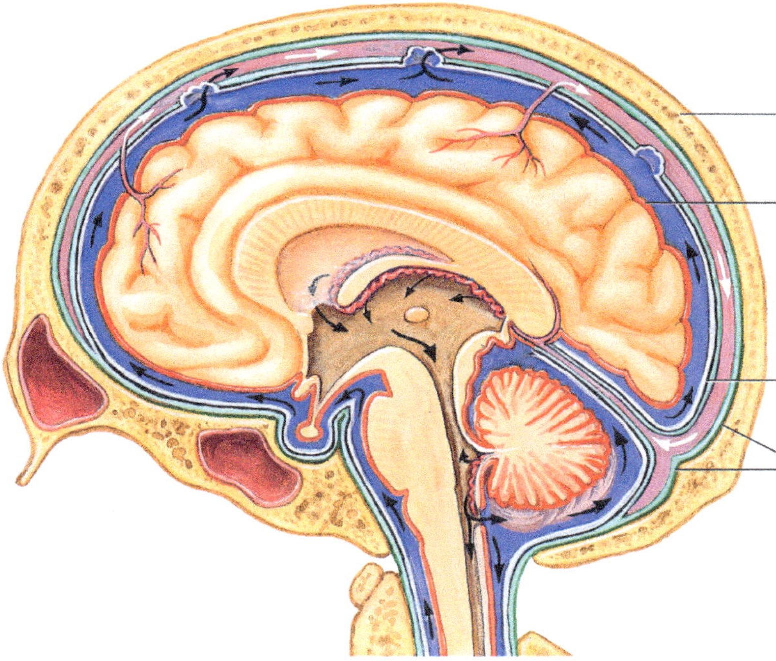

FIGURE 26-8 The internal components of the head

The complexity of surgical treatment of skull base lesions often demands the skills of more than one surgeon during the same session. When one surgeon provides one portion of the procedure and another surgeon a different portion, each surgeon only uses the code for the surgical procedure he or she performed.

Typically, the segments of the procedure include the following:

1. The *approach* describes the tactic of the procedure, such as craniofacial, orbitocranial, or transcochlear:
   a. Anterior cranial fossa, 61580–61586
   b. Middle cranial fossa, 61590–61592
   c. Posterior cranial fossa, 61595–61598
2. The *definitive* describes the procedure itself, such as resection, excision, repair, biopsy, or transection:
   a. Base of anterior cranial fossa, 61600–61601
   b. Base of middle cranial fossa, 61605–61613
   c. Base of posterior cranial fossa, 61615–61616
3. The *repair/reconstruction* identifies a secondary repair, such as
   a. Extensive dural grafting
   b. Cranioplasty
   c. Local or regional myocutaneous pedicle flaps
   d. Extensive skin grafts

If one surgeon performs more than one of the procedures, each segment should be reported separately, with the second (and third, if applicable) appended with modifier 51 to indicate that multiple procedures were performed at the same session by the same physician.

GUIDANCE CONNECTION

Read the additional explanations in the in-section guidelines within the **Surgery** section, subhead **Nervous System**, subsection **Surgery of Skull Base**, directly above code 61580 in your CPT book.

When a surgeon embeds a neurostimulator electrode array and performs microelectrode recording, the recording is included in the implantation code and shouldn't be coded separately.

Code 62263 includes the following:

- Percutaneous insertion of an epidural catheter.
- Removal of the catheter several days later.
- Procedure injections.
- Fluoroscopic guidance and localization.
- Multiple adhesiolysis sessions over the course of 2 or more days.

CODING BITES

If multiple treatments are provided all in 1 calendar day, then use code 62264.

The code should be used only once to represent the entire series.

62263 **Percutaneous lysis of epidural adhesions using solution injection (e.g., hypertonic saline, enzyme) or mechanical means (e.g., catheter) including radiologic localization (includes contrast when administered), multiple adhesiolysis sessions; 2 or more days**

62264 **1 day**

Spinal Cord Injury Repair

Injury to the spinal cord is almost always the result of trauma. This damage can result in changes to the patient's strength, sensations, and other bodily functions that are regulated by these nerves, impacting virtually every aspect of life. The extent of the patient's ability to control his or her limbs will be determined by the location (specific site along the spine) and the severity of the damage. The location is identified by the lowest (most distal) segment of the spine that is unaffected by the injury.

At this time, treatments of spinal cord injuries are directed at pain control and stabilization of the spine to prevent additional irritation or damage to the nerves.

Methylprednisolone acetate (brand name Medrol) is an anti-inflammatory with immunosuppressive properties. Some spinal cord injury patients find that it can reduce the damage to the nerve cells as well as reduce inflammation near the site of the injury, decreasing pain and discomfort. This is an off-label use of this drug but has been found to be beneficial for these cases.

When the trauma causes something to press against the spinal cord, this compression can interfere with the transmission of impulses within the nerves. Surgical decompression of a nerve is typically provided by a neurosurgeon performing a procedure known as a neuroplasty. This procedure may be reported with, for example, CPT code 64713 Neuroplasty, major peripheral nerve, arm, or leg, open; brachial plexus or 64714 Neuroplasty, major peripheral nerve, arm, or leg, open; lumbar plexus.

Functional electrical stimulation (FES), also termed neuromuscular electric stimulation (NMES), may be used to support the restoration of neuromuscular function, sensory function, or autonomic function (e.g., bladder, bowel, or respiratory function) by employing electrical currents to activate damaged nerves within the spinal cord. Procedures focused on the use of spinal neurostimulator systems, reported with CPT codes 63650, 63655, and 63661–63664 (for insertion, revision, replacement, and/or removal), include the implanted neurostimulator, an external controller, an extension, and multiple contacts (also known as electrodes). These contacts may be located on a lead, similar to a catheter, or on a plate-shaped or paddle-like surface. Percutaneous stereotaxis (stereotactic surgery) may be used to stimulate the spinal cord by locating specific points in the brain that may be identified for additional therapy. This would be reported with CPT code 63610 Stereotactic stimulation of spinal cord, percutaneous, separate procedure not followed by other surgery.

Pain Management

Virtually everyone knows what pain feels like, and this is a very personal evaluation. Medically speaking, pain is an unpleasant sensation often initiated by tissue damage, resulting in impulses transmitted to the brain via specific nerve fibers. Most health care facilities use some type of pain scale from 0 to 10, with 0 indicating no pain at all and 10 representing excruciating, intolerable pain. In most instances, each number on the scale is accompanied by an illustration to help patients accurately communicate what they are feeling. This numeric scale (no illustrations), provided by the National Institutes of Health, can help improve communication with patients (**Table 26-5**).

When the documentation indicates that an encounter is prompted by a patient's need for pain management, especially when the pain is noted as acute and/or chronic, there are several options for treatment.

Electrical Reprocessing

Researchers are consistently searching for new ways to help patients manage their pain. Transcutaneous electrical modulation pain reprocessing (TEMPR), also referred to as scrambler therapy, administers electrical impulses designed to interrupt pain

TABLE 26-5 Numeric Rating Scale for Pain

0	=	No pain
1-3	=	Mild pain (nagging, annoying, interfering little with ADL*)
4-6	=	Moderate pain (interferes significantly with ADL*)
7-10	=	Severe pain (disabling; unable to perform ADL*)

*ADL = activities of daily living
Source: National Institute of Health.

signals. Although this experimental procedure uses a type of transcutaneous electrical nerve stimulation (TENS), it is not the same procedure. Each session lasts about an hour, with the physician making adjustments approximately every 10 minutes. Each treatment session is reported with Category III code 0278T.

0278T **Transcutaneous electrical modulation pain reprocessing (e.g., scrambler therapy), each treatment session (includes placement of electrodes)**

Epidural/Intrathecal Medication Administration

Medication administered intrathecally (directly into the cerebrospinal fluid via the subarachnoid space in the spinal cord) may be used for chronic pain management. This methodology typically uses pumps, devices that can provide continual delivery of the drug, biologicals, or genetically engineered encapsulated cells. This route of administration has been found to be less invasive for the patient and enables treatment of a larger portion of the central nervous system utilizing the cerebrospinal fluid circulation pathways. Epidural administration tenders the medication into the dura mater of the spinal cord rather than the subarachnoid space.

EXAMPLES

62350 Implantation, revision, or repositioning of tunneled intrathecal or epidural catheter, for long-term medication administration via an external pump or implantable reservoir/infusion pump; without laminectomy

62360 Implantation or replacement of device for intrathecal or epidural drug infusion; subcutaneous reservoir

62362 Implantation or replacement of device for intrathecal or epidural drug infusion; programmable pump, including preparation of pump, with or without programming

99601 Home infusion/specialty drug administration, per visit (up to 2 hours)

Intravenous Therapy

This may be the administration route with which you are most familiar. The medication enters the body via the patient's vein, most often using a point inside the patient's antecubital fossa (elbow). If the condition is chronic, a peripherally inserted central catheter (PICC) line may be inserted and used for the administration of the medication for the duration of the therapy.

EXAMPLE

36568 Insertion of peripherally inserted central venous catheter (PICC), without subcutaneous port or pump, without imaging guidance; younger than 5 years of age

36569 Insertion of peripherally inserted central venous catheter (PICC), without subcutaneous port or pump, without imaging guidance; 5 years or older

96365 Intravenous infusion, for therapy, prophylaxis, or diagnosis (specify substance or drug); initial, up to 1 hour

CODING BITES

Whenever you report the administration of a drug, you will need the code for the administration, such as implantation of a pump or infusion, as well as a code to report the specific drug that is administered. Most often, the codes used to report the specific drug come from the HCPCS Level II code set. See the chapter ***HCPCS Level II*** in this textbook for more information on these codes.

LET'S CODE IT! SCENARIO

Gerald Rosen, a 63-year-old male, was admitted for the implantation of a cerebral cortical neurostimulator. Dr. Grumman performed a craniotomy and then successfully implanted the electrodes.

Let's Code It!

Dr. Grumman first performed a *craniotomy*. Let's go to the Alphabetic Index and look. Below *craniotomy*, you will see the listing for *implant of neurostimulators*. That matches our notes, so let's go to the numeric listing and check the descriptions for 61850–61875, as suggested. Read through the codes and their descriptions in this section. Do you agree that the following matches our notes the best?

61860 Craniectomy or craniotomy for implantation of neurostimulator electrodes, cerebral, cortical

It does!

Endovascular Therapy

Included in this category of neurologic procedures are balloon angioplasties and intravascular stents. You learned about these types of procedures in the ***Cardiovascular System*** section of this chapter. However, the codes *here* report these procedures when done intracranially (within the skull) and not intracardially (within the heart).

An intra-arterial mechanical embolectomy or thrombectomy is most often performed to treat an acute ischemic stroke (when a thrombus or embolus blocks blood flow to the brain).

LET'S CODE IT! SCENARIO

Alvin Bartholemew, a 71-year-old male, was admitted through the ED with signs of a stroke. He was taken into surgery immediately and Dr. Newton performed a percutaneous transluminal mechanical thrombectomy in the anterior parietal artery. Fluoroscopic guidance was used, and the thrombus was removed and Alteplase 0.9 mg/kg (a thrombolytic agent) was injected.

Let's Code It!

What did Dr. Newton do for Alvin? A *transluminal mechanical thrombectomy* was performed. Turn to the Alphabetic Index in your CPT code book to

Thrombectomy

There is a lengthy list below this term, so review them and read the scenario again and see if you can match any words in common . . .

Thrombectomy

Percutaneous

Intracranial artery 61645

Mechanical arterial 37184-37186

These both match but are in very different subsections of the **Surgery** section. Let's investigate these codes. Remember, you must review all of them before you can determine which is the most accurate.

(continued)

61645 Percutaneous arterial transluminal mechanical thrombectomy and/or infusion for thrombolysis, intracranial, any method, including diagnostic angiography, fluoroscopic guidance, catheter placement, and intraprocedural pharmacological thrombolytic injection(s)

37184 Primary percutaneous transluminal mechanical thrombectomy, noncoronary, non-intracranial, arterial or arterial bypass graft, including fluoroscopic guidance and intraprocedural pharmacological thrombolytic injection(s); initial vessel [*NOTE:* Codes 37185 and 37186 are both add-on codes, so we can focus our analysis on this first code in this series. Then, if 37184 is the right code for this procedure, we can come back and analyze these add-on codes to determine if they are needed.]

Hmm. These two descriptions are very close. However, did you notice that code 61645 specifically states "intracranial," whereas code 37184 specifically states "non-intracranial."

Go back to the documentation. It does not state "intracranial" or "non-intracranial." It does state the thrombectomy was performed on the "*anterior parietal artery.*"

According to my medical dictionary, the *anterior parietal artery* is one of the branches of the middle cerebral artery, distributed to the front or forward part of the parietal lobe of the brain.

OK, so if the thrombectomy was performed to remove a thrombus from the anterior parietal artery, and you know that this artery is in the brain, this means that this procedure was "intracranial" [remember, the cranium is the skull].

Now you know exactly which code to report for this procedure:

61645 Percutaneous arterial transluminal mechanical thrombectomy and/or infusion for thrombolysis, intracranial, any method, including diagnostic angiography, fluoroscopic guidance, catheter placement, and intraprocedural pharmacological thrombolytic injection(s)

Good job!

26.13 The Optical and Auditory Systems

Optical System

Loss of sight, or even the reduction of vision, has both a social and an economic impact on a patient and his or her family. In the United States, it is estimated that 14 million people aged 12 and over have some type of visual impairment, and about 61 million adults are believed to be at high risk for acute vision loss.

There are two recesses in the human skull, each known as an orbit, or eye socket. Within this bony conical orbit sits the contents of the eye and its ancillary parts (muscles, nerves, blood vessels). The optical system is the most complex organ system of the human body (**Figure 26-9**).

Ophthalmologists diagnose and treat problems and concerns of the eye and ocular adnexa (anatomical parts and sites adjacent to an organ). Most commonly, cataracts are corrected and foreign materials are removed.

Glaucoma Surgery

Glaucoma is a malfunction of the fluid pressure within the eye; the pressure rises to a level that can cause damage to the optic disc and nerve. Treatment can successfully prevent blindness or any vision loss from resulting. When eye drops, oral medication, or laser treatments have failed to control the patient's glaucoma condition, a trabeculectomy may be performed. This procedure treats glaucoma with an incision into the trabecular tissue of the eye to drain the excess fluid that has accumulated. In some cases, a drainage tube is inserted.

EXAMPLES

65850 Trabeculectomy ab externo

66170 Fistulization of sclera for glaucoma; trabeculectomy ab externo in absence of previous surgery

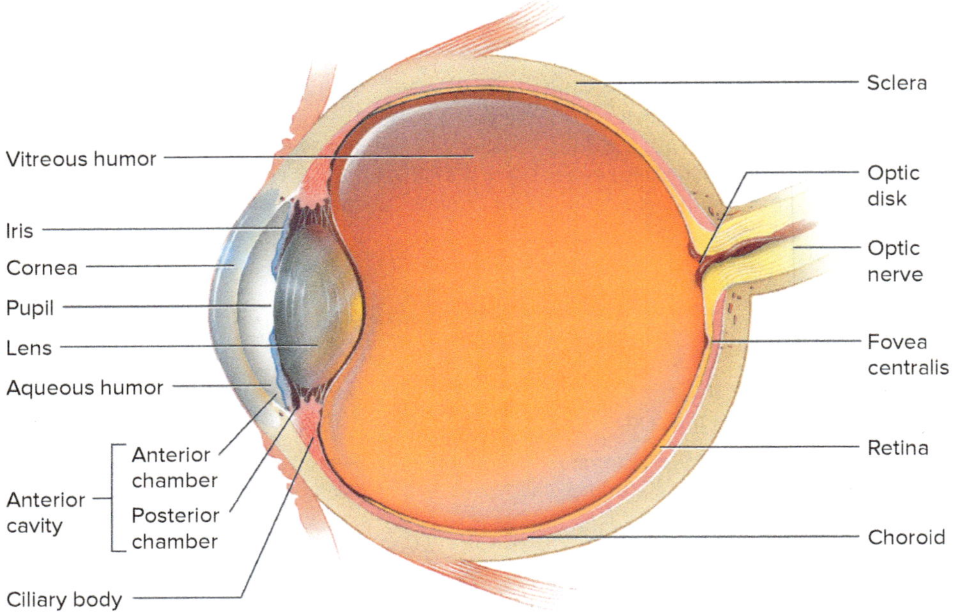

FIGURE 26-9 An illustration of the components of the optical system

Vitrectomy

Patients diagnosed with diabetes mellitus are at risk for ophthalmic manifestations of their abnormal glucose levels. Diabetic retinopathy is the most common; it is a condition that causes damage to the tiny blood vessels inside the retina. In cases where the bleeding in the eye is severe, a vitrectomy, the surgical removal of vitreous gel from the center of the eye, may be necessary.

EXAMPLES

65810 Paracentesis of anterior chamber of eye (separate procedure); with removal of vitreous and/or discission of anterior hyaloid membrane, with or without air injection

67005 Removal of vitreous, anterior approach (open sky technique or limbal incision); partial removal

Foreign Object in Eye

We all know . . . things happen. Tiny specks of dirt, gravel, debris, etc. can fly into one's eyes and may need to be surgically removed. In those cases where the foreign body is difficult to remove, the patient may be admitted to the hospital to have a surgical extirpation. Read the documentation carefully to identify the specific part of the eye from which the object is removed, as well as the direction of the approach.

EXAMPLES

65205 Removal of foreign body, external eye; conjunctival superficial

67413 Orbitotomy without bone flap (frontal or transconjunctival approach); with removal of foreign body

67430 Orbitotomy with bone flap or window, lateral approach (e.g., Kroenlein); with removal of foreign body

68530 Removal of foreign body or dacryolith, lacrimal passages

Dacryocystorhinostomy

Nasolacrimal duct (NLD) stenosis is a condition that may be congenital or acquired. A patient may acquire an NLD stenosis as a result of a granulomatous disease, such as sarcoidosis; a sinus condition; or the formation of dacryoliths (calculus in the lacrimal duct or sac). A dacryocystorhinostomy (DCR) is the standard of care for an NLD obstruction. DCR can be performed using a percutaneous approach by way of a facial incision, or the approach may be via the natural opening of the nose endoscopically. The procedure is designed to bypass the obstructed nasolacrimal duct and enable tear drainage directly into the nose from the lacrimal sac.

EXAMPLES

68801 Dilation of lacrimal punctum, with or without irrigation

68815 Probing of nasolacimal duct, with or without irrigation; with insertion of tube or stent

Fornix
The conjunctival fornix is the area between the eyelid and the eyeball. The superior fornix is between the upper lid and eyeball; the inferior fornix is between the lower lid and the eyeball [plural: fornices].

LET'S CODE IT! SCENARIO

Delores Leon was diagnosed with a herniated orbital mass, OD (right inferior orbit). Dr. Marconi performed an excision of the mass and repair. From his notes, "The lower lid was everted and the inferior ***fornix*** *examined. The herniating mass was viewed and measured at 0.81 cm in diameter. Westcott scissors were used to incise the conjunctival fornices. The herniating mass was then clamped, excised, and cauterized. It appeared to contain mostly fat tissue, which was sent to pathology. The inferior fornix was repaired using running suture of 6-0 plain gut. Bacitracin ointment was applied to the eye followed by an eye pad."*

Let's Code It!

The procedure performed was "*excision of the mass and repair, right inferior orbit.*"

In the CPT Alphabetic Index, turn to *excision* and review the long list of anatomical sites below. What did Dr. Marconi excise? Not the eye (that would be removal of the eyeball). He removed a "*mass* from the eye orbit" and then "*repaired* the orbit."

There is no listing for *mass*, but you should remember from medical terminology class (or look it up in a medical dictionary) that another term for *mass* is *lesion*. In the Alphabetic Index, find:

Excision . . . Lesion . . . another long list. On your scratch pad, write down the codes suggested next to the word *Orbit*—61333, 67412, 67420—so that you can check them out. However, while you are here, also write down the codes suggested for *Conjunctiva*—68110–68130. Why? Because in the body of the notes, it states "*incise the conjunctival fornices.*" This is why it is so important to read the complete notes and not just code from the procedure statement at the top.

Now, let's turn to the main portion of the CPT and find the complete code descriptions:

61333 Exploration of orbit (transcranial approach); with removal of lesion

67412 Orbitotomy without bone flap (frontal or transconjunctival approach); with removal of lesion

67420 Orbitotomy with bone flap or window, lateral approach (e.g., Kroenlein); with removal of lesion

68110 Excision of lesion, conjunctiva; up to 1 cm

68115 Excision of lesion, conjunctiva; over 1 cm

68130 Excision of lesion, conjunctiva; with adjacent sclera

Which code description matches the physician's notes accurately? **68110**. Good work!

YOU CODE IT! CASE STUDY

Ronald Jackson, a 49-year-old male, was working in a metal shop. As he was trimming a steel bar, some metal splinters got into his eye. Fortunately, Dr. Draman found that the metal pieces presented superficial damage and had not embedded themselves in Ronald's conjunctiva. Dr. Draman removed all the metal pieces and placed a patch over Ronald's eye.

You Code It!

Go through the steps and determine the procedure code(s) that should be reported for this encounter between Dr. Draman and Ronald Jackson.

Step #1: Read the case carefully and completely.
Step #2: Abstract the scenario. Which key words or terms describe what service the physician provided to the patient during this encounter?
Step #3: Are there any details missing or incomplete for which you would need to query the physician? [If so, ask your instructor.]
Step #4: Determine the correct CPT procedure code or codes to explain the details about what was provided to the patient during this encounter.
Step #5: Check for any relevant guidance, including reading all of the symbols and notations.
Step #6: Do you need to append any modifiers to ensure complete and accurate information is provided?
Step #7: Double-check your work.

Answer:

Did you determine this to be the correct code?

65205 Removal of foreign body, external eye; conjunctival superficial

Good for you!

The Auditory System

The auditory system of the human body is referenced in three sections (**Figure 26-10**).

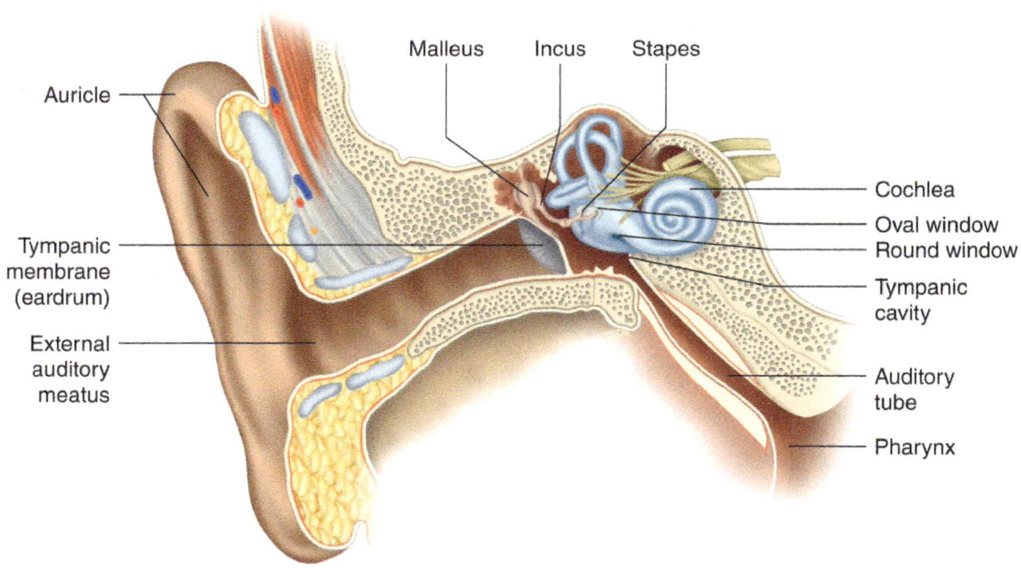

FIGURE 26-10 The auditory system

The Outer Ear

- Auricle (pinna).
- External acoustic meatus (also known as the external auditory canal).
- Eardrum (the tympanic membrane).

EXAMPLES

69100	Biopsy external ear
69209	Removal of impacted cerumen using irrigation/lavage, unilateral
69310	Recontruction of external auditory canal (meatoplasty) (e.g., for stenosis due to injury, infection) (separate procedure)

The Middle Ear

- Auditory ossicles: malleus, incus, and stapes.
- Oval window.
- Eustachian tube (auditory tube), which connects the middle ear to the nasopharynx (throat).

EXAMPLES

69421	Myringotomy, including aspiration and/or eustachian tube inflation requiring general anesthesia
69535	Resection temporal bone, external approach

The Inner Ear

- Semicircular canals.
- Cochlea.

EXAMPLE

69801	Labyrinthotomy, with perfusion of vestibuloactive drug(s), transcanal
69905	Labyrinthectomy; transcanal

Tympanostomy

When a patient has a middle ear infection (otitis media), pressure caused by the buildup of fluid or pus in the middle ear compresses the eardrum, causing pain and decreasing the patient's ability to hear. A lack of treatment can result in a perforation of the tympanic membrane. Tympanostomy (ear tube surgery) is a relatively common procedure performed on about 2 million children each year in the United States. It involves the insertion of a ventilating tube into the opening of the tympanum to relieve the pressure.

When reporting a tympanostomy, you need to know what type of anesthesia was provided to the patient: local or general anesthesia.

69433 **Tympanostomy (requiring insertion of ventilating tube), local or topical anesthesia**

69436 **Tympanostomy (requiring insertion of ventilating tube), general anesthesia**

These codes report the insertion of the tube into one ear only. When the physician performs this for both ears at the same encounter, you will need to append modifier 50 Bilateral procedure to the correct procedure code.

Sometimes, over a period of time, the tubes naturally fall out. However, when the physician must go in and surgically remove the tubes under general anesthesia, this procedure will be reported separately:

69424 Ventilating tube removal requiring general anesthesia

YOU CODE IT! CASE STUDY

Anna Mendoza, a 33-year-old female, has been deaf since she was 11. She is admitted today for Dr. Eberhardt to put a cochlear implant in her left ear. It is expected that Anna will gain back much of her hearing.

You Code It!

Go through the steps, and determine the procedure code(s) that should be reported for this encounter between Dr. Eberhardt and Anna Mendoza.

Step #1: Read the case carefully and completely.
Step #2: Abstract the scenario. Which key words or terms describe what service the physician provided to the patient during this encounter?
Step #3: Are there any details missing or incomplete for which you would need to query the physician? [If so, ask your instructor.]
Step #4: Determine the correct CPT procedure code or codes to explain the details about what was provided to the patient during this encounter.
Step #5: Check for any relevant guidance, including reading all of the symbols and notations.
Step #6: Do you need to append any modifiers to ensure complete and accurate information is provided?
Step #7: Double-check your work.

Answer:

Did you determine this to be the correct code?

69930 Cochlear device implantation, with or without mastoidectomy

26.14 Organ Transplantation

Lung Transplantation

Allotransplantation
The relocation of tissue from one individual to another (both of the same species) without an identical genetic match.

Transplantation
The transfer of tissue from one site to another.

Special guidelines help you report any lung transplant. However, as soon as you begin to read the notation shown before codes 32850–32856, you will see that the editors of the CPT book use the term lung **allotransplantation** in addition to **transplantation**. These words have a very similar meaning.

A lung transplant requires three steps, which can be performed by a single physician or a team of physicians, with each physician submitting his or her own claim. Each step has its own code.

Cadaver Donor Pneumonectomy

Because a human cannot live without lungs, the donor has to be deceased (a cadaver) prior to the harvesting of the organ. This portion of the transplant, or allotransplantation, procedure should be identified with the code

32850 Donor pneumonectomy(s) (including cold preservation), from cadaver donor

Backbench Work

The actual preparation of the cadaver lung allograft prior to the transplant procedure is known as *backbench work*. The actual preparation of the cadaver donor lung allograft prior to the transplant procedure is coded by using either of the following:

32855 Backbench standard preparation of cadaver donor lung allograft prior to transplantation . . . ; unilateral

or

32856 Backbench standard preparation of cadaver donor lung allograft prior to transplantation . . . ; bilateral

GUIDANCE CONNECTION

Read the additional explanations in the in-section guidelines within the **Surgery** section, subhead **Respiratory System**, subsection **Lung Transplantation**, directly above code 32850 in your CPT book.

Recipient Lung Allotransplantation

The final code for the entire operation identifies the placement of the allograft in the patient (the recipient). The selection of a code from the range 32851–32854 is determined by whether the procedure is performed unilaterally or bilaterally and with or without a cardiopulmonary bypass.

32851 Lung transplant, single; without cardiopulmonary bypass

32852 with cardiopulmonary bypass

32853 Lung transplant, double (bilateral sequential or en bloc); without cardiopulmonary bypass

32854 with cardiopulmonary bypass

LET'S CODE IT! SCENARIO

Abbey Reason, a 15-year-old female, was diagnosed 3 years ago with idiopathic pulmonary fibrosis, a chronic interstitial pulmonary disease. Corticosteroid therapy has not improved her condition, so Dr. Flemming admitted her today for a double-lung transplantation. The harvesting of the allograft and the preparation of the cadaver donor double-lung allograft were done by Dr. Orenge. Dr. Flemming only performed the actual lung transplant, en bloc, along with a cardiopulmonary bypass. Abbey tolerated the procedure well and has an excellent prognosis.

Let's Code It!

The notes indicate that Dr. Flemming performed only one of the three steps. Therefore, you will have only one code on his claim form for Abbey's surgery.

Let's go to the Alphabetic Index and look for *transplant*. Read down until you find *lung*. You know that Abbey received a *double-lung* transplant, *en bloc, with a bypass*. That information leads to the suggested code 32854. Now go to the numeric listing to check the complete code description.

32854 Lung transplant, double (bilateral sequential or en bloc); with cardiopulmonary bypass

Terrific! This code matches the notes.

Heart/Lung Transplantation

Similar to the components of the lung transplantation that we reviewed earlier, a heart transplant, with or without a lung allotransplantation, requires three steps to be performed by a single physician or a team of physicians. Each step has its own codes.

Cadaver Donor Cardiectomy with or without a Pneumonectomy

A human cannot live without a heart or lungs, so the donor has to be deceased (a cadaver) prior to any organ harvesting. This portion of the transplant or allotransplantation procedure is identified with the code 33930 (heart and lungs) or 33940 (heart alone):

33930 **Donor cardiectomy-pneumonectomy (including cold preservation)**

or

33940 **Donor cardiectomy (including cold preservation)**

Backbench Work

The actual preparation of the cadaver donor heart, or heart and lung, allograft prior to the transplant procedure is known as *backbench work*. The second portion of the transplant is coded by using either of the following:

33933 **Backbench standard preparation of cadaver donor heart/lung allograft to transplantation, including dissection of allograft from surrounding soft tissues to prepare aorta, superior vena cava, inferior vena cava, and trachea for implantation**

or

33944 **Backbench standard preparation of cadaver donor heart allograft to transplantation, including dissection from surrounding soft tissues to prepare aorta, superior vena cava, inferior vena cava, pulmonary artery, and left atrium for implantation**

Recipient Heart with or without Lung Allotransplantation

The third code for the entire operation identifies the placement of the allograft into the patient (the recipient). Select the code from either of the following:

33935 **Heart-lung transplant with recipient cardiectomy-pneumonectomy**

or

33945 **Heart transplant with or without recipient cardiectomy**

The codes for the insertion of the transplanted organs include the removal of the damaged or diseased organs.

Liver Transplantation

Again, the components that we have reviewed for the other organ transplants are involved with a liver allotransplantation.

Donor Hepatectomy

A human can live without a portion of the liver, so the donor can be either deceased (a cadaver) or living. The best code for this portion of the transplant process is determined by whether or not the donor is living, and if living, what percentage or portion of the liver is donated.

47133 **Donor hepatectomy (including cold preservation), from cadaver donor**

or

47140 **Donor hepatectomy (including cold preservation), from living donor; left lateral segment only (segments II and III)**

or

47141 **Donor hepatectomy (including cold preservation), from living donor; total left lobectomy (segments II, III, and IV)**

or

47142 **Donor hepatectomy (including cold preservation), from living donor; total right lobectomy (segments V, VI, VII, and VIII)**

Backbench Work

The actual preparation of the whole liver graft prior to the transplant procedure is coded with

47143 **Backbench standard preparation of cadaver donor whole liver graft prior to allotransplantation, including cholecystectomy, if necessary, and dissection and removal of surrounding soft tissues to prepare the vena cava, portal vein, hepatic artery, and common bile duct for implantation; without trisegment or lobe split**

47144 **with trisegment split of whole liver graft into 2 partial liver grafts (i.e., left lateral segment [segments II and III] and right trisegment [segments I and IV through VIII])**

47145 **with lobe split of whole liver graft into 2 partial liver grafts (i.e., left lobe [segments II, III, and IV] and right lobe [segments I and V through VIII])**

In certain cases, and almost always if the donor is living, some reconstruction of the liver will be required prior to the transplantation. If the notes indicate that a venous and/or arterial anastomosis was also performed, then you will need to use

47146 **Backbench reconstruction of cadaver or living donor liver graft prior to allotransplantation; venous anastomosis, each**

Recipient Liver Allotransplantation

The third code for the entire operation identifies the placement of the allograft in the patient (the recipient): orthotopic (normal position) or heterotopic (other than normal position).

47135 **Liver allotransplantation; orthotopic, partial or whole, from cadaver or living donor, any age**

Pancreas Transplantation

Again, the components that we have reviewed for the other organ transplants are involved with a pancreatic allotransplantation.

Cadaver Donor Pancreatectomy

A pancreas graft has to come from a deceased (a cadaver) donor.

48550 **Donor pancreatectomy (including cold preservation), with or without duodenal segment for transplantation**

Backbench Work

When the preparation of the pancreas graft prior to the transplant procedure is routine, you use the following code:

48551 **Backbench standard preparation of cadaver donor pancreas allograft prior to transplantation, including dissection of allograft from surrounding soft tissues, splenectomy, duodenotomy, ligation of bile duct, ligation of mesenteric vessels, and Y-graft arterial anastomoses from iliac artery to superior mesenteric artery and to splenic artery**

However, in certain cases, some reconstruction of the pancreas will be required prior to the transplantation. If the notes indicate that a venous and/or arterial anastomosis was performed, then you have to use

48552 **Backbench reconstruction of cadaver donor pancreas allograft prior to allotransplantation; venous anastomosis, each**

Recipient Pancreatic Allotransplantation

The final code for the entire operation identifies the placement of the allograft in the patient (the recipient). For this, use the following code:

48554 **Transplantation of pancreatic allograft**

> **GUIDANCE CONNECTION**
>
> Read the additional explanations in the in-section guidelines within the **Surgery** section, subhead **Digestive System**, subsection **Pancreas Transplantation**, directly above code 48550 in your CPT book.

Renal (Kidney) Transplantation

The same three components exist for renal transplantation as for the other organ transplants.

Donor Nephrectomy

A human can live without one kidney, so the donor can be either deceased (a cadaver) or living.

50300 Donor nephrectomy (including cold preservation); from cadaver donor, unilateral or bilateral

or

50320 Donor nephrectomy (including cold preservation); open, from living donor

or

50547 Laparoscopy, surgical; donor nephrectomy (including cold preservation), from living donor

Backbench Work

Performing the routine preparation of the allograft is coded differently, depending upon whether the donor is living or a cadaver.

50323 Backbench standard preparation of cadaver donor renal allograft prior to transplantation, including dissection and removal of perinephric fat, diaphragmatic and retroperitoneal attachments, excision of adrenal gland, and preparation of ureter(s), renal vein(s), and renal artery(s), ligating branches, as necessary

or

50325 Backbench standard preparation of living donor renal allograft prior to transplantation, including dissection and removal of perinephric fat, diaphragmatic and retroperitoneal attachments, excision of adrenal gland, and preparation of ureter(s), renal vein(s), and renal artery(s), ligating branches, as necessary

In certain cases, some reconstruction of the kidney will be required prior to the transplantation. If the notes indicate that a venous, arterial, and/or ureteral anastomosis was performed, then you have to use one of the following codes:

50327 Backbench reconstruction of cadaver or living donor renal allograft prior to allotransplantation; venous anastomosis, each

or

50328 Backbench reconstruction of cadaver or living donor renal allograft prior to allotransplantation; arterial anastomosis, each

or

50329 Backbench reconstruction of cadaver or living donor renal allograft prior to allotransplantation; ureteral anastomosis, each

Recipient Renal Allotransplantation

The final code for the entire operation identifies the placement of the allograft in the patient (the recipient). Choose the code by whether or not a recipient nephrectomy (the removal of the organ being replaced) is performed at the same time by the same physician:

50360 Renal allotransplantation; implantation of graft; without recipient nephrectomy

or

50365 Renal allotransplantation; implantation of graft; with recipient nephrectomy

GUIDANCE CONNECTION

Read the additional explanations in the in-section guidelines located within the **Surgery** section, subhead **Urinary System**, subsection **Renal Transplantation**, directly above code 50300 in your CPT book.

YOU CODE IT! CASE STUDY

PATIENT: Ethan Norwood IV

PROCEDURE PERFORMED: Percutaneous kidney transplant biopsy.

DESCRIPTION OF PROCEDURE: After informed written consent was obtained from the patient, he was taken to the ultrasound suite and placed in the supine position on the stretcher with the left side propped up slightly with towels for optimal exposure of the transplant. The kidney transplant was localized in the left iliac fossa with ultrasound and a point overlying the lower pole was marked on the skin. The area was then prepped with Betadine and covered with a sterile fenestrated drape. Lidocaine 1% was infiltrated at the mark superficially and then to less than 1 cm, as indicated by ultrasound, to the surface of the kidney. A small incision was made at the anesthetized site with a #11 blade. A 16-gauge Monopty biopsy gun was then introduced through the incision to a depth of less than 1 cm and fired. A core tissue was obtained and placed in 10% formalin. The procedure was repeated once more, again yielding a core tissue. It was divided between formalin and Michel's solution. The procedure was then terminated. Firm pressure was applied to the biopsy site after each pass including 5 minutes after the last pass. A Band-Aid was then placed over the incision. A final ultrasound scan showed no obvious evidence of hematoma. A pressure dressing was applied. The patient tolerated the procedure well. There were no apparent complications. He has been returned to the floor in satisfactory condition and orders have been written for frequent vital signs, hematocrit, exam parameters.

Ava Ferrer, MD

You Code It!

Read the details about the biopsy that Dr. Ferrer performed and determine the most accurate way to report it.

Step #1: Read the case carefully and completely.
Step #2: Abstract the scenario. Which key words or terms describe what service the physician provided to the patient during this encounter?
Step #3: Are there any details missing or incomplete for which you would need to query the physician? [If so, ask your instructor.]
Step #4: Determine the correct CPT procedure code or codes to explain the details about what was provided to the patient during this encounter.
Step #5: Check for any relevant guidance, including reading all of the symbols and notations.
Step #6: Do you need to append any modifiers to ensure complete and accurate information is provided?
Step #7: Double-check your work.

Answer:

Did you determine these to be the codes?

50200 **Renal biopsy; percutaneous, by trocar or needle**

76942 **Ultrasonic guidance for needle placement (e.g., biopsy, aspiration, injection, localization device), imaging supervision and interpretation**

Did you find the radiology code for the ultrasound, too? You will learn more about coding for radiology services in our next chapter of this textbook. However, to get to this code, all you had to do is read the guideline notation beneath code 50200.

(For radiological supervision and interpretation, see 76942, 77002, 77012, 77021)

This notation not only told you how to report the ultrasound service for this biopsy; it also informed you that it was not already included in the 50200 code.

26.15 Operating Microscope

When a surgeon performs microsurgery, he or she has to use an operating microscope. In such cases, you must code the use of the microscope (69990) in addition to the procedure in which the microscope is used.

+69990 Microsurgical techniques, requiring use of operating microscope (List separately in addition to code for primary procedure.)

There are two guidelines with regard to this add-on code:

1. Do not append modifier 51 Multiple Procedures to the code for the microscope. It is not an additional procedure. Code 69990 indicates the use of a special technique or tool, making modifier 51 incorrect.
2. There are some codes that already include the use of the operating microscope. Therefore, adding code 69990 is redundant. The tough part here is that none of the codes that already include use of the operating microscope include this information in their description. Following, and in many CPT books above the code description, is the list of codes to which you are *not* permitted to add code 69990 because it is already included:

15756–15758	31531	49906
15842	31536	61548
19364	31541	63075–63078
19368	31545	64727
20955–20962	31546	64820–64823
20969–20973	31571	64912–64913
22551–22552	43116	65091–68850
22856–22861	43180	0184T
26551–26554	43496	0308T
26556	46601	0402T
31526	46607	0583T

EXAMPLE

19364 Breast reconstruction with free flap
(Do not report code 69990 in addition to code 19364.)

As you can see, the codes involved are throughout the ***Surgery*** section of the CPT. You might want to go through and mark or highlight the codes, should you be coding for a physician who works with an operating microscope.

GUIDANCE CONNECTION

Read the additional explanations in the in-section guidelines within the **Surgery** section, subhead **Operating Microscope**, directly above code 69990 in your CPT book.

LET'S CODE IT! SCENARIO

PATIENT: Olivia Prima

PREOPERATIVE DIAGNOSIS: Right vocal cord lesion

POSTOPERATIVE DIAGNOSIS: Respiratory papilloma

PROCEDURE: Microscopic laryngoscopy with biopsy and papilloma shave

SURGEON: Serita Frapenstein, MD

ASSISTANT: Morris Bershic, MD

(continued)

ANESTHESIA: General endotracheal

COMPLICATIONS: None

SPECIMENS REMOVED: Biopsy samples sent from the anterior commissure of the vocal cord

INDICATION FOR PROCEDURE: The patient is a 37-year-old female with a 6-month history of isolated hoarseness with a vocal cord lesion on direct laryngoscopy, who presents for biopsy of the vocal cord lesion.

DESCRIPTION OF PROCEDURE: The patient was brought to the operating room, and an appropriate plane of anesthesia was obtained via endotracheal intubation.

The head of the bed was turned 90 degrees. The Dedo laryngoscope was used to visualize the base of tongue, the bilateral vallecula, both surfaces of the epiglottis, the aryepiglottic folds, the bilateral pyriform sinuses, and hypopharynx. All of these areas were clear of any lesions or mucosal abnormalities. The true vocal cords were noted to have papillomatous lesions on the right inferior aspect of the cord and the anterior commissure. The false cords and ventricles were clear.

The patient's larynx was suspended via the laryngoscope. Biopsy samples were taken for frozen and permanent specimens from the anterior commissure lesion. This came back to confirm papilloma. Next, the operating microscope was brought into the field to obtain a detailed visualization of the vocal cord lesion. A straight shaver was then utilized to remove the papillomatous tissue on the right vocal cord. Care was taken to preserve the mucosa on that side and not injure the vocal cord. This was done unilaterally again on the right. Appropriate hemostasis was obtained.

The patient tolerated the procedure well. The operating microscope was removed from the field. The patient was extubated and taken to recovery in stable condition with no immediate complications.

Let's Code It!

As you read in the operative reports, Dr. Frapenstein performed a *laryngoscopy* using an operating microscope. First, you must determine the code for the laryngoscopy. Find this in the CPT Alphabetic Index.

Laryngoscopy

with Operating Microscope or Telescope 31526, 31531, 31536, 31541, 31545, 31546, 31561, 31571

Turn to the main section and find the codes suggested. Remember, you are obligated to read ALL of these code descriptions to determine which one is most accurate.

31526 Laryngoscopy direct, with or without tracheoscopy; diagnostic, with operating microscope or telescope

31531 Laryngoscopy direct, operative, with foreign body removal; with operating microscope or telescope

31536 Laryngoscopy direct, operative, with biopsy; with operating microscope or telescope

31541 Laryngoscopy direct, operative, with excision of tumor and/or stripping of vocal cords or epiglottis; with operating microscope or telescope

31545 Laryngoscopy direct, operative, with operating microscope or telescope, with submucosal removal of non-neoplastic lesion(s) of vocal cord; reconstruction with local tissue flap(s)

31546 Laryngoscopy direct, operative, with operating microscope or telescope, with submucosal removal of non-neoplastic lesion(s) of vocal cord; reconstruction with graft(s) (includes obtaining autograft)

31561 Laryngoscopy direct, operative, with arytenoidectomy; with operating microscope or telescope

31571 Laryngoscopy direct, operative, with injection into vocal cord(s), therapeutic; with operating microscope or telescope

Now that you know, specifically, what these codes report, go back to the operative notes and abstract the details, beyond laryngoscopy + operating microscope.

The documentation reads, "*Biopsy samples were taken.*" . . . This leads you to code 31536. However, the documentation also states,

"*A straight shaver was then utilized to remove the papillomatous tissue on the right vocal cord.*"
[*NOTE:* Use your medical dictionary if you don't already know that papillomatous tissue is benign.]

. . . This might lead to code 31545 or 31546, except there is documentation that "*Care was taken to preserve the mucosa*," so you know that submucosal tissue was not removed. And there is no mention of a reconstruction being performed.

(continued)

So, you can confidently report code 31536. One more thing to check . . . do you need to report a second code for the use of the operating microscope? Turn to code 69990 and read the guideline carefully. Code 31536 is included in the "*Do not report 69990*" notation.

You also know that code 31536 includes the specific detail that an operating microscope was used, therefore meaning that this tells the whole story and reporting 69990 would just be repetitive. Now, you know the accurate way to report this procedure:

31536 **Laryngoscopy direct, operative, with biopsy; with operating microscope or telescope**

Good job!

Chapter Summary

When coding surgical procedures, you have the challenge of determining which services are included in the procedure code, which services are part of the global package, and which services must be coded separately.

In addition, it is important to remember that the ***Surgery*** section of the CPT book not only includes codes for reporting services provided in an OR under general anesthesia but also includes codes for reporting simple and small procedures such as removing a splinter.

When reporting surgical procedures, it is important to (1) identify the components of the operation and (2) determine which services are included in the code's description and which services require a separate code. The ***Surgery*** section of the CPT book is divided into subsections identified by the body system upon which the technique was performed.

CODING BITES

CPT Surgical Package

- Subsequent to the decision for surgery, one related E/M encounter on the date immediately prior to or on the date of the procedure (including history and physical).
- Local infiltration, metacarpal/metatarsal/digital block, or topical anesthesia.
- The procedure itself.
- Immediate postoperative care, including dictating operative notes and talking with the family and other physicians/health care professionals.
- Writing orders.
- Evaluation of the patient in the postanesthesia recovery area.
- Typical postoperative follow-up care.

You Interpret It! Answers

1. Diagnostic, **2.** Therapeutic, **3.** Therapeutic, **4.** Prophylactic, **5.** Open, **6.** Percutaneous, **7.** Endoscopic, **8.** Included, **9.** Not included; report separately, **10.** Not included; report separately, **11.** 90 days, **12.** Zero days, **13.** 90 days, **14.** Zero days, **15.** Zero days

CHAPTER 26 REVIEW
CPT Surgery Section

Mc Graw Hill connect

Enhance your learning by completing these exercises and more at mcgrawhillconnect.com!

Let's Check It! Terminology

Match each key term to the appropriate definition.

Part I

1. **LO 26.2** The length of time allotted for postoperative care included in the surgical package, which is generally accepted to be 90 days for major surgical procedures and up to 10 days for minor procedures.
2. **LO 26.5** The process of taking skin or tissue (on the same body or another).
3. **LO 26.5** The area or part of the body from which skin or tissue is removed with the intention of placing that skin or tissue in another area or body.
4. **LO 26.1** The methodology or technique used by the physician to perform the procedure, service, or treatment.
5. **LO 26.2** The accepted principles of conduct, services, or treatments that are established as the expected behavior.
6. **LO 26.5** A method of sealing an opening in the skin involving a multilayered closure and a reconstructive procedure such as scar revision, debridement, or retention sutures.
7. **LO 26.5** The full-thickness removal of a lesion, including margins; includes (for coding purposes) a simple closure.
8. **LO 26.5** The area, or site, of the body receiving a graft of skin or tissue.
9. **LO 26.5** A multilevel method of sealing an opening in the skin involving one or more of the deeper layers of the skin.
10. **LO 26.5** A method of sealing an opening in the skin (epidermis or dermis), involving only one layer. It includes the administration of a local anesthesia and/or chemical or electrocauterization of a wound not closed.
11. **LO 26.5** A measure that extends from the epidermis to the connective tissue layer of the skin.

A. Complex Closure
B. Donor Area
C. Excision
D. Full-Thickness
E. Global Period
F. Harvesting
G. Intermediate Closure
H. Recipient Area
I. Simple Closure
J. Standard of Care
K. Surgical Approach

Part II

1. **LO 26.6** Surgically opening the fracture site, or another site in the body nearby, in order to treat the fractured bone.
2. **LO 26.6** The treatment of a fracture without surgically opening the affected area.
3. **LO 26.6** The insertion of fixation instruments (such as pins) placed across the fracture site. It may be done under x-ray imaging for guidance purposes.
4. **LO 26.6** The surgical removal of a vertebral posterior arch.
5. **LO 26.8** Either of the two major veins in the leg that run from the foot to the thigh near the surface of the skin.
6. **LO 26.14** The relocation of tissue from one individual to another (both of the same species) without an identical genetic match.
7. **LO 26.14** The transfer of tissue from one site to another.
8. **LO 26.6** The immobilization of a joint using a surgical technique.
9. **LO 26.6** The attempted return of the fracture or dislocation to its normal alignment manually by the physician.
10. **LO 26.13** The area between the eyelid and the eyeball.

A. Allotransplantation
B. Arthrodesis
C. Closed Treatment
D. Fornix
E. Laminectomy
F. Manipulation
G. Open Treatment
H. Percutaneous Skeletal Fixation
I. Saphenous Vein
J. Transplantation

CPT

Let's Check It! Concepts

Choose the most appropriate answer for each of the following questions.

Part I

1. **LO 26.2** The global surgical package includes all *except*
   a. preprocedure evaluation and management.
   b. general anesthesia.
   c. the procedure.
   d. follow-up care.
2. **LO 26.3** The global period is determined by
   a. the type of anesthesia provided.
   b. the size of the excision.
   c. the location of the donor site.
   d. the standard of care.
3. **LO 26.1** Which of the following is an example of a diagnostic test not included in the global package?
   a. Closure **b.** Local infiltration **c.** Biopsy **d.** Metacarpal block
4. **LO 26.2** When a procedure is planned as a series of procedures, each service after the first should be appended with the modifier
   a. 76 **b.** 79 **c.** 58 **d.** 59
5. **LO 26.4** When a surgeon does not provide preoperative or postoperative care to the patient upon whom he or she operates, the procedure code should be appended with modifier
   a. 54 **b.** 55 **c.** 56 **d.** 77
6. **LO 26.5** Excision of lesions is reported
   a. with total measurement of all lesions removed in one code.
   b. with only the largest lesion coded.
   c. with each lesion coded separately.
   d. as a part of the total surgical procedure.
7. **LO 26.5** The code for excision of a lesion includes this type of repair.
   a. Intermediate **b.** Complex **c.** None **d.** Simple
8. **LO 26.5** If the surgeon performs a reexcision of a lesion during a later encounter with the patient, append the procedure code with modifier
   a. 58 **b.** 59 **c.** 51 **d.** 77
9. **LO 26.5** If multiple wounds located on the same anatomical site are repaired with the same complexity, report this procedure by
   a. coding each wound separately.
   b. coding only the largest wound.
   c. adding all the lengths together and coding the total.
   d. coding the average of all the wounds repaired.
10. **LO 26.5** The elements of determining the most accurate code for a skin graft include all *except*
    a. the size of the recipient area.
    b. the type of donor.
    c. the location of the recipient area.
    d. the type of graft.

Part II

1. **LO 26.6** Codes within the musculoskeletal subsection include
   a. x-rays. **b.** casts. **c.** medications. **d.** shoes.
2. **LO 26.13** Which of the following is/are part of the inner ear?
   a. Auditory ossicles **b.** Oval window **c.** Eustachian tube **d.** Semicircular canals

3. **LO 26.7** Thoracotomy, with biopsy of pleura, would be coded

   a. 32096 **b.** 32097 **c.** 32098 **d.** 32400

4. **LO 26.14** Backbench work during a transplant process is

   a. the harvesting of an organ from a donor. **b.** the implantation of the new organ.
   c. the documentation of the surgery. **d.** the preparation of the organ.

5. **LO 26.8** When an arterial graft is performed, which of the following codes, in addition to the code for the bypass procedure, would be assigned if the graft is harvested from the femoropopliteal vein?

   a. 35600 **b.** 35500 **c.** 35572 **d.** 35601

6. **LO 26.11** Vulvectomy, radical, partial; with unilateral inguinofemoral lymphadenectomy would be coded

   a. 56620 **b.** 56630 **c.** 56631 **d.** 56632

7. **LO 26.8** The code for an endovascular repair of an iliac aneurysm includes all *except*

   a. introduction of graft. **b.** stent deployment. **c.** balloon angioplasty. **d.** pacemaker.

8. **LO 26.9** A laparoscopy, surgical, gastric restrictive procedure; with gastric bypass and Roux-en-Y gastroenterostomy of 145 cm would be coded

   a. 43846 **b.** 43847 **c.** 43644 **d.** 43645

9. **LO 26.12** Code 62263 includes all of the following *except*

   a. percutaneous insertion of an epidural catheter.
   b. extensive dural grafting.
   c. procedure injections.
   d. multiple adhesiolysis sessions over the course of 2 or more days.

10. **LO 26.10** A physician who only interprets the results of a urodynamic procedure must append the code with

   a. modifier 32 **b.** modifier 26 **c.** modifier 53 **d.** modifier 51

Let's Check It! Guidelines

Refer to the Surgery Guidelines and fill in the blanks accordingly.

concomitant	supervision	session	independently	Follow-up
component	Introduction	technique	therapeutic	integral
usually	guidelines	"separate procedure"	management	guidance
59	date	modifiers	itself	diagnostic
addition	one	Radiology	Evaluation and Management	surgical
designated	only	destruction	separately	post-operative

1. Guidelines to direct general reporting for services are presented in the ____.
2. Services rendered in the office, home, or hospital, consultations, and other medical services are listed in the ____ Services section.
3. ____ care for diagnostic procedures includes ____ that care related to recovery from the diagnostic procedure itself.
4. Care of the condition for which the ____ procedure was performed or of other ____ conditions is not included and may be listed ____.
5. Follow-up care for ____ surgical procedure includes only that care which is ____ a part of the ____ service.
6. When more than ____ procedure/service is performed on the same ____, same ____ or during a ____ period, several CPT ____ may apply.
7. The codes designated as ____ should not be reported in ____ to the code for the total procedure or service of which it is considered an ____ component.

8. However, when a procedure or service that is ___ as a "separate procedure" is carried out ___ or considered to be unrelated or distinct from other procedures/services provided at that time, it may be reported by ___, or in addition to other procedures/services by appending modifier ___ to the specific "separate procedure" code to indicate that the procedure is not considered to be a ___ of another procedure, but is a distinct, independent procedure.
9. When imaging ___ or imaging ___ and interpretation is included in a surgical procedure, ___ for image documentation and report, included in the guidelines for ___, will apply.
10. Surgical ___ is a part of a surgical procedure and different methods of destruction are not ordinarily listed separately unless the ___ substantially alters the standard ___ of a problem or condition.

Let's Check It! Rules and Regulations

Please answer the following questions from the knowledge you have gained after reading this chapter.

1. **LO 26.1** Explain the difference between prophylactic, diagnostic, and therapeutic treatments.
2. **LO 26.4** What does the notation "Separate Procedure" tell a professional coder?
3. **LO 26.5** What is the formula to find the correct coded size of an excised lesion?
4. **LO 26.5** Differentiate between intermediate closure repair and complex closure repair.
5. **LO 26.15** When a surgeon performs microsurgery, he or she has to use an operating microscope. What code identifies the use of the microscope?

ICD-10-CM

YOU CODE IT! Basics

First, identify the procedural main term in the following statements; then code the procedure or service.

Example: Dr. Slaughter drains an ovarian cyst, vaginal approach:

a. main term: Drainage b. procedure: 58800

1. Dr. Ladd performs a fine-needle aspiration using ultrasound-guidance imaging; first lesion:
   a. main term:______ b. procedure:______
2. Dr. Dingle performs paring of six soft corn lesions:
   a. main term:______ b. procedure:______
3. Dr. Gunter removes 10 skin tags:
   a. main term: ______ b. procedure:______
4. Dr. Strobel performs an insertion of a nonbiodegradable drug delivery contraception implant:
   a. main term:______ b. procedure:______
5. Dr. Amerson performs cryotherapy for acne:
   a. main term:______ b. procedure:______
6. Mark Latham was accidentally shot in the arm; Dr. Quattlebaum explores and enlarges the wound to remove the bullet. Code the exploration of the wound:
   a. main term:______ b. procedure:______
7. Dr. Hunter applies a uniplane external fixation device for temporary stabilization of a radial fracture:
   a. main term: ______ b. procedure:______
8. Dr. Preston performs an arthroscopic repair of a rotator cuff tear:
   a. main term: ______ b. procedure:______
9. Roy has an implanted single-chamber pacemaker; Dr. Terrence removes the existing pulse generator, tests the existing lead, and inserts a new dual-chamber system for an upgrade:
   a. main term: ______ b. procedure:______
10. Dr. Shumpert performs a infratentorial craniotomy to remove a hematoma; intracerebellar:
    a. main term: ______ b. procedure:______
11. Dr. Wattel performs an epidermal facial chemical peel:
    a. main term: ______ b. procedure:______
12. Dr. Rudner performs a breast reconstruction with free flap:
    a. main term: ______ b. procedure:______

(continued)

13. Dr. Payton excises a malignant lesion from the neck that measured 2.9 cm with margins:

a. main term: ______ **b.** procedure:______

14. Dr. Charne excises an ischial pressure ulcer with a primary suture:

a. main term:______ **b.** procedure:______

15. Dorothy Loman had a small partial-thickness burn on her hand. Dr. Beariman performed a debridement and dressing of the injury:

a. main term:______ **b.** procedure:______

YOU CODE IT! Practice

Using the techniques described in this chapter, carefully read through the case studies and determine the most accurate surgery CPT code(s) and modifier(s), if appropriate, for each case study.

1. Jack Friedman, a 41-year-old male, was in a fight at a soccer game and was hit in the head with a bottle, which caused some deep lacerations in his scalp. Dr. Girald performed a layered closure of the wounds: one 2.0 cm, one 4.5 cm, and two lacerations that were 1.0 cm each in length.
2. Bobby Sherman, a 36-year-old male, cut his left thumb at work on a construction site 2 weeks ago. He did not get any treatment for the wound, which became infected. Today, Dr. Ravenell admitted Bobby to Westward Hospital and amputated the thumb. The procedure is made more complicated by the spread of the infection to the surrounding tissues, as Dr. Ravenell fights to save as much of the hand as possible.
3. Patricia Atkins, a 31-year-old female, has been diagnosed with pleural effusion. Patricia is having difficulty breathing and is admitted to the hospital, where Dr. Jamison performs a percutaneous pleural drainage and inserts an indwelling catheter. Dr. Jamison is aided by image guidance. Patricia tolerates the procedure well and is breathing easier.
4. Kevin Benchley, a 52-year-old male, has been diagnosed with benign prostatic hyperplasia (BPH). Kevin and Dr. Derek, his urologist, have discussed the options, and Kevin has elected to proceed with a TURP. Kevin is taken to the OR, where he is placed under general anesthesia and the transurethral electrosurgical resection of prostate, complete, is performed without complication. Code the TURP procedure.
5. Dr. Albertson performed a lumbar laminectomy, 2 vertebral segments, for decompression on Grace James on September 15. One month later, as originally planned, Dr. Albertson brought Grace back into the OR to implant an epidural drug infuser with a subcutaneous reservoir. Code both procedures.
6. Bridgette Smith found a sore on her neck. The lab test identified it as a malignant lesion, and Dr. Payas excised the lesion, which measured 2.9 cm with margins.
7. Alice Milton, a 39-year-old female, was diagnosed with an abdominal wall incisional hernia, which was repaired using prosthetic mesh. Alice has had recurrent infections. Alice is taken to the OR, where Dr. Gilroy debrides the infected subcutaneous tissue and removes the prosthetic mesh.
8. Samantha DaVita, a 74-year-old female, has a permanent subcutaneous implanted defibrillator system, which is not functioning properly. Samantha is taken to the OR, where Dr. Meetze removes and replaces the implanted defibrillator pulse generator and subcutaneous electrode; 25 minutes of moderate sedation was achieved. The new defibrillator system is tested and is working within normal limits. The nurse monitored Samantha's vital signs during the procedure. Samantha tolerated the procedure well.
9. Having trouble hearing, Ruth Ann Marcelle, a 73-year-old female, came to see Dr. Assiss, an otolaryngologist. After examination, Dr. Assiss uses a curette to remove the impacted earwax from both ears. Ruth Ann was amazed at the improvement in her hearing and left the office feeling much better.
10. One week ago, Dr. Alden performed a ureteroneocystostomy with cystoscopy and ureteral stent placement laparoscopically on Brad Vitalli. Brad is admitted to the hospital today because Dr. Alden must perform an open procedure to drain a renal abscess that was discovered. Dr. Alden drained the abscess. Brad tolerated the procedure well. Code the drainage of Brad's renal abscess.

(continued)

11. Frank Chestnut, a 17-year-old male, came to see Dr. Quartermain for the first time. He was in a fight at school and got punched in the jaw, dislocating his temporomandibular joint. Dr. Quartermain performed a closed treatment of the temporomandibular dislocation. The dislocation did not require any wiring or fixation.
12. Dr. Quinn ordered a catheter aspiration with fiberscope of Stephan's tracheobronchial tree. The procedure was performed at Stephan's bedside in his hospital room. The patient received 15 minutes of conscious sedation. Stephan is a 34-year-old male.
13. Colleen Sizmauski, a morbidly obese 27-year-old female, was admitted for a gastric restrictive procedure. In addition to the gastric bypass performed by Dr. Lafferty, Colleen's small intestine was reconstructed to limit absorption.
14. Dr. Macintosh performed the backbench preparation of a cadaver donor heart allograft prior to Dr. Gantt's performing the transplantation. Code for Dr. Mackintosh's work.
15. Hannah Lopez, a 53-year-old female, hurt her eye in an accident. Dr. Dawson examined her and noticed that her cornea was scratched. It was not a perforating laceration. Dr. Dawson repaired the laceration of the cornea in the office.

CPT HCPCS Level II

YOU CODE IT! Application

The following exercises provide practice in the application of abstracting the physicians' notes and learning to work with documentation from our health care facility, Prader, Bracker, & Associates. These case studies are modeled on real patient encounters. Using the techniques described in this chapter, carefully read through the case studies and determine the most accurate surgery CPT code(s) and modifier(s), if appropriate, for each case study.

PRADER, BRACKER, & ASSOCIATES

A Complete Health Care Facility

159 Healthcare Way • SOMEWHERE, FL 32811 • 407-555-6789

PATIENT: PENNETTA, OSCAR

ACCOUNT/EHR #: PENNOS001

Preoperative DX: Lacerations of arm, hand, and leg

Postoperative DX: Same

Procedure: Layered closure of leg laceration; simple closure of arm and hand lacerations

Surgeon: Gregg Wilson, MD

Assistant: None

Anesthesia: General

INDICATIONS: The patient is a 4-year-old male brought to the emergency room by his mother. He was helping his father install a new window when the window fell and shattered. Oscar suffered lacerations on his left hand, left arm, and left leg.

PROCEDURE: The patient was placed on the table in supine position. Satisfactory anesthesia was obtained. The area was prepped, and attention to the deeper laceration of the left thigh, right above the patella, was first. A layered closure was performed, and the 5.1-cm laceration was closed successfully with sutures. The lacerations on the upper extremity, a 2-cm laceration on the left hand at the base of the fifth metacarpal and the 3-cm laceration on the left arm, just below the joint capsule in the posterior position, were successfully closed with 4-0 Vicryl, as well. Patient tolerated the procedures well and was transported to the recovery room.

Determine the most accurate surgery CPT code(s) and modifier(s), if appropriate.

(continued)

WESTON HOSPITAL

629 Healthcare Way • SOMEWHERE, FL 32811 • 407-555-6541

PATIENT: DRESDEN, NELDA

ACCOUNT/EHR #: DRESNE001

Preoperative DX: Toxic epidermal necrolysis

Postoperative DX: Same

Procedure: Xenograft

Surgeon: William Dresser, MD

Assistant: None

Anesthesia: Local

INDICATIONS: The patient is a 9-year-old female with a diagnosis of toxic epidermal necrolysis as a result of a reaction to procainamide, previously prescribed by a physician no longer in attendance.

PROCEDURE: The patient was placed on the table in supine position. Local anesthesia was administered. As soon as patient stated a complete loss of feeling in the left forearm, the dermal xenograft proceeded. Procedure was repeated for right forearm.

A total of 150 sq. cm of grafting was successfully completed.

Bandages were applied. A prescription for Darvocet N100 po q4–6h prn was given to the patient before discharge.

Follow-up appointment in office scheduled for 10 days.

Determine the most accurate surgery CPT code(s) and modifier(s), if appropriate.

WESTON HOSPITAL

629 Healthcare Way • SOMEWHERE, FL 32811 • 407-555-6541

PATIENT: APPON, CYNTHIA

ACCOUNT/EHR #: APPOCY001

Attending Physician: Regina Glasser, MD

Preoperative DX: C5 compression fracture

Postoperative DX: Same

Procedure: C5 corpectomy and fusion fixation with fibular strut graft and Atlantis plate

Anesthesia: General endotracheal

This is a 31-year-old female status post assault. The patient sustained a C5 compression fracture. MRI scan showed compression with evidence of posterior ligamentous injury. The patient was subsequently set up for the surgical procedure. The procedure was described in detail, including the risks. The risks included but were not limited to bleeding, infection, stroke, paralysis, death, CSF leak, loss of bladder and bowel control, hoarse voice, paralyzed vocal cord, death, and damage to adjacent nerves and tissues. The patient understood the risks. The patient also understood that bank bone instrumentation would be used and that the bank bone could collapse and the instrumentation could fail or break, or the screws could pull out. The patient provided consent.

The patient was taken to the OR. The patient was induced. An endotracheal tube was placed. A Foley was placed. The patient was given preoperative antibiotics. The patient was placed in slight extension. The right neck was prepped and draped in the usual manner. A linear incision was made over the C5 vertebral body. The platysma was divided. Dissection was continued medial to the sternocleidomastoid to the prevertebral fascia. This was cauterized and divided. The longus colli was cauterized and elevated. The fracture was visualized. A spinal needle was used to verify the location using fluoroscopy. The C5 vertebral body was drilled out. The bone was saved. The disks above and below were removed. The posterior longitudinal ligament was removed. The bone was quite collapsed and

(continued)

fragmented. Distraction pins were then packed with bone removed from the C5 vertebral body prior to implantation. A plate was then placed with screws in the C4 and C6 vertebral bodies. The locking screws were tightened. The wound was irrigated. Bleeding was helped with the bipolar. The retractors were removed. The incision was approximated with simple interrupted Vicryl. The subcutaneous tissue was approximated, and skin edges were approximated subcuticularly. Steri-Strips were applied. A dressing was applied. The patient was placed back in an Aspen collar. The patient was extubated and transferred to recovery.

Determine the accurate surgery CPT code(s) and modifier(s), if appropriate.

WESTON HOSPITAL

629 Healthcare Way • SOMEWHERE, FL 32811 • 407-555-6541

PATIENT: WHEATON, MARLA

ACCOUNT/EHR #: WHEAMA001

Preoperative DX: High-grade squamous intraepithelial lesion of the cervix

Postoperative DX: Same

Operation: Loop electrosurgical excision procedure (LEEP) and endocervical curettage (ECC)

Surgeon: Ralph L. Goff, MD

Assistant: None

Anesthesia: General by LMA

Findings: Large ectropion, large nonstaining active cervix essentially encompassing the entire active cervix

Specimens: To pathology

Disposition: Stable to recovery room

PROCEDURE: The patient was taken to the OR, where she was placed in the supine position and administered general anesthesia. She was then placed in candy cane stirrups and prepped and draped in the usual fashion. Her vaginal vault was not prepped. The coated speculum was then placed and the cervix exposed. It was then painted with Lugol and the entire active cervix was nonstaining with the clearly defined margins where the stain began to be picked up. The cervix was injected with approximately 7 cc of lidocaine with 1% epinephrine. Using a large loop, the anterior cervix was excised, and then the posterior loop was excised in separate specimens. Because of the size of the lesion, one piece in total was not accomplished. Prior to the excision, the endocervical curettage was performed, and specimens were collected. All specimens were sent to pathology. The remaining cervical bed was cauterized and then painted with Monsel for hemostasis. The case was concluded with this. Instruments were removed. The patient was taken down from candy cane stirrups, awakened from the anesthesia, and taken to the recovery room in stable condition.

Determine the accurate surgery CPT code(s) and modifier(s), if appropriate.

WESTON HOSPITAL

629 Healthcare Way • SOMEWHERE, FL 32811 • 407-555-6541

PATIENT: UPTON, MAXINE

ACCOUNT/EHR #: UPTOMA001

Diagnosis: Medulloblastoma

Procedure: Central Venous Access Device (CVAD) insertion

Physician: Vincent Hoyt, MD

Anesthesia: Conscious sedation

(continued)

PROCEDURE: Patient is a 4-year-old female, with a recent diagnosis of malignancy. Due to an upcoming course of chemotherapy, the CVAD is being inserted to ease administration of the drugs. The patient was placed on the table in supine position and 1 mg of Versed was administered IM; moderate sedation was achieved, 13 minutes. Maxine's vital signs were monitored by the nurse. The incision was made to insert a central venous catheter, centrally. During the placement of the catheter, a short tract (nontunneled) was made as the catheter was advanced from the skin entry site to the point of venous cannulation. The catheter tip was set to reside in the subclavian vein. The patient was gently aroused from the sedation and was awake when transported to the recovery room.

Determine the accurate surgery CPT code(s) and modifier(s), if appropriate.

27

CPT Radiology Section

Key Terms

Angiography
Arthrography
Computed Tomography (CT)
Computed Tomography Angiography (CTA)
Fluoroscope
Magnetic Resonance Arthrography (MRA)
Magnetic Resonance Imaging (MRI)
Nuclear Medicine
Radiation
Sonogram
Venography

Learning Outcomes

After completing this chapter, the student should be able to:

LO 27.1 Distinguish the different types of imaging.
LO 27.2 Abstract the different reasons for imaging services.
LO 27.3 Identify the technical components from professional components.
LO 27.4 Apply the guidelines accurately regarding the number of views.
LO 27.5 Apply the guidelines to determine how to code the administration of contrast materials.
LO 27.6 Recognize diagnostic radiologic services.
LO 27.7 Interpret accurately into CPT codes to report mammography services.
LO 27.8 Discern how to report bone and joint studies.
LO 27.9 Decide when to code radiation treatments.
LO 27.10 Determine how to accurately report nuclear medicine services.

STOP! Remember, you need to follow along in your CPT code book for an optimal learning experience.

27.1 Types of Imaging

Health care professionals use medical imaging technologies to see inside the body to support medical decision making and accurate diagnostics. Radiologic services, also known as *interventional radiology*, can be used to investigate a potential condition (diagnostically), measure the progress of a disease or condition, or aid in the actual reduction or prevention of disease or other condition (therapeutically).

Many, many years ago, radiology was simply known as x-ray because this was the extent of the equipment. Now, technology has made tremendous advancements in the science of imaging, and health care professionals can screen, diagnose, monitor, and treat patients much more effectively and efficiently.

X-Rays (Radiography)

Radiography is the term that describes the use of x-rays to visualize the visceral aspects (internal structures) of the human body. An x-ray tube emits a type of electromagnetic radiation that is passed through and recorded on the opposite side of the anatomical site being investigated by a digital detector (the digital version of film). Radiologists can identify bone, muscle, and soft tissue on the image because each absorbs the radiation at differing levels. The resulting contrast records a two-dimensional image for evaluation and analysis.

Clinical Applications

- Chest x-rays are most commonly used to analyze aspects of the lungs.
- Skeletal x-rays are frequently used to identify and diagnose fractures, dislocations, and other abnormalities of the bones.
- Abdominal x-rays are used to determine obstructions in any organs within the cavity, or to illuminate the presence of air or fluid.
- Dental x-rays are employed to detect abnormalities such as dental caries or abscesses.

Computed Tomography (CT) Scans

A computed tomography (CT) scanner is similar to radiography in that it is constructed of an x-ray tube and detectors. During a CT scan, an x-ray beam is emitted, aimed through the anatomical site being studied, and recorded by the detectors, which reconstruct the emissions in order to create a two- or three-dimensional image that results in a cross-sectional slice through the patient at that point. Each consecutive image is acquired at a slightly different angle, providing a more complete picture of the internal aspects. Other types of CT scans include: Computed tomography angiography (CTA) which is focused on the visualization of arteries and veins of a specific anatomical site; and perfusion computed tomography (CT perfusion) used to investigate blood flow parameters.

Contrast media may be used to enable differentiation of the various structures of similar density throughout the body. The contrast materials enable the identification of various abnormalities, including hemorrhaging and malignant tissue.

Clinical Applications

- Brain function
- Neck/head
- Vascular system

Magnetic Resonance Imaging (MRI)

Magnetic resonance imaging (MRI) provides three-dimensional views of internal body organs, in real time, with greater visibility of variations within soft tissues, making visualization of brain, spine, muscles, joints, and other structures more informative. The images are captured utilizing a multiplanar modality (various body planes without changing the position of the patient). Similarly to CT scans, contrast materials may be used to illuminate specific visceral aspects.

Clinical Applications

- Measuring volumes of brain structures.
- Measurement of brain tissue.
- Soft tissue damage.

Positron Emission Tomography (PET)

Unlike CT or MRI, PET studies metabolic activity and/or body function. A radioactive medication is administered via IV enabling the areas of abnormal metabolism as well as the detection of tumors and other dysfunctions, not typically detectable by other means, to be captured.

Clinical Applications

- Detection and staging of cancer.
- Diagnosis of certain dementias such as Alzheimer's disease.
- Evaluation of coronary artery disease.

Nuclear Medicine

Nuclear medicine employs the administration of radioactive tracers to enable images of internal organs. The radioactive tracer produces gamma radiation, enabling a gamma camera to capture two-dimensional or three-dimensional images.

Nuclear medicine might also be used for therapeutic purposes. For instance, a larger dose of therapeutic radiation (a radiopharmaceutical specific to the particular diagnosis) may be used to eradicate malignant cells.

Clinical Applications

- Assessing the metabolic activity of a skeletal structure.
- Comparing blood flow to the myocardium at exercise and rest.
- Determining renal perfusion and drainage.
- Comparing pulmonary ventilation and perfusion.
- Assessing the thyroid gland's appearance and function.

Fluoroscopy

Fluoroscopy also utilizes x-rays to visualize internal organ structure and function. The emission of the x-ray beams is continuous, producing a real-time, dynamic image. High-density contrast agents, such as barium, might be administered to enable comparative data.

Clinical Applications

- Hysterosalpingography (HSG).
- Retrograde urethrogram.
- Micturating cysto-urethrogram.
- Fistulography.
- Guidance for procedures, such as the reduction of a fracture.

Ultrasound (Sonography)

Ultrasound, also known as sonography, uses high-frequency sound waves to capture cross-sectional images of visceral organs, including the arteries, veins, and lymph nodes. There are several different types of ultrasound:

- *A-mode* indicates a one-dimensional ultrasonic measurement procedure.
- *M-mode* is also a one-dimensional ultrasonic measurement procedure; however, it includes the movement of the trace so that there can be a recording of both amplitude and velocity of the moving echo-producing structures.
- *B-scan* indicates a two-dimensional ultrasonic scanning procedure with a two-dimensional display.
- *Real-time scan* indicates that a two-dimensional ultrasonic scanning procedure with a display was performed, and included both the two-dimensional structure and motion with time.

Ultrasound also may be used as a visual guide for percutaneous surgical procedures.

Clinical Applications

- Abdominal cavity.
- Pelvic area [*NOTE:* Codes are different for an obstetrical ultrasound vs. nonpregnant pelvic area].
- Cardiovascular structures, i.e., (echocardiography).

Angiography

During an angiography, x-rays are used to identify obstruction or stenosis of an artery or vein, as well as other problems with the cardiovascular system. Contrast dyes may be administered to illuminate a specific vessel to enable visualization of blood flow and blockages.

Clinical Applications

- Tracking blood flow through arteries.
- Identifying blood vessel malformations (thrombi, aneurysms).
- Discovering arteriosclerosis.

CPT

LET'S CODE IT! SCENARIO

PATIENT: Bonnie Suzett-Ellenton

REFERRING PHYSICIAN: Lawrence Chorino, MD

RE: MRI OF THE LUMBAR SPINE

Comparison is made to an earlier exam.

TECHNIQUE: Multiplanar images were obtained using multiple pulse sequences to the lumbar spine. Because of the post-operative nature of the lumbar spine, additional axial and sagittal postgadolinium T1-weighted images were obtained.

(continued)

Plain films are not available for comparison; therefore, it will be assumed there is a normal complement of lumbar vertebrae. Scanning was performed on 0.3-Tesla open bore scanner.

FINDINGS: The examination shows lumbar vertebrae to be in normal overall alignment with preservation in vertebral body heights and normal signal within the marrow. For descriptive purposes of this study, a fairly small disc is noted at the S1–S2 interspace. The tip of the conus lies near the lower body of L1; we believe this nomenclature is the same as that used on the prior exam.

Transaxial images show postsurgical changes from prior right semi-hemilaminectomy at the S1 vertebra. Examination does show the presence of a small annular disc bulge and perhaps some early annular spurring; however, the traversing S1 nerve roots are unimpeded, and there is no evidence of recurrent focal disc herniation. There is some normal enhancement seen involving the soft tissues, presumably of a postoperative nature.

At the L4–L5 level, there is likewise no evidence of focal disc herniation or significant central spinal stenosis.

The L3–L4 interspace shows trace annular bulging without focal disc herniation or stenosis. L1–L2 and L2–L3 interspaces show a normal appearance on sagittal imaging.

IMPRESSION: MR examination of the lumbar spine with postsurgical changes from previous right semi-hemilaminectomy at L5-S1 level on the right.

While there may be some minimal annular bulging and annular spurring at this level, there is no discrete focal disc herniation, and traversing S1 nerve roots are not compromised.

The remainder of the lumbar interspaces may show some very minimal disc bulging; however, there is no focal disc herniation or central spinal stenosis. The cause of the patient's right lower extremity radicular symptoms cannot easily be explained on the basis of findings.

Jason Kunerreth, MD

Chief of Radiology

Let's Code It!

Dr. Kunerreth supervised and analyzed the MRI of Bonnie's lumbar spine. Turn to the Alphabetic Index of CPT and look for the term that MRI stands for . . .

Magnetic Resonance Imaging (MRI)

Go back and read the documentation to determine if the MRI was done for diagnostic purposes or as guidance for another procedure. This was to determine the patient's current condition; therefore, it is a diagnostic procedure.

Magnetic Resonance Imaging (MRI)

Diagnostic

Spine

Cervical 72141, 72142, 72156

Lumbar 72148, 72149, 72158

Thoracic 72146, 72147, 72157

What part of Bonnie's spine was examined? Her *lumbar* spine. Now, you need to turn to the *Main Section* and check out all three of the suggested codes.

72148 **Magnetic resonance (e.g., proton) imaging, spinal canal and contents, lumbar; without contrast material**

72149 **Magnetic resonance (e.g., proton) imaging, spinal canal and contents, lumbar; with contrast material**

72158 **Magnetic resonance (e.g., proton) imaging, spinal canal and contents, without contrast material, followed by contrast material(s) and further sequences; lumbar**

Does the documentation mention the use of contrast materials? Yes, it does. See the sentence in the section titled **TECHNIQUE**:

"*Because of the postoperative nature of the lumbar spine, additional axial and sagittal postgadolinium T1-weighted images were obtained.*"

(continued)

Gadolinium is a contrast material. *Postgadolinium* means after the contrast material was introduced. "*Additional . . . images*" tells you that both without contrast and with contrast images were captured.

Now you know how to report Dr. Kunerreth's services . . .

72158 **Magnetic resonance (e.g., proton) imaging, spinal canal and contents, without contrast material, followed by contrast material(s) and further sequences; lumbar**

27.2 Purposes for Imaging

Screening or Diagnostic

Identifying whether an imaging service is performed as a screening or a diagnostic tool can be important in determining the correct code for the procedure. This designation refers to the reason the physician ordered the test.

A screening image is typically performed as part of a regular preventive checkup. This is ordered because the standard of care and the calendar have matched up. For example, a screening mammogram will be ordered the same time every year for a woman over the age of 50. There are no signs or symptoms that would prompt the test. It is just the wise thing to do to make certain all is fine.

A diagnostic image is taken to assist in the identification and/or confirmation of a suspected condition or diagnosis. In these cases, the physician would identify specific signs or symptoms that led him or her to decide this test was needed.

There are times when an imaging session for a patient begins as a screening test and becomes a diagnostic test while the patient is still there. With technology providing instant imaging, the radiologist can review the images almost immediately after they have been taken, while the patient is still on the premises. This eliminates a patient's needing to come back at another time to retake an image that was not clear or the technician's having to take additional views because the radiologist identified a suspicious element. When a screening test turns into a diagnostic test, report only the diagnostic imaging service because that will include the screening aspect of the procedure.

EXAMPLES

74261 Computed tomography (CT) colonography, diagnostic, including image postprocessing; without contrast material

74263 Computed tomography (CT) colonography, screening, including image postprocessing

Image Guidance

When a procedure is conducted percutaneously, the physician cannot see into the body. Therefore, in order to ensure that the needle or scalpel finds the correct spot on an internal organ, image guidance will be used. This may be as simple as a fine needle aspiration to a biopsy to a more complex surgical procedure.

In some cases, the CPT book will provide you with a code that includes the imaging guidance; for example:

10007 **Fine needle aspiration biopsy, including fluoroscopic guidance; first lesion**

10009 **Fine needle aspiration biopsy, including CT guidance; first lesion**

10021 **Fine needle aspiration biopsy, without imaging guidance; first lesion**

33289 **Transcatheter implantation of wireless pulmonary artery pressure sensor for long-term hemodynamic monitoring, including . . . radiological supervision and interpretation, and pulmonary artery angiography, when performed**

Often, the CPT book will alert you to the need for a second code to report this additional service with a notation below the code, such as

(For radiological supervision and interpretation, see 76942, 77002, 77012, 77021)

And more code options can be found in the ***Radiology*** section of CPT:

- Ultrasonic Guidance Procedures: 76930-76965
- Other Procedures: 76970-76999
- Fluoroscopic Guidance: 77001-77003
- Computed Tomography Guidance: 77011-77014
- Magnetic Resonance Imaging Guidance: 77021-77022

YOU CODE IT! CASE STUDY

Every year, Margarette Sanchez gets a mammogram the week before her birthday. She feels fine and no lumps were noted during her gynecologist's manual exam. Margarette arrives at the Women's Imaging Center for her annual exam.

You Code It!

Determine the correct code or codes to report the provision of Margarette's annual mammogram.

Step #1: Read the case carefully and completely.
Step #2: Abstract the scenario. Which key words or terms describe what service the physician provided to the patient during this encounter?
Step #3: Are there any details missing or incomplete for which you would need to query the physician? [If so, ask your instructor.]
Step #4: Determine the correct CPT procedure code or codes to explain the details about what was provided to the patient during this encounter.
Step #5: Check for any relevant guidance, including reading all of the symbols and notations.
Step #6: Do you need to append any modifiers to ensure complete and accurate information is provided?
Step #7: Double-check your work.

Answer:

Did you determine this to be the correct code?

77067 Screening mammography, bilateral (2-view study of each breast), including computer-aided detection (CAD) when performed

Good job!

27.3 Technical vs. Professional

Essentially, there are two primary components of any radiologic procedure: the technical and the professional (referred to as supervision and interpretation in the CPT). This is not to say that radiologic technicians are not professionals. The designation is merely to divide the services provided so that it can be determined which facility or practitioner should be paid for what.

EXAMPLE

Jerod Paley, a 41-year-old male, was sent to the Kinsey Imaging Center to get an x-ray, three views, of his skull after he was hit in the head by a bat at a softball game.

The x-ray equipment is owned by the facility. Kris Chappel, the x-ray technician who will operate the equipment, is a member of the facility's staff, and Dr. Briscoe, a board-certified radiologist who will interpret the films and send a report of this evaluation to Jerod's physician, is also a staff member of the center. Therefore, Kinsey Imaging's coding specialist will ask the insurance company for reimbursement for both the technical procedure (the use of the equipment, materials, and the staff to work and maintain that equipment) and the professional aspect (the cost and work to supervise and interpret the films). For Jerod's case, the code to be reported is **70250 Radiologic examination, skull; less than 4 views**.

CODING BITES

You learned in medical terminology class that the suffix *-graphy* means the recording of an image and the suffix *-scopy* means to look or view. We tend to think of all these procedures and services as radiology. However, not all of them are coded from the *Radiology* section of the CPT book.

For example, cardiography is listed in the *Medicine* section. Therefore, always use the Alphabetic Index to help point you toward the correct area of the book. It will save you time in the long run.

Purchasing (or leasing) and maintaining imaging equipment is very expensive and cannot be supported by every health care facility. In addition, physicians who are specially trained radiologists are not necessarily staff members of all health care facilities with the equipment. Therefore, circumstances may arise when the technical procedure and the professional service must be billed separately. In those cases, the coder who is responsible for charging for the professional services must use modifier 26 to identify the separation of the components.

26 **Professional Component:** *Certain procedures are a combination of a physician component and a technical component. When the physician component is reported separately, the service may be identified by adding modifier 26 to the usual procedure number.*

CODING BITES

Technical component: coded to gain reimbursement for the facility that owns and maintains the equipment used, amortized cost of the machine, supplies, maintenance, overhead (electricity and so on), and the technician.

Professional component: coded to gain reimbursement for the health care professional, radiologist, or physician who supervises and interprets the images taken.

CODING BITES

If the third-party payer accepts HCPCS Level II, append modifier **TC Technical Component** to the CPT code, when appropriate.

CODING BITES

Some third-party payers will determine the TC and PC components for payment without the modifier by the place of service code shown on the claim form.

EXAMPLE

Walter Wasser, a 31-year-old male, was brought into the emergency department of a small hospital near his farm after he fell off a ladder onto his back while working in the barn. The physician sent Walter to radiology for x-rays of his entire thoracic, lumbar, and sacral spine (two views). The hospital does not have a staff radiologist, so Dr. Chen is brought over to evaluate the x-rays and write the report for the physician.

The hospital, which owns the equipment and pays the salary of the technician, will bill the insurance carrier for the technical portion of the examination, using code 72082-TC.

Dr. Chen's coding specialist will send in a claim for Dr. Chen's interpretation only, the professional services he provided. In order to make this clear on the claim form, the modifier **26 Professional Component** will be appended to the code for the radiologic examination; the code that will be reported on his claim form will be 72082-26.

As you have already learned, sometimes the CPT book will save you work. Certain radiologic examination codes distinguish the technical component and professional component of services for you. One of the easiest ways to identify such cases is by the notation within the code's description that specifies the code is for radiologic supervision and interpretation only.

EXAMPLE

70015 Cisternography, positive contrast, radiological supervision and interpretation

From the example, you can see that code 70015 excludes the technical component. If you are coding for the physician's services only, that makes it easy. If you are coding for the facility for the technical aspect, you need to add modifier TC Technical Component. After a while, you will learn the details about the procedures performed by all of the professionals in your health care facility, and you will be able to identify the components easily. It just takes some practice.

CPT HCPCS Level II

LET'S CODE IT! SCENARIO

Roland Dellman, an 8-year-old male, is brought into the emergency department by ambulance. He was skateboarding off a homemade ramp and fell on his neck and shoulder. Dr. Tyner suspects a broken clavicle and orders a complete radiologic exam of the area. This facility does not have a radiologist on staff at this time, so the facility took the x-ray and the digital images were electronically sent to Radiology Associates in another state. Dr. Neuman reads the films and sends a report to Dr. Tyner confirming the fracture. Code for Dr. Neuman.

Let's Code It!

The physician's notes state that a *radiologic exam* of Roland's *clavicle* was performed. Let's turn to the Alphabetic Index under *radiology*. Note that the choices are not going to satisfy our needs. Therefore, let's try an alternate term for radiology: x-ray. Turn to *x-ray*, and you find a long list of anatomical sites. Next to the word *clavicle* you see only one suggested code. Let's go to the numeric listing and read the complete description:

73000 Radiologic examination; clavicle, complete

This is exactly what Dr. Tyner ordered for Roland. And the facility only provided the technical component, so the coder would report:

73000-TC Radiologic examination; clavicle, complete, technical component

The coder for Radiology Associates would report **73000-26** to be reimbursed for Dr. Neuman's work.

Good job!

CPT

LET'S CODE IT! SCENARIO

Jalyssa Miland, a 35-year-old female, is 10 weeks pregnant. This is her first pregnancy, and twins run in her family. In order to determine how many fetuses there are, Dr. Ruber orders a **sonogram**. *Iona Appell is the technician at the imaging center next door to Dr. Ruber's office. The Kinsey Imaging Center performs Jalyssa's real-time transabdominal exam and sends the documentation to Dr. Ruber so that he can read and interpret the results. A single fetus was observed.*

Let's Code It!

You are Dr. Ruber's coder, and his notes state that a sonogram of Jalyssa was performed at the imaging center. We know that she is pregnant, and this is why she is having the test done, so the anatomical site of the examination is her *pregnant uterus*.

Turn to the Alphabetic Index under *sonography*, and the CPT book tells you to *see echography*, which is the type of technology that sonograms use. Turn to *echography* (caution—not echo*cardio*graphy; this is not of Jalyssa's heart), and find a list of anatomical sites. Looking for *pregnant uterus*, you see a range of suggested codes. Let's go to the numeric listing and read the complete description of the first one.

76801 Ultrasound, pregnant uterus, real time with image documentation, fetal and maternal evaluation, first trimester (<14 weeks 0 days), transabdominal approach; single or first gestation

Great! The very first code seems to match the notes perfectly. However, to make certain you are using the best, most appropriate code, you will want to read through all the suggested codes.

Remember, you are coding for Dr. Ruber. With regard to Jalyssa's radiologic exam, he provided the interpretation—the professional component only. Therefore, the claim form you prepare should show this code as **76801-26**.

Sonogram
The use of sound waves to record images of internal organs and tissues; also called an *ultrasound.*

27.4 Number of Views

Throughout the ***Radiology*** section of the CPT book, radiologic examinations are often described by the number of views taken by the technician.

EXAMPLE

73060 Radiologic examination, humerus, minimum of 2 views

The "two views" refers to the number of angles, or perceptions, from which the images were taken, such as anterior and posterior. Such codes represent the norm, or standard, in imaging when it comes to these certain anatomical sites.

The most common angles, or pathways, of imaging include:

AP *Anteroposterior:* Front to back.

PA *Posteroanterior:* Back to front.

O *Oblique:* At an angle.

RAO *Right anterior oblique:* At an angle from the right front.

LAO *Left anterior oblique:* At an angle from the left front.

LPO *Left posterior oblique:* At an angle from the left back.

Lat *Lateral (lat):* From one side to the other side.

In those cases when the radiologist takes fewer than the minimum number of views included in the description, you have to append the radiologic code with modifier 52 Reduced Services.

52 Reduced Services: Under certain circumstances a service or procedure is partially reduced or eliminated at the physician's discretion. Under these circumstances, the service provided can be identified by its usual procedure number and the addition of modifier 52, signifying that the service is reduced. This provides a means of reporting reduced services without disturbing the identification of the basic service.

YOU CODE IT! CASE STUDY

Carly-Ann Price, an 18-month-old female, is brought into the office of her pediatrician, Dr. Lattel. She fell off the couch onto a hard tile floor and it appears that her hip is painful to her. Dr. Lattel has his staff take an x-ray of the pelvis and hip to determine if there is a fracture. He orders only the anteroposterior view to be taken. He does not subject his patients to radiology exposure unnecessarily, and he believes that the one view will tell him what he needs to know. The x-ray confirms a hairline fracture, and he applies a cast.

You Code It!

Go through the steps, and determine the code(s) that should be reported for the radiologic service Dr. Lattel provided to Carly-Ann.

Step #1: Read the case carefully and completely.

Step #2: Abstract the scenario. Which key words or terms describe what service the physician provided to the patient during this encounter?

Step #3: Are there any details missing or incomplete for which you would need to query the physician? [If so, ask your instructor.]

Step #4: Determine the correct CPT procedure code or codes to explain the details about what was provided to the patient during this encounter.

(continued)

Step #5: Check for any relevant guidance, including reading all of the symbols and notations.
Step #6: Do you need to append any modifiers to ensure complete and accurate information is provided?
Step #7: Double-check your work.

Answer:

Did you determine this to be the correct code?

73501 Radiologic examination, hip, unilateral, with pelvis when performed; 1 view

Good job!

27.5 Procedures with or without Contrast

Some imaging examinations use contrast materials to gain a clearer picture of an organ or anatomical site. The phrase "with contrast" means that the technician or physician gave the patient a substance to enhance the image. For example, arthrography is used to identify abnormalities that may be present within a joint (wrist, hip, shoulder, knee). Gadolinium is injected into the joint that is to be visualized to provide better-quality images of the patient's condition. In other procedures, different substances are injected. For example, when myelography is done to examine a patient's spinal cord and nerves, an injection of x-ray dye may be used to more clearly visualize a patient's disc herniation, bone spurs, or vertebral stenosis.

Arthrography
The recording of a picture of an anatomical joint after the administration of contrast material into the joint capsule.

Fluoroscope
A piece of equipment that emits x-rays through a part of the patient's body onto a fluorescent screen, causing the image to identify various aspects of the anatomy by density.

Computed Tomography (CT)
A specialized computer scanner with very fine detail that records imaging of internal anatomical sites; also known as computerized axial tomography (CAT).

Computed Tomography Angiography (CTA)
A CT scan using contrast materials to visualize arteries and veins all over the body.

Magnetic Resonance Arthrography (MRA)
MR imaging of an anatomical joint after the administration of contrast material into the joint capsule.

Magnetic Resonance Imaging (MRI)
A three-dimensional radiologic technique that uses nuclear technology to record pictures of internal anatomical sites.

GUIDANCE CONNECTION

Read the additional explanations in the **Radiology Guidelines (Including Nuclear Medicine and Diagnostic Ultrasound)**, subhead **Administration of Contrast Material(s)**, in your CPT book directly in front of the Radiology section that lists all the codes.

1. When radiographic **arthrography** is performed, use an additional code for the supervision and interpretation of the appropriate joint. This includes the use of a **fluoroscope**.

EXAMPLE

Dr. Horace, a radiologist, supervised a radiographic arthrography of Porter Maison's ankle; later the interpreted results were reported with this code:

73615 Radiologic examination, ankle, arthrography, radiological supervision and interpretation

2. Imaging "with contrast" has some guidelines that you have to know in order to code accurately.
   a. If the code description includes the term "with contrast," such as **computed tomography (CT)** with contrast, **computed tomography angiography (CTA)** with contrast, **magnetic resonance arthrography (MRA)** with contrast, or **magnetic resonance imaging (MRI)** with contrast, the injection of the contrast materials, when administered intravenously, is already included in the code and should *not* be reported separately.
   b. If the contrast material is injected intra-articularly (into a joint) or intrathecally (into a tendon or sheath), an additional code is reported for the appropriate injection.
   c. Providing contrast materials orally and/or rectally alone does not constitute an exam "with contrast."

EXAMPLE

Dr. Groder injected Vincent Speck's elbow intrathecally with contrast materials to do a radiographic arthrography for his tennis elbow. This is reported with these codes:

73085	Radiologic examination, elbow, arthrography, radiological supervision and interpretation
20550	Injection(s); single tendon sheath, or ligament, aponeurosis (e.g., plantar "fascia")

3. When a CT or MR arthrography is performed without radiographic arthrography, you will need three different codes:
   a. A code for the injection of the contrast material into the specific joint.
   b. A code for the appropriate CT or MR.
   c. A code for the imaging guidance (fluoroscopy) of the placement of the needle to inject the contrast material.

EXAMPLE

Felicia Hanson is experiencing pain in her pelvic region. Dr. Alvarez orders an MRA of her hip/pelvis with contrast. The material is injected intra-articularly. This is reported using these codes:

27093	Injection procedure for hip arthrography; without anesthesia
72198	Magnetic resonance angiography, pelvis; with or without contrast material(s)
+77002	Fluoroscopic guidance for needle placement (e.g., biopsy, aspiration, injection, localization device)

Other types of radiologic procedures include

- *Positron emission tomography (PET):* Uses a variety of radiopharmaceuticals that mimic natural sugars, water, proteins, and oxygen and collect in various tissues and organs. It is a time-exposure picture of cellular biologic activities.
- *Bone density scan (DEXA):* Used most often for osteoporosis screenings; enables assessment of bone minerals in spine, hip, and other skeletal sites.
- *Nuclear medicine scan:* Used to assess organ system function.

LET'S CODE IT! SCENARIO

Mark Silver, an 81-year-old male, has been having problems with his memory and his walking. After an extensive examination, his neurologist, Dr. Chernuchin, orders an MRI, brain, with and without contrast, to determine if Mark is suffering from hydrocephalus.

Let's Code It!

This is very straightforward. Mark had an *MRI* of his *brain* taken. Let's go to the Alphabetic Index and look this up. Under *magnetic resonance imaging (MRI),* you see the list of anatomical sites, including *brain*, which suggests code range 70551–70553. (*NOTE: Intraoperative*, indented below *brain*, means that the MRI was performed during surgery. This was not the case for Mark, according to the physician's notes.) Let's go to the numeric listing and read the descriptions.

70551	**Magnetic resonance (e.g., proton) imaging, brain (including brain stem); without contrast material**
70552	**with contrast material(s)**
70553	**without contrast material, followed by contrast material(s) and further sequences**

(continued)

Dr. Chernuchin's notes state that the MRI is *with and without contrast.* That means both types of imaging were done. Code 70551 describes without contrast, and code 70552 includes the contrast. When you keep reading, you see that code 70553 is the correct code because, as the notes state, it includes both sequences: without the contrast followed by with contrast materials. Of course, you also will add the appropriate HCPCS Level II codes to report the contrast materials used.

CODING BITES

Appropriate HCPCS Level II codes from the range Q9951–Q9969, based on the number of units, should be assigned to report the contrast materials supplied.

27.6 Diagnostic Radiology

Diagnostic Angiography

The coding of the process of imaging the body's blood vessels, diagnostic **angiography**, carries certain guidelines affecting the use of the codes.

Angiography
The imaging of blood vessels after the injection of contrast material.

1. In some cases, interventional coding guidelines don't permit you to report a diagnostic angiography when it is performed at the same time as a therapeutic interventional procedure. This rule applies when the patient has already been diagnosed and has scheduled a therapeutic intervention to correct the problem. As you have already learned, you must read the guidelines and the code descriptions carefully.

EXAMPLE

Dr. Victoria performed a left internal and external carotid arterial angiography to check for blockage and immediately performed an intervention procedure. You would report this by using codes

36224 Selective catheter placement, internal carotid artery, unilateral, with angiography of the ipsilateral intracranial carotid circulation and all associated radiological supervision and interpretation, includes angiography of the extracranial carotid and cervicocerebral arch, when performed

+36227 Selective catheter placement, external carotid artery, unilateral, with angiography of the ipsilateral external carotid circulation and all associated radiological supervision and interpretation (List separately in addition to code for primary procedure.)

2. In other cases, the diagnostic angiography *should be coded separately* even though it is done at the same session as an interventional procedure. This is true if one of the following conditions has been met:
   - **a.** A full diagnostic study is done, no prior catheter-based angiographic study is available, and the decision to intervene is determined by the diagnostic study.
   - **b.** The patient's condition has changed since a previously done study.
   - **c.** The patient's condition changes during the interventional procedure that requires a diagnostic procedure to look at vessels outside of the area.
   - **d.** The prior diagnostic angiography did not show the applicable anatomy and/or pathology being treated at the session.

EXAMPLE

Thelma Hadid had a diagnostic angiography of her adrenal gland 1 year ago. Since then, her condition has deteriorated. Therefore, Dr. Carnicki first performs a diagnostic procedure. Because this shows changes, at the same session, he performs an interventional procedure.

GUIDANCE CONNECTION

Read the additional explanations in the in-section guidelines within the **Radiology** section, subhead **Vascular Procedures**, subsection **Aorta and Arteries**, directly above code 75600 in your CPT book.

3. Diagnostic angiography is included with the code for an interventional procedure and should *not* be coded separately when that diagnostic angiography is performed for any of the following:
   a. Vessel measurement.
   b. Postangioplasty or stent angiography.
   c. Contrast injections, angiography, road mapping, and/or fluoroscopic guidance for the interventional procedure.

LET'S CODE IT! SCENARIO

Alene Ransom, a 61-year-old female, has had two mild heart attacks in the past 2 years. Today, Alene is at the Beyers Ambulatory Surgical Center for a diagnostic angiography to quantify the degree of blockage suspected in her left renal artery. Dr. Black performs the procedure, which includes placing the catheter directly in the renal artery. Later that day, Dr. Black dictates a report indicating that Alene's left renal artery is 50% blocked.

Let's Code It!

The notes indicate that a *left renal angiography* was performed on Alene. Let's go to the Alphabetic Index and look up *angiography.* You know that Alene's renal artery was examined, and the Alphabetic Index suggests codes 36251–36254. Let's check the complete descriptions in the numeric listings:

36251 **Selective catheter placement (first-order), main renal artery and any accessory renal artery(s) for renal angiography, including arterial puncture and catheter placement(s), fluoroscopy, contrast injection(s), image postprocessing, permanent recording of images, and radiological supervision and interpretation, including pressure gradient measurements when performed, and flush aortogram when performed; unilateral**

36252 **bilateral**

The difference between these two code descriptions is that 36251 is for a unilateral procedure and 36252 is for a bilateral procedure. Alene had only her left renal artery examined. One side is unilateral, leading us to the correct code of **36251**.

Venography
The imaging of a vein after the injection of contrast material.

Diagnostic Venography

The codes for reporting diagnostic **venography** have guidelines similar to those for diagnostic angiography.

1. Some interventional procedure codes include the diagnostic venography when done at the same time as the procedure. You must read the descriptions carefully to determine if this is the case.
2. Diagnostic venography done at the same time as an interventional procedure *should be coded separately* if one of the following conditions has been met:
   a. A full diagnostic study is done, no prior catheter-based venographic study is available, and the decision to intervene is determined by this diagnostic study.
   b. The patient's condition has changed since a previously done study.
   c. The patient's condition changes during the interventional procedure and requires a diagnostic procedure to look at vessels outside of the area.
   d. The prior diagnostic venography did not show the applicable anatomy and/or pathology being treated at the session.

3. Diagnostic venography is included with the code for an interventional procedure and should *not* be coded separately when that diagnostic venography is performed for any of the following:
   a. Vessel measurement.
   b. Postangioplasty or stent venography.
   c. Contrast injections, venography, road mapping, and/or fluoroscopic guidance for the interventional procedure.

GUIDANCE CONNECTION

Read the additional explanations in the in-section guidelines within the **Radiology** section, subhead **Vascular Procedures**, subsection **Veins and Lymphatics**, directly above code 75801 in your CPT book.

LET'S CODE IT! SCENARIO

Charles Baseman, a 55-year-old male, flew in yesterday from Australia, a 26-hour airplane ride. Since getting off the plane, he has been having pain in his right calf. Dr. Vernon performed a diagnostic venography to determine if Charles has deep vein thrombosis (DVT). After completing the procedure, he wrote a report with his interpretation, which was sent to Charles's internist.

Let's Code It!

Dr. Vernon performed a *diagnostic venography* of Charles's *right leg*. Let's go to the Alphabetic Index and find *venography*. Beneath *venography*, you see the anatomical site *leg* with the suggested code range 75820–75822. Let's look at the code descriptions in the numeric listings:

75820 Venography, extremity, unilateral, radiological supervision and interpretation

75822 Venography, extremity, bilateral, radiological supervision and interpretation

The difference between these two codes is that 75820 is a unilateral procedure and 75822 is a bilateral procedure. Charles had only his right leg examined, making it a unilateral procedure and making **75820** the correct code.

Transcatheter Procedures

Therapeutic transcatheter radiologic supervision and interpretation codes, when associated with intervention, already include

1. Vessel measurement.
2. Postangioplasty or stent venography.
3. Contrast injections, angiography/venography, road mapping, and/or fluoroscopic guidance for the interventional procedure.

Transcatheter therapeutic radiologic and interpretation services *are* separately reportable from diagnostic angiography/venography done at the same time *unless* they are specifically included in the code descriptor.

GUIDANCE CONNECTION

Read the additional explanations in the in-section guidelines within the **Radiology** section, subhead **Vascular Procedures**, subsection **Transcatheter Procedures**, directly above code 75894 in your CPT book.

LET'S CODE IT! SCENARIO

Dr. Grubman is in the OR today to perform a transcatheter placement of an intravascular stent, percutaneously, in Olivia Samuel's common iliac.

Let's Code It!

You are Dr. Grubman's coding specialist, so you are going to code only the radiologic supervision and interpretation of the *transcatheter* procedure, as well as the placement of the stent itself. Let's go to *transcatheter* in the Alphabetic Index. You will notice that, if you go to *placement* under *transcatheter*, you see *intravascular stents* indented below. Here, the Alphabetic Index suggests some Category III codes (0075T, 0076T) along with code ranges 37215–37218, 37236–37239, and 92928–92929.

When you turn to the codes, you realize that they are in the ***Surgery*** section, not ***Radiology***. However, they are the only codes offered by the Alphabetic Index, so let's take a look at them all. Notice

37236 Transcatheter placement of an intravascular stent(s) (except lower extremity artery(s) for occlusive disease, cervical carotid, extracranial vertebral or intrathoracic carotid, intracranial or coronary), open or percutaneous, including radiological supervision and interpretation and including all angioplasty within the same vessel, when performed; initial artery

But we are coding for Dr. Grubman's radiologic supervision and interpretation for the procedure as well as the stent placement. Notice that the description for code 37236 includes "radiological supervision and interpretation."

Perfect!

Magnetic Resonance (MR) Safety Implants

Magnetic resonance (MR) imaging provides important insights into the human body and its condition. It is noninvasive while creating high-resolution pictures of the patient's organs, tissues, and skeletal system illuminating details critical to an accurate diagnosis or exclusion of a potential diagnosis. At the same time, there are serious contraindications for performing magnetic resonance imaging on a patient. When a patient has a medical device implant, such as a pacemaker, or a foreign body is present within, it can cause serious harm to the body within the MR chamber.

Codes 76014–76019 provide the ability to report MR safety protocols and the time spent by a trained clinician or health care professional to determine if the implant has an FDA-approved specification for the safe use of MR imaging on this patient, or other ways to reduce or eliminate the danger. All of these safety determinations require a written report of the findings.

Diagnostic Ultrasound

When reporting diagnostic ultrasound services, you need to abstract specific details about the anatomical sites viewed. As the coding specialist, you must read the report and pay attention to whether the exam was "complete" or "limited" and choose the correct code. The description of an ultrasound exam as being "complete" is determined by the specific number of elements, such as organs or areas, that are surveyed during the test. However, sometimes the full list is not visualized. For example, an organ may have been previously removed surgically, or another organ may be blocking the view. The report that is submitted for the patient's record, after the exam, should note everything that was studied–as well as those elements that should have been but were not, along with why they were not.

CODING BITES

If the reason that an organ was not visible is documented in the patient's record, you are permitted to code this as "complete."

You will find information regarding what is included in a complete exam in the guidelines shown below each of the ultrasound subheadings: **Abdomen and Retroperitoneum**, **Pelvis—Obstetrical**, **Pelvis—Nonobstetrical**.

Should an ultrasound exam be performed *without* a thorough evaluation of an organ or anatomical region *and* recording of the image *and* a final, written report, you are not permitted to code the procedure separately.

EXAMPLE

Abdomen and Retroperitoneum

A complete ultrasound examination of the abdomen (76700) consists of real-time scans of the liver, gallbladder, common bile duct, pancreas, spleen, kidney, and the upper abdominal aorta and inferior vena cava including any demonstrated abdominal abnormality.

GUIDANCE CONNECTION

Read the additional explanation in the in-section guidelines within the **Radiology** section, subhead **Diagnostic Ultrasound**, directly above code 76506 in your CPT book.

Let's say an ultrasound examination is done on Herman Smith's abdomen. The documentation includes the physician's (radiologist's) interpretation of all organs except the gallbladder. The patient had his gallbladder removed 1 year prior to this ultrasound exam. As long as this fact is also documented, code 76700 for a complete ultrasound examination of the abdomen is accurate.

You already know that an ultrasound may be called a *sonogram*. However, other definitions are important for you to know so that you can determine the best, most appropriate code. The following terms identify the type of scan:

- *A-mode* indicates a one-dimensional ultrasonic measurement procedure.
- *M-mode* is also a one-dimensional ultrasonic measurement procedure; however, it includes the movement of the trace so that there can be a recording of both amplitude and velocity of the moving echo-producing structures.
- *B-scan* indicates a two-dimensional ultrasonic scanning procedure with a two-dimensional display.
- *Real-time scan* indicates that a two-dimensional ultrasonic scanning procedure with a display was performed and included both the two-dimensional structure and motion with time.

CODING BITES

Ultrasound services are especially dangerous to code from superbills instead of notes. Make certain you get the complete documentation before choosing a code.

If the report indicates that a Doppler evaluation of vascular structures, or another diagnostic vascular ultrasound study, was performed, it should be coded separately with the codes from the **Noninvasive Vascular Diagnostic Studies** subsection, codes 93880–93998.

YOU CODE IT! CASE STUDY

Eriq Taleni, a 57-year-old male, was sent to the Kinsey Imaging Center by Dr. Rayman to have an ophthalmic biometry by ultrasound echography, A-scan. After performing the exam, Dr. Turner, the radiologist, wrote in his report that a second test using intraocular lens power calculation might be necessary to further clarify the condition of the eye. Dr. Rayman determined that Eriq should wait before having the second test.

You Code It!

Go through the steps, and determine the codes that should be reported for the service provided to Eriq Taleni by Dr. Turner.

Step #1: Read the case carefully and completely.
Step #2: Abstract the scenario. Which key words or terms describe what service the physician provided to the patient during this encounter?
Step #3: Are there any details missing or incomplete for which you would need to query the physician? [If so, ask your instructor.]
Step #4: Determine the correct CPT procedure code or codes to explain the details about what was provided to the patient during this encounter.
Step #5: Check for any relevant guidance, including reading all of the symbols and notations.
Step #6: Do you need to append any modifiers to ensure complete and accurate information is provided?
Step #7: Double-check your work.

(continued)

Answer:

Did you determine this to be the correct code?

76516 Ophthalmic biometry by ultrasound echography, A-scan

Good job!

27.7 Mammography

Until researchers can find a way to prevent breast cancer, the best weapon in the health care arsenal is early detection—finding the malignancy when it is tiny and easier to eradicate. Mammography, low-dose radiology, is considered the best method for identifying a small, otherwise undetectable lump or microcalcification. Mammography employs low-energy x-rays specifically designed to take and record images of breast tissue for the discovery of breast lesions.

77065 Diagnostic mammography, including computer-aided detection (CAD) when performed; unilateral

77066 Diagnostic mammography, including computer-aided detection (CAD) when performed; bilateral

77067 Screening mammography, bilateral (2-view film study of each breast), including computer-aided detection (CAD) when performed

At times, computer-aided detection (CAD) is used in conjunction with the x-ray imaging. CAD transitions the x-ray image into a digital image, which is then scanned by a computer, searching for anything that might be abnormal.

YOU CODE IT! CASE STUDY

Every year, Donna Simmons, a 47-year-old female, came in for her annual well-woman exam, and then would go over to the Imaging Center for her screening mammogram. This year, Dr. Douglas felt a lump during Donna's manual exam, so he ordered a diagnostic mammogram for the left breast and a screening mammogram for the right. These mammograms were provided the next day at the Imaging Center.

You Code It!

Read the case study of Donna's encounter at the Imaging Center, and determine the correct code or codes.

Step #1: Read the case carefully and completely.
Step #2: Abstract the scenario. Which key words or terms describe what service the physician provided to the patient during this encounter?
Step #3: Are there any details missing or incomplete for which you would need to query the physician? [If so, ask your instructor.]
Step #4: Determine the correct CPT procedure code or codes to explain the details about what was provided to the patient during this encounter.
Step #5: Check for any relevant guidance, including reading all of the symbols and notations.
Step #6: Do you need to append any modifiers to ensure complete and accurate information is provided?
Step #7: Double-check your work.

Answer:

Did you determine these to be the correct codes?

77065 Diagnostic mammography, including computer-aided detection (CAD) when performed; unilateral

77067-52 Screening mammography, bilateral (2-view film study of each breast), including computer-aided detection (CAD) when performed, reduced services

Good job!

27.8 Bone and Joint Studies

There are many reasons a physician may need information about a patient's bone structure and strength, and several imaging techniques that could be used to provide the most accurate data.

- Bone age studies enable the physician to identify the degree of maturation of a child's bones.
- CT scanography has surpassed orthoroentgenogram in the last decade to determine leg length discrepancies.
- Osseous survey is a radiologic procedure used to identify fractures, tumors, and degenerative conditions of the bone.
- Bone mineral density (BMD) scanning, also called dual-energy x-ray absorptiometry (DXA or DEXA) or bone densitometry, is an enhanced form of x-ray technology that is used to measure bone loss.

GUIDANCE CONNECTION

The **United States Preventive Services Task Force** recommends screening for osteoporosis in women aged 65 years and older and in younger women whose fracture risk is equal to or greater than that of a 65-year-old white woman who has no additional risk factors.

YOU CODE IT! CASE STUDY

Rachel VanHeusen, a 65-year-old female, arrived at the Kinsey Imaging Center to have a DEXA bone density study, both axial and appendicular skeleton. Dr. Underwood, the staff radiologist, analyzed the images and wrote a report.

You Code It!

The Kinsey Imaging Center performed a DEXA bone density study for both the axial and appendicular skeleton of Rachel VanHeusen. Review the details, and determine the code or codes for this service.

Step #1: Read the case carefully and completely.
Step #2: Abstract the scenario. Which key words or terms describe what service the physician provided to the patient during this encounter?
Step #3: Are there any details missing or incomplete for which you would need to query the physician? [If so, ask your instructor.]
Step #4: Determine the correct CPT procedure code or codes to explain the details about what was provided to the patient during this encounter.
Step #5: Check for any relevant guidance, including reading all of the symbols and notations.
Step #6: Do you need to append any modifiers to ensure complete and accurate information is provided?
Step #7: Double-check your work.

Answer:

Did you accurately determine these to be the codes?

77080 **Dual-energy X-ray absorptiometry (DXA), bone density study, 1 or more sites; axial skeleton (e.g., hips, pelvis, spine)**

77081-59 **Dual-energy X-ray absorptiometry (DXA), bone density study, 1 or more sites; appendicular skeleton (peripheral) (e.g., radius, wrist, heel), Distinct procedural service**

27.9 Radiation Oncology

Radiation oncology is performed to treat malignant neoplasms and other carcinomas, commonly known as cancer.

Radiation
The high-speed discharge and projection of energy waves or particles.

GUIDANCE CONNECTION

Read the additional explanations in the in-section guidelines within the **Radiology** section, subhead **Radiation Oncology**, directly above code 77261 in your CPT book.

The codes in this subsection already include certain services:

- Initial consultation.
- Clinical treatment planning.
- Simulation.
- Medical radiation physics.
- Dosimetry (the determination of the correct dosage).
- Treatment devices.
- Special services.
- Clinical treatment management procedures.
- Normal follow-up care during treatment and for 3 months following the completion of the treatment.

Radiation oncology services may be provided in varying degrees of intensity and are usually determined in the planning process. Therefore, the preparation for the sequence of treatments must be coded accurately. Some professionals may describe the planning as simple, intermediate, or complex. However, others may provide the detail, leaving you to match the components performed with the level of service.

Here are the specifics involved in each level:

- *Simple planning* involves one treatment area with one port, or parallel opposed ports, with simple or no blocking.
- *Intermediate planning* involves two separate treatment areas, three or more converging ports, multiple blocks, or special time-dose constraints.
- *Complex planning* involves three or more separate treatment areas, highly complex blocking, custom shielding blocks, tangential ports, special wedges or compensators, rotational or special beam consideration, or a combination of therapeutic methods.

Just to keep you on your toes, you will find the same terms *(simple, intermediate, complex)* also used to describe the simulation applied, with different definitions. The good news is that the same terms relate to the same elements involved in the process.

CODING BITES

Interventional radiologic services, such as radiation oncology, are typically provided in a series over a span of time. Make certain to code dates of service accurately.

With simulation, there is one additional descriptor:

- *Simple simulation:* a single treatment area with either a single port or parallel opposed ports, simple or no blocking.
- *Intermediate simulation:* three or more converging ports, two separate treatment areas, multiple blocks.
- *Complex simulation:* tangential portals, three or more treatment areas, rotation or arc therapy, complex blocking, custom shielding blocks, brachytherapy source verification, hyperthermia probe verification, any use of contrast materials.
- *Three-dimensional computer-generated:* reconstruction of the size and mass of the tumor and the normal tissues that surround the tumor site.

If you work in a facility that provides proton beam treatments and/or clinical brachytherapy for patients, you will note that the CPT book has different definitions for the same three terms: simple, intermediate, and complex.

LET'S CODE IT! SCENARIO

PATIENT: Craig Bennington

PREOPERATIVE DIAGNOSIS: Adenocarcinoma of the prostate

POSTOPERATIVE DIAGNOSIS: Adenocarcinoma of the prostate

PROCEDURE PERFORMED: Prostate brachytherapy

SURGEON: Carlos Arias, MD

ANESTHESIA: General anesthesia via LMA

COMPLICATIONS: None

(continued)

DRAINS: One 18-French Foley catheter per urethra

INDICATIONS FOR PROCEDURE: This patient has a new diagnosis of adenocarcinoma of the prostate diagnosed due to a very slowly rising PSA. His current PSA level is only 2.0, but prostate ultrasound biopsies were performed showing adenocarcinoma of the prostate at the left base of the prostate, and two biopsies were positive out of eight with a Gleason score of 6. Treatment options have been discussed, and he wishes to proceed with prostate brachytherapy. Informed consent has been obtained.

DESCRIPTION OF PROCEDURE: The patient was placed on the operating table in the supine position. General anesthesia was administered via LMA. He was then placed in the dorsal lithotomy position and sterilely prepped and draped in the usual fashion. The prostate ultrasound was inserted. The prostate was visualized using the preplanned study as a guide. Intracavitary application of prostate brachytherapy was performed. The patient tolerated the procedure well and had no immediate intraoperative or postoperative complications.

We implanted a total of 54 iodine-125 radioactive seeds through 12 needles with each seed containing 0.373 millicurie per seed. During the procedure, the patient received 4 mg of Decadron IV and 400 mg of Cipro IV. Subsequent fluoroscopy showed good distribution of the seeds throughout the prostate. The patient will have a CAT scan of the pelvis and simulation for his seed localization. Total target dose is 14,500 cGy.

The patient will be discharged with prescriptions for Cardura 1 mg a day for a month with two refills; Tylenol No. 3 one t.i.d. p.r.n. for pain, a total of 20; Pyridium Plus one b.i.d. for 10 days; Cipro 500 mg b.i.d. for 5 days; and prednisone 10 mg t.i.d. for a week.

Discharge instructions were explained to the patient and his wife. He will return to see Dr. Ferguson, his oncologist, in 2 weeks and Dr. Victors, his urologist, in 4 weeks for a follow-up.

Let's Code It!

Dr. Arias performed brachytherapy, so turn to this term in the CPT Alphabetic Index.

Brachytherapy

Read down the listing of the types of brachytherapic methods. Notice the documentation states, "*Intracavitary application of prostate brachytherapy was performed*," which leads you to

Intracavitary Application 0395T, 77761-77763

Now, look up each of these codes and read each complete description to find the one that matches:

0395T **High dose rate electronic brachytherapy, interstitial or intracavitary treatment, per fraction, includes basic dosimetry, when performed**

77761 **Intracavitary radiation source application; simple**

77762 **Intracavitary radiation source application; intermediate**

77763 **Intracavitary radiation source application; complex**

Analyze each of these codes' descriptions. Code 0394T or 0395T cannot be accurate for this encounter because there is no mention of electronic brachytherapy being used. Codes 77761, 77762, and 77763 are essentially the same except for the level of intensity: simple, intermediate, or complex.

Do you know which level is described in the documentation? No, so you need to query the physician. The physician responds by adding a notation in the patient's chart that this was a low-dose (simple) application. Now you have what you need to report:

77761 **Intracavitary radiation source application; simple**

Good work!

The delivery of external beam radiation treatments each have specific descriptions that will direct you to the accurate CPT code:

- Superficial and orthovoltage x-rays
- Electron beams
- Neuron beams
- Proton beans
- Magavoltage photons

Surface radiation therapy (SRT) is also a type of external radiation therapy, using low-energy radiation which restricts the area of penetration. SRT is reported with a code from the 77436 through 77439 range.

27.10 Nuclear Medicine

> **Nuclear Medicine**
> Treatment that includes the injection or digestion of isotopes.

Nuclear medicine uses tiny quantities of radioactive material, also known as tracers, in conjunction with a scintillation or gamma camera to record the emissions from the tracers to create an image of the anatomical site. Several types of nuclear medicine tests are used to identify a health concern:

- Bone scans are used to investigate injuries (fractures, sprains, and strains) as well as tumors.
- Thyroid uptake scans are used to assess thyroid function and record the structure of the gland.
- Lung scans are used to determine the presence of blood clots. In addition, scans can be valuable to calculate the flow of air into and out of the lungs.
- Hepatobiliary scans can provide information to evaluate the function of the liver and the gallbladder.
- Gallium scans can be used to identify the presence of infection and some types of tumors.

In addition to the diagnostic benefits of nuclear medicine, this methodology also can be used therapeutically to treat hyperthyroidism and thyroid cancer and to help to correct blood imbalances.

One important point that you have to know as a coding specialist working with nuclear medicine procedures is that the codes presented in the CPT book do not include diagnostic or therapeutic radiopharmaceuticals (the drugs or isotopes used in the treatments). Therefore, you have to code them separately. If the insurance carrier accepts HCPCS Level II codes, you will use them. You will learn all about HCPCS Level II codes in **Part IV** of this textbook.

Radiopharmaceutical therapy, the administration of nuclear drugs, whether given to the patient orally, intravenously, intracavitarily, interstitially, or intra-arterially, are reported with codes 79005–79999.

Also note that any chemical pathology or chemical analysis done in connection with the provision of nuclear medicine treatments should be coded separately from the ***Pathology and Laboratory*** section of the CPT book.

YOU CODE IT! CASE STUDY

Nadya Bartlett, a 43-year-old female, had gained a great deal of weight recently, with no change in her diet or exercise regimen. After a thorough examination, Dr. Posner ordered nuclear imaging of her thyroid, with uptake. Radiopharmaceuticals were administered intravenously. The report came back to Dr. Posner with the multiple determinations of Nadya's exam.

You Code It!

Go through the steps of coding, and determine the radiology code or codes that should be reported for this encounter between Dr. Posner and Nadya Bartlett.

Step #1: Read the case carefully and completely.
Step #2: Abstract the scenario. Which key words or terms describe what service the physician provided to the patient during this encounter?
Step #3: Are there any details missing or incomplete for which you would need to query the physician? [If so, ask your instructor.]
Step #4: Determine the correct CPT procedure code or codes to explain the details about what was provided to the patient during this encounter.
Step #5: Check for any relevant guidance, including reading all of the symbols and notations.
Step #6: Do you need to append any modifiers to ensure complete and accurate information is provided?
Step #7: Double-check your work.

Answer:

Did you determine this to be the correct code?

78014 Thyroid imaging (including vascular flow, when performed); with single or multiple uptake(s) quantitative measurement(s) (including stimulation, suppression, or discharge, when performed)

Great job!

Chapter Summary

Health care technology has advanced tremendously in the area of radiology and imaging. It is important that, as a coding specialist, you understand the differences among the types of radiologic methods, as well as the components of each. Procedures with contrast and without contrast, CT scans, MRIs, sonograms, and so many more enable professionals to look inside the patient in a noninvasive manner, and it is your job to obtain the correct reimbursement for every procedure.

CODING BITES

Isotopes Used in Nuclear Medicine

Lutetium-177	A therapeutic radioisotope with just enough gamma to enable imaging.
Yttrium-90	Treatment of cancer, particularly non-Hodgkin's lymphoma and liver cancer, and it is being used more widely, including for arthritis treatment.
Iodine-131	Treats thyroid for malignancy and other abnormal conditions such as hyperthyroidism (overactive thyroid).
Phosphorus-32	Controls an excess of red blood cells (RBCs).
Caesium-131, Palladium-103, Iodine-125, and Radium-223	Used for brachytherapy.

CHAPTER 27 REVIEW
CPT Radiology Section

Let's Check It! Terminology

Match each key term to the appropriate definition.

1. **LO 27.6** The imaging of a vein after the injection of contrast material.
2. **LO 27.3** The use of sound waves to record images of internal organs and tissues; also called an *ultrasound.*
3. **LO 27.6** The imaging of blood vessels after the injection of contrast material.
4. **LO 27.5** A piece of equipment that emits x-rays through a part of the patient's body onto a fluorescent screen, causing the image to identify various aspects of the anatomy by density.
5. **LO 27.5** A three-dimensional radiologic technique that uses nuclear technology to record pictures of internal anatomical sites.
6. **LO 27.5** A specialized computer scanner with very fine detail that records imaging of internal anatomical sites.
7. **LO 27.9** The high-speed discharge and projection of energy waves or particles.
8. **LO 27.5** The recording of a picture of an anatomical joint after the administration of contrast material into the joint capsule.
9. **LO 27.10** Treatment that includes the injection or digestion of isotopes.
10. **LO 27.5** MR imaging of an anatomical joint after the administration of contrast material into the joint capsule.
11. **LO 27.5** A CT scan using contrast materials to visualize arteries and veins all over the body.

A. Angiography
B. Arthrography
C. Computed Tomography (CT)
D. Computed Tomography Angiography (CTA)
E. Fluoroscope
F. Magnetic Resonance Arthrography (MRA)
G. Magnetic Resonance Imaging (MRI)
H. Nuclear Medicine
I. Radiation
J. Sonogram
K. Venography

Let's Check It! Concepts

Choose the most appropriate answer for each of the following questions.

1. **LO 27.3** The professional component of radiologic services includes
   a. repair of the equipment.
   b. interpretation of the imaging.
   c. supplies.
   d. training.
2. **LO 27.1** Interventional radiologic services are provided with the intent of all *except*
   a. diagnosing a condition.
   b. preventing the spread of a disease.
   c. measuring the progress of a disease.
   d. testing the equipment.
3. **LO 27.10** Dani Thompson presents for a thyroid carcinoma metastases imaging; limited area (neck and chest only). What radiology code would you assign?
   a. 78012
   b. 78013
   c. 78014
   d. 78015
4. **LO 27.5** The phrase "with contrast" means that the technician or radiologist
   a. administered a substance to enhance the image.
   b. used a black background behind the patient.
   c. took the image a second time, to compare to the first.
   d. used a blue background beneath the patient.
5. **LO 27.4** If the code description includes the phrase "two views" and the radiology reports show that only one view was taken, you should code the service
   a. with that code alone.
   b. with that code plus the modifier 52.
   c. with that code plus the modifier 53.
   d. with that code plus the modifier 22.
6. **LO 27.6** Therapeutic transcatheter radiologic supervision and interpretation codes, when associated with intervention, include all of the following *except*
   a. vessel measurement.
   b. postangioplasty or stent venography.
   c. catheter placement.
   d. contrast injections, angiography/venography, road mapping, and/or fluoroscopic guidance for the interventional procedure.
7. **LO 27.4** RPO stands for
   a. right procedure operation.
   b. regional protocol obstetric.
   c. right posterior oblique.
   d. right preventive oblique.
8. **LO 27.9** Radiation for the treatment of a malignant neoplasm is most often used for
   a. diagnostic purposes.
   b. therapeutic purposes.
   c. research purposes.
   d. prevention purposes.
9. **LO 27.1** An x-ray is the same as
   a. a CTA.
   b. a CT.
   c. an MRI.
   d. a radiologic exam.
10. **LO 27.10** Nuclear medicine uses tiny quantities of radioactive material, also known as ___, in conjunction with a scintillation or gamma camera to record the emissions from the ___ to create an image of the anatomical site.
    a. isotopes, tracers
    b. tracers, isotopes
    c. tracers, tracers
    d. tracers, drugs

Let's Check It! Guidelines

Refer to the Radiology Guidelines and fill in the blanks accordingly.

Imaging	joint	arthrography	new
contrast	surgical	not	Medicine
injection	analog	MR	integral
access	"with contrast"	rarely	enhancement
descriptors	intravascular	signed	without
qualify	included	needle	service

1. A service that is ___ provided, unusual, variable, or ___ may require a special report.
2. ___ may be required during the performance of certain procedures or certain imaging procedures may require surgical procedures to ___ the imaged area.
3. Many services include image guidance, and imaging guidance is ___ separately reportable when it is included in the base service.
4. When imaging is not included in a ___ procedure or procedure from the ___ section, image guidance codes or codes labeled "radiological supervision and interpretation" may be reported for the portion of the ___ that requires imaging.
5. The phrase ___ used in the codes for procedures performed using contrast for imaging ___ represents contrast material administered intravascularly, intra-articularly, or intrathecally.
6. For intra-articular injection, use the appropriate ___ injection code.
7. If radiographic ___ is performed, also use the arthrography supervision and interpretation code for the appropriate joint.
8. If computed tomography or magnetic resonance arthrography are performed ___ radiographic arthrography, use the appropriate joint ___ code, the appropriate CT or ___ code, and the appropriate imaging guidance code for ___ placement for contrast injection.
9. Injection of ___ contrast material is part of the "with contrast" CT, computed tomographic angiography, magnetic resonance imaging and magnetic resonance angiography procedure.
10. Oral and/or rectal ___ administration alone does not ___ as a study "with contrast."
11. A written report ___ by the interpreting individual should be considered an ___ part of a radiologic procedure or interpretation.
12. With regard to CPT ___ for imaging services, "images" must contain anatomic information unique to the patient for which the imaging service is provided. "images" refer to those acquired in either an ___ or digital manner.

Let's Check It! Rules and Regulations

Please answer the following questions from the knowledge you have gained after reading this chapter.

1. **LO 27.3** Differentiate between the technical component and professional component and identify the modifiers that represent each component.
2. **LO 27.2** What is the difference between a screening image and a diagnostic image? Why is it important for the professional coder to know the difference?
3. **LO 27.2** When a screening test turns into a diagnostic test, what service(s) should be reported?
4. **LO 27.9** What is radiation oncology? What do the codes in this subsection already include?
5. **LO 27.10** What are the types of nuclear medicine tests that are used to identify a health concern?

YOU CODE IT! Basics

First, identify the procedural main term in the following statements; then code the procedure or service.

Example: Dr. Bradford performs a CT scan of the brain without contrast material:

a. main term: *CT* **b.** procedure: *70450*

1. Dr. Gray takes an eye x-ray for detection of foreign body:

   a. main term:______ **b.** procedure:______

2. Dr. Robertson takes a CT scan of the pelvis with contrast:

   a. main term:______ **b.** procedure:______

3. Dr. Banks performs a renal ultrasound, complete, real-time with image documentation:

   a. main term:______ **b.** procedure:______

4. Dr. Hicks takes a panoramic x-ray:

   a. main term:______ **b.** procedure:______

(continued)

5. Dr. Louche administers brachytherapy, intracavitary radiation, 8 sources:
   a. main term: ______ b. procedure:______
6. Dr. Pullets performs a liver SPECT (single photon emission computed tomography) with vascular flow tomography:
   a. main term: ______ b. procedure:______
7. Dr. Roof completes PET imaging of a heart:
   a. main term:______ b. procedure:______
8. Dr. Darby performs a ureteral reflux study:
   a. main term: ______ b. procedure:______
9. Dr. Allister takes a unilateral x-ray of ribs, 2 views:
   a. main term: ______ b. procedure:______
10. Dr. Alexander completes kidney imaging morphology:
   a. main term: ______ b. procedure:______
11. Dr. Steiner performs a DXA scan, hips:
   a. main term: ______ b. procedure:______
12. Dr. Smyth completes a radiopharmaceutical localization of inflammatory process; whole body:
   a. main term:______ b. procedure:______
13. Dr. Benton performs radiopharmaceutical therapy by intra-articular administration:
   a. main term:______ b. procedure:______
14. Dr. Gilbert completes an angiography, extremity (arm), bilateral, radiological supervision and interpretation:
   a. main term:______ b. procedure:______
15. Dr. Johannson performs an MRI, spinal canal and contents, lumbar; without contrast material:
   a. main term: ______ b. procedure:______

CPT ICD-10-CM

YOU CODE IT! Practice

Using the techniques described in this chapter, carefully read through the case studies and determine the most accurate radiology CPT code(s) and modifier(s), if appropriate, for each case study.

1. Edith Shapin, a 24-year-old female, is pregnant for the first time and is at approximately 11 weeks gestation. She is brought into the diagnostic center for a fetal biophysical profile with nonstress testing.
2. William Browne, a 15-year-old male, is brought into Dr. Jenkins's office with severe right leg pain. Dr. Jenkins takes x-rays of his right femur, AP and PA, to determine whether or not Bill's leg is fractured.
3. Martha Lightfood, an 82-year-old female, was brought into Dr. Morrison's office by her daughter because Martha was complaining of a sharp pain in her chest. After a negative EKG, Dr. Morrison had a quantitative differential pulmonary perfusion and ventilation study performed, which confirmed a pulmonary embolism. Martha was taken immediately by ambulance to the hospital. Code the quantitative differential pulmonary perfusion and ventilation study only.
4. Dr. Logan saw Jason Miolo, a 38-year-old male, with a swollen right eye and loss of vision. Dr. Logan ordered a CT with contrast of the right eye and area, which revealed marked proptosis of the right orbit, thrombosis, and enlargement of the right superior ophthalmic vein.
5. Carl Gadsden, a 66-year-old male, was diagnosed with intrinsic laryngeal cancer, supraglottic T1 tumor. With the tumor confined to one subsite in the supraglottis, Dr. Yoshihashi provided radiation treatment delivery, with a single port, simple block, of 4.5 MeV.
6. Olivia Kane, a 33-year-old female, came into Kinsey Imaging Center for her annual screening mammogram. Due to her family history of malignant neoplasms of the breast (both her mother and sister have been diagnosed), the mammogram was ordered with computer-aided detection (CAD).
7. Brianna Haralson, a 24-year-old female, is brought into Dr. Duncan's office with sharp pains in her lower right abdomen, shooting across to the left side. Dr. Duncan ordered some blood work and an MRA to confirm the suspected diagnosis of acute appendicitis. Code the MRA.

(continued)

8. Charles Gresham, a 40-year-old male, was in training at Cape Canaveral when he hit his head in a weightlessness simulator, causing him to lose consciousness for 3 minutes. Charles was transported to the nearest hospital, where Dr. Neumours, the ED on-call physician, took a skull x-ray, three views, and did an MRI without contrast of Charles's brain.
9. Jonelle Graybar, a 73-year-old female, was experiencing pain in her back that radiated around her trunk. She was also suffering with spastic muscle weakness. Dr. Maxwell ordered a radioisotope bone scan of Jonelle's lumbar spinal area. The scan identified a metastatic invasion of L1-L3.
10. Maxine Zeigleman, newly diagnosed with metastatic lumbar spinal tumors, has been referred to Dr. Appleton for the creation of a simple radiation therapy plan.
11. Vernon Unger had been diagnosed with a malignancy and came today for intravenous radiopharmaceutical therapy.
12. Before beginning a series of treatments, Anna Hogan came to the Diagnostic Imaging Center for a metabolic evaluation PET scan of her brain. The radiologist read the scan and sent their report to the ordering physician, Dr. Ellis.
13. Ira Morgan, a 16-month-old male, was brought to radiology for a real-time, limited, static ultrasound of his hips.
14. Xavier Pollack, a 62-year-old male, arrived at the Kinsey Imaging Center to have a SPECT (single photon emission computed tomography) performed on his left kidney.
15. Dr. Astrone performed a complete ultrasound evaluation of Alden Roberts's pelvis. The procedure included evaluation and measurement of Alden's urinary bladder, evaluation of his prostate and seminal vesicles, and pathology of his enlarged prostate.

ICD-10-CM

YOU CODE IT! Application

The following exercises provide practice in the application of abstracting the physicians' notes and learning to work with documentation from our Kinsey Imaging Center. These case studies are modeled on real patient encounters. Using the techniques described in this chapter, carefully read through the case studies and determine the most accurate radiology CPT code(s) and modifier(s), if appropriate, for each case study. You are coding for the radiologist.

KINSEY IMAGING CENTER

951 SYDNEY STREET • SOMEWHERE, FL 32811 • 407-555-3573

PATIENT: SAVOY, MARCELLA

ACCOUNT/EHR#: SAVOMA001

Procedure Performed: MRI, Spinal canal, thoracic, 3 views CT, abdomen/pelvis

Radiologist: Keith Robbins, MD

Referring Physician: Oscar R. Prader, MD

INDICATIONS: Probable metastatic disease, T1–T3, asymptomatic; metastatic mucinous adenocarcinoma of unknown primary

IMPRESSIONS: MRI scans also showed edema at T1, T2, and T3, but no obvious metastatic disease. In the course of her evaluation, a CT of the abdomen and pelvis showed some mild common bile duct dilation, but no obvious primary malignancy.

Keith Robbins, MD

Determine the most accurate radiology CPT code(s) and modifier(s), if appropriate.

(continued)

KINSEY IMAGING CENTER

951 SYDNEY STREET • SOMEWHERE, FL 32811 • 407-555-3573

PATIENT: JAQUARD, JOEL

ACCOUNT/EHR#: JAQUJO001

Procedure Performed: X-rays, skull, two views
CT, soft tissue of neck, with contrast
MRI, brain stem

Radiologist: Robyn Campbell, MD

Referring Physician: Renee O. Bracker, MD

INDICATIONS: Concussion, after fall from ladder

IMPRESSIONS:

1. Full muscle and tendon retraction of the supraspinatus and infraspinatus structures.
2. Bruising and possible microfractures to the skull at occipital base.
3. Other partial tearing of the superior aspect of the semispinalis capitis

Determine the most accurate radiology CPT code(s) and modifier(s), if appropriate.

KINSEY IMAGING CENTER

951 SYDNEY STREET • SOMEWHERE, FL 32811 • 407-555-3573

PATIENT: BURMAN, CECILIA

ACCOUNT/EHR#: BURMCE001

Procedure Performed: MRI, brain, no contrast
MRA, brain, no contrast
MRA, neck, no contrast

Radiologist: Eryn Alberts, MD

Clinical Information: Evaluate for VP shunt
No prior studies available for a comparison

TECHNICAL INFORMATION: The examination was performed without the use of intravenous contrast material.

INTERPRETATION: Evaluation of the posterior fossa demonstrates hydrocephalus versus low pressure communicating hydrocephalus.

Eryn Alberts, MD

Determine the most accurate radiology CPT code(s) and modifier(s), if appropriate.

KINSEY IMAGING CENTER

951 SYDNEY STREET • SOMEWHERE, FL 32811 • 407-555-3573

PATIENT: TREMONT, GARETT

ACCOUNT/EHR#: TREMGA001

EXAMINATION: Chest and abdomen

(continued)

CLINICAL HISTORY: Fever

CHEST: AP supine and lateral films demonstrate no evidence of alveolar infiltrate or consolidation or pleural effusion. The mediastinal structures are not enlarged. There is very mild increase in central bronchovascular markings. There is no evidence of focal destructive bone lesion.

IMPRESSION: No infiltrate.

ABDOMEN: Supine and erect films demonstrate mild to moderate dilatation of loops of small bowel with short air/fluid levels on the erect film. The large bowel is within normal limits in size but is visualized to the level of the splenic flexure. There is no air visualized in the remainder of the colon. The findings are not specific but consistent with ileus. Further clinical correlation is advised. There is no evidence of focal destructive bone lesion. There is no suspicious calcification in the upper abdomen.

IMPRESSIONS: Abdominal bowel pattern, not specific, consistent with ileus.

Milton Harrison, MD

Determine the most accurate radiology CPT code(s) and modifier(s), if appropriate.

KINSEY IMAGING CENTER

951 SYDNEY STREET • SOMEWHERE, FL 32811 • 407-555-3573

PATIENT: WILLARD, NADINE

ACCOUNT/EHR#: WILLNA001

Procedure Performed: CT angiography of the head, without contrast and with contrast

Radiologist: Kevin Linnard, MD

Referring Physician: Renee O. Bracker, MD

INDICATIONS: Left CVA

IMPRESSIONS: The current study is compared with the previous one of 05-25-14. Compared with the previous study, there is a focal area of hypodensity present in the right posterior cerebral arterial distribution adjacent to the falx, a finding suspicious for a small acute infarction, nonhemorrhagic, most likely the parieto-occipital branch. No other abnormality detected. There are no intra- or extra-axial hemorrhages. There is no significant midline shift or hydrocephalus. Small new area as described above is suspicious for an area of acute infarction in the right posterior cerebral arterial distribution, likely the occipital branch. Please clinically correlate.

Kevin Linnard, MD

Determine the most accurate radiology CPT code(s) and modifier(s), if appropriate.

28

CPT Pathology & Lab Section

Key Terms

Cytology
Etiology
Gross Examination
Laboratory
Microscopic Examination
Pathology
Qualitative
Quantitative
Specimen
Surgical Pathology

Learning Outcomes

After completing this chapter, the student should be able to:

LO 28.1 Recognize key factors involved in pathology testing.
LO 28.2 Identify testing methodologies and sources.
LO 28.3 Report panel codes when qualified.
LO 28.4 Analyze blood test reports to ensure accurate reporting.
LO 28.5 Discern clinical chemistry studies.
LO 28.6 Interpret details about molecular diagnostic testing.
LO 28.7 Distinguish immunologic, microbiologic, and cytopathologic testing.
LO 28.8 Abstract the correct details to report surgical pathology testing.
LO 28.9 Append the correct modifier, when required.
LO 28.10 Accurately interpret the abbreviations used most often in pathology and laboratory reports.

STOP! Remember, you need to follow along in your CPT code book for an optimal learning experience.

28.1 Specimen Collection and Testing

Laboratory
A location with scientific equipment designed to perform experiments and tests.

Pathology
The study of the nature, etiology, development, and outcomes of disease.

Etiology
The original source or cause for the development of a disease; also, the study of the causes of disease.

As physicians and health care professionals work to help their patients, very often they need medical science to guide them. The guidance frequently comes from tests performed by professionals working in a **laboratory**, studying the evolution of a patient's disease. This type of study is called **pathology**, which includes **etiology**.

Pathology and lab testing help detect the early presence of disease, ruling out or confirming conditions that might have similar symptoms yet need to be treated differently. The results of these tests also may predict the occurrence of disease in the future. You probably already know from your own experiences the importance of such work. Your annual physical has possibly included blood tests to measure your cholesterol. Physicians order blood work to confirm pregnancy or a urinalysis to determine if a symptom could be the result of an infection. Testing takes time and the expertise of professionals educated in interpreting the results. It also takes materials and resources.

A specimen sent to the lab for testing may be from any number of different sources:

- Blood
- Urine
- Other bodily fluids, such as
  - sputum
  - sperm
  - mucus
- Tissue
- An organ

CODING BITES

Every pathology or lab test requires specimens to examine. In some cases, you may need to report the collection of the specimen separately.

For example:

36415 Collection of venous blood by venipuncture

83930 Osmolality; blood

Be alert to the fact that the collection of the specimen may be provided at a separate facility from the lab, in which case, each facility would report the code for the part performed.

As a coding specialist, you may work for a health care organization that has a laboratory within its facilities, a billing company that codes everything, or an independent facility that does nothing other than taking and analyzing **specimens**. In any case, you should understand the different aspects of pathology and lab testing and procedures, as well as the guidelines involved in coding the services.

Specimen
A small part or sample of any substance obtained for analysis and diagnosis.

CODING BITES

When you code pathology and laboratory work, you may be reporting the work provided by the professional performing the test and interpreting the results (the pathologist), or you may be reporting for the facility that provided the testing.

LET'S CODE IT! SCENARIO

Cynthia Cardamen, a 33-year-old female, was not feeling well, so she went to see her family physician, Dr. Slater. After talking with her and performing an exam, Dr. Slater began to suspect that Cynthia had diabetes mellitus, type 2. Reagan Dram, the nurse, obtained a specimen of capillary blood from Cynthia's left index finger and took it to Abbey Carmichael, who ran their in-house lab, for a glucose test to be performed. She used a reagent strip to perform the test and delivered the results to Dr. Slater.

Let's Code It!

There are two steps to this test: the collection of the specimen and the testing of that blood to determine Cynthia's glucose level.

Let's turn to the CPT Alphabetic Index, and find

Collection and Processing

Specimen

Capillary Blood 36416

Now, turn to the *Main Section* of CPT and find

36416 Collection of capillary blood specimen (e.g., finger, heel, ear stick)

Now, we must report the test that Abbey will perform on this blood specimen. Dr. Slater ordered a blood glucose test. Turn in the Alphabetic Index to

Glucose

Blood Test 82947, 82948, 82950

(continued)

This time, we have three different codes to investigate.

82947 Glucose; quantitative, blood (except reagent strip)

82948 Glucose; blood, reagent strip

82950 Glucose; post glucose dose (includes glucose)

Compare the details in these code descriptions to the details you have in the documentation. Code 82948 matches.

36416 Collection of capillary blood specimen (e.g., finger, heel, ear stick)

82948 Glucose; blood, reagent strip

Good work!

28.2 Testing Methodology and Desired Results

Although no one expects you, as the coding specialist, to be completely knowledgeable about the details of laboratory and pathology testing, you will need certain information about how the tests are performed in order to code them correctly. This may begin with exactly what type of properties are needed, going beyond just the name of the test itself.

Types of Test Results

Quantitative
The counting or measurement of something.

Qualitative
The determination of character or essential element(s).

Two of the types of results that lab tests can evidence are **quantitative** and **qualitative**. These details can support a physician's medical decision making, especially when trying to determine an accurate diagnosis or identify the success of a treatment, or lack of success of a treatment.

For example, serum calcium tests are used to assess parathyroid function and calcium metabolism. The quantitative results (total amount of calcium in the blood) also can be used to check on patients with renal failure.

Other tests you may be familiar with are white blood cell (WBC) count (quantitative) and differential count (qualitative and quantitative) tests. These tests are part of routine blood testing. The quantitative totals can provide important diagnostic details–for example, an increased white blood cell count usually identifies the presence of an infection, inflammation, tissue necrosis, or leukemic neoplasia, while a decreased total white blood cell count can be present due to bone marrow failure, indicating a potential immunocompromised patient.

EXAMPLES

Calcium

82310 Calcium; total

82330 Calcium; ionized

82331 Calcium; after calcium infusion test

82340 Calcium; urine quantitative, timed specimen

White Blood Cell

85004 Blood count; automated differential WBC count

85007 Blood count; blood smear, microscopic examination with manual differential WBC count

85008 Blood count; blood smear, microscopic examination without manual differential WBC count

85009 Blood count; manual differential WBC count, buffy coat

The guidelines tell you that, if the documentation does not specify, you may assume that the examination performed was quantitative. However, remember that documentation is absolute in the health care industry. Therefore, it is recommended that you query the lab technician or pathologist and request that the report include this important detail.

Testing Methodologies

For other testing, you might see the details about the methodology of the testing. Some of the terms you will notice in test descriptions and their codes include

- By dipstick.
- Automated or nonautomated.
- With or without microscopy.
- Visual or gross inspection.

These terms refer to the methods that the lab technicians use to test the specimen and obtain the results.

LET'S CODE IT! SCENARIO

Margaret O'Hanahan came to see Dr. Marinson. She states that she has been feeling a stinging pain when she urinates. She confirms some lower back aches but denies hematuria. Dr. Marinson asks Margaret to go into the bathroom and provide a urine sample, which is then tested in the office by dipstick, automated without microscopy.

Let's Code It!

Dr. Marinson is performing a *urinalysis, by dipstick, automated.* Turn to *urinalysis* in your CPT Alphabetic Index.

Urinalysis

Automated 81001, 81003

These two listings fit the details according to the documentation, so turn to the *Main Section* and read these code descriptions.

81000 Urinalysis, by dip stick or tablet reagent for bilirubin, glucose, hemoglobin, ketones, leukocytes, nitrite, pH, protein, specific gravity, urobilinogen, any number of these constituents; nonautomated, with microscopy

81001 Urinalysis, by dip stick or tablet reagent for bilirubin, glucose, hemoglobin, ketones, leukocytes, nitrite, pH, protein, specific gravity, urobilinogen, any number of these constituents; automated, with microscopy

81002 Urinalysis, by dip stick or tablet reagent for bilirubin, glucose, hemoglobin, ketones, leukocytes, nitrite, pH, protein, specific gravity, urobilinogen, any number of these constituents; nonautomated, without microscopy

81003 Urinalysis, by dip stick or tablet reagent for bilirubin, glucose, hemoglobin, ketones, leukocytes, nitrite, pH, protein, specific gravity, urobilinogen, any number of these constituents; automated, without microscopy

Go back to the scenario and abstract the details about the test. The documentation states, "*dipstick, automated without microscopy.*" When you read all of these code descriptions, you can see that only one accurately reports this specific test:

81003 **Urinalysis, by dip stick or tablet reagent for bilirubin, glucose, hemoglobin, ketones, leukocytes, nitrite, pH, protein, specific gravity, urobilinogen, any number of these constituents; automated, without microscopy**

Good work!

CODING BITES

All the details regarding the specimen and the testing are important. There are times when the code descriptions include the type of test, the type of specimen, or both.

In addition to how the test is performed, you must also know the type of specimen involved in the testing and, sometimes, how many specimens or sources are involved. The type of specimen being tested may change the code. Consider a physician ordering a potassium test. Let's go to the Alphabetic Index for *potassium*.

EXAMPLE

Potassium 84132

Urine 84133

The first code in the example, listed next to the word *potassium*, is code 84132, but it does not contain any additional descriptors. However, the second code, listed under *potassium*, indicates that it would be the code used if the potassium were tested from the patient's urine rather than blood (serum). When you look at the codes' complete descriptions in the numeric listing, you see the details shown.

EXAMPLE

84132 Potassium; serum, plasma, or whole blood

84133 urine

The listings clearly show that there is a difference as to which code is correct based on the source of the specimen.

In certain circumstances, an analysis may be performed on multiple specimens collected at different times or from different sources. In these cases, the guidelines tell you to code each source and each specimen separately. However, be certain to always read the code descriptions carefully. Some codes already include multiple tests and/or multiple sources.

LET'S CODE IT! SCENARIO

Gilian Morrison, RN, performs a rapid influenza test using a commercial test kit in the office to determine if Hester Childs has the virus. This way the results can be provided while Hester is still in with Dr. Alberts. When complete, Nurse Morrison visually reads the result as positive.

Let's Code It!

For this scenario, you are going to focus only on reporting the provision of the rapid influenza test. The first place you look in the CPT Alphabetic Index is under the word *Test*. However, there is nothing there, so let's look up the term *Influenza*. There are several choices. Let's analyze them.

The first two choices are titled *Influenza A* and *Influenza B*. There is nothing in the notes about which this might be. Before querying the nurse or doctor, let's keep reading.

The next listing is *Influenza Vaccine*. There is nothing in the notes stating that Hester was given a vaccination, so this is not applicable to this encounter.

The last listing category is titled *Influenza Virus*. This could be possible because the notes state the test was given to "determine if Hester has the virus." Two codes are suggested here:

Antibody 86710

Detection

by Immunoassay with Direct Optical Observation 87804

by Nucleic Acid 87501–87503

(continued)

Let's turn to the *Main Section* of CPT, look for these two possible codes in the ***Pathology and Laboratory*** section, and read the complete code descriptions.

86710 Antibody; influenza virus

87804 Infectious agent antigen detection by immunoassay with direct optical observation; influenza

When you read the scenario and the complete code description, you can see how code **87804** matches accurately.

28.3 Panels

A pathology report, such as the one shown in **Figure 28-1**, will typically itemize the tests performed for the patient along with the results of each test.

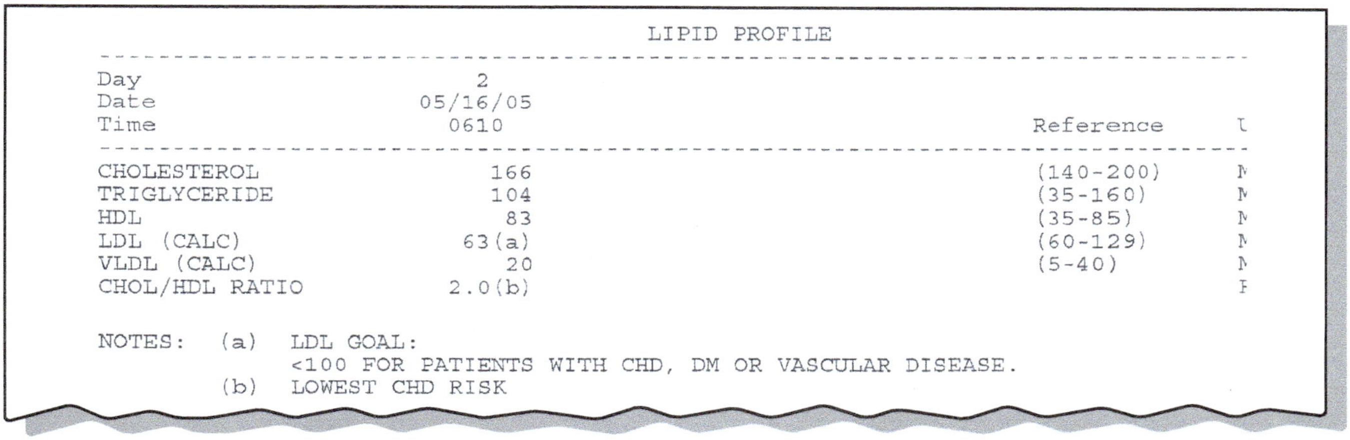

LIPID PROFILE

		Reference	U
Day	2		
Date	05/16/05		
Time	0610		
CHOLESTEROL	166	(140-200)	M
TRIGLYCERIDE	104	(35-160)	M
HDL	83	(35-85)	M
LDL (CALC)	63(a)	(60-129)	M
VLDL (CALC)	20	(5-40)	M
CHOL/HDL RATIO	2.0(b)		F

NOTES: (a) LDL GOAL:
<100 FOR PATIENTS WITH CHD, DM OR VASCULAR DISEASE.
(b) LOWEST CHD RISK

FIGURE 28-1 Sample lab report showing the tests run as part of a lipid profile

When you turn to the ***Pathology and Laboratory*** section of the CPT book, you will notice that many codes include a long list of tests within one code's description. These groupings of tests commonly performed at the same time are called *panels*.

EXAMPLE

80051 Electrolyte panel

This panel must include the following:

Carbon dioxide (82374)

Chloride (82435)

Potassium (84132)

Sodium (84295)

This example shows you that, in order for you to report code 80051 legally and accurately, the lab must have performed all four tests: carbon dioxide, chloride, potassium, and sodium.

If the lab performed fewer than *all* the tests listed in a panel, you must report the code for each test separately; you are *not* permitted to use the panel code.

Again, the CPT book will help you. Should you have to code any of the tests separately, each test code is given in parentheses right next to the name of the test listed there. From our example, next to carbon dioxide, you can see the number 82374. Turn to code 82374, and you will see that it is the code for testing carbon dioxide alone.

CODING BITES

Remember that the codes for testing a specimen do not include collecting the specimen. Collection, such as performing a biopsy, venipuncture, or fine-needle aspiration, is coded separately by the coder for the professional who performed the collection.

CODING BITES

When all the included tests of a panel are performed, you must use the panel code. Coding the tests individually is considered unbundling. Unbundling is unethical and illegal. If fewer tests are performed, using a panel code with the modifier **52 Reduced Services** is ***not*** permitted. You must code the tests individually.

Let's say, instead of fewer tests than those listed in a panel, the lab performs more tests. The guidelines state that you are to report those additional tests, those not included in the panel code, separately and additionally.

LET'S CODE IT! SCENARIO

Concerned that Keisha Evans, a 51-year-old female, might be suffering from hypercholesterolemia, Dr. Rawlins ordered blood work, including a total cholesterol serum test, lipoprotein (direct measurement of high-density lipoprotein), and triglycerides. He also added a potassium serum test to the order.

Let's Code It!

The lab performed four tests: *total cholesterol serum test, lipoprotein (direct measurement of high-density lipoprotein), triglycerides*, and *potassium serum*. When you look up the tests individually, you are directed to codes for each. However, when it comes to pathology and laboratory coding, you must take an extra step.

Turn to the numeric listings at the beginning of the ***Pathology and Laboratory*** section, where you find the standardized panels listed. Review the list of tests included in each of the panels and match it with the list of tests Dr. Rawlins ordered. You see that code **80061 Lipid Panel** includes three of the four tests performed.

80061 Lipid Panel

Since none of the panels includes all four tests, you use the lipid panel code and code the potassium test additionally, code 84132.

84132 Potassium; serum, plasma, or whole blood

Therefore, you have two codes for the lab work's claim: 80061 and 84132.

Good job!

CODING BITES

Experience and practice will help you learn the components of panels. After working at a lab or for a facility with a lab, you will recognize the lab tests that are typically performed together and possibly have a panel code grouping them. Should a test not be in a panel, the Alphabetic Index will direct you to the correct individual code for that test.

CODING BITES

Remember, you are only permitted to report a code, legally, when you are coding for the individual or facility that actually did the work.

When a physician documents ordering a test to be done (by an outside lab), this is part of the E/M service.

GUIDANCE CONNECTION

Read the additional explanations in the in-section guidelines located within the **Pathology and Laboratory** section, subhead **Organ or Disease-Oriented Panels**, directly above code 80047 in your CPT book.

28.4 Blood Test Documentation

Determining the code for a blood test can be complex, as you are learning in this chapter. The lab report (see **Figure 28-2**) is an important part of the documentation you will have to report the performing of the tests.

- *Bicarbonate:* Kidneys and lungs keep bicarbonate balanced to maintain homeostatic pH levels (ensure a balance of acid and alkali levels). Abnormal levels can indicate dysfunction of these organs (kidneys and lungs).
- *Blood culture:* This test measures the presence of bacteria or yeast in the blood, which is used to confirm (or deny) a suspected infection or sepsis.
- *Blood differential (Diff):* This test measures numbers of WBCs, which are used to identify presence of infection. Normal is less than 20%.
- *Blood urea nitrogen (BUN):* This test measures kidney function. A low count might indicate malnutrition, while a high count may identify the presence of heart failure, kidney disease, or liver disease. Normal range: 7–20 milligrams per deciliter (mg/dL).
- *Creatinine:* This test measures levels of this chemical excreted by the kidneys. It is used to determine muscle damage, dehydration, and/or kidney dysfunction. Normal range: 0.8–1.4 mg/dL.

Mon Mar 31 10:10:27

LABORATORIES

Augusta, GA.	Orlando, FL	Tampa, FL
Tel:	Tel:	Tel:
Fax:	Fax:	Fax:

Patient:		Collecting Time:	03/26/22	08:27	PHYSICIAN	P96
DOB:	Age: Yrs Sex:	Log in DT/TM:	03/27/22	00:57	550	
PID:		Report DT/TM:	03/27/22	05:02		
Phone:		Reprint DT/TM:	03/31/22	10:07		
Episode:		FASTING: Y	Priority: R		Physician:	
Notes:						
Copy to:						

TEST NAME		RESULT	UNITS	REF RANGE	LAB
COMPREHENSIVE METABOLIC PANEL WITH eGFR					ORL
Sodium		139	mEq/L	(133–146)	
Potassium		3.9	mEq/L	(3.5–5.4)	
Chloride		101	mEq/L	(97–110)	
Carbon Dioxide		31	mEq/L	(21–33)	
Anion Gap		7.0	mEq/L	(5.0–15.0)	
Glucose		96	mg/dL	(65–100)	
BUN		11	mg/dL	(8–25)	
Creatinine		0.64	mg/dL	(0.6–1.4)	
eGFR African American		113	mL/min	(>60)	
eGFR Non-African Am.		98	mL/min	(>60)	
BUN/Creatinine Ratio		17		(6–28)	
Calcium		9.3	mg/dL	(8.2–10.6)	
Total Protein		7.2	g/dL	(6.0–8.3)	
Albumin		4.5	g/dL	(3.5–5.7)	
Globulin		2.7	g/dL	(1.6–4.2)	
A/G Ratio		1.7		(0.9–2.5)	
Bilirubin Total		0.5	mg/dL	(0.1–1.30	
Alkaline Phosphatase		87	U/L	(35–126)	
AST (SGOT)		17	U/L	(5–43)	
ALT (SGPT)		11	U/L	(7–56)	
TSH		4.199	uIU/mL	(0.550–4.780)	ORL
Free T4		1.16	ng/dL	(0.89–1.76)	ORL
LIPID PANEL					
Cholesterol	H	243	mg/dL	(80–199)	
Triglycerides		188	mg/dL	(30–150)	
HDL Cholesterol		55	mg/dL	(40–110)	
LDL Cholesterol Calc		141	mg/dL	(30–130)	
VLDL Cholesterol Calc		28	mg/dL	(10–60)	
Risk Ratio (CHOL/HDL)		3.6	Ratio	(0.0–5.0)	
Non-HDL Cholesterol		145	mg/dL		

Cholesterol/HDL	Ratio	Interpretation:	
Gender	CVD	Risk Category	
Female			
		Average Risk	4.4
		Twice Average Risk	71

Printed at: 03/31 10:07 "CONTINUED REPORT"

FIGURE 28-2 Pathology report showing a list of all of the individual blood tests run for the patient, including results and reference ranges

- *Erythrocyte sedimentation rate (ESR):* This test measures the speed with which red blood cells cling together, fall, and settle in the bottom of a glass tube within 60 minutes. It is used to detect inflammatory, neoplastic, infectious, and necrotic processes. When inflammation is present, the higher the rate, the greater the amount of inflammation. Normal range: male = up to 15 millimeters per hour (mm/h); female = up to 20 mm/h.

- *Glucose:* This test measures the level of sugar in the blood. Low levels may indicate hypoglycemia or liver disease, whereas high levels may indicate hyperglycemia (diabetes) or hyperthyroidism. Normal range: 70–99 mg/dL.
- *Hematocrit (HCT):* This test identifies the percentage of RBCs, which is used to identify anemia. Low counts may indicate bone marrow damage or vitamin deficiency, while high counts may indicate congenital heart disease, renal problems, or pulmonary disease. Normal range: 34%–45%.
- *Hemoglobin (Hgb):* This test measures oxygen being carried by the RBCs. Low counts may indicate bone marrow damage or vitamin deficiency, while high counts may indicate congenital heart disease, renal problems, or pulmonary disease. Normal range: 11.5–15.5 grams per deciliter (g/dL).
- *Mean corpuscular hemoglobin (MCH):* This test measures the amount of hemoglobin in RBCs. A low number may indicate an iron deficiency, whereas a high number may indicate a vitamin deficiency. Normal range: 27–34 picograms (pg).
- *Mean corpuscular volume (MCV):* This test identifies the average size of the RBCs. Small size may indicate an iron deficiency, whereas a large reading may indicate a vitamin deficiency. Normal range: 80–100 femtoliters (fL).
- *Partial thromboplastin time (PTT):* This test measures factors I (fibrinogen), II (prothrombin), V, VIII, IX, X, XI, and XII. Inadequate quantities of these factors cause the PTT to be prolonged, a delay in the clotting of the blood that increases the opportunity for the patient to hemorrhage. Normal PTT: 60–70 seconds.
- *Platelet count:* Low platelet counts can indicate a clotting disorder, putting the patient at risk for hemorrhage. Low levels may indicate pernicious anemia, lupus, or a viral infection, while high levels may identify leukemia. Normal range: 150–400 thousand per microliter (K/mcL).
- *Potassium:* This test measures levels of potassium in the blood. Low potassium levels can cause muscle cramps and/or weakness; abnormal levels (too high or low) can result in an abnormal heartbeat. Low levels can identify use of corticosteroids or diuretics, while high levels may signify kidney failure, diabetes, or Addison's disease. Normal range: 3.7–5.2 milliequivalents per liter (mEq/L).
- *Prothrombin time (PT):* This test evaluates the clotting ability of factors I (fibrinogen), II (prothrombin), V, VII, and X. Low quantities of these clotting factors result in a prolonged PT. PT results include the use of the international normalized ratio (INR) value as well as absolute numbers. Normal PT result: 85%–100% in 11–12.5 seconds and an INR of 0.8–1.1.
- *Sodium:* This test determines if the balance between sodium and liquid in the blood is at the correct proportion. Low levels of sodium can identify the use of diuretics or adrenal insufficiency, while high levels may indicate dehydration or kidney dysfunction. High levels of sodium can lead to hypertension. Normal range: 136–144 mEq/L.

YOU CODE IT! CASE STUDY

Rosalyn Alvarez, an 84-year-old female, complained to Dr. Files that she was having severe cramps in her legs and hands. She said it has been getting worse the last few months. In Rosalyn's chart, it notes that she has been on diuretics, so Dr. Files orders blood work to quantify her creatinine levels to check on her kidney function. Thelma Brooks, RN, performed the venipuncture and sent the blood specimen to the lab.

You Code It!

Determine the code for the pathology lab testing Rosalyn's blood to quantify the potassium levels.

Step #1: Read the case carefully and completely.
Step #2: Abstract the scenario. Which key words or terms describe what service the physician provided to the patient during this encounter?
Step #3: Are there any details missing or incomplete for which you would need to query the physician? [If so, ask your instructor.]
Step #4: Determine the correct CPT procedure code or codes to explain the details about what was provided to the patient during this encounter.
Step #5: Check for any relevant guidance, including reading all of the symbols and notations.
Step #6: Do you need to append any modifiers to ensure complete and accurate information is provided?
Step #7: Double-check your work.

(continued)

Answer:

Did you determine this to be the code?

82565 Creatinine; blood

Good job!

28.5 Clinical Chemistry

The lab tests that are most commonly performed use chemical processes to distinguish qualities and quantities of elements in the specimens provided. Typically, the specimens are samples of a patient's blood or urine. Tests with which you might be familiar include the following:

- *Blood glucose* (sugar) is used to diagnose conditions such as diabetes mellitus (hyperglycemia) or hypoglycemia.
- *Electrolytes* are used to diagnose metabolic or kidney disorders.
- *Enzymes* can be released into the bloodstream by a damaged or diseased organ. The presence of creatine kinase can indicate damage after a heart attack, or amylase and lipase elevations may be a sign of cancer of the pancreas and/or pancreatitis.
- *Hormones*, such as cortisol, in quantities too high or too low might indicate the malfunction of the patient's adrenal glands.
- *Lipids* (fatty substances) can signal coronary heart disease or liver disease.
- *Metabolic substances*, such as uric acid, at incorrect levels can identify the presence of gout.
- *Proteins* identified at the wrong levels on electrophoresis can point to malnutrition or certain infections.

GUIDANCE CONNECTION

Read the additional explanations in the in-section guidelines located within the **Pathology and Laboratory** section, subhead **Chemistry**, directly above code 82009 in your CPT book.

Many tests can be easily performed in the physician's office with a small amount of blood or urine. Companies have created kits that make measuring such elements as simple as dipping a little slip of special paper into the patient's specimen. It means that you have a much greater opportunity to code any number of tests.

YOU CODE IT! CASE STUDY

Charles Endicott, a 31-year-old male, is an up-and-coming stockbroker who does not pay much attention to a proper diet. He came to see his physician, Dr. Falacci, because he has been experiencing episodes of light-headedness. Dr. Falacci asks his assistant, Carla Falco, to do a quantitative blood glucose test. Carla takes a blood sample, goes to the back, and checks the specimen. The results indicate that Charles has hypoglycemia.

You Code It!

Go through the steps, and determine the pathology/lab code(s) that should be reported for this encounter.

Step #1: Read the case carefully and completely.
Step #2: Abstract the scenario. Which key words or terms describe what service the physician provided to the patient during this encounter?
Step #3: Are there any details missing or incomplete for which you would need to query the physician? [If so, ask your instructor.]
Step #4: Determine the correct CPT procedure code or codes to explain the details about what was provided to the patient during this encounter.
Step #5: Check for any relevant guidance, including reading all of the symbols and notations.
Step #6: Do you need to append any modifiers to ensure complete and accurate information is provided?
Step #7: Double-check your work.

(continued)

Answer:

Did you determine this to be the correct code?

82947 Glucose; quantitative, blood (except reagent strip)

Good work!

28.6 Molecular Diagnostics

Molecular diagnostic tests investigate infectious disease, oncology concerns (malignant neoplasms), hematology (the study of blood and its disorders), neurology, and inherited disorders (genetics).

Specifically, genetic testing involves the analysis of specimens to identify any presence of a genetic disorder. Research and technology have developed testing methodologies for more than 2,000 diseases that can be performed to provide peace of mind, or early detection of diseases and conditions that are passed from parents to child via their genes.

The ability for parents-to-be to determine if they have any conditions that might be passed on to their future children has been found to be an important part of family planning. After conception, embryos and fetuses can be tested to reassure parents, to enable physicians to treat some conditions in utero, or to enable the family to be prepared with accommodations before the baby arrives.

Adults with a family or personal history of a genetic disorder may be tested to provide the option for preventive health care services or treatment as early as possible.

Pharmacogenomic Testing

Physicians are trained to determine the correct medication and dosage to prescribe for their patients based on several factors, including age, weight, personal history, general health, and allergies/sensitivities. In recent years, researchers have discovered that an individual's genes also may affect the efficacy of a specific drug, explaining why one version of a drug may really help one patient while having no or little benefit to another. Evolving from these discoveries has been the development of pharmacogenomic tests to provide specific information that will assist the physician with a more accurate and effective prescription.

YOU CODE IT! CASE STUDY

Parker Thomasini, a 4-year-old male, has a cousin who was diagnosed with cystic fibrosis last year. Recently, he has been wheezing and has a dry, nonproductive cough. The fact that his cousin has cystic fibrosis means that Parker has a 25% chance of carrying the disease. Therefore, Dr. Preston ordered a molecular diagnostic test for the mutation of delta F 508 deletion in his DNA by sequencing, single segment.

You Code It!

Go through the steps, and determine the pathology/lab code(s) that should be reported for this encounter.

Step #1: Read the case carefully and completely.
Step #2: Abstract the scenario. Which key words or terms describe what service the physician provided to the patient during this encounter?
Step #3: Are there any details missing or incomplete for which you would need to query the physician? [If so, ask your instructor.]
Step #4: Determine the correct CPT procedure code or codes to explain the details about what was provided to the patient during this encounter.
Step #5: Check for any relevant guidance, including reading all of the symbols and notations.
Step #6: Do you need to append any modifiers to ensure complete and accurate information is provided?
Step #7: Double-check your work.

(continued)

Answer:

Did you determine this to be the correct code?

81220 **CFTR (cystic fibrosis transmembrane conductance regulator) (e.g., cystic fibrosis) gene analysis; common variants (e.g., ACMG/ACOG guidelines)**

Good job!

GUIDANCE CONNECTION

Read the additional explanations in the in-section guidelines located within the **Pathology and Laboratory** section, subhead **Molecular Pathology**, on the pages directly before code 81170 in your CPT book.

28.7 Immunology, Microbiology, and Cytopathology

Immunology

Immunology is the study of the body's immune system—how it works and what can go wrong. Immunologic tests identify problems that may occur when a disease causes the body's defense system to attack itself (called an *autoimmune disease*) or when a disease causes a malfunction of the body's immune system (called an *immunodeficiency disorder*). The tests also can evaluate the compatibility of tissues and organs for transplantation.

Conditions and diseases that you may be familiar with, which fall into this category, include rheumatoid arthritis, allergies, and, of course, human immunodeficiency virus (HIV).

GUIDANCE CONNECTION

Read the additional explanations in the in-section guidelines located within the **Pathology and Laboratory** section, subhead **Microbiology**, directly above code 87003 in your CPT book.

LET'S CODE IT! SCENARIO

Nigel Winthrope, a 19-year-old male, was diagnosed with hemophilia many years ago. As a result of a blood transfusion, he contracted HIV. He has come today for lab work to check on his T-cell count, an indicator of whether the HIV is progressing.

Let's Code It!

Nigel is having a test to determine the *count* of *T cells* in his blood. Let's turn to the Alphabetic Index to the letter *T*.

Are you surprised at the many listings with *T cell* in the heading? Read through them all carefully. Remember that Nigel does not have leukemia; he has HIV. Keep going down the list to *T Cells*, under which you see *Count*, with the suggested code 86359.

The complete code description in the numeric listing shows us

86359 **T cells; total count**

Good job!

Coding for COVID-19 Testing

As you all know, Coronavirus 2, aka COVID-19, is the first pandemic on earth in many decades. In order to track pathological testing being done to identify COVID-19 throughout the United States, and the world, new codes have been implemented. These are codes used to report the provision of the actual testing (by the laboratory) to determine if a patient has the virus or if the patient had the virus and now has antibodies. The antibody codes can also be reported for testing to confirm the efficacy of the vaccines.

86328 **Immunoassay for infectious agent antibody(ies), qualitative or semiquantitative, single-step method (e.g., reagent strip); severe acute respiratory syndrome coronavirus 2 (SARS-CoV-2) (Coronavirus disease [COVID-19])**

86413 **Severe acute respiratory syndrome coronavirus 2 (SARS-CoV-2) (Coronavirus disease [COVID-19]) antibody, quantitative**

86769 **Antibody; severe acute respiratory syndrome coronavirus 2 (SARS-CoV-2) (Coronavirus disease [COVID-19])**

87426 **Infectious agent antigen detection by immunoassay technique (e.g., enzyme immunoassay [EIA], enzyme-linked immunosorbent assay [ELISA], fluorescence immunoassay [FIA], immunochemiluminometric assay [IMCA]) qualitative or semiquantitative; severe acute respiratory syndrome coronavirus (e.g., SARSCoV, SARS-CoV-2 [COVID-19])**

87636 **Infectious agent detection by nucleic acid (DNA or RNA); severe acute respiratory syndrome coronavirus 2 (SARS-CoV-2) (Coronavirus disease [COVID-19]) and influenza virus types A and B, multiplex amplified probe technique**

87637 **Infectious agent detection by nucleic acid (DNA or RNA); severe acute respiratory syndrome coronavirus 2 (SARS-CoV-2) (Coronavirus disease [COVID-19]), influenza virus types A and B, and respiratory syncytial virus, multiplex amplified probe technique**

87811 **Infectious agent antigen detection by immunoassay with direct optical (i.e., visual) observation; severe acute respiratory syndrome coronavirus 2 (SARS-CoV-2) (Coronavirus disease [COVID-19])**

Microbiology

Microbiologic tests use many different methods to study bacteria, fungi, parasites, and viruses. The specimens used in the tests might be blood, urine, sputum (mucus, also called *phlegm*), feces (stool), cerebrospinal fluid (CSF), and other bodily fluids. Blood cultures are used to diagnose bacterial infections of the blood, sputum cultures can identify respiratory infections like pneumonia, and stool cultures can confirm the presence of pinworms and other parasites.

Code descriptions in this subsection may include some specific terms, such as

- *Presumptive identification.* This is the pathologic identification of colony morphology; growth on selective media (such as a culture or slide); gram stains; or other tests such as catalase, oxidase, indole, or urease. For example: 87081 Culture, presumptive, pathogenic organisms, screening only.
- *Definitive identification.* This is the pathologic identification of the genus or species that requires additional testing, such as biochemical panels or slide cultures. For example: 87106 Culture, fungi, definitive identification, each organism, yeast.

LET'S CODE IT! SCENARIO

Sally Tong, a 5-year-old female, went to a picnic at the park with her playgroup and had a hamburger, cooked very rare. Later that evening, her parents rushed her to the hospital because she was vomiting and had severe diarrhea. Dr. Warner ordered an infectious agent antigen enzyme immunoassay for E. coli *O157. Fortunately, the test was negative, and it turned out that she just had eaten too much ice cream and milk.*

Let's Code It!

Dr. Warner ordered "*an infectious agent antigen enzyme immunoassay*" for Sally to determine if she was suffering from *Escherichia coli (E. coli).* Let's go to the Alphabetic Index to *immunoassay* and find *infectious agent* below it, with the suggested codes 86317–86318, 87449–87451. Let's go to the numeric listings and read the complete code descriptions.

(continued)

86317 **Immunoassay for infectious agent antibody, quantitative, not otherwise specified (For immunoassay techniques for antigens, see 83516, 83518, 83519, 83520, 87301–87450, 87810–87899)**

The code description states *antibody*, but the notes say *antigen*. Luckily, the CPT book is guiding you via the parenthetical notation below the code description, which directs you to a long list of codes. The descriptions for 83516, 83518, 83519, and 83520 do not come any closer to Dr. Warner's notes. Let's turn to the next set of suggested codes:

87301 **Infectious agent antigen detection by immunoassay technique (e.g., enzyme immunoassay [EIA], enzyme-linked immunosorbent assay [ELISA], immunochemiluminometric assay [IMCA]), qualitative or semiquantitative, multiple-step method; adenovirus enteric types 40/41**

Read down the list a little farther:

87335 **Escherichia coli O157**

When you read the complete description, you get the following:

87335 **Infectious agent antigen detection by immunoassay technique (e.g., enzyme immunoassay [EIA], enzyme-linked immunosorbent assay [ELISA], immunochemiluminometric assay [IMCA]), qualitative or semiquantitative, multiple-step method; Escherichia coli O157**

Sometimes, even with the CPT book pointing at codes, it may take a lot of reading to be certain you have the best, most appropriate code.

Cytopathology and Cytogenetic Studies

Cytology
The investigation and identification of cells.

Cytology is the study of one cell at a time to discover abnormal cells present in tissue or bodily fluids. Cytologic testing is used to detect cancer cells and infectious organisms and to screen for fetal abnormalities.

Specimens used in cytopathologic testing are obtained by fine-needle aspirations (as in amniocentesis), scraping of tissue surfaces (as in Pap smears), and collection of bodily fluids (as with sputum or seminal fluid, or sperm).

LET'S CODE IT! SCENARIO

Rosalie Panesca, a 47-year-old female, came to see Dr. Sizemore for her annual well-woman checkup. In addition to the examination, Dr. Sizemore took a Pap smear, to be examined using cytopathological testing, specifically, the Bethesda reporting system with manual screening. Rosalie's examination showed she was completely healthy.

Let's Code It!

Dr. Sizemore took a *smear* of tissue for a cytopathologic examination of Rosalie's cervical cells using *the Bethesda reporting system.*

Let's go to the Alphabetic Index to *cytopathology, smears, cervical or vaginal,* with five more choices as to the type: Automated Screen, Hormone Evaluation, Manual Screen, Partially Automated Screen, and Physician Interpretation—each with its own suggested codes. Go back to the documentation and see if you can find any terms that will help you narrow this down. The notes state, "*Bethesda reporting system with manual screening.*" In the Alphabetic Index, you can see that cytopathology, smears, cervical or vaginal, manual screen suggests 88150, 88153, 88164, 88165. Let's go to the *Main Section* and read the complete code descriptions.

Before you begin reading all the code descriptions, read the paragraph of instructions directly before code 88141. You will note that these instructions tell you to "Use codes 88164–88167 to report Pap smears that are examined using the Bethesda System of reporting." That saves you quite a lot of time. Reading that one small paragraph directs you to the four best codes:

(continued)

88164 **Cytopathology, slides, cervical or vaginal (the Bethesda System); manual screening under physician supervision**

88165 **Cytopathology, slides, cervical or vaginal (the Bethesda System); with manual screening and rescreening and under physician supervision**

88166 **Cytopathology, slides, cervical or vaginal (the Bethesda System); with manual screening and computer-assisted rescreening under physician supervision**

88167 **Cytopathology, slides, cervical or vaginal (the Bethesda System); with manual screening and computer-assisted rescreening using cell selection and review under physician supervision**

Which of these four codes most accurately describes the pathology test done for Rosalie? No rescreening or computer-assisted rescreening is documented. This means the most accurate code for this test is

88164 **Cytopathology, slides, cervical or vaginal (the Bethesda System); manual screening under physician supervision**

Great job!

28.8 Surgical Pathology

Surgical Pathology
The study of tissues removed from a living patient during a surgical procedure.

When a biopsy is taken during a surgical procedure (or is the surgical procedure itself), the specimen is sent to the lab for testing. The testing, typically performed immediately upon receipt from the OR, is called **surgical pathology**. Its purpose, much like that of other testing and studies, is to provide the information necessary to diagnose a disease or condition and to set forth a treatment plan. In such cases, all the steps (taking the specimen, testing, diagnosis, and treatment) may occur during one surgical session. The benefit of this quick and immediate process is that there is less trauma for the patient, who has to undergo anesthesia and an invasive procedure only once. In addition, it saves money for the patient, the facility, and the third-party payer.

Gross Examination
The visual study of a specimen (with the naked eye).

Microscopic Examination
The study of a specimen using a microscope (under magnification).

Codes 88300–88309 represent six levels of surgical pathologic testing. The codes include accession, the testing itself, and the written report from the pathologist. The codes (with the exception of 88300) also include both **gross examination** (also known as macroscopic examination) of the specimen and **microscopic examination**.

The first level, code 88300, is applicable for any and all specimens that are examined only by visual, or gross, examination. It means that the sample has not been looked at under a microscope.

88300 **Level I – Surgical pathology, gross examination only**

GUIDANCE CONNECTION

Read the additional explanations in the in-section guidelines located within the **Pathology and Laboratory** section, subhead **Surgical Pathology**, directly above code 88300 in your CPT book.

Codes 88302–88309 recognize the various amounts of work required by the pathologist or physician doing the examination to determine the accurate condition of the specimen. Don't worry—you don't have to study pathology to decide which level to use properly to represent the work done. Each code level is determined by the anatomical site from where the specimen was taken. Under each, the sites are listed in alphabetic order. However, you have to know what happened in the OR to find the correct code because that will change the level involved.

Reading the Lab Report

You may find a report, such as the one shown in **Figure 28-3**, that shows the results of the surgical pathology along with the pathologist's interpretation.

HILL MCGRAW PATHOLOGY LABORATORIES INC.
Warren R. Mulford, MD,. Director
123 Learning Way • Academia, FL 12345

PATIENT INFORMATION	PHYSICIAN INFORMATION
Name: NICOLE GABRINI Sex: Female D.O.B: 09/07/01 Patient ID: 55899 Patient Phone: 555-456-5555	JOSE MARKETTEN, MD 456 Healing Lane Suite 505 Academia, FL 12345 555-399-5555

SPECIMEN INFORMATION

COLLECTED: 04/29/26 Reported: 05/01/26 Received: 04/30/26	Accession # IF_16_6971 Other Accession (IC):

PATHOLOGY REPORT

CLINICAL INFORMATION

A. Right upper extremity—Scabies vs Eczema
B. Left lower extremity—Scabies vs Eczema
C. Right lower extremity—Scabies vs Eczema

Terrell Rodriguez, PA-C

SPECIMEN DATA

GROSS DESCRIPTION:

A. The specimen is a punch biopsy received in immunofluorescence transport medium that measures 0.1 × 0.4 × 0.1 cm. The specimen is flash frozen and multiple 4 micron sections are cut for manual immunof uorescence staining. The sections are probed with fluorescein labeled antihuman antibodies against IgG, IgA, IgM, C3, C5b-9, and fibrinogen.

B. Received is a 0.2 cm punch biopsy of skin, submitted complete. The specimen is received in formalin.

C. Received is a 0.2 cm punch biopsy of skin, submitted complete. The specimen is received in formalin.

MICROSCOPIC DESCRIPTION:
All positive and negative controls stained appropriately as required.

RESULTS

DIAGNOSIS:

A. DIRECT IMMUNOFLUORESCENCE, RIGHT UPPER EXTREMITY—NEGATIVE (See Note)
Note: There is no IgG, IgA, IgM, C3, C5b-9, and fibrinogen deposition seen in this specimen. There is no immunof uorescence evidence of connective tissue, vasculitis, dermatitis herpetiformis, porphyria cutanea tarda, pseudoporphyria, or autoimmune blistering disease; however, clinical histologic and, if pertinent, serologic correlation is recommended. Multiple immunoreactant dilutions and sections were performed.

B. PUNCH BIOPSY, LEFT LOWER EXTREMITY—STASIS ECZEMA, TRAUMATIZED AND IMPETIGINIZED
Note: PAS is negative for fungus. Multiple deeper sections have been reviewed and no mite or mite elements identified. There is an impetiginized ulcer with bacterial colonization of the stratum corneum containing neutrophils and serum exudate. The papillary dermis contains a capillary proliferation, a few neutrophils, rare eosinophils and dermal cicatrix. These histopathologic features are consistent with traumatized and impetiginized stasis eczema. There is no evidence of scabies.

C. PUNCH BIOPSY, RIGHT LOWER EXTREMITY—STASIS ECZEMA, TRAUMATIZED AND IMPETIGINIZED
Note: PAS is negative for fungus. Multiple deeper sections have been reviewed and no mite or mite elements identified. There is an impetiginized ulcer with bacterial colonization of the stratum corneum containing neutrophils and serum exudate. The papillary dermis contains a capillary proliferation, a few neutrophils, rare eosinophils and dermal cicatrix. These histopathologic features are consistent with traumatized and impetiginized stasis eczema. There is no evidence of scabies.

Noah W. Wegner, MD Dermatopathologist (electronic signature)

FINAL REPORT

FIGURE 28-3 Sample pathology report showing details and analysis of a surgical specimen

The physician's operative report may state a tissue biopsy was taken; however, you may need more details from the pathologist's report so you can code this accurately. Remember, when you are reporting a code or codes from the ***Pathology and Laboratory*** section of CPT, you are reporting *for the pathologist*, not the surgeon. The code from the ***Surgery*** section of CPT will report the *collection* of the specimen, while the code from the ***Pathology and Laboratory*** section will report the *testing* of the specimen.

YOU CODE IT! CASE STUDY

Hildy French, an 11-year-old female, was taken to the OR to have her tonsils removed. However, due to additional symptoms, Dr. Anachino did a biopsy and sent a specimen of Hildy's tonsils to the lab for surgical pathologic examination. The report came back from the lab that Hildy had a malignant neoplasm of her tonsils. Dr. Anachino surgically removed additional sections to be certain that the entire tumor had been removed. Hildy tolerated the procedure well and was taken to the recovery room.

You Code It!

Go through the steps, and determine the pathology/lab code(s) that should be reported for this encounter.

Step #1: Read the case carefully and completely.
Step #2: Abstract the scenario. Which key words or terms describe what service the physician provided to the patient during this encounter?
Step #3: Are there any details missing or incomplete for which you would need to query the physician? [If so, ask your instructor.]
Step #4: Determine the correct CPT procedure code or codes to explain the details about what was provided to the patient during this encounter.
Step #5: Check for any relevant guidance, including reading all of the symbols and notations.
Step #6: Do you need to append any modifiers to ensure complete and accurate information is provided?
Step #7: Double-check your work.

Answer:

Did you determine this to be the correct code?

88305 Level IV – Surgical pathology, gross and microscopic examination; Tonsil, biopsy

Good work!

Pathologic Testing on Bone Marrow

Medical Necessity for Bone Marrow Testing

Although not performed as commonly as blood tests or urinalysis (because obtaining the specimen is complex), pathologic examination of a patient's bone marrow has many possible uses, including:

- To serve as a diagnostic tool for suspected myeloma, leukemia, myelodysplastic syndromes, and myeloproliferative disorders.
- To assess a current diagnosis of thrombocytopenia, anemia, or leukopenia.
- To measure quantities of stored iron and marrow cellularity.
- To determine neoplasm, infection, fibrosis, or other infiltrative bone disease.
- To enable staging of lymphoma and/or other malignant neoplasms.

A patient may have abnormal blood counts for which an explanation has yet to be identified, or the patient may have other abnormal cells evidenced in circulating blood. These, as well as a current diagnosis of a bone marrow-related disease (such as lymphoma) or indications that a malignancy has metastasized into the marrow, are standard-of-care justifications to obtain and study a bone marrow specimen.

Collection of the Specimen

Typically, the specimen is taken from the posterior superior iliac spine of the pelvis to acquire a sampling of the blood-forming cells in the marrow space. Evaluation of a specimen taken by biopsy is considered to be more accurate than one obtained by aspiration because the quantity of material gathered is greater and therefore more likely to provide a representative sampling of a wider scope.

When coding for bone marrow biopsy, the first procedure to be reported is for obtaining the specimen, using either 38220 Bone marrow; aspiration only or 38221 Bone marrow, biopsy, needle or trocar.

Note that the abstraction of bone marrow from a patient is not performed solely for the lab. Therefore, it is very important to identify, from the documentation, not only how the bone marrow was taken but also for what purpose. For example, bone marrow aspiration for platelet-rich stem cell injections are not reported with 38220 but with code 0232T Injection(s), platelet-rich plasma, any site, including image guidance, harvesting and preparation when performed. Harvesting bone marrow for transplantation is reported with either 38230 Bone marrow harvesting for transplantation; allogeneic or 38232 Bone marrow harvesting for transplantation; autologous.

When both a bone marrow biopsy and a bone marrow aspiration are performed on a Medicare beneficiary during the same encounter, do not report code 38220. Instead, use code G0364 Bone marrow aspiration performed with bone marrow biopsy through the same incision on the same date of service.

Pathologic Testing

Next, the specimen will be sent to the laboratory for analysis. A bone marrow specimen, obtained by either biopsy or aspiration, can enable a hematologist/pathologist to investigate the patient's hematopoiesis (the process of forming blood cells), as well as the shape, size, and quantity of red and white blood cells and megakaryocytes (very large bone marrow cells that produce blood platelets). Blood cell formation is primarily the responsibility of the red bone marrow, specifically in the sternum, ribs, and iliac bones (pelvis).

Code 88305 Level IV – Surgical pathology, gross and microscopic examination reports both evaluation of the bone marrow biopsy specimen by the naked eye (gross examination) and visualization of the specimen using a microscope. When the documentation states that the specimen was obtained by aspiration, instead of 88305, the analysis is reported with 85097 Bone marrow; smear interpretation.

It is not uncommon for a decalcification procedure and/or iron staining to be performed at the same time as the surgical pathologic examination. When documentation confirms this, report these procedures separately using +88311 Decalcification procedure (list separately in addition to code for surgical pathology examination) and/or 88313 Special stain including interpretation and report; Group II, all other (e.g., iron, trichrome) except stain for microorganisms, stains for enzyme constituents, or immunocytochemistry and immunohistochemistry.

Per CPT parenthetical instruction, you should report one unit of 88313 for each special stain on each surgical pathologic block, cytologic specimen, or hematologic smear. Check documentation or query the pathologist performing the testing to ensure that the notes are clear as to how many blocks, specimens, or smears are tested so that you can report the accurate number of codes.

Immunophenotyping by flow cytometry provides the identification of cell-specific antibodies, enabling a more accurate determination of cell percentages as well as identification of abnormal cell patterns. Report this test using 88184 Flow cytometry, cell surface, cytoplasmic, or nuclear marker, technical component only; first marker and +88185 each additional marker, as appropriate.

Because 88184 and 88185 are specifically limited to the technical component only, you will need a code to report the interpretation service separately. Note that no modifiers (neither TC nor 26) are necessary because these details are already included in the code descriptors, as follows:

88187 **Flow cytometry, interpretation; 2 to 8 markers**

88188 **Flow cytometry, interpretation; 9 to 15 markers**

88189 **Flow cytometry, interpretation; 16 or more markers**

Fluorescent in situ hybridization (FISH) analysis (88365 In situ hybridization [e.g., FISH], per specimen; initial single probe stain procedure) is usually performed after the analysis of the bone marrow, the results of which will direct the specific DNA probes to be conducted. FISH analysis is better than an overall karyotype test because it can find smaller pieces of chromosomes that may be missing or may have extra copies.

YOU CODE IT! CASE STUDY

Danielle Lee, a 37-year-old female, has a history of chronic myeloid leukemia (CML) and came to our facility today for a bone marrow aspiration, right side posterior iliac crest. Dr. Hansen used a 15-gauge needle to obtain the aspirate including an aspirate clot. The patient tolerated the procedure well.

(continued)

You Code It!

Part 1: *Go through the steps of coding, and determine the code or codes that should be reported for this encounter between Dr. Hansen and Danielle Lee.*

Step #1: Read the case carefully and completely.
Step #2: Abstract the scenario. Which key words or terms describe what service the physician provided to the patient during this encounter?
Step #3: Are there any details missing or incomplete for which you would need to query the physician? [If so, ask your instructor.]
Step #4: Determine the correct CPT procedure code or codes to explain the details about what was provided to the patient during this encounter.
Step #5: Check for any relevant guidance, including reading all of the symbols and notations.
Step #6: Do you need to append any modifiers to ensure complete and accurate information is provided?
Step #7: Double-check your work.

Answer:

Did you determine this to be the correct code for obtaining the bone marrow specimen?

38220 Diagnostic bone marrow; aspiration(s)

Part 2: *Dr. Uker, a certified pathologist, wrote this report after testing the bone marrow.*

PATHOLOGY REPORT:

The following specimens were reviewed:

- peripheral smear of bone marrow aspirate and clot section
- iron stain

Determine the code or codes that should be reported for Dr. Uker.

Answer:

Did you determine these to be the correct codes for the pathology testing?

85097 Bone marrow; smear interpretation

88313 Special stain including interpretation and report; Group II, all other (e.g., iron, trichrome) except stain for microorganisms, stains for enzyme constituents, or immunocytochemistry and immunohistochemistry

28.9 Modifiers for Laboratory Coding

If your health care facility uses an outside laboratory that bills your office, you include the charges for the lab work on the claim form that you file. In such instances, you must append the CPT code for the lab test with modifier 90. If the outside lab bills the patient's insurance directly, you will not include the test code or modifier on the claim form you submit.

90 **Reference (Outside) Laboratory:** When laboratory procedures are performed by a party other than the treating or reporting physician, the procedure may be identified by adding modifier 90 to the usual procedure number.

Also on occasion, you may find that a lab test has to be repeated, on the same day for the same patient, in order to get several readings of a level or measurement. When this is documented, append modifier 91:

91 **Repeat Clinical Diagnostic Laboratory Test:** In the course of treatment of the patient, it may be necessary to repeat the same laboratory test on the same day to obtain subsequent (multiple) test results. Under these circumstances, the laboratory test performed can be identified by its usual procedure number and the addition of modifier 91. (**Note**: This modifier may not be used when tests are rerun to confirm initial results; due to testing problems with specimens or equipment; or for any other reason when a normal, one-time, reportable result is all that is required. This modifier may not be used when other code[s] describe a series of test results [e.g., glucose tolerance tests, evocative/suppression testing]. This modifier may only be used for laboratory test[s] performed more than once on the same day on the same patient.)

The use of testing kits is increasing in health care facilities because they make it easier to obtain fast, accurate results. When a testing kit is being used, append modifier 92.

92 **Alternative Laboratory Platform Testing:** when laboratory testing is being performed using a kit or transportable instrument that wholly or in part consists of a single use, disposable analytical chamber, the service may be identified by adding modifier 92 to the usual laboratory procedure code (HIV testing 86701–86703, and 87389). The test does not require permanent dedicated space, hence by its design may be hand carried or transported to the vicinity of the patient for immediate testing at that site, although location of the testing is not in itself determinative of the use of this modifier.

YOU CODE IT! CASE STUDY

Dr. Georges is implementing a new treatment protocol for Priscilla Roper. He ordered that qualitative urinalysis be performed first thing in the morning, again at noon, and again at 5:00 p.m. Erline Cutter, RN, collected the specimens from Priscilla's catheter and sent them to the lab for each of the tests.

You Code It!

Review the scenario, and report the appropriate code or codes for the pathology lab's work.

Step #1: Read the case carefully and completely.
Step #2: Abstract the scenario. Which key words or terms describe what service the physician provided to the patient during this encounter?
Step #3: Are there any details missing or incomplete for which you would need to query the physician? [If so, ask your instructor.]
Step #4: Determine the correct CPT procedure code or codes to explain the details about what was provided to the patient during this encounter.
Step #5: Check for any relevant guidance, including reading all of the symbols and notations.
Step #6: Do you need to append any modifiers to ensure complete and accurate information is provided?
Step #7: Double-check your work.

Answer:

Did you determine this to be the code?

81005-91 x 3 **Urinalysis; qualitative or semiquantitative, except immunoassays, repeat clinical diagnostic laboratory test, three tests**

Proprietary Laboratory Analyses

New diagnostic laboratory tests have been adopted to investigate the presence of very specific elements, such as colorectal adenomatous polyps or Helicobacter pylori detection and antibiotic resistance. These codes are unusual for the CPT code set, in that they are all alphanumeric and end with the letter "U." Find these codes at the end of the Pathology and Laboratory section.

For example:

0005U **Oncology (prostate) gene expression profile by real-time RT-PCR of 3 genes (ERG, PCA3, and SPDEF), urine, algorithm reported as risk score**

28.10 Pathology and Lab Abbreviations

Abbreviations for pathology and laboratory tests are used in reports from labs all over the country. Some of the most common are shown in **Table 28-1**.

TABLE 28-1 Abbreviations and Acronyms for Most Common Diagnostic and Laboratory Tests

ABG	Arterial blood gases
ACE	Angiotensin-converting enzyme
ACT	Activated clotting time
AFP	Alpha-fetoprotein
A/G	Albumin/globulin ratio
AIT	Agglutination inhibition test
ALP	Alkaline phosphatase
ALT	Alanine aminotransferase
AMA	Antimitochondrial antibody
ANA	Antinuclear antibody
APTT	Activated partial thromboplastin time
AST	Aspartate aminotransferase
BASO	Basophiles
BMC	Bone mineral content
BMD	Bone marrow density
BST	Blood serologic test
BUN	Blood urea nitrogen
CBC	Complete blood count
CEA	Carcinoembryonic antigen
CK	Creatine kinase
CMV	Cytomegalovirus
CO_2	Carbon dioxide
CPK	Creatine phosphokinase
DIC	Disseminated intravascular coagulation
DIFF	Differential
EIA	Enzyme immunoassay
EOS	Eosinophil count
ESR	Erythrocyte sedimentation rate
FBS	Fasting blood sugar
GTT	Glucose tolerance test
HCT	Hematocrit
HDL	High-density lipoprotein
HGB	Hemoglobin
HPF	High-power field
INR	International normalization ratio
LD	Lactic dehydrogenase
LDL	Low-density lipoprotein
LFT	Liver function tests
LPF	Low-power field
LYMPHS	Lymphocytes
MCH	Mean corpuscular hemoglobin
MCHC	Mean corpuscular hemoglobin concentration

(continued)

MCV	Mean corpuscular volume
MONO	Monocyte count
MPV	Mean platelet volume
NEUT	Neutrophils
PAP	Prostatic acid phosphatase
PH	Hydrogen ion concentration
PLT	Platelet
PSA	Prostate-specific antigen
PT	Prothrombin time
PTT	Partial thromboplastin time
RBC	Red blood cells
RDW	Red cell distribution width
RF	Rheumatoid factor
RPR	Rapid plasma reagin test
SEGS	Segmented neutrophils
SGOT	Serum glutamicoxaloacetic transaminase
SGPT	Serum glutamicpyruvic transaminase
SMA	Sequential multiple analyzer
SP GRAV	Specific gravity
STS	Serologic test for syphilis
T&C	Type and crossmatch
TSH	Thyroid-stimulating hormone
UA	Urinalysis
WBC	White blood cell

Chapter Summary

Pathology and laboratory tests provide health care professionals with definitive evidence as to the condition that may be interfering with a patient's good health. That proof will help direct the physician toward a more accurate diagnosis and a beneficial treatment plan. Lab tests are an invaluable part of the health care toolbox and must be coded accurately.

CODING BITES

Common Abbreviations Used in Pathology Testing

PT	=	Prothrombin time, which is used to evaluate bleeding and clotting disorders
CBC	=	Complete blood count, which includes the following tests:
WBC	=	White blood cell count
RBC	=	Red blood cell count
PLT	=	Platelet count, which is used to diagnose or monitor bleeding and clotting disorders
HCT	=	Hematocrit
HGB	=	Hemoglobin concentration, which is the concentration of the oxygen-carrying pigment in red blood cells
DIFF	=	Differential blood count

Remember that the CBC includes the WBC, RBC, HCT, HGB, platelet count, and differential count. Therefore, you are not to code those tests separately.

CHAPTER 28 REVIEW
CPT Pathology & Lab Section

McGraw Hill connect
Enhance your learning by completing these exercises and more at mcgrawhillconnect.com!

Let's Check It! Terminology

Match each key term to the appropriate definition.

1. **LO 28.7** The investigation and identification of cells.
2. **LO 28.2** The counting or measurement of something.
3. **LO 28.8** The study of tissues removed from a living patient during a surgical procedure.
4. **LO 28.8** The study of a specimen using a microscope (under magnification).
5. **LO 28.1** A location with scientific equipment designed to perform experiments and tests.
6. **LO 28.1** The study of the nature, etiology, development, and outcomes of disease.
7. **LO 28.8** The visual study of a specimen (with the naked eye).
8. **LO 28.1** The study of the causes of disease.
9. **LO 28.1** A small part or sample of any substance obtained for analysis and diagnosis.
10. **LO 28.2** The determination of character or essential element(s).

A. Cytology
B. Etiology
C. Gross Examination
D. Laboratory
E. Microscopic Examination
F. Pathology
G. Qualitative
H. Quantitative
I. Specimen
J. Surgical Pathology

Let's Check It! Concepts

Choose the most appropriate answer for each of the following questions.

1. **LO 28.10** What is the correct abbreviation for a liver function test?
   a. INR **b.** LDL **c.** LPF **d.** LFT
2. **LO 28.7** What code(s) would you assign for a blood compatibility test by incubation technique, 2 units?
   a. 86920 **b.** 86921, 86921 **c.** 86921 **d.** 86922, 86921
3. **LO 28.1** A specimen can be
   a. blood. **b.** urine. **c.** sputum. **d.** all of these.
4. **LO 28.3** When not all of the tests listed in a panel are performed, you should
   a. code the panel with modifier 52. **b.** code the panel alone.
   c. code the tests individually. **d.** code the panel with modifier 53.
5. **LO 28.2** The guidelines tell you that, if the documentation does not specify, you may assume that the examination performed was
   a. qualitative **b.** measured **c.** quantitative **d.** none of these
6. **LO 28.5** The lab test most commonly performed using a chemical process to identify hyperglycemia uses
   a. hormones. **b.** blood glucose. **c.** electrolytes. **d.** lipids.
7. **LO 28.9** What modifier would you append to a CPT code for a lab test that has to be repeated, on the same day for the same patient, in order to get several readings of a level or measurement?
   a. 99 **b.** 90 **c.** 92 **d.** 91
8. **LO 28.4** This test identifies the percentage of RBCs, which is used to identify anemia.
   a. BUN **b.** ESR **c.** Hgb **d.** HCT

9. **LO 28.8** Surgical pathology may include
   a. gross examination. **b.** microbiology. **c.** genetic testing. **d.** nuclear medicine.
10. **LO 28.6** ___ testing involves the analysis of specimens to identify any presence of a genetic disorder.
   a. Infectious **b.** Oncology **c.** Genetic **d.** Hematology

Let's Check It! Guidelines

Refer to the Pathology and Laboratory Guidelines and fill in the blanks accordingly.

multiple	rarely	same
definition	technologists	special
separate	effort	85999
extent	may	physician

1. Services in Pathology and Laboratory are provided by a physician or by ___ under responsible supervision of a ___.
2. It is appropriate to designate ___ procedures that are rendered on the ___ date by ___ entries.
3. Unlisted hematology and coagulation procedure is represented by code ___.
4. A service that is ___ provided, unusual, variable, or new ___ require a ___ report.
5. Pertinent information should include an adequate ___ or description of the nature, ___, and need for the procedure; and the time, ___, and equipment necessary to provide the service.

Let's Check It! Rules and Regulations

Please answer the following questions from the knowledge you have gained after reading this chapter.

1. **LO 28.1** Differentiate between pathology and etiology.
2. **LO 28.2** What is the difference between *quantitative* and *qualitative*?
3. **LO 28.7** What is cytopathology? What is cytologic testing used for, and how are specimens obtained?
4. **LO 28.8** What are the purpose and benefit of surgical pathology?
5. **LO 28.9** If your health care facility uses an outside laboratory that bills your office, and you include the charges for the lab work on the claim form, what modifier must you append?

YOU CODE IT! Basics

First, identify the procedural main term in the following statements; then code the procedure or service.

Example: Dr. Gleason performs a definitive drug test for barbiturates:

a. main term: *Drug Assay* **b.** procedure: *80345*

1. Dr. McElory completes a drug monitoring of total digoxin:
   a. main term:_____ **b.** procedure:_____
2. Dr. Gavin performs a bleeding time test:
   a. main term:_____ **b.** procedure:_____
3. Dr. Kaufmann completes a tuberculosis skin test:
   a. main term: _____ **b.** procedure:_____
4. Dr. Lovece performs an HLA crossmatch test, first dilution:
   a. main term: _____ **b.** procedure:_____
5. Dr. Sox completes a blood typing compatibility test by spin technique:
   a. main term:_____ **b.** procedure:_____
6. Dr. Dickenson performs a urine bacterial culture quantitative colony count:
   a. main term:_____ **b.** procedure:_____
7. Dr. Campos performs an HBsAg (hepatitis B surface antigen) immunoassay test:
   a. main term:_____ **b.** procedure:_____

(continued)

8. Dr. Hearon performs a forensic necropsy:
   a. main term:_____ b. procedure:_____
9. Dr. Busby completes a mature oocytes cryopreservation:
   a. main term:_____ b. procedure:_____
10. Dr. Klausing performs a blood cell count with automated differential WBC count:
    a. main term: _____ b. procedure:_____
11. Dr. Reilly completed a creatine kinase, total:
    a. main term:_____ b. procedure:_____
12. Dr. Flemington performs an RPR syphilis test:
    a. main term:_____ b. procedure:_____
13. Dr. Jensen completes a CMV (cytomegalovirus) antibody IgM:
    a. main term: _____ b. procedure:_____
14. Dr. Vance performs a bilirubin, total; direct test:
    a. main term: _____ b. procedure:_____
15. Dr. Humphrey completes a direct Coombs test:
    a. main term:_____ b. procedure:_____

CPT

YOU CODE IT! Practice

Using the techniques described in this chapter, carefully read through the case studies and determine the most accurate pathology and laboratory CPT code(s) and modifier(s), if appropriate, for each case study.

1. Walter Winegarten, a 42-year-old male, was feeling rundown and tired all the time. So, Dr. Stevenson, thinking that Walter might have anemia, ordered a complete CBC, automated with an automated differential WBC count.
2. Deidra Lowe, a 23-year-old female, has been living on the street and in shelters and comes to the free clinic for a checkup because she is 5 months pregnant. Dr. Ashton orders a complete CBC, automated and appropriate manual differential WBC count, hepatitis B surface antigen, rubella antibody, qualitative syphilis test, RBC antibody screening, blood typing ABO, and Rh factor.
3. Vivian Praxis, a 3-year-old female, is at the office of her pediatrician, Dr. Ashley, for her regular checkup. Dr. Ashley notices that Vivian is very small for her age and orders a growth hormone stimulation panel to be done.
4. Jay Zeeman, a 36-year-old male, went to the shore with his friends and feasted on raw oysters and beer. About 7 hours later, after getting home, he began to cough and vomit, and he found blood in his stool. He went to the walk-in clinic, where Dr. Lanahan ran a smear test for ova and parasites, particularly *Anisakis*.
5. Gregg Abernathy, a 41-year-old male, was diagnosed with prostate cancer last week. Before beginning radiation treatments, which will make him unable to have children, he comes today to submit his sperm for cryopreservation.
6. Rudy Porter, a 71-year-old male, has a history of gastrointestinal problems, including intestinal polyps. After taking a special kit home, he submits fecal specimens for an occult blood test by immunoassay.
7. Tiffany Matheson, a 28-year-old female, just got a new job with the space industry. As a condition of her employment, she came to the lab today for a presumptive drug test for alcohol, amphetamines, and barbiturates. The test was performed and the results were read by direct optical observation; they confirmed negative outcomes for all drugs.
8. Caitlyn Deloach, a 21-year-old female, was found unconscious by her roommate and brought into the emergency department by ambulance. The roommate stated that Caitlyn was very depressed, and she feared that Caitlyn might have taken an overdose of her medication. Dr. Leroy ordered a therapeutic drug assay for phenobarbital.
9. Rulon Cutler, a 25-year-old male, is overweight, bordering on obese, and Dr. Jacobs is concerned that he may be developing diabetes, so he orders an insulin tolerance panel for adrenocorticotropic hormone (ACTH) insufficiency.
10. Shawn McCully, a 51-year-old female, goes to her physician, Dr. Kahlil, for her annual checkup, which includes a nonautomated urinalysis with microscopy for glucose, ketones, and leukocytes. Dr. Kahlil's assistant, Donna, performs the test, by dipstick, in the office. The results are normal.
11. Margaret Calhoun, a 23-year-old female, got drunk at a party and had unprotected sex. She came into the clinic today for an HIV-1 and HIV-2 single assay test.
12. At the doctor's suggestion, Margaret Calhoun (previous scenario) also was tested for syphilis, qualitative (VDRL).

(continued)

13. Georgia Stuart, a 37-year-old female, is pregnant for the first time. Dr. Ferguson performed an amniocentesis to do a chromosome analysis, count 15 cells, 1 karyotype, with banding. The results showed that the baby is fine.
14. Sean Olin, a 61-year-old male, was in the operating room for Dr. Tanger to perform a subtotal resection of his pancreas. Surgical pathology showed no malignancy.
15. Chad Snell, a 22-day-old male, was born at 33 weeks gestation, and there is concern that he may have hyperbilirubinemia. Therefore, Dr. Bateman performed a total transcutaneous bilirubin.

YOU CODE IT! Application

The following exercises provide practice in the application of abstracting the physicians' notes and learning to work with documentation from our health care facility, Millard Pathology & Diagnostic Labs. These case studies are modeled on real patient encounters. Using the techniques described in this chapter, carefully read through the case studies and determine the most accurate pathology and laboratory CPT code(s) and modifier(s), if appropriate, for each case study. You are coding for the pathologist.

MILLARD PATHOLOGY & DIAGNOSTIC LABS

753 LITTLE WEST RD • SOMEWHERE, FL 32811 • 407-555-9371

PATIENT: MEDFORD, ROBERT

ACCOUNT/EHR #: MEDFRO001

Procedure Performed: Comprehensive metabolic panel

Pathologist: Derrick Castel, MD

Referring Physician: Oscar R. Prader, MD

INDICATIONS: Routine physical exam

IMPRESSIONS:

Albumin 3.9

Bilirubin Small*

Calcium 8.9

Carbon dioxide (CO_2) 28

Chloride 96 L C

Creatinine 1.2

Glucose 102

Phosphatase, alkaline 90

Potassium 3.9

Protein, total 30*

Sodium 138

Transferase, alanine amino (ALT) (SGPT) 30

Transferase, aspartate amino (AST) (SGOT) 29

Urea nitrogen (BUN) 18

* = Abnormal, L = Low, H = High

Derrick Castel, MD

Determine the most accurate pathology and laboratory CPT code(s) and modifier(s), if appropriate.

(continued)

MILLARD PATHOLOGY & DIAGNOSTIC LABS

753 LITTLE WEST RD • SOMEWHERE, FL 32811 • 407-555-9371

PATIENT: INGER, TERRENCE

ACCOUNT/EHR #: INGETE001

Procedure Performed: Tissue, skin, head, mutation identification

Pathologist: Peter Havner, MD

Referring Physician: Oscar R. Prader, MD

INDICATIONS: Suspected melanoma

IMPRESSIONS: Abnormal cells present, by surgical pathology, gross and microscopic examination

Peter Havner, MD

Determine the most accurate pathology and laboratory CPT code(s) and modifier(s), if appropriate.

MILLARD PATHOLOGY & DIAGNOSTIC LABS

753 LITTLE WEST RD • SOMEWHERE, FL 32811 • 407-555-9371

PATIENT: WALLER, FELIX

ACCOUNT/EHR #: WALLFE001

Procedure Performed: Surgical pathology, gallbladder, gross and microscopic examination

Pathologist: Peter Havner, MD

Referring Physician: Renee O. Bracker, MD

INDICATIONS: R/O malignancy

IMPRESSIONS: All tissues unremarkable
Surgical pathology, gross and microscopic examination of gallbladder

Peter Havner, MD

Determine the most accurate pathology and laboratory CPT code(s) and modifier(s), if appropriate.

MILLARD PATHOLOGY & DIAGNOSTIC LABS

753 LITTLE WEST RD • SOMEWHERE, FL 32811 • 407-555-9371

PATIENT: DALTON, ANGELA

ACCOUNT/EHR #: DALTAN001

Procedure Performed: Rectal biopsies, gross and microscopic examination

Pathologist: Walter Alchemy, MD

Referring Physician: Matthew Appellet, MD

INDICATIONS: Inflammatory bowel disease

IMPRESSIONS: All tissues normal
Surgical pathology, gross and microscopic examination, colon biopsy

Walter Alchemy, MD

Determine the most accurate pathology and laboratory CPT code(s) and modifier(s), if appropriate.

(continued)

MILLARD PATHOLOGY & DIAGNOSTIC LABS

753 LITTLE WEST RD • SOMEWHERE, FL 32811 • 407-555-9371

PATIENT: PRIMERO, GINO

ACCOUNT/EHR #: PRIMGI001

Procedure Performed: Mass (fat tissue), upper eyelid gross and microscopic examination

Pathologist: Derrick Castel, MD

Referring Physician: Renee O. Bracker, MD

INDICATIONS: Herniated orbital fat pad, OD

IMPRESSIONS: Carcinoma in situ
Surgical pathology, gross and microscopic examination, soft tissue tumor, extensive resection

Derrick Castel, MD

Determine the most accurate pathology and laboratory CPT code(s) and modifier(s), if appropriate.

29

CPT Medicine Section

Key Terms

Ablation
Catheter
Duplex Scan
Immunization
Infusion
Injection
Ophthalmologist
Optometrist
Otorhinolaryngology
Push

Learning Outcomes

After completing this chapter, the student should be able to:

LO 29.1 Interpret the guidelines for coding the administration of immunizations.
LO 29.2 Apply the guidelines to accurately report injections and infusions.
LO 29.3 Determine the correct coding parameters for reporting psychiatric services.
LO 29.4 Abstract physicians' notes to accurately report dialysis and gastroenterology services.
LO 29.5 Identify specifics to correctly report ophthalmology and otorhinolaryngologic services.
LO 29.6 Determine how to accurately report cardiovascular services.
LO 29.7 Recognize the details required for accurately reporting pulmonary function testing.
LO 29.8 Report accurately the provision of immunology services.
LO 29.9 Interpret the specifics for accurately reporting neurologic services.
LO 29.10 Abstract the required details for reporting physical medical and rehabilitation services.
LO 29.11 Employ the guidelines to accurately report alternative medicine services: acupuncture, osteopathic, and chiropractic treatments.
LO 29.12 Abstract documentation for reporting special and other services.

STOP! Remember, you need to follow along in your CPT code book for an optimal learning experience.

29.1 Immunizations

Immunization
To make someone resistant to a particular disease by vaccination.

GUIDANCE CONNECTION

Read the additional explanations in the in-section guidelines located within the **Medicine** section, subheads **Immune Globulins, Serum or Recombinant Products**, directly above code 90281; **Immunization Administration for Vaccines/Toxoids**, directly above code 90460; and **Vaccines, Toxoids**, directly above code 90476, all in your CPT book.

Immunizations, also known as vaccinations, are developed to train a patient's immune system against a specific pathogen. Immunization sera work to build immune memory by creating antibodies, similar to special forces, that are ready to battle should a specific bacterium or virus invade. This system is designed to prevent, or at least limit, the damage done by invading pathogens. Immunization of a patient includes two parts: the medication itself and the administration of the medication. Each part is coded separately.

The medication may be an immune globulin, an antitoxin, a vaccine, or a toxoid. Codes 90281-90399 and 90476-90756 are available for you to identify specific drugs. You must be diligent and read all of the options for the specific vaccines because there may be several choices with small differences that are still important to accuracy. For example, there are actually 24 different codes (90653-90689) to report an influenza virus vaccine, each identifying a different version. The physician's documentation should provide you with the specifics you need to identify the version that was used. If not, you must query so you can report the correct code. On occasion, a clinician may discuss immunization(s) with the patient, reviewing priorities and options, and the patient will leave to think about it without any vaccinations being administered. When this counseling is documented, report this with a code from 90482, 90483, or 90484, based on the time spent counseling.

LET'S CODE IT! SCENARIO

Phillip Landstone, a 21-year-old male, came in so Dr. Micah can administer a flu vaccine before he starts volunteering at Community Hospital. Dr. Micah documents that the vaccine was trivalent, split virus, 0.5 mL dosage, administered IM.

Let's Code It!

The documentation states that Dr. Micah administered a *trivalent, split virus* influenza vaccination to Phillip. Turn to the CPT Alphabetic Index and find

Vaccination

Vaccine Administration

See Immunization Administration

Vaccines and Toxoids

See Vaccines and Toxoids

This is great! The Alphabetic Index is reminding you that, when reporting the administration of a vaccination (or other injection), you will need two codes: one for the administration + one for the serum (what is inside that syringe).

As long as you are here, let's find the suggestion(s) for the serum—the influenza vaccine itself.

Vaccines and Toxoids

Read down the list until you find something that matches what you abstracted from the documentation. Do you see . . .

Influenza

Read down the indented list below *Influenza* to find

Influenza

Trivalent, Split Virus (IIV3) 90654–90658, 90660, 90673

for Intradermal Use 90654

for Intramuscular Use 90655–90658

Increased Antigen Content 90662

The documentation states, "*trivalent, split virus, administered IM.*" This matches, so turn to the suggested codes to read the entire code descriptions.

90655 Influenza virus vaccine, trivalent (IIV3), split virus, preservative free, 0.25 mL dosage, for intramuscular use

90656 Influenza virus vaccine, trivalent (IIV3), split virus, preservative free, 0.5 mL dosage, for intramuscular use

90657 Influenza virus vaccine, trivalent (IIV3), split virus, 0.25 mL dosage, for intramuscular use

90658 Influenza virus vaccine, trivalent (IIV3), split virus, 0.5 mL dosage, for intramuscular use

As you read these four code descriptions, you can see that there are two differences: preservative free or not + the dosage. There is no mention that the vaccine was preservative free, so this narrows down the options to 90657 and 90658. What was the dosage? The documentation states, "*0.5 mL dosage.*" Now, you can determine the accurate code for this vaccine is

90658 Influenza virus vaccine, trivalent (IIV3), split virus, 0.5 mL dosage, for intramuscular use

(continued)

Now, you need to go back to the Alphabetic Index, this time to the main term "Immunization Administration."

Immunization Administration

Each Additional Vaccine/Toxoid 90472, 90474

with Counseling 90461

One Vaccine/Toxoid 90471, 90473

with Counseling 90460

Dr. Micah documented only one vaccine was administered; there is no documentation of any counseling. Turn to the *Main Section* to code 90471 so you can read the entire code description:

90471 **Immunization administration (includes percutaneous, intradermal, subcutaneous, or intramuscular injections); 1 vaccine (single or combination vaccine/toxoid)**

90473 **Immunization administration by intranasal or oral route; 1 vaccine (single or combination vaccine/toxoid)**

Go back to the documentation to check what route of administration was used. The documentation states, "*administered IM.*" IM is the abbreviation for *intramuscular*. This fact eliminates 90473 as an option, and you know what code to report. Good job! You now can report codes **90471** and **90658** for Dr. Micah's service to Phillip with confidence!

If more than one vaccine was administered during the same encounter, there may be a combination code available for those vaccinations that are typically provided together, such as the MMR (Measles, Mumps, Rubella) or the DTaP (Diphtheria, Tetanus toxoids, and Acellular Pertussis vaccines). It is illegal to report these vaccines individually if they are administered in a combination.

Medications can be given, or administered, to the patient in several different ways: percutaneous, intradermal, subcutaneous (SC), or intramuscular (IM) injections; intranasal (INH) or oral (ORAL); intra-arterial (IA) or intravenous (IV). The method of administration will help you find the correct administration codes 90460-90461 and 90471-90474.

When more than one vaccine is provided on the same date, use the add-on codes for the administration of the additional injections. You will find that most of the codes are offered in sets: the first injection, administration, or hour and then the add-on code for each additional injection, administration, or hour.

LET'S CODE IT! SCENARIO

Isaac Nelson, a 5-year-old male, came to Dr. Rubino for his MMR vaccine so that he can start kindergarten next month. Dr. Rubino administered an injection subcutaneously. Dr. Rubino met face-to-face with Isaac's mother and discussed the importance of the vaccine, as well as indications of a reaction that she should watch for. Isaac chose a red balloon as his prize for being a good patient.

Let's Code It!

Dr. Rubino gave Isaac *one subcutaneous injection* of the *MMR vaccine*. Do you know what *MMR* stands for? Even if you don't know that it is an acronym for *measles, mumps, and rubella*, you can look it up in the Alphabetic Index under *MMR shots*. The suggested code is 90707. The numeric listing confirms

90707 **Measles, mumps, and rubella virus vaccine (MMR), live, for subcutaneous use**

The description matches Dr. Rubino's notes exactly. However, the code will reimburse Dr. Rubino's office only for the drug itself, not Dr. Rubino's time and expertise in administering the injection and counseling the family. You could go back to the Alphabetic Index, or you could read the instructional paragraph at the beginning of the **Vaccines, Toxoids** subsection (where you found the code 90707). You will see that this paragraph tells you that you must use these codes "in addition to an immunization administration code(s) 90460–90474." Let's turn to the first code, 90460, and read the description:

(continued)

90460 **Immunization administration through 18 years of age via any route of administration, with counseling by physician or other qualified health care professional; first or only component of each vaccine or toxoid administered**

+90461 **each additional vaccine or toxoid component administered (list separately in addition to code for primary procedure)**

Now, you have the codes to reimburse Dr. Rubino for the MMR vaccine, as well as his time and expertise in administering the injection and talking with Isaac's mother. Remember, the MMR vaccine is a combination vaccine with three components. So, you will need to report four codes:

90707, 90460, 90461, 90461

Good job!!

NOTE: If Dr. Rubino had not spent time face-to-face with Isaac and his mother, 90460 and 90461 would not be used. Instead you would use codes 90471, +90472, +90472, which do not include the phrase "when the physician counsels the patient/family" in the code description.

Reporting COVID-19 Immunizations

New Vaccines, Toxoids have been created to specifically report the administration of the COVID-19 vaccines. These three codes differ by the quantity of the dosage. Remember: these codes only report the sera that was in the syringe.

91300 **Severe acute respiratory syndrome coronavirus 2 (SARS-CoV-2) (Coronavirus disease [COVID-19]) vaccine, mRNA-LNP, spike protein, preservative free, 30 mcg/0.3 mL dosage, diluent reconstituted, for intramuscular use**

91301 **Severe acute respiratory syndrome coronavirus 2 (SARS-CoV-2) (Coronavirus disease [COVID-19]) vaccine, mRNA-LNP, spike protein, preservative free, 100 mcg/0.5 mL dosage, for intramuscular use**

91302 **Severe acute respiratory syndrome coronavirus 2 (SARS-CoV-2) (COVID-19) vaccine, DNA, spike protein, chimpanzee adenovirus Oxford 1 (ChAdOx1) vector, preservative-free, 5x10^{10} viral particles/0.5 mL dosage, for intramuscular use**

As you are learning here, you will always need an additional code to report the actual administration services. These new codes are authorized for all COVID-19 vaccine sera approved by the FDA [Food and Drug Administration]. At this time, there are three sets of codes. Each set has one code for the first dose, the second dose, and a third dose (often referred to as a booster shot).

0001A **Immunization administration by intramuscular injection of severe acute respiratory syndrome coronavirus 2 (SARS-CoV-2) (Coronavirus disease [COVID-19]) vaccine, mRNA-LNP, spike protein, preservative free, 30 mcg/0.3 mL dosage, diluent reconstituted; first dose**

0002A **Immunization administration by intramuscular injection of severe acute respiratory syndrome coronavirus 2 (SARS-CoV-2) (Coronavirus disease [COVID-19]) vaccine, mRNA-LNP, spike protein, preservative free, 30 mcg/0.3 mL dosage, diluent reconstituted; second dose**

0003A **Immunization administration by intramuscular injection of severe acute respiratory syndrome coronavirus 2 (SARS-CoV-2) (coronavirus disease [COVID-19]) vaccine, mRNA-LNP, spike protein, preservative free, 30 mcg/0.3 mL dosage, diluent reconstituted; third dose**

0011A **Immunization administration by intramuscular injection of severe acute respiratory syndrome coronavirus 2 (SARS-CoV-2) (Coronavirus disease [COVID-19]) vaccine, mRNA-LNP, spike protein, preservative free, 100 mcg/0.5 mL dosage; first dose**

0012A **Immunization administration by intramuscular injection of severe acute respiratory syndrome coronavirus 2 (SARS-CoV-2) (Coronavirus disease [COVID-19]) vaccine, mRNA-LNP, spike protein, preservative free, 100 mcg/0.5 mL dosage; second dose**

0013A **Immunization administration by intramuscular injection of severe acute respiratory syndrome coronavirus 2 (SARS-CoV-2) (Coronavirus disease [COVID-19]) vaccine, mRNA-LNP, spike protein, preservative free, 100 mcg/0.5mL dosage; third dose**

0021A **Immunization administration by intramuscular injection of severe acute respiratory syndrome coronavirus 2 (SARS-CoV-2) (coronavirus disease [COVID-19]) vaccine, DNA, spike protein, chimpanzee adenovirus Oxford 1 (ChAdOx1) vector, preservative free, 5x10^{10} viral particles/0.5 mL dosage; first dose**

0022A **Immunization administration by intramuscular injection of severe acute respiratory syndrome coronavirus 2 (SARS-CoV-2) (coronavirus disease [COVID-19]) vaccine, DNA, spike protein, chimpanzee adenovirus Oxford 1 (ChAdOx1) vector, preservative free, 5x10^{10} viral particles/0.5 mL dosage; second dose**

29.2 Injections and Infusions

> **CODING BITES**
>
> When a drug is provided to a patient, two types of codes are reported: one for the administration—being discussed here—plus one for the drug itself—discussed in the chapter *HCPCS Level II*.

The administration of fluids (such as saline solution to hydrate a patient suffering from dehydration), pharmaceuticals (such as medications for treatment or preventive purposes), or dyes (such as those used for diagnostic testing) is coded from the **Injections and Infusions** subsection, which includes codes 96360-96379.

Some of these terms may sound familiar to you because we discussed them earlier when reviewing the various ways drugs can be administered into the body. In **Figure 29-1**, do you see how the needle illustrating an *intradermal* injection has its tip pointing into the dermis (*intra* = within + *dermal* = dermis)? The injection that is delivered *subcutaneously* has the tip of the needle all the way down into the fatty tissue layer. And the *intramuscular* (*intra* = within + *muscular* = muscle) injection leads down to the layer of muscle that lies below the fatty tissue layer.

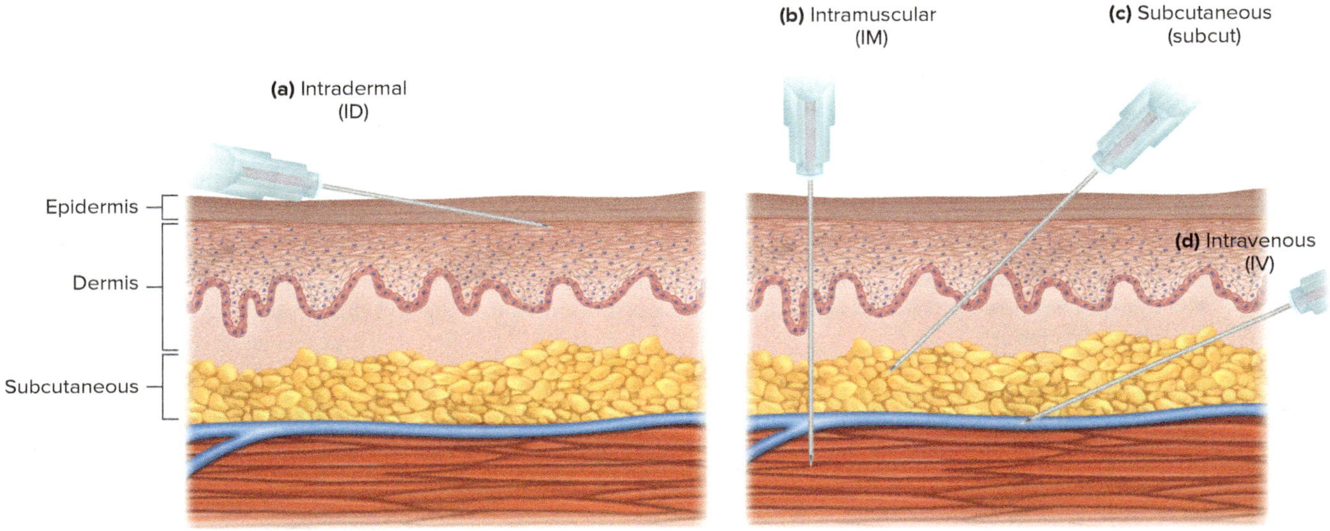

FIGURE 29-1 An illustration showing various injection routes

> **Infusion**
> The introduction of a fluid into a blood vessel.

> **Injection**
> Compelling a fluid into tissue or cavity.

> **CODING BITES**
>
> The administration of chemotherapy drugs is *not* coded from the **Injections and Infusions** subsection, but from the **Chemotherapy Administration** subsection, codes 96401-96549.

The **infusion** and **injection** codes include certain standard parts involved in administering liquids. Services included and therefore not reported separately are

- The administration of a local anesthetic.
- The initiation of the IV.
- Accessing an indwelling IV, subcutaneous catheter, or port.
- Flushing the line at the completion of the infusion.
- The appropriate supplies: tubing, syringes, and so on.

The guidelines for coding injections and infusions provide further direction when coding these services:

- When more than one infusion is provided into one IV site, report only the first service.
- Should more than one IV site be used, report the appropriate services for each site.
- Report different drugs or materials and that service separately.
- Report infusion time as the actual time the fluid is provided.

An IV or intra-arterial **push** is described by the CPT guidelines as

- An injection administered to the patient and then observed continuously by the health care professional who administered the drug.

or

- An infusion that lasts 15 minutes or less.

Push
The delivery of an additional drug via an intravenous line over a short period of time.

Multiple Administrations

When more than one injection or infusion is provided to a patient at the same encounter, there is a specific order in which you need to report the codes. The sequencing guidelines are different for those reporting physician services than for those reporting for the facility.

When you are reporting for the physician's, or other health care professional's, services, you must read the notes carefully to determine the main diagnosis or reason for the treatment. The primary reason for the injection or infusion should be reported first, as the "initial" service, no matter in what order the injections were administered.

EXAMPLE

Wendy comes to see her physician because she has been vomiting a lot over the last several days. Dr. Kilmer identifies that she has become dehydrated due to this excessive vomiting. Dr. Kilmer gives Wendy an intramuscular (IM) injection of an antiemetic (a drug to stop vomiting) and then gives her an IV infusion, 45 minutes, of normal saline for hydration. The primary reason for the encounter is Wendy's excessive vomiting; therefore, the injection of the antiemetic is the "initial" service, followed by the hydration infusion service.

96372 Therapeutic, prophylactic, or diagnostic injection; subcutaneous or intramuscular

96360 Intravenous infusion, hydration; initial, 31 minutes to 1 hour

NOTE: Remember, you will also need an additional code for the specific antiemetic medication that was inside that injection, as well as an additional code for the saline.

When you are reporting services on behalf of a facility rather than the providing professional, the order is determined by the type of service provided as well as the reason for that service:

1. Chemotherapy service.
2. Therapeutic, prophylactic, and diagnostic services.
3. Hydration services.

Then, the specific service hierarchy is

1. Infusions.
2. Pushes.
3. Injections.

GUIDANCE CONNECTION

Read the additional explanations in the in-section guidelines located within the **Medicine** section, subheads **Hydration**, directly above code 96360, and **Therapeutic, Prophylactic, Diagnostic Injections and Infusions (Excludes Chemotherapy and Other Highly Complex Drug or Highly Complex Biologic Agent Administration)**, directly above code 96365, both in your CPT book.

LET'S CODE IT! SCENARIO

Melissa Fusion, a 51-year-old female, postmastectomy for malignant neoplasm of the breast, has been having chemotherapy treatments. She was seen today for nausea and vomiting as a result of this therapy. Dr. Saludo ordered an antiemetic 10 mg IV push and another antiemetic IV infusion over 30 minutes.

(continued)

Let's Code It!

Melissa received two medications via two different routes of administration: *IV push* and *IV infusion*. Therefore, you need two codes.

The notes report that an intravenous push, which is an injection given intravenously, was given. Let's turn to the Alphabetic Index and look up *injection, intravenous*.

Injection

Intravenous 96379

Keep reading below that and you will see

Injection

Intravenous push 96374–96376

That looks perfect. Turn to the numeric listing and read the complete descriptions. You see that 96374 matches the notes:

96374 Therapeutic, prophylactic or diagnostic injection (specify substance or drug); intravenous push, single or initial substance/drug

You also know that Melissa was given an *infusion, intravenously*, and that it was for *therapeutic* reasons—to eliminate her nausea and vomiting. Let's go to the Alphabetic Index and look up *infusion, intravenous, therapeutic*.

Infusion

Intravenous

Diagnostic/Prophylactic/Therapeutic 96365–96368, 96379

Hydration 96360, 96361

When you turn to the numeric listing to check the code descriptions, you see that codes 96360–96361 are for hydration only. Look through the complete descriptions for the next grouping, 96365–96368, and you see that the best, most accurate code is

96367 Intravenous infusion, for therapy, prophylaxis, or diagnosis (specify substance or drug); additional sequential infusion of a new drug/substance, up to 1 hour

The notes indicate that Melissa was given the infusion after the first (sequentially) for 30 minutes. Excellent!

Therefore, the claim form for this encounter with Melissa will show **96374** and **96367**.

Great job!

Chemotherapy Administration

Codes 96401-96549 cover the different methods of chemotherapy dispensation that may be used with one patient. Each method (such as steroidal agents and biologic agents) and/or each technique (such as infusion or IV push) should be coded separately. The codes include the following services:

- The administration of a local anesthetic.
- The initiation of the IV.
- Accessing an indwelling IV, subcutaneous catheter, or port.
- Flushing the line at the completion of the infusion.
- The appropriate supplies: tubing, syringes, and so on.
- The preparation of the chemotherapy agent(s).

GUIDANCE CONNECTION

Read the additional explanations in the in-section guidelines located within the **Medicine** section, subhead **Chemotherapy and Other Highly Complex Drug or Highly Complex Biologic Agent Administration**, directly above code 96401 in your CPT book.

YOU CODE IT! CASE STUDY

Andrew Gitner is admitted today for his chemotherapy, which consists of an antineoplastic drug, 500 mg IV infusion over 3 hours. Dr. Munch is in attendance during Andrew's treatment.

You Code It!

Go through the steps, and determine the code(s) that should be reported for this encounter between Dr. Munch and Andrew Gitner.

Step #1: Read the case carefully and completely.
Step #2: Abstract the scenario. Which key words or terms describe what service the physician provided to the patient during this encounter?
Step #3: Are there any details missing or incomplete for which you would need to query the physician? [If so, ask your instructor.]
Step #4: Determine the correct CPT procedure code or codes to explain the details about what was provided to the patient during this encounter.
Step #5: Check for any relevant guidance, including reading all of the symbols and notations.
Step #6: Do you need to append any modifiers to ensure complete and accurate information is provided?
Step #7: Double-check your work.

Answer:

Did you determine these to be the correct codes?

96413 **Chemotherapy administration, intravenous infusion technique; up to 1 hour, single or initial substance/drug**

+96415 **each additional hour (List separately in addition to code for primary procedure) [for second hour]**

+96415 **each additional hour (List separately in addition to code for primary procedure) [for third hour]**

29.3 Psychiatry, Psychotherapy, and Biofeedback

Sometimes we become so focused on physical health care issues that we forget the health care professionals who treat mental health concerns. This area is a great opportunity for coding specialists because more and more health care plans cover psychotherapy and psychiatric services. Codes 90785–90911 provide details on such services.

Psychiatry services are categorized as:

- Interactive Complexity
- Psychiatric Diagnostic Procedures
  - Psychotherapy
  - Psychotherapy for Crisis
  - Other Psychotherapy
  - Other Psychiatric Services or Procedures

Once the type of therapy is determined, the next factor to consider is how much time the provider spent face-to-face with the patient.

There is a difference between *psychiatric* E/M and *medical* E/M, so, lastly, you must abstract from the documentation whether the physician or therapist provided *medical* E/M services in addition to the therapy session at the same time or on the same day.

When medical E/M services are provided at the same time or on the same date, and are documented as separately identified–specifically different from those issues covered by the therapy–then a code from the ***Evaluation and Management (E/M)*** section of the CPT book may be appropriate.

GUIDANCE CONNECTION

Read the additional explanations in the in-section guidelines located within the **Medicine** section, subhead **Psychiatry**, directly above code 90785 in your CPT book

LET'S CODE IT! SCENARIO

Taylor Loeb, a 32-year-old male, was sent to Dr. Panjab for psychotherapy to deal with anger management issues. Dr. Panjab spent 45 minutes with Taylor in her office.

Let's Code It!

Taylor saw Dr. Panjab in *her office* for psychotherapy for *45 minutes.* Let's look in the Alphabetic Index under *psychotherapy*, beneath which you see *family* of patient, for crisis, group other than multifamily, individual patient, and several more, as choices. The notes indicate that Taylor had an individual psychotherapy session. The Alphabetic Index suggests codes 90832–90834 and 90836–90838. Let's look at the numeric listing and see which of these matches Dr. Panjab's notes.

90834 **Psychotherapy, 45 minutes with patient**

+90836 **Psychotherapy, 45 minutes with patient when performed with an evaluation and management service (List separately in addition to the code for primary procedure.)**

The next issue to consider is whether Dr. Panjab provided medical E/M services at the same time. According to her notes, she did not. This means that code 90834 is the code to report.

Great job!

Telemedicine Synchronous Services

Several codes within the **Psychiatry** subsection qualify to be provided using telemedicine synchronous audio/video services, as noted by the star (★) symbol to the left of the code: 90791, 90792, 90832, 90833, 90834, 90836, 90837, 90838, 90845, 90846, 90847, and 90863. Telemedicine services provided in an audio only format are designated with a speaker (🔈) symbol.

As you learned in the chapter ***CPT and HCPCS Level II Modifiers*** in the section ***Service-Related Modifiers***, the documentation for these encounters must confirm that the content of the physician/patient meeting is sufficient to meet the requirements for the code to be reported whether the service was provided face-to-face or with the use of synchronous telemedicine services (as indicated by appending modifier 93 for audio only or modifier 95 for audio/video).

YOU CODE IT! CASE STUDY

Adam has been acting out, often losing his temper and getting violent, since his parents divorced. After individual sessions, Dr. Eisenberg holds a family psychotherapy session with Adam and his parents. As Adam's mother had moved about 1 hour away, and Adam's father was at work, Dr. Eisenberg used Skype to connect the whole family for the 50-minute session. Dr. Eisenberg's notes indicate good progress was made.

(continued)

You Code It!

Dr. Eisenberg used encrypted audio/video technology to have one session with an entire family. Determine the appropriate code to report this service.

Step #1: Read the case carefully and completely.
Step #2: Abstract the scenario. Which key words or terms describe what service the physician provided to the patient during this encounter?
Step #3: Are there any details missing or incomplete for which you would need to query the physician? [If so, ask your instructor.]
Step #4: Determine the correct CPT procedure code or codes to explain the details about what was provided to the patient during this encounter.
Step #5: Check for any relevant guidance, including reading all of the symbols and notations.
Step #6: Do you need to append any modifiers to ensure complete and accurate information is provided?
Step #7: Double-check your work.

Answer:

Did you determine this to be the correct code?

90847-95 **Family psychotherapy (conjoint psychotherapy) (with patient present), 50 minutes, synchronous telemedicine service rendered via a real-time interactive audio and video telecommunications system**

29.4 Dialysis and Gastroenterology Services

Dialysis

Dialysis is an artificial process used to clean the blood by removing excess water and waste products when the individual's body cannot do this. In addition to hospitals providing this service, independent centers and home health agencies help patients receive treatment. The correct code for reporting dialysis service is determined by the patient's age, where the services are provided, and the level of physician services during the encounters.

Physician services provided during a dialysis month included in these codes are

- Determination of the dialysis cycle.
- Outpatient E/M of the dialysis visits.
- Telephone calls.
- Patient management.
- Face-to-face visit with the patient.

Hemodialysis

Hemodialysis is a process that uses a mechanical dialyzer to extract blood via an intravenous catheter to filter out waste products and excess fluids, and returns the "cleaned" blood back into the patient via an intra-arterial catheter. Typically, three sessions a week are provided.

Prior to beginning ongoing hemodialysis treatments, the nephrologist will order the insertion of either an arteriovenous fistula (AVF) or an arteriovenous graft (AVG). For more information on these procedures, see the additional explanations in the in-section guidelines located within the ***Surgery*** section, subhead **Dialysis Circuit**, directly above code 36901 in your CPT book.

Hemodialysis procedures are reported with one of two codes determined by the number of evaluations provided by the physician during the encounter:

90935 **Hemodialysis procedure with single evaluation by a physician or other qualified physician or other health care professional**

90937 **Hemodialysis procedure requiring repeated evaluation(s) with or without substantial revision of dialysis prescription**

When the hemodialysis services are performed by a nonphysician health care professional in the patient's residence, including a private home, assisted living center, group home, nontraditional provider home, custodial care facility, or a school, use this code:

99512 Home visit for hemodialysis

When hemodialysis is provided via an AV fistula, graft, or catheter, there are Category II codes to report this service:

4052F Hemodialysis via functioning arteriovenous (AV) fistula [ESRD]

4053F Hemodialysis via functioning arteriovenous (AV) graft [ESRD]

4054F Hemodialysis via catheter [ESRD]

Access flow studies may be provided to determine the effectiveness of the dialysis process.

90940 Hemodialysis access flow study to determine blood flow in grafts and arteriovenous fistulae by an indicator method

93990 Duplex scan of hemodialysis access (including arterial inflow, body of access and venous outflow)

GUIDANCE CONNECTION

Read the additional explanations in the in-section guidelines located within the **Medicine** section, subhead **Dialysis**, subsections **Hemodialysis**, directly above code 90935; **Miscellaneous Dialysis Procedures**, directly above code 90945; and **End-Stage Renal Disease Services**, directly above code 90951, all in your CPT book.

Other Renal Therapies

There are other types of dialysis provided to patients with renal failure, including

- *Peritoneal dialysis*, which uses a catheter connected to the abdominal cavity, using the peritoneal membrane to filter the blood.
- *Hemofiltration*, which is a process that uses mechanical filtration circuit to clean the blood of waste products and excess fluid using a convection process.

These types of renal therapies are reported with one of two codes:

90945 Dialysis procedure other than hemodialysis, with single evaluation by a physician or other qualified physician or other health care professional

90947 Dialysis procedure other than hemodialysis, requiring repeated evaluation(s) by a physician or other qualified health care professional, with or without substantial revision of dialysis prescription

When these services are provided at the patient's home by a nonphysician professional, use these:

99601 Home infusion/specialty drug administration, per visit (up to 2 hours)

+99602 each additional hour (List separately in addition to code for primary procedure.)

End-Stage Renal Disease (ESRD)

When a patient is diagnosed with end-stage renal disease (ESRD), dialysis services are reported on a monthly basis, rather than for each individual encounter, with a code from the range 90951–90966. The correct code for reporting dialysis service is determined by

- *Patient's age:* Grouped into ranges: younger than 2 years of age, 2–11 years of age, 12–19 years of age, and 20 years of age and older.
- *Where the services are provided:* Outpatient facility or home dialysis.
- *Level of physician services:* Number of face-to-face visits by a physician.

If a facility does not provide a full month of services to a patient, for whatever reason, then you should use one code from the range 90967–90970, determined by the age of the patient, multiplied by each day of service.

LET'S CODE IT! SCENARIO

Glory Anders, a 61-year-old female, was diagnosed with ESRD 6 months ago. She has just moved to Springfield to be closer to her daughter and began her daily dialysis on June 20 at the Southside Dialysis Center. Prepare the claim for dialysis services for June.

Let's Code It!

Glory has *ESRD* and has received *dialysis* as an *outpatient* from Southside Dialysis Center. Let's look up *dialysis* in the Alphabetic Index. You can see in the listing for *end-stage renal disease*, there is a reference: "*See* End-Stage Renal Disease Services, Dialysis." Let's turn, in the Alphabetic Index, to this listing. Under this header, you will see Dialysis with the suggested code range of 90951–90970, with further clarification by the location at which the dialysis service was provided. What does the documentation state? "*. . . at the Southside Dialysis Center.*" This helps narrow down the suggested codes to Outpatient . . . 90951–90962.

When you turn to the numeric listing, you read that codes 90951–90962 are only for a full month of treatment. Glory received *11 days* of treatment from the facility (June 20 through June 30 is 11 days), so you have to find the code to report each day of service to Glory. Codes 90967–90970 report dialysis "less than a full month of service, per day" and are broken down by the patient's age. Glory is *61 years old*, bringing us to the following code:

90970 End-stage renal disease (ESRD) related services for dialysis less than a full month of service, per day; for patients 20 years of age and over

Great! So the code will read **90970 × 11**.

Gastroenterology Services

A limited number of tests and services for the gastroenterological system–from the patient's mouth down the esophagus to the stomach through the intestinal tract to the rectum–are included in the ***Medicine*** section of the CPT book. The Alphabetic Index will guide you to the best, most appropriate code in the best section, depending upon the service provided.

YOU CODE IT! CASE STUDY

Paulina Porter, a 39-year-old female, has been battling with indigestion for over a year. After trying virtually every over-the-counter medication possible, she came to see Dr. Dahl, who decided to administer an esophageal acid reflux test. The test was administered in the office using a nasal catheter intraluminal impedance electrode. The 45-minute test was recorded and analyzed and interpreted by Dr. Dahl.

You Code It!

Go through the steps, and determine the procedure code(s) that should be reported for the test provided by Dr. Dahl to Paulina Porter.

Step #1: Read the case carefully and completely.
Step #2: Abstract the scenario. Which key words or terms describe what service the physician provided to the patient during this encounter?
Step #3: Are there any details missing or incomplete for which you would need to query the physician? [If so, ask your instructor.]
Step #4: Determine the correct CPT procedure code or codes to explain the details about what was provided to the patient during this encounter.
Step #5: Check for any relevant guidance, including reading all of the symbols and notations.
Step #6: Do you need to append any modifiers to ensure complete and accurate information is provided?
Step #7: Double-check your work.

(continued)

Answer:

Did you determine this to be the correct code?

91037 **Esophageal function test, gastroesophageal reflux test with nasal catheter intraluminal impedance electrode(s) placement, recording, analysis and interpretation**

29.5 Ophthalmology and Otorhinolaryngologic Services

Ophthalmology

Ophthalmologist
A physician qualified to diagnose and treat eye disease and conditions with drugs, surgery, and corrective measures.

Optometrist
A professional qualified to carry out eye examinations and to prescribe and supply eyeglasses and contact lenses.

CODING BITES

Codes for ophthalmologic services include attention to both eyes. Therefore, if only one eye is addressed by the physician, you should include modifier **52 Reduced Services** with the code.

Ophthalmologists are commonly called *eye doctors* or *vision specialists*. However, be careful not to confuse them with **optometrists**, who are eyeglass specialists.

The **Ophthalmology** subsection of the CPT book reports services provided by an ophthalmologist. General services, codes 92002–92014, are divided in two ways:

1. *The relationship between the patient and the physician: new patient or established patient.* Remember this from E/M coding? As a reminder, a new patient is one who has not received any services or treatments from the ophthalmologist (or any other physician with the same specialty in the same group practice) within the last 3 years.
   a. *The level of service: intermediate or comprehensive.* An intermediate service is similar to a problem-focused evaluation. That is, the patient has a new or existing specific condition to be addressed by the physician. The comprehensive service is more of a general evaluation of the patient's entire visual system.

It is important to remember that these general services include both technical examinations and medical decision-making services. Therefore, it is not appropriate to code any of those services separately.

However, special services may be coded separately if provided at the same time as general services or E/M services. The documentation must be specific in its identification of the additional services. (Of course, special services can be provided alone and coded as such.) Codes 92015–92499 are used to report other ophthalmologic services.

LET'S CODE IT! SCENARIO

Warren Preston, a 61-year-old male, has been having a problem with blurred vision and pain in his eyes. His father has glaucoma, which makes Warren at high risk for the disease. Therefore, Dr. Coreley is going to perform a bilateral visual field examination and a serial tonometry with multiple measurements. None of these services is done as a part of a general ophthalmologic service provided to Warren.

Let's Code It!

Dr. Coreley is giving Warren a "*bilateral visual field examination and a serial tonometry*" today. Let's go to the Alphabetic Index and look at *visual field, exam.* The Alphabetic Index suggests codes 92081–92083. Let's take a look at the numeric listing's code description:

92081 **Visual field examination, unilateral or bilateral, with interpretation and report; limited examination (e.g., tangent screen, Autoplot, arc perimeter, or single stimulus level automated test, such as Octopus 3 or 7 equivalent)**

(continued)

It matches the notes. Now, you need to code the second test, the tonometry. You see that the Alphabetic Index shows *tonometry, serial* and suggests code 92100. Let's take a look at the complete code description:

92100 Serial tonometry (separate procedure) with multiple measurements of intraocular pressure over an extended time period with interpretation and report, same day (e.g., diurnal curve or medical treatment of acute elevation of intraocular pressure)

That's great! You are ready to create the claim form for Warren's tests: codes **92081** and **92100**. Good job!

GUIDANCE CONNECTION

Read the additional explanations in the in-section guidelines located within the **Medicine** section, subhead **Ophthalmology**, directly above code 92002 in your CPT book.

Otorhinolaryngologic Services

Otorhinolaryngology
The study of the human ears, nose, and throat (ENT) systems.

In the **Special Otorhinolaryngologic Services** portion of the ***Medicine*** section are codes for special services that are not usually included in an office visit or evaluation encounter in the field of **otorhinolaryngology**.

Throughout the listings for codes 92502–92700, you will see all types of tests and services that can help health care professionals diagnose and treat conditions relating to a patient's ears, nose, and throat and their functions.

YOU CODE IT! CASE STUDY

Darlene Watson came with her husband, Albert, to see Dr. Hudman because of the problems Albert has been having sleeping. Darlene noticed that Albert snores terribly during the night and has, at times, abruptly stopped making noise. She is concerned that he may have actually stopped breathing during one of his episodes. Dr. Hudman performed a nasopharyngoscopy with an endoscope to check Albert's adenoids and lingual tonsils. The results of the exam indicated that Albert is suffering from sleep apnea.

You Code It!

Go through the steps, and determine the code(s) that should be reported for this test provided by Dr. Hudman to Albert Watson.

Step #1: Read the case carefully and completely.
Step #2: Abstract the scenario. Which key words or terms describe what service the physician provided to the patient during this encounter?
Step #3: Are there any details missing or incomplete for which you would need to query the physician? [If so, ask your instructor.]
Step #4: Determine the correct CPT procedure code or codes to explain the details about what was provided to the patient during this encounter.
Step #5: Check for any relevant guidance, including reading all of the symbols and notations.
Step #6: Do you need to append any modifiers to ensure complete and accurate information is provided?
Step #7: Double-check your work.

Answer:

Did you determine this to be the correct code?

92511 Nasopharyngoscopy with endoscope (separate procedure)

That is exactly what Dr. Hudman did. In addition, he did not perform it as a part of any other service, so it was a separate procedure. Excellent!

GUIDANCE CONNECTION

Read the additional explanations in the in-section guidelines located within the **Medicine** section, subhead **Special Otorhinolaryngologic Services**, directly above code 92502 in your CPT book.

29.6 Cardiovascular Services

When reporting cardiovascular services from the ***Medicine*** section of CPT, you will find both diagnostic and therapeutic services for conditions of the heart and its vessels. As you look through the descriptions of the codes in this section, you might think that some appear to be surgical in nature (an atherectomy), while others appear to be imaging (radiologic), such as an echocardiogram. Regardless of what you think, the CPT book is structured the way it is, and it is your job as a coding specialist to find the best, most appropriate code to represent the service or treatment provided by the physician or other health care professional for whom you are reporting. Again, this is why it is so important that you take nothing for granted, read all notations and instructions carefully, and use the Alphabetic Index to guide you through the numeric listings.

Cardiovascular Therapeutic Services

A variety of procedures relating to the heart are included in the **Cardiovascular** subsection ***Therapeutic Services and Procedures*** that might seem more appropriate for other places in the CPT book. For example, the inclusion of intravascular ultrasound and percutaneous transluminal coronary balloon angioplasty illustrates the importance of using the Alphabetic Index to locate the correct range of codes for the procedures performed.

YOU CODE IT! CASE STUDY

Ransom Sweeney was in Dr. Plenmen's office when Ransom went into cardiac arrest. Dr. Plenmen immediately performed cardiopulmonary resuscitation (CPR). The nurse called 911, and Ransom was taken to the hospital after regaining consciousness and being stabilized.

You Code It!

Go through the steps, and determine the code(s) that should be reported for the service provided by Dr. Plenmen for Ransom Sweeney.

Step #1: Read the case carefully and completely.
Step #2: Abstract the scenario. Which key words or terms describe what service the physician provided to the patient during this encounter?
Step #3: Are there any details missing or incomplete for which you would need to query the physician? [If so, ask your instructor.]
Step #4: Determine the correct CPT procedure code or codes to explain the details about what was provided to the patient during this encounter.
Step #5: Check for any relevant guidance, including reading all of the symbols and notations.
Step #6: Do you need to append any modifiers to ensure complete and accurate information is provided?
Step #7: Double-check your work.

Answer:

Did you determine this to be the correct code?

92950 Cardiopulmonary resuscitation (e.g., in cardiac arrest)

It matches the notes perfectly. Good work!

Cardiography

The electronic measurement of heart rhythms very often uses an electrocardiograph (ECG, also called an EKG, machine). Services involving an electrocardiogram are coded from the **Cardiography** subsection.

> **EXAMPLE**
>
> Deliah Munroe experienced a rapid heartbeat and mild pain in her chest. Dr. Donaldson took a 12-lead routine ECG to rule out a heart attack. He interpreted the tracing and wrote a report for the file. The code is
>
> 93000 Electrocardiogram, routine ECG with at least 12 leads; with interpretation and report

Implantable and Wearable Cardiac Device Evaluations

Technology has provided physicians with the ability to monitor a person's heart function under various circumstances. You learned how to code the implantation of these devices in the ***CPT Surgery Section*** chapter of this book, subsection ***Cardiovascular System***.

These incredible measuring devices must be programmed, and then data must be gathered by using in-person and/or remote transmission and interpreted by the physician. The codes in this subsection report these services.

> **EXAMPLE**
>
> Henriette had a dual-lead pacemaker implanted 3 days ago by Dr. Rasmussen. She is here to have him do the evaluation and programming.
>
> 93286 Peri-procedural device evaluation (in person) and programming of device system parameters before or after a surgery, procedure, or test with analysis, review, and report by a physician or other qualified health care professional; single, dual, or multiple lead pacemaker system, or leadless pacemaker system

Echocardiography

Echocardiography is different from electrocardiography. As the name indicates, an echocardiogram uses ultrasound (sound waves to produce an echo), rather than a measurement by electronic impulses, as with the ECG.

When coding echocardiography, the codes already include

- The exam (the recording of the images of the organ or anatomical areas being studied).
- The interpretation and report of the findings.

You are not permitted to use these codes for echocardiograms that have been taken when no interpretation or report has been done.

Cardiac Catheterization

The codes available for reporting cardiac catheterization include the following:

- The introduction of the **catheter(s)**.
- The positioning and repositioning of the catheter(s).
- Recording of the intracardiac and intravascular pressure.
- Obtaining blood samples for the measurement of blood gases, dilution curves, and/or cardiac output with or without electrode catheter placement.
- Final evaluation and report of the procedure.

> **Catheter**
> A thin, flexible tube, inserted into a body part, used to inject fluid, to extract fluid, or to keep a passage open.

CODING BITES

The provision of a cardiac catheterization may require as many as five codes. The determination of how many of these codes you are responsible for reporting will depend upon for whom you are coding (which professional or facility):

1. The professional service for the catheterization . . . procedure code + modifier 26.
2. The administration of the dye . . . procedure code + modifier 51.
3. The radiologist's supervision and interpretation for the guidance for the injection of the dye . . . procedure code + modifier 26.
4. The procedure itself, such as coronary artery angiography.
5. The radiologist's supervision and interpretation of the images.

LET'S CODE IT! SCENARIO

Mason Franks, a 4-month-old male, was experiencing cyanotic episodes, known as "blue" spells. Dr. Zahn, his pediatrician, performed a transthoracic echocardiogram, which identified a ventricular septal defect and hypertrophied walls of the right ventricle. He then performed a right cardiac catheterization of the normal native connections, that confirmed a diagnosis of a tetralogy of Fallot.

Let's Code It!

Dr. Zahn performed two tests on little Mason: first, a *transthoracic echocardiogram* and, second, a *right cardiac catheterization.* Let's go to the Alphabetic Index and look for the echocardiogram or echocardiography. Beneath *echocardiography,* you see *transthoracic* with a series of suggested codes. But before you go on, take a look at the indented listing below *transthoracic* for *congenital cardiac anomalies.* Mason is only 4 months old, and his heart problems are congenital; therefore, those are likely the more accurate codes. Let's take a look at the complete descriptions in the numeric listing for the suggested codes 93303 and 93304.

93303 Transthoracic echocardiography for congenital cardiac anomalies; complete

This matches the notes. Now, we must code the catheterization. In the Alphabetic Index, under *catheterization,* you find *cardiac,* and indented below that you find a notation, "*See* Cardiac Catheterization." Therefore, look back and find this header in the Alphabetic Index.

Under the *Cardiac Catheterization* header, read down to find *congenital cardiac anomalies* . . . 93530–93533. Let's take a look at the complete description:

93593 Right heart catheterization for congenital heart defect(s) including imaging guidance by the proceduralist to advance the catheter to the target zone; normal native connections

93594 Right heart catheterization for congenital heart defect(s) including imaging guidance by the proceduralist to advance the catheter to the target zone; abnormal native connections

93596 Right and left heart catheterization for congenital heart defect(s) including imaging guidance by the proceduralist to advance the catheter to the target zone(s); normal native connections

93597 Right and left heart catheterization for congenital heart defect(s) including imaging guidance by the proceduralist to advance the catheter to the target zone(s); abnormal native connections

Excellent. Now, you can see how terms you learned from coding the first procedure—congenital cardiac anomalies—make coding the second procedure easier. From all of those code choices, there is only one that matches the documentation:

93593 Right heart catheterization for congenital heart defect(s) including imaging guidance by the proceduralist to advance the catheter to the target zone; normal native connections

It is a small example of how practice and experience will make the entire coding process go more smoothly for you.

Electrophysiologic Procedures

Intracardiac electrophysiologic studies (EPS) codes include

- The insertion of the electrode catheters (usually performed with two or more catheters).
- The repositioning of the catheters.
- Recording of electrograms both before and during the pacing or programmed stimulation of multiple locations of the heart.
- Analysis of the recorded electrograms.
- Report of the procedure and the findings.

There are cases when a diagnostic EPS is followed by treatment (**ablation**) of the problem at the same encounter. When ablation is done at the same time as an EPS, you must code it separately.

Ablation
The destruction or eradication of tissue.

GUIDANCE CONNECTION

Read the additional explanations in the in-section guidelines located within the **Medicine** section, subhead **Cardiovascular**, subsections **Cardiography**, directly above code 93000; **Cardiovascular Monitoring Services**, directly above code 93224; **Implantable, Insertable, and Wearable Cardiac Device Evaluations**, directly above code 93264; **Echocardiography**, directly above code 93303; **Cardiac Catheterization**, directly above code 93451; and **Intracardiac Electrophysiological Procedures/Studies**, directly above code 93600, all in your CPT book.

Noninvasive Vascular Studies

Codes 93880–93998 are provided for reporting noninvasive vascular studies of the arteries and veins of a patient and include the following:

- Preparation of the patient for the testing.
- Supervision of the performance of the tests.
- Recording of the study.
- Interpretation and report of the findings.

Codes are chosen by the type of study done: noninvasive physiologic, transcranial Doppler (TCD), or **duplex scan**.

CODING BITES

If the device used does *not* record the test, then you may not use a separate code for the service.

Duplex Scan
An ultrasonic scanning procedure to determine blood flow and pattern.

YOU CODE IT! CASE STUDY

Dr. Robbins was giving Teena Salazar her annual physical examination. She had a low-grade fever, and swelling and cyanosis were evident on her lower right leg. Concerned that she might have deep-vein thrombophlebitis, he performed a duplex Doppler ultrasonogram to study the arteries in her leg.

You Code It!

Go through the steps, and determine the code(s) that should be reported for this test performed on Teena Salazar.

Step #1: Read the case carefully and completely.
Step #2: Abstract the scenario. Which key words or terms describe what service the physician provided to the patient during this encounter?
Step #3: Are there any details missing or incomplete for which you would need to query the physician? [If so, ask your instructor.]

(continued)

Step #4: Determine the correct CPT procedure code or codes to explain the details about what was provided to the patient during this encounter.
Step #5: Check for any relevant guidance, including reading all of the symbols and notations.
Step #6: Do you need to append any modifiers to ensure complete and accurate information is provided?
Step #7: Double-check your work.

Answer:

Did you determine this to be the correct code?

93926 Duplex scan of lower extremity arteries or arterial bypass grafts; unilateral or limited study

Good job!

29.7 Pulmonary

Codes 94002–94799 in the **Pulmonary** subsection identify procedures and tests on the pulmonary system and include

- The exam and/or laboratory procedure.
- Interpretation of the findings.

Pulmonary Function Testing

Pulmonary function testing is performed to measure the ability of the patient's lungs to inspire (bring air into the lungs) and expire (expel gases from the body) as well as measure the efficacy of the lungs to transfer oxygen into the circulatory system of the body.

Spirometry

Spirometry, the basis of pulmonary function testing, measures the quantity of airflow during expiration (exhaling), as well as the speed of this action. The results of this assessment can provide indications of a wide range of lung diseases.

94010 Spirometry, including graphic record, total and timed vital capacity, expiratory flow rate measurement(s), with or without maximal voluntary ventilation

94060 Bronchodilation responsiveness, spirometry as in 94010, pre- and post-bronchodilator administration

Lung Volume Measurement

Measurement of lung volumes can be done in several ways:

- Plethysmography is used to determine total lung capacity, residual volume, functional residual capacity, and airway resistance.
- Helium dilution and/or nitrogen washout are used to measure lung volumes, distribution of ventilation, and closing volume.

Diffusing Capacity

A test for diffusing capacity uses an inhaled tracer gas and is measured during expiration. The comparison between the amount of gas acquired during inspiration and the amount exhaled evidences the effectiveness of air and gases moving from the lungs into the blood.

+94729 Diffusing capacity (e.g., carbon monoxide, membrane)

GUIDANCE CONNECTION

Read the additional explanations in the in-section guidelines located within the **Medicine** section, subhead **Pulmonary**, subsection **Pulmonary Diagnostic Testing and Therapies**, directly above code 94010 in your CPT book.

YOU CODE IT! CASE STUDY

Carmine Allen, a 2-day-old male, was born at 35 weeks gestation, with a birth weight of 1,450 g. After exhibiting hypotension, peripheral edema, and oliguria, Carmine was diagnosed by Dr. Yanger with respiratory distress syndrome. Dr. Yanger performed the initiation of continuous positive airway pressure ventilation (CPAP).

You Code It!

Go through the steps, and determine the code(s) that should be reported for this treatment provided to Carmine.

Step #1: Read the case carefully and completely.

Step #2: Abstract the scenario. Which key words or terms describe what service the physician provided to the patient during this encounter?

Step #3: Are there any details missing or incomplete for which you would need to query the physician? [If so, ask your instructor.]

Step #4: Determine the correct CPT procedure code or codes to explain the details about what was provided to the patient during this encounter.

Step #5: Check for any relevant guidance, including reading all of the symbols and notations.

Step #6: Do you need to append any modifiers to ensure complete and accurate information is provided?

Step #7: Double-check your work.

Answer:

Did you determine this to be the correct code?

94660 Continuous positive airway pressure ventilation (CPAP) initiation and management

Excellent!

29.8 Allergy and Clinical Immunology

Codes 95004–95199 cover allergy and clinical immunology procedures. Allergies can be responsible for many different reactions in the human body. Beyond the typical sneezing and watery eyes, outcomes can cause anything from hives and rashes to behavioral problems, sleeplessness, and even death.

Often, when there is concern or suspicion that a patient may be suffering from an allergic reaction, the physician will begin with allergy sensitivity tests. In these cases, small yet potent samples of the suspected allergen are given to the patient in one of a number of methods: percutaneously (scratch, puncture, or prick), intracutaneously (intradermal), inhalation, or ingestion. Then the patient is watched, and the body's reaction to the allergen is documented. The results of the tests tell the physician to which elements the patient is considered allergic.

Once an allergy is identified, immunotherapy may be provided. The therapy is a way of retraining the patient's immune system, or desensitizing it, so that the body no longer views the particles as a threat.

EXAMPLE

Dr. Bagg conducted percutaneous scratch testing with immediate reactions on Shelley to identify the cause of her asthma. He tested her for a dozen common allergens. Report this with **95004 Percutaneous tests × 12** tests.

CODING BITES

The process of desensitizing can take weeks, months, or years, so pay close attention to the dates of service.

LET'S CODE IT! SCENARIO

PATIENT: Marina Louongo

REASON FOR VISIT: Skin testing to environmental allergens.

HISTORY OF PRESENT ILLNESS: The patient was a long-standing patient of Dr. Yeager in Masonville, her previous hometown in the north side of the state, and had received immunotherapy for the past several years. She was referred to us by her new neighbor.

She had been getting injections for grass/ragweed/plantain, cat/dog/mold, dust mite, and trees. She states she has been having some difficulty with local reactions and swelling to the tree injection. She is using Tylenol before and after injections along with ice, which has helped somewhat. She gets injections every 3 weeks. Patient states she had an episode one time where her arms swelled significantly and she required oral prednisone. She typically has allergy symptoms in February, March, November, and December with rhinitis, congestion, and itchy eyes. She was going to get dust covers for her pillow and mattress but hasn't gotten around to it. Her bedroom is carpeted. She denies smoking.

CURRENT MEDICATIONS: Flonase and Clarinex prior to injections.

PHYSICAL EXAMINATION: She is a healthy-appearing, well-nourished, well-developed 27-year-old female in no acute distress.

Skin testing via prick was positive to birch 2+, beech 2+, ash 0/1+, hickory 1+, mite DF 2+, mite DP 2+, histamine 3+, grass 3+, mugwort 1+, oak 4+, and maple 3+.

IMPRESSION: Seasonal and perennial allergic rhinitis.

RECOMMENDATIONS:

1. Continue immunotherapy here with birch/oak/maple, mite DF/DP, grass/mugwort.
2. Continue Flonase two sprays per nostril daily during the spring and fall.
3. Environmental control measures regarding dust and pollen.
4. Report was sent to Dr. Yeager, along with patient's signed Release of Information form so we can get copies of her previous medical records.

Alvin Birchwood, MD

Let's Code It!

Dr. Birchwood did percutaneous skin prick testing on Marina. Turn in the CPT Alphabetic Index and find

Allergy Tests

Skin Tests

Allergen Extract 95004, 95024, 95027

Turn to the *Main Section* of CPT and read carefully the complete code descriptions for all three of these suggestions.

95004 **Percutaneous tests (scratch, puncture, prick) with allergenic extracts, immediate type reaction, including test interpretation and report, specify number of tests**

95024 **Intracutaneous (intradermal) tests with allergenic extracts, immediate type reaction, including test interpretation and report, specify number of tests**

95027 **Intracutaneous (intradermal) tests, sequential and incremental, with allergenic extracts for airborne allergens, immediate type reaction, including test interpretation and report, specify number of tests**

Which of these is supported by Dr. Birchwood's documentation? Did you determine . . .

95004 **Percutaneous tests (scratch, puncture, prick) with allergenic extracts, immediate type reaction, including test interpretation and report, specify number of tests**

Correct! Now, how many tests were performed? The documentation states: "birch, beech, ash, hickory, mite DF, mite DP, histamine, grass, mugwort, oak, maple."

A total of 11 tests were performed, so you can report **95004 × 11** with confidence.

Good work!

29.9 Neurology and Neuromuscular Procedures

As with so many other headings in this section, the neurology and neuromuscular procedure codes (95782–96020) include the recording of the test as well as the physician's interpretation and report of the findings.

GUIDANCE CONNECTION

Read the additional explanations in the in-section guidelines located within the **Medicine** section, subhead **Neurology and Neuromuscular Procedures**, directly following code 95251 in your CPT book.

Acronyms often seen in this arena of health care services include:

EEG	Electroencephalogram
EMG	Electromyogram
EOG	Electrooculogram
MEG	Magnetoencephalography

LET'S CODE IT! SCENARIO

Ian Ellington, a 47-year-old male, was having a hard time staying awake during the day and asleep during the night. Dr. Bruse sent him down the hall to have a polysomnography, with three additional parameters, to rule out sleep apnea.

Let's Code It!

Dr. Bruse ordered a *polysomnography* on Ian to see if he has *sleep apnea*. Let's turn to the Alphabetic Index and find

Polysomnography 95782, 95783, 95808–95811

As you read through the complete code descriptions in the numeric listing, you will see that, because Dr. Bruse ordered *three additional parameters*, the best code is

95808 **Polysomnography; any age, sleep staging with 1–3 additional parameters of sleep, attended by a technologist**

Excellent!

Central Nervous System Assessments

When a patient exhibits problems with cognitive processes, testing may evaluate the extent of the condition so that a treatment plan can be established. It is expected that the results of the tests in the **Central Nervous System** subsection (codes 96105–96146) will be formulated into a report to be used in the creation of a treatment plan.

GUIDANCE CONNECTION

Read the additional explanations in the in-section guidelines located within the **Medicine** section, subhead **Central Nervous System Assessments/Tests** (e.g., **Neuro-Cognitive, Mental Status, Speech Testing**), directly above code 96105 in your CPT book.

YOU CODE IT! CASE STUDY

Oliver Gates, a 3-year-old male, does not appear to be meeting certain milestones. Dr. Saunders performed a developmental test known as an Early Language Milestone Screening and spent 85 minutes assessing his motor skills, social, and language functions. Once the test was interpreted, he sent his report and contacted a speech therapist to consult on a treatment plan.

You Code It!

Go through the steps, and determine the code(s) that should be reported for this screening test performed on Oliver.

Step #1: Read the case carefully and completely.
Step #2: Abstract the scenario. Which key words or terms describe what service the physician provided to the patient during this encounter?
Step #3: Are there any details missing or incomplete for which you would need to query the physician? [If so, ask your instructor.]
Step #4: Determine the correct CPT procedure code or codes to explain the details about what was provided to the patient during this encounter.
Step #5: Check for any relevant guidance, including reading all of the symbols and notations.
Step #6: Do you need to append any modifiers to ensure complete and accurate information is provided?
Step #7: Double-check your work.

Answer:

Did you determine this to be the correct code?

96112 Developmental testing administration (including assessment of fine and/or gross motor, language, cognitive level, social, memory and/or executive functions by standardized developmental instruments when performed) by physician or other qualified health care professional, with interpretation and report, first hour

+96113 each additional 30 minutes

Good work!

29.10 Physical Medicine and Rehabilitation

Physiatrists are health care professionals who specialize in physical medicine and rehabilitation, focusing their skills and knowledge to evaluate and treat traumatic injuries, illnesses, and resulting disabilities affecting components of the nervous system and musculoskeletal systems. The goals of these health care encounters are most often centered around maximizing the patient's physical function and improving quality of life.

Physical therapy focuses on working with patients who have been injured or disabled by an illness, with the goal of helping them restore their mobility. These sessions educate patients with methodologies to manage their physical situations, promote healing, and prevent further deterioration of physical abilities.

Occupational therapy connects patients with activities they can participate in to improve their quality of life, and sometimes independence. The positive outcomes of these therapies include disabled students gaining inclusion in school and social events, as well as working with patients to function despite cognitive or physical changes.

Throughout the **Physical Medicine and Rehabilitation** subsection and its components, note that some groups of codes require the provider to have direct (face-to-face) contact with the patient during the course of the treatment and others do not.

CODING BITES

Codes 97010–97799 are used to report each distinct procedure provided to the patient. Modifier 51 cannot be used with any of these codes.

YOU CODE IT! CASE STUDY

DATE OF PHYSICAL THERAPY EVALUATION: 05/31/2026

DATE OF INJURY: 03/18/2026

HISTORY OF PRESENT ILLNESS: The patient is a 19-year-old male who was the driver in an MVA. He was struck from behind by a tractor trailer, causing his car to fishtail, landing beneath the truck's trailer. He is single and lives with his parents while he finishes college. His injuries have halted his education for now, but he is determined to reenroll at a future date. He depends, right now, on someone to transport him to our facility.

ASSESSMENT AND PLAN: The patient is a 19-year-old male, status post multiple trauma.

For full assessment notes, including exam and clinical presentation of characteristics, see attached notes.

1. Rehabilitation: Toe-touch weightbearing, left lower extremity. Weightbearing as tolerated, left upper extremity. PT, OT, speech language pathology, therapeutic recreation, and psychology to see and treat.
2. Deep venous thrombosis prophylaxis: The patient is on Fragmin. The patient is to have his Dopplers repeated.
3. Gastrointestinal prophylaxis: The patient is not on anything but complains of systemic nausea. We will start Pepcid 20 mg b.i.d.
4. Bowel and bladder: Overflow urinary incontinence. We will place Foley and start Urecholine 12.5 mg p.o. t.i.d.
5. Pain: Not well controlled. Start Oramorph 15 mg with Percocet for breakthrough and schedule before therapies.

DISPOSITION: The patient will likely be discharged to home with any equipment and modifications PRN.

You Code It!

Dr. Gerald Foxglove was called in to perform a predischarge physical therapy evaluation.

Step #1: Read the case carefully and completely.
Step #2: Abstract the scenario. Which key words or terms describe what service the physician provided to the patient during this encounter?
Step #3: Are there any details missing or incomplete for which you would need to query the physician? [If so, ask your instructor.]
Step #4: Determine the correct CPT procedure code or codes to explain the details about what was provided to the patient during this encounter.
Step #5: Check for any relevant guidance, including reading all of the symbols and notations.
Step #6: Do you need to append any modifiers to ensure complete and accurate information is provided?
Step #7: Double-check your work.

Answer:

Did you determine this to be the correct code?

97163 Physical therapy evaluation; high complexity, requiring these components: a history of present problem with 3 or more personal factors and/or comorbidities that impact the plan of care; an examination of body systems using standardized tests and measures addressing a total of 4 or more elements from any of the following: body structures and functions, activity limitations, and/or participation restrictions; a clinical presentation with unstable and unpredictable characteristics; and clinical decision-making of high complexity using standardized patient assessment instrument and/or measurable assessment of functional outcome.

29.11 Acupuncture, Osteopathic, and Chiropractic Treatments

Acupuncture

GUIDANCE CONNECTION

Read the additional explanations in the in-section guidelines located within the **Medicine** section, subhead **Acupuncture**, directly above code 97810 in your CPT book.

The health care industry is always evolving and incorporating new techniques into its accepted methods for helping patients. The techniques of acupuncture (codes 97810–97814) are thousands of years old but are newly accepted by Western medicine and health insurance payers.

Acupuncture services are measured in 15-minute increments of direct provider-patient contact. While the needles may be in place for a longer period of time, you are permitted to report only the time actually spent with the patient.

LET'S CODE IT! SCENARIO

Josie Rossini, a 57-year-old female, was having a problem with menopause. Because of the reported concerns about hormone replacement therapy (HRT), she decided to try acupuncture. After discussing her symptoms and a treatment plan, Dr. Kini inserted several needles. The needles were removed 20 minutes later. Dr. Kini reviewed the follow-up plan and made an appointment for Josie's next visit. Dr. Kini spent 30 minutes in total face-to-face with Josie, who reported marked improvement.

Let's Code It!

Dr. Kini's treatment of Josie included *30 minutes face-to-face time* and *several needles* during the *acupuncture* treatment. Let's turn to the Alphabetic Index and look up *acupuncture*.

Acupuncture

with Electrical Stimulation 97813–97814

without Electrical Stimulation 97810–97811

There is no mention of electrical stimulation being used in Josie's treatment, so turn to the codes recommended for *without electrical stimulation*.

97810 **Acupuncture, 1 or more needles; without electrical stimulation, initial 15 minutes of personal one-on-one contact with the patient**

+97811 **without electrical stimulation, each additional 15 minutes of personal one-on-one contact with the patient, with reinsertion of needles(s) (List separately in addition to code for primary procedure.)**

The first code, 97810, reports Dr. Kini's services, but only for the first 15 minutes. You have to add the second code, 97811, to report the remainder of the time so that the doctor can be reimbursed for the total 30 minutes for the session.

Osteopathic Manipulative Treatments

Codes 98925–98929, to report osteopathic manipulative treatments (OMT), are defined by the number of body regions involved in the encounter. Ten regions are identified with the codes:

- Head
- Cervical
- Thoracic

- Rib cage
- Upper extremities
- Lumbar
- Sacral
- Abdominal/visceral
- Pelvic
- Lower extremities

GUIDANCE CONNECTION

Read the additional explanations in the in-section guidelines located within the **Medicine** section, subhead **Osteopathic Manipulative Treatment**, directly above code 98925 in your CPT book.

Chiropractic Manipulative Treatment

Similar to the osteopathic treatment codes, chiropractic manipulative treatment (CMT) codes 98940–98943 are determined by the number of regions treated during an encounter. The codes use spinal or extraspinal descriptions and are identified as follows:

Spinal Regions

- Cervical, including atlanto-occipital joint.
- Thoracic, including costovertebral and costotransverse joints.
- Lumbar.
- Sacral.
- Pelvic, including the sacroiliac joint.

Extraspinal Regions

- Head, including temporomandibular joint (but not the atlanto-occipital).
- Upper extremities.
- Rib cage, excluding costotransverse and costovertebral joints.
- Abdomen.
- Lower extremities.

GUIDANCE CONNECTION

Read the additional explanations in the in-section guidelines located within the **Medicine** section, subhead **Chiropractic Manipulative Treatment**, directly above code 98940 in your CPT book.

YOU CODE IT! CASE STUDY

Evan LaVelle, a 37-year-old male who is 6 ft. 6 in. tall, has pain in his neck and spine. Dr. Eisenberg, a chiropractor, provides CMT to his cervical, thoracic, lumbar, sacral, and pelvic regions to alleviate Evan's pain.

You Code It!

Go through the steps, and determine the code(s) that should be reported for this CMT encounter.

Step #1: Read the case carefully and completely.

(continued)

Step #2: Abstract the scenario. Which key words or terms describe what service the physician provided to the patient during this encounter?
Step #3: Are there any details missing or incomplete for which you would need to query the physician? [If so, ask your instructor.]
Step #4: Determine the correct CPT procedure code or codes to explain the details about what was provided to the patient during this encounter.
Step #5: Check for any relevant guidance, including reading all of the symbols and notations.
Step #6: Do you need to append any modifiers to ensure complete and accurate information is provided?
Step #7: Double-check your work.

Answer:

Did you determine this to be the correct code?

98942 Chiropractic manipulative treatment (CMT); spinal, five regions

Good job!

29.12 Other Services Provided

Education and Training for Patient Self-Management

Technological and other health care treatment and pharmaceutical advancements have made it easier for the average patient to care for him- or herself or for a caregiver to administer treatments formerly provided exclusively by a physician. Of course, this is not something that should be done without guidance, so it is important that the patient or caregiver is taught how to administer treatment properly. Education and training for patient self-management are reported by using codes 98960–98962.

EXAMPLE

- Teaching a diabetic patient how to self-administer insulin injections.
- Teaching a caregiver how to change a dressing.

Non-Face-to-Face Nonphysician Services

GUIDANCE CONNECTION

Read the additional explanations in the in-section guidelines located within the **Medicine** section, subhead **Non-Face-to-Face Nonphysician Services**, directly above code 98966 in your CPT book.

Nurses and allied health care professionals extend the ability of a physician to communicate with patients. When a qualified nonphysician member of the health care team provides an assessment and management service to an established patient via telephone or online electronic contact, this service is reported with a code from 98966–98969.

Special Services, Procedures, and Reports

There are times when a health care professional is required to provide a service or write a report that is outside the normal realm of his or her responsibilities or outside of the scope of other codes in the CPT book. In those cases, match the circumstance to one of the descriptions in the Special Services, Procedures, and Reports subsection (codes 99000–99091). Each code identifies a different special situation.

GUIDANCE CONNECTION

Read the additional explanations in the in-section guidelines located within the **Medicine** section, subhead **Special Services, Procedures and Reports**, directly above code 99000 in your CPT book.

EXAMPLE

Dr. Schnering comes into the office to meet Jason Carter on Thanksgiving because Jason was bitten by his nephew's pet snake and Dr. Schnering has the only antidote for that species. You would use the following code in addition to the codes needed to report the specific services Dr. Schnering provided:

99050 Services provided in the office at times other than regularly scheduled office hours, or days when the office is normally closed (e.g., holidays, Saturday or Sunday), in addition to basic service

Medication Therapy Management Services

When a patient is prescribed multiple medications, especially when ordered by multiple providers, a pharmacist may step in to assess the list and intervene as necessary. The pharmacist can provide insights into potential drug interactions and duplications caused by secondary ingredients.

Medication Therapy Management Services (MTMS) codes can be reported when the following has been documented:

- Review of the pertinent patient history.
- Review of the medication profile for prescription and nonprescription drugs and herbal supplements.
- Specific recommendations for improving patient health outcomes.
- Recommendations to support the patient's treatment compliance.

The codes available to report these services are

99605 Medication therapy management service(s) provided by a pharmacist, individual, face-to-face with patient, with assessment and intervention, if provided; initial 15 minutes, new patient

99606 Medication therapy management service(s) provided by a pharmacist, individual, face-to-face with patient, with assessment and intervention, if provided; initial 15 minutes, established patient

+99607 each additional 15 minutes (List separately in addition to code for primary service.)

As stated in the CPT guidelines, these codes should not be used to report the provision of product-specific information at the time the product is provided to the patient or any other routine dispensing-related activities.

Home Health Procedures/Services

In the chapter ***CPT Evaluation and Management Coding***, you learned about codes 99341–99350 for services provided by a physician at the patient's home. However, occasionally a health care professional in your facility *other than the physician* provides services to a patient at his or her home. The person may be a nurse or therapist, for example. For nonphysician clinical professionals, you must use the codes 99500–99602 from the **Home Health Procedures/Services** subsection in the ***Medicine*** section.

EXAMPLE

Shawn Webber, RN, stopped by Beatrice Mulligan's home to give her an injection of morphine sulfate, 10 mg, IM, for pain management. Report Nurse Webber's visit with **99506 Home visit for intramuscular injections**.

GUIDANCE CONNECTION

Read the additional explanations in the in-section guidelines located within the **Medicine** section, subhead **Home Health Procedures/Services**, directly above code 99500 in your CPT book.

YOU CODE IT! CASE STUDY

Eliot Sharpton is a Certified Diabetes Educator (CDE) and is meeting today with Robyn Wu. She was just diagnosed with type 2 diabetes mellitus. Eliot spends 30 minutes with her, using the standardized curriculum, to help Robyn adjust her diet, get some exercise in her routine, and answer questions about her medication.

You Code It!

Determine the correct code or codes to report Eliot Sharpton, CDE's training of Robyn Wu.

Step #1: Read the case carefully and completely.
Step #2: Abstract the scenario. Which key words or terms describe what service the physician provided to the patient during this encounter?
Step #3: Are there any details missing or incomplete for which you would need to query the physician? [If so, ask your instructor.]
Step #4: Determine the correct CPT procedure code or codes to explain the details about what was provided to the patient during this encounter.
Step #5: Check for any relevant guidance, including reading all of the symbols and notations.
Step #6: Do you need to append any modifiers to ensure complete and accurate information is provided?
Step #7: Double-check your work.

Answer:

Did you determine this to be the code?

98960 **Education and training for patient self-management by a qualified, nonphysician health care professional using a standardized curriculum, face-to-face with the patient (could include caregiver/family) each 30 minutes; individual patient**

Fantastic!

Chapter Summary

Many services provided by physicians, therapists, chiropractors, and other trained health care professionals deserve to receive reimbursement. The *Medicine* section contains information about these services. The variety of services included in the *Medicine* section emphasizes the fact that finding the correct code begins in the Alphabetic Index and culminates in the numeric listings.

CODING BITES

As you have read in this chapter, the ***Medicine*** section of the CPT book has codes for services that are supplied by health care professionals but not represented in any other sections. Services reported using codes from the ***Medicine*** section include these:

- Flu shots
- Vaccinations for the kids to go back to school
- Allergy shots
- Chiropractic services
- Psychotherapy
- Dialysis
- Hearing evaluations
- Vision checks
- Chemotherapy
- Acupuncture

Wherever you work as a coding specialist, there is an excellent chance you will be using this section.

CHAPTER 29 REVIEW
CPT Medicine Section

Let's Check It! Terminology

Match each key term to the appropriate definition.

1. **LO 29.2** The introduction of a fluid into a blood vessel.
2. **LO 29.6** The destruction or eradication of tissue.
3. **LO 29.2** The delivery of an additional drug via an intravenous line over a short period of time.
4. **LO 29.6** A thin, flexible tube, inserted into a body part, used to inject fluid, to extract fluid, or to keep a passage open.
5. **LO 29.5** A professional qualified to carry out eye examinations and to prescribe and supply eyeglasses and contact lenses.
6. **LO 29.2** Compelling a fluid into tissue or cavity.
7. **LO 29.5** A physician qualified to diagnose and treat eye disease and conditions with drugs, surgery, and corrective measures.
8. **LO 29.6** An ultrasonic scanning procedure to determine blood flow and pattern.
9. **LO 29.5** The study of the human ears, nose, and throat (ENT) systems.
10. **LO 29.1** To make someone resistant to a particular disease by vaccination.

A. Ablation
B. Catheter
C. Duplex scan
D. Immunization
E. Infusion
F. Injection
G. Ophthalmologist
H. Optometrist
I. Otorhinolaryngology
J. Push

Let's Check It! Concepts

Choose the most appropriate answer for each of the following questions.

1. **LO 29.1** When an immunization is given, you will need
   a. one code for administering the immunization.
   b. two codes: one for the administration and one for the drug.
   c. one code for the medication or drug.
   d. one HCPCS Level II code.
2. **LO 29.2** When a patient receives infusion therapy via more than one IV site, code
   a. only the first site. **b.** all appropriate services for each site.
   c. infusion time instead of number of sites. **d.** only when chemotherapy is infused.
3. **LO 29.3** Which of the following codes identifies an encounter for psychotherapy, 60 minutes with patient?
   a. 90832 **b.** 90834 **c.** 90836 **d.** 90837
4. **LO 29.4** Dialysis codes are reported by
   a. the patient's age. **b.** the number of days treated.
   c. the location of treatment (inpatient or outpatient). **d.** all of these.
5. **LO 29.5** An optometrist is qualified to
   a. diagnose and treat serious eye diseases.
   b. supply glasses and contact lenses.
   c. write prescriptions for the treatment of serious eye diseases.
   d. perform surgery.
6. **LO 29.6** What code would you assign for a duplex scan of the left radial artery?
   a. 93925 **b.** 93926 **c.** 93930 **d.** 93931

7. **LO 29.12** Medication Therapy Management Services (MTMS) codes can be reported when all of the following have been documented *except*
   a. review of the pertinent patient examination.
   b. review of medication profile for prescription and nonprescription drugs and herbal supplements.
   c. specific recommendations for improving patient health outcomes.
   d. recommendations to support the patient's treatment compliance.
8. **LO 29.11** Chiropractic treatment codes are chosen by
   a. the time spent face-to-face with the patient.
   b. the total number of treatments in a month.
   c. the number of regions treated.
   d. the age of the patient.
9. **LO 29.9** Kinney Harris, a 41-year-old male, was in an automobile accident and was transported to the nearest hospital, unconscious. The ED physician, Dr. Alexander, attempted to awaken Kinney with stimulants without success. Dr. Alexander performs an EEG due to Kinney's comatose condition. What is the correct code for the EEG?
   a. 95812
   b. 95816
   c. 95822
   d. 95824
10. **LO 29.10** Betty Cannon receives an acupuncture treatment, two needles, for a total of 45 minutes of face-to-face time with Dr. Hamilton. What is/are the correct code(s) for this procedure?
   a. 97810
   b. 97810, 97811
   c. 97813, 97814
   d. 97810, 97811, 97811

Let's Check It! Guidelines

Refer to the Medicine Guidelines and fill in the blanks accordingly.

99070	not	Medicine	assessment
add-on	identified	itself	16 minutes
"Special Report"	"separate procedure"	independent	
independently	59	integral	
99600	Introduction	supply	
nomenclature	"Unlisted Procedure"	exempt	

1. In addition to the definitions and commonly used terms present in the ___, several other items unique to this section on ___ are defined or identified here.
2. All ___ codes found in the CPT codebook are ___ from the multiple procedure concept.
3. Add-on codes in the CPT codebook can be readily ___ by specific descriptor ___ which includes phrases such as "each additional" or "(List separately in addition to primary procedure.)"
4. The codes designated as ___ should not be reported in addition to the code for the total procedure or service of which it is considered an ___ component.
5. However, when a procedure or service that is designated as a "separate procedure" is carried out ___ or considered to be unrelated or distinct from other procedures/services provided at the time, it may be reported by ___, or in addition to other procedures/services by appending modifier ___ to the specific "separate procedure" code to indicate that the procedure is not considered to be a component of another procedure, but is a distinct, ___ procedure.
6. Supplies and materials over and above those usually included with the procedure(s) rendered are reported separately using code ___ or a specific ___ code.
7. A service or procedure may be provided that is ___ listed in this edition of the CPT code book. When reporting such a service, the appropriate ___ code may be used to indicate the service, identifying it by ___.
8. Unlisted home visit service or procedure is reported with code ___.
9. The psychotherapy services codes 90832–90838 include ongoing ___ and adjustment of psychotherapeutic interventions, and may include involvement of informants in the treatment process.
10. Do not report psychotherapy of less than ___ duration.

Let's Check It! Rules and Regulations

Please answer the following questions from the knowledge you have gained after reading this chapter.

1. **LO 29.1** List five ways medication can be administered to a patient.
2. **LO 29.2** Explain the *standard parts* included in infusion and injection codes.
3. **LO 29.3** What are the categories of psychotherapy?
4. **LO 29.4** What physician services are included in the codes during a dialysis month?
5. **LO 29.6** What do the available codes for reporting a cardiac catheterization include?

YOU CODE IT! Basics

First, identify the procedural main term(s) in the following statements; then code the procedure or service.

Example: Alan Capshaw, PA, completes a home visit for mechanical ventilation care.

a. main term: *Ventilation Assist* **b.** procedure: *99504*

1. Dr. Jameson performs a psychotherapy session with the patient, 45 minutes:

   a. main term:______ **b.** procedure:______

2. Dr. Graban completes a therapeutic repetitive transcranial magnetic stimulation (TMS), initial treatment:

   a. main term: ______ **b.** procedure:______

3. Dr. Kantsiper performs biofeedback training, anorectal:

   a. main term:______ **b.** procedure:______

4. Dr. Abernethy completes a diagnostic transcutaneous electrogastrography:

   a. main term: ______ **b.** procedure:______

5. Dr. Shutter fits a contact lens for management of keratoconus, initial fitting:

   a. main term:______ **b.** procedure:______

6. Dr. Sanning completes a positional nystagmus test:

   a. main term: ______ **b.** procedure:______

7. Dr. Foldings performs a tympanometry and reflex threshold measurements:

   a. main term:______ **b.** procedure:______

8. Dr. Edge completes a right heart catheterization including measurement of oxygen saturation and cardiac output:

   a. main term: ______ **b.** procedure:______

9. Dr. Pugh performs a duplex scan of lower extremity arteries; complete bilateral study:

   a. main term: ______ **b.** procedure:______

10. Dr. McKee completes nitric oxide expired gas determination:

    a. main term: ______ **b.** procedure:______

11. Dr. Middleton performs an unattended sleep study with simultaneous recording of heart rate, oxygen saturation, respiratory analysis, and sleep time:

    a. main term:______ **b.** procedure:______

12. Dr. Trezevant completes a manual muscle testing with report of extremity:

    a. main term: ______ **b.** procedure:______

13. Dr. Reese performs a chemotherapy administration, intra-arterial; infusion technique, 45 minutes:

    a. main term:______ **b.** procedure:______

14. Dr. Kemper performs an anogenital (perineum) examination, magnified in childhood for suspected trauma:

    a. main term: ______ **b.** procedure:______

15. Pam Guinyard, a home health RN, completes a home visit for prenatal monitoring and assessment including fetal heart rate and nonstress test:

    a. main term:______ **b.** procedure:______

YOU CODE IT! Practice

Using the techniques described in this chapter, carefully read through the case studies and determine the most accurate Medicine section CPT code(s) and modifier(s), if appropriate, for each case study.

1. Marlene Overton, a 59-year-old female, has been suffering from bronchitis off and on for 2 years. Dr. Turner has ordered a cardiopulmonary exercise test for her. Dr. Turner notes that he wants her CO_2 and O_2 uptake measured during the test as well as an electrocardiogram to be recorded.
2. Grant Hughes, a 74-year-old male, has uncontrolled diabetes and comes into the emergency department complaining of signs of hyperglycemia. Dr. Hawkins gives him insulin subcutaneous and IV push to bring his blood sugar down. Code injection administration only.
3. After finding relief nowhere else, Rasheem Conner, a 42-year-old female, goes to Dr. Johnston, an acupuncturist, for treatment of her osteoarthritic knee. Dr. Johnston spends 15 minutes with the patient reviewing history and symptoms, palpating, and locating the points to treat, and inserts the needles and applies electrical stimulation. Rasheem is asked to rest. Dr. Johnston comes back in about 10 minutes later and spends 5 minutes monitoring the patient and restimulating the needles. Ten minutes later, Dr. Johnston sees that the pain and swelling in Rasheem's knee have reduced, removes the needles, and instructs Rasheem on home care measures. Dr. Johnston spent a total of 30 minutes in direct contact with Rasheem.
4. Darlene Overton, an 8-year-old female, is brought to Dr. Mackinaw by her mother after a referral from the school counselor and her pediatrician. Darlene is having difficulties with classwork. Mrs. Overton also tells Dr. Mackinaw that Darlene has a problem understanding speech in noisy environments. Darlene may have a hearing deficiency that has not shown up in hearing tests before, and it may account for her declining work in class. Dr. Mackinaw performs a central auditory function evaluation, which takes 1 hour, with report.
5. Kent Egerton, a 13-year-old male, suffered from a severe asthma attack while at the playground. He was rushed to the clinic, where he was given a nebulizer treatment (nonpressurized inhalation).
6. Kenya Cantrell, a 41-year-old female, broke out in a rash, which would not go away. After trying multiple over-the-counter treatments, she went to Dr. Beech, who did a series of 11 allergenic extract scratch tests to see if he could identify an allergen. The tests pointed to an allergy to her new kitten.
7. Kenya (previous scenario) didn't want to give away her new kitten, so Dr. Beech prepared the allergenic extract and began immunotherapy injections. She received the first injection today.
8. Paul Kensington, a 51-year-old male, is beginning chemotherapy today with the administration of methotrexate, via IV push. Code administration only.
9. Darren Pinchot, a 24-year-old male, is a lifeguard at the beach and came into the emergency clinic with uncontrolled nausea and vomiting. Darren told Dr. Valentine that he was on the beach for 12 hours straight with no breaks because his replacement didn't show up. Dr. Valentine diagnosed him with severe dehydration and ordered 20 minutes of Zofran, IV infusion, and then saline for 4 hours.
10. Robin Gerstein, a 32-year-old female, comes to Duane Nettles, a licensed massage therapist, as prescribed by Dr. Luellen. Robin is pregnant and has been suffering from acute lower back pain for over a month. Duane performs therapeutic massage with effleurage on the left side and kneading on the iliac band, nerve stroking, and light compression on the gluteus for a total of 15 minutes.
11. Robert Kini, a 9-day-old male, was born prematurely, and Dr. Martin is concerned about Robert's heart. He performs a left heart catheterization including intraprocedural injection for left ventriculography by transseptal puncture through intact septum. Dr. Martin provides conscious sedation, 15 minutes, while the nurse monitors Robert's status during the procedure.
12. Felicia Gardener, a 6-year-old female, comes to see Dr. Kaplan for an evaluation of her cochlear implant. Dr. Kaplan reprograms the implant to improve Felicia's reception.
13. Alice Heath, a 73-year-old female, came to see Dr. Browne, her ophthalmologist, for an annual checkup of her eyes. Dr. Browne does a comprehensive evaluation of Alice's complete visual system.
14. Jalal Kalisz, a 68-year-old male, came to see Dr. McDaniel because he was having chest pain. Dr. McDaniel performed a routine ECG with 15 leads. After talking with Jalal and reviewing the ECG results, Dr. McDaniel determined that Jalal was having a bout of indigestion.

(continued)

15. Cecil Rossini, an 18-year-old female, is a professional gymnast who pulled a muscle in her shoulder. Today, Dr. Salton measured her range of motion in the shoulder to confirm that the area has healed completely. Dr. Salton then wrote and signed the report.

YOU CODE IT! Application

The following exercises provide practice in the application of abstracting the physicians' notes and learning to work with documentation from our health care facilities. These case studies are modeled on real patient encounters. Using the techniques described in this chapter, carefully read through the case studies and determine the most accurate Medicine section CPT code(s) and modifier(s), if appropriate, for each case study.

WESTON HOSPITAL

629 Healthcare Way • SOMEWHERE, FL 32811 • 407-555-6541

PATIENT: HAUPTON, NICHOLAS

ACCOUNT/EHR #: HAUPNI001

Attending Physician: Jessica P. Turner, MD

PATIENT SERVICES:

IV fluid replacement for dehydration, intravenous, 58 minutes

Continuous pulse oximetry

Therapeutic warm water enema for intussusception

Robin P. Moss, RN

Determine the most accurate Medicine section CPT code(s) and modifier(s), if appropriate.

SPELLING CHIROPRACTIC CENTER

A Complete Health Care Facility

159 Healthcare Way • SOMEWHERE, FL 32811 • 407-555-6789

PATIENT: CARMICHAEL, ABIGAIL

ACCOUNT/EHR #: CARMAB001

Attending Physician: Philip M. Osburn, DC

Diagnosis: Lumbar stenosis, sciatica

Procedure: CMT; traction, manual

PROCEDURE: The patient was placed on the table.

Chiropractic manipulative treatment: spinal, thoracic

Chiropractic manipulative treatment: lower extremity, left

Manual traction: cervical & lumbar regions × 30 minutes

Determine the most accurate Medicine section CPT code(s) and modifier(s), if appropriate.

(continued)

NORTHSIDE PHYSICAL THERAPY CENTER

955 East Main Ave. • SOMEWHERE, FL 32811 • 407-555-1191

PATIENT: TRAULER, CASIE

ACCOUNT/EHR #: TRAUCA001

Attending Physician: Laverne Aspiras, MD

Physical Therapist: Harvey Shaw

DX: Postsurgical carpal tunnel (CT) release LT

TYPE OF THERAPY: Occupational therapy (hand) BIW × 3 weeks

VISIT # 1/6:

Reported Pain Level: 6/10

Patient reports: "I am still having pain in my hand and fingers."

1. Ultrasound for 10 minutes, 3 mgHz, 0.4 u/cm2 100% to scar at LT CT area
2. Massage: Retrograde, 4 minutes to LT hand
3. Manual therapy: Soft tissue mobilization, 7 minutes to scar at LT wrist
4. AROM and stretching, 4 minutes
5. Therapeutic exercise: 12 minutes, tendon glides, joint blocking, digit extension, median nerve glides, and desensitization with cold towels (tolerated up until #5)

Pain level: 4–5/10. Pt still with heavy scar tissue adhesions in CT area. Pt still having pain in fingertips and numbness, reportedly up arm and into his neck.

Harvey Shaw

Determine the most accurate Medicine section CPT code(s) and modifier(s), if appropriate.

PRADER, BRACKER, & ASSOCIATES

A Complete Health Care Facility

159 Healthcare Way • SOMEWHERE, FL 32811 • 407-555-6789

PATIENT: PASTNERNAC, ELSA

ACCOUNT/EHR #: PASTEL001

Attending Physician: Walter P. Henricks, MD

Referring Physician: Renee O. Bracker, MD

Pt is a 69-year-old female who recently had a stroke. She is here on referral from Dr. Bracker for an assessment of her aphasia.

Assessment of expressive and receptive speech and language function; language comprehension, speech production ability, reading, spelling, writing, using Boston Diagnostic Aphasia Examination.

Interpretation and report to follow.

Total time: 60 minutes

Walter P. Henricks, DC

Determine the most accurate Medicine section CPT code(s) and modifier(s), if appropriate.

(continued)

RAILS RADIOLOGY

A Complete Health Care Facility

159 Healthcare Way • SOMEWHERE, FL 32811 • 407-555-6789

PATIENT: CRESSENA, FRANCIE

ACCOUNT/EHR #: CRESFR001

Attending Physician: James I. Cipher, MD

Radiologist: Rhonda E. Beardall, MD

Reason for Exam: MD order—pre-op clearance

EXAMINATION:

1. Chest two views

Chest—AP and lateral views.

Clinical history states evaluation: kidney stone with obstruction.

Slightly elongated thoracic aorta. Prominent left ventricle. No pulmonary vascular congestion. No acute inflammatory infiltrates in the lungs.

2. ECG, 12 leads

Unremarkable.

Rhonda E. Beardall, MD

Determine the most accurate Medicine section CPT code(s) and modifier(s), if appropriate.

30

Physicians' Services Capstone

Learning Outcomes

After completing this chapter, the student should be able to:

LO 30.1 Determine the correct procedure codes, using the CPT code set, for these case studies.

Patients come to a physician for help to feel better, or to maintain good health. You have learned that CPT codes are one of three code sets used to report WHAT the physician did for the patient during a specific encounter. Now, this chapter provides you with case studies so you can get some hands-on practice using CPT to report physician services.

For each of the following case studies, read through the documentation, and determine:

- Which code or codes report WHAT the physician did for this patient.
- If any modifiers are necessary, and if so, which modifiers, and in what order.
- If more than one code is required, the sequence in which to report the codes.

Remember, the notations, symbols, and Official Guidelines—both before each section as well as those in some subsections—are there to help you get it correct.

CASE STUDY #1: PAUL HENDRICKS

Marlena Hendricks brought her 13-year-old son, Paul, into my office as a walk-in. Paul stated that he fell through a sliding glass door, while chasing his brother, and sustained three lacerations: left knee, right knee, and left hand.

After physical examination, Dr. Smyth determined that the wounds of both knees and left hand required debridement and suture repair using 1% lidocaine for topical anesthetic.

Left knee: 5.5 cm laceration involving deep subcutaneous tissue and fascia, repaired with layered closure. Some debridement was performed.

Right knee: 7.2 cm laceration repaired with a single-layer closure.

Left hand: 2.5 cm laceration of the dermis, repaired with simple closure.

Plan: Instructions for keeping bandages and area clean, and change of bandages provided to Mrs. Hendricks. Follow-up in 10 days for suture removal. Call office PRN any problems or complications.

CASE STUDY #2: MARIA CURRY

Maria Curry, a 39-year-old female, status post right knee arthroplasty, was referred to our rehabilitation clinic for a physical therapy evaluation by Dr. Hanson, her orthopedic surgeon. Patient was diagnosed with degenerative osteoarthritis approximately 2 years ago. As part of my evaluation, I completed a range of motion measurement on both legs. The physician was provided with a copy of my evaluation and a written report was developed.

CASE STUDY #3: SABRINA BARBARA

Sabrina Barbara, a 23-year-old gravida 1 para 1 by cesarean delivery, presented to the emergency department in active labor. She is at 38 weeks gestation and was visiting her parents here in town. She lives 250 miles away in another state. Patient delivered vaginally in the elevator on the way up to obstetrics. The emergency services physician, Dr. Zebbria, delivered the baby. The patient will follow up with her obstetrician for postpartum care.

CASE STUDY #4: ROGER FORCHETTA

Roger Forchetta, a 33-year-old male, came in to our ophthalmology office today. I last saw him 6 years ago when he had a corneal ulcer on his right eye. This is now cleared. He states that over the last few weeks, his vision is "a bit off."

I began with a complete, interval history. He denied any specific trauma or problems with his eyes prior to this latest concern. Overall, this patient is a healthy male with an admitted diet filled with a great deal of fast food and restaurant food.

His external ocular and adnexal areas were unremarkable, free from injury or infection. The patient has a normal corneal anterior chamber and iris but with very slow dilating pupils. Ophthalmoscopy shows there is no pseudoexfoliation, but there are dense juvenile nuclear cataracts on both eyes, the right greater than the left.

I counseled him regarding cataract surgery of this right eye first, and then the left eye; the need for postop correction; a 4- to 6-week recovery time; and the type of procedure. He agreed to schedule the procedure for next Friday. Kathy, my assistant, obtained the appropriate consent form signatures.

CASE STUDY #5: CAMILLE FIELDS

Camille Fields, a 67-year-old female, came into our Allergy & Immunology Clinic with urticarial rash over a large portion of her body.

Patient has a history of hysterectomy at age 35. She has current diagnoses of generalized osteoporosis, severe bone pain, and risk of bone fractures. After failure of prior treatments for osteoporosis (bisphosphonates, alendronate, and risedronic acid) and experiencing major side effects—gastrointestinal erosion with bisphosphonates and alendronate, and severe gastrointestinal bleeding, severe muscle and joint pain, fever, flu symptoms, conjunctivitis, episcleritis, and uveitis with risedronic acid—she was referred to Dr. Lantana for alternate therapies of her condition. All symptoms were intense and persistent. Dr. Lantana prescribed denosumab. He administered Prolia, 60 mg subq into abdomen and told her to come back in 6 months.

On the day after the first administration of denosumab, the patient developed a generalized urticarial rash (thighs, abdomen, bilateral breast area, back) accompanied by bilateral facial angioedema and pruriginous injuries in the area of drug administration (the abdomen). The symptoms started 2 hours after the first administration and resolved completely after 15 days with the administration of antihistamines and oral corticoids and the application of local corticoids.

She came here, to our office, to determine if the denosumab was the instigator of the allergic reaction, or if other sources were to blame. She agreed to a skin prick test (SPT) with denosumab, along with house dust mites, cat and dog dander, olive, grass pollen, and latex, which we performed today.

A positive reaction was defined as a wheal with a diameter at least 3 mm larger than that obtained by a negative control, shown at the test spot of denosumab.

We discussed a rapid desensitization protocol and she agreed. We began with an initial subcutaneous dose of 0.005 mg, which will gradually be increased in an 8-hour cycle until a cumulative dose of 60 mg.

CASE STUDY #6: BELINDA PETTAWAY

Oscar Pettaway brought his unconscious 3-year-old daughter, Belinda, into the emergency department after finding her on the floor of the bathroom. An empty bottle of his wife's thyroid medication, Synthroid, was lying by her side. Oscar told the physician on call, Dr. Rubinstein, that his wife had just refilled the prescription.

Dr. Rubinstein immediately evaluated Belinda's condition and, after obtaining permission from Oscar, ordered a gastric aspiration and lavage be done immediately, due to the poisoning.

CASE STUDY #7: JOSEPH GREESON

PATIENT: Joseph Greeson

S: The last time I saw this 29-year-old male was 6 months ago for his annual checkup. He came in today stating that he has been feeling feverish × 3 days and noticed increased redness on his arm last night and this morning. He denies joint pain. He explained that yesterday he was playing with his girlfriend's new dog and it bit him on the right forearm. The dog is a stray and has had no shots, and the patient states that he believes he accidentally provoked the dog by getting too rough with it.

O: Temp 99.2 degrees, pulse 68, resp 20, weight 142. Right arm reveals four puncture wounds with secondary cellulitis around the area. The area is warm to the touch and is erythematous.

A: Infected dog bite.

P: Patient is given 1 gram of Rocephin IM today. Follow up in 24 hours. A bandage was applied. He was given a rabies immune globulin (RIG), human, IM. Tylenol is recommended PRN for pain. The patient is given a prescription for Erythromycin 333 mg t.i.d. for 10 days.

CASE STUDY #8: MONIQUE KENNARD

Monique Kennard, a 17-year-old female, came into our office today. She is accompanied by her mother, who is very worried about her daughter. Patient states she has been experiencing wheezing × 10 days. She states the symptoms are worse at night. She was seen a week ago at this clinic and started on a 5-day course of azithromycin without improvement. Yesterday she was seen at an urgent care clinic and prescribed an albuterol inhaler, amoxicillin/clavulanic acid, and methylprednisolone. Symptoms continued to worsen throughout the day. Patient reports chest pain attempting to swallow the amoxicillin/clavulanic acid tablets. Chest pain involves her left upper chest; it does not radiate. The quality is "heavy."

VS: 97.9°F, HR 85, RR 25, BP 144/101, SaO_2 97%

HEAD/NECK: She is awake and alert, NAD (no apparent distress), HEENT (head, eyes, ears, nose, throat), NC/AT (normocephalic and atraumatic), EOMI (extraocular movements intact). Left EAC (external auditory canal) is swollen shut; right is occluded with cerumen. Oropharynx is pink and moist.

HEART: RRR (regular rate and rhythm)

LUNGS: No wheezing, but patient is stridorous

ABDOMEN: Benign/unremarkable

EXTREMITIES: Normal pulses × 4, CN II–XII grossly intact

INTEGUMENTARY: Dermatologic exam reveals no rash

ALLERGIES: NKDA (no known drug allergies)

PMHx (Past Medical History): Unremarkable

SocHx (Social History): Patient denies EtOH (ethanol, alcohol). Denies smoking but states positive for secondhand tobacco exposure.

PLAN: Orders written for CXR (chest x-ray) to be done at imaging center across the road. Nurse to perform venipuncture for specimens for comprehensive metabolic panel; CBC complete, automated; and automated differential WBC count.

Patient to return once results are in.

CASE STUDY #9: HARRISON PARKER

Harrison Parker, a 69-year-old right-handed male, was referred to me for a neurologic evaluation by his internist, Dr. Brady, for a tremor that has been present for approximately 20 years.

Patient states that the tremor began insidiously and has progressed gradually. It now involves both hands and affects his handwriting, drinking coffee and other liquids with a cup, and general work that requires manual dexterity. Other people occasionally notice a tremor in his head.

(continued)

He is otherwise healthy, although he feels his balance is not quite as good as it used to be. A glass of beer or wine markedly decreases the tremor severity. His mother and daughter also have tremor. Patient denies smoking.

On examination, he has a rather regular tremor of approximately 8 cycles per second (Hz) with his hands extended and also on finger-nose-finger maneuver. Mild regular "waviness" is seen when writing or drawing spirals. His tone is normal, although when performing voluntary movements with one hand there is a "ratchety" quality felt in the tone of the contralateral arm. Occasional tremor is also noted in the head and voice.

Diagnosis: Probable essential tremor (ET)

Next diagnostic step: MRI of brain and cervical spine + Labs (CBC + TSH) done in our facility today.

Nurse Montana drew blood specimens.

Next step in therapy: Primidone or propranolol

CASE STUDY #10: TORI BENSIO

PATIENT: Tori Bensio

Preop Diagnosis: Acute cholecystitis, cholelithiasis

Postop Diagnosis: Acute cholecystitis, cholelithiasis

Procedure: Laparoscopic cholecystectomy

Surgeon: Anthony DeTaglia, MD

Assistant: Robyn Acculo, MD

Anesthesiologist: Benjamin Sullivan, MD

Anesthesia: General endotracheal

Findings at Surgery: Pericholecystic adhesions, large gallstones

DESCRIPTION OF OPERATION: This otherwise healthy patient was brought to the OR and after the induction of general endotracheal anesthesia, the patient's abdomen was prepped and draped in the usual sterile manner and a small infraumbilical incision was made in the skin and carried down to the linea alba, which was grasped with a clamp and incised in a vertical manner. The peritoneum was entered under direct vision. Stay sutures were placed in the fascia. The Hasson introducer was placed. Pneumoperitoneum was established, and following this, three additional trocars were placed in the abdomen: one in the left epigastrium and two in the right upper quadrant, all 5 mm. Following this, the gallbladder was grasped with cephalad retraction of the gallbladder fundus and lateralward retraction of the gallbladder infundibulum. The dissector was employed to take down the peritoneum overlying the gallbladder infundibulum and cystic duct junction. When this was well delineated on both the anterior and posterior surfaces of the cystic duct, the 5-mm endoscopic clip applier was inserted and two clips were placed on the patient's side, on the gallbladder side of the cystic duct, which was transected. Further dissection in the triangle of Calot revealed the cystic artery, which was handled in an identical manner. The remainder of the dissection was performed by using the Bovie spatula cautery, and the liver bed was dry. A 10- to 15-mm camera change-out was performed, and the camera was inserted into the left epigastric port. A toothed clamp was passed through the umbilicus to grasp the gallbladder, which was then removed through the umbilicus in a standard manner. Following this, the operative field was copiously irrigated with saline and the return was clear. All three upper abdominal ports were seen to exit the abdomen under direct vision, and with the Hasson introducer removed, the fascial incision was closed with a 2-0 Vicryl figure-of-eight suture. The skin at the umbilicus was closed with a 4-0 Maxon subcuticular suture. Steri-strips were applied at all sites. The patient tolerated the procedure well.

ADDENDUM: There were three cystic artery branches; each was doubly clipped and transected.

Code for both Dr. DeTaglia and Dr. Sullivan.

CASE STUDY #11: ENID REYNOLDS

EMERGENCY DEPARTMENT

HISTORY OF PRESENT ILLNESS: The patient came in today for possible reaction to immunotherapy. She has been seeing Dr. Oligby for allergic rhinitis and asthma. She states that she is currently building on immunotherapy and yesterday received injections with oak/birch/maple 100 PNU 0.3 mL, grass and ragweed 100 BAU 0.3 mL, cat/dog 50 BAU 0.3 mL,

(continued)

and mite and mold mix 100 units 0.3 mL. The patient tells me after the immunotherapy, she went home and within hours felt some chest tightness. The patient used her albuterol inhaler, but the chest tightness got worse and she ended up taking her Symbicort 160/4.5 two puffs as well as some Claritin. She continued to feel lethargic and out of breath. She also had an itchy area on her left arm where she received the cat/dog injection. She was able to go to sleep that night but woke twice due to wheezing and used her albuterol inhaler and went back to sleep. When she woke up this morning, she was very tired and dizzy and could not catch her breath. She used her albuterol inhaler once or twice this morning as well as the Symbicort and took a tablet of Zyrtec. Then, around 9 or 9:30, when she was at work, she felt her tongue swelling. During this time, she felt she couldn't breathe normally. The albuterol inhaler did not have any benefit; neither did the other medications she tried. She tells me she had no rash, hives, or vomiting and is not coughing. She tells me she has not been sick this week. No fever. She has been off of her Symbicort since November because she felt her asthma is fine. She has had no recent trouble with asthma. No recent exposure to animals, dust, or other allergens. She is on no new medications. She has no pets at home and continues to avoid turkey and chicken and has no new foods during this time. She has a history of anxiety and panic attacks and does feel she is having one now.

MEDICATIONS: Topamax for migraine headaches, Lexapro

ALLERGIES: NKDA

PHYSICAL EXAMINATION:

GENERAL: The patient is a healthy-appearing, well-nourished, well-developed 45-year-old female in no acute distress but does appear to be breathing heavy and very shaky and panicky.

VITAL SIGNS: Height is 63 inches. Weight is 132 pounds. Blood pressure is 106/70.

HEENT: Tympanic membranes are normal. Throat is clear. I did not appreciate any swelling of the tongue or angioedema.

NECK: Supple without adenopathy

LUNGS: Completely clear

HEART: Regular rate and rhythm without murmur

STUDIES: I administered spirometry when she was a little bit more relaxed and achieved an FEV1 of 3.1 liters or 88% of predicted, FEF25–75 is 118% of predicted. Graphic record was placed in patient's chart.

IMPRESSION:

1. The patient appears to be having some anxiety and panic now. It is hard to say whether this started with some mild asthma symptoms as a result of her immunotherapy or if this is purely an anxiety issue.
2. Allergic asthma
3. Allergic rhinitis

RECOMMENDATIONS:

1. We recommend a cutback of the dose of immunotherapy at the next visit to oak/birch/maple 100 PNU at 0.2 mL, grass and ragweed 100 BAU at 0.2 mL, cat/dog 50 BAU at 0.2 mL, and mite and mold mix 100 units at 0.2 mL
2. Restart Symbicort 160/4.5 two puffs twice daily
3. Zyrtec 10 mg daily for the next week and prior to immunotherapy
4. Albuterol two puffs every 4 hours as needed
5. The patient should follow up if symptoms do not clear in the next day or two
6. Report to be sent to Dr. Oligby
7. Patient discharged at 16:55

CASE STUDY #12: ARNOLD TITLEMAN

OPERATION: Colonoscopy to the cecum

DESCRIPTION OF PROCEDURE: The patient was taken to the outpatient endoscopy suite where he was monitored for pulse oximetry and blood pressure monitoring. He was turned to the left side and given 50 mg of Demerol with 2 mg of Versed, IV, titrated during the procedure; the nurse monitored Arnold's vital signs for a total of 28 minutes.

An Olympus video colonoscope was inserted in the patient's anus and directed up to the rectum, sigmoid colon, descending colon, around the splenic flexure, through the transverse colon, around the hepatic flexure, ascending colon, and cecum. The ileocecal area was inspected and appeared grossly normal.

Terminal ileum was cannulated, appeared grossly normal. The scope was then slowly withdrawn back through the entire colon, rectum, and anus and no gross abnormality or lesion was identified. Mucosa pattern appeared normal. The patient tolerated the procedure well. He will be discharged home with instructions to follow up for a surveillance colonoscopy.

CASE STUDY #13: DARLIN EVERSTANG

OPERATIONS:

1. Flexible bronchoscopy
2. Cervical mediastinoscopy with biopsy and thyroid isthmusectomy

PROCEDURE: This otherwise normally healthy patient was brought to the operative suite and placed in supine position. After satisfactory induction of general endotracheal anesthesia, a flexible Olympus bronchoscope was passed through the endotracheal tube visualizing the distal trachea, carina, and right and left main stem bronchi of the primary and secondary divisions. No evidence of any endobronchial tumor was noted. The scope was then withdrawn.

The patient was then prepped and draped in the usual sterile fashion. A shoulder roll was placed. A curvilinear incision was made above the suprasternal notch in the line of a skin crease. Dissection was carried down through the subcutaneous tissue down through the platysma muscle. The strap muscles were next identified and laterally retracted. We continued our dissection down to the pretracheal space. A thyroid isthmusectomy was done without any problems; this gave me clear access to the pretracheal space. A pretracheal plane was next developed. A mediastinoscope was placed. I saw multiple, firm right paratracheal lymph nodes. After first aspirating these structures to make sure they are not vascular in nature, generous biopsies were taken and sent to pathology for examination. Frozen section analysis revealed these to be consistent with lymphoma. Excellent hemostasis was obtained. The wound was irrigated using warm antibiotic saline solution. The wound was then closed in layers using Vicryl sutures. Dressings were applied. Marcaine 0.25% was used as a regional block. The patient tolerated the procedure and was sent to the recovery room in stable condition.

CASE STUDY #14: DAVIDA PRAGER

PROCEDURE: Needle-localized biopsy, right breast

DESCRIPTION OF PROCEDURE: After proper consent was obtained, the patient (48-year-old female) was brought to the operating room and placed on the table in a supine position. Patient was given 2 mg of midazolam HCL, IV, titrated during the procedure; the nurse monitored Davida's vital signs for a total of 15 minutes.

The right breast area was prepped and draped in a sterile manner. Plain Marcaine 0.5% solution was injected for local anesthesia in the perioperative region. A curvilinear incision was made medial to the insertion site of the wire, as the wire was noted to pass medially in the breast. The preoperative localization films were reviewed, noting that the clip was posterior to the wire. The dissection was carried out with cautery to remove a core of tissue around the wire, being more generous on the posterior aspect around the wire and especially near the end of the wire, taking a very generous area of tissue posteriorly; in fact, it was all the way down to the pectoralis fascia at that site. The specimen was removed, noting that the wire was within the mid portion of removed tissue with a large amount of surrounding tissue. This was submitted for radiographic analysis and the wire was noted to be within the large specimen. However, the clip could not be visualized. For this reason, the operative area was inspected with fluoroscopy with diligence and there was no evidence of any residual clip within the right breast tissue or within the drapes around the right breast. The Ray-Tec sponge was also evaluated with fluoroscopy and direct inspection and no clip was noted. The suction canister and tubing were also evaluated with fluoroscopy and no clip was noted. At this point, due to the generous size of the biopsy specimen, decision was made to not blindly remove any further breast tissue. I suspect that the clip may have become stuck to a Ray-Tec sponge or other instrument during this procedure and came out of the wound and fell out of the field of dissection. The operative area was irrigated, noted to hemostatic, and closed in layers using interrupted #3-0 Vicryl suture to close deep dermis and running #4-0 subcuticular Vicryl suture to close the skin. Benzoin, Steri-Strips, and sterile gauze dressings were placed. The patient had her sedation stopped and she was taken to the recovery area.

CASE STUDY #15: HENRY SYSTONA

OPERATION: Orbitotomy on the right with biopsy of right lacrimal gland

DESCRIPTION OF OPERATION: The patient was brought to the major operating room where general endotracheal anesthesia was induced. Lateral lid crease of the right eye was marked, and I marked the incision to extend lateral to the lateral canthus in case a lateral orbitotomy became necessary, pending the biopsy. The area of the lateral upper lid, beyond the lateral canthus, was injected with approximately 5 cc of 50:50 mix of 2% Xylocaine with 1:100,000 epinephrine, 0.75% Marcaine with 1:100,000 epinephrine. He was prepped and draped in the usual manner for sterile oculoplastic surgery.

(continued)

Attention was turned to the right upper lid. A lateral lid crease incision was made with a 15 blade. Dissection was carried down through the orbicularis to the superior orbital rim using the Colorado needle. The periosteum of the superior and lateral orbital rim was incised with the Colorado needle. Freer elevator was then used to reflect the periorbital off the lateral orbital wall and lateral orbital roof. Prior to proceeding with the orbital dissection, a 4-0 silk suture was placed on the insertion of the lateral rectus muscle for traction to better identify lateral rectus if an orbitotomy became necessary.

It was obvious, as the periorbital and lacrimal gland were lifted off the superotemporal orbit, that the lacrimal gland was enlarged with an infiltrative mass. Periosteum was opened near the posterior third of the mass and a modest biopsy was taken. It was then opened at the anterior edge and a biopsy was taken from this portion. Clinically, the biopsies looked like a lymphomatous infiltrate. These were sent for frozen section, and frozen section did reveal lymphomatous infiltrate consistent with non-Hodgkin lymphoma. Because of the need for special studies, more tissue was excised and as much of the infiltrative mass that was safely excisable was excised.

Bleeders were cauterized with the Colorado needle and the use of cottonoids saturated with 1:100,000 epinephrine. After adequate hemostasis was obtained, the 4-0 silk was removed from the lateral rectus muscle. The periosteum was closed with 2 interrupted 5-0 Vicryl, and the skin was closed with a running 5-0 fast-absorbing gut. Polysporin ointment was placed in the right eye and along the wound. The patient was awakened and taken to the recovery room in good condition. Estimated blood loss less than 10 cc. He tolerated the procedure well without complications.

PART IV

DMEPOS & TRANSPORTATION

There is another portion to the procedure coding system that professional coding specialists use to report services and treatments. HCPCS (pronounced "hick-picks") is the acronym for Healthcare Common Procedure Coding System. You have learned about the CPT codes used to report physician services and outpatient facility services. This part of this textbook will give you the opportunity to learn about HCPCS Level II codes (referred to as HCPCS codes).

DMEPOS is a combination abbreviation that stands for

- *DME = Durable Medical Equipment*
- *P = Prosthetics*
- *O = Orthotics*
- *S = Supplies*

Transportation refers to moving a patient from one point to another, such as ambulance services.

31
HCPCS Level II

Key Terms

- Advanced Life Support (ALS)
- Basic Life Support (BLS)
- Chelation Therapy
- DMEPOS
- Durable Medical Equipment (DME)
- Durable Medical Equipment Regional Carrier (DMERC)
- Enteral
- Not Otherwise Specified (NOS)
- Orthotic
- Parenteral
- Prosthetic
- Self-Administer
- Specialty Care Transport (SCT)

Learning Outcomes

After completing this chapter, the student should be able to:

LO 31.1 Abstract physician's notes to identify the category of HCPCS Level II codes needed.
LO 31.2 Employ the Alphabetic Index to find suggested HCPCS Level II codes.
LO 31.3 Distinguish the types of services, products, and supplies reported with HCPCS Level II codes.
LO 31.4 Follow the directions supplied by the notations and symbols.
LO 31.5 Utilize the additional information provided by Appendices.

STOP!

Remember, you need to follow along in your HCPCS Level II code book for an optimal learning experience.
Different publishers may vary regarding content of the Alphabetic Index and other elements, such as symbols and notations. Please understand that listings in this text may not perfectly match your HCPCS Level II coding manual. All of the codes and descriptions, however, match universally.

31.1 HCPCS Level II Categories

HCPCS Level II codes and modifiers are listed in their own book and are used to report services, procedures, and supplies that are not properly described in the CPT book. There are almost 5,000 HCPCS codes, each represented by five characters: one letter followed by four numbers.

EXAMPLES

C9460 Injection, cangrelor, 1 mg
R0076 Transportation of portable EKG to facility or location, per patient

HCPCS Level II codes cover specific aspects of health care services, including

- Durable medical equipment
  - e.g., a wheelchair or a humidifier
- Pharmaceuticals administered by a health care provider
  - e.g., a saline solution or a chemotherapy drug
- Medical supplies provided for the patient's own use
  - e.g., an eye patch or gradient compression stockings

- Dental services
    - e.g., all services provided by a dental professional
- Transportation services
    - e.g., ambulance services
- Vision and hearing services
    - e.g., trifocal spectacles or a hearing screening
- **Orthotic** and **prosthetic** procedures
    - e.g., scoliosis braces or postsurgical fitting

Orthotic
A device used to correct or improve an orthopedic concern.

Prosthetic
Fabricated artificial replacement for a damaged or missing part of the body.

Not all insurance carriers accept HCPCS Level II codes, but Medicare and Medicaid want you to use them. It is your responsibility as a coding specialist to find out whether each third-party payer with which your facility works accepts HCPCS Level II codes. If not, you have to ask for the payer's policies on reporting the services and supplies covered by HCPCS Level II.

EXAMPLES

Medicare accepts HCPCS Level II codes and therefore requires you to code an injection of tetracycline, 200 mg, with two codes (for administration of the shot and the drug inside the syringe).

96372 Therapeutic, prophylactic or diagnostic injection (specify substance or drug injected); subcutaneous or intramuscular

J0120 Injection, tetracycline, up to 250 mg

Yankee Health Insurance does not accept HCPCS Level II codes. This payor includes reimbursement for the drug in the CPT code for the actual injection. Therefore, you would only report the one code to get paid for both the service (the giving of the shot) and the material (the drug inside the syringe).

96372 Therapeutic, prophylactic or diagnostic injection (specify substance or drug injected); subcutaneous or intramuscular

The process for using HCPCS Level II codes is the same as coding from the CPT book. You abstract the key words from the physician's notes regarding the services and procedures, look those key words up in the Alphabetic Index of the appropriate book (CPT or HCPCS), confirm the code in the numeric listing, and report the service using that code. You know how to do this already! However, there are specific elements unique to HCPCS Level II coding that you need to know.

Understanding how to use HCPCS codes accurately will open new employment opportunities for you. In addition to hospitals, physician's offices, and outpatient clinics, nursing homes, home health care agencies, health care equipment and supply companies, and other facilities use these codes quite extensively.

LET'S CODE IT! SCENARIO

Carole Shelton, a 47-year-old female, came to see Dr. Giardino, a podiatrist recommended by her primary care physician, complaining of acute pain in the ball of her left foot. She states that the pain has been ongoing for about 2 months. After examination, and an x-ray of the foot, two views, Dr. Giardino took a walking boot, non-pneumatic, from the storage room and placed it on her foot. He instructed Carole to wear the boot at all times, except while in bed, for 6 weeks, and return for a follow-up evaluation.

(continued)

Let's Code It!

Review the information in the scenario and abstract the services that Dr. Giardino provided: he evaluated her condition, took x-rays, and provided her with the boot (durable medical equipment).

You have learned about CPT coding, so you can determine that these two codes will be reported for this encounter:

99202 **Office visit, new patient, straightforward medical decision-making**

73620 **Radiologic examination, foot; 2 views**

Now, you need to report the provision of the boot. It is only right that Dr. Giardino be reimbursed for providing this to the patient for her use at home. Turn in your HCPCS Level II code book to the Alphabetic Index, and find:

Walking splint, L4386

Go back to the documentation, which states, "*walking boot.*" Is a splint the same as a boot? I don't know, so turn in the Main Section of HCPCS Level II so you can read the complete code description.

L4386 **Walking boot, non-pneumatic, with or without joints, with or without interface material, prefabricated item that has been trimmed, bent, molded, assembled, or otherwise customized to fit a specific patient by an individual with expertise.**

Go back to the documentation. Is there any mention of customization, as mentioned in the description for code L4386? No, there is not. And the documentation does state that the boot came right out of Dr. Giardino's storage room. There are three other codes that describe a walking boot in this subsection of *Ancillary Orthotic Services*. Take a look at the full descriptions for L4360, L4361, and L4387 to see if any of these match the documentation. Aha! L4387 matches!

Now, you can report the three codes for this encounter with confidence: the two CPT codes + this one HCPCS Level II code.

L4387-LT **Walking boot, non-pneumatic, with or without joints, with or without interface material, prefabricated, off-the-shelf, left foot**

Good work!

CODING BITES

A physiatrist is a health care professional who uses physical methodologies to treat illness or injury.

These methodologies include electrical stimulation, heat/cold, light, water, exercise, manipulation, and mechanical devices.

CODING BITES

Never, never, never, never, never code from the Alphabetic Index. Always confirm the code in the Alphanumeric Listing before deciding which code to report.

31.2 The Alphabetic Index

Like the other coding books, the HCPCS Level II book has an Alphabetic Index as well as an Alphanumeric Listing.

The Alphabetic Index lists the Level II code descriptions in alphabetic order from A to Z. After abstracting the key terms from the provider's notes, you can look up key words in the Alphabetic Index by using the following:

- Brand name of the drug
- Generic name of the drug
- Medical supply item
- Orthotic
- Prosthetic
- Service
- Surgical supply

The Alphabetic Index will suggest a code or a range of codes, similarly to CPT's Alphabetic Index. Then, as you have done before, you look the suggestions up in the Alphanumeric Listing, read the complete description(s) and all of the symbols and notations, and determine the best, most accurate code. (*NOTE:* The Alphabetic Index in the HCPCS Level II book does not list *all* the codes included in the Alphanumeric Listing. So if you can't find what you are looking for in the Alphabetic Index, you might want to find something closely related to get you to the appropriate section of the book and then look around.)

This index includes many alternate terms identified by notations in the Alphanumeric Listings:

> **EXAMPLE**
>
> In the Alphabetic Index, you will see
>
> Abciximab, J0130
>
> In the Table of Drugs, you will see
>
> ReoPro, J0130
>
> In the Alphanumeric Listing, you will see:
>
> J0130 Injection, abciximab, 10 mg
>
> Other: ReoPro

Deleted code descriptions are not included in the Alphabetic Index. However, the new code(s) that is to be used instead of the deleted code is listed:

> **EXAMPLE**
>
> In the Alphabetic Index, you will see
>
> **Ventilator**
>
> Home ventilator, any type, E0465, E0466
>
> used with invasive interface, E0465
>
> In the Alphanumeric Listing, you will see:
>
> E0465 Home ventilator, any type, used with invasive interface, (e.g., tracheostomy tube)

The Alphanumeric Listing shows a notation to use one code with another code.

> **EXAMPLE**
>
> In the Alphanumeric Listing, you will see
>
> D2953 Each additional indirectly fabricated post–same tooth
>
> *To be used with D2952*

HCPCS Level II codes are listed in sections, grouped by the type of service, the type of supply item, or the type of equipment they represent. However, you should not assume that a particular item or service is located only in that specific section. Use the Alphabetic Index to direct you to the correct category in the Alphanumeric Listing of the book. One type of service or procedure might be located under several different categories depending upon the details.

> **EXAMPLE**
>
> Transportation services may be identified by A, Q, R, or V codes.
>
> Transportation
>
> Ambulance, A0021–A0999, Q3019, Q3020
>
> Corneal tissue, V2785
>
> EKG equipment, portable, R0076

31.3 The Alphanumeric Listing Overview

The Alphanumeric Listing presents the codes in alphabetic order by the first letter and then numeric order beginning with the first number of that code. Let's go through all the sections together so you can get a general idea of the procedures, services, and supplies that are reported using these codes.

A0000–A0999 Transportation Services Including Ambulance

If a severely ill or injured individual must be moved, whether from home or an accident scene, to a health care facility or from one health care facility to another, transportation arrangements are made. The patient may need to be lying down or receiving continuous IV therapy. The health care professional may have to monitor the patient's vital signs and other issues constantly. The room for additional personnel, the ability to keep special equipment secure and functional, and the configuration of the seating so that everyone involved can be kept safe during the ride are all concerns that demand more than the average vehicle.

HCPCS Level II codes A0021-A0999 report the following transportation services:

- Ground ambulances
- Air ambulances (often a helicopter but not exclusively)
- Nonemergency transportation, such as a special van, a taxi cab, a car, or even a bus
- Additional or secondary related costs and fees

Coding Components

Advanced Life Support (ALS)
Life-sustaining, emergency care provided, such as airway management, defibrillation, and/or the administration of drugs.

Basic Life Support (BLS)
The provision of emergency CPR, stabilization of the patient, first aid, control of bleeding, and/or treatment of shock.

Specialty Care Transport (SCT)
Continuous care provided by one or more health professionals in an appropriate specialty area, such as respiratory care or cardiovascular care, or by a paramedic with additional training.

The transportation section codes are determined by the answers to these questions:

1. What type of vehicle was used to transport the patient?
   - Ground (ambulance, taxi, bus, minibus, van, etc.)
   - Air–fixed wing (such as an airplane)
   - Air–rotary wing (such as a helicopter)
2. What type of services did the patient need?
   - Emergency
   - Nonemergency
   - **Advanced life support** (ALS)
   - **Basic life support** (BLS)
   - **Specialty care transport** (SCT)
3. Did the ambulance have to wait?
4. How many miles did the ambulance have to travel from origin to destination?
5. Were extra personnel required?

Determining the answers to these five questions from the documentation will direct you to the best, most appropriate code or codes needed to properly report transportation services for a patient.

GUIDANCE CONNECTION

Read the guidelines within section **A**, subhead **Transportation Services Including Ambulance A0000-A0999** in your HCPCS Level II book.

EXAMPLE

EMTs Garret Tyson and Peter Gromine were asked by Jason Aeronson to travel over the state line to the Morrison Nursing Center and transport his mother, Melinda Donner, a 93-year-old female, to the Bramington Nursing Center back near their home base and Jason's home. Ms. Donner requires ALS services during the ambulance transport. Upon arrival at Morrison Nursing Center, they had to wait 30 minutes for the staff to process Melinda out and release her to their care. The round trip was 52 miles. Pre-approval from Medicaid was documented.

A0021 x 52	Ambulance service, outside state per mile, transport, 52 miles round trip
A0420	Ambulance waiting time (ALS or BLS), one-half (1/2) hour increments

LET'S CODE IT! SCENARIO

Priscilla DeLucca, an emergency medical technician (EMT), was called in as an extra ambulance attendant for the ALS ground transportation of Willow Lawarence, a 12-year-old autistic female.

Let's Code It!

Priscilla was called in as an *extra ambulance attendant*. When you look in the Alphabetic Index of the HCPCS Level II book, notice that this does not match any of the listings under *Ambulance* or *Attendant*. So let's turn to the range shown next to the term *Ambulance* in the index: A0021–A0999.

Although reading down the listing will take time, sometimes it is the best way to find the code you need. Fortunately, you won't have to read too far to reach:

A0424 **Extra ambulance attendant, ground (ALS or BLS) or air (fixed or rotary winged); (requires medical review)**

Transportation Codes in Other Sections

A few transportation codes in the HCPCS Level II book are in sections other than the A codes. This, of course, is an excellent example of why you should use the Alphabetic Index to find the best code in the Alphanumeric Listing–because there may be a better, more appropriate code in a section you might not otherwise examine. In all cases of temporary codes, you must confirm the acceptance of the temporary code by the third-party payer to whom you are billing.

The S series (S0000–S9999) consists of temporary codes and is not accepted by Medicare, according to the HCPCS Level II book. Medicaid programs and some private insurers, such as Blue Cross and Blue Shield Association, do accept S codes. You must check with the organization or association in your state to confirm the acceptance of S codes. Here are two of the S codes that relate to transportation:

S0215 **Non-emergency transportation; mileage, per mile**

S9992 **Transportation costs to and from trial location and local transportation costs (e.g., fares for taxicab or bus) for clinical trial participant and one caregiver/companion**

The T codes (T1000–T9999) are used by Medicaid state agencies to report services, procedures, and other items for which there are no permanent national codes. You must communicate with the third-party payer to whom you are sending the claim to ensure that it accepts T codes. Here are some transportation services that may be reported using T codes:

T2001 **Non-emergency transportation; patient attendant/escort**

T2002 **Non-emergency transportation; per diem**

T2003 **Non-emergency transportation; encounter/trip**

T2004 **Non-emergency transport; commercial carrier, multi-pass**

T2005 **Non-emergency transportation; stretcher van**

T2007 **Transportation waiting time, air ambulance and non-emergency vehicle, one-half (1/2) hour increments**

T2049 **Non-emergency transportation; stretcher van, mileage; per mile**

LET'S CODE IT! SCENARIO

Barry Camacho, a 79-year-old male, had a stroke 3 weeks ago. He has now improved sufficiently to be discharged from the hospital. However, he is not completely well. Barry is being transferred to a short-term rehabilitation facility to help him regain use of his legs and right arm. Ira Waxen, from Flomenhoff Ambulance Services, drove the wheelchair van to take Barry from McGraw Hospital to Flowers Nursing and Rehabilitation Center, a 12-mile ride.

(continued)

Let's Code It!

Ira, the driver, will submit the documentation to you. He noted that he drove a *wheelchair van* to transport Barry from the hospital to the nursing facility. The notes also indicate that Barry is being discharged from the hospital and there is no indication that this is an emergency. In addition, the wheelchair van does not contain emergency equipment, so we know that this is a *non-emergency* trip.

Let's go to the Alphabetic Index and turn to *Wheelchair*. Go down the list to the indented term *Van, nonemergency*, A0130. Turn to the Alphanumeric Listing to check out the complete description of the code:

A0130 Non-emergency transportation: wheelchair van

This matches Ira's documentation, doesn't it? Yes. In addition, it is the only code shown for that portion of the service. However, you might also look in the Alphabetic Listing under *Transportation, nonemergency*, A0080–A0210, T2001–T2005. Once you review the complete descriptions of the suggested codes, you will see rather quickly that A0130 is the most specific and accurate.

Now, you must include a code for the mileage traveled by the van. Under *Transportation, non-emergency, wheelchair van*, you get the suggestion for codes A0130 and S0209. We already know that A0130 reports the use of the van itself. Let's find out what the description is for S0209:

S0209 Wheelchair van, mileage, per mile

also note just below this . . .

S0215 Non-emergency transportation; mileage per mile

You also might notice:

A0380 BLS mileage (per mile)

A0390 ALS mileage (per mile)

A0425 Ground mileage, per statute mile

Five different codes appear applicable to reporting the mileage component of the service. Look at S0209 versus S0215 versus A0380, A0390, and A0425. You can see that the descriptions of A0380 and A0390 do not match your notes and would be considered upcoding! S0209 is more accurate and more specific in its description of the type of vehicle involved in the transportation. Therefore, as long as the insurance carrier accepts S codes, the claim form should show these codes:

A0130 Non-emergency transportation: wheelchair van

S0209 Wheelchair van, mileage, per mile; Number of miles: twelve (12)

Great job!

Ambulance Origin/Destination

When reporting transportation services to insurance carriers, you have to identify the *origin of service* and the *destination of service*. The most common modifiers for the origin and the destination of service are one-letter codes that categorize locations.

D Diagnostic or therapeutic site other than P or H when these are used as origin codes

E Residential, domiciliary, custodial facility (other than 1819 facility)

G Hospital-based ESRD facility

H Hospital

I Site of transfer (e.g., airport or helicopter pad) between modes of ambulance transport

J Free-standing ESRD facility

N Skilled nursing facility (SNF) (1819 facility)

P Physician's office

R **Residence**

S **Scene of accident or acute event**

X **Intermediate stop at physician's office on way to hospital (destination code only)**

A4000–A8004 Medical and Surgical Supplies and A9000–A9999 Administrative, Miscellaneous and Investigational

These codes cover medical supplies, surgical supplies, and some services related to **durable medical equipment (DME)**.

In almost every health care encounter, materials and supplies are used. The paper used to cover the examination table and the disposable cover on the digital thermometer are good examples. Such medical supplies are used by the health care facility itself. However, they are *not* the types of medical and surgical supplies to which the HCPCS Level II book refers. The codes in the HCPCS Level II book are for reporting supplies given to a patient to **self-administer** health care at home.

> **Durable Medical Equipment (DME)**
> Apparatus and tools that help individuals accommodate physical frailties, deliver pharmaceuticals, and provide other assistance that will last for a long time and/or be used to assist multiple patients over time.

> **Self-Administer**
> To give medication to oneself, such as a diabetic giving herself an insulin injection.

A Codes and B Codes

Let's begin by reviewing the subheadings throughout the A code and B code sections to get a good idea of which items are covered.

- **Miscellaneous Supplies:** The supplies used by a physician in the course of treatment (syringes, alcohol wipes, urine test strips, and so on) are included in the amount reimbursed for the provision of that treatment or service. The codes in miscellaneous supplies (HCPCS Level II) are used to report, and be reimbursed for, supplies provided to patients for their own use at home. For example, if a diabetic patient requires a daily insulin shot at home, he or she would need to have syringes available.
- **Vascular Catheters:** These codes report the use of a disposable drug delivery system (DDS) as well as implantable access catheters. The codes are not for reporting the physician's work to implant the catheter but for the facility to be reimbursed for the cost of the catheter itself.
- **Incontinence Appliances and Care Supplies** and **External Urinary Supplies:** The sections **Incontinence Appliances and Care Supplies** and **External Urinary Supplies** cover urinary supplies that a patient uses when he or she has been diagnosed with permanent, or chronic, incontinence.
- **Ostomy Supplies:** Patients who have had surgery to create an ostomy need supplies every day to make their medical situation easier to deal with and to enable them to live their lives more normally.

EXAMPLES

A4245	Alcohol wipes, per box
A4452	Tape, waterproof, per 18 sq. in.
A4490	Surgical stocking above knee length, each
A4637	Replacement, tip, cane, crutch, or walker, each

You will also find codes in this section for

- Nonprescription drugs (also known as over-the-counter drugs)
- Exercise equipment
- Radiopharmaceutical diagnostic imaging agents
- Noncovered items and services

(*NOTE:* An item or service may be noncovered with regard to national standards but covered by your state or other third-party carrier. Never take anything for granted. Always ask!)

EXAMPLES

A9280 Alert or alarm device, not otherwise classified

A9505 Thallium T1-201, thallous chloride, diagnostic, per millicurie

LET'S CODE IT! SCENARIO

Teresa Baum, a 55-year-old female, has been diagnosed with malignant neoplasm of the liver. She has lost all her hair because of the chemotherapy and radiation treatments. Dr. Colter prescribed a wig to help lift her spirits and self-esteem.

Let's Code It!

You have to submit a claim to Medicare for the wig. Let's go to the Alphabetic Index of the HCPCS Level II book and find the W section. Beneath this, find

Wig, A9282

Go to the Alphanumeric Listing to confirm it is the best code:

A9282 Wig, any type, each

B4000–B9999 Enteral and Parenteral Therapy

Enteral
Within, or by way of, the gastrointestinal tract.

Parenteral
By way of anything other than the gastrointestinal tract, such as intravenous, intramuscular, intramedullary, or subcutaneous.

The B codes cover supplies, formulas, nutritional solutions, and infusion pumps for **enteral** and **parenteral** therapy. These codes report the supply of items related to providing nutrition to a patient by alternate means–other than by mouth and/or the digestive tract.

EXAMPLES

B4083 Stomach tube–Levine type

B9006 Parenteral nutrition, infusion pump, stationary

C1000–C9999 CMS Hospital Outpatient Payment System

Codes from the ***Temporary Hospital Outpatient PPS*** category are used to report drugs, biologicals, devices for transitional pass-through payments for hospitals, and items classified in new-technology ambulatory payment classifications.

GUIDANCE CONNECTION

Read the guidelines within section **C**, subhead **CMS Hospital Outpatient Payment System (C1000–C9999)** in your HCPCS Level II book.

EXAMPLES

C1724 Catheter, transluminal atherectomy, rotational

C2636 Brachytherapy linear source, non-stranded, Palladium-103, per 1 mm

C9364 Porcine implant, Permacol, per square centimeter

D0000–D9999 Dental Procedures

The **Dental Procedures** category is the ***Dental Procedures and Nomenclature (CDT)*** code set, copyrighted by the American Dental Association.

The codes are used to report dental services, such as x-rays (**Figure 30-1**).

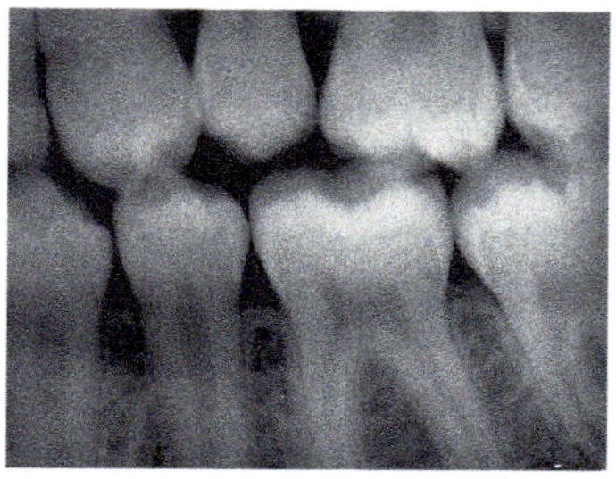

FIGURE 30-1 An x-ray of teeth (bitewing view) is one type of dental service

Design Pics Inc./Alamy Stock Photo

EXAMPLES

D0240	Intraoral–occlusal radiographic image
D1110	Prophylaxis–adult
D3310	Endodontic therapy, anterior tooth (excluding final restoration)

NOTE: Prophylaxis is also known as a dental cleaning, and *anterior (excluding final restoration)* is one of the codes that can be used to report root canal therapy.

LET'S CODE IT! SCENARIO

Alvin Tunney, an 81-year-old male, came to Dr. Kahn for a complete maxillary denture. His old one was broken beyond repair, so Alvin needed something immediately.

Let's Code It!

Dr. Kahn provided Alvin with a *complete maxillary denture*. Let's go to the HCPCS Level II Alphabetic Index:

Dentures D5110–D5899

As you read the full list, you see that the reference matches Dr. Kahn's notes. Next, turn to the Alphanumeric Listing to see which code is the most accurate.

D5110	**Complete denture—maxillary**
D5120	**Complete denture—mandibular**
D5130	**Immediate denture—maxillary**
D5140	**Immediate denture—mandibular**

Is there additional information in the notes that will help us determine the best code? They state that Alvin needed the denture *immediately*. It leads us directly to this code:

D5110 **Complete denture—maxillary**

Excellent!

E0100–E8002 Durable Medical Equipment

The E codes are used to identify certain pieces of durable medical equipment (DME) provided to a patient.

Science and technology have provided our society with great innovations that make life easier and more functional. Canes, walkers, and wheelchairs, among other items, help individuals move from one place to another without further assistance. Portable oxygen, humidifiers, vaporizers, and other equipment assist breathing, and pacemakers and electrical nerve stimulators help keep a heart beating. Some items are so commonplace that we take them for granted, yet only 10 years ago, patients would be forced to stay home all day every day. Other products, such as wheelchairs, have evolved into more convenient and accommodating pieces of equipment. Each item and every accessory costs money to build. Therefore, the health care facility or company should be reimbursed for giving, renting/leasing, or selling equipment. HCPCS Level II codes for DME are used in the reimbursement process.

Durable Medical Equipment

Durable medical equipment (DME) includes such items as canes, wheelchairs, and ventilators. However, to be accurate, Medicare has four qualifiers to determine whether an item can be classified as DME. These qualifiers are

1. The item can withstand repeated use.
2. The item is primarily used for medical purposes.
3. The item is used in the patient's home (rather than only in a health care facility).
4. The item would not be used if the individual were not ill or injured.

DMEPOS
Durable medical equipment, prosthetic, and orthotic supplies.

Durable Medical Equipment Regional Carrier (DMERC)
A company designated by the state or region to act as the fiscal intermediary for all DME claims.

Most often, **DMEPOS** dealers supply DME to the patient. Such companies submit their claims not to Medicare or the state's Medicare fiscal intermediary (FI) but to their assigned **durable medical equipment regional carrier (DMERC)**, which is contracted by Centers for Medicare and Medicaid Services (CMS).

HCPCS E Code Subheadings

The DME E code section, codes E0100–E8002, is divided into subheadings. It is not the only section in the HCPCS Level II book having codes related to DME services and supplies; however, it is the section dedicated to them. Take a minute to look through its subheadings, and you should gain a clearer understanding of the items and services included here.

EXAMPLES

Walking Aids and Attachments (E0100–E0159)

- Canes
- Crutches
- Walkers

CODING BITES

Be careful not to confuse the HCPCS Level II E codes with ICD-10-CM E codes, which report endocrinological diagnoses.

E0980 Safety vest, wheelchair

Letter followed by four numbers (from HCPCS Level II)

E09.8 Drug or chemical induced diabetes mellitus with unspecified complications

Letter followed by two numbers, a period, and possibly additional numbers or letters (from ICD-10-CM)

CODING BITES

Remember that a coding specialist's job is to report with the greatest specificity. There will be times when you will need a code from this section because it provides more specificity than a code from the CPT.

EXAMPLES

E0105 Cane, quad or three prong, includes canes of all materials, adjustable or fixed, with tips

E0156 Seat attachment, walker

E0242 Bathtub rail, floor base

G0000–G9999 Temporary Procedures/Professional Services

Codes from this section are used to report services and procedures that do not have an accurate code description in the main portion of the CPT book.

EXAMPLES

G0102 Prostate cancer screening; digital rectal examination

G0151 Services performed by a qualified physical therapist in the home health or hospice setting, each 15 minutes

G0268 Removal of impacted cerumen (one or both ears) by physician on same date of service as audiologic function testing

CODING BITES

Throughout section **G** are codes grouped as *Quality Measures*. These codes are used to report services related to the **Physician Quality Reporting System (PQRS)** and are only used when an appropriate CPT Category II code is not available.

H0001–H9999 Behavioral Health and/or Substance Abuse Treatment Services

When alcohol and drug treatment, as well as some other mental health services, is provided, some state Medicaid agencies will have you use codes from the ***Behavioral Health and/or Substance Abuse Treatment*** category.

EXAMPLES

H0005 Alcohol and/or drug services; group counseling by a clinician

H0038 Self-help/peer services, per 15 minutes

H2020 Therapeutic behavioral services, per diem

J0100–J8999 Drugs Other Than Chemotherapy Drugs and J9000–J9999 Chemotherapy Drugs

This ***Drugs Administered*** section provides you with codes to identify the specific drugs that are given to the patient by a health care professional in any way. This includes immunosuppressive drugs, inhalation solutions, and other miscellaneous drugs and solutions. These codes have nothing to do with the writing of a prescription or when a patient self-administers medication.

EXAMPLES

J0207 Injection, amifostine, 500 mg

J7100 Infusion, dextran 40, 500 mL

J7610 Albuterol, inhalation solution, compounded product, administered through DME, concentrated form, 1 mg

You will find that drugs identified in the code descriptions are most often the chemical, or generic, name of the pharmaceutical. At times the brand, or trade, name is listed in the Alphabetic Index and/or in the Table of Drugs in an appendix of your HCPCS Level II book. If your provider notes refer to a name that you cannot find in this book, you might need to look in the *Physician's Desk Reference* (PDR) to find an alternate name for the drug.

EXAMPLE

Dr. Valentine asked the nurse to administer a 250 mg tablet, CellCept, PO, to Benjamin Rudon.

CellCept, generic name mycophenolate mofetil, is classified as an immunosuppressant.

- Neither name is listed in the Alphabetic Index of HCPCS.
- CellCept is listed in the **Table of Drugs**.
- Mycophenolate mofetil is listed in the **Table of Drugs**.

J7517 Mycophenolate mofetil, oral, 250 mg

> **CODING BITES**
>
> If you do not have access to a Drug Directory, such as *Physician's Desk Reference* (PDR), you can find all the necessary information on pharmaceuticals at https://www.pdr.net/browse-by-drug-name.

In the chapter ***CPT Medicine Section***, you learned about coding for the administration of pharmaceuticals (drugs). Those codes are used for reporting the services–the labor–of the health care professional who gives the patient the drug. You may remember that the different methods of administering drugs include

IA	**Intra-arterial administration**
IV	**Intravenous administration (e.g., gravity infusion, injections, and timed pushes)**
IM	**Intramuscular administration**
IT	**Intrathecal**
SC	**Subcutaneous administration**
INH	**Inhaled solutions**
VAR	**Various routes for drugs that are commonly administered into joints, cavities, tissues, or topical applications, as well as other parenteral administrations**
ORAL	**Administered orally**
OTH	**Other routes of administration, such as suppositories or catheter injections**

The codes in HCPCS Level II enable you to report and gain reimbursement for the actual drug or medication, as well as the syringe or IV bag used. The codes cover the pharmaceutical materials only–*not* the administration of the drug.

In some cases, you may find DME has been supplied to the patient to provide medication, or drugs. When the equipment is made available to an individual, it may need to be reported separately from the drug itself.

LET'S CODE IT! SCENARIO

Janine Howell, a 55-year-old female, came in for her chemotherapy treatment. She is given Adriamycin, 30 mg/m^2, IV daily, as treatment for malignant lymphoma. She tolerates the treatment well, and is discharged home.

Let's Code It!

You learned in the ***CPT Medicine Section*** chapter that you will need one code for the administration of this drug therapy and a second code from HCPCS Level II to identify the specific drug administered.

Let's begin determining the code for the Adriamycin. Open your HCPCS Level II code book to the *Table of Drugs*. Did you find it listed? It is there but listed as *Adriamycin, PFS, RDF*. Is this the same? Check the HCPCS Level II code book's *Alphabetic Index*. It is not there. You know there must be a code for this, so adriamycin may be an alternate name. You will need to check the PDR. [*NOTE:* If you do not have access to the PDR, you can use PDR.net or Drugs.com.]

You will see in the listing for Adriamycin that:

Therapeutic Classification: Antineoplastics

Common Name: Doxorubicin hydrocholoride

Go back to the HCPCS Level II code book's *Table of Drugs*. Can you find it using the common name?

Doxorubicin HCL 10 MG IV J9000

Now, let's go into the Alphanumeric Listing and find the specific code and its full description.

J9000 Injection, doxorubicin HCL, 10 mg

Perfect! However, this code only reports the provision of 10 mg. The documentation states, "*30 mg.*" Therefore, you will need a multiplier.

J9000 x 3 Injection, doxorubicin HCL, 10 mg × 3

(continued)

If you have your CPT code book nearby, try to determine the code for the administration of this medication. Did you determine this to be the correct code?

96413 **Chemotherapy administration, intravenous infusion technique; up to 1 hour, single or initial substance/drug**

Good work!

K0000–K9999 Temporary Codes Assigned to DME Regional Carriers

Durable Medical Equipment Regional Carrier (DMERC)
A company designated by the state or region to act as the fiscal intermediary for all DME claims.

The K codes were developed for **durable medical equipment regional carriers (DMERCs)** to report services that are not currently identified by other codes.

EXAMPLES

K0001 Standard wheelchair

K0462 Temporary replacement for patient-owned equipment being repaired, any type

L0100–L4999 Orthotics and L5000–L9999 Prosthetics

The codes included in the ***Orthotic Procedures and Devices*** and ***Prosthetic Procedures and Devices*** categories identify orthotic devices, orthopedic shoes, prosthetic devices, prosthetic implants, and scoliosis equipment.

An *orthotic* is a device used to correct or improve the function of a musculoskeletal concern or abnormality, whereas a *prosthetic* is an artificial replacement for a damaged or missing part of the body (see **Figure 30-2**).

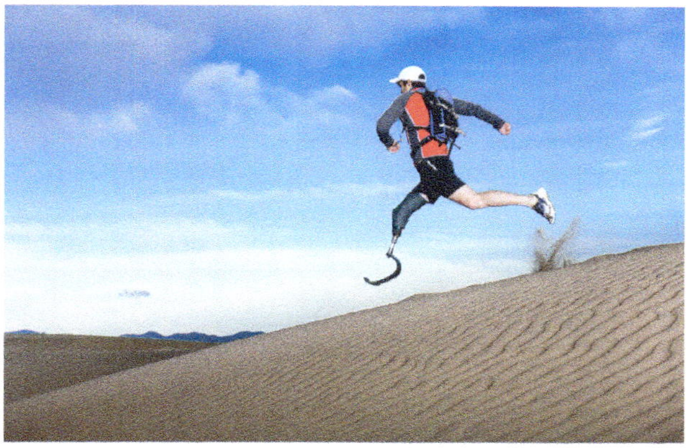

FIGURE 30-2 Man with prosthetic leg running in the desert

Michael Svoboda/Vetta/the Agency/Getty Images

EXAMPLES

ORTHOTICS

L0170 Cervical, collar, molded to patient model

L0984 Protective body sock, prefabricated, off-the-shelf, each

L3809 Wrist-hand-finger orthosis (WHFO), without joint(s), prefabricated, off-the-shelf, any type

(continued)

PROSTHETICS

L5100	Below knee, molded socket, shin, SACH foot
L6100	Below elbow, molded socket, flexible elbow hinge, triceps pad
L8020	Breast prosthesis, mastectomy form

SACH = Solid-Ankle Cushioned Heel

Chelation Therapy
The use of a chemical compound that binds with metal in the body so that the metal will lose its toxic effect. It might be done when a metal disc or prosthetic is implanted in a patient, eliminating adverse reactions to the metal itself as a foreign body.

M0000–M1149 Other Medical Services

The codes in the ***Other Medical Services*** category cover cellular therapy, prolotherapy, intragastric hypothermia, intravenous **chelation therapy**, and fabric wrapping of an abdominal aneurysm (MNP).

EXAMPLES

M0075	Cellular therapy
M1021	Patient had only urgent care visits during the performance period

P0000–P9999 Laboratory Services

HCPCS Level II codes in the ***Pathology and Laboratory Services*** category include codes for services not listed in the CPT book, including chemistry, toxicology, microbiology, screening Papanicolaou (Pap) procedures, and numerous blood products.

EXAMPLES

P2031	Hair analysis (excluding arsenic)
P7001	Culture, bacterial, urine; quantitative, sensitivity study
P9051	Whole blood or red blood cells, leukocytes reduced, CMV-negative, each unit

CODING BITES

Remember that you must always choose the code with the greatest specificity.

Q0000–Q9999 Temporary Codes Assigned by CMS

The Q codes replace the less specific codes that you may find elsewhere in the coding process for casting and splinting supplies when a health care professional cares for a patient with a fracture. The section also includes codes for certain drugs and services having nothing to do with the management of a fracture.

EXAMPLES

Q0113	Pinworm examinations
Q2017	Injection, teniposide, 50 mg
Q4049	Finger splint, static

R0000–R9999 Diagnostic Radiology Services

The codes in the ***Diagnostic Radiology Services*** section are used to report the hauling of portable radiologic equipment.

EXAMPLES

R0070	Transportation of portable X-ray equipment and personnel to home or nursing home, per trip to facility or location, one patient seen
R0075	Transportation of portable X-ray equipment and personnel to home or nursing home, per trip to facility or location, more than one patient seen
R0076	Transportation of portable EKG to facility or location, per patient

S0000–S9999 Temporary National Codes Established by Private Payers

The ***Temporary National Codes*** section was developed by the Health Insurance Association of America (HIAA) and the Blue Cross Blue Shield Association (BCBSA) for use by the Medicaid program and other third-party payers. The codes cover supplies, services, and drugs for which there are no other codes.

CODING BITES

Be certain to ask the third-party payer if it accepts "S" codes and, if not, ask how to report these services and provisions.

EXAMPLES

S0081	Injection, piperacillin sodium, 500 mg
S0317	Disease management program; per diem
S2060	Lobar lung transplantation
S9024	Paranasal sinus ultrasound

T1000–T9999 Temporary National Codes Established by Medicaid

Planned for use by state agencies that administer Medicaid programs, the T codes are used to report services not otherwise described by any other code. Services represented in this category include nursing facility and home health-related services, substance abuse treatment, and training-related procedures.

EXAMPLES

T1013	Sign language or oral interpretive services, per 15 minutes
T2022	Case management, per month
T2045	Hospice general inpatient care; per diem

V0000–V9999 Vision, Hearing, Speech-Language Pathology Services

V0000–V2999 Vision Services

If not represented by any other codes, ophthalmic and optometric services and supplies may be coded from this V code category, including contact lenses, intraocular lenses, miscellaneous lenses, prostheses, spectacles, and other vision-related supplies.

EXAMPLES

V2118	Aniseikonic lens, single vision
V2321	Lenticular lens, per lens, trifocal
V2530	Contact lens, scleral, gas impermeable, per lens

V5000–V9999 Hearing Services

Services related to hearing and speech-language pathology are included in this V code category and cover hearing tests, repair of augmentative communicative system, speech-language pathology screenings, and other hearing test-related supplies and equipment.

EXAMPLES

V5008	Hearing screening
V5100	Hearing aid, bilateral, body worn
V5364	Dysphagia screening

YOU CODE IT! CASE STUDY

Alfonzo Doyle, a 20-year-old male, lost his eye in a skiing accident and has come to see Dr. Durran to receive his prosthetic eye. It is a custom-made, plastic prosthesis. Code for the prosthesis only.

You Code It!

Go through the steps of coding, and determine the code(s) that should be reported for the prosthetic provided by Dr. Durran to Alfonzo Doyle.

Step #1: Read the case carefully and completely.
Step #2: Abstract the scenario. Which key words or terms describe what service the physician provided to the patient during this encounter?
Step #3: Are there any details missing or incomplete for which you would need to query the physician? [If so, ask your instructor.]
Step #4: Determine the correct HCPCS Level II code or codes to explain the details about what was provided to the patient during this encounter.
Step #5: Check for any relevant guidance, including reading all of the symbols and notations.
Step #6: Do you need to append any modifiers to ensure complete and accurate information is provided?
Step #7: Double-check your work.

Answer

Did you find this to be the correct code?

V2623 Prosthetic eye, plastic, custom

Good job!

Specialized Codes: COVID-19 Related Services

The people of the United States have needed so many healthcare-related services due to COVID-19. An important part of medical coding is to enable the tracking of the use of medications and services. Therefore, beginning January 2021, new HCPCS Level II codes were established.

Two new codes for the collection of specimens for testing to determine if the patient has been infected by COVID-19:

- G2023 Specimen collection for severe acute respiratory syndrome coronavirus 2 (SARS-CoV-2) (Coronavirus disease [COVID-19]), any specimen source
- G2024 Specimen collection for severe acute respiratory syndrome coronavirus 2 (SARS-CoV-2) (Coronavirus disease [COVID-19]), from an individual in a SNF or by a laboratory on behalf of an HHA, any specimen source

Due to the specific location stated in the description of G2024, it is important to remember that this code should only be reported for those patients whose stays are not covered by Medicare. Skilled Nursing Facility (SNF) residents whose specimen has been collected during a Medicare-covered stay will have these, and other lab services and tests, covered under Part A's SNF benefit. [FYI: HHA = Home Health Agency]

The work provided by the laboratory processing these specimens will also have specific codes to report, depending upon the details of the testing.

- U0001 CDC 2019-nCoV Real-Time RT-PCR Diagnostic Panel
- U0002 2019-nCoV Coronavirus, SARS-CoV-2/2019-nCoV (COVID-19), any technique, multiple types or subtypes (includes all targets), non-CDC

Four new codes for drugs used to treat patients with a confirmed diagnosis of COVID-19, one for an injection and another for infusion:

- Q0239 Injection, Bahamanian-xxxx, 700 mg
- Q0243 Injection, casirivimab and imdevimab, 2,400 mg

It should be noted that, according to CMS, those providers who receive this drug for free should not report either code Q0239 or Q0243. If the administration of this drug is being tracked for purposes, other than reimbursement, the code can be reported with a price of Zero or $0.01 (one cent).

- M0239 Intravenous infusion, bamlanivimab-xxxx, includes infusion and post-administration monitoring
- M0243 Intravenous infusion, casirivimab and imdevimab includes infusion and post-administration monitoring

31.4 Symbols and Notations

Throughout many versions of a HCPCS Level II code book, you may see notations that will help you use the codes correctly and determine the best, most appropriate code available. Check the front of your code book for meanings.

GUIDANCE CONNECTION

Read the guidelines in the **Introduction** and **HCPCS Level II Use and Convention** sections in your HCPCS Level II book.

HCPCS quarterly updates are posted on the website when available: https://www.cms.gov/medicare/coding/hcpcsreleasecodesets/hcpcs-quarterly-update.html.

Symbols

● Bullet

A large bullet (●), or solid circle, shown next to a code indicates that it is the first year that the code is included in this code set. That is, it marks a new code.

EXAMPLES

● J1306	Injection, inclisiran, 1 mg
● K1032	Non-pneumatic sequential compression garment, full leg

▲ Solid Triangle

A solid triangle (▲) shown next to a code lets you know that the code's description has been changed or revised since last year or that a rule or guideline regarding the code has changed.

EXAMPLES

▲ A9276	Sensor, invasive (e.g., subcutaneous), disposable, for use with non-durable medical equipment interstitial continuous glucose monitoring system, one unit = 1 day supply
▲ G2199	Patient not screened for unhealthy alcohol use using a systematic screening method

○ Open Circle

An open circle (○) next to a code identifies that the code had been deleted but now has been restored (reinstated).

EXAMPLES

○ J3090	Injection, tedizolid phosphate, 1 mg
○ J3380	Injection, vedolizumab, 1 mg

⃠ Circle with Slash

CODING BITES

In CPT, the symbol ⃠ means that the code may not be used with modifier 51. In HCPCS Level II, this same symbol means not covered under SNFPPS.

CODING BITES

Should the provider administer less than the amount in the code descriptor, report the code.

When more than the quantity in the code description is indicated, report the appropriate code in the proper number. For example, the provider gave the patient 2 mg of decitabine, report J0894 ×2 to indicate two units.

A circle with a slash through it (⃠), also known as the Forbidden Symbol in the HCPCS Level II book, identifies a code that is not covered under the skilled nursing facility (SNF) prospective payment system (PPS).

EXAMPLES

⃠ L5970	All lower extremity prostheses, foot, external keel, SACH foot
⃠ L7367	Lithium ion battery, rechargeable, replacement

☑ Box with Check Mark

A check mark inside a square box (☑) marks a code description that identifies a specific quantity of material or supply. It is a reminder for you to check the detail in the notes and report the code not only for the item it represents but for the amount as well.

EXAMPLES

☑ J0894	Injection, decitabine, 1 mg
☑ K0073	Caster pin lock, each

♂ Male Symbol

The male symbol (♂) is placed next to codes that identify procedures, services, and equipment that can *only* be performed or used on a male patient.

EXAMPLES

L3219 Orthopedic footwear, man's shoes, Oxford, each ♂

L8330 Truss, addition to standard pad, scrotal pad ♂

♀ Female Symbol

The female symbol (♀) identifies codes used to report procedures, services, and equipment that can *only* be performed or used on a female patient.

EXAMPLES

A4286 Locking ring for breast pump, replacement ♀

L8600 Implantable breast prosthesis, silicone or equal ♀

A Capital Letter A

The A symbol highlights the fact that a code is used only for procedures, services, and equipment that are performed or used on a patient of a certain age group. Read the code description carefully to ensure the age limitation of the code matches the patient.

EXAMPLES

A A4280 Adhesive skin support attachment for use with external breast prosthesis, each

A A4561 Pessary, rubber, any type

M Capital Letter M

The M symbol is used to remind you that the code describes maternity procedures, services, and equipment that are performed or used on a pregnant female 12–55 years of age.

EXAMPLES

M A4284 Breast shield and splash protector for use with breast pump, replacement

M S9001 Home uterine monitor with or without associated nursing services

~~Z1111~~ Any Code with a Line Through It

A line through the center of a code and its description means that the code has been deleted and may no longer be used.

EXAMPLES

~~G6018~~ ~~Ileoscopy, through stoma; with transendoscopic stent placement (includes predilation)~~

~~S9015~~ ~~Automated EEG monitoring~~

Notations

Just as in the CPT book, you will find notations (below code descriptions in the Alphanumeric Listing) that guide you on the proper use of HCPCS Level II codes.

Always Report Concurrent to the xxx Procedure

This notation directs you to always report this code with a code for another specific procedure. The notation is similar to the "code also" instruction found in CPT or ICD-10-CM.

> **EXAMPLE**
>
> A4262 Temporary, absorbable lacrimal duct implant, each
>
> ***Always report concurrent to the implant procedure.***
>
> A4263 Permanent, long-term, non-dissolvable lacrimal duct implant, each
>
> ***Always report concurrent to the implant procedure.***

In the previous example, the "A" code is for the implant itself, and the note reminds you that you have to code the physician's services for putting the implant into the patient.

See Also Code Z1111

The *see also code* notation cross-references this code with another code that may be similar in description. The notation serves as a reminder for you to double-check that you are using the most accurate code.

> **EXAMPLES**
>
> A4450 Tape, non-waterproof, per 18 square inches
> ***See also code A4452***
>
> A4452 Tape, waterproof, per 18 square inches
> ***See also code A4450***

Clarifications of Coverage

Clarifications of coverage notations are worded differently from code to code but indicate when to use or *not* use the code. However, always check with the specific payer to whom you will be sending the claim.

> **EXAMPLES**
>
> A4570 Splint
>
> **Dressings applied by a physician are included as part of the professional service.**
>
> A6260 Wound cleansers, any type, any size
>
> **Surgical dressings applied by a physician are included as part of the professional service. Surgical dressings obtained by the patient to perform homecare as prescribed by the physician are covered.**

Report in Addition to Code Z1111

When one code is to be reported with other codes, a notation *Report in addition to* (a particular *code*) will identify those circumstances. It not only tells you the circumstances but also tells you which code to use. You may notice that it is similar to an add-on code in CPT.

EXAMPLE

D2953 Each additional indirectly fabricated post—same tooth
Report in addition to code D2952

To Report, See Code Z1111

When a code has been deleted, you may find a notation that directs you to another HCPCS Level II code that can be used instead.

EXAMPLES

~~J0560~~ ~~Injection, penicillin G benzathine, up to 600,000 units~~
To report, see J0561

~~C9026~~ ~~Injection, vedolizumab, 1 mg~~
To report, see J3380

See Code(s): 00000

The notation *See* (a particular *code*) refers you to a CPT code for a description that is *potentially* better and may be more specific for reporting what was actually done or given to the patient.

EXAMPLES

E1130 Standard wheelchair; fixed full-length arms, fixed or swing-away, detachable footrests
See code(s): K0001

E1086 Hemi-wheelchair detachable arms, desk or full-length, swing-away, detachable footrests
See code(s): K0002

Determine If an Alternative HCPCS Level II or a CPT Code Better Describes . . .

You will see the notation *Determine if an alternative HCPCS Level II or a CPT code better describes* beneath each miscellaneous, unlisted, unclassified, not otherwise classified (NOC), not otherwise listed, or **not otherwise specified (NOS)** code. The notation serves as a warning to you to make certain that there is no better or more specific code in either the CPT or elsewhere in this HCPCS Level II book that correctly reports the services or procedures performed.

Not Otherwise Specified (NOS)
The absence of additional details documented in the notes.

EXAMPLES

L0999 Addition to spinal orthosis, not otherwise specified

Determine if an alternative HCPCS Level II or a CPT code better describes the service being reported. This code should be used only if a more specific code is unavailable.

J8999 Prescription drug, oral, chemotherapeutic, NOS

Determine if an alternative HCPCS Level II or a CPT code better describes the service being reported. This code should be used only if a more specific code is unavailable.

Use This Code for . . .

The notation *Use this code for* provides you with alternative names, brand names, and other terms that are also represented by the code's description.

> **EXAMPLES**
>
> J0585 Injection, onabotulinumtoxinA, 1 unit
> *Use this code for Botox, Botox Cosmetic*
>
> J1160 Injection, digoxin, up to 0.5 mg
> *Use this code for Lanoxin*

Pertinent Documentation to Evaluate Medical Appropriateness Should Be . . .

Some procedures are not automatically accepted as being medically necessary. The notation *Pertinent documentation to evaluate medical appropriateness should be* warns you up-front that you should include the proper documentation along with the claim *the first time* you submit it, rather than wait to be asked by the third-party payer, which would delay payment.

> **EXAMPLES**
>
> D2980 Crown repair, by report
> *Pertinent documentation to evaluate medical appropriateness should be included when this code is reported.*
>
> V2399 Specialty trifocal (by report)
> *Pertinent documentation to evaluate medical appropriateness should be included when this code is reported.*

Do Not Use This Code to Report . . .

The notation *Do not use this code to report* warns you of circumstances when you are not permitted to use a code.

> **EXAMPLE**
>
> D3220 Therapeutic pulpotomy (excluding final restoration)—removal of pulp coronal to the dentinocemental junction and application of medicament
> *Do not use this code to report the first stage of root canal therapy.*

Medicare Covers . . .

Throughout the HCPCS Level II book, you will see notations giving you information about coverage, particularly Medicare and Medicaid coverage. You should note that the book covers the entire nation and that both programs are state-administered. This means that you should still confirm the terms and policies of what is covered with your own state's fiscal intermediary (FI)–the agency or organization that is in charge of reimbursement for your state's program. Also check with other third-party payers to see if they will cover this item or service.

EXAMPLES

E0607 Home blood glucose monitor

Medicare covers home blood-testing devices for diabetic patients when the devices are prescribed by the patient's physicians. Many commercial payers provide this coverage to non–insulin dependent diabetics as well.

Q0174 Thiethylperazine maleate, 10 mg, oral, FDA approved prescription antiemetic, for use as a complete therapeutic substitute for an IV antiemetic at the time of chemotherapy treatment, not to exceed a 48-hour dosage regimen

Medicare covers at the time of chemotherapy if regimen doesn't exceed 48 hours. Submit on the same claim as the chemotherapy.

Code with Caution

When you see the notation *Code with caution* beneath a code, you need to go back and double-check the provider's notes carefully. If this is what was actually done, then be certain to attach documentation explaining why that method was used instead of the newer technique because it is surely going to be questioned.

EXAMPLES

M0301 Fabric wrapping of abdominal aneurysm

Code with caution: This procedure has largely been replaced with more effective treatment modalities. Submit documentation.

P2028 Cephalin flocculation, blood

Code with caution: This test is considered obsolete. Submit documentation.

CODING BITES

When you determine from the documentation that a different code may be more accurate than one indicated by the physician, you should query the physician to have him or her document complete accurate details.

YOU CODE IT! CASE STUDY

Dr. Principe modified Miriam Collins's left orthopedic shoe by inserting a between-sole metatarsal bar wedge to accommodate Miriam's shrinking Achilles tendon. Dr. Principe checked off the code L3649 on the superbill. As the professional coding specialist, is this the best code available?

You Code It!

Go through the steps of coding, and determine the code(s) that should be reported for this product between Dr. Principe and Miriam Collins.

Step #1: Read the case carefully and completely.
Step #2: Abstract the scenario. Which key words or terms describe what service the physician provided to the patient during this encounter?
Step #3: Are there any details missing or incomplete for which you would need to query the physician? [If so, ask your instructor.]
Step #4: Determine the correct HCPCS Level II code or codes to explain the details about what was provided to the patient during this encounter.
Step #5: Check for any relevant guidance, including reading all of the symbols and notations.
Step #6: Do you need to append any modifiers to ensure complete and accurate information is provided?
Step #7: Double-check your work.

(continued)

Answer

Did you find this to be the correct code?

L3410 Metatarsal bar wedge, between sole

Now that's a much more specific code. Good job!

LET'S CODE IT! SCENARIO

Rita Warren came with her husband, Ryan, to see Dr. Capshaw because of the problems Ryan was having sleeping. Dr. Capshaw had performed a nasopharyngoscopy and diagnosed Ryan with sleep apnea. At this encounter, Dr. Capshaw provided Ryan with an apnea monitor, complete with a recording feature, so that more data could be collected and Dr. Capshaw could further evaluate his condition.

Let's Code It!

Dr. Capshaw has supplied Ryan with an *apnea monitor with a recording feature.* This machine is considered durable medical equipment (DME). Ryan's insurance carrier accepts HCPCS Level II codes. Therefore, we have determined the code so that Dr. Capshaw can be reimbursed for the machine. Let's go to the Alphabetic Index and look up the word *monitor* because that is the key word that best describes this item. Beneath the word *monitor*, indented slightly, you see the word *apnea*, and the suggestion for the codes E0618 and E0619. This seems to be exactly what Dr. Capshaw described in his notes, so let's turn to the Alphanumeric Listing to read the complete description of the codes.

E0618 Apnea monitor, without recording feature

This matches the notes with one big exception. The code description specifically states *without* recording feature. Dr. Capshaw documented giving Ryan a monitor *with* a recording feature. Let's look at the other suggested code:

E0619 Apnea monitor, with recording feature

Excellent! It matches perfectly.

LET'S CODE IT! SCENARIO

Dr. Bettesh provided Lauren Martins, a 79-year-old female, with a quad cane, after putting on a new handgrip. Code for the supply only.

Let's Code It!

When you pull out the key words that describe the items for which Dr. Bettesh should be reimbursed, you see that Lauren was provided with a *quad cane* and *new handgrip*.

It wouldn't be out of line to think that the codes are automatically going to be listed in the ***Durable Medical Equipment*** section, codes E0100–E8002. If you turned to that section directly, you would find the code for the quad cane rather quickly. It's right in the front. However, you could examine and search through the entire listing of 7,902 possible codes in the section and never find the correct code for the replacement handgrip. When you look these key words up in the Alphabetic Index first, you see very quickly, and more efficiently, that the codes you need are these:

E0105 Cane, quad or three prong, includes canes of all materials, adjustable or fixed, with tips

A4636 Replacement, handgrip, cane, crutch, or walker, each

It's great when the process works, isn't it? You bet!

31.5 Appendices

The HCPCS Level II book provides you with additional information in the back of the book to help you code more accurately (see **Table 31-1**).

TABLE 31-1 List of most common Appendices found in HCPCS Level II code books.

Appendices	Description
Table of Drugs	This is an alphabetic listing of drug names, along with the standard unit of administration, a particular method of administration, and a reference to its HCPCS Level II code.
Modifiers	This is an alphabetic list of all HCPCS Level II modifiers. You will learn more about these modifiers in Appendix B of this text.
Abbreviations and Acronymns	Abbreviations and acronyms are used throughout the health care industry. This appendix lists those used in HCPCS Level II descriptions to help you better understand the meaning of the codes.
CMS References	Certain components of the coding system change from time to time. Up-to-date manuals and information can be found online in the Centers for Medicare and Medicaid Services (CMS) manual system found at www.cms.hhs.gov/manuals. Included in each annual edition of some printed HCPCS Level II books are references to national coverage determinations made just prior to publication. As a student, this may be outside the scope of your studies. As you mature in your career, this reference will be very handy.
New, Changed, Deleted, and Reinstated HCPCS Codes	This appendix lists all HCPCS Level II codes that have experienced a change since the previous year's printed book. As a student, this will have little relevance for you. But when the new book comes out, it serves as an excellent reference for someone who may use the same code or codes over and over again.
Place of Service and Type of Service Codes	This appendix offers you a thorough explanation of each place of service (POS) and type of service (TOS) code required for boxes 24B and 24C of the CMS 1500 claim form.
Deleted Code Crosswalk	This is a list of all deleted codes from last year to this, and includes the new codes to use to report the service, when available.
Glossary	Key terms used throughout this code set are listed here, along with their definitions.
Physician Quality Reporting System (PQRS)	This appendix provides up-to-date details about codes used in this program.

CODING BITES

NOTE: The content of appendices may vary depending upon the publisher of the HCPCS Level II book used.

You may find additional details at https://www.cms.gov/medicare/coding-billing/healthcare-common-procedure-system/quarterly-update

CODING BITES

The list in ***Abbreviations and Acronyms*** appendix is not inclusive of all abbreviations and acronyms used in the health care industry. It is a good idea to keep a medical dictionary close by to reference those abbreviations not included in this appendix.

Chapter Summary

HCPCS Level II codes are updated quarterly and are officially effective January 1 of each year, with no grace period. Most printed versions of the book are published with those codes posted by the Centers for Medicare and Medicaid Services (CMS) as of November 1. Read the following notation in the introduction of the HCPCS Level II book:

> *"Because of the unstable nature of HCPCS Level II codes, everything has been done to include the latest information available at print time. Unfortunately, HCPCS Level II codes, their descriptions, and other related information change throughout the year. Consult the patient's payer and the CMS website to confirm the status of any HCPCS Level II code. The existence of a code does not imply coverage under any given payment plan."*

CODING BITES

Some of the Health Care Services/Items Reported with HCPCS Level II Codes

- Patient Transportation
- Enteral and Parenteral Therapy
- Durable Medical Equipment
- Pharmaceuticals Administered by a Health Professional
- Orthotics
- Prosthetics

CHAPTER 31 REVIEW HCPCS Level II

connect

Enhance your learning by completing these exercises and more at mcgrawhillconnect.com!

Let's Check It! Terminology

Match each key term to the appropriate definition.

1. **LO 31.3** The provision of emergency CPR, stabilization of the patient, first aid, control of bleeding, and/or the treatment of shock.
2. **LO 31.3** A company designated by the state or region to act as the fiscal intermediary for all DME claims.
3. **LO 31.3** By way of anything other than the gastrointestinal tract, such as intravenous, intramuscular, intramedullary, or subcutaneous.
4. **LO 31.4** An indication that more detailed information is not available from the physician's notes.
5. **LO 31.1** A device used to correct or improve an orthopedic concern.
6. **LO 31.3** Life-sustaining, emergency care is provided, such as airway management, defibrillation, and/or the administration of drugs.
7. **LO 31.3** Apparatus and tools that help individuals accommodate physical frailties, provide pharmaceuticals, and provide other assistance that will last for a long time and/or be used to assist multiple patients over time.
8. **LO 31.3** Within, or by way of, the gastrointestinal tract.
9. **LO 31.1** Fabricated artificial replacement for a damaged or missing part of the body.
10. **LO 31.3** The use of a chemical compound that binds with metal in the body so that the metal will lose its toxic effect. It might be done when a metal disc or prosthetic is implanted in a patient, eliminating adverse reactions to the metal itself as a foreign body.
11. **LO 31.3** Continuous care provided by one or more health professionals in an appropriate specialty area, such as respiratory care or cardiovascular care, or by a paramedic with additional training.

A. Advanced Life Support (ALS)
B. Basic Life Support (BLS)
C. Chelation Therapy
D. Durable Medical Equipment (DME)
E. Durable Medical Equipment Regional Carrier (DMERC)
F. Enteral
G. Not Otherwise Specified (NOS)
H. Orthotic
I. Parenteral
J. Prosthetic
K. Specialty Care Transport

Let's Check It! Concepts

Choose the most appropriate answer for each of the following questions.

1. **LO 31.4** The symbol of a circle with a line through it ⃠ means
   - **a.** a new code.
   - **b.** a revised code.
   - **c.** a code exempt from a particular modifier.
   - **d.** a service not covered under the skilled nursing facility payment system.
2. **LO 31.4** The box with a check mark in it ☑ indicates a code description that
   - **a.** includes a quantity measurement.
   - **b.** is always covered by Medicare.
   - **c.** is approved for reimbursement at a higher rate.
   - **d.** includes refills.
3. **LO 31.3** The J codes are used to bill insurance carriers for
   - **a.** prescription drugs patients get at the drugstore.
   - **b.** drugs administered by a health care professional.
   - **c.** nothing. They are deleted codes.
   - **d.** items not accepted by Medicaid in any state for any reason.
4. **LO 31.1** HCPCS Level II codes are used, most often, to report all except
   - **a.** drugs used for treatment of a patient.
   - **b.** equipment provided to a patient.
   - **c.** anesthesia administered by an anesthesiologist.
   - **d.** dental services.
5. **LO 31.3** The acronym DME stands for
   - **a.** determination of medical effectiveness.
   - **b.** durable medical equipment.
   - **c.** donated medical equipment.
   - **d.** diluted medicine equivalent.
6. **LO 31.1** HCPCS Level II codes are presented as
   - **a.** five numbers.
   - **b.** one letter followed by four numbers.
   - **c.** four numbers followed by one letter.
   - **d.** five letters.
7. **LO 31.1** HCPCS is an acronym that stands for
   - **a.** Health Care Professional Classification Systems.
   - **b.** Health and Caretaker Providers Coding Series.
   - **c.** Home Care Providers Coding System.
   - **d.** Healthcare Common Procedure Coding System.
8. **LO 31.3** The code D1110 is an example of a
   - **a.** HCPCS Level I code, also known as a CPT code.
   - **b.** HCPCS Level II code.
   - **c.** HCPCS Level III code.
   - **d.** HCPCS Level IV code.
9. **LO 31.3** The D0000–D9999 codes are created and maintained by the
   - **a.** American Medical Association.
   - **b.** American Dental Association.
   - **c.** Centers for Medicare and Medicaid Services.
   - **d.** Department of Health and Human Services.
10. **LO 31.2** You can look up key words in the HCPCS Alphabetic Index by using which of the following?
    - **a.** Generic name of the drug.
    - **b.** Medical supply item.
    - **c.** Orthotic.
    - **d.** All of these.
11. **LO 31.3** The E codes shown in the HCPCS Level II book are
    - **a.** an expansion of the E codes in the ICD-10-CM book.
    - **b.** used to identify DME provided to a patient.
    - **c.** not accepted by Medicaid.
    - **d.** always first listed on a claim form.
12. **LO 31.3** An example of DME is
    - **a.** an injection of Demerol.
    - **b.** a prosthetic ankle.
    - **c.** a three-prong cane.
    - **d.** home infusion therapy.

13. **LO 31.4** A deleted code in the HCPCS Level II book means
    - **a.** the procedure is obsolete.
    - **b.** the service is no longer reimbursable.
    - **c.** the code is reinstated.
    - **d.** the code is no longer available to represent the service or item.

14. **LO 31.3** Alcohol intervention treatment might be coded in the range
    - **a.** H0001-H2037
    - **b.** H5000-H9999
    - **c.** F1000-F9999
    - **d.** G0000-G9999

15. **LO 31.4** A code with a capital "A" or A next to it means that
    - **a.** a drug was administered intravenously.
    - **b.** the machine can only be used for infusion therapy.
    - **c.** the service is limited to a specific age group.
    - **d.** the equipment is illegal in some states.

Let's Check It! Symbols and Notations

Part I

Match each HCPCS Level II symbol to the appropriate HCPCS Level II description

1. **LO 31.4** The female symbol.
2. **LO 31.4** Indicates that it is the first year that the code is included in this code set.
3. **LO 31.4** Lets you know that the code's description has been changed or adjusted since last year or that a rule or guideline regarding the code has changed.
4. **LO 31.4** Means that the code has been deleted and may no longer be used.
5. **LO 31.4** Identifies that the code had been deleted but now has been restored (reinstated).
6. **LO 31.4** Reminds you that the code describes maternity procedures, services, and equipment that are performed or used on a pregnant female 12–55 years of age.
7. **LO 31.4** The male symbol.
8. **LO 31.4** Identifies a specific quantity of material or supply. It is a reminder for you to check the detail in the notes and report the code not only for the item it represents but for the amount as well.
9. **LO 31.4** Highlights the fact that a code is used only for procedures, services, and equipment that are performed or used on a patient of a certain age group.
10. **LO 31.4** Identifies a code that is not covered under the skilled nursing facility (SNF) prospective payment system (PPS).

- **A.** ●
- **B.** ▲
- **C.** ○
- **D.** ⊘
- **E.** ☑
- **F.** ♂
- **G.** ♀
- **H.** 🅰
- **I.** Ⓜ
- **J.** ~~Z1111~~

Part II

Match each HCPCS Level II notation to the appropriate notation description.

1. **LO 31.4** This notation cross-references this code with another code that may be similar in description. The notation serves as a reminder for you to double-check that you are using the most accurate code.
2. **LO 31.4** Refers you to a CPT code for a description that is potentially better and may be more specific for reporting what was actually done or given to the patient.
3. **LO 31.4** When one code is to be reported with other codes, a notation to "Report in addition to" (a particular code) will identify those circumstances. It not only tells you the circumstances but also tells you which code to use.
4. **LO 31.4** This notation directs you to always report this code with a code for another specific procedure.

- **A.** Always report concurrent to the *xxx* procedure
- **B.** *See also code . . .*
- **C.** Clarifications of coverage
- **D.** *Report in addition to code . . .*
- **E.** *See code(s): . . .*

5. **LO 31.4** This notation indicates when to use or not use the code.
6. **LO 31.4** Serves as a warning to you to make certain that there is no better or more specific code in either the CPT or elsewhere in this HCPCS Level II book that correctly reports the services or procedures performed.
7. **LO 31.4** This notation warns that you need to go back and double-check the provider's notes carefully. If this is what was actually done, then be certain to attach documentation explaining why that method was used instead of the newer technique because it is surely going to be questioned.
8. **LO 31.4** Warns you of circumstances when you are not permitted to use a code.
9. **LO 31.4** Provides you with alternative names, brand names, and other terms that are also represented by the code's description.
10. **LO 31.4** This notation giving you information about coverage, particularly Medicare and Medicaid coverage.
11. **LO 31.4** Warns you up-front that you should include the proper documentation along with the claim the first time you submit it, rather than wait to be asked by the third-party payer, which would delay payment.

F. Determine if an alternative HCPCS Level II or a CPT code better describes . . .
G. *Use this code for . . .*
H. Pertinent documentation to evaluate medical appropriateness should be . . .
I. Do not use this code to report . . .
J. Medicare covers . . .
K. *Code with caution*

Let's Check It! Rules and Regulations

Please answer the following questions from the knowledge you have gained after reading this chapter.

1. **LO 31.1** List four HCPCS Level II codes specific to aspects for health care services.
2. **LO 31.1** Do all insurance carriers accept HCPCS Level II codes? What is the responsibility of the coding specialist with regards to billing third-party payers?
3. **LO 31.2** List five ways to look up the key words after abstracting them from the provider's notes.
4. **LO 31.3** What HCPCS Level II codes represent Procedures and Professional Services (Temporary)?
5. **LO 31.4** What does the notation "*Use this code for . . .*" indicate?

YOU CODE IT! Basics

First, identify the HCPCS Level II main term in the following statements; then code the procedure or service.

Example: Airlift by helicopter, one-way:

a. main term: *Ambulance* **b.** procedure: *A0431*

Example: A 5 mL injection, IM, of Robaxin:

a. main term: *Robaxin* **b.** procedure: *J2800*

1. A bottle of 50 blood glucose reagent strips:
   a. main term:______ **b.** procedure:______
2. Johannsen Health Care delivered 1000 mL of distilled water for use with nebulizer:
   a. main term:______ **b.** procedure:______
3. Youth-sized disposable incontinence brief, one:
   a. main term:______ **b.** procedure:______
4. Arterial blood tubing:
   a. main term:______ **b.** procedure:______
5. Neonate ambulance transport, one-way, base rate:
   a. main term:______ **b.** procedure:______
6. Ambulance ride with oxygen administered along with other advanced life support (ALS) services:
   a. main term:______ **b.** procedure:______
7. Nonemergency transportation by stretcher van:
   a. main term:______ **b.** procedure:______
8. A 200-mg injection IM of chloroquine hydrochloride:
   a. main term:______ **b.** procedure:______
9. An injection SC of 30 mg of codeine phosphate:
   a. main term:______ **b.** procedure:______
10. Dr. Longwell ordered Fosphenytoin, with an initial dose of 50 mg:
    a. main term:______ **b.** procedure:______

(continued)

11. A 25-mg injection of lepirudin:
    a. main term:______ b. procedure:______
12. A seat attachment for a Starke's walker:
    a. main term:______ b. procedure:______
13. One heel protector:
    a. main term:______ b. procedure:______
14. Portable noninvasive ventilator:
    a. main term:______ b. procedure:______
15. Prostate cancer screening, antigen test:
    a. main term:______ b. procedure:______

YOU CODE IT! Practice

Using the techniques described in this chapter, carefully read through the case studies and find the most accurate HCPCS Level II code(s) and modifier(s) if appropriate for each case study.

NOTE: All insurance carriers and third-party payers for the patients accept HCPCS Level II codes and modifiers.

1. Daisha Kurucz, a 23-year-old female, has severe asthma. Dr. Benton ordered a nebulizer, with compressor, for her to use at home. Code for the home health agency that supplied the equipment.
2. Daniel Hair, a 56-year-old male with end-stage renal disease (ESRD), was fitted for a reciprocating peritoneal dialysis system. Code the supply of the equipment.
3. Due to his condition, Daniel Hair (previous case study) had an unscheduled dialysis treatment at the nearest hospital outpatient department; this hospital is not certified as an ESRD facility.
4. Muddy Hambaugh, a 27-year-old female with a history of bipolar disorder, was given an injection IM of Thorazine, 45 mg. Code for the drug.
5. Allen Jeter, a 48-year-old male, was being prepared for his kidney transplant. The nurse administered 100 mg of Zenapax, IV, parenteral. Code the drug.
6. After Allen Jeter (previous case study) received his kidney transplant, the nurse gave him an oral dose of 250 mg of CellCept (mycophenolate mofetil) in the hospital. Code the drug.
7. Shirley Loveichelle, an 82-year-old female, was having trouble eating for such a long period of time that she was exhibiting signs of malnutrition. Therefore, Dr. Milliner ordered enteral formula (Ensure) to be administered through a feeding tube at 500 calories per day. Code for the nutritional supplement only.
8. Keith Pawley, a 34-year-old male, came to see Dr. Praylow, his dentist, for an implant-supported porcelain crown on his back tooth.
9. Johnette Potash, a 13-year-old female, lost her maxillary retainer at camp. She is at Dr. Rivera's office to get a replacement.
10. Clifton Beckman, a 15-year-old male, sat in poison ivy while camping in the woods. Dr. Gregg prescribed a portable sitz bath for him to use at home.
11. Roberta Henthorne, a 52-year-old female, was recuperating from surgery to repair a complex fracture of her tibia and a compound fracture of her ankle. To help her be more comfortable, Dr. Locklear ordered a fixed-height hospital bed, without side rails and with a mattress, for her to use at home. Code for the DME only.
12. Kenneth Paynter, a 68-year-old male, was on complete bed rest while recuperating from surgery. Because his skin was very sensitive, he was particularly prone to decubitus ulcers. Dr. Roche prescribed a lamb's wool sheepskin pad to help prevent any ulcers from forming.
13. Dr. Sloan provided a complete set of dentures, maxillary and mandibular, for Cheryl Delaney.
14. Dennis Lederrick, a 39-year-old male, had surgery on his left foot. To enable him to take a shower safely, Dr. Willrodt gave him a tub stool to sit on.
15. Scott Zamcho came home from serving in the Marines a double amputee, having had both legs damaged badly in a suicide bomber's attack. Dr. Lovell supplied him with an amputee wheelchair, desk height, with detachable arms and no footrests or leg rests.

(continued)

YOU CODE IT! Application

On the following pages, you will see physicians' notes documenting encounters with patients at our textbook's health care facility, Prader, Bracker, & Associates. Carefully read through the notes, and find the best code or codes from the HCPCS Level II book for each of the cases.

NOTE: All insurance carriers and third-party payers for the patients accept HCPCS Level II codes and modifiers.

PRADER, BRACKER, & ASSOCIATES

A Complete Health Care Facility

159 Healthcare Way • SOMEWHERE, FL 32811 • 407-555-6789

PATIENT: ADDLER, ANNETTE

ACCOUNT/EHR #: ADDLAN001

Representative: Elizabeth Alexander

Attending Physician: Renee O. Bracker, MD

The Pt is a 27-year-old female who recently returned from working in Africa. She was diagnosed with variola and has been on a gastric feeding tube to increase her fluids, electrolytes, and calories because the pharyngeal lesions make swallowing difficult. Nasogastric tubing without a stylet was supplied for this patient.

A: Variola

P: Service number given to caregiver

Elizabeth Alexander

Determine the best, most appropriate HCPCS Level II code(s).

BRACKER DURABLE MEDICAL EQUIPMENT

A Complete Health Care Facility

159 Healthcare Way • SOMEWHERE, FL 32811 • 407-555-6789

PATIENT: CARLYLE, JOY

ACCOUNT/EHR #: CARJAY001

Representative Technician: LuAnn Hallmark

Attending Physician: Renee O. Bracker, MD

The Pt is a 72-year-old female diagnosed with adult kyphosis caused by poor posture. Dr. Bracker prescribed bed rest on a firm mattress with pelvic traction attached to the footboard. At 5:00 p.m. on this date, I delivered a bed board and the traction frame to Ms. Carlyle's home. I placed the bed board underneath the existing mattress in order to create a firm surface upon which the patient could sleep. I then attached the traction frame to the footboard of the existing bed. I spent 45 minutes instructing the patient, her family, and caretaker on the proper use of the equipment, how to properly get into and out of the traction, and the expected sensations.

A: Adult kyphosis

P: Follow up in 2 weeks to see if patient has any questions or concerns.

LuAnn Hallmark

Determine the best, most appropriate HCPCS Level II code(s).

(continued)

PRADER ONCOLOGY

A Complete Health Care Facility

159 Healthcare Way • SOMEWHERE, FL 32811 • 407-555-6789

PATIENT: BALMORAL, MARK

ACCOUNT/EHR #: BALMAR001

Attending Physician: Oscar R. Prader, MD

Pt is a 61-year-old male with metastatic testicular tumors. He comes in today for the administration of cisplatin solution, IV, 20 mg. It is the first of five treatments he will receive this week.

IV infusion given over 7 hours.

Patient reports mild nausea. Refuses any pharmaceutical treatment for that side effect of this treatment.

Patient discharged at 4:15 p.m.

Determine the best, most appropriate HCPCS Level II code(s).

VICTORS AMBULANCE SERVICE

159 Healthcare Way • SOMEWHERE, FL 32811 • 407-555-6789

PATIENT: CUTTER, WILIMENA

ACCOUNT/EHR #: CUTTWI001

Attending Physician: Renee O. Bracker, MD

EMT/Attendant: Lance H. Reynoso, EMT

Pt is a 78-year-old female who appears to have suffered a myocardial infarction in her nursing home's day room. Pt complained of numbness and tingling in the left arm and sharp pains in her chest. EKG showed abnormal activity. Pulse and respiration were abnormal.

While preparing the patient for transport, she went into arrest. Defibrillator restored heartbeat. ALS1-emergency services were administered, and patient was transported immediately to Barton Hospital.

Routine disposable supplies were used.

Ambulance service was provided under arrangement by a provider of services.

Total Mileage: 4.5

Lance H. Reynoso, EMT

Determine the best, most appropriate HCPCS Level II code(s).

PRADER, BRACKER, & ASSOCIATES

A Complete Health Care Facility

159 Healthcare Way • SOMEWHERE, FL 32811 • 407-555-6789

PATIENT: VANCE, TOMIKA

ACCOUNT/EHR #: VANTOM001

Attending Physician: Salvatore L. Bloome, MD

Indications: Ulcerative enterocolitis

Procedure: Colonoscopy

Instrument: Olympus video colonoscope CF 100L

Anesthesia: Versed 4 mg; Demerol 75 mg MAC < 30 min

(continued)

HISTORY: This is a 71-year-old female admitted to the ambulatory surgical center for a colonoscopy. Due to her chronic enterocolitis, she is at high risk for a malignancy of the colon, and, therefore, this screening is being done. She has been informed of the nature of the procedure, the risks, and the consequences, as well as told of alternative procedures. She consents to the procedure.

PROCEDURE: The patient is placed in the left lateral decubitus position. The rectal exam reveals normal sphincter tone and no masses. A colonoscope is introduced into the rectum and advanced to the distal sigmoid colon. Due to a marked fixation and severe angulation of the rectosigmoid colon, the scope could not be advanced any further and the procedure was aborted. On withdrawal, no masses or polyps are noted, and the mucosa is normal throughout. Retroflexion in the rectal vault is unremarkable.

DISPOSITION: The patient tolerated the procedure and was discharged from the minor operating department in satisfactory condition.

IMPRESSIONS: Normal colonoscopy, only to the distal sigmoid colon

PLAN: Strong recommendation for a barium enema

Salvatore L. Bloome, MD

Determine the best, most appropriate HCPCS Level II code(s).

32

DMEPOS and Transportation Capstone

Learning Outcomes

After completing this chapter, the student should be able to:

LO 32.1 Determine the correct codes for these case studies using the HCPCS Level II code set.

The health care team extends beyond the physician's office or hospital. Home care services are on the increase as a greater number of patients prefer care in their residences, whenever possible. The provision of these services enables patients greater comfort and lowers costs, especially for those with chronic conditions.

In addition, transportation of patients should be recorded and reported for reimbursement purposes, as well as the provision of orthotics and prosthetics. And, as you learned in previous chapters about CPT coding, the provision of medication (drugs) by a health care professional also must be recorded and reimbursed.

For each of the following case studies, read through the documentation and determine

- What medical supply, equipment, or other item or service was provided to this patient. Do not code the procedure.
- Whether any modifiers are necessary, and, if so, which modifiers and in what order.
- Whether more than one code is required, and, if so, the sequence in which to report the codes.

Remember, read carefully and completely.

CASE STUDY #1: RHONDA SYNCOWSKI

Rhonda Syncowski is a 64-year-old female with a long-standing history of a seizure disorder. She also has hypertension (high blood pressure) and chronic obstructive pulmonary disease (COPD). She is no stranger to the hospital because of her health issues. At home, she takes a number of medications, including three for her COPD and three—levetiracetam, lamotrigine, and valproate sodium—to help control seizures.

The patient went to see Dr. Bushera, her family physician, last week because she was wheezing and having trouble breathing. Dr. Bushera conducted a physical examination that yielded signs of an acute worsening of her COPD—including FEV1 of less than 50% predicted value plus respiratory failure.

PLAN: Orders written for flunisolide 160 mcg, b.i.d. via nebulizer; portable oxygen (gaseous) with 1-month supply. Follow up with physician in 3 weeks, or PRN.

Joshua Medical Supplies and Equipment was called by the patient to provide the equipment and medications to the patient's home. As per physician's orders:

1. Nebulizer with compressor
2. Flunisolide inhalation solution 1 mg
3. Portable oxygen system (gaseous), rental, cannula
4. Portable O_2 contents, gaseous, 1 unit

CASE STUDY #2: RYAN MCNAULTY

Ryan McNaulty, a 6-year-old male with a defect in bowel function, was hospitalized for severe constipation. He was given a dose of neostigmine methylsulfate 0.4 mg, IM. Code for the drug, one date of service, only.

CASE STUDY #3: NADIYA LONGSTEP

Nadiya Longstep was rescued from her apartment building, which was engulfed in a two-alarm fire. The firemen carried her out, and she was handed over to the EMTs, who immediately began to examine the burns on 45% of her body. She was having trouble breathing and was given oxygen. She lost consciousness. CPR was started immediately, followed by external defibrillation at 200 joules until normal sinus rhythm was reestablished. Orders came through to take her to the MacHill Burn Center unit of Mulford Hospital immediately.

CASE STUDY #4: SONIA GRASSO

Sonia Grasso, an 11-year-old female, was diagnosed with idiopathic adolescent scoliosis.

Joshua Medical Supplies and Equipment was referred by Dr. Karpel, her orthopedist, to provide a Milwaukee brace: cervical/thoracic/lumbar/sacral orthotic.

CASE STUDY #5: DANIEL BISHOP

Daniel Bishop, an 18-year-old male, was in an MVA and subsequently diagnosed with whiplash, resulting in pain in C2–C4. Dr. Samman recommended traction for his cervical region, which he could attach to the headboard of his bed at home. Dr. Samman told Daniel to spend at least 5 hours each night in the traction device for 3 weeks. Follow-up appointment in 2 weeks.

CASE STUDY #6: MALIK HUMISTON

Malik Humiston, a 16-year-old male, suffered a displaced (comminuted) fracture of the right tibial shaft during his high school football game. Dr. Peterson prescribed articulating, spring-assisted underarm crutches for him upon postsurgical discharge. Joshua Medical Supplies and Equipment provided him with a pair and spent approximately 30 minutes fitting him and teaching him how to use them properly.

CASE STUDY #7: ZIVAH MASTRIANI

Zivah Mastriani, a 41-year-old female, was diagnosed with type 2 diabetes mellitus, and Dr. Ross wrote a prescription for her to obtain a home glucose disposable monitor. Zivah brought the order to Roxone Home Medical Supplies, where a monitor and test strips were provided. Harold Carter spent about 20 minutes teaching her how to use it correctly.

CASE STUDY #8: VICTOR JEFFRIES

Victor Jeffries, a 71-year-old male, weighs 320 pounds and is currently bedridden due to a fractured hip. In an effort to prevent any pressure ulcers or decubitus ulcer development, Dr. Abreen ordered an air pressure mattress pad for his bed at home.

CASE STUDY #9: ANNA CHENG

Anna Cheng, an 83-year-old female, has been exhibiting dysphagia (problems swallowing), resulting in her no longer wanting to eat. Dr. Baldwin inserted a standard gastrostomy/jejunostomy tube to enable enteral nutrition for 10 days.

CASE STUDY #10: CECIL DENOSO

Cecil Denoso, a 27-year-old male, was admitted to the Masters Behavioral Health Center due to his current manic state. Dr. Levine ordered Haloperidol 5 mg IM t.i.d. Code for the drug, one date of service, only.

CASE STUDY #11: COURTNEE CALLAHAN

SUBJECTIVE FINDINGS: This patient is a 55-year-old white female with pain in her lumbosacral spine, extending into her buttocks bilaterally. She describes the pain as being sharp and sometimes intense. She states it diminishes to an achy feeling. She rates its intensity at 10/10 at its worst. Normally, she states it is 6–7/10. She describes the pain as being ever-present, varying in intensity, increasing with activities and decreasing with rest. She is using pain medications currently and is able to sleep through the night.

HISTORY: This patient initially injured her back by catching a falling bookcase. She had immediate pain that was disabling. The pain was resolved with occasional recurrence. She sought intervention last year from doctors, who diagnosed degenerative disc disease and arthritis. She had a course of physical therapy with some resolution, but recurrence of pain occurred in June secondary to bending over while washing her hands. She was referred here.

OBJECTIVE FINDINGS:

Observation: This patient appears as a normally developed white female of stated age. She reports moving with forward flexed posture and an occasional antalgic gait on the right when the pain is increasing. She currently postures and moves normally.

Palpation: Positive over L5 and S1 and paravertebral muscles at that same level.

Lumbosacral range of motion: Forward flexion 35 degrees with pain at the end of range. Right side bending 30 degrees with pain at the end of range. Left side bending 35 degrees. Extension 0 degree with pain at the end of range.

Resisted motion: Positive in all directions

DTRs: Hyperreflexive bilaterally

Lasègue's sign: Positive at 25 degrees bilaterally

Cram test: Positive at 25 degrees bilaterally

Cervical range of motion:

1. Right side bending: Within normal limits, painful
2. Left side bending: Within normal limits
3. Forward flexion: 45 degrees with pain at the end of range
4. Extension: Within normal limits

Radiculopathy: Positive with pain down the left arm and occasional tingling and numbness

TREATMENT PLAN: We would like to see the patient three times per week to initiate exercises and modalities to decrease pain and increase range of motion and function.

GOALS: The purpose of physical therapy intervention is to

1. Increase range of motion to normal limits.
2. Decrease pain to zero.
3. Increase strength and function to normal.

RECOMMENDATION: I discussed with the patient the benefit of using a transcutaneous electrical nerve stimulation device on her lumbar area. I suggested that she rent the unit from us to give her the opportunity to try it out and see if it helps to reduce pain at L5–S1. She agreed, and we provided her with a 2-lead unit. Instructions were for her to use it every day, 15 minutes, b.i.d., first thing in the morning after getting out of bed and immediately prior to bed. Richard Penuto, my associate, taught her how to apply the leads and use the machine. Appointment made for her to return in 2 weeks for evaluation.

Code for the provision of the transcutaneous electrical nerve stimulation device only.

CASE STUDY #12: ARTHUR PAIGE

HISTORY OF PRESENT ILLNESS: This patient is a 43-year-old male with pain in his cervical spine. He states that the pain extends over the entire posterior neck and into the right shoulder, including the upper trapezius. He rates that at a level of 7–8 on a scale of 10 currently. He states that at its least it is 3–4 on a scale of 10. The patient is using a cervical collar with good results. He also uses ibuprofen at night.

This patient was involved in an MVA 5 years ago resulting in a fracture of C5. He had manipulation approximately 3 years ago resulting in pain for approximately 5 months. He had neck pain develop again approximately 18 months ago resulting in bilateral shoulder surgery. The pain has remained the same, although the numbness is better for approximately 1 year. He currently has complaints of a radial distribution into his left hand, which caused him enough concern to seek intervention from Dr. Furmenn. The patient was then referred here.

PHYSICAL EXAMINATION:

Observation: This patient is a normally developed male of stated age. He gaits normally without apparent guarding or splinting.

Palpation: Positive over the right upper trapezius

Range of motion: Right rotation is 50 degrees, left rotation is 45 degrees, right side bending 30 degrees with pain at the end of range, left side bending 30 degrees, forward flexion 35 degrees, and extension 25 degrees.

Resisted motion: Negative

Radiculopathy: Positive in the left shoulder extending down to the left hand into his thumb and digits 2 and 3.

Sensation: Some decreased sensation over the left hand to pinprick, particularly over the radial digits.

TREATMENT PLAN: We would like to see the patient three times per week as per instructions for cervical traction and exercises.

GOALS: The purpose of physical therapy intervention is to

1. Increase range of motion to normal limits.
2. Increase pain-free function to normal.
3. Decrease pain generally to zero.

RECOMMENDATION: To encourage healing, I discussed with the patient using traction equipment at home, for beneficial outcomes in between appointments. Petra Zoztrev, our trainer, worked with Arthur to show him how to set up the equipment, put it on, and take it off. Instructions for use are every night to sleep in the equipment until we determine he has made sufficient progress. I also gave him a sheet with exercises—diagrammed out, for him to do at home also. Petra helped him carry the box out to his car.

Code for the provision of the traction equipment only.

CASE STUDY #13: WILLETTA FREEMAN

HISTORY: The patient is a 23-year-old black female professional athlete who, last month, fell on her left elbow while reaching for a ball during a tennis game, sustaining a left distal humerus fracture. The patient states the following day she had surgery to stabilize the fracture. The patient was unsure if the surgery performed was for plates and screws.

PAST MEDICAL HISTORY: The patient fractured her right wrist approximately a year ago.

CHIEF COMPLAINT: The patient reports left elbow pain, currently 8/10, at best 7/10, and at worst 10/10. The patient states she is taking her pain medications, which provide minimal relief but affect her performance on the court. The patient reports she does have numbness in the left upper extremity, along the ulnar nerve distribution. The patient states she does use some ice or heat; it provides minimal relief. The patient is left-hand dominant.

PHYSICAL EXAMINATION: Left elbow AROM 35–120 degrees. Left elbow PROM 30–135 degrees. Left shoulder AROM within normal limits. Left wrist AROM within functional limits. Left elbow strength 3–4/5. Left shoulder strength grossly 4/5. Left wrist strength grossly 4/5. Left grip strength is 30 pounds. Right grip strength is 55 pounds.

Palpation: The patient is tender to palpation in the posterolateral aspect of the left elbow. The incision is healed. No signs of infection. No swelling in the left elbow, no bruising.

(continued)

GOALS:

1. Increase left elbow AROM and PROM to within normal limits.
2. Increase left elbow strength to within normal limits.
3. Eliminate pain.
4. Independent with home exercise program.
5. Return function to normal.

TREATMENT PLAN: We would like to see the patient three times a week to initiate and advance range of motion, stretching, and strengthening program to left elbow; may use modalities as needed for pain control.

RECOMMENDATIONS: To ensure progress to help this patient recover more completely, I recommend a static progressive stretch elbow device with a range of motion adjustment for her use at home. I discussed a workout plan, using the equipment, with Willetta and her coach. They left with the device and instructions. Appointment is made for her to return in 1 week to begin regular treatment.

Code for the provision of the device only.

CASE STUDY #14: GARY ELLIOTT

SUBJECTIVE FINDINGS: The patient said that he slept well last night.

OBJECTIVE FINDINGS:

General: The patient is a well-developed, obese male in no apparent distress.

Vital signs: Temperature 98.6 degrees, pulse 72, respirations 18, and blood pressure 158/80.

HEENT: Head is normocephalic

Neck: Supple to palpation

Extremities: Examination of the extremities shows incision site to be healing well without any sign of infection or skin breakdown. Peripheral pulses are intact. Minimal edema in the left lower extremity. Homans sign is absent.

FUNCTIONAL STATUS: Functionally, the patient is able to demonstrate improvement with full range of motion, −5 to 80 degrees of flexion actively and 86 degrees passively. His functional gait has advanced 200 feet with the use of front-wheel walker with supervision. He is supervised level with his bedside commode transfers and contact guard assistance with shower chair transfers. He is modified independent level with his eating and set up with his grooming skills. He requires moderate assistance with lower body dressing.

IMPRESSION:

1. Polyarthritis
2. Left total knee arthroplasty
3. Status post coronary artery bypass graft
4. Chronic obstructive pulmonary disease

PLAN: We provided the patient with a Continuous Positive Airway Pressure (CPAP) machine with headgear and instructed both Gary and his wife on how to use it properly. Instructions are provided in writing. I emphasized the importance of using the CPAP machine every night. Continue with current treatment program. We will continue to monitor the patient's hypertension, which is still out of control.

Code for the provision of the CPAP machine with headgear.

CASE STUDY #15: PAULA BARKIN

Paula, a 4-year-old female, was referred for speech therapy by her school after discussion about parents' concerns over her difficulties pronouncing certain speech sounds. These irregular pronunciations were making it challenging for those outside her family to understand Paula when she spoke to them. Paula had suffered from hearing loss and had grommets inserted at age 3.

(continued)

An initial assessment was performed to look at her current speech profile and to provide information as to whether intervention was needed and, if so, what kind. Assessment results revealed that Paula had difficulties with the 't' and 'd' sounds and was replacing these with 'k' and 'g,' so 'letter' was 'lekker' and 'bed' was "beg." I explained to the parents that this is called "backing," whereby sounds that should be produced at the front of the mouth are produced at the back of the mouth instead. This is not a process found in typically developing speech and therefore would be targeted in therapy.

Paula also showed difficulties with other early developing sounds 's' and 'v.' These sounds that are produced with a long flow of air were being cut short so 'f' was 'p'—therefore, 'fish' was 'pish.' This process is called stopping, which is expected to have resolved by the age of 3 years and so was also targeted in therapy.

Paula was set up for individual therapy sessions at her home, by me, for 30 minutes each visit. The sessions will be focused on developing Paula's awareness and production of the above speech sounds and processes. For each sound, visual materials including a picture card with the grapheme and cued articulation (similar to a gesture/sign) are used to help Paula learn them. Before asking Paula to produce any of the sounds she had difficulties with, Paula was provided with many opportunities to hear these sounds being produced correctly (this is known as auditory bombardment). Paula then completed tasks in which she had to discriminate between a target sound, e.g., 't,' and the sound that she replaced it with, e.g., 'k,' to ensure she could tell the two apart.

Therapy will then move to production. How each of the sounds is produced in the mouth will be explained to Paula using words accompanied by diagrams. The first step is to get Paula to try to produce her new sounds in isolation (e.g., 't') and then combined with a vowel (e.g., 'tee'). The next steps are to practice new sounds at the start of words (e.g., 'tiger'), followed by at the end of words (e.g., 'boat') and then in the middle of words (e.g., 'bottle') and finally onto sentences. These will be incorporated into fun games. Parents will be given activities to practice in between weekly sessions; in addition, advice on how to support Paula's new speech sounds in natural conversations will also be provided. For example, if Paula made an error with one of her new speech sounds, others will be able to provide her with options, e.g., is it a 'kiger' or a 'tiger,' emphasizing the correct sound.

PLAN: In addition to the 30-minute sessions at her home, I supply software with 30 minutes of prerecorded sounds and messages so the parents can work with her in between our sessions.

Code for the one 30-minute home visit by the speech-language pathologist + the speech software.

PART V

INPATIENT (HOSPITAL) REPORTING

Reporting inpatient (hospital) and outpatient encounters requires the same foundational knowledge and skill: anatomy, physiology, and medical terminology. Part V of this text provides you with the next layer of your learning about coding health care.

In these chapters, you will learn how to employ ICD-10-PCS (International Classification of Diseases-10th revision-Procedure Coding System), *the code set used to report the procedures, services, and treatments provided by the* acute care facility (hospital) *to inpatients (those who have been admitted).*

33

Introduction to ICD-10-PCS

Key Terms

Approach
Axis of Classification
Body Part
Body System
Device
Qualifier
Root Operation Term

Learning Outcomes

After completing this chapter, the student should be able to:

LO 33.1 Explain the purpose of ICD-10-PCS codes.
LO 33.2 Identify the structure of ICD-10-PCS codes.
LO 33.3 Recognize the proper ways to use the Alphabetic Index and Tables in ICD-10-PCS.
LO 33.4 Discern the general conventions for using ICD-10-PCS.
LO 33.5 Determine the principal ICD-10-PCS code and proper sequencing for multiple procedure codes.

STOP! **Remember, you need to follow along in your ICD-10-PCS code book for an optimal learning experience.**

33.1 The Purpose of ICD-10-PCS

The *International Classification of Diseases-10th revision-Procedure Coding System* (ICD-10-PCS) was implemented in the United States on October 1, 2015, for the reporting of procedures, services, and treatments provided to a patient who has been admitted into an inpatient facility.

Earlier in **Part III** of this book, you learned how to use the CPT code set to report physician's services in any facility. And you learned that CPT codes are also used to report services provided by an outpatient facility, during the care of the patient. Now, you will learn to use the ICD-10-PCS code set to report the inpatient facility's participation in providing these services.

When patients are provided with room and food, in addition to medical care, and stay overnight in the facility, they are considered "inpatients." This means that acute care hospitals, as well as skilled nursing facilities, long-term care facilities, and short-term care facilities, may use this code set.

The structure of this code set is very different, as you will learn in this and the next few chapters. Rather than looking up the code and determining the correct choice from a list, you will build the code from the details shown in the tables of ICD-10-PCS (see **Figure 33-1**). Each table contains details about procedures pertaining to that particular type of procedure and that particular body system and body part.

33.2 The Structure of ICD-10-PCS Codes

The main purpose of creating the *International Classification of Diseases-10th Revision-Procedure Coding System* (ICD-10-PCS) was to give you, the professional coder, an easier way to determine the best, most accurate, and most specific code to report procedures, services, and treatments provided to an inpatient (a patient admitted to an acute care hospital or other inpatient facility). That purpose has led to a new structure for the codes. In this code set, you will actually build the code.

CODING BITES

ICD-10-PCS codes may include any letter of the alphabet *except* the letters *O* and *I*. This is done to avoid any confusion between the letter *O* and the number 0 (zero), as well as any mix-up between the letter *I* and the number 1 (one).

Section	**0**	Medical and Surgical	
Body System	**2**	Heart and Great Vessels	
Operation	**4**	Creation: Putting in or on biological or synthetic material to form a new body part that to the extent possible replicates the anatomic structure or function of an absent body part	
Body Part Character 4	*Approach Character 5*	*Device Character 6*	*Qualifier Character 7*
F Aortic Valve	**0** Open	**7** Autologous Tissue Substitute **8** Zooplastic Tissue **J** Synthetic Substitute **K** Nonautologous Tissue Substitute	**J** Truncal Valve
G Mitral Valve **J** Tricuspid Valve	**0** Open	**7** Autologous Tissue **8** Zooplastic Tissue **J** Synthetic Substitute **K** Nonautologous Tissue Substitute	**2** Common Atrioventricular Valve

FIGURE 33-1 An example from the Medical and Surgical Tables of 2026 ICD-10-PCS

Seven Characters

Every ICD-10-PCS code is made up of seven (7) alphanumeric characters, and each character position has its own specific meaning–a specific piece of information relating to the procedure, service, or treatment provided. You must read carefully because each section has its own particular use for the character. As always, in coding, you can never assume!

Let's begin with the first, and largest, section of the ICD-10-PCS code set . . . ***Medical and Surgical*** section, just as an example. You will learn all the details about this and all of the other code set sections in the chapters that follow this one. In this section, the seven characters describe, in order, the:

1. *Section* of the ICD-10-PCS code set.
2. *Body system* upon which the procedure or service was performed.
3. *Root operation*, which explains the category or type of procedure.
4. *Body part*, which identifies the specific anatomical site involved in the procedure.
5. *Approach*, which reports which method was used to perform the service or treatment.
6. *Device*, which reports, when applicable, the type of device involved in the service or procedure.
7. *Qualifier*, which adds any additional detail.

Let's go through each of these character positions, one by one, to understand what each represents. To help illustrate these data points, we are going to use a snippet from an operative report and build the code as an ongoing example:

Laparoscopic bypass, radial vein to ulnar vein, left, using autologous tissue substitute

Using this short statement as an example to work with, you are going to build the ICD-10-PCS code as you make your way through this chapter. You will learn how each character reports a part of the whole story about the specific procedure or service. This should then help you understand how to build a code on your own.

Section (First Character)

The first character in the seven-character sequence identifies the section of the ICD-10-PCS code set in which the procedure is listed. There are 17 section titles:

0 Medical and Surgical

1 Obstetrics

2 Placement

3 Administration

4 Measurement and Monitoring

5 Extracorporeal or Systemic Assistance and Performance

6 Extracorporeal or Systemic Therapies

7 Osteopathic

8 Other Procedures

9 Chiropractic

B Imaging

C Nuclear Medicine

D Radiation Therapy

F Physical Rehabilitation and Diagnostic Audiology

G Mental Health

H Substance Abuse Treatment

X New Technology

EXAMPLES

An ankle x-ray is an imaging procedure—Section **B**

A breech extraction is an obstetrics procedure—Section **1**

An amputation is a surgical procedure—Section **0**

CODING BITES

Using our example . . . ***Laparoscopic bypass***

You can tell from the description that this is a surgical procedure, so this code is reported from within the **Medical and Surgical** section of ICD-10-PCS.

First character = 0

0 Medical and Surgical

Body System (Second Character)

The second character of the code reports the **body system** upon which the procedure, service, or treatment was performed. The classes you took in anatomy will be very important to your accuracy in determining the correct character to report. Plus, you need to pay careful attention due to greater specificity than typically defined by standard anatomy classifications. There are 31 body systems used for clarification and identification by the second character of codes reporting a medical or surgical procedure or service:

Body System
The physiological system, or anatomical region, upon which the procedure was performed.

0 Central Nervous System and Cranial Nerves

1 Peripheral Nervous System

2 Heart and Great Vessels

3 Upper Arteries

4 Lower Arteries

5 Upper Veins

6 Lower Veins

7 Lymphatic and Hemic Systems

8 Eye

9 Ear, Nose, Sinus

B Respiratory System

C Mouth and Throat

D Gastrointestinal System

F Hepatobiliary System and Pancreas

G Endocrine System

H Skin and Breast

J Subcutaneous Tissue and Fascia

K Muscles

L Tendons

M Bursae and Ligaments

N Head and Facial Bones

P Upper Bones

Q Lower Bones

R Upper Joints

S Lower Joints

T Urinary System

U Female Reproductive System

V Male Reproductive System

W Anatomical Regions, General

X Anatomical Regions, Upper Extremities

Y Anatomical Regions, Lower Extremities

The other sections of the code set describe the body systems that are appropriate to those services. Take a look at **Table 33-1**, The Other Sections of ICD-10-PCS and Their Body Systems.

TABLE 33-1 The Other Sections of ICD-10-PCS and Their Body Systems

SECTION	BODY SYSTEM(S)
1 Obstetrics	**0** Pregnancy
2 Placement	**W** Anatomical Regions **Y** Anatomical Orifices
3 Administration	**0** Circulatory **C** Indwelling Device **E** Physiological Systems & Anatomical Regions
4 Measurement and Monitoring	**A** Physiological Systems **B** Physiological Devices
5 Extracorporeal or Systemic Assistance and Performance	**A** Physiological Systems
6 Extracorporeal or Systemic Therapies	**A** Physiological Systems
7 Osteopathic	**W** Anatomical Regions
8 Other Procedures	**C** Indwelling Device **E** Physiological Systems & Anatomical Regions
9 Chiropractic	**W** Anatomical Regions
B Imaging	[See *Medical and Surgical* body systems]
C Nuclear Medicine	[See *Medical and Surgical* body systems]
D Radiation Therapy	[See *Medical and Surgical* body systems]
F Physical Rehabilitation and Diagnostic Audiology	**0** Rehabilitation* **1** Diagnostic Audiology
G Mental Health	**Z** None
H Substance Abuse	**Z** None
X New Technology	**0** Nervous System **2** Cardiovascular System **D** Gastrointestinal System **F** Hepatobiliary System and Pancreas **H** Skin, Subcutaneous Tissue, Fascia and Breast **K** Muscles, Tendons, Bursae and Ligaments **N** Bones **R** Joints **T** Urinary System **W** Anatomical Regions **X** Physiological Systems **Y** Extracorporeal

*The **Rehabilitation and Diagnostic Audiology** section identifies the body system with the fourth character rather than the second as with other sections. The same 31 body systems used for the **Medical and Surgical** section apply here, as well.

CODING BITES

Using our example . . . ***radial vein to ulnar vein***

Remember learning this in anatomy class? Don't worry if you don't; use that anatomy resource now. Then, you will know, for certain, that these veins are located in the arm (upper extremity). Therefore, your second character will report a procedure that was performed on the patient's *upper veins*.

First character = 0

Second character = 5

0 Medical and Surgical

5 Upper veins

Root Operation (Third Character)

The third character in the ICD-10-PCS code reports the **root operation term**—the central aspect of the procedure or service being provided. Just as you learned when reporting procedures using CPT, you are essentially looking for the term that describes WHAT the physician did for the patient. You can see that these terms are, for the most part, familiar to you. Notice that once again the ***Medical and Surgical*** section has 31 different root operations.

Root Operation Term
The category or classification of a particular procedure, service, or treatment.

0 Alteration

1 Bypass

2 Change

3 Control

4 Creation

5 Destruction

6 Detachment

7 Dilation

8 Division

9 Drainage

B Excision

C Extirpation

D Extraction

F Fragmentation

G Fusion

H Insertion

J Inspection

K Map

L Occlusion

M Reattachment

N Release

P Removal

Q Repair

R Replacement

S Reposition

T Resection

U Supplement

V Restriction

W Revision

X Transfer

Y Transplantation

This is a long list. But don't worry. You will learn about each of these root operation terms, and more used in other sections, in the upcoming chapters. Most importantly, they are in your code book, along with their descriptions. So, no memorization is required . . . just reading carefully and completely.

The other sections may use some of the same terms as the ***Medical and Surgical*** section in addition to some terms specific to their area. Try not to get overwhelmed by all these terms. You have time to learn about these procedures, look them up in a medical dictionary, and become familiar with them. And remember, they are always right there, at your fingertips, in the ICD-10-PCS code book.

CODING BITES

In ICD-10-PCS, the word *operation* has nothing to do with surgery.

CODING BITES

Using our example . . . ***bypass***

Yes, sometimes it really is this easy. The physician uses the same term for the procedure as the ICD-10-PCS code book does.

First character = 0

Second character = 5

Third character = 1

0 Medical and Surgical

5 Upper veins

1 Bypass

NOTE: They are not all this easy. More to help you interpret root operation terms in the upcoming chapters.

Body Part (Fourth Character)

Body Part
The anatomical site upon which the procedure was performed.

The fourth character of the ICD-10-PCS code provides information regarding the specific **body part**, anatomical site, or body region upon which the procedure, service, or treatment was performed. These characters, and what they represent, vary, determined by the section and body system. This is one of the reasons the Alphabetic Index will not usually reach this level of specificity.

CODING BITES

Using our example . . . ***radial vein to ulnar vein, left***

You can see how the details are built into the code.

The radial and ulnar veins are both specifically grouped into the category of brachial veins. Again, if you did not know this offhand, don't worry. Check your medical dictionary or anatomy reference. This is one of the wonderful aspects of being a coder; you can always use your resources to ensure accuracy.

Character 4 will provide the more specific detail, including laterality (right or left).

First character = 0

Second character = 5

Third character = 1

Fourth character = A

0 Medical and Surgical

5 Upper veins

1 Bypass

A Brachial vein, left

Approach (Fifth Character)

Approach
The specific technique used for the procedure.

The term **approach**, as reported by the fifth character, reports the technique or methodology used during the procedure, such as open or laparoscopic. This character explains how the physician got to the anatomical site upon which the procedure was performed.

NOTE: Other sections use this character position (character 5) to report a different detail, such as single or multiple duration for extracorporeal therapy. The ***Imaging*** section uses this position to report the use of contrast materials. Again, don't worry; the ICD-10-PCS code book will share this information with you. All you have to do is read carefully and completely.

CODING BITES

Using our example . . . ***Laparoscopic***

This detail must be provided by the physician in his or her operative notes. ***The words may not be identical, so you will have to understand the meaning so you can interpret.***

A laparoscope is an *endoscope* inserted through an incision in the abdominal wall (*percutaneously*), used to visualize the interior of the peritoneal cavity. Therefore, you would interpret this as a PERCUTANEOUS ENDOSCOPIC approach.

First character = 0

Second character = 5

Third character = 1

Fourth character = A

Fifth character = 4

(continued)

0 Medical and Surgical

5 Upper veins

1 Bypass

A Brachial vein, left

4 Percutaneous endoscopic

More about the specific approaches coming up in the following chapters.

Device (Sixth Character)

Some of the sections use the sixth character to identify a **device** used in the procedure. To some, this term may conjure up pictures of hard, metal equipment. However, in ICD-10-PCS, the term *device* is used in a more general sense to mean any item that will remain in or with the body after the procedure is complete. So it might mean equipment, such as a pacemaker, or it may report the use of a graft.

Device
The identification of any materials or appliances that may remain in or on the body after the procedure is completed.

CODING BITES

Using our example . . . ***using autologous tissue substitute***

For the sixth character, you need to read the notes to determine if any devices, substances, or other components were used. First, check your ICD-10-PCS section to familiarize yourself with what type of details this character, in this table, will report. Then, you will know what to look for in the documentation.

Here, in our example code, you have already determined that you are working with the 051 Table in ICD-10-PCS. In this table, the sixth character reports a device, something that will remain in, or with, the patient after the procedure is completed. Look at the options you have for the sixth character in this table: tissue substitutes of various origins. *Autologous tissue substitute* was used during the bypass to support the rerouting of the vein.

First character	=	0
Second character	=	5
Third character	=	1
Fourth character	=	A
Fifth character	=	4
Sixth character	=	7

0 Medical and Surgical

5 Upper veins

1 Bypass

A Brachial vein, left

4 Percutaneous endoscopic

7 Autologous tissue substitute

Some sections of ICD-10-PCS, such as the ***Administration*** section, will have you report a category of substance, such as anti-inflammatory or antineoplastic, with the sixth character. When you are working in that section, keep your pharmacology reference close at hand.

More about this in the following chapters.

Qualifier (Seventh Character)

The seventh character of the ICD-10-PCS code, the **qualifier**, is like a wild card, reporting whatever additional information may be needed. Because the coding system is designed for future expansion, there will be cases where a specific procedure does not currently have the details to require all seven characters. In such cases, the letter Z is used to indicate that nothing in that position was applicable to the particular procedure.

Qualifier
Any additional feature of the procedure, if applicable.

CODING BITES

Using our example . . . ***to ulnar vein***

In this case, there is one more detail that must be explained . . . *to* what anatomical site was the radial vein rerouted, or bypassed "to"—a different upper vein.

As you have seen throughout this textbook, **GUIDANCE CONNECTION** icons direct you to official guidelines that will help you make accurate determinations for each character. For this case, Guideline B3.6a directs you to specify the body part bypassed *from* for the fourth character and the body part bypassed *to* for the seventh character. In this table, you only have one choice. However, there may be occasions in the future where this reminder will come in handy. Good thing these guidelines are always right there, in the front of your code book.

First character	=	0
Second character	=	5
Third character	=	1
Fourth character	=	A
Fifth character	=	4
Sixth character	=	7
Seventh character	=	Y

0 Medical and Surgical

5 Upper veins

1 Bypass

A Brachial vein, left

4 Percutaneous endoscopic

7 Autologous tissue substitute

Y Upper vein

Again, you will need to look at the table within the section of ICD-10-PCS first to discover what detail or type of detail this character of this code will report. As you read earlier, sometimes there is nothing left to share, so you will use the letter **Z No Qualifier**.

Don't worry. More about this all coming in the next chapters.

Placeholder Characters

The letter ***Z*** means "not applicable" or "none." The Z placeholder will be used most often as the seventh character; however, it can be used in any of the seven character positions, when needed. It also can be used in multiple positions in one code.

EXAMPLE

Dr. McCoy performed a biopsy on Clark's neck. The ICD-10-PCS code to report this would be 0WB6XZX . . .

0	=	Medical and Surgical
W	=	Anatomical regions, general
B	=	Excision
6	=	Neck
X	=	External
Z	=	No device
X	=	Diagnostic

There is no device, so there is nothing to report in the sixth character position. But you can't leave that part of the code out. So you put a *Z* in that spot and report that there is no device.

EXAMPLE

Dr. Rothwell used a percutaneous endoscope in an attempt to control post-procedural bleeding in Isaac's colon, after several polyps had been removed. The ICD-10-PCS code to report this would be 0W3P4ZZ . . .

0 = Medical and Surgical

W = Anatomical regions, general

3 = Control

P = Gastrointestinal tract

4 = Percutaneous endoscope

Z = No device

Z = No qualifier

There is no device, so there is nothing to report in the sixth character position. There is no qualifier, so there is nothing to report in the seventh character position either. By placing a *Z* in both positions, you are explaining exactly that. By the way, this is not a decision you have to make. In this subsection of the ICD-10-PCS tables, **Z No Device** and **Z No Qualifier** are the only choices on the chart for those two character positions.

33.3 The ICD-10-PCS Book

The ICD-10-PCS book is divided into three parts: the Alphabetic Index, the Tables, and the Appendixes. *NOTE:* The Appendixes are filled with great descriptions and examples to help you better understand and use this code set. More detail coming up.

The Alphabetic Index

The Alphabetic Index's entries are primarily sorted by root operation terms.

- Root operation term

A root operation term identifies the specific service or type of treatment that is the basis of the entire procedure.

EXAMPLES

Root operation terms include *bypass*, *drainage*, *excision*, and *insertion*.

After you find the root operation term, as stated in the documentation, there are subentries listed by the following:

- Body system

EXAMPLES

Digestive system

Musculoskeletal system

- Body part

EXAMPLES

Arm, leg, hand, foot

- Common procedure names and eponyms

The Alphabetic Index also lists common terms for some procedures and eponyms.

> ## EXAMPLES
>
> *Hysterectomy* is listed and then cross-referenced to *resection* (a root operation term) and *female reproductive system* (body system).
>
> *Roux-en-Y* operation is listed and then cross-referenced to *bypass* (a root operation term) and *gastrointestinal system* or *hepatobiliary system and pancreas* (both are body systems).

The Alphabetic Index will usually give you only the first three or four characters of the seven-character procedure code. You then must go to the Tables to find the additional characters. You won't have to be reminded to *never code from the Alphabetic Index* with ICD-10-PCS. Often, you won't be able to code from the Alphabetic Index alone anymore!

> ## EXAMPLE
>
> Fragmentation
>
> Bladder 0TF8-

For the most part, you will find that the Alphabetic Index will include information relating to the first three characters. This information will enable you to turn to the correct page in the Tables and determine the rest of the characters for the code. As you have seen, virtually all of the sections are consistent with the first three elements. However, as you get to the last four characters, the information represented by these characters may change, depending upon what type of procedure was performed or upon what body system a procedure was performed. This is a major aspect of the flexibility of the ICD-10-PCS system.

The Tables

The Tables are divided by body systems. Of course, like all the other code sets, each section is in order by the first character in the code. Within each section's body system division, the list continues in order by the root operation term for that procedure. Each section of the list has a grid that specifies the assigned meaning to each letter or number along with its position in the seven-character code. (See an example in **Figure 33-2**.)

You will go through the grid and construct the correct code based on the physician's notes. As you have already learned, <u>*all*</u> ICD-10-PCS codes are seven characters. Therefore, you will build the code in this order, as directed by the grid.

- First character: Section (such as ***Medical and Surgical, Mental Health***, or ***Imaging***)
- Second character: **Body system**
- Third character: **Root operation**
- Fourth character: **Body part** or region
- Fifth character: **Approach**
- Sixth character: **Device**
- Seventh character: **Qualifier**

Therefore, when you review the information in **Figure 33-2**, you can see that the correct ICD-10-PCS code for *Dilation of one site of a Coronary Artery, using an open approach with an Intraluminal device* is 02700DZ.

Section	**0**	Medical and Surgical
Body System	**2**	Heart and Great Vessels
Operation	**7**	Dilation: Expanding an orifice or the lumen of a tubular body part

Body Part Character 4	*Approach Character 5*	*Device Character 6*	*Qualifier Character 7*
0 Coronary Artery, One Artery **1** Coronary Artery, Two Arteries **2** Coronary Artery, Three Arteries **3** Coronary Artery, Four or More Arteries	**0** Open **3** Percutaneous **4** Percutaneous Endoscopic	**4** Intraluminal Device, Drug-eluting **5** Intraluminal Device, Drug-eluting, Two **6** Intraluminal Device, Drug-eluting, Three **7** Intraluminal Device, Drug-eluting, Four or More **D** Intraluminal Device **E** Intraluminal Device, Two **F** Intraluminal Device, Three **G** Intraluminal Device, Four or More **T** Intraluminal Device, Radioactive **Z** No Device	**6** Bifurcation **Z** No Qualifier
F Aortic Valve **G** Mitral Valve **H** Pulmonary Valve **J** Tricuspid Valve **K** Ventricle, Right **L** Ventricle, Left **P** Pulmonary Trunk **Q** Pulmonary Artery, Right **S** Pulmonary Vein, Right **T** Pulmonary Vein, Left **V** Superior Vena Cava **W** Thoracic Aorta, Descending **X** Thoracic Aorta, Ascending/Arch	**0** Open **3** Percutaneous **4** Percutaneous Endoscopic	**4** Intraluminal Device, Drug-eluting **D** Intraluminal Device **Z** No Device	**Z** No Qualifier
R Pulmonary Artery, Left	**0** Open **3** Percutaneous **4** Percutaneous Endoscopic	**4** Intraluminal Device, Drug-eluting **D** Intraluminal Device **Z** No Device	**T** Ductus Arteriosus **Z** No Qualifier

FIGURE 33-2 Table 027 from the Medical and Surgical Section 2026 ICD-10-PCS

LET'S CODE IT! SCENARIO

Jahlil Browne was playing football in the park with his friends. A player on the other team hit him at full force in the chest when he ran to catch a pass. Jahlil was taken to the ED by ambulance and admitted into the hospital with an open fracture of the third rib, right side. Dr. Wolf operated on Jahlil to insert an internal fixation device, using a percutaneous endoscopic approach to secure the fractured bone together with the fourth rib, so it can heal properly.

Let's Code It!

What did the doctor do for Jahlil? Dr. Wolf *inserted an internal fixation device* on Jahlil's fractured rib. It is always wise to begin with the actual term that the physician used in his or her notes, so let's go to the Alphabetic Index and look up the term *insertion.*

Below the main term, *insertion*, is a list. None of these terms seem to go with this situation. Wait a minute. Right below this is a main term that does fit: *Insertion of device in.* Beneath this is a list of anatomical sites. What anatomical site did the fixation device go onto? *Rib.* Then, check the documentation to identify how many ribs were involved in the procedure. Find

Insertion of device in

Rib

1 to 2 0PH1

3 or more 0PH2

These four characters are a good start. Remember, all ICD-10-PCS codes require seven (7) characters. You must go to the Tables to confirm this is correct.

In the Tables, turn to the ***Medical and Surgical*** section: 0PH. Look carefully at the second row.

Section	**0**	Medical and Surgical
Body System	**P**	Upper Bones
Operation	**H**	Insertion

Body Part	*Approach*	*Device*	*Qualifier*
1 Ribs, 1 to 2 **2** Ribs, 3 or more **3** Cervical Vertebra **4** Thoracic Vertebra **5** Scapula, Right **6** Scapula, Left	**0** Open **3** Percutaneous **4** Percutaneous Endoscopic	**4** Internal Fixation Device	**Z** No Qualifier

OK, let's build a code:

The section:	**0 Medical and Surgical** (Dr. Wolf performed surgery on Jahlil)
The body system:	**P Upper Bones** (the ribs are in the upper half of the body)
The root operation:	**H Insertion** (Dr. Wolf inserted a fixation device)
The body part:	**1 Ribs, 1 to 2** (as per the physician's documentation)
The approach:	**4 Percutaneous Endoscopic** (the documentation states this approach)

(continued)

The device: **4 Internal Fixation Device** (this equipment will stay on Jahlil's rib after the procedure until it is healed)

The qualifier: **Z No Qualifier**

The ICD-10-PCS code to report the repair of Jahlil's rib is **0PH144Z.**

Good job!

LET'S CODE IT! SCENARIO

Montell was in a car accident and his right knee hit against the steering column. He was admitted into the hospital, and Dr. Tompkins took a high osmolar x-ray of his knee.

Let's Code It!

What did Dr. Tompkins do for Montell? He *x-rayed his knee.*

In the Alphabetic Index, look up *x-ray*. The Alphabetic Index suggests

X-ray—see Plain Radiography

OK, so turn to *Plain Radiography* in the Alphabetic Index. Beneath this main term is a long list of anatomical sites, so read down and find

Plain Radiography

Knee

Left BQ08

Right BQ07

The Alphabetic Index provided only four of the seven needed characters of this suggested code, so turn to the Tables to complete the code and confirm its correctness.

In the Tables, turn to the *Imaging* section: BQ0.

Section	**B**	Imaging
Body System	**Q**	Non-Axial Lower Bones
Type	**0**	Plain Radiology: Planar display of an image developed from the capture of external ionizing radiation on photographic or photoconductive plate

Body Part	*Approach*	*Device*	*Qualifier*
0 Hip, Right **1** Hip, Left	**0** High Osmolar **1** Low Osmolar **Y** Other Contrast	**Z** None	**Z** None
0 Hip, Right **1** Hip, Left	**Z** None	**Z** None	**1** Densitometry **Z** None
3 Femur, Right **4** Femur, Left	**Z** None	**Z** None	**1** Densitometry **Z** None

(continued)

7 Knee, Right **8** Knee, Left **G** Ankle, Right **H** Ankle, Left	**0** High Osmolar **1** Low Osmolar **Y** Other Contrast **Z** None	**Z** None	**Z** None
D Lower leg, Right **F** Lower leg, Left **J** Calcaneus, Right **K** Calcaneus, Left **L** Foot, Right **M** Foot, Left **P** Toe(s), Right **Q** Toe(s), Left **V** Patella, Right **W** Patella, Left	**Z** None	**Z** None	**Z** None
X Foot/Toe Joint, Right **Y** Foot/Toe Joint, Left	**0** High Osmolar **1** Low Osmolar **Y** Other Contrast	**Z** None	**Z** None

OK, let's build the code:

The section: **B Imaging** (you know that x-rays are a type of imaging)

The body system: **Q Non-axial lower bones** (*non-axial* means away from the central part of the body, and you know that the knee is a lower bone)

The root operation: **0 Plain Radiography** (also known as x-ray)

The body part: **7 Knee, Right** (as per the physician's notes)

The contrast: **0 High Osmolar** (as per the physician's notes)

The qualifier: **Z None**

The qualifier: **Z None**

The ICD-10-PCS code to report the x-ray of Montell's knee is **BQ070ZZ**.

Good work!

Appendices

> **CODING TIP**
>
> Different publishers may place Appendices in a different order.

The information shared in the appendices of your ICD-10-PCS code book can be very valuable as you abstract documentation to interpret to the correct character as you build your code. In addition to the definitions for each of the major components of the ICD-10-PCS code, there are also examples, which may help your understanding. And . . . they are right there in the back of your ICD-10-PCS code book!

Appendices

Components of the Medical and Surgical Approach Definitions

Root Operation Definitions

Comparison of Medical and Surgical Root Operations

Body Part Key

Body Part Definitions

Device Key and Aggregation Table

Device Definitions

Substance Key/Substance Definitions

Sections B-H Character Definitions

Hospital Acquired Conditions

Answers to Coding Exercises

Procedure Combination Tables

Use the information in these appendices to support your determination of the accurate characters and the correct ICD-10-PCS code.

CODING BITES

Various publishers of ICD-10-PCS code books may present these appendices in a different order, and some may not include all. Don't worry. If your coding manual does not include appendices, you can download the Definitions, included within the file titled *2026 ICD-10-PCS Addendum*, from https://www.cms.gov/files/zip/2026-icd-10-pcs-addendum.zip

33.4 ICD-10-PCS General Conventions

The ICD-10-PCS code set has its own set of guidelines, of course. The following list contains the general conventions of how the codes are constructed and how to use the Tables.

GUIDANCE CONNECTION

In the front of your ICD-10-PCS code book, look for the page titled **ICD-10-PCS Official Guidelines for Coding and Reporting**. Then, follow along as we discuss the first section, **Conventions**.

Read through these guidelines to get a strong start to accurately reporting inpatient procedures. But don't worry about memorizing them because they are right there, in the front of your code book.

A1. ICD-10-PCS codes are composed of seven characters. Each character is an **axis of classification** that specifies information about the procedure performed. Within a defined code range, a character specifies the same type of information in that axis of classification.

Axis of Classification
A single meaning within the code set; providing a detail.

This convention is explaining that all ICD-10-PCS codes must have seven (7) characters—no more, no less—and that each character position (axis of classification) has a specific meaning.

EXAMPLE

The third character of the code specifies the *root operation term.*

A2. One of 34 possible values can be assigned to each axis of classification in the seven-character code: they are the numbers 0 through 9 and the letters of the alphabet (except I and O because they are easily confused with the numbers 1 and 0). The number of unique values used in an axis of classification differs as needed.

When this convention refers to "34 possible values," it is referring to the fact that this code set uses letters of the American alphabet (letters A to Z minus O and I, so 26 letters minus 2 = 24 possible letters) plus 10 possible numbers (0–9) = 34 possibilities for each position in each code. And while there may be 34 possibilities, only what is needed is used at this time. This means that this code set has lots of room to grow and include new codes as they become a part of our standards of care.

EXAMPLE

Where the fifth character specifies the approach, seven different approach values are currently used to specify the approach.

A3. The valid values for an axis of classification can be added to as needed.

This convention means that this code set has lots of room to grow and include new codes as they become a part of our standards of care.

> **EXAMPLE**
>
> If a significantly distinct type of device is used in a new procedure, a new device value can be added to the system.

A4. As with words in their context, the meaning of any single value is a combination of its axis of classification and any preceding values on which it may be dependent.

This convention tells you to interpret each meaning, not only according to each specific character's definition, but also in combination with the meanings of the other characters that are in that table, in that row. It is the total meaning that you must look at, as well as each individual character. So, if once you put all seven characters together, something doesn't make sense, you need to read again.

> **EXAMPLE**
>
> The meaning of a body part value in the ***Medical and Surgical*** section is always dependent on the body system value. The body part value 0 in the Central Nervous body system specifies Brain; the body part value 0 in the Peripheral Nervous body system specifies Cervical Plexus.

A5. As the system is expanded to become increasingly detailed, over time more values will depend on preceding values for their meaning.

This convention means that they will continue to expand the system and ensure that new characters added will not overlap or duplicate the meanings of characters that already exist in that table, in the row.

> **EXAMPLE**
>
> In the Lower Joints body system:
>
> - Under the root operation *Insertion*: *Table 0SH*
>
>   Device character 6: value 3 specifies "Infusion Device"
>
> - Under the root operation *Replacement*: *Table 0SR*
>
>   Device character 6: value 3 specifies "Synthetic Substitute, Ceramic"

A6. The purpose of the Alphabetic Index is to locate the appropriate table that contains all information necessary to construct a procedure code. The PCS Tables should always be consulted to find the most appropriate valid code.

Essentially, this convention is telling you what you may have learned when coding from other code sets. *Never* report a code from the Alphabetic Index. *Always* refer to the tables and double-check the meaning for each and every character in that table, in that row.

A7. It is not required to consult the Index first before proceeding to the tables to complete the code. A valid code may be chosen directly from the tables.

This takes convention A6 a little further in telling you that you are NOT required to ever look in the Alphabetic Index. As you gain more experience, and you are on the job, you may learn your way through this code set. So, if you are coding for the labor and delivery services to a pregnant woman, you can go directly to the ***Obstetrics*** tables without looking in the Alphabetic Index if you don't need the suggestion. And if you are coding for a psychiatrist providing care to a patient in a behavioral health hospital, you can go directly to the ***Mental Health*** tables.

A8. All seven characters must be specified to be a valid code. If the documentation is incomplete for coding purposes, the physician should be queried for the necessary information.

Every character in every code must report the facts, as supported by the physician's documentation. If any detail is missing, and you are not able to determine the correct character, then you must query the physician to have the documentation amended. You can *never* assume and never guess.

A9. Within a PCS table, valid codes include all combinations of choices in characters 4 through 7 contained in the same row of the table. In the example below, 0HTWXZZ is a valid code, and 0HTW0ZZ is **not** a valid code.

Section	**0**	Medical and Surgical
Body System	**H**	Skin and Breast
Operation	**T**	Resection: Cutting out or off, without replacement, all of a body part

Body Part	*Approach*	*Device*	*Qualifier*
Q Finger Nail **R** Toe Nail **W** Nipple, Right **X** Nipple, Left	**X** External	**Z** No Device	**Z** No Qualifier
T Breast, Right **U** Breast, Left **V** Breast, Bilateral **Y** Supplemental Breast	**0** Open	**Z** No Device	**Z** No Qualifier

This convention tells you how to read the table to build your code. Once you find the table with the correct first three characters (section, body system, root operation term), then go down the column to find the correct 4th character. Once you determine this accurate character, you can only go across in that one row. If you determine that the procedure was done on the right nipple (character **W** in the first row), then you only have one option for the approach: **X External**. If the documentation states an open approach was used, then you cannot put **0 Open** with **W Nipple, Right** because they are on two different rows. This would highlight to you that you need to go back to the documentation because you can't build this code from more than one row.

A10. "And," when used in a code description, means "and/or," except when used to describe a combination of multiple body parts for which separate values exist for each body part (e.g., Skin and Subcutaneous Tissue used as a qualifier, where there are separate body part values for "Skin" and "Subcutaneous Tissue").

Take a look at an example: *Knee Bursa and Ligament*. You would interpret this as

Knee Bursa and Ligament

Knee Bursa

Knee Ligament

EXAMPLE

Lower Arm and Wrist Muscle means lower arm and/or wrist muscle.

A11. Many of the terms used to construct PCS codes are defined within the system. It is the coder's responsibility to determine what the documentation in the medical record equates to in the PCS definitions. The physician is not expected to use the terms used in PCS code descriptions, nor is the coder required to query the physician when the correlation between the documentation and the defined PCS terms is clear.

This convention tells you, directly, that it is your responsibility to interpret the terms and phrases used by the physician in the documentation. For example, if the physician documents that he performed a *biopsy*, you, as the coder, must interpret that to the ICD-10-PCS root operation term *excision*, and if the physician documents that she manipulated the dislocated shoulder back into position, you, as the coder, must interpret this into the ICD-10-PCS root operation term *reposition*.

EXAMPLE

When the physician documents "cauterization," the coder can independently correlate "cauterization" to the root operation "destruction" without querying the physician for clarification.

33.5 Selection of Principal Procedure

Similar to CPT and HCPCS Level II coding, ICD-10-PCS has its guidelines for determining the sequencing when reporting more than one procedure provided during an encounter. This is always going to be determined in coordination with the diagnosis codes being reported to identify the medical necessity for performing these procedures. Here are the Official Guidelines for ICD-10-PCS code sequencing:

The following instructions should be applied in the selection of principal procedure and clarification on the importance of the relation to the principal diagnosis when more than one procedure is performed:

1. Procedure performed for definitive treatment of both principal diagnosis and secondary diagnosis.

   a. Sequence procedure performed for definitive treatment most related to principal diagnosis as principal procedure.

2. Procedure performed for definitive treatment and diagnostic procedures performed for both principal diagnosis and secondary diagnosis.

   a. Sequence procedure performed for definitive treatment most related to principal diagnosis as principal procedure.

3. A diagnostic procedure was performed for the principal diagnosis and a procedure is performed for definitive treatment of a secondary diagnosis.

   a. Sequence diagnostic procedure as principal procedure, since the procedure most related to the principal diagnosis takes precedence.

4. No procedures performed that are related to principal diagnosis; procedures performed for definitive treatment and diagnostic procedures were performed for secondary diagnosis.

   a. Sequence procedure performed for definitive treatment of secondary diagnosis as principal procedure, since there are no procedures (definitive or nondefinitive treatment) related to principal diagnosis.

Source: ICD-10-PCS *Official Guidelines for Coding and Reporting,* 2026.

CODING BITES

You learned about the different types of procedures in the chapter ***Introduction to the Languages of Coding***, the section titled **Procedure Coding**.

As you read through these four guidelines to determine how multiple ICD-10-PCS procedure codes should be sequenced, notice that you must refer to the diagnosis codes, and the sequencing of those codes, as part of your decision-making process. In addition, you must understand why each procedure was performed—not only for the intended outcome, but also to understand if the procedure was done for diagnostic or therapeutic purposes.

GUIDANCE CONNECTION

Read the **ICD-10-PCS Official Guidelines for Coding and Reporting**, section **Selection of Principal Procedure**.

CODING BITES

Additional information about ICD-10-PCS can be found at:

https://www.cms.gov/medicare/coding-billing/icd-10-codes

Chapter Summary

The purpose of this chapter is to provide an overview of ICD-10-PCS, giving you an idea of what to expect, and to help you establish a comfort level so that you are not apprehensive about the new system. This chapter shared with you the distinct benefits of this code set. Then, step by step, the chapter differentiated the way the codes look and are constructed. The notations and explanations, exclusive to ICD-10-PCS, are all reviewed. Examples are provided to illustrate the concepts and elements throughout the chapter.

CHAPTER 33 REVIEW
Introduction to ICD-10-PCS

Let's Check It! Terminology

Match each key term to the appropriate definition.

1. **LO 33.3** The identification of any materials or appliances that may remain in or on the body after the procedure is completed.
2. **LO 33.3** The category or classification of a particular procedure, service, or treatment.
3. **LO 33.3** The anatomical site upon which the procedure was performed.
4. **LO 33.3** Any additional feature of the procedure, if applicable.
5. **LO 33.3** The physiological system, or anatomical region, upon which the procedure was performed.
6. **LO 33.3** The specific technique used for the procedure.
7. **LO 33.4** A single meaning within the code set; providing a detail.

A. Approach
B. Axis of Classification
C. Body Part
D. Body System
E. Device
F. Qualifier
G. Root Operation Term

Let's Check It! Concepts

Choose the most appropriate answer for each of the following questions.

1. **LO 33.1** In ICD-10-PCS, the initials *PCS* stand for
   a. Popular Coding System. **b.** Procedure Coding System.
   c. Possible Coding Solutions. **d.** Proper Coding System.
2. **LO 33.2** The Alphabetic Index's entries are primarily sorted by
   a. root operation terms. **b.** the approach. **c.** the device. **d.** the body system.
3. **LO 33.2** The structure of ICD-10-PCS codes includes
   a. three numbers. **b.** five numbers. **c.** seven characters. **d.** up to nine characters.
4. **LO 33.2** ICD-10-PCS codes include
   a. only numbers. **b.** only letters.
   c. one letter followed by numbers. **d.** letters and numbers.
5. **LO 33.2** An example of a root operation term is
   a. bypass. **b.** x-ray. **c.** obstetrics. **d.** hysterectomy.
6. **LO 33.2** Digestive system is an example of a
   a. body part. **b.** root operation term. **c.** medical procedure. **d.** body system.
7. **LO 33.2** The 17 sections of ICD-10-PCS are identified by
   a. numbers 1–17. **b.** numbers 0–9, then letters *B–H* and *X*.
   c. letters *A–Z*. **d.** alphabetic order by the name of the section.
8. **LO 33.2** Placeholders are indicated in ICD-10-PCS with
   a. the number 0. **b.** the letter *X*. **c.** the letter *Z*. **d.** the number 9.
9. **LO 33.2** An example of an approach is
   a. open. **b.** ileostomy. **c.** pacemaker. **d.** ventricular.
10. **LO 33.2** An example of a device, for purposes of ICD-10-PCS coding, is
    a. ablation. **b.** laparoscopy. **c.** pacemaker. **d.** allotransplantation.

11. **LO 33.2** The ICD-10-PCS code for the provision of a cesarean section would be found in

a. Section 2 Placement. **b.** Section 1 Obstetrics.
c. Section B Imaging. **d.** Section 6 Extracorporeal Therapies.

12. **LO 33.2** Coding a chiropractic manipulative treatment would begin in

a. Section 0 Medical and Surgical. **b.** Section 4 Measurement and Monitoring.
c. Section 7 Osteopathic. **d.** Section 9 Chiropractic.

13. **LO 33.2** What is the letter or number that represents the device in code 2W22X4Z?

a. 2 **b.** W **c.** 4 **d.** X

14. **LO 33.2** What is the letter or number that represents the approach in code 3E00X3Z?

a. E **b.** X **c.** 0 **d.** Z

15. **LO 33.2** What is the letter or number that represents the root operation in code 3E1S38Z?

a. 1 **b.** S **c.** 8 **d.** E

16. **LO 33.2** What is the letter or number that represents the section in code 2W10X7Z?

a. 2 **b.** W **c.** 1 **d.** 0

17. **LO 33.2** What is the letter or number that represents the qualifier in code 3E0Y70M?

a. 0 **b.** Y **c.** 7 **d.** M

18. **LO 33.3** The Alphabetic Index will usually give you only the first ________ or ________ characters of the seven-character procedure code.

a. one, two **b.** two, three **c.** three, four **d.** five, six

19. **LO 33.4** Which ICD-10-PCS general convention states that within a PCS table, valid codes include all combinations of choices in characters 4 through 7 contained in the same row of the table?

a. A1 **b.** A3 **c.** A6 **d.** A9

20. **LO 33.5** ICD-10-PCS does not have guidelines for determining the sequencing when reporting more than one procedure provided during an encounter.

a. True **b.** False

Let's Check It! Rules and Regulations

Please answer the following questions from the knowledge you have gained after reading this chapter.

1. **LO 33.2** ICD-10-PCS codes may include any letter of the alphabet *except* the letter(s) ________; include why these letters are avoided.
2. **LO 33.2** List the related pieces of information for the seven ICD-10-PCS character positions.
3. **LO 33.3** How are the ICD-10-PCS tables divided?
4. **LO 33.4** What are the 11 ICD-10-PCS General Convention guidelines? Include a brief description of each.
5. **LO 33.5** What are the instructions for selection of the principal procedure when more than one procedure is performed?

YOU CODE IT! Application

The following exercises provide practice in abstracting physicians' notes and learning to work with documentation from our health care facility, Westward Hospital. These case studies are modeled on real patient encounters. Using the techniques described in this chapter, carefully read through the case studies and determine the most accurate answers for each case study.

(continued)

WESTWARD HOSPITAL

591 Chester Road

Masters, FL 33955

PATIENT: WELLINGTON, ALISHA

DATE OF ADMISSION: 03/13/26

DATE OF SURGERY: 03/13/26

DATE OF DISCHARGE: 03/14/26

PREOPERATIVE DX: Right ureteral obstruction secondary to colon cancer

POSTOPERATIVE DX: Same

PROCEDURE: Cystoscopy
Right retrograde pyelogram
Removal and replacement of double-J stent

ANESTHESIA: General

HISTORY/INDICATIONS: This is a 39-year-old female with a history of colon cancer and secondary right ureteral obstruction who had a stent inserted a number of months ago. At this time, she is in the hospital and it is time for a stent change. Consequently, the patient presents for the procedure.

PROCEDURE: The patient was taken to the operating room and there she was given general anesthetic, positioned in the dorsal lithotomy position, the genitalia scrubbed and prepped with Betadine. Sterile towels and sheets were utilized to drape the patient in the usual fashion. A cystoscope was introduced into the bladder. The ureteral catheter was identified. It was grabbed and removed without any difficulty. Subsequently, the cystoscope was reinserted into the bladder and the right ureteral orifice was identified over a Pollack catheter. A glide wire was inserted into the right collecting system. Some contrast was injected and a hydronephrotic right side was noted. Then, the wire was placed through the Pollack catheter. With the wire in position, over the wire a 7 French 26 cm double-J stent was inserted. Excellent coiling was noted fluoroscopically in the kidney and distally with a cystoscope. The bladder was then drained and again it was inspected prior to removal. There was no evidence of any tumors or lesions in the bladder. The stent was in good position. The cystoscope was removed and the patient was taken to the recovery room awake and in stable condition.

Benjamin Johnston, MD

In Dr. Johnston's documentation of Alisha Wellington's procedure, what is/are the root operation term(s)?

a. Replacement

b. Fluoroscopy

c. Removal, Insertion and fluoroscopy

d. Removal

WESTWARD HOSPITAL

591 Chester Road

Masters, FL 33955

PATIENT: FIELDING, STEPHEN

DATE OF ADMISSION: 07/15/26

DATE OF SURGERY: 07/15/26

DATE OF DISCHARGE: 07/16/26

PREOPERATIVE DX: Superior canalicular laceration

POSTOPERATIVE DX: Same

PROCEDURE: Superior canalicular repair

This patient is a 3-year-old male who is admitted into the Pediatric Unit with a dog bite to left side of face.

(continued)

HPI: Approximately 3 hours ago, patient was playing with a large dog, the pet of a neighbor. Family witnessed the dog make a single lunge at the boy's face. Due to the adults' attempts to intervene, only the top jaw made contact. The dog did not attack further, and the incomplete bite to the left face was the only injury sustained. Ophthalmology called in for consult.

POH/PMH/SH: No past ocular history. No past medical history. No current medications or allergies. Well-adjusted preschool child lives at home with both parents. Childhood immunizations are up-to-date, according to the mother.

OCULAR EXAM:

- VA 20/25 OD and OS without correction
- Extraocular motility and IOP were normal, OU
- CVF: Full OD, OS
- Lids: Right side—Normal
- Lids: Left side—2 lacerations on the left upper lid, the larger and deeper of the lacerations passes just medial to the upper punctum. Initial exploration of laceration raises concerns for probable canalicular involvement, but further detailed examination in this anxious pediatric patient was unable to be accomplished.
- Continuation of the examination in the operating suite revealed that the remainder of the anterior segment examination and DFE were normal.

TREATMENT: Primary surgical repair of the lacerated or avulsed canaliculus using pigtail probes is performed immediately. The patient was taken to the operating suite for examination under general anesthesia (EUA) and laceration repair, likely to include canalicular repair.

DX: Superior canalicular laceration

Roxan Kernan, MD

In Dr. Kernan's documentation of the procedure on Stephen Fielding, what is the root operation term?

a. Repair
b. Eyelid
c. Canalicular
d. Bite

WESTWARD HOSPITAL

591 Chester Road

Masters, FL 33955

PATIENT: O'LEARY, KEVIN

DATE OF ADMISSION: 03/05/26

DATE OF DISCHARGE: 03/17/26

PREOPERATIVE DX: Third-degree burn, neck

POSTOPERATIVE DX: Same

PROCEDURE: Skin graft

ANESTHESIA: General

This patient is a 43-year-old male who works as a county firefighter. He is recovering from third-degree burns on his neck. He was admitted today for the first session of skin grafting. Patient is brought into the surgical suite and general anesthesia is administered by Dr. Rambeau. Once the patient is unconscious, he is prepped and draped in the usual, sterile fashion. A split-thickness autograft, which contains the dermis with only a portion of the epidermis, is taken from a donor site on the patient's inner thigh, left. The graft harvested is 11/1000ths of an inch in thickness, using a derma-tome. The graft is carefully spread on the bare area and held in place with surgical staples. Plasmatic imbibition is initiated. The graft is meshed with lengthwise rows of short, interrupted cuts, each a few millimeters long, with each row offset by half a cut length. The area is covered with derma-surgical gauze. Patient is awakened and taken to recovery.

Benjamin Johnston, MD

(continued)

What is/are the root operation term(s), as documented in Dr. Johnston's procedure notes for Kevin O'Leary?

a. Excision
b. Excision and replacement
c. Replacement and neck
d. Neck

WESTWARD HOSPITAL
591 Chester Road
Masters, FL 33955

PATIENT: SWANSONN, HANS

DATE OF ADMISSION: 05/23/26

DATE OF DISCHARGE: 05/23/26

PREOPERATIVE DX: Rule out bladder tumor

POSTOPERATIVE DX: Same

PROCEDURE: Cystoscopy, biopsy, and fulguration of bladder

ANESTHESIA: Spinal

INDICATIONS: The patient is a 67-year-old male with a history of grade II superficial transitional cell carcinoma of the bladder. Cystoscopy showed a suspicious erythematous area on the right trigone. He presented today for cystoscopy, biopsy, and fulguration. Findings: the urethra was normal; the bladder was 1+ trabeculated; the mid and right trigone areas were slightly erythematous and hypervascular. No papillary tumors were noted; no mucosal abnormalities were noted.

PROCEDURE: The patient was placed on the table in supine position. Satisfactory spinal anesthesia was obtained. He was placed in dorsal lithotomy position and prepped sterilely with Hibiclens and draped in the usual manner. A #22 French cystoscopy sheath was passed per urethra in atraumatic fashion. The bladder was resected with the 70-degree lens with findings as noted above. Cup biopsy forceps were placed and three biopsies were taken of the suspicious areas of the trigone. These areas were fulgurated with the Bugby electrode; no active bleeding was seen. The scope was removed; the patient was returned to recovery having tolerated the procedure well. Estimated blood loss was minimal.

PATHOLOGY REPORT: Chronic cystitis (cystica) with squamous cell metaplasia.

Roxan Kernan, MD

What is the root operation term identified in Dr. Kernan's procedure notes about Hans Swansonn?

a. Diagnostic
b. Excision
c. Bladder
d. Endoscopic

WESTWARD HOSPITAL
591 Chester Road
Masters, FL 33955

PATIENT: ZANDER, MARISSA

DATE OF ADMISSION: 02/16/26

DATE OF DISCHARGE: 02/18/26

PREOPERATIVE DX: Delivery

(continued)

POSTOPERATIVE DX: Same

PROCEDURE: Cesarean section, classical

In the 40th week of her first pregnancy, a 29-year-old female arrived at labor and delivery at 0830 for a planned induction of labor due to mild, pregnancy-induced hypertension. After intra-vaginal placement of misoprostol, the nurse observed her briefly and, at 1100, discharged her from the unit. She went for a walk with her husband in a park next to the hospital. Patient's membranes spontaneously ruptured and she readmitted to the labor and delivery unit. The nurse admitted the patient, took her vital signs, and checked the fetal heart rate. The mother's blood pressure was 176/95, but the nurse thought this was related to nausea, vomiting, and discomfort from the contractions. The resident examined the mother, determined that her cervix was 5–6 cm, 90% effaced, and the vertex was at 0 station. An internal fetal heart monitor was placed because the mother's vomiting and discomfort caused her to move around too much in the bed, making it hard to record the fetal heart rate with an external monitor. The internal monitor revealed a steady fetal heart rate of 120 and no decelerations. The mother continued to complain of painful contractions and requested an epidural. Shortly after placement of the epidural, the monitor recorded a prolonged fetal heart rate deceleration. The heart rate returned slowly to the baseline rate of 120 as the nurse repositioned the mother, increased her intravenous fluids, and administered oxygen by mask. An epidural analgesia infusion pump was started. The fetal heart rate strip indicated another deceleration that recovered to baseline. The nurse informed the resident, who checked the tracing and told her to "keep an eye on things." The primary nurse noted in the labor record that the baseline fetal heart rate was "unstable, between 100–120," but she did not report this to the resident. The nurse recorded that the fetal heart rate was "flat, no variability." As the nurse was documenting this as a non-reassuring fetal heart rate pattern, the patient expressed a strong urge to push and the nurse called for an exam. A resident came to the bedside, examined the mother, and noted that she was fully dilated with the caput at +1. A brief update was written in the chart, but the clinician who had performed the exam was not noted. The mother was repositioned and began pushing. The fetal heart rate suddenly dropped and remained profoundly bradycardic for 11 minutes. The resident was called and attempted a vacuum delivery since the fetal head was at +2 station. The attending then entered and attempted forceps delivery. An emergency classical cesarean delivery was performed; the baby was stillborn. The physician identified a uterine rupture that required significant blood replacement. Whole blood transfusion, nonautologous, was performed, via peripheral vein.

Roxan Kernan, MD

In Dr. Kernan's documentation on the procedure performed on Marissa Zander, identify the root operation term(s).

a. Extraction

b. Transfusion

c. Percutaneous

d. Extraction and transfusion

34

ICD-10-PCS Medical and Surgical Section

Key Terms

Approach
Character
Root Operation Term

Learning Outcomes

After completing this chapter, the student should be able to:

LO 34.1 Identify the section and body systems used in Medical and Surgical section codes.

LO 34.2 Interpret the procedure to determine the accurate root operation term used in Medical and Surgical section codes.

LO 34.3 Utilize knowledge of anatomy to determine the body part treated to be used in Medical and Surgical section codes.

LO 34.4 Identify the approach used to accomplish the procedure used in Medical and Surgical section codes.

LO 34.5 Distinguish the type of device implanted, when applicable, for Medical and Surgical section codes.

LO 34.6 Select the appropriate qualifier character for Medical and Surgical section codes.

LO 34.7 Determine the correct way to report multiple and discontinued procedures for Medical and Surgical section codes.

LO 34.8 Analyze all of the details to build an accurate seven-character code for Medical and Surgical section codes.

STOP! Remember, you need to follow along in your ICD-10-PCS code book for an optimal learning experience.

34.1 Medical/Surgical Section/Body Systems: Characters 1 and 2

As you learned earlier, every ICD-10-PCS code has seven characters, and each **character** position has a meaning. While all of these codes have the same number of characters, each section uses each character position differently. So let's review the meanings for the ***Medical and Surgical*** section characters:

Character
A letter or number component of an ICD-10-PCS code.

Character Position	Character Meaning
1	Section of the ICD-10-PCS book
2	Body system being treated
3	Root operation term
4	Body part (specific anatomical site)
5	Approach used by physician
6	Device
7	Qualifier

Character Position 1: Medical and Surgical Section 0 (Zero)

Character Position	Character Meaning
1	**Section of the ICD-10-PCS book**
2	Body system being treated
3	Root operation term
4	Body part (specific anatomical site)
5	Approach used by physician
6	Device
7	Qualifier

All of the codes reporting a medical or surgical procedure will begin with a zero. ***Medical and Surgical*** is the first section of the Tables, after the Alphabetic Index. When you look up a procedure in the Alphabetic Index and see that the suggested code begins with a zero, you will know immediately that you will find the rest of this code in the ***Medical and Surgical*** Tables.

Character Position 2: Body System

Character Position	Character Meaning
1	Section of the ICD-10-PCS book
2	**Body system being treated**
3	Root operation term
4	Body part (specific anatomical site)
5	Approach used by physician
6	Device
7	Qualifier

In this code set, the body systems are broken down into further detail than the organ systems you learned in your anatomy and physiology course. The body systems and their corresponding characters are:

0 Central Nervous System and Cranial Nerves

1 Peripheral Nervous System

2 Heart and Great Vessels

3 Upper Arteries

4 Lower Arteries

5 Upper Veins

6 Lower Veins

7 Lymphatic and Hemic Systems

8 Eye

9 Ear, Nose, Sinus

B Respiratory System

C Mouth and Throat

D Gastrointestinal System

F Hepatobiliary System and Pancreas

G Endocrine System

H Skin and Breast

J Subcutaneous Tissue and Fascia

K Muscles

L Tendons

M Bursae and Ligaments

N Head and Facial Bones

P Upper Bones

Q Lower Bones

R Upper Joints

S Lower Joints

T Urinary System

U Female Reproductive System

V Male Reproductive System

W Anatomical Regions, General

X Anatomical Regions, Upper Extremities

Y Anatomical Regions, Lower Extremities

Notice that, in this list, there is a 0 (zero) and a number 1 (one) but no letter *O* or letter *I*. The creators of this code set did this purposely to avoid confusion.

Take a look at body system **5** Upper Veins and **6** Lower Veins. As explained in the guidelines, the imaginary transverse line is at the diaphragm, dividing the body into top (upper) and bottom (lower). A procedure performed on the brachial vein, located in the arm, will be reported with body system character 5, and a procedure performed on the gastric vein, located in the stomach, is reported with body system character 6. Similarly, the same applies for characters 3 and 4 (Upper and Lower Arteries), P and Q (Upper and Lower Bones), and R and S (Upper and Lower Joints).

GUIDANCE CONNECTION

Read the ICD-10-PCS Official Guidelines for Coding and Reporting, **Medical and Surgical Section Guidelines (Section 0)**, subhead **B2. Body system**, paragraphs **B2.1a** and **B2.1b**.

Now, let's look at body system characters W, X, and Y, which report anatomical regions instead of a specific body section or system. These should be used only when the documentation identifies that the procedure was performed on an anatomical cavity rather than an individual body part. You must read carefully to distinguish the details. To illustrate this, let's look at a case of a patient diagnosed with ascites (a buildup of fluid in the abdominal cavity). The physician drains this excess fluid from the abdominal cavity; therefore, it will require a character of W for the body system: Anatomical Regions, General.

You do not need to worry about remembering that the liver is part of the hepatobiliary system or that a pacemaker generator is inserted into the subcutaneous tissue and fascia and its leads are inserted into the heart. The Alphabetic Index will help you, as will the listings for body part (character position 4).

EXAMPLE

Dr. Franklin inserted a neurostimulator lead into Matthew Short's cerebrum, during an open procedure.
The Body System is reported: Central Nervous System and Cranial Nerves with a 0 (zero) character.

YOU INTERPRET IT!

Identify which body system this anatomical site would report for the second character.

1. Umbilical artery: _______
2. Cervical lymph node: _______
3. Cornea: _______
4. Pharynx: _______
5. Stomach: _______
6. Deltoid muscle: _______
7. Zygomatic process of frontal bone: _______
8. Coccyx: _______
9. Elbow joint: _______
10. Trachea: _______

34.2 Medical/Surgical Root Operations: Character 3

Character Position	Character Meaning
1	Section of the ICD-10-PCS book
2	Body system being treated
3	**Root operation term**
4	Body part (specific anatomical site)
5	Approach used by physician
6	Device
7	Qualifier

Root Operation Term
The category or classification of a particular procedure, service, or treatment.

GUIDANCE CONNECTION

Read the ICD-10-PCS Official Guidelines for Coding and Reporting, **Medical and Surgical Section Guidelines (Section 0)**, subsection **B3. Root Operation**, paragraphs **B3.1a** through **B3.17**.

The ***Medical and Surgical*** section uses 31 **root operation terms** to describe what procedure was performed for the patient during this encounter. Don't worry–the definitions are listed in the ICD-10-PCS code book. However, you still need to learn and understand them so that you can abstract the operative report or procedure notes accurately and completely from the documentation. Remember that you are required to use the ICD-10-PCS term definition in its entirety. Also, just as in reporting with CPT procedure codes, it is important that you understand all of the components of a specific root operation or procedure. You don't want to code inclusive components separately or miss a second code because a component is not part of that procedure automatically. Using the root operation term is the most efficient way of using the Alphabetic Index as well.

Alteration

Alteration: Modification of a natural anatomic structure of a body part without affecting the function of the body part . . . Character: **0 (zero)**

EXAMPLE

Alteration is a procedure most often performed for cosmetic purposes, to improve the patient's appearance, such as a face lift.

Rhytidectomy (face lift surgery) is a procedure performed to alter the look of the skin on the face. Liposuction and breast augmentation are also examples of this type of procedure.

0J013ZZ Alteration of subcutaneous tissue and fascia, face, percutaneous approach

Bypass

Bypass: Altering the route of the contents of a tubular body part . . . Character: **1**

Bypass procedures are coded by identifying the body part bypassed "from," identified by character **4** (Body Part), and the body part bypassed "to," identified by character **7** (Qualifier).

GUIDANCE CONNECTION

Read the ICD-10-PCS Official Guidelines for Coding and Reporting, **Medical and Surgical Section Guidelines (Section 0)**, subsection **B3. Root Operation**, subhead **Bypass procedures**, paragraphs **B3.6a**, **B3.6b**, and **B3.6c**.

EXAMPLE

A *bypass* can be performed only on a tubular body part, such as a vein or an artery, the esophagus, lymphatic vessel, or the intestines. A colostomy formation is another example of a bypass.

02114Z8 Coronary artery bypass, one site, percutaneous endoscopic approach, rerouted to internal mammary, right side

07120Z4 Lymphatic vessel bypass, open approach, from left neck to central vein

Change

Change: Taking out or off a device from a body part and putting back an identical or similar device in or on the same body part without cutting or puncturing the skin or a mucous membrane . . . Character: **2**

EXAMPLE

Change is a root operation used only when a device is involved in the procedure—a device that stays with the patient after the procedure is complete. A urinary catheter change and a gastronomy tube change are good examples. Often, this term will actually be used in the documentation.

0020X0Z Changing a drainage device in the brain, external approach

Control

Control: Stopping, or attempting to stop, postprocedural or other acute bleeding . . . Character: **3**

The root operation term *Control* is used only when the only action taken during this procedure is the intent to achieve homeostasis (balance) beyond that which is already a part of the procedure itself, utilizing cautery, suturing, ligation, clipping, etc. that does not align with a more specific operation root term. If another specific root operation was performed to accomplish this task, such as excision or resection, then report the code for *that* root operation *instead* of Control. You will not report both.

GUIDANCE CONNECTION

Read ICD-10-PCS Official Guidelines for Coding and Reporting, **Medical and Surgical Section Guidelines (Section 0)**, subsection **B3. Root Operation**, subhead **Control vs. more definitive root operations**, paragraph **B3.7**.

EXAMPLE

Control is a procedure to stop massive bleeding (hemorrhaging).

0W3B0ZZ Control post-procedural bleeding in the pleural cavity, left side, open approach

Creation

Creation: Putting in or on biological or synthetic material to form a new body part that to the extent possible replicates the anatomic structure or function of an absent body part . . . Character: **4**

This procedure is used when the physician actually makes a new structure, such as creation of an artificial vagina during a male-to-female procedure in a gender reassignment surgery, procedures to correct congenital anomalies, or replacement of a dysfunctional heart valve.

EXAMPLES

Creation of a body part, such as a penis or a heart valve, is reported with this root operation term.

0W4N0J1 Creation of an artificial penis using synthetic substitute, open approach

024G082 Creation of a mitral valve using zooplastic tissue, open approach

Destruction

Destruction: Physical eradication of all or a portion of a body part by the direct use of energy, force, or a destructive agent . . . Character: **5**

Several methodologies are reported as destruction, such as fulguration, the application of high-frequency electrical current, also known as electrofulguration, when it is used to destroy tissue (typically malignant neoplasm). Chemical agents, such as salicylic acid, can also be used to destroy tissue.

EXAMPLE

Destruction is used to describe when the tissue is no longer in existence, and there is no specimen to send to pathology. Terms that may be used in the documentation include *fulguration*, *cauterization*, and *cryosurgery*.

0U5B8ZZ Fulguration of endometrium, vaginal endoscopic approach

Detachment

Detachment: Cutting of all or a portion of the upper or lower extremities . . . Character: **6**

This is the root operation term for *amputation* of an arm or a leg, in whole or in part.

EXAMPLE

Detachment is only used to report the amputation of an arm or a leg, no other body part.

0Y6J0Z1 Amputation, directly below knee, left leg, open approach

Dilation

Dilation: Expanding an orifice or the lumen of a tubular body part . . . Character: **7**

Remember, an orifice is a natural body opening (such as vagina or anus) and the lumen of a tubular body part (*lumen* = "space within the tube"). Blood vessels are tubular body parts, as are a woman's fallopian tubes.

EXAMPLES

Dilation is the process of opening a closed tubular body part.

037H34Z Dilation of right common carotid artery, with drug-eluting intraluminal device, percutaneous approach

0U7C7ZZ Dilation of the cervix, via natural opening

Division

Division: Cutting into a body part, without draining fluids and/or gases from the body part, in order to separate or transect a body part . . . Character: **8**

EXAMPLE

Division is the separation of body parts.

An episiotomy, an osteotomy, and spinal cordotomy are all good examples.

0K820ZZ Division of sternocleidomastoid muscle, right side, open approach

Drainage

Drainage: Taking or letting out fluids and/or gases from a body part . . . Character: **9**

EXAMPLE

Drainage is, as it sounds, the process of helping gases or fluids escape.

0W9B30Z Drainage of excess air from left pleural cavity, percutaneous approach

Excision

Excision: Cutting out or off, without replacement, a portion of a body part . . . Character: **B**

Pay close attention to this description of excision. This term has a narrower meaning in ICD-10-PCS than it does in CPT and in many physicians' notes. Excision is used in ICD-10-PCS only when a segment is cut out. This includes obtaining a tissue biopsy, performing a lumpectomy, and cutting out a bone spur. However, if the entire organ or body part is removed, the root operation term used is *resection* (even if the physician documents that an organ was excised–you must interpret it).

GUIDANCE CONNECTION

Read the ICD-10-PCS Official Guidelines for Coding and Reporting, **Medical and Surgical Section Guidelines (Section 0)**, subsection **B3. Root Operation**, subhead **Excision vs. Resection**, paragraph **B3.8**, and **Excision for Graft**, paragraph **B3.9**.

EXAMPLE

Excision is the surgical removal of a part or portion of a body part, not the entire organ.

0FB13ZX Excision, liver, right lobe, percutaneous approach, diagnostic procedure

Extirpation

Extirpation: Taking or cutting out solid matter from a body part . . . Character: **C**

This reference to "solid matter" may indicate a blood clot or gallstones when surgically removed.

EXAMPLE

Extirpation is the surgical removal of a solid formation from within the body.

Some good examples are thrombectomy (surgical removal of a blood clot attached to the wall of a vein or artery) and cholelithotomy (surgical removal of gallstones).

04CL0ZZ Extirpation of thrombus, femoral artery, left side, open approach

Extraction

Extraction: Pulling or stripping out or off all or a portion of a body part by the use of force . . . Character: **D**

EXAMPLE

Extraction may be done by scraping (curettage), pulling, suction, or other process.

Vein stripping, D&C (dilation and curettage), and a cesarean section (extracting a baby from the womb) are all good examples.

0UDB8ZZ Suction extraction of endometrium, via natural opening, endoscopic approach

Fragmentation

Fragmentation: Breaking solid matter in a body part into pieces . . . Character: **F**

An example of fragmentation is lithotripsy—the use of shock waves to break kidney stones (renal lithiasis) into smaller pieces with the hope that the body will be able to pass them naturally.

> **EXAMPLE**
>
> *Fragmentation* is the process of breaking up something in the body into smaller pieces, such as the procedure of lithotripsy.
>
> 0TFCXZZ Fragmentation of stones in the bladder neck, using external approach

Fusion

Fusion: Joining together portions of an articular body part rendering the articular body part immobile . . . Character: **G**

> **GUIDANCE CONNECTION**
>
> Read the ICD-10-PCS Official Guidelines for Coding and Reporting, **Medical and Surgical Section Guidelines (Section 0)**, subsection **B3. Root Operation**, subhead **Fusion procedures of the spine**, paragraphs **B3.10a**, **B3.10b**, and **B3.10c**.

Arthrodesis, the surgical immobilization of a joint, such as of the spine, is one type of fusion (*articular* = "joint").

> **EXAMPLE**
>
> *Fusion* is a procedure that is the opposite of *division*.
>
> 0RG40A0 Fusion of cervicothoracic vertebral joint, open procedure, anterior approach, anterior column, using an interbody fusion device

Insertion

Insertion: Putting in nonbiological appliance that monitors, assists, performs, or prevents a physiological function but does not physically take the place of a body part . . . Character: **H**

This is another opportunity for reading very carefully. In ICD-10-PCS, this root operation applies only to the placement into the body of a medical device, such as a pacemaker, that will remain in the body after the procedure is completed.

> **EXAMPLE**
>
> *Insertion* is the placing of a device into the body.
>
> 05H933Z Insertion of catheter (infusion device) into right brachial vein, percutaneous approach

> **GUIDANCE CONNECTION**
>
> Read the ICD-10-PCS Official Guidelines for Coding and Reporting, **Medical and Surgical Section Guidelines (Section 0)**, subsection **B3. Root Operation**, subhead **Inspection procedures**, paragraphs **B3.11a**, **B3.11b**, and **B3.11c**.

Inspection

Inspection: Visually and/or manually exploring a body part . . . Character: **J**

This root operation term is limited to the physician's looking at the body part.

> **EXAMPLE**
>
> *Inspection* in this case is just like the English word . . . to look at.
>
> 09JEXZZ Inspection of the left inner ear, external approach

Map

Map: Locating the route of passage of electrical impulses and/or locating functional areas in a body part . . . Character: **K**

Cardiac conduction mapping and brain mapping are two illustrations of this root operation. Note that this root operation term reports the examination only.

> **EXAMPLE**
>
> *Map* is a methodology that enables the physician to obtain a record of the function of a specific anatomical part.
>
> 00K03ZZ Mapping of brain function, percutaneous approach

Occlusion

Occlusion: Completely closing an orifice or lumen of a tubular body part . . . Character: **L**

There are times when an opening, such as a fistula, or a tubular body part, such as a fallopian tube, is purposely closed off or blocked.

> **GUIDANCE CONNECTION**
>
> Read the ICD-10-PCS Official Guidelines for Coding and Reporting, **Medical and Surgical Section Guidelines (Section 0)**, subsection **B3. Root Operation**, subhead **Occlusion vs. Restriction for vessel embolization procedures**, paragraph **B3.12**.

> **EXAMPLE**
>
> *Occlusion* is the opposite of *dilation*.
>
> 0VLH4ZZ Occlusion of spermatic cords, bilaterally, percutaneous endoscopic approach, no device

Reattachment

Reattachment: Putting back in or on all or a portion of a separated body part to its normal location or other suitable location . . . Character: **M**

This word is the same as the term most often used by physicians for this procedure, such as reattaching a finger after it has been severed during an accident.

> **EXAMPLE**
>
> *Reattachment* is reported for anatomical sites only.
>
> 0XMP0ZZ Reattachment of left index finger, open approach

Release

Release: Freeing a body part from an abnormal physical constraint by cutting or by use of force . . . Character: **N**

The procedure reported with this root operation term involves cutting or separation only, such as tendon lengthening, in order to free a body part from some type of restriction.

GUIDANCE CONNECTION

Read the ICD-10-PCS Official Guidelines for Coding and Reporting, **Medical and Surgical Section Guidelines (Section 0)**, subsection **B3. Root Operation**, subhead **Release procedures**, paragraph **B3.13**, and **Release vs. Division**, paragraph **B3.14**.

EXAMPLE

Release is similar to *division*, so be careful to read the descriptions and the documentation very carefully.

0LNS0ZZ Release of right ankle tendon, open approach

Removal

Removal: Taking out or off a device from a body part . . . Character: **P**

Read this carefully: As the description specifically states "device," this can be used only for this type of procedure–to remove a previously inserted device. As you abstract the physician's notes, be cautious of the use of this term in documentation. The removal of a mole, for example, is really an excision, not a removal.

EXAMPLE

Removal is only used when a device has been removed.

0QP304Z Removal of internal fixation device from left pelvic bone, open approach

Repair

Repair: Restoring, to the extent possible, a body part to its normal anatomic structure and function . . . Character: **Q**

EXAMPLE

Repair is often the therapeutic process of correcting an abnormality.

0CQV8ZZ Repair of left vocal cord, via natural opening, endoscopic approach

Replacement

Replacement: Putting in or on biological or synthetic material that physically takes the place and/or function of all or a portion of a body part . . . Character: **R**

Essentially, this is the placement of a prosthetic device, such as a hip replacement or a prosthetic heart valve.

GUIDANCE CONNECTION

Read the ICD-10-PCS Official Guidelines for Coding and Reporting, **Medical and Surgical Section Guidelines (Section 0)**, subsection **B3. Root Operation**, subhead **Reposition for fracture treatment**, paragraph **B3.15**.

EXAMPLE

Replacement is directly related to the use of internal prosthetics.

02RG0JZ Replacement of mitral valve with synthetic prosthesis, open approach

Reposition

Reposition: Moving to its normal location or other suitable location all or a portion of a body part . . . Character: **S**

> **EXAMPLE**
>
> *Reposition* is the correction that is usually employed with a patient who has a dislocation.
>
> 0PSFXZZ Reposition humeral shaft, right side, external approach

Resection

Resection: Cutting out or off, without replacement, all of a body part . . . Character: **T**

Remember how this differs from *excision*. When the entire body part is surgically removed, it is reported as a resection. If only a portion of the body part is removed, it is reported as an excision.

> **GUIDANCE CONNECTION**
>
> Read the ICD-10-PCS Official Guidelines for Coding and Reporting, **Medical and Surgical Section Guidelines (Section 0)**, subsection **B3. Root Operation**, subhead **Excision vs. Resection**, paragraph **B3.8.**

> **EXAMPLE**
>
> *Resection* is the root operation term used for the surgical removal of an entire organ.
>
> 0FT44ZZ Resection of gallbladder, percutaneous endoscopic approach

Restriction

Restriction: Partially closing an orifice or lumen of a tubular body part . . . Character: **V**

Compare this with the root operation term *occlusion*. Restriction is a partial closure, and occlusion is a complete closure.

> **EXAMPLE**
>
> *Restriction* is a surgical methodology for limiting the function, or malfunction, of an anatomical site.
>
> 0DV44CZ Restriction of esophagogastric junction, using extraluminal device, percutaneous endoscopic approach

Revision

Revision: Correcting, to the extent possible, a portion of a malfunctioning device or the position of a displaced device . . . Character: **W**

Again, pay careful attention to the word *device*. This root operation term can only be used when a medical device is being fixed.

> **EXAMPLE**
>
> *Revision* is correcting the internal positioning of a device.
>
> 02WA0MZ Revision of cardiac lead, open approach

Supplement

Supplement: Putting in or on biological or synthetic material that physically reinforces and/or augments the function of a portion of a body part . . . Character: **U**

NOTE: In the Tables section, *supplement* is in alphabetic order by its character *U*, not by the term *supplement*, so it falls between *resection* and *restriction*.

EXAMPLES

Supplement, just as in English, is something that provides support.

0TUB4JZ Supplementation of bladder, percutaneous endoscopic approach, using synthetic mesh

0YUA47Z Use of autologous tissue substitute mesh to repair an inguinal hernia laparoscopically, bilateral

Transfer

GUIDANCE CONNECTION

Read the ICD-10-PCS Official Guidelines for Coding and Reporting, **Medical and Surgical Section Guidelines (Section 0)**, subsection **B3. Root Operation**, subhead **Transfer procedures using multiple tissue layers**, paragraph **B3.17**.

Transfer: Moving, without taking out, all or a portion of a body part to another location to take over the function of all or a portion of a body part . . . Character: **X**

EXAMPLE

Transfer is the process when the body part transferred still remains connected to its original vascular and nervous supply.

0JX03ZB Transfer of skin and subcutaneous tissue, scalp, percutaneous approach

Transplantation

GUIDANCE CONNECTION

Read the ICD-10-PCS Official Guidelines for Coding and Reporting, **Medical and Surgical Section Guidelines (Section 0)**, subsection **B3. Root Operation**, subhead **Transplantation vs. Administration**, paragraph **B3.16**.

Transplantation: Putting in or on all or a portion of a living body part taken from another individual or animal to physically take the place and/or function of all or a portion of a similar body part . . . Character: **Y**

ICD-10-PCS uses this term in the same manner that physicians do. However, this includes more than just organ transplant procedures.

EXAMPLE

Transplantation is the implanting of a donor body organ into a recipient.

0TY00Z0 Transplant of an allogeneic right kidney, open approach

Adjusting Your Interpretations

As you abstract the physician's documentation, you may need to adjust some of your interpretative processes for reporting procedures using ICD-10-PCS. The root operation term is based on the objective of the procedure. You are seeking the word describing the action, such as *excision* or *drainage*. Combination terms with which you are very familiar, such as *colonoscopy*, *liver biopsy*, or *appendectomy*, may describe the procedure; however, these terms do not specifically explain the action of the physician, or do they? Let's take a closer look at these terms and interpret them into the root operation terms:

Colonoscopy: *colon* = "large intestine" (anatomical site) + *-oscopy* = "to view"

In ICD-10-PCS, you would use the root operation term *Inspection: Visually and/or manually exploring a body part.*

Liver biopsy: *liver* = anatomical site + *biopsy* = "excision of tissue for diagnostic purposes"

In ICD-10-PCS, you would use the root operation term *Excision: Cutting out or off, without replacement, a portion of a body part.* In just a bit, you will learn about adding a qualifier in the character 7 position to include the detail that this was a diagnostic excision.

Appendectomy: *append* = "appendix" (anatomical site) + *-ectomy* = "surgical removal"

In ICD-10-PCS, you would use the root operation term *Resection: Cutting out or off, without replacement, all of a body part.*

With some procedures, you will use your knowledge of the specific procedure and what it is expected to accomplish. For example, you will need to remember that lithotripsy is performed for *Fragmentation: Breaking solid matter in a body part into pieces*, which is done when a patient has kidney stones. Another example is thoracentesis (*thora* = "thorax [chest]" + *-centesis* = "puncture"), performed for *Drainage: Taking or letting out fluids and/or gases from a body part.*

CODING BITES

Review *Appendix: Root Operation Definitions* in the back of your ICD-10-PCS code book.

YOU INTERPRET IT!

Practice interpreting from the common procedure terms used to reference the ICD-10-PCS root operation term. The Root Operation Definitions Appendix may help you.

11. Colostomy formation: _______
12. Cautery of skin lesion: _______
13. Transluminal angioplasty: _______
14. Choledocholithotomy: _______
15. Free skin graft: _______
16. Adhesiolysis: _______
17. Fallopian tube ligation: _______
18. Diagnostic arthroscopy: _______
19. Ankle arthrodesis: _______
20. Total nephrectomy: _______
21. Esophagogastric fundoplication: _______

34.3 Medical/Surgical Body Parts: Character 4

Character Position	Character Meaning
1	Section of the ICD-10-PCS book
2	Body system being treated
3	Root operation term
4	**Body part (specific anatomical site)**
5	Approach used by physician
6	Device
7	Qualifier

The fourth character position identifies the specific body part that is the focus of a procedure. The operative report or the procedure notes should be clear about these details. However, sometimes it can be a challenge to match the documentation to the choices offered in the tables. Following are some guidelines to help you determine the accurate code in ICD-10-PCS.

General Guidelines

There may be times when the notes are more specific than the code character specifics. If the physician documents that the procedure was performed on a specific anatomical site, such as the biceps femoris muscle, yet the listing of body parts under Muscles (Body System character K) does not provide this detail, you will need to code to the body part that includes this anatomical site. In this case, you would report Upper Leg Muscle.

Bilateral Procedures

If the documentation identifies that a procedure was performed on both a right body part and a left body part, and a Body Part code character is available to report the bilateral procedure, that is the one code to report. However, if there is no code character available to report a bilateral procedure, then you will need to report two codes: one for each procedure.

EXAMPLES

0HRV3KZ Replacement of breasts, bilateral, percutaneous approach

0CNT8ZZ Release of right vocal cord, via natural opening endoscopic

0CNV8ZZ Release of left vocal cord, via natural opening endoscopic

Coronary Arteries

While the coronary arteries are represented by one code character, there are additional characters to report when more than one site is treated in this one set of arteries.

EXAMPLE

Dr. Forreau performed an angioplasty in the left anterior descending coronary artery in two distinct sites with two intraluminal, drug-eluting stents placed.

027135Z Dilation of coronary artery, two sites, percutaneous approach with two intraluminal devices, drug-eluting

Joints and Muscles

Many body systems provide individual code characters for body parts specific to a joint or a muscle. There are some cases when the Body Part characters may not be as specific as the physician's notes. The guidelines provide direction in determination of a code character to report the body part. When a procedure is performed on the skin, the subcutaneous tissue, or the fascia that is lying over a joint,

- Shoulder is reported as Upper Arm.
- Elbow is reported as Lower Arm.
- Wrist is reported as Lower Arm.
- Hip is reported as Upper Leg.
- Knee is reported as Lower Leg.
- Ankle is reported as Foot.

For an on-the-spot reminder, see Guideline B4.6.

When a body system does not include a separate Body Part code character for fingers or toes,

- Finger is reported as Hand.
- Toe is reported as Foot.
  For an on-the-spot reminder, see Guideline B4.7.

Gastrointestinal Body System

Certain areas within the gastrointestinal Body System tables group the individual body parts of the intestinal tract into upper and lower. For these cases, the Upper Intestinal Tract includes the esophagus, stomach, and small intestine, up to and including the duodenum. The Lower Intestinal Tract includes the jejunum, ileum, cecum, and large intestine, all the way to and including the anus.

The ***Body Part Key Appendix*** in ICD-10-PCS also can help you when a specific anatomical site is documented and the Body Part components are not as specific. For instance, Stensen's duct is reported as the parotid duct, and the superior gluteal nerve is described in ICD-10-PCS as the lumbar plexus.

GUIDANCE CONNECTION

Read the ICD-10-PCS Official Guidelines for Coding and Reporting, **Medical and Surgical Section Guidelines (Section 0)**, subsection **B4. Body Part**, paragraphs **B4.1a** through **B4.8**.

CODING BITES

Review ***Appendix: Body Part Key*** and ***Appendix: Body Part Definitions*** in the back of your ICD-10-PCS code book. Various publishers of ICD-10-PCS code books may present these appendices in a different order, and some may not include all. Don't worry. If your coding manual does not include appendices, you can download the Definitions, included within the file titled *2026 ICD-10-PCS Addendum*, from https://www.cms.gov/medicare/coding-billing/icd-10-codes

YOU INTERPRET IT!

Practice using the Body Part Key Appendix and fill in the descriptions used by ICD-10-PCS for coding.

22. Superior olivary nucleus: _______

23. Sigmoid vein: _______

24. Right suprarenal vein: _______

25. Ulnar notch: _______

26. Ventricular fold: _______

27. Sweat gland: _______

28. Optic disc: _______

29. Oropharynx: _______

30. Nasal concha: _______

31. Manubrium: _______

32. Ischium: _______

34.4 Medical/Surgical Approaches: Character 5

Character Position	Character Meaning
1	Section of the ICD-10-PCS book
2	Body system being treated
3	Root operation term
4	Body part (specific anatomical site)
5	Approach used by physician
6	Device
7	Qualifier

As you continue to build a code, you can see that you are telling a story. The first four characters explain what the physician did and the anatomical site upon which he or she worked. Now, with the fifth character, you are going to explain how the physician got to the anatomical site to perform the procedure. This is known as the **approach**, and seven approaches are used within the ***Medical and Surgical*** section.

Approach
The path the physician took to access the body part upon which the treatment or procedure was targeted.

GUIDANCE CONNECTION

Read the ICD-10-PCS Official Guidelines for Coding and Reporting, **Medical and Surgical Section Guidelines (Section 0)**, subhead **B5. Approach**, paragraphs **B5.2**, **B5.3a**, **B5.3b**, and **B5.4**.

Open

Open: Cutting through the skin or mucous membrane and any other body layers necessary to expose the site of the procedure . . . Character: **0**

An open procedure is the traditional approach when the physician makes an incision into the body to access an internal organ. The operative notes should include the details of the incision, providing open access to the internal organ that needs the treatment.

EXAMPLES

You might see documentation that states:

> *". . . Attention was then turned to the patient's lower abdomen. Incision was made from symphysis pubis to umbilicus, midline. The incision was carried down through the dermis, subcutaneous fat, and linea alba using electrocautery. Preperitoneal fat was incised using electrocautery. Peritoneum was grasped with pickups. . . ."*

You can see that the physician describes the incision made, cutting through the subcutaneous and adipose layers to the peritoneum (the membrane that lines the abdominal cavity).

> *". . . The patient was taken to the operating room after being administered an epidural anesthetic, placed in the supine position, prepped and draped in a sterile fashion with a wedge under the right hip. A Pfannenstiel skin incision was made and carried down through layers along the old incision line. . . ."*

In this excerpt from an operative report, the physician states this process more simply, but you can still understand that the patient is being cut into.

GUIDANCE CONNECTION

Read the ICD-10-PCS Official Guidelines for Coding and Reporting, **Medical and Surgical Section Guidelines (Section 0)**, subsection **B5. Approach**, subhead **Open approach with percutaneous endoscopic assistance**, paragraph **B5.2**.

Percutaneous

Percutaneous: Entry, by puncture or minor incision, of instrumentation through the skin or mucous membrane and any other body layers necessary to reach the site of the procedure . . . Character: **3**

When a percutaneous approach is used, the physician cannot see inside the body. Often, a radiologist will provide imaging guidance (which would be reported separately). A needle aspiration and needle biopsy are good illustrations of a percutaneous approach.

EXAMPLE

You might see documentation that states:

> *". . . The patient was prepped and draped in the usual fashion. A long, thin needle is inserted through the patient's abdominal wall, periumbilical quadrant, passed into the amniotic sac. Ultrasound guidance is used. When puncture into the sac is confirmed, a small sample of amniotic fluid is extracted and sent to the lab. . . ."*

A needle is inserted through the dermis (percutaneously) all the way into the amniotic sac. The fact that ultrasound guidance was used supports the fact that the physician could not see where the point of the needle was going (no scope to see inside; no internal visualization).

Percutaneous Endoscopic

<u>Percutaneous Endoscopic</u>: Entry, by puncture or minor incision, of instrumentation through the skin or mucous membrane and any other body layers necessary to reach and visualize the site of the procedure . . . Character: **4**

In this type of approach, a scope is placed through the incision or puncture. A laparoscopic procedure is a good example.

EXAMPLES

You might see documentation that states:

> *" . . . The patient was positioned supine on the operating room table. . . . A small umbilical incision allowed for introduction of the Veress needle and inflation of the abdomen to 15 cm of water pressure using carbon dioxide gas. The 0 degree, 5-mm laparoscope was introduced through a 5-mm port at the umbilicus and 3 additional ports were placed in the usual anatomic positions. The liver was found to be markedly enlarged. . . ."*

A percutaneous endoscopic approach also can be described as a laparoscopic procedure. This approach also can be recognized by the description of a "small" incision, which only needs to be large enough to fit the endoscope through, typically about one inch long (2.54 cm).

Via Natural or Artificial Opening

<u>Via Natural or Artificial Opening</u>: Entry of instrumentation through a natural or artificial external opening to reach the site of the procedure . . . Character: **7**

The natural openings to the body include the nose, mouth, ear, vagina, urethra, and anus. An artificial opening includes a stoma (an opening that has been surgically created).

EXAMPLE

> *" . . . A weighted speculum was placed in the posterior vaginal wall and the right-angle retractor used to visualize the cervix. The cervix was grasped across the anterior lip with a single-toothed tenaculum. . . . The cervix was circumferentially excised with the scalpel. . . ."*

This excerpt is from the operative notes for a vaginal hysterectomy. Just the name tells you that the approach was via the patient's vagina, but you know that the name is insufficient upon which to support a code. As you read the description of what the physician did, you know you have the documentation to support the reporting of this hysterectomy being performed using a vaginal (natural opening) approach.

Via Natural or Artificial Opening Endoscopic

<u>Via Natural or Artificial Opening Endoscopic</u>: Entry of instrumentation through a natural or artificial external opening to reach and visualize the site of the procedure . . . Character: **8**

Note that the difference between this approach and "via natural or artificial opening" is the use of an endoscope to visualize the anatomical site upon which the procedure will be performed.

EXAMPLES

You might see documentation that states:

> *" . . . The patient was placed in the dorsolithotomy position on a cystoscopy table, prepped and draped in the usual fashion. A #21 French cystoscope was passed through the urethra into the bladder. . . ."*

(continued)

The urethra is the anatomical tube that leads from the urinary bladder to the outside of the body. This is a natural opening into visceral organs, such as the bladder, ureters, and kidneys. The insertion of the cystoscope through the urethra is an endoscope being used to see inside the body via a natural opening.

> "*. . . The patient was brought to the operative suite, placed in the supine position. After satisfactory induction of general endotracheal anesthesia, a flexible Olympus bronchoscope was passed through the endotracheal tube, visualizing the distal trachea, carina, right and left main stem bronchus with primary and secondary divisions. . . .*"

Your understanding of anatomy will help you identify this natural opening—the pharynx is the medical term for the throat. The bronchoscope was threaded through the patient's mouth, down the throat, into the bronchi.

Via Natural or Artificial Opening with Percutaneous Endoscopic Assistance

<u>Via Natural or Artificial Opening with Percutaneous Endoscopic Assistance</u>: Entry of instrumentation through a natural or artificial external opening and entry, by puncture or minor incision, of instrumentation through the skin or mucous membrane and any other body layers necessary to aid in the performance of the procedure . . . Character: **F**

This approach is kind of a combination endoscopic (laparoscopic) approach along with the use of a natural or artificial opening.

EXAMPLE

You might see documentation that states:

> "*. . . The endoscope is inserted into the esophagus and down into the esophogastric junction. The anterior aspect of the gastric lining is visualized. A 2.5-cm incision is made into the right lateral aspect of the abdominal wall to allow for the insertion of the gastrostomy tube. . . .*"

This excerpt from the documentation of the placement of a feeding tube (also known as a G-tube) uses a percutaneous endoscopic gastrostomy (PEG) approach along with the natural opening approach of the mouth for the esophagogastro-duodenoscope (EGD).

External

<u>External</u>: Procedure performed directly on the skin or mucous membrane and procedures performed indirectly by the application of external force through the skin or mucous membrane . . . Character: **X**

EXAMPLES

You might see documentation that states:

> "*. . . Used the McIvor mouth gag to retract the tongue and endotracheal tube inferiorly, giving good exposure to the oropharynx. The tonsils were visualized. . . .*"

As you read this physician's description, it clearly indicates that the patient's mouth was held open so the *tonsils were visualized* . . . seen by the naked eye. There were no incisions or penetrations through the tissues, neither was any type of scope used.

> "*. . . Upper eyelid incision was performed in the skin with 15 blade scalpel. . . .*"

The eyelid is right there, on the outside (external) part of the body. Again, no incisions, penetrations through the tissues, or any type of scope was necessary.

GUIDANCE CONNECTION

Read the ICD-10-PCS Official Guidelines for Coding and Reporting, **Medical and Surgical Section Guidelines (Section 0)**, subsection **B5. Approach**, subhead **External approach**, paragraphs **B5.3a** and **B5.3b**.

CODING BITES

As you abstract the documentation and interpret the way the physician describes how the procedure was performed, you may find ***Appendix: Components of the Medical and Surgical Approach Definitions*** or ***Approach Table*** in your ICD-10-PCS code book helpful. Various publishers of ICD-10-PCS code books may present these appendices in a different order, and some may not include all. Don't worry. If your coding manual does not include appendices, you can download the Definitions, included within the file titled *2026 ICD-10-PCS Addendum*, from https://www.cms.gov/medicare/coding-billing/icd-10-codes

YOU INTERPRET IT!

Practice using the Medical and Surgical Approach Definitions Appendix or the Approach Table and fill in the approach used by ICD-10-PCS for coding.

33. Liposuction: _______

34. Sigmoidoscopy: _______

35. Laparoscopic hysterectomy: _______

36. Fracture manipulation (closed): _______

37. Traditional cholecystectomy: _______

38. Foley catheter placement: _______

39. Lumbar puncture: _______

40. Breast biopsy with guidance: _______

41. Endoscopy: _______

42. Cesarean section: _______

43. Blepharotomy: _______

34.5 Medical/Surgical Devices: Character 6

Character Position	Character Meaning
1	Section of the ICD-10-PCS book
2	Body system being treated
3	Root operation term
4	Body part (specific anatomical site)
5	Approach used by physician
6	**Device**
7	Qualifier

As you can see, a character placed in the sixth position will identify a device that will remain with the patient after the procedure has been completed. ICD-10-PCS qualifies these generalized types of devices:

- Grafts
- Prostheses
- Implants
- Simple or mechanical appliances
- Electronic appliances

GUIDANCE CONNECTION

Read the ICD-10-PCS Official Guidelines for Coding and Reporting, **Medical and Surgical Section Guidelines (Section 0)**, subsection **B6. Device**, paragraphs **B6.1a**, **B6.1b**, **B6.1c**, and **B6.2**.

Reading through the ***Medical and Surgical*** section, with a focus on some of the options for the sixth character, you will find a limited number of descriptors. Let's take a closer look at these:

Grafts

Autologous Tissue . . . Character: **7**
Autologous Venous Tissue . . . Character: **9**
Autologous Arterial Tissue . . . Character: **A**

This refers to a graft made with tissue from the patient's own body.

Synthetic Substitute . . . Character: **J**

This explains that the graft material may be carbon fibers, polypropylene, or other nonhuman substance.

Nonautologous Tissue Substitute . . . Character: **K**

This graft is made from materials other than the patient's own tissue.

Zooplastic Tissue . . . Character: **8**

This identifies that the graft was made with tissue from a species other than human.

GUIDANCE CONNECTION

Read the ICD-10-PCS Official Guidelines for Coding and Reporting, **Medical and Surgical Section Guidelines (Section 0)**, subsection **B6. Device**, subhead **General guidelines**, paragraphs **B6.1a**, **B6.1b**, and **B6.1c**, as well as subhead **Drainage device**, paragraph **B6.2**, for more details.

Simple or Mechanical Appliances	Character
Drainage Device	0
Monitoring Device	2
Monitoring Device, Pressure Sensor	0
Infusion Device	3
Extraluminal Device	C
Intraluminal Device	D
Intraluminal Device, Two	E
Intraluminal Device, Three	F
Intraluminal Device, Four or More	G
Intraluminal Device, Drug-Eluting	4
Intraluminal Device, Drug-Eluting, Two	5
Intraluminal Device, Drug-Eluting, Three	6
Intraluminal Device, Drug-Eluting, Four or More	7
Bioactive Intraluminal Device	B
Intraluminal Device, Radioactive	T

Implants and Electronic Appliances	Character
Stimulator (Cardiac) Lead	M
Cardiac Lead, Pacemaker	J
Intracardiac Pacemaker	N
Implantable Heart Assist System	Q
External Heart Assist System	R
Radioactive Element	1
No Device	Z

CODING BITES

Review *Appendix: Device Key and Aggregation Table* and *Appendix: Device Definitions* in your ICD-10-PCS code book.

In operative reports and procedure notes, when a device is placed into the patient, the notes will identify the brand name and details, rather than "synthetic substitute" or "intraluminal device." For instance, an AxiaLIF® System is an interbody fusion device used in lower joints, or Ultrapro plug is a synthetic substitute. Don't panic. You don't have to memorize these brand names. Just bookmark ***Appendix: Device Key and Aggregation Table*** in your ICD-10-PCS code book.

EXAMPLES

How can you determine if a device was implanted into the patient? The documentation will state something like one of these surgical notes excerpts.

". . . A Kapandji technique was also used for intrafocal pinning, taking a 0.062 K-wire in both the radial and ulnar aspects of the distal fragment and elevating it, followed by reducing it, controlling the distal fragment. . . ."

". . . A Palmaz Blue Genesis stent, 6 x 80 mm was used. It was deployed across the left renal artery stenosis in good position. . . ."

". . . A stylet (a thin wire) is inserted inside the center channel of the pacemaker lead to make it more rigid, and the lead-stylet combination is then inserted into the sheath and advanced under fluoroscopy to the appropriate heart chamber. . . ."

YOU INTERPRET IT!

Practice using the Device Key Appendix and fill in the device description used by ICD-10-PCS for coding.

44. Bovine pericardial valve: _______

45. Acuity Steerable Lead: _______

46. Embolization coil(s): _______

47. Tissue bank graft: _______

48. Pump reservoir: _______

49. Lap-Band® Adjustable Gastric Banding System: _______

50. Prestige cervical disc: _______

51. Versa: _______

52. Novacor Left Ventricular Assist Device: _______

53. EndoSure® sensor: _______

54. Brachytherapy seeds: _______

34.6 Medical/Surgical Qualifiers: Character 7

Character Position	Character Meaning
1	Section of the ICD-10-PCS book
2	Body system being treated
3	Root operation term
4	Body part (specific anatomical site)
5	Approach used by physician
6	Device
7	**Qualifier**

This seventh character is required. In many cases, there may be no more details to add, so you will use the placeholder **Z** No Qualifier—the equivalent of "not applicable."

You will find that, depending on the procedure provided, you may need to check the documentation for applicable details. For instance, when an excision is performed, you may find a Qualifier character option to explain that this was a biopsy (for diagnostic purposes . . . character **X**).

Earlier in this chapter, in the section that discussed root operation terms, you learned that bypass procedures are coded by identifying the body part bypassed "from," identified by character 4 (Body Part), and the body part bypassed "to," identified by character 7 (Qualifier). This is just a reminder that, in some cases, the Qualifier character will partner with the Body Part character to explain the whole story about the procedure.

EXAMPLE

0D164JA Gastric bypass, percutaneous endoscopic approach, rerouted from stomach to jejunum

LET'S CODE IT! SCENARIO

Callie MacDonald, a 2-year-old female, was admitted to the hospital by her ophthalmologist, Dr. Epps. Her right lacrimal duct was occluded. After sedation was administered, Dr. Epps probed her nasolacrimal duct and inserted a transluminal balloon catheter to expand the duct. The balloon was deflated and removed. She tolerated the procedure well.

Let's Code It!

Let's go through the steps of coding for ICD-10-PCS and determine the code or codes that should be reported for this encounter between Dr. Epps, an ophthalmologist, and Callie MacDonald.

First character: Section: Medical and Surgical . . . 0

Second character: Body System: Eye . . . 8

What root operation term would be most accurate? Read through the scenario carefully. Dr. Epps "expanded" the duct. The description of the term "dilation" is to expand an orifice or the lumen of a tubular body part.

Third character: Root Operation: Dilation . . . 7

Now, which "tubular body part" was dilated? The scenario states, "*Her right lacrimal duct . . .*"

You may have been tempted to think "eye"; however, when you get to the table for Eye, Dilation . . . 087, you will see that "eye" is the Body System and not an option for Body Part.

Fourth character: Body Part: Lacrimal Duct, Right . . . X

Dr. Epps inserted the catheter directly into the duct (this opening is how our tears flow from our eyes). Therefore, he used a natural opening.

Fifth character: Approach: Via Natural or Artificial Opening . . . 7

Dr. Epps inserted a *transluminal balloon catheter*, however, then the documentation states, "*The balloon was deflated and removed.*" Therefore, there is no Device reported in this position.

Sixth Character: Device: No Device . . . Z

Seventh Character: Qualifier: No Qualifier . . . Z

The ICD-10-PCS code you will report is

087X7ZZ Dilation, lacrimal duct, right, via natural or artificial opening

Good job!

34.7 Multiple and Discontinued Procedures in Medical and Surgical Cases

Multiple Procedures

Just because the physician performs more than one procedure does not necessarily mean you will report more than one code. The Official Guidelines provide four illustrations of cases when you will report multiple procedures:

a. *The same root operation is performed on different body parts as defined by distinct values of the body part character.* Two codes are reported.

GUIDANCE CONNECTION

Read the ICD-10-PCS Official Guidelines for Coding and Reporting, **Medical and Surgical Section Guidelines (Section 0)**, subsection **B3. Root Operation**, subhead **Multiple procedures**, paragraph **B3.2**.

b. *The same root operation is repeated at different body sites that are included in the same body part value.* You will report the same code twice. It is recommended that a report to explain is appended.

c. *Multiple root operations with distinct objectives are performed on the same body part.* Two codes are reported, one for each root operation.

d. *The intended root operation is attempted using one approach but is converted to a different approach.* One code will report what was actually accomplished with the first approach, and a second code will report the second approach.

LET'S CODE IT! SCENARIO

Ronald Markum, a 21-year-old male, was riding his motorcycle when he skidded out. The bike fell on top of him and his left ankle was dislocated. He was admitted into the hospital, and Dr. Traub tried to manually realign the tarsal bone to its rightful position. Unfortunately, he was unable to accomplish this and had to take Ronald to the OR to perform an open procedure.

Let's Code It!

Let's go through the steps of coding for ICD-10-PCS and determine the code or codes that should be reported for this encounter between Dr. Traub and Ronald Markum.

First code:

First character: Section: Medical and Surgical . . . 0

What is the body system? The documentation states, "*tarsal bone.*" That is in the ankle . . . therefore, **Lower Bones**.

Second character: Body System: Lower Bones . . . Q

What did the physician actually do? The documentation states, "*manually realign the tarsal bone to its rightful position.*" Read the definitions of the root operation terms. This matches **Reposition**.

Third character: Root Operation: Reposition . . . S

What body part was treated? The documentation states, "*his left ankle*" + "*the tarsal bone.*"

Fourth character: Body Part: Tarsal, Left . . . M

What was the approach? Did the physician go into the body? No, treatment was done from the outside.

Fifth character: Approach: External . . . X

Was any device inserted into the patient and left there? There is no mention of this.

Sixth Character: Device: No Device . . . Z

No details left to report.

Seventh Character: Qualifier: No Qualifier . . . Z

The ICD-10-PCS code you will report is

0QSMXZZ Reposition, left tarsal bone, externally

Remember the guideline about multiple procedures, B3.2, part d. You will need a second code to report the second attempt to realign Ronald's ankle. Notice the differences between the first attempt and the second attempt. The only difference is that the procedure was changed from an EXTERNAL approach to an OPEN approach.

Second code:

First character: Section: Medical and Surgical . . . 0
Second character: Body System: Lower Bones . . . Q
Third character: Root Operation: Reposition . . . S
Fourth character: Body Part: Tarsal, Left . . . M
Fifth character: Approach: Open . . . 0
Sixth character: Device: No Device . . . Z
Seventh character: Qualifier: No Qualifier . . . Z

(continued)

The ICD-10-PCS code you will report is

0QSM0ZZ Reposition, left tarsal bone, open approach

Finally, consider in what sequence you will report these two codes. The rule is that the most intense procedure will be reported first, so you should report the open procedure first, followed by the external approach.

0QSM0ZZ Reposition, left tarsal bone, open approach

0QSMXZZ Reposition, left tarsal bone, externally

Good job!

Discontinued Procedures

GUIDANCE CONNECTION

Read the ICD-10-PCS Official Guidelines for Coding and Reporting, **Medical and Surgical Section Guidelines (Section 0)**, subsection **B3. Root Operation**, subhead **Discontinued or incomplete procedures**, paragraph **B3.3**, for more details.

It has happened: The physician begins a procedure and for some reason must stop before accomplishing the goal originally planned. Should this occur, you are directed to report those root operations that were actually done.

EXAMPLE

Dr. Zander has planned a laparoscopic cholecystectomy. The incisions are made and the scope is inserted. The gallbladder can be visualized. However, before the organ can be surgically removed, the patient has a seizure. Dr. Zander stops the procedure and closes the incisions.

0FJ44ZZ Inspection of gallbladder, percutaneous endoscopic approach

YOU CODE IT! CASE STUDY

Nita Yessa has been in the hospital with a compound fracture of the leg, and she was brought into the procedure room to have her two-lead pacemaker replaced. Dr. Balthazar was able to remove her current pacemaker easily. However, there was a problem with the new device and he did not want to insert it. He closed the incision and sent Nita back to her room. He told Rita Holsman, his assistant, to notify him as soon as a new pacemaker was available.

You Code It!

Dr. Balthazar intended to replace Nita's pacemaker, but he couldn't complete the procedure. Using your ICD-10-PCS code book, determine the correct code to report this procedure.

Step #1: Read the case carefully and completely.

Step #2: Abstract the scenario. Which key words or terms describe what service the physician provided to the patient during this encounter?

Step #3: Are there any details missing or incomplete for which you would need to query the physician? [If so, ask your instructor.]

Step #4: Build the correct ICD-10-PCS procedure code or codes to explain the details about what was provided to the patient during this encounter.

Step #5: Check for any relevant guidance.

Step #6: Double-check your work.

Answer:

Did you determine this to be the correct code?

02PA3QZ Removal of implantable heart assist system, percutaneous approach

(continued)

As Guideline B3.3 directs you, when an intended procedure is discontinued, you need to code for what was actually completed. Dr. Balthazar was able to remove the old pacemaker, so you must code for the removal. You cannot code for the insertion of the new pacemaker because this was not done.

Good work!

GUIDANCE CONNECTION

Read the ICD-10-PCS Official Guidelines for Coding and Reporting, **Medical and Surgical Section Guidelines (Section 0)**, subsection **B6. Device**, subhead **General guidelines**, paragraph **B6.1a**, which addresses how to report the discontinuation of inserting a device. This guideline directs that if a device is intended to be inserted to remain after the procedure, and instead is removed before the end of the procedure (e.g., the device does not fit or a complication develops), you need to report both the ICD-10-PCS code for the insertion along with the code for the removal.

34.8 Medical/Surgical Coding: Putting It All Together

LET'S CODE IT! SCENARIO

PATIENT: Randolph Joy

HISTORY OF PRESENT ILLNESS: Patient was admitted to the Medical/Surgical floor last evening with acute upper abdominal pain and dyspnea. Blood work results were inconclusive, as was x-ray. Today, we are going to perform an EGD to investigate further.

PROCEDURE PERFORMED: Esophagogastroduodenoscopy

MEDICATIONS: Fentanyl 50 mcg, Versed 4 mg.

DESCRIPTION OF PROCEDURE: Informed consent was obtained. The patient was then placed in the left lateral decubitus position. IV sedation was started in a sequential fashion until the appropriate level of consciousness was achieved. Hurricaine spray was applied to the back of the throat and the endoscope was then advanced under direct visualization over the tongue, the esophagus, stomach, and duodenum. It was slowly withdrawn and the mucosa was carefully evaluated. Duodenal mucosal abnormalities were not visualized. Antegrade and retrograde views of the stomach did demonstrate some mild nonerosive gastritis, predominantly in the antrum. Portal gastropathy was noted throughout the gastric body, cardia, and fundus. Thickened gastric folds were noted and biopsied. Retroflexed view as well demonstrated no signs of a gastric varix; no coffee grounds or red blood was seen in the gastric lumen either. The scope was then withdrawn through the GE junction and careful examination did demonstrate shallow esophageal ulceration distally; biopsies were obtained. The suspicion of Barrett's esophagus noted with two salmon tongues of mucosa emanating 1 cm proximal to the GE junction. Careful examination of the remainder of the esophagus did demonstrate a hyperemic esophagus without further ulceration. The scope was then withdrawn from the patient and the procedure terminated. It was well tolerated and there were no immediate complications.

POST-PROCEDURE DIAGNOSES:

1. Probable Barrett's esophagus
2. Distal esophageal ulceration
3. Thickened hypertrophied gastric folds
4. Portal gastropathy and nonerosive gastritis

IMPRESSION AND PLAN: I suspect this patient's upper GI bleed is likely related to the ulcerations noted on this examination. As we await results of biopsies, I will change his proton pump inhibitor from an IV drip to oral and begin oral feeding as well. Hemoglobin and hematocrit will continue to be followed and, if stable, discharge may take place tomorrow.

(continued)

Let's Code It!

Dr. Ferrante performed an EGD to visually inspect Randolph's interior stomach to determine the cause of the pain and respiratory issues.

First character: Section: Medical and Surgical . . . 0

An esophagogastroduodenoscopy was performed. What body system does this involve? You learned about this in medical terminology class. *Esopha-* = esophagus + *-gastro-* = stomach + *-duoden-* = duodenum. To what body system do these anatomical sites belong?

Second character: System: Gastrointestinal System . . . D

Dr. Ferrante performed an EGD to visually inspect Randolph's interior stomach to determine the cause of the pain. This would point to the root operation term *inspection*. However, then tissue biopsies were taken, which points to the root operation term *excision*. Do you report two ICD-10-PCS codes? Let's analyze this. They are two different reasons for the procedure; however, while an inspection could be done without any excisions, the fact is that the biopsies could not be acquired without the inspection. Therefore, you only need one code, using the root operation term *Excision*.

Third character: Root Operation: Excision . . . B

From what anatomical site were the biopsies taken? The documentation states, "*esophageal ulceration distally; biopsies were obtained.*"

Fourth character: Body Part/Region: Esophagus, Lower . . . 3

How did Dr. Ferrante get to the distal (lower) esophagus? The documentation states, "*the endoscope was then advanced under direct visualization. . . .*"

Fifth character: Approach: Via Natural or Artificial Opening Endoscopic . . . 8

Sixth character: Device: No Device . . . Z

Our last character will explain the essential reason for this procedure. Was it to gather details to support a diagnosis (i.e., diagnostic)? Or was it to repair or fix a problem (i.e., therapeutic)?

Seventh character: Qualifier: Diagnostic . . . X

Now, you can put all of these characters together to report the ICD-10-PCS code, with confidence:

0DB38ZX Esophagogastroduodenoscopy, with biopsies, diagnostic

Good work!

LET'S CODE IT! SCENARIO

PATIENT: Gary Salton

PREOPERATIVE DIAGNOSIS: Subdural hematoma, traumatic

HISTORY OF PRESENT ILLNESS: This is a 17-year-old male, legally blind since birth, admitted after an assault. During the assault, he suffered extensive subarachnoid hemorrhage, LeFort fracture of the face, right arm venous phlebitis, and subdural hematoma. He was maintained on SICU, prophylaxis Dilantin, because of extensive subarachnoid hemorrhage. He went to the OR for facial ORIF. His course was complicated by ventricular tachycardia, but he was ruled out for MI at that time. He was started on amiodarone for the rate control. He also suffered a mandibular fracture so PEG was placed because of his inability to eat. No mention is made of acute seizure in this patient. There is no report of MRIs anywhere in the documentation. Preadmission summary states intracerebral hemorrhage and subdural hematoma, although they do not state where. He had to be emergently intubated due to hypoxemia. Other complications, during his hospital course, include cellulitis around the trach site, FUOs, and sinusitis. He has phlebitis in his right forearm. Repeat head CT showed increased bilateral frontal subdural hygroma and subarachnoid hemorrhage. He also developed hyphema of the right eye.

PAST MEDICAL HISTORY: Hypertension

(continued)

FAMILY HISTORY: Hypertension and stroke

SOCIAL HISTORY: He smokes a pack a day and occasional alcohol. Otherwise, independent prior to the admission.

MEDICATIONS: Prednisone, bacitracin topical cream, amiodarone, vancomycin, methadone b.i.d., dalteparin subcu daily, BuSpar 10 mg b.i.d., metoprolol 50 mg b.i.d., Pepcid, and Percocet.

PROCEDURE: Patient was taken to the OR for excision of frontal subdural hygroma and subarachnoid hemorrhage for evacuation. Once endotracheal administration of anesthesia was accomplished, patient was prepped and draped in the usual fashion, in a supine position. Using the drill, one small hole was made in the skull to relieve pressure and allow blood and fluids to be drained from the anterior cerebral vein. This was accomplished, and suction was applied to ensure the area was cleaned thoroughly. The area was bandaged and the patient was aroused successfully.

Scott Taucher, MD

Let's Code It!

Dr. Taucher drained Gary Salton's anterior cerebral vein. Let's analyze the documentation and build the code.

First character: Section: Medical and Surgical . . . 0

What specific body system was operated upon? The documentation states, "*anterior cerebral vein.*" The body system, therefore, would be the cerebrovascular system. However, there is not one character to cover this. Instead, you have four: **3** Upper Arteries; **4** Lower Arteries; **5** Upper Veins; and **6** Lower Veins. In which of these does the "*anterior cerebral vein*" fit? Cerebral indicates the brain, and, therefore, Upper Veins.

Second character: System: Upper Veins . . . 5

What did Dr. Taucher actually do in this procedure? The documentation states, "*allow blood and fluids to be drained.*"

Third character: Root Operation: Drainage . . . 9

Now, turn to the 059 Table in the Tables section. Read carefully through the options listed for the fourth character. Can you find "*anterior cerebral vein*"? You can see it with a broader descriptor . . .

Fourth character: Body Part: Intracranial Vein . . . L

Do you see the specific type of approach used in this procedure? The documentation states, "*Using the drill, one small hole was made in the skull.*"

Fifth character: Approach: Open . . . 0

Go back to the notes. Was a device placed into the patient and left there after the procedure ended?

Sixth character: Device: No Device . . . Z

Did Dr. Taucher do this to gather information to determine a diagnosis, or was this to fix or repair a problem?

Seventh character: Qualifier: No Qualifier . . . Z

Now you can put all of these characters together to report this ICD-10-PCS code, with confidence:

059L0ZZ Drainage of intracranial vein, open approach

Good work!

LET'S CODE IT! SCENARIO

PATIENT: Anabelle Preston

DATE OF OPERATION: 10/18/2026

PREOPERATIVE DIAGNOSIS: Bilateral urolithiasis

POSTOPERATIVE DIAGNOSIS: Bilateral urolithiasis

(continued)

OPERATIONS PERFORMED:

1. Cystoscopy
2. Right retrograde pyelogram
3. Right ureteral stent placement
4. Right percutaneous nephrolithotripsy

SURGEON: Sonia Petrosky, MD

ANESTHESIA: Laryngeal mask general

ANESTHESIOLOGIST: Matthew Sorensten, MD

ESTIMATED BLOOD LOSS: Minimal

IV FLUIDS: 2.5 liters crystalloid

DRAINS: A #5-French x 28 cm right double-pigtail ureteral stent and #18-French Foley catheter

COMPLICATIONS: None

INDICATIONS: The patient is a 63-year-old female, admitted last night through the ED with acute right flank pain, who denies prior history of kidney stones. She underwent parathyroidectomy 3 years ago. She stated that over the past few weeks she had intermittent right flank pain. An ultrasound showed mild dilation of the right collecting system with an 11-mm stone. Smaller stones were noted in the left kidney without any hydronephrosis. This was confirmed on her KUB showing an 11-mm stone in the right mid kidney and three stones on the left measuring 3–6 mm. She has had follow-up testing showing a 24-hour urine calcium output of only 90 mg. Her serum calcium level is normal.

DESCRIPTION OF THE PROCEDURE: The patient was brought to the lithotripsy suite. After induction of laryngeal mask general anesthesia, she was placed in dorsal lithotomy position. Perineum and introitus were prepped and draped. A #22-French rigid cystoscope was passed per urethra with obturator. The bladder was drained and then inspected with 12- and 70-degree lenses. She has a central cystocele. Both orifices appear normal. Minimal squamous metaplasia in the bladder neck area and no suspicious mucosal changes elsewhere. No trabeculation noted. Pollack catheter was threaded into the right ureter and dilute contrast was used to perform segmental pyelogram images on the right. Distally, multiple pelvic calcifications are lateral to the ureter consistent with phleboliths. No obvious filling defects seen. There is mild dilation of the majority of the collecting system above the pelvic brim. The stone appeared to be free floating within the renal pelvis.

Sensor guidewire was threaded up into the kidney. The Pollack catheter was inserted over the wire and the ureteral length was estimated. The contrast in the kidney was also allowed to drain to improve visualization of the stone for lithotripsy. The guidewire was then replaced and the Pollack catheter removed. A #5-French x 28-cm Polaris double-pigtail stent was then inserted with good pigtail formation on both ends. Cystoscope was removed and replaced with an #18-French Foley catheter.

Next, we performed a percutaneous nephrolithotripsy on the right kidney stone in the ureteropelvic junction. The stone appeared to fragment well. Periodic AP and oblique fluoroscopy was used. The patient was awakened, extubated, and transported to the recovery room in stable condition.

Let's Code It!

Dr. Petrosky completed two procedures on Annabelle during this session: insertion of a stent + the percutaneous nephrolithotripsy. Let's begin with the nephrolithotripsy:

First character: Section: Medical and Surgical . . . 0

These procedures were performed on Annabelle's kidneys. Therefore, the body system is the

Second character: System: Urinary System . . . T

What exactly does a nephrolithotripsy do? This procedure is performed to remove kidney stones by breaking them up. A good clue is in the documentation, where it states, "The stone appeared to fragment well."

Third character: Root Operation: Fragmentation . . . F

Read the options listed in the Body Part (character 4) column of this Table. The documentation states, "*in the ureteropelvic junction*." There is an additional descriptor under Kidney Pelvis, which also matches the documentation, which states, "*The stone appeared to be free floating within the renal pelvis*" and "*on the right kidney stone*."

Fourth character: Body Part/Region: Kidney Pelvis, Right . . . 3

(continued)

What approach was used to access the kidney stone to fragment it? The documentation states, "*percutaneous.*"

Fifth character: Approach: Percutaneous . . . 3

The options for the sixth and seventh characters are straightforward.

Sixth character: Device: No Device . . . Z

Seventh character: Qualifier: No Qualifier . . . Z

Now, you can put all of these characters together to report this ICD-10-PCS code, with confidence:

0TF33ZZ Nephrolithotripsy, percutaneous, kidney pelvis, right.

Good work!

Chapter Summary

This chapter showed you that building a code in ICD-10-PCS may require you to become familiar with a different perspective and way of interpreting the physician's notes. However, it all fits together, even though you will be using your knowledge in a slightly different way.

The ICD-10-PCS is used for reporting procedures performed in hospital inpatient health care settings only. And the ***Medical and Surgical Section*** code components are necessary for the largest percentage of procedures provided to patients while admitted to a hospital.

CODING BITES

Medical and Surgical Section character positions and their meanings:

Character Position	Character Meaning
1	Section of the ICD-10-PCS book
2	Body system being treated
3	Root operation term
4	Body part (specific anatomical site)
5	Approach used by physician
6	Device
7	Qualifier

You Interpret It! Answers

1. Lower Arteries, **2.** Lymphatic and Hemic Systems, **3.** Eye, **4.** Mouth and Throat, **5.** Gastrointestinal System, **6.** Muscles, **7.** Head and Facial Bones, **8.** Lower Bones, **9.** Upper Joints, **10.** Respiratory System, **11.** Bypass, **12.** Destruction, **13.** Dilation, **14.** Extirpation, **15.** Replacement, **16.** Release, **17.** Occlusion, **18.** Inspection, **19.** Fusion, **20.** Resection, **21.** Restriction, **22.** Pons, **23.** Inferior Mesenteric Vein, **24.** Inferior Vena Cava, **25.** Radius, **26.** Larynx, **27.** Skin, **28.** Retina, **29.** Pharynx, **30.** Nasal Turbinate, **31.** Sternum, **32.** Pelvic Bone, **33.** Percutaneous, **34.** Via Natural or Artificial Opening Endoscopic, **35.** Via Natural or Artificial Opening with Percutaneous Endoscopic Assistance, **36.** External, **37.** Open, **38.** Via Natural or Artificial Opening, **39.** Percutaneous, **40.** Percutaneous, **41.** Via Natural or Artificial Opening Endoscopic, **42.** Open, **43.** External, **44.** Zooplastic Tissue, **45.** Cardiac Lead, **46.** Intraluminal Device, **47.** Nonautologous Tissue Substitute, **48.** Infusion Device, Pump, **49.** Extraluminal Device, **50.** Synthetic Substitute, **51.** Pacemaker, Dual Chamber, **52.** Implantable Heart Assist System, **53.** Monitoring Device, Pressure Sensor, **54.** Radioactive Element

CHAPTER 34 REVIEW
ICD-10-PCS Medical and Surgical Section

Let's Check It! Terminology

Match each key term to the appropriate definition.

1. **LO 34.1** A letter or number component of an ICD-10-PCS code.
2. **LO 34.4** The path the physician took to access the body part upon which the treatment or procedure was targeted.
3. **LO 34.2** The term used to describe the function or purpose of the procedure.

A. Approach
B. Character
C. Root Operation Term

Let's Check It! Concepts

Choose the most appropriate answer for each of the following questions.

1. **LO 34.1** Character position 4 represents which of the following?
   a. The body system being treated **b.** The approach used by the physician
   c. The body part (specific anatomical site) **d.** A device
2. **LO 34.1** Character position 2: Body Systems: The endocrine system is identified by what number or letter?
   a. 2 **b.** G **c.** 7 **d.** S
3. **LO 34.1** What letters are *not* found in the list of body systems?
   a. B and H **b.** C and W **c.** K and Q **d.** O and I
4. **LO 34.2** According to the Official Guidelines for Coding and Reporting paragraph B2.1a, the example "Control of postoperative hemorrhage" is coded to the ________ "Control" found in the general anatomical regions body systems.
   a. root operation **b.** approach **c.** device **d.** qualifier
5. **LO 34.1** According to the Official Guidelines for Coding and Reporting paragraph B2.1b, the example "Vein body parts above the diaphragm" is found in the ________ body system.
   a. Heart and Great Vessels **b.** Upper Veins
   c. Anatomical Regions, Upper Extremities **d.** Upper Arteries
6. **LO 34.2** Which character position does the root operation term represent?
   a. 1 **b.** 3 **c.** 5 **d.** 7
7. **LO 34.2** Creation of a vagina in male perineum with nonautologous tissue substitute, open approach, would be coded with which of the following?
   a. 0W4M070 **b.** 0W4N071 **c.** 0W4M0K0 **d.** 0W4N0K1
8. **LO 34.2** According to the Official Guidelines for Coding and Reporting paragraph B3.7, the example "Resection of spleen to stop post-procedural bleeding" is coded to
   a. resection. **b.** control. **c.** excision. **d.** incision.
9. **LO 34.2** Extraction of the right cornea, external approach, would be coded with which of these?
   a. 08D9XZX **b.** 08DJ3ZZ **c.** 08DK3ZZ **d.** 08D8XZZ
10. **LO 34.2** The complete closing of an orifice or a lumen of a tubular body part is known as
   a. map. **b.** occlusion. **c.** fusion. **d.** detachment.

11. **LO 34.2** According to the Official Guidelines for Coding and Reporting paragraph B3.14, the example "Severing a nerve root to relieve pain" is coded to the root operation term

    a. release. b. reposition. c. division. d. restriction.

12. **LO 34.2** A diagnostic arthroscopy would be interpreted as

    a. bypass. b. extirpation. c. resection. d. inspection.

13. **LO 34.2** An esophagogastric fundoplication would be interpreted as

    a. fusion. b. restriction. c. resection. d. dilation.

14. **LO 34.1** The ileum is part of which body system?

    a. Upper Intestinal Tract b. Upper Leg c. Lower Intestinal Tract d. Lower Leg

15. **LO 34.3** The appendix that helps you when a specific anatomical site is documented and the body part components are not as specific is entitled

    a. *Definition Key.* b. *Body Part Key.*
    c. *Device Key.* d. *Device Aggregation Table.*

16. **LO 34.4** The approach to a procedure was entry, by puncture or minor incision, of instrumentation through the skin or mucous membrane and any other body layers necessary to reach the site of the procedure and is identified with the character 3. What type of approach was used?

    a. Open b. External
    c. Percutaneous d. Via natural or artificial opening

17. **LO 34.4** Endoscopic repair of the urethra via natural opening would be coded with which of these?

    a. 0TQC8ZZ b. 0TQD7ZZ c. 0TQD4ZZ d. 0TQD8ZZ

18. **LO 34.5** A cardiac lead, pacemaker implant device is represented by what sixth character?

    a. M b. J c. K d. R

19. **LO 34.6** A diagnostic qualifier is identified by what letter?

    a. X b. Z c. B d. F

20. **LO 34.5** Single upper tooth drainage device implant, open approach, would be coded with which of the following?

    a. 0C9W000 b. 0C9XX02 c. 0C9W0Z1 d. 0C9W001

Let's Check It! Guidelines

Refer to the Official ICD-10-PCS Medical and Surgical Section Guidelines and fill in the blanks accordingly.

only	Open	Percutaneous
root operations	overlapping	Release
Inspection	device	coded
after	deepest	not
Reposition	separate	autograft
fused	freed	External
indirectly	drainage	bypassed

1. Biopsy procedures are coded using the _________ Excision, Extraction, or Drainage and the qualifier Diagnostic.
2. If the root operations Excision, Repair or Inspection are performed on _________ layers of the musculoskeletal system, the body part specifying the _________ layer is coded.
3. If multiple coronary arteries are _________, a separate procedure is coded for each coronary artery that uses a different device and/or qualifier.
4. If an _________ is obtained from a different procedure site in order to complete the objective of the procedure, a separate procedure is coded.
5. If multiple vertebral joints are _________, a separate procedure is coded for each vertebral joint that uses a different device and/or qualifier.

6. ________ of a body part(s) performed in order to achieve the objective of a procedure is not coded separately.
7. In the root operation ________, the body part value coded is the body part being ________ and not the tissue being manipulated or cut to free the body part.
8. Reduction of a displaced fracture is coded to the root operation ________ and the application of a cast or splint in conjunction with the Reposition procedure is ________ coded separately.
9. If a body system does not contain a ________ body part value for fingers, procedures performed on the fingers are coded to the body part value for the hand.
10. Procedures performed using the open approach with percutaneous endoscopic assistance are coded to the approach ________.
11. Procedures performed ________ by the application of external force through the intervening body layers are coded to the approach ________.
12. Procedures performed percutaneously via a ________ placed for the procedure are coded to the approach ________.
13. A device is coded only if a device remains ________ the procedure is completed.
14. Procedures performed on a device ________ and not on a body part are specified in the root operations Change, Irrigation, Removal and Revision, and are ________ to the procedure performed.
15. A separate procedure to put in a ________ device is coded to the root operation Drainage with the device value Drainage Device.

Let's Check It! Rules and Regulations

Please answer the following questions from the knowledge you have gained after reading this chapter.

1. **LO 34.1** List the seven character positions of an ICD-10-PCS Medical and Surgical section code; include each character's meaning.
2. **LO 34.3** If the notes state a bilateral procedure was performed and there is no code character available to report a bilateral procedure, how would you report this procedure accurately?
3. **LO 34.3** What is the title of the appendix that helps you when a specific anatomical site is documented and the body part components are not as specific?
4. **LO 34.4** List the seven approaches used within the Medical and Surgical section; explain each approach.
5. **LO 34.7** The Official Guidelines provide four illustrations of cases when you will report multiple procedures. What are the four cases?

Let's Check It! Anatomical Term: ICD-10-PCS Value

Refer to the ICD-10-PCS Appendix entitled "Body Part Key" and identify the ICD-10-PCS value for each anatomical term.

Example: *Abdominal aortic plexus:*

a. ICD-10-PCS value: *Abdominal Sympathetic Nerve*

1. Apneustic center:
   a. ICD-10-PCS value: ________
2. Columella:
   a. ICD-10-PCS value: ________
3. Dural venous sinus:
   a. ICD-10-PCS value: ________
4. Fifth cranial nerve:
   a. ICD-10-PCS value: ________
5. Gastroduodenal artery:
   a. ICD-10-PCS value: ________

6. Genitofemoral nerve:
   a. ICD-10-PCS value: ________
7. Inferior cardiac nerve:
   a. ICD-10-PCS value: ________
8. Mammillary body:
   a. ICD-10-PCS value: ________
9. Palatine gland:
   a. ICD-10-PCS value: ________
10. Recurrent laryngeal nerve:
    a. ICD-10-PCS value: ________
11. Stylopharyngeus muscle:
    a. ICD-10-PCS value: ________
12. Tympanic nerve:
    a. ICD-10-PCS value: ________
13. Ventricular fold:
    a. ICD-10-PCS value: ________
14. Xiphoid process:
    a. ICD-10-PCS value: ________
15. Zygomaticus muscle:
    a. ICD-10-PCS value: ________

YOU CODE IT! Practice

Using the techniques described in this chapter, carefully read through the case studies and determine the most accurate ICD-10-PCS code(s) for each case study.

1. Theron Patel, a 12-year-old male, is experiencing obstructive sleep apnea. Dr. Pascal admits Theron to the hospital and performs an adenoidectomy, open approach.
2. Juanita Keane, a 38-year-old female, was admitted to Westwood Hospital yesterday. Dr. Chavez performs a laparoscopic cholecystectomy today.
3. Tom Gilbert, a 29-year-old male, is admitted to Weston Hospital due to severe hypertension. Dr. Benton notes left kidney atrophy and performs an endoscopic left renal artery biopsy.
4. Bella Cable, a 62-year-old female, has severe pain in her right foot when she walks. Upon examination her right big toe has turned toward the second toe. Bella is admitted to the hospital, where Dr. Meltzer performs a bunionectomy, open approach, with a soft tissue correction.
5. Richard McMillan, a 26-year-old male, has had a bad cough for the last 3 months. Therefore, Dr. Skenes admitted him into the hospital and performed a diagnostic fiberoptic bronchoscopy with hopes of determining the cause of the irritation.
6. Merle Sims, a 34-year-old female, is a professional runner and has won three marathons. Today, she is admitted to the hospital for a total arthroplasty (replacement) of her right knee, nonautologous tissue substitute, open approach.
7. Carolyn Bulwark, a 21-year-old female, feels she has "big ears." Carolyn was admitted to the hospital, where her external ears were altered bilaterally, percutaneous approach.

(continued)

8. Harry Matthews, a 48-year-old male, was admitted to Westwood Hospital yesterday. Harry was diagnosed with esophageal cancer. A middle esophagus bypass, percutaneous endoscopic approach, rerouted to stomach, was performed today.
9. John Andrews, a 46-year-old male, was admitted to the hospital, where he underwent urinary bladder surgery 2 days ago. Today, John's urinary bladder drainage device is changed, external approach.
10. Annie Campbell, a 28-year-old female, was admitted to Westwood Hospital. The patient closed the car door on her foot and severely injured her left foot. Annie's left 5th toe is completely amputated.
11. Wilburn Backwinkel, a 54-year-old male, has had left upper quadrant pain radiating to his back. Dr. Dix admits Wilburn to Westwood Hospital, where he performs an endoscopic (via natural opening) inspection of the pancreatic duct.
12. Lynda Dibble, a 39-year-old female, gave birth to her fourth child 6 months ago. The patient presents today requesting tubal ligation. Lynda is admitted to Westwood Hospital, where Dr. Connell performs a bilateral fallopian tube ligation, percutaneous endoscopic approach.
13. Mike Raval, a 53-year-old male, underwent an abdominal procedure this morning at Westwood Hospital. After the procedure was completed, Mike began to hemorrhage. Dr. Scott performed a control of postoperative bleeding in the abdominal wall, open approach.
14. Lee Spigner, an 83-year-old male, cannot swallow his food and has lost a substantial amount of weight. Lee is admitted to the hospital, where Dr. Ubaldo inserts a feeding device in Lee's stomach, percutaneous endoscopic approach.
15. Vickie Turner, a 24-year-old female, has a history of uncontrolled motor movements and some uncontrolled eye movement. Vickie is admitted to the hospital, where Dr. Allen performs a mapping of Vickie's basal ganglia signals, percutaneous approach.

ICD-10-PCS

YOU CODE IT! Application

The following exercises provide practice in abstracting physicians' notes and learning to work with documentation from our health care facility, Westward Hospital. These case studies are modeled on real patient encounters. Using the techniques described in this chapter, carefully read through the case studies and determine the most accurate ICD-10-PCS code(s), if appropriate, for each case study.

WESTWARD HOSPITAL

591 Chester Road

Masters, FL 33955

OPERATIVE REPORT

PATIENT: FASCHEL, MARTIN

DATE OF ADMISSION: 11/15/26

DATE OF SURGERY: 11/16/26

DATE OF DISCHARGE: 11/19/26

ADMITTING DIAGNOSIS: Uncontrolled epilepsy

DISCHARGE DIAGNOSIS: Uncontrolled epilepsy

PROCEDURE PERFORMED: Left vagal nerve stimulator insertion.

SURGEON: Kevin Mulford, MD

ASSISTANT: Denny Granger, MD

ANESTHESIA: General endotracheal

ESTIMATED BLOOD LOSS: Less than 10 mL

(continued)

COMPLICATIONS: None

DRAINS: None

OPERATIVE FINDINGS: A model 102 generator with 2-mm electrodes was utilized.

INDICATION FOR PROCEDURE: The patient is a 6-year-old child who was found to have progressive epilepsy. It was recommended that a vagal nerve stimulator be placed. We discussed the options, the risks, and benefits with the child's parents, and their questions were welcomed and answered. The procedure and potential risks of surgery include, but are not limited to, vagal nerve injury, vascular damage, stroke, inoperability, malfunction, the need for continuous monitoring and evaluations, the possible need for further surgical interventions, among others. With the family's understanding and permission, the child was brought to the operating room for this procedure.

DESCRIPTION OF PROCEDURE: After suitable general endotracheal anesthesia was obtained, the patient was placed in the supine position and the head immobilized in a donut. The skin was prepared using Betadine scrub and solution and a suitable surgical drape. Marcaine with epinephrine was infiltrated.

Initially, we made a 2.5-cm incision along the neck crease, and the platysma muscle was divided. The sternocleidomastoid muscle was retracted and dissected medially, and we identified the carotid sheath. The carotid sheath was opened and we identified the vagal nerve. This was then isolated with vessel loops.

We then attached the two electrodes in the grounding mechanism using 2-mm size coils. These were found to be securely placed and a small loop was left for anchoring.

We then prepared the pocket while making a 6-cm curvilinear incision just medial to the axilla. A subcutaneous pocket was created over the pectoralis muscle, and the area was irrigated.

We then used the tunneling device from the cervical to the chest incisions, and the electrodes were placed in the subcutaneous tunnel. The model 102 generator was then connected to the electrodes. An impedance test was done and was found to be 1.

The electrode in the subclavian was left with a small loop for growth, and this was anchored to the fascia using a Vicryl suture.

Subsequently, the generator was turned on at the 0.25 mA at 30 Hz, on 30 seconds, off for 5 minutes, with a magnet strength of 0.5 for 60 seconds.

The wounds were then irrigated and subsequently painted with Betadine solution. They were then closed using 3-0 Vicryl sutures for the deep layer. The skin was approximated using 4-0 Vicryl suture in a running subcuticular fashion. Steri-Strips were applied, and the patient was awakened and transported to the recovery room, having tolerated the procedure well.

We discussed the operation, the findings, and the potential implications and complications with the patient's family. Their questions were welcomed and answered, and they expressed understanding of the situation.

Determine the most accurate ICD-10-PCS code(s).

WESTWARD HOSPITAL

591 Chester Road

Masters, FL 33955

OPERATIVE REPORT

PATIENT: TUTTLE, BARBIE

DATE OF ADMISSION: 05/07/26

DATE OF SURGERY: 05/08/26

DATE OF DISCHARGE: 05/11/26

ADMITTING DIAGNOSIS: Avascular necrosis with severe collapse, total head involvement, left hip.

DISCHARGE DIAGNOSIS: Avascular necrosis with severe collapse, total head involvement, left hip.

OPERATION PERFORMED: Left total hip arthroplasty.

(continued)

SURGEON: Gerard Brighton, MD

ASSISTANT: Peter Alfredson, MD

ANESTHESIA: General.

INDICATIONS FOR OPERATION: This 55-year-old female was noted to have progressively worsening hip pain. She was noted to have on x-ray avascular necrosis with severe collapse and loss of sphericity of the femoral head, Ficat grade 4. The risks and benefits of total hip arthroplasty were discussed in detail, and the patient signed surgical consent.

DESCRIPTION OF OPERATION: The surgical site was signed. The patient was prepped and draped in a routine sterile manner. The IV antibiotics were given prior to the procedure. The surgical team used space suits for added sterility. A posterolateral approach to the hip was made. The fascia was identified and split in line of its fibers. The short external rotators were identified. A T-capsulotomy was performed. The hip was dislocated. The femoral neck was cut using a reciprocating saw. The cut was made based on intraoperative and preoperative templating.

Once the neck was cut, the patient's anteversion was noted, and bone wax was placed on the neck cut to decrease bleeding. The acetabular retractors were placed, a cobra retractor anteriorly, and a posterior-inferior retractor placed into the obturator foramen after an inferior radial capsulotomy. The acetabulum was exposed. The soft tissues, including the labrum and pulvinar, were removed from the acetabulum, and then the acetabulum was progressively reamed from a size 50 up to a size 56. Using a Zimmer M/L Taper Hip Prosthesis, 16.5 mm, ceramic on polyethylene, with a Zimmer head diameter of 12/14 internal taper, a 57-mm Converge cup was then impacted into place at position of 45 degrees of abduction and 20 degrees of anteversion. The overhanging osteophytes were removed. The 38-mm liner was snapped into the cup. A lap sponge was used to protect the cup.

The acetabular retractors were removed. A proximal femoral retractor was placed. The proximal femur was machined first with a cookie cutter osteotome, then a lateralizing reamer, and then progressive broaches. The broaches were taken up to a size 13.5. This initially had good fit. X-rays were taken with a 13.5-mm stem and a neutral ball.

Of note, intraoperative x-rays did note that there was residual room at the lateral aspect of the femur. This was likely secondary to scarred bone from her prior cord decompression. The trial stem was then removed, and using a large curette, the lateral bone was removed. We then again machined from a size 13.5 up to a size 16.25 stem. The 16.25 had excellent fit, kept the equal leg length at the same level as the intraoperative x-ray, taken with the 13.5, but had better canal fill. The real stem was then placed. A neutral ball was placed.

The hip was then tested for range of motion, noted to be quite stable with flexion to 90 degrees, internal rotation to 70, and no instability with extension, external rotation. The capsule was then repaired with #2 FiberWire. The short external rotators were repaired with #2 FiberWire to the trochanter. The fascia was closed with 0 PDS, the subcutaneous tissue was closed with 0 Vicryl, a running 3-0 Monocryl was placed at the subcuticular region. Dermabond was placed at the skin.

The patient was taken to recovery room in stable condition. Estimated blood loss was 150 mL. Sponge and needle counts were correct.

Determine the most accurate ICD-10-PCS code(s).

WESTWARD HOSPITAL

591 Chester Road

Masters, FL 33955

OPERATIVE REPORT

PATIENT: LATCHMAN, VICTOR

DATE OF ADMISSION: 03/05/26

DATE OF DISCHARGE: 03/17/26

ADMITTING DIAGNOSIS: Dislocation, right humeroulnar joint

PROCEDURE: Open Reposition

(continued)

Patient is a 31-year-old male, admitted via the ED with acute pain in his right arm. Patient is a landscaper and tree trimmer and was hit by a falling tree limb. X-rays show dislocation of the humeroulnar joint, right side.

Patient was taken into the operating room and placed in the supine position. General anesthesia was administered. The area was opened with a 9-cm incision point to the distal aspect of the joint. Once the dislocation was visualized, manipulation was employed to reconfigure the tendons, muscles, and bones back to normal position.

The incision was closed using 4.0 silk; bandage and cast were applied. The patient was taken into the recovery room, having tolerated the procedure well.

Benjamin Johnston, MD

Determine the most accurate ICD-10-PCS code(s).

WESTWARD HOSPITAL

591 Chester Road

Masters, FL 33955

OPERATIVE REPORT

PATIENT: MAGGUIOTT, FELIX

DATE OF ADMISSION: 08/15/26

DATE OF DISCHARGE: 08/17/26

ADMITTING DIAGNOSIS: Inguinal hernia, left

PROCEDURE: Herniorrhaphy, with synthetic substitute

OPERATION: Left inguinal hernia repair with mesh

DESCRIPTION OF OPERATION: The patient was taken to the operating room and placed supine on the operating room table. After general anesthesia was induced, the left inguinal area was prepped with Betadine solution and sterilely draped in the usual manner for procedure in this area. The skin and subcutaneous tissues of the left inguinal area were anesthetized, and an incision beginning at the left pubic tubercle and extending laterally along natural skin lines was created. The incision was extended through the subcutaneous tissues to the aponeurosis of the external oblique. Hemostasis was obtained with the Bovie cautery. The subaponeurotic tissues were anesthetized.

The aponeurosis of the external oblique was incised along the length of its fibers. Care was taken to avoid the ilioinguinal nerve. At the level of the pubic tubercle, the spermatic cord was bluntly dissected from its surrounding structures and encircled with a 0.25-inch Penrose drain. The direct hernia sac was dissected off of the cord structures and invaginated into the preperitoneal space. A search for an indirect component proved fruitless.

A large Marlex mesh "plug" was placed in the preperitoneal space, reducing the direct inguinal hernia. It was anchored to the conjoint tendon and the shelving edge of the Poupart's ligament and the pubic tubercle with 2-0 PDS sutures. The onlay portion was placed over the floor of the inguinal canal, while it was anchored to the shelving edge of the Poupart's ligament to the conjoint tendon and laterally to the internal oblique with interrupted 2-0 PDS sutures. The Marlex mesh plug was attached to the onlay portion with a 3-0 Prolene suture. The aponeurosis of the external oblique was closed with a running suture of 3-0 PDS. Subcutaneous tissues were approximated with interrupted sutures of 3-0 PDS. The skin was closed with subcuticular suture of 4-0 PDS. A 0.5-inch Steri-Strip tape was applied. A sterile occlusive dressing was applied over this.

The patient tolerated the procedure well and was transferred to the recovery room in stable condition. Estimated blood loss was 5 cc. Sponge, needle, and instrument counts were correct.

Kenzi Bloomington, MD

Determine the most accurate ICD-10-PCS code(s).

(continued)

WESTWARD HOSPITAL

591 Chester Road

Masters, FL 33955

OPERATIVE REPORT

PATIENT: KENSINGTON, LOUIS

DATE OF ADMISSION: 10/07/26

DATE OF DISCHARGE: 10/09/26

ADMITTING DIAGNOSIS: Chronic anal fissure and anal stenosis.

DISCHARGE DIAGNOSIS: Chronic anal fissure and anal stenosis.

OPERATIONS:

1. V-Y anoplasty.
2. Lateral internal sphincterotomy with fissurectomy.
3. Flexible sigmoidoscopy.

ESTIMATED BLOOD LOSS: 30 mL.

SPECIMENS: No specimens.

DRAINS: A 0.25-inch Penrose to the flap.

COMPLICATIONS: None.

DESCRIPTION OF OPERATION: After informed consent was obtained, the patient was taken to the OR. He was placed in the prone jackknife position and IV sedation was given by the anesthesiologist. The buttocks were taped laterally, exposing the perianal area. I began with the lubricated scope. The videoscope was inserted into the rectum and advanced through the colon to about 40 cm. At 40 cm, there was some angulation and some looping of the scope, and I elected not to proceed beyond this point. I then began to slowly withdraw the scope, carefully inspecting the lumen. The prep was adequate up to this point. I withdrew the scope. I noted no tumors or polyps. There was no evidence of colitis or proctitis and no diverticular disease was noted. I then desufflated the colon and rectum and removed the scope.

The perianal area was then prepped with Betadine and draped in the usual fashion. I then used a solution of 0.5% Marcaine with epinephrine and injected about 30 mL perianally as well as intramuscularly to achieve some relaxation of the sphincter muscles. After adequate analgesia was obtained, the small Ferguson retractor was inserted and the anal canal was inspected. The anterior fissure was very chronic appearing and measured about 1 × 0.5 cm in size. The anal canal was rather small and there seemed to be spasm of the distal edge of the internal sphincter muscle.

I then inserted the Buie retractor and opened it to expose the right lateral anal canal. An incision was made over the anoderm in the right lateral position and then I dissected down to the distal edge of the internal sphincter muscle, which was easily palpable as a tight band. I used a hemostat to dissect underneath it and elevated and divided it for a length of less than 1 cm. This did achieve relaxation of the sphincter muscle.

Then at this point, I was able to remove the Buie retractor and inserted the Chelsea-Eaton retractor. There was a definite release of the spasm of the sphincter muscle. However, there was also now obvious evidence of stenosis of the anal canal and there was no way to bring the mucosal edges together to cover the sphincterotomy wound without putting tension on the anal canal. Because of this, I did elect to go ahead with the anoplasty.

I used a marking pen to outline a house-shaped flap on the perianal skin in the right lateral position. I then anesthetized this area. I used a #15 blade scalpel to incise the skin edges. I then mobilized the flap by dissecting laterally to give the flap a very broad base. With the lateral dissection, I was then able to mobilize the flap down into the anal canal to cover up the lateral internal sphincterotomy wound.

The area was irrigated. Then the flap was sewed into place using interrupted sutures, using combination of #3-0 Vicryl and #4-0 Vicryl sutures, using the #3-0 Vicryl primarily on the tension points of the flap. Once the proximal edge of the flap was sewed to the dentate line, I then came up the anterior and posterior sides of the flap, suturing again in an interrupted fashion to the cut mucosal edges. I then used a scalpel to make a small incision in the right posterior position about 1 centimeter or 2 away from the flap and then used the stab incision to bring a 0.25-inch Penrose through the skin and positioned it underneath the flap. It was sutured to the skin with a single #3-0 Vicryl

(continued)

suture. The excess drain was then cut away, leaving about 2 or 3 cm protruding and the remainder positioned underneath the flap. I then used #2-0 Vicryl and a mattress suture to perform the long portion of the Y of the flap. This was done on the distal edge of the incision, bringing the two skin edges together with two of these mattress sutures to form the Y.

At this point, I now just had the remainder of the bottom of the Y portion of the flap to close and this was done again using a combination of interrupted #3-0 and #4-0 Vicryl sutures. At this point, I had good hemostasis throughout the flap and the flap appeared to be viable. There was no tension on it. There was a good color with no blanching noted.

I then directed my attention back toward the anal fissure in the anterior position. The small anterior tag was excised. That was a small hypertrophied anal papilla. I then mobilized the mucosal side of the fissure, elevating the mucosa, and a very small amount of muscle as well and then used a #4-0 Vicryl suture to bring this mucosal edge about halfway up the fissure to partially cover it and facilitate the healing process. There was a small amount of bleeding that was controlled with the #3-0 Vicryl figure-of-eight suture.

At this point, I had good release of the anal stenosis and good hemostasis throughout. On further examination, there was a very small posterior anal fissure, which was simply coagulated with the electrocautery. At this point, the retractor was removed. A roll of Gelfoam was placed in the anal canal and then a fluffy gauze dressing was placed over the Gelfoam.

The patient was then returned to the supine position and taken to the recovery area in stable condition.

Phillip Carlsson, MD

Determine the most accurate ICD-10-PCS code(s).

35
Obstetrics Section

Key Terms

Abortifacient
Laminaria
Products of Conception

Learning Outcomes

After completing this chapter, the student should be able to:

LO 35.1 Recognize the details reported in the Obstetrics section of ICD-10-PCS.
LO 35.2 Interpret the procedure to determine the accurate Obstetrics root operation term.
LO 35.3 Employ your knowledge of anatomy to determine the body part treated in Obstetrics coding.
LO 35.4 Determine the approach used for the Obstetrics procedure.
LO 35.5 Identify any devices that will stay with the body after an Obstetrics procedure.
LO 35.6 Utilize the details required to report the correct qualifier for an Obstetrics code.
LO 35.7 Analyze all of the details to build an accurate seven-character Obstetrics code.

STOP! Remember, you need to follow along in your ICD-10-PCS code book for an optimal learning experience.

35.1 Obstetrics Section/Body System: Characters 1 and 2

Obstetrics is the medical specialty that focuses on the care of pregnant women. The relationship between the physician—the obstetrician—and the patient often begins prior to conception and lasts all the way through gestation through delivery to the postpartum period. The entire scope of this care is *not* an issue for coders in a hospital. However, there will be times when a pregnant woman might be admitted into a hospital requiring acute care. These are the procedures and services reported from this section.

GUIDANCE CONNECTION

Read the ICD-10-PCS Official Guidelines for Coding and Reporting, **Obstetrics Section Guidelines (Section 1)**, subsection **C. Obstetrics Sections**, paragraphs **C1** and **C2**.

So let's review the meanings for the ***Obstetrics*** section characters:

Character Position	Character Meaning
1	Section of the ICD-10-PCS book
2	Body system being treated (Pregnancy)
3	Root operation term
4	Body part (Products of Conception)
5	Approach used by physician
6	Device
7	Qualifier

At this time, there are only two Official Guidelines to support your reporting from the ***Obstetrics*** section in ICD-10-PCS. You should become familiar with them both.

Character Position 1: Obstetrics Section 1

Character Position	Character Meaning
1	**Section of the ICD-10-PCS book**
2	Body system being treated (Pregnancy)
3	Root operation term
4	Body part (Products of Conception)
5	Approach used by physician
6	Device
7	Qualifier

All of the codes reporting an obstetrics procedure provided to a pregnant woman who has been admitted into a hospital will begin with the number one (1).

Character Position 2: Body System: 0

Character Position	Character Meaning
1	Section of the ICD-10-PCS book
2	**Body system being treated (Pregnancy)**
3	Root operation term
4	Body part (Products of Conception)
5	Approach used by physician
6	Device
7	Qualifier

In this section there is only one body system, that is, the gestational term:

Pregnancy . . . Character: **0**

From conception to delivery, procedures, services, and treatments provided to the products of conception within a woman who is pregnant and has been admitted into a hospital are reported with codes from this section to report the hospital (facility) care. Before conception or after the baby is born, the services will be reported from a different section of this code set.

35.2 Obstetrics Root Operations: Character 3

Character Position	Character Meaning
1	Section of the ICD-10-PCS book
2	Body system being treated (Pregnancy)
3	**Root operation term**
4	Body part (Products of Conception)
5	Approach used by physician
6	Device
7	Qualifier

The ***Obstetrics*** section uses 12 root operation terms to describe the specific procedure provided during this encounter. Some interpretation may be necessary so you can understand what terms to abstract from the operative report or procedure notes accurately and completely. Using the root operation term is the most efficient way of using the Alphabetic Index, as well.

As you learned in previous chapters, the root operation term is based on the objective of the procedure. You are seeking the word describing the action, such as *extraction* or *delivery*. Terms with which you are very familiar, such as cesarean section (c-section) or amniocentesis, may name the procedure; however, these terms do not specifically explain the action of the physician, or do they? Let's take a closer look at these two terms, as examples, and interpret them into the root operation terms:

Cesarean section: What precisely is this procedure? The extraction of the baby via surgical incision. This explanation leads you to the root operation term used in ICD-10-PCS, *extraction*.

Amniocentesis: What specifically is done during this procedure? Using a needle, the physician takes out (drains) some of the amniotic fluid. Understanding this, you can interpret that the root operation term *drainage* describes this perfectly.

With some procedures, you will use your knowledge of the specific procedure and what it is expected to accomplish. For example, you will need to remember that the physician supporting the natural process of a vaginal delivery is reported with the root operation term *delivery*. That one works very well in translation, doesn't it?

Now, let's go over each of the 12 root operation terms used in this section of ICD-10-PCS and look at some examples, to help you understand what each reports.

Abortion

Abortion: Artificially terminating a pregnancy . . . Character: **A**

Note, this is not typically reporting a voluntary abortion. Those are most often performed on an *out*patient basis. This root operation term refers to a procedure performed for medical necessity only.

GUIDANCE CONNECTION

Read the ICD-10-PCS Official Guidelines for Coding and Reporting, **Obstetrics Section Guidelines (Section 1)**, subsection **C. Obstetrics Section**, subhead **Procedures following delivery or abortion**, paragraph **C2**.

EXAMPLES

Deena Wolff has been in a coma for a week, as a the result of being raped and beaten. Blood work shows she is pregnant and her injuries make the pregnancy not viable. Dr. Owens performed an abortion, vaginal approach, using a vacuum method.

10A07Z6 Abortion of products of conception via natural or artificial opening using vacuum

The patient was pregnant with monochorionic twins (twins that share a common placenta) and there was a problem. Evidence of unbalanced flow of blood from one twin to the other twin caused twin–twin transfusion syndrome. Because she was only at 13 weeks, a pregnancy termination was determined to be the best option for the mother's health and a future opportunity to get pregnant again. He performed a dilation and curettage.

10A08ZZ Abortion of products of conception via natural or artificial opening

Change

Change: Taking out or off a device from a body part and putting back an identical or similar device in or on the same body part without cutting or puncturing the skin or a mucous membrane . . . Character: **2**

EXAMPLE

Two days ago, Dr. Conners inserted a fetal scalp electrode on Jenna's 27-gestational-week-old fetus. Today, Jenna is admitted into the hospital to monitor her and the fetus, and to change the current electrode to a new one.

102073Z Changing a monitoring device for the products of conception via natural or artificial opening

Delivery

Delivery: Assisting the passage of the products of conception from the genital canal . . . Character: **E**

GUIDANCE CONNECTION

Read the ICD-10-PCS Official Guidelines for Coding and Reporting, **Obstetrics Section Guidelines (Section 1)**, subsection **C. Obstetrics Section**, subhead **Procedures following delivery or abortion**, paragraph **C2**.

EXAMPLE

The patient is a 31-year-old G2, P0 female at 38 weeks and 5 days estimated gestational age who presented in labor. On vaginal examination, the patient was found to be 4 cm dilated, 70% effaced, and –3 station, and the fetal heart tracing at that time was in the 140s with minimal long-term variability. She was admitted to Labor and Delivery for Pitocin augmentation and amniotomy. She continued to have a good labor pattern and proceeded to deliver a viable 6-pound, 12-ounce male infant over an intact perineum with Apgars of 8 and 9 at 1 and 5 minutes. There were no nuchal cords and no true knots, and the number of vessels in the cord was three. Her postpartum course was uncomplicated, and the patient was discharged to home in stable and satisfactory condition.

10E0XZZ Delivery of a neonate (products of conception), external approach

NOTE: The administration of the Pitocin, IV, would be reported separately (you will learn about these codes in the ***Placement through Chiropractic Sections*** chapter, section ***Reporting Services from the Administration Section***).

Drainage

Drainage: Taking or letting out fluids and/or gases from a body part . . . Character: **9**

EXAMPLES

Maria Lettio was 39 years old when Dr. Platt confirmed she was pregnant. Today, she has been admitted into the hospital for a gastroesophageal fundoplication. While here, Dr. Lowenthal performed an amniocentesis to check the fetus for genetic abnormalities.

10903ZU Drainage of amniotic fluid, percutaneous approach, for diagnostic purposes

Concern for the existence of alloimmune thrombocytopenia, fetal blood sampling to assess the baby's platelet count is performed.

10903Z9 Drainage, fetal blood sampling, percutaneously

The patient's uterus is compressing due to an overabundance of amniotic fluid. Therefore, today we will perform an amnioreduction to decompress the womb to prevent preterm delivery. A needle is inserted into the amniotic cavity and the excess fluid is removed.

10903ZC Drainage of amniotic fluid, percutaneous approach, for therapeutic purposes

Extraction

Extraction: Pulling or stripping out or off all or a portion of a body part by the use of force . . . Character: **D**

A great example of an extraction is a cesarean section, which is not a separate root operation because the intention is to *extract* the baby from the mother's body. However, it is not the only type of procedure reported with this root operation.

GUIDANCE CONNECTION

Read the ICD-10-PCS Official Guidelines for Coding and Reporting, **Obstetrics Section Guidelines (Section 1)**, subsection **C. Obstetrics Section**, subhead **Procedures following delivery or abortion**, paragraph **C2**.

EXAMPLES

Dr. Traucher determined that Petricka's pregnancy was ectopic. He used an endoscopic method, via her vagina, to remove the fertilized egg from her fallopian tube.

10D28ZZ Extraction of ectopic products of conception via natural or artificial opening, endoscopic

The patient was admitted on the morning of her scheduled surgery. Detailed informed consent was again reobtained. All consents were signed. Under spinal anesthesia, uncomplicated repeat low transverse cesarean section was performed. A viable male infant with Apgars of 9 and 9 with birth weight of 8 pounds 6 pounds was delivered. The patient's postoperative course was uneventful.

10D00Z1 Extraction of products of conception, open approach, using a low cervical incision

Insertion

Insertion: Putting in nonbiological appliance that monitors, assists, performs, or prevents a physiological function but does not physically take the place of a body part . . . Character: **H**

This is another opportunity for reading very carefully. In ICD-10-PCS, this root operation, *insertion*, applies only to the placement into the body of a medical device, such as a monitoring device, that will remain in the body after the procedure is completed.

EXAMPLE

Concerned about the fetus's sustainability, Dr. Franklin placed a scalp electrode while Mei Lynn was still in the hospital for another issue.

10H073Z Insertion of monitoring electrode via natural or artificial opening

Inspection

Inspection: Visually and/or manually exploring a body part . . . Character: **J**

This root operation term is limited to the physician's looking.

EXAMPLE

Using a scope via a percutaneous incision, Dr. Klotzky viewed the fetus's position using an operative fetoscopy.

10J04ZZ Inspection of productions of conception, percutaneous endoscopic approach

Removal

Removal: Taking out or off a device from a body part . . . Character: **P**

Read this carefully: As the description specifically states "device," this can only be used for this type of procedure, to remove a previously inserted device. As you abstract the physician's notes, be cautious of the use of this term in documentation. The removal of a mole, for example, is really an excision, not a removal.

EXAMPLE

After gathering the data he needed, Dr. Abernathy removed the electrode that had been placed on the fetus's scalp.

10P003Z Removal of monitoring electrode, open approach

Repair

Repair: Restoring, to the extent possible, a body part to its normal anatomic structure and function . . . Character: **Q**

EXAMPLES

Dr. Atlante determined that Geena Simpson's fetus has indications of spina bifida. He performed a repair of the skin over the spinal opening, in utero, with hopes of enabling the child to be born without disability.

10Q03ZQ Repair of skin, percutaneous approach

Aortic stenosis may be relieved in utero by performing an aortic balloon valvuloplasty. This is accomplished by inserting a needle into the fetal heart through which the balloon catheter is passed.

10Q03ZF Repair of cardiovascular system, percutaneous approach

Reposition

Reposition: Moving to its normal location or other suitable location all or a portion of a body part . . . Character: **S**

EXAMPLE

Rae-Ann was in the last stage of labor and ready to deliver when Dr. Bornstine realized the baby was breech. Externally, he manually manipulated the position of the baby, and a 7 lb. 3 oz. boy was delivered a short time later.

10S0XZZ Reposition of fetus, external approach

Resection

Resection: Cutting out or off, without replacement, all of a body part . . . Character: **T**

Remember how this differs from excision. When the entire body part is surgically removed, it is reported as a resection. If only a portion of the body part is removed, it is reported as an excision.

EXAMPLE

Dr. Peterson determined that Ursula's fertilized egg was stuck in her left fallopian tube and was growing. He had to surgically remove the fallopian tube before it burst.

10T28ZZ Resection of fallopian tube for ectopic products of conception, via natural or artificial opening, endoscopic

Transplantation

Transplantation: Putting in or on all or a portion of a living body part taken from another individual or animal to physically take the place and/or function of all or a portion of a similar body part . . . Character: **Y**

ICD-10-PCS uses this term in the same manner that physicians do, when a donor organ is placed in lieu of a natural organ that is malformed or dysfunctional. Technology has enabled some organ transplants to be performed on a fetus (in utero).

EXAMPLE

A percutaneous bone marrow transplant was performed on a 25-gestational-week-old fetus.

10Y03ZG Transplantation, percutaneous, lymphatics and hemic

YOU INTERPRET IT!

Practice interpreting from the common term used to reference the ICD-10-PCS root operation term.

1. Amniocentesis: _______
2. Chorionic villus sampling: _______
3. Surgical treatment of ectopic pregnancy: _______
4. Cerclage of cervix during pregnancy: _______
5. Intrauterine cordocentesis (percutaneous umbilical cord blood sampling): _______
6. Fetal shunt placement: _______
7. Induced abortion, by dilation and curettage: _______
8. Uterine evacuation and curettage: _______
9. In utero fetal kidney transplant: _______
10. Vaginal delivery: _______
11. Hysterorrhaphy: _______

35.3 Obstetrics Body Parts: Character 4

Character Position	Character Meaning
1	Section of the ICD-10-PCS book
2	Body system being treated (Pregnancy)
3	Root operation term
4	**Body part (Products of Conception)**
5	Approach used by physician
6	Device
7	Qualifier

Products of Conception
The zygote, embryo, or fetus, as well as the amnion, umbilical cord, and placenta.

The only procedures reported from this section are those performed on the **products of conception**: zygote, embryo, or fetus, as well as the amnion, umbilical cord, and placenta.

When a sperm fertilizes an oocyte (egg), a zygote is created. Two weeks later (after fertilization), the zygote becomes an embryo. At week 8, the embryo, about 1 inch in length, is considered a fetus.

The ***Obstetrics*** section focuses on three body parts, which are not specific anatomical sites with which you are familiar:

GUIDANCE CONNECTION

Read the ICD-10-PCS Official Guidelines for Coding and Reporting, **Obstetrics Section Guidelines (Section 1)**, subsection **C. Obstetrics Section**, subhead **Products of conception**, paragraph **C1**.

Products of conception . . . Character: **0 (zero)**

Products of conception, retained . . . Character: **1**

Products of conception, ectopic . . . Character: **2**

In the simplest terms, the products of conception are fertilized ova (zygote, embryo, or fetus) along with the components that accompany, including amnion (the inmost membrane, also known as the *amniotic sac*, that encloses the fetus in utero and the amniotic fluid), umbilical cord, and placenta. The change in the character will designate if these components are ectopic (outside of the uterus) or retained (still inside).

There are times when placental tissue remnants or fetal tissue may remain inside the uterus after a miscarriage, planned pregnancy termination, or a successful delivery. This is known as retained products of conception (RPOC).

A zygote (fertilized egg) usually travels through the fallopian tube and plants itself into the wall of the uterus to begin to grow. When there is a narrowing or other blockage preventing the completion of the journey into the uterus, the zygote may begin to develop outside the uterus. This condition can be life-threatening to the mother and is known as an ectopic pregnancy.

35.4 Obstetrics Approaches: Character 5

Character Position	Character Meaning
1	Section of the ICD-10-PCS book
2	Body system being treated (Pregnancy)
3	Root operation term
4	Body part (Products of Conception)
5	**Approach used by physician**
6	Device
7	Qualifier

As you continue to build a code, you can see that you are telling a story. The first four characters explain what the physician did and the anatomical site upon which he or she worked. Now, with the fifth character, you are going to explain how the physician got to the anatomical site to perform the procedure. You learned in previous chapters that this is known as the *approach*.

Open

Open: Cutting through the skin or mucous membrane and any other body layers necessary to expose the site of the procedure . . . Character: **0**

An open procedure is the traditional approach when the physician makes an incision into the body to access an internal organ.

EXAMPLE

10D00Z1 Cesarean section, low cervical, open incision

Percutaneous

Percutaneous: Entry, by puncture or minor incision, of instrumentation through the skin or mucous membrane and any other body layers necessary to reach the site of the procedure . . . Character: **3**

EXAMPLE

10903Z9 Drainage of fetal blood, percutaneous approach

Percutaneous Endoscopic

Percutaneous Endoscopic: Entry, by puncture or minor incision, of instrumentation through the skin or mucous membrane and any other body layers necessary to reach and visualize the site of the procedure . . . Character: **4**

EXAMPLE

10Q04ZT Repair of the female reproductive system, products of conception, via percutaneous endoscopic approach

CODING BITES

In utero procedures can be performed on the fetus by percutaneous endoscopic approach using a fetoscope.

Via Natural or Artificial Opening

Via Natural or Artificial Opening: Entry of instrumentation through a natural or artificial external opening to reach the site of the procedure . . . Character: **7**

EXAMPLE

10J17ZZ Inspection of retained products of conception, vaginal approach

Via Natural or Artificial Opening Endoscopic

Via Natural or Artificial Opening Endoscopic: Entry of instrumentation through a natural or artificial external opening to reach and visualize the site of the procedure . . . Character: **8**

EXAMPLE

10S28ZZ Reposition of products of conception from fallopian tube to uterus, via vaginal endoscopic approach

External

External: Procedure performed directly on the skin or mucous membrane and procedures performed indirectly by the application of external force through the skin or mucous membrane . . . Character: **X**

EXAMPLE

10E0XZZ Delivery of neonate, vaginal delivery, no assistance

YOU INTERPRET IT!

Interpret these statements from physicians' documentation on the approach used to determine the ICD-10-PCS approach term.

12. Endoscope was inserted into vagina and into the uterus: _______

13. Needle aspiration of amniotic fluid: _______

14. Transverse incision: _______

15. Vaginal delivery: _______

16. Laparoscopic entry into uterus for in vitro surgery: _______

35.5 Obstetrics Devices: Character 6

Character Position	Character Meaning
1	Section of the ICD-10-PCS book
2	Body system being treated (Pregnancy)
3	Root operation term
4	Body part (Products of Conception)
5	Approach used by physician
6	Device
7	Qualifier

As you can see, a character placed in the sixth position will identify a device that will remain with the patient after the procedure has been completed. Remember, the patient for whom the device is involved in care–in this section of ICD-10-PCS–is the fetus . . . *not* the mother.

Monitoring Electrode . . . Character: **3**

Other Device . . . Character: **Y**

No Device . . . Character: **Z**

Fetal monitoring can be performed either internally or externally. When done internally, the physician will place an electrode (electronic transducer) directly onto the scalp of the fetus, typically using a natural opening approach (through the vagina/cervix), with the intention of directly and continuously evaluating the fetal heart rate as well as its variability between beats, particularly in relation to the uterine contractions of labor. Another device, called an internal uterine pressure monitor (IUPM), may be used in conjunction with internal fetal heart rate monitoring. Using a catheter inserted via the vagina/cervix, an IUPM is placed inside the uterus, next to the fetus, to transmit the readings of the contraction pressure to a nearby monitor.

External fetal heart rate monitoring can be accomplished with a handheld electronic Doppler ultrasonic device, most often used at outpatient prenatal visits. Continuous electronic fetal heart monitoring, typically used during labor and delivery, consists of placing an ultrasound transducer on the mother's abdomen, where it can transfer the sounds of the fetal heart to a computer. The computer is able to show the heart pattern on a screen as well as print it out on paper similar to that used during an EKG.

35.6 Obstetrics Qualifiers: Character 7

Character Position	Character Meaning
1	Section of the ICD-10-PCS book
2	Body system being treated (Pregnancy)
3	Root operation term
4	Body part (Products of Conception)
5	Approach used by physician
6	Device
7	**Qualifier**

The seventh character is required. In some cases, there may be no more details to add, so you will use the placeholder letter **Z** No Qualifier–the equivalent of "not applicable."

Extraction Procedures

During a delivery, if the physician uses forceps or another assisting mechanism, this delivery becomes an *extraction*, and the additional detail will be reported with a Qualifier character:

Low Forceps . . . Character: **3**

Mid Forceps . . . Character: **4**

High Forceps . . . Character: **5**

Vacuum . . . Character: **6**

Internal Version . . . Character: **7**

Other . . . Character: **8**

- *Low forceps:* The physician uses forceps to help the neonate the last short way out of the birth canal; the baby's head is visible from the outside.
- *Mid forceps:* Forceps are used to help the baby before the head has reached the lower part of the birth canal.
- *High forceps:* A very unusual situation where forceps are used to delivery the baby through the birth canal prior to engagement.
- *Vacuum:* The physician places a cup, attached to a vacuum pump, on the baby's head to guide the neonate through the birth canal.
- *Internal version:* The physician manually turns the fetus using his hand or fingers through the dilated cervix.

Earlier you learned that a cesarean delivery is reported in ICD-10-PCS using the root operation term *extraction*. For this procedure, the Qualifier character will report

High (Classical c-section incision) . . . Character: 0

Low Cervical . . . Character: 1

Extraperitoneal . . . Character: 2

- *High:* Incision is made vertically, from the naval to the pubic line.
- *Low:* Incision is made transversely just above the pubic line; also known as the bikini cut.
- *Extraperitoneal:* Incision is made into the lowest part of the anterior aspect of the uterus.

EXAMPLES

You may read these words in the physician's documentation:

"*. . . low transverse cesarean section . . .*"

"*. . . Lower uterine segment was then scored in a curvilinear fashion . . .*" [extraperitoneal]

"*. . . A vertical incision was made in the umbilicus . . .*" [classical]

Drainage Procedures

CODING BITES

Read carefully! There are two different characters available to report the drainage of amniotic fluid . . . therapeutic or diagnostic. Check the documentation to determine why the amniocentesis was done.

During amniocentesis, or any other drainage procedure performed on a pregnant woman, the Qualifier character will explain exactly *what* was drained:

Fetal Blood . . . Character: **9**

Fetal Cerebrospinal Fluid . . . Character: **A**

Fetal Fluid, Other . . . Character: **B**

Amniotic Fluid, Therapeutic . . . Character: **C**

Fluid, Other . . . Character: **D**

Amniotic Fluid, Diagnostic . . . Character: **U**

EXAMPLES

You might see these phrases and descriptions in physician documentation:

"*. . . second trimester amniocentesis . . .*" [drainage of amniotic fluid for diagnostic/genetic testing]

"*. . . serial vesicocenteses will be performed to check the kidney function (measuring urinary electrolytes in the fetus's urine). A needle is inserted into the fetal bladder and the urine is entirely removed . . .*" [drainage of fetal fluid, other]

"*. . . fetal blood sampling will be done to collect specimens for testing . . .*" [drainage of fetal blood]

Laminaria
Thin sticks of kelp-related seaweed, used to dilate the cervix, that can induce abortive circumstance during the first 3 months of pregnancy.

Abortifacient
A drug used to induce an abortion.

Abortive Procedures

When the artificial termination of a pregnancy (abortion) is performed, the Qualifier character will report the methodology:

Vacuum . . . Character: **6**

Laminaria . . . Character: **W**

Abortifacient . . . Character: **X**

- *Vacuum:* The use of aspiration using a cannula (tube) inserted into the uterus; also known as suction curettage.
- *Laminaria:* A small rod, created of dehydrated types of kelp, is inserted into the cervix for the purposes of dilation.
- *Abortifacient:* A substance, using a pharmaceutical, used to induce expulsion of the products of conception.

In Utero Procedures

The Qualifier character will report the body system that was repaired or transplanted during an in utero procedure performed on the fetus (root operation *repair* or *transplantation*).

Nervous System . . . Character: **E**

Cardiovascular System . . . F

Lymphatics and Hemic . . . G

Eye . . . H

Ear, Nose, and Sinus . . . J

Respiratory System . . . K

Mouth and Throat . . . L

Gastrointestinal System . . . M

Hepatobiliary and Pancreas . . . N

Endocrine System . . . P

Skin . . . Q

Musculoskeletal System . . . R

Urinary System . . . S

Female Reproductive System . . . T

Male Reproductive System . . . V

Other Body System . . . Y

ICD-10-PCS

LET'S CODE IT! SCENARIO

PATIENT: Elicia Moralise

HISTORY OF PRESENT ILLNESS: The patient is a 26-year-old G1, P0 at 39-3/7 weeks with an EDD of 06/01/2026 based on a 6-week ultrasound. The patient presented to labor and delivery with complaints of contractions every 3 minutes and leaking of fluid since 0400 on 05/28/2026. The patient reports positive fetal movement and denies vaginal bleeding. Prenatal care began at 9 weeks × 15 visits. Total weight gain was 37 pounds. The patient is A positive, rubella immune, GBS positive. She has no known drug allergies.

Upon admission, vaginal exam was 1, 80%, and −1 station per the RN. Fetal heart tones were 124, positive long-term variability, positive acceleration, and no decelerations. Uterine contractions every 2 to 3 minutes, 60 to 80 seconds and moderate to palpation.

PLAN: Admit the patient to the labor and delivery unit. Dr. Lorrantz informed and agrees with plan. GBS protocol, ampicillin. The patient encouraged to ambulate, shower, use the birth ball. Reassess in 3 to 4 hours or p.r.n.

LABOR PROGRESS: At 0900, the patient was pushing with contractions. She was feeling pressure but was still comfortable with the epidural. The patient stated that she was exhausted. The Pitocin was restarted at 2 mU as the RN realized that the catheter had come loose from the patient's IV and the Pitocin was not being delivered to the patient. Pitocin currently now at 18 mU per minute. Contractions were every 2 to 6 minutes, 50 to 60 seconds long. Fetal heart tones were 125, average variability, 15 × 15 accelerations with mild variable decelerations with good return to baseline. Vaginal exam at 0830 hours was complete, 100%, with the head at the 0 station and the caput at +2 station. The patient appeared to be making some progress with pushing; however, Dr. Lorrantz was consulted and was asked by the CNM to assess the patient after leaving an OR case. The plan was that the patient would continue pushing provided fetal heart tones remained stable until Dr. Lorrantz was able to get out of the OR to evaluate her. The plan was to consider vacuum extraction.

DELIVERY NOTE: The patient pushed extremely well and through excellent maternal efforts and frequent position changes, the infant rotated and descended and normal spontaneous vaginal delivery occurred at 0950 hours in the LOA position over intact perineum. Meconium-stained fluid was noted as the head came over the perineum and Neonatology was called to the room. The mouth and nose were bulb suctioned on the perineum by the CNM. The shoulders delivered easily and a nuchal cord loose x1 was noted and reduced with the delivery of the body. The cord was immediately clamped x2 and cut by the father of the baby and the infant was taken to the warmer for evaluation by Neonatology. The placenta delivered spontaneously at 0958 hours, was complete, had a 3-vessel cord, and was in the Schultz fashion. Estimated blood loss was 200 mL. Pitocin was run open after the delivery of the placenta. The vagina was inspected and a first-degree vaginal and left first-degree labial laceration were repaired with 2-0 chromic and 3-0 Vicryl, respectively. The fundus was firm, midline, and −2. There was light lochia. Infant's Apgars were 6, 8, and 9. Weight was 6 pounds 9 ounces. The mother and the infant were left in stable condition.

(continued)

Let's Code It!

Congratulations! A healthy baby was born. Now, let's determine the accurate ICD-10-PCS code for the delivery.

From which section would you report the delivery of this baby? The baby is a product of conception, therefore, ***Obstetrics***.

First character: Section: Obstetrics . . . 1

Only one option for the body system . . .

Second character: System: Pregnancy . . . 0

This is also straightforward. The documentation states, "*normal spontaneous vaginal delivery*."

Third character: Root Operation: Delivery . . . E

The rest of this code will come together easily because there is only one option for each of the last four characters:

Fourth character: Body Part: Products of Conception . . . 0

Fifth character: Approach: External . . . X

Sixth character: Device: No Device . . . Z

Seventh character: Qualifier: No Qualifier . . . Z

Now put it all together and report, with confidence, this ICD-10-PCS code:

10E0XZZ Natural, spontaneous vaginal delivery

Good job!

35.7 Obstetrics Coding: Putting It All Together

Throughout this chapter, you have learned about each of the seven components of an ICD-10-PCS code used to report a procedure, service, or treatment on a pregnant woman. Now, let's put it all together and determine some codes all the way through.

LET'S CODE IT! SCENARIO

LaToya Donner, a 37-year-old female, is pregnant, G1 P0, second trimester (15 weeks, 3 days), and has been admitted to have some tests, including an amniocentesis. Because she is categorized as elderly primigravida, Dr. Brummel is performing this test to determine the health and well-being of the fetus.

Let's Code It!

Let's go through the steps of coding for ICD-10-PCS and determine the code or codes that should be reported for this encounter between Dr. Brummel and LaToya Donner.

First character: Section: Obstetrics . . . 1
Second character: Body System: Pregnancy . . . 0
Third character: Root Operation: Drainage . . . 9

Remember the meaning and purpose of this procedure: amniocentesis (puncturing of the amnion) to drain amniotic fluid.

Fourth character: Body Part: Products of Conception . . . 0
Fifth character: Approach: Percutaneous . . . 3
Sixth character: Device: No Device . . . Z
Seventh character: Qualifier: Amniotic Fluid, Diagnostic . . . U

(continued)

What is being drained? Amniotic fluid. Why? To test (diagnostics).

The ICD-10-PCS code you will report is

10903ZU Amniocentesis for prenatal testing

Good job!

ICD-10-PCS

LET'S CODE IT! SCENARIO

PATIENT NAME: Yessina Catina

PHYSICIAN: Travis Jonquin, MD

DATE OF ADMISSION: 05/28/2026

DATE OF DISCHARGE: 05/29/2026

ADMITTING DIAGNOSIS: Intrauterine pregnancy at 38 weeks and 5 days. Presented with contractions, leakage of fluid, and decreased fetal movements that day.

HISTORY OF PRESENT ILLNESS/HOSPITAL COURSE: The patient is a 31-year-old G2, P0 female at 38 weeks and 5 days estimated gestational age who presented in labor. On vaginal examination, the patient was found to be 4 cm dilated, 70% effaced, and –3 station, and the fetal heart tracing at that time was in the 140s with minimal long-term variability. She was admitted to Labor and Delivery for Pitocin augmentation and amniotomy. She continued to have a good labor pattern and proceeded to deliver a viable 6-pound, 12-ounce male infant over an intact perineum with Apgars of 8 and 9 at 1 and 5 minutes. There were no nuchal cords and no true knots, and the number of vessels in the cord was three. Her postpartum course was uncomplicated, and the patient was discharged to home in stable and satisfactory condition.

PROCEDURES PERFORMED: Normal spontaneous delivery and Pitocin augmentation.

COMPLICATIONS: None.

FINAL DIAGNOSIS: Status post normal spontaneous vaginal delivery at 38 weeks and 5 days.

DISCHARGE INSTRUCTIONS: Call for increased pain, fever, or increased bleeding.

DIET: Advance as tolerated.

ACTIVITY: Advance as tolerated. Pelvic rest for 6 weeks. Nothing to be inserted into the vagina for 6 weeks, i.e., no tampons, douche, or sex.

Code for the delivery.

Let's Code It!

Let's go through the steps of ICD-10-PCS coding and determine the code to report for Dr. Jonquin's support in the delivery of Yessina's baby.

First character: Section: Obstetrics . . . 1
Second character: Body System: Pregnancy . . . 0

This was documented as a vaginal delivery.

Third character: Root Operation: Delivery . . . E

The neonate was delivered, and this boy is a product of conception.

Fourth character: Body Part: Products of Conception . . . 0

There is only one option for each of the following three characters.

Fifth character: Approach: External . . . X
Sixth character: Device: No Device . . . Z
Seventh character: Qualifier: None . . . Z

(continued)

Put the seven characters together to get the code to report:

10E0XZZ **Delivery of products of conception, vaginally**

Good work!

LET'S CODE IT! SCENARIO

PATIENT: Isabelle Calaveri

DATE: 11/15/2026

PROCEDURE: Primary low segment transverse cesarean section

DESCRIPTION OF OPERATION: Due to concern that the umbilical cord was around the fetus's neck, the patient was brought to the operating room and placed on the table in supine position, and after adequate epidural anesthesia, she was prepped and draped in the usual sterile fashion.

A Pfannenstiel incision was made with a clean scalpel. The incision was taken down the fascial layer with a clean second knife. The fascial layer was incised transversely to the full length of the primary incision. The underlying muscle bellies were dissected with blunt and sharp dissection. The muscle belly was split in the midline. The peritoneum was then grasped between 2 Kelly clamps and elevated. After ensuring no adherent bowel or bladder, the peritoneum was nicked between clamps. The abdominal cavity was thus entered. The bladder flap was formed with blunt and sharp dissection and then the uterus was scored in the lower uterine segment in transverse fashion, and the incision was enlarged in elliptical fashion with bandage scissors. The infant was found to be in face presentation with nuchal cord x1. Mouth and nose were suctioned prior to delivery of rest of the body. The cord was slipped over the shoulders and then the infant was delivered. It was a living female with Apgars of 8 and 9. There was meconium, but it was not thick. Cord pH was 7.30. The cord was doubly clamped, cut between the clamps, and the infant was handed away to the pediatrician, Dr. Toliver. Cord bloods were taken.

The placenta was then manually separated. The edges of the uterine incision were then reapproximated with continuous running suture of #1 chromic catgut. The second imbricating layer was also sewn using #1 chromic catgut. Good hemostasis was noted. The abdomen was cleaned of blood and clots. Tubes and ovaries were inspected and found to be normal. Then, the abdomen was closed in layers after correct sponge, needle, and instrument counts. The peritoneum was closed with continuous running suture of 0 chromic catgut. The muscle bellies were closed with interrupted sutures of 0 chromic catgut. The fascia was closed with 2 continuous running sutures of 0 Vicryl beginning at either angle of the incision intermittently overlapping the midline. The subcutaneous tissue was closed with continuous running suture of 3-0 plain catgut, and the skin was closed with surgical staples. A sterile pressure dressing was applied. Sponge, needle, and instrument counts were correct at the end of the procedure.

Matthew Ansara, MD

Let's Code It!

Dr. Ansara performed a c-section to deliver Isabelle's baby.

First character: Section: Obstetrics . . . 1

Second character: Body System: Pregnancy . . . 0

This was documented as a c-section. You have learned that ICD-10-PCS uses the term *extraction*.

Third character: Root Operation: Extraction . . . D

What has been extracted? The fetus, which is a *product of conception*.

Fourth character: Body Part: Products of Conception . . . 0

What was the approach the physician used? The documentation states, "*A Pfannenstiel incision was made with a clean scalpel.*" This tells you the approach was *open*.

Fifth character: Approach: Open . . . 0

(continued)

Was there a device involved in this procedure? No.

Sixth character: Device: No Device . . . Z

The Qualifier will report the type of incision used by the physician. The documentation states, "*The fascial layer was incised transversely.*" You learned about the different incisions, and that this is known as a "low cervical."

Seventh character: Qualifier: Low Cervical . . . 1

Put all seven characters together to get the code to report:

10D00Z1 Extraction of products of conception, open approach using low cervical incision

Good job!

Chapter Summary

The services, procedures, and treatments reported with codes from the ***Obstetrics Section*** of ICD-10-PCS are all provided in a pregnant inpatient. The most important thing to remember is that, for these procedures, the patient is the product of conception–what is inside a pregnant patient.

CODING BITES

The Products of Conception

- The **fertilized ovum**:
  - Zygote: 0 to 2 weeks
  - Embryo: 2 to 8 weeks
  - Fetus: 8 weeks to birth
- **Amnion**: the innermost membrane, also known as the *amniotic sac*, that encloses the fetus in utero and the amniotic fluid.
- **Umbilical cord**
- **Placenta**

You Interpret It! Answers

1. Drainage, **2.** Extraction, **3.** Resection, **4.** Insertion, **5.** Drainage, **6.** Insertion, **7.** Abortion, **8.** Extraction, **9.** Transplantation, **10.** Delivery, **11.** Repair, **12.** Via natural or artificial opening endoscopic, **13.** Percutaneous, **14.** Open, **15.** External, **16.** Percutaneous endoscopic

CHAPTER 35 REVIEW
Obstetrics Section

McGraw Hill connect

Enhance your learning by completing these exercises and more at mcgrawhillconnect.com!

Let's Check It! Terminology

Match each key term to the appropriate definition.

1. LO 35.6 A drug used to induce an abortion.

2. LO 35.3 The zygote, embryo, or fetus, as well as the amnion, umbilical cord, and placenta.

3. LO 35.6 Thin sticks of special seaweed used to dilate the cervix that can induce abortive circumstance during the first 3 months of pregnancy.

A. Abortifacient

B. Laminaria

C. Products of Conception

Let's Check It! Concepts

Choose the most appropriate answer for each of the following questions.

1. **LO 35.4** Within the Obstetric Section, character position 5 represents which of the following?
   a. Body system **b.** Root operation term **c.** Approach **d.** Device
2. **LO 35.1** All of the codes reporting an Obstetrics procedure will begin with which section number?
   a. 5 **b.** 4 **c.** 2 **d.** 1
3. **LO 35.3** The products of conception include
   a. zygote and embryo. **b.** amnion and umbilical cord.
   c. placenta. **d.** all of these.
4. **LO 35.2** All of the following are root operation terms in the Obstetrics Section *except*
   a. abortion. **b.** delivery. **c.** irrigation. **d.** inspection.
5. **LO 35.2** Within the Obstetrics Section, character position 5 Approach, the approach to an intrauterine cordocentesis would be which of the following?
   a. Via natural or artificial opening **b.** Percutaneous endoscopic
   c. External **d.** Open
6. **LO 35.4** Inspection of retained products of conception, vaginal approach, would be coded
   a. 10J17ZZ **b.** 10J18ZZ **c.** 10J13ZZ **d.** 10J00ZZ
7. **LO 35.5** Within the Obstetrics Section, character position 6 represents
   a. body system being treated. **b.** root operation.
   c. device. **d.** qualifier.
8. **LO 35.6** During a delivery, the physician uses mid forceps for the extraction. This will be reported with the qualifier character
   a. 6 **b.** 4 **c.** 5 **d.** 3
9. **LO 35.6** The qualifier character that reports an in-utero procedure performed on the fetus's eye is
   a. E. **b.** N. **c.** M. **d.** H.
10. **LO 35.1** Within the Obstetrics Section, what is the character that reports the body system representing the gestational term?
    a. 1 **b.** 0 **c.** 3 **d.** 5

Let's Check It! Root Operation Definitions—Obstetrics

Refer to the ICD-10-PCS Appendix entitled "Root Operation Definitions." Look for Root Operation Definitions for Other Sections, Obstetrics, and match the ICD-10-PCS value for each Operation, Character 3, to its definition.

1. Delivery	**A.** A
2. Removal	**B.** D
3. Resection	**C.** E
4. Abortion	**D.** H
5. Inspection	**E.** J
6. Insertion	**F.** P
7. Repair	**G.** Q
8. Reposition	**H.** S
9. Transplantation	**I.** T
10. Extraction	**J.** Y

Let's Check It! Guidelines

Refer to the Official ICD-10-PCS Obstetrics Section Guidelines and fill in the blanks accordingly.

Amniocentesis	retained	obstetric
all	therapeutic	pregnant
Obstetrics	Medical and Surgical	postpartum
delivery	Endometrium	Extraction

1. Procedures performed on the products of conception are coded to the ________ section.
2. Procedures performed on the ________ female other than the products of conception are coded to the appropriate root operation in the ________ section.
3. ________ is coded to the products of conception body part in the Obstetrics section. Repair of ________ urethral laceration is coded to the urethra body part in the Medical and Surgical section.
4. Procedures performed following a ________ or abortion for curettage of the endometrium or evacuation of ________ products of conception are ________ coded in the Obstetrics section, to the root operation ________ and the body part Products of Conception, Retained.
5. Diagnostic or ________ dilation and curettage performed during times other than the ________ or post-abortion period are all coded in the Medical and Surgical section, to the root operation Extraction and the body part ________.

Let's Check It! Rules and Regulations

Please answer the following questions from the knowledge you have gained after reading this chapter.

1. **LO 35.2** Explain the difference between delivery and extraction; include the character that represents each.
2. **LO 35.3** The Obstetrics section character position 4 focuses on three body parts, which are not specific anatomical sites. List the three body parts; include the character that identifies each.
3. **LO 35.4** List the six approaches used in the Obstetrics section of ICD-10-PCS, explain each approach, and include the character that identifies each approach.
4. **LO 35.6** What does the Obstetrics section seventh character position present, and is it required?
5. **LO 35.6** Explain what a cesarean section procedure is and include the root operation term used in ICD-10-PCS.

YOU CODE IT! Practice

Using the techniques described in this chapter, carefully read through the case studies and determine the most accurate ICD-10-PCS code(s) for each case study.

1. Candy Moss, a 31-year-old female, is G1 P0, 8 weeks gestation. Candy requests an abortion due to genetic problems in the fetus. She is admitted to the hospital, where a vacuum abortion is performed, via natural opening.
2. Keren Medlin, a 29-year-old female, is admitted to Westward Hospital at 12 weeks gestation. Dr. Hanks performs a repair to the fetus's urinary system endoscopically, via natural opening.
3. Annie Charles, a 23-year-old female, G2 P1, at 40 weeks gestation in active labor, is admitted to Westward Hospital. Dr. Downs assisted in a vaginal delivery, low forceps over midline episiotomy.
4. Loretta Smith, a 36-year-old female, G3 P2 at 38 weeks gestation, is admitted to Westward Hospital. Dr. McWhirter changes a monitor electrode, vaginal approach.
5. Debbie Slay, a 29-year-old female, G1 P0, is admitted to Westward Hospital in labor. Dr. Atkinson inserts an intrauterine pressure catheter, vaginal approach, to evaluate contractions.
6. Rhonda Hart, a 19-year-old female, is admitted to Westward Hospital in labor at 41 weeks gestation, G1 P0. AROM is performed and spontaneous vaginal delivery with intact perineum occurs 1 hour later, manually assisted delivery.
7. Laura McMillan, a 28-year-old female, at 39 weeks gestation, is admitted to Westward Hospital in labor; a vaginal delivery occurs 6 hours later, vacuum assisted.

(continued)

8. Latoya Medlin, an 18-year-old female, G1 P0, is admitted to Westward Hospital at 18 weeks gestation. Latoya is requesting termination of pregnancy due to confirmed fetal anencephaly. Pregnancy was terminated by a luminaria stick, which produced a complete abortion.
9. Sherry Moore, a 29-year-old female, is admitted to Westward Hospital for an open in utero fetal mouth repair.
10. Janie Knight, a 16-year-old female, G1 P0, is admitted to Westward Hospital and Dr. Gifford performs an amniotic fluid test, open approach, for therapeutic purposes.
11. Sharon Heyward, a 24-year-old female, G2 P1 at 40 weeks gestation, is admitted to Westward Hospital. Dr. Jessup performs a pelvic examination revealing an open, soft cervix.
12. Kristi Williams, a 31-year-old female, is admitted to Westward Hospital in active labor at 41 weeks gestation. Dr. Gerald assisted with a vaginal delivery, with high forceps, 4 hours later.
13. Keyana Haulbrook, a 17-year-old female, G1 P0, 12 weeks gestation, is admitted to Westward Hospital to terminate pregnancy due to a genetic defect in the fetus. Abortion was performed by hysterotomy technique.
14. Natalie Phillips, a 32-year-old female, 37.5 weeks gestation, G2 P1, is admitted to Westward Hospital for a fetal spinal tap, percutaneous.
15. Eleanor Coaxum, a 26-year-old female, G1 P0, 32 weeks gestation, is admitted to Westward Hospital for a fetal skin transplantation, via natural opening.

YOU CODE IT! Application

The following exercises provide practice in abstracting physicians' notes and learning to work with documentation from our health care facility, Westward Hospital. These case studies are modeled on real patient encounters. Using the techniques described in this chapter, carefully read through the case studies and determine the most accurate ICD-10-PCS code(s) for each case study.

WESTWARD HOSPITAL

591 Chester Road

Masters, FL 33955

DISCHARGE SUMMARY

PATIENT: ALBERTS, SERITA

DATE OF ADMISSION: 03/05/26

DATE OF DISCHARGE: 03/17/26

ADMITTING DIAGNOSIS: 1. Intrauterine pregnancy at 40 plus weeks.
2. Active labor.
3. History of two previous cesarean sections.

DISCHARGE DIAGNOSIS: 1. Intrauterine pregnancy at 40 plus weeks.
2. Active labor.
3. History of two previous cesarean sections.

OPERATION: Repeat low transverse cesarean section.

FLUIDS: 2,500 mL lactated Ringer.

ESTIMATED BLOOD LOSS: 300 mL.

URINE OUTPUT: 125 mL, clear and yellow.

DESCRIPTION OF OPERATION: The patient was identified and taken to the operating room. Appropriate anesthesia was administered. The patient was placed in the dorsal supine position with a leftward tilt and prepped and draped in the usual sterile fashion. Following that, a low Pfannenstiel skin incision was made with a #10 scalpel. This incision was carried down to the underlying layer of fascia with the scalpel. The fascia was then nicked in the midline with the scalpel. This fascial incision was then extended laterally with the Mayo scissors and pickups with teeth.

(continued)

Following that, the superior aspect of the fascial incision was grasped with straight Kocher clamps x2, tented up from the rectus muscles below and dissected away sharply with the scalpel and Mayo scissors. This was repeated similarly to the inferior aspect of the fascial incision. Following that, the peritoneum was identified below, grasped with hemostat x2, and entered sharply with Metzenbaum scissors. After appropriate visualization of the bowel and bladder, the peritoneal incision was extended superiorly and inferiorly. The bladder blade was then placed inferiorly and the vesicouterine peritoneum tented up with the smooth pickups, incised with the Metzenbaum scissors, and this incision was extended laterally.

Following that, the bladder blade was replaced deflecting the bladder anteriorly and inferiorly. The #10 scalpel was taken in hand again, and a 3-cm low transverse area incision was then made. This incision was then extended laterally. Following that, the infant's vertex was mobilized and delivered through the incision in a direct OP position. The infant's nasopharynx was suctioned with the bulb syringe and then the rest of the infant was delivered along with fundal pressure.

Following that, the infant's cord was clamped and cut and the infant was handed off to the awaiting pediatricians. Following that, the placenta was spontaneously expressed. The uterus was then exteriorized and cleared of all clots and debris. The uterine incision was repaired with #1 chromic in a running-locking fashion. The uterus was then returned to the abdominal cavity, and the abdominal cavity was cleared of all clots and debris.

The uterine incision and the pelvic cavity were reinspected and excellent hemostasis was noted overall. The fascial incision was reapproximated with #0 Vicryl in a running fashion x2. Following that, the skin was reapproximated with staples. The instrument, needle, and sponge counts were correct x2.

Benjamin Johnston, MD

Determine the most accurate ICD-10-PCS code(s) for the c-section.

WESTWARD HOSPITAL

591 Chester Road

Masters, FL 33955

OPERATIVE REPORT

PATIENT: HUDSON, LYNN

ACCOUNT/EHR #: HUDSLY001

DATE OF ADMISSION: 17 March 2026

ATTENDING PHYSICIAN: Denny Stewart, MD

ANESTHESIA: EPIDURAL TYPE OF DELIVERY: NSVD

CONDITION OF PERINEUM: MLE

EPISIOTOMY: Midline performed

VAGINA/CERVIX: Intact

DELIVERED: Live, single-born female, weight 7 lb. 2 oz. @ 02:17

TYPE OF STIMULATION: Mouth suction

CONDITION: Good

BIRTH INJURY: None

APGAR RATING: 1 min. = 9 . . . 5 min. = 9

Denny Stewart, MD

Determine the most accurate ICD-10-PCS code(s) for the delivery.

(continued)

WESTWARD HOSPITAL

591 Chester Road

Masters, FL 33955

OPERATIVE REPORT

PATIENT: CARROLL, DAWN

ACCOUNT/EHR #: CARRDA001

DATE OF ADMISSION: 21 March 2026

ATTENDING PHYSICIAN: Steven Phifer, MD

In the 40th week of her first pregnancy, a 34-year-old woman arrived at Labor and Delivery at 5:00 a.m. for a planned induction of labor due to mild, pregnancy-induced hypertension. After intravaginal placement of misoprostol, the nurse observed her briefly and, at 9:00 a.m., discharged her from the unit. She went for a walk with her husband in a park next to the hospital.

Patient's membranes spontaneously ruptured, and she returned to the Labor and Delivery unit. Patient's vital signs were taken, and the fetal heart rate checked. The mother's blood pressure was 182/97, but the nurse thought this was related to nausea, vomiting, and discomfort from the contractions.

The resident examined the mother, determined that her cervix was 5–6 cm, 90 percent effaced, and the vertex was at 0 station. An internal fetal heart monitor was placed because the mother's vomiting and discomfort caused her to move around too much in the bed, making it hard to record the fetal heart rate with an external monitor. The internal monitor revealed a steady fetal heart rate of 120 and no decelerations.

The mother continued to complain of painful contractions and requested an epidural. Shortly after placement of the epidural, the monitor recorded a prolonged fetal heart rate deceleration. The heart rate returned slowly to the baseline rate of 120 as the nurse repositioned the mother, increased her intravenous fluids, and administered oxygen by mask.

An epidural analgesia infusion pump was started. The fetal heart rate strip indicated another deceleration that recovered to baseline. The nurse informed the resident, who checked the tracing and told her to "keep an eye on things."

The primary nurse noted in the labor record that the baseline fetal heart rate was "unstable, between 100–120," but she did not report this to the resident.

The nurse recorded that the fetal heart rate was "flat, no variability." As the nurse was documenting this as a nonreassuring fetal heart rate pattern, the patient expressed a strong urge to push and the nurse called for an exam.

A resident came to the bedside, examined the mother, and noted that she was fully dilated with the caput at +1. A brief update was written in the chart, but the clinician who had performed the exam was not noted.

The mother was repositioned and began pushing.

The fetal heart rate suddenly dropped and remained profoundly bradycardic for 11 minutes. The resident was called and attempted a vacuum delivery because the fetal head was at +2 station. The attending then entered and attempted forceps delivery.

An emergency cesarean delivery was performed; the baby was stillborn. The physician identified a uterine rupture that required significant blood replacement.

Steven Phifer, MD

Determine the most accurate ICD-10-PCS code(s) for the c-section.

WESTWARD HOSPITAL

591 Chester Road

Masters, FL 33955

OPERATIVE REPORT

PATIENT: FAULDS, MAGGIE

ACCOUNT/EHR #: FAULMA001

(continued)

DATE OF ADMISSION: 25 November 2026

ATTENDING PHYSICIAN: Sandra Lindler, MD

ANESTHESIA: General

Patient is in her 12th week of pregnancy. She presented to the emergency department with severe cramping and vaginal bleeding. After examination the patient was diagnosed with an incomplete early spontaneous abortion and a D&C was recommended. The patient was fully counseled as to the risks and benefits of the D&C and admitted to the hospital. The patient agreed to the procedure.

The patient was then taken to the operating room and placed in a supine position on the operating room table. General endotracheal anesthesia was administered, and once adequate anesthesia was demonstrated, the patient's legs were then placed in candy cane stirrups. The patient was then prepped and draped in the standard D&C surgical fashion.

The patient was placed in 10 degrees of Trendelenburg. The patient was given 100 mg of doxycycline. The bladder was then decompressed and approximately 45 mL of urine was produced. A weighted speculum was placed in the posterior vagina and the cervix was grasped with single-tooth tenaculum. Uterus sounded to 8.2 cm. The cervix was then serially dilated with Hanks dilator. An 8-cm straight suction curette was then introduced and a suction curettage was performed. Once all products of conception were evacuated, a sharp curettage was performed until a gritty surface was appreciated on all four quadrants of the uterus. No further bleeding was noted. Products of conception were then examined on the back table, which was grossly consistent with products of conception.

The patient tolerated the procedure and anesthesia well, was awakened from anesthesia without complications, and was transported to the recovery room in stable condition.

Sandra Lindler

Determine the most accurate ICD-10-PCS code(s) for the extraction.

WESTWARD HOSPITAL

591 Chester Road

Masters, FL 33955

OPERATIVE REPORT

PATIENT: HOFFMEIER, KATHLEEN

ACCOUNT/EHR #: HOFFKA001

DATE OF ADMISSION: 28 December 2026

ADMITTING DIAGNOSIS: Right tubal ectopic pregnancy

PROCEDURE: Operative laparoscopy, right salpingectomy

SURGEON: William G. Cohen, MD

ANESTHESIA: General

This 28-year-old female presents to the emergency room with vaginal bleeding and belly pain that gets worse with movement. Patient states she is pregnant at approximately 8 weeks gestation, G1 P0. Ultrasound report showed a mass near the cul-de-sac. The patient denies any medical or surgical history. No known allergies. Family history is noncontributory. The patient was admitted to the hospital.

The patient was taken to the OR, where general anesthesia was easily obtained. The patient was then prepped and draped in a sterile fashion and placed in dorsal lithotomy position. A weighted speculum was introduced into the patient's vagina for cervical visualization. Once the cervix was visualized, a single-toothed tenaculum was applied to the upper lip of the cervix, and acorn manipulator was introduced into the patient's cervix.

Attention was then drawn to the abdomen, where a 10-mm horizontal incision was done below the umbilicus and carried down all the way to the fascia. Under direct visualization, a 10-mm trocar was introduced into the patient's abdomen. Once intraperitoneal placement was confirmed, pneumoperitoneum was started. Opening pressure was 3 mmHg; pneumoperitoneum was obtained.

(continued)

Once pneumoperitoneum was obtained, a second port was put two fingerbreadths above the pubic symphysis, and under direct visualization, a 5-mm trocar was then introduced into the patient's abdomen. The patient was placed in Trendelenburg position. Pelvic structures were revealed; ampullary ectopic was noted on the right side with some amount of hemoperitoneum and moderate amount of free fluid.

Attention was focused on the right fallopian tube, which initially was incised where the ectopic pregnancy was and products of conception were removed. Since no hemostasis was able to be obtained from the incision site from the salpingostomy and due to the amount of dense adhesions on that fallopian tube, decision was then made to proceed with right salpingectomy, so the IP ligament was identified and fallopian tube was then grasped by the fimbria and incised from the mesosalpinx. Good hemostasis was noted from the fallopian tube sites and the operative site. Specimen was then removed from the patient's abdomen. Copious irrigation was done and all clots and debris were removed from the patient's abdomen. Once good hemostasis was noted from the patient's abdomen, pneumoperitoneum was deflated and all trocars were removed. Infraumbilical fascia was closed with 0 Vicryl and interrupted suture. The skin was closed with 4-0 Vicryl. The right infrapubic and suprapubic ports were closed with 0 Vicryl in running fashion, and third port, which was introduced two fingerbreadths above the pubis symphysis and 6 cm in the midaxillary line, under direct visualization, was also closed with 4-0 Monocryl. Sponge, lap, and needle counts were correct x2. The patient was taken to the recovery room in stable condition.

DIET: As tolerated.

PHYSICAL ACTIVITY: No heavy lifting. Pelvic rest.

William G. Cohen, MD

Determine the most accurate ICD-10-PCS code(s) for the salpingectomy.

36

Placement through Chiropractic Sections

Key Terms

Administration
Extra-articular
Extracorporeal
Measurement
Placement
Somatic

Learning Outcomes

After completing this chapter, the student should be able to:

LO 36.1 Recognize the details reported in the Placement—Anatomical Regions section and Placement—Anatomical Orifices section.
LO 36.2 Evaluate the details to determine the services reported from the Administration section.
LO 36.3 Determine the specifics required to build a code from the Measurement and Monitoring section.
LO 36.4 Interpret the documentation to report a service from the Extracorporeal or Systemic Assistance and Performance section.
LO 36.5 Abstract the documentation to determine a code for a service reported from the Extracorporeal or Systemic Therapies section.
LO 36.6 Utilize knowledge to report a code from the Osteopathic section.
LO 36.7 Identify the details necessary to build a code from the Other Procedures section.
LO 36.8 Distinguish the services provided to determine reporting a code from the Chiropractic section.
LO 36.9 Analyze the documentation to build a complete and accurate code(s) in ICD-10-PCS for sections 2–9.

STOP! Remember, you need to follow along in your ICD-10-PCS code book for an optimal learning experience.

36.1 Reporting Services from the Placement Section

Character Definitions

The meanings for the ***Placement*** section characters are in the following table:

Character Position	Character Meaning
1	Section of the ICD-10-PCS book
2	Anatomical region/orifices
3	Root operation term
4	Body region/orifice
5	Approach used by physician
6	Device
7	Qualifier

You might have noticed that these are slightly different meanings for characters 2 and 4 than those in the ***Medical and Surgical*** and ***Obstetrics*** sections.

Character Position 1: Placement Section 2

Character Position	Character Meaning
1	**Section of the ICD-10-PCS book**
2	Anatomical region/orifices
3	Root operation term
4	Body region/orifice
5	Approach used by physician
6	Device
7	Qualifier

The procedures reported with codes from this section explain the location of a device either in or on a body region for protection, immobilization, stretching, compression, or packing. These procedures are some that you are familiar with, such as application of a splint to immobilize or a traction device to stretch a muscle. For the most part, the devices in this section are "off the shelf," so to speak, and not customized fabrications. (More about these devices will be discussed when we get to that character position.)

Character Position 2: Anatomical Region/Orifices

Character Position	Character Meaning
1	Section of the ICD-10-PCS book
2	**Anatomical region/orifices**
3	Root operation term
4	Body region/orifice
5	Approach used by physician
6	Device
7	Qualifier

CODING BITES

Remember, an anatomical orifice is a natural opening into the body; for example, mouth, nose, urethra.

There are only two body system options:

Anatomical Regions . . . Character: **W**

Anatomical Orifices . . . Character: **Y**

Character Position 3: Root Operation

Character Position	Character Meaning
1	Section of the ICD-10-PCS book
2	Anatomical region/orifices
3	**Root operation term**
4	Body region/orifice
5	Approach used by physician
6	Device
7	Qualifier

The codes from the ***Placement*** section only report procedures that are noninvasive, meaning that the outer layer of the skin is not punctured and no incision is made.

Change

Change: Taking out or off a device from a body part and putting back an identical or similar device in or on the same body part without cutting or puncturing the skin or a mucous membrane . . . Character: **0**

Caution! This root operation term means the same as it does in the ***Medical and Surgical*** and the ***Obstetrics*** sections; however, the character used to report this in the ***Placement*** section is different.

EXAMPLE

2W05X3Z Change external back brace

Compression

Compression: Putting pressure on a body region . . . Character: **1**

EXAMPLE

2W1RX7Z Placement of intermittent pressure device on lower left leg

Dressing

Dressing: Putting material on a body region for protection . . . Character: **2**

EXAMPLE

2W2EX4Z Placement of bandage on right hand

Immobilization

Immobilization: Limiting or preventing motion of an external body region . . . Character: **3**

EXAMPLES

2W3KX1Z Application of a splint to a left finger

2W35X3Z Back brace placed on patient

Packing

Packing: Putting material in a body region or orifice . . . Character: **4**

EXAMPLES

2W48X5Z Packing to wound on right upper extremity

2Y41X5Z Packing of nasal cavities due to epistaxis

Removal

Removal: Taking out or off a device from a body part . . . Character: **5**

Read this carefully: As the description specifically states "device," this can be used only for this type of procedure–to remove a previously placed device. As you abstract the physician's notes, be cautious of the use of this term in documentation.

Caution! This root operation term means the same as it does in the ***Medical and Surgical*** and the ***Obstetrics*** sections; however, the character used to report this in the ***Placement*** section is different.

> **EXAMPLES**
>
> 2W5MX3Z Removal, G3 XL post-op knee brace, left leg
>
> 2W5TX0Z Removal of traction apparatus from left foot

Traction

Traction: Exerting a pulling force on a body region in a distal direction . . . Character: **6**

Notice that *Traction* is presented as a root operation term as well as traction apparatus that is offered as an option for the device used.

> **EXAMPLE**
>
> 2W62X0Z Traction apparatus placed at neck

Character Position 4: Body Region/Orifice

Character Position	Character Meaning
1	Section of the ICD-10-PCS book
2	Anatomical region/orifices
3	Root operation term
4	**Body region/orifice**
5	Approach used by physician
6	Device
7	Qualifier

The two body systems in this section (Anatomical Regions and Anatomical Orifices) each has a list of applicable body regions and their characters.

Anatomical Regions

Head . . . Character: **0**

Face . . . 1

Neck . . . 2

Abdominal Wall . . . 3

Chest Wall . . . 4

Back . . . 5

Inguinal Region, Right . . . 6

Inguinal Region, Left . . . 7

Upper Extremity, Right . . . 8

Upper Extremity, Left . . . 9

Upper Arm, Right . . . A

Upper Arm, Left . . . B

Lower Arm, Right . . . C

Lower Arm, Left . . . D

Hand, Right . . . E

Hand, Left . . . F

Thumb, Right . . . G

Thumb, Left . . . H

Finger, Right . . . J

Finger, Left . . . K

Lower Extremity, Right . . . L

Lower Extremity, Left . . . M

Upper Leg, Right . . . N

Upper Leg, Left . . . P

Lower Leg, Right . . . Q

Lower Leg, Left . . . R

Foot, Right . . . S

Foot, Left . . . T

Toe, Right . . . U

Toe, Left . . . V

Anatomical Orifices

Mouth and Pharynx . . . 0

Nasal . . . 1

Ear . . . 2

Anorectal . . . 3

Female Genital Tract . . . 4

Urethra . . . 5

Character Position 5: Approach

Character Position	Character Meaning
1	Section of the ICD-10-PCS book
2	Anatomical region/orifices
3	Root operation term
4	Body region/orifice
5	**Approach used by physician**
6	Device
7	Qualifier

This one is easy; there is only one choice. Remember that all procedures reported from the ***Placement*** section do not involve incisions or punctures. This means all of these devices are external.

External Approach . . . Character: **X**

Character Position 6: Device

Character Position	Character Meaning
1	Section of the ICD-10-PCS book
2	Anatomical region/orifices
3	Root operation term
4	Body region/orifice
5	Approach used by physician
6	**Device**
7	Qualifier

It makes sense that there are several options for the character to report a device because that is really the primary activity of this section: **placement** of a device.

> **Placement**
> To put a device in or on an anatomical site.

Traction Apparatus . . . Character: **0**

Splint . . . Character: **1**

Cast . . . Character: **2**

Brace . . . Character: **3**

Bandage . . . Character: **4**

Packing Material . . . Character: **5**

Pressure Dressing . . . Character: **6**

Intermittent Pressure Device . . . Character: **7**

Wire . . . Character: **9**

Other Device . . . Character: **Y**

No Device . . . Character: **Z**

EXAMPLES

You might see phrases such as these in the documentation:

". . . and a short arm splint, right side, was applied. . . ."

(continued)

2W38X1Z Immobilization using a splint, upper extremity, right

"*. . .The new Philadelphia collar was removed. . . .*"

2W52X3Z Removal of neck brace

Character Position 7: Qualifier

Character Position	Character Meaning
1	Section of the ICD-10-PCS book
2	Anatomical region/orifices
3	Root operation term
4	Body region/orifice
5	Approach used by physician
6	Device
7	**Qualifier**

There are no details reported by the Qualifier position, so the only option is **Z** No Qualifier.

ICD-10-PCS

LET'S CODE IT! SCENARIO

Michael Shinto, a 31-year-old male, was in a fight at a bar and was punched in the face. Along with other injuries, Michael's lower jaw was dislocated. Dr. Northrop admitted Michael into the hospital due to internal bleeding. Once in his room, Dr. Northrop took Michael to the procedure room to wire his jaw to immobilize it and permit it to heal.

Let's Code It!

Let's go through the steps of coding for ICD-10-PCS and determine the code or codes that should be reported for this encounter between Dr. Northrop and Michael Shinto.

Which section will provide you with the details to report this procedure? Let's think this through. Dr. Northrop wired Michael's jaw. Therefore, he placed wire . . . the ***Placement*** section.

First character: Section: Placement . . . 2

You have two choices for body system: Anatomical Regions or Anatomical Orifices. The jaw is not an orifice, so the decision is straightforward.

Second character: Body Region: Anatomical Regions . . . W

What was the purpose of placing the wire? The documentation states, "*to immobilize it.*"

Third character: Root Operation: Immobilization . . . 3

Read the options in the Body Region column carefully. Which anatomical site comes closest because *jaw* is not listed? Yes, the jaw is a part of the head, but it is also part of the face. Hmm. In this circumstance, we need to read ahead a little bit to the list shown in the column to the right for Device. You know for certain that *wire* was used, and there is only an option for Wire on the row with Face, not Head. Therefore, you can tell which to report.

Fourth character: Body Region: Face . . . 1

It is logical that the wire was placed externally, and this is the only option you have for the fifth character. Nice.

Fifth character: Approach: External . . . X

You know that the device is Wire because the documentation states, "*wire his jaw.*"

Sixth character: Device: Wire . . . 9

There is only one option for the qualifier for this row on this Table.

Seventh character: Qualifier: No Qualifier . . . Z

(continued)

The ICD-10-PCS code you will report is

2W31X9Z **Wire jaw**

Good job!

36.2 Reporting Services from the Administration Section

Character Definitions

The meanings for the ***Administration*** section characters are shown in the following table:

Character Position	Character Meaning
1	Section of the ICD-10-PCS book
2	Physiological system or anatomical region
3	Root operation term
4	Body system or region
5	Approach used by physician
6	Substance
7	Qualifier

For the most part, these character positions have different meanings than the other sections you have already learned about.

Character Position 1: Administration Section 3

Character Position	Character Meaning
1	**Section of the ICD-10-PCS book**
2	Physiological system or anatomical region
3	Root operation term
4	Body system or region
5	Approach used by physician
6	Substance
7	Qualifier

Procedures reported from the ***Administration*** section will all begin with the number **3**.

Character Position 2: Physiological System/Anatomical Region

Character Position	Character Meaning
1	Section of the ICD-10-PCS book
2	**Physiological system or Anatomical region**
3	Root operation term
4	Body system or region
5	Approach used by physician
6	Substance
7	Qualifier

There are only three options for the second character:

Circulatory . . . Character: **0** [*This is used for transfusion procedures.*]

Indwelling Device . . . Character: **C**

Physiological Systems and Anatomical Regions . . . Character: **E**

EXAMPLE

Roy Shearmann, a 47-year-old male, was diagnosed with myelodysplastic syndrome several months ago when he presented with progressive pancytopenia. Since admission, he has undergone treatment with antibiotics and has received transfusion of nonautologous packed RBCs, administrated via peripheral vein, IV. The patient continues on weekly Procrit. Code for the blood transfusion.

30233N1 Transfusion, nonautologous red blood cells, peripheral vein, percutaneously

Character Position 3: Root Operation

Character Position	Character Meaning
1	Section of the ICD-10-PCS book
2	Physiological system or anatomical region
3	**Root operation term**
4	Body system or region
5	Approach used by physician
6	Substance
7	Qualifier

There are only three root operation terms used to report procedures in this section:

Introduction: Putting in or on a therapeutic, diagnostic, nutritional, physiological, or prophylactic substance except blood or blood products . . . Character: **0**

Irrigation: Putting in or on a cleansing substance . . . Character: **1**

Transfusion: Putting in blood or blood products . . . Character: **2**

EXAMPLE

Illanya Sibgame, a pleasant 55-year-old female patient, is admitted to undergo treatment for a non-Hodgkin lymphoma. While admitted, intrathecal chemotherapy, DepoCyt 50 mg (a low-dose interleukin-2 drug), was administered. She did tolerate all treatments well with no complication noted, and once stable, was made ready for discharge home.

3E0R303 Introduction of low-dose interleukin-2 antineoplastic, intrathecal

Character Position 4: Body System/Region

Character Position	Character Meaning
1	Section of the ICD-10-PCS book
2	Physiological system or anatomical region
3	Root operation term
4	**Body system or region**
5	Approach used by physician
6	Substance
7	Qualifier

Specifically for this section, the fourth character position will report the anatomical site into which the substance is administered. Be careful. This may be different from the site expected to benefit from the ultimate effect of this substance. For example, if the substance is administered intradermally (such as an intradermal patch), the body system/region would be skin and mucous membrane, whereas an IM (intramuscular) injection would be reported as the muscle in this character position. IA (intra-arterial) or IV (intravenous) **administrations** would be reported to the peripheral artery or peripheral vein, respectively. However, if a catheter is used—for example, to travel to administer the substance directly to a clot—this would be reported as a central artery or central vein, per the documentation.

> **Administration**
> To introduce a therapeutic, prophylactic, protective, diagnostic, nutritional, or physiological substance.

Oddly, there is an exception. When an irrigating substance (such as saline solution) is administered into an indwelling device (reported as body system **C** Indwelling Device), the body system/region will be **Z** None.

Character Position 5: Approach

Character Position	Character Meaning
1	Section of the ICD-10-PCS book
2	Physiological system or anatomical region
3	Root operation term
4	Body system or region
5	**Approach used by physician**
6	Substance
7	Qualifier

> **CODING BITES**
>
> If you want a refresher on the different approaches, you can revisit the **ICD-10-PCS Medical and Surgical Section** chapter, section **Medical/Surgical Approaches: Character 5**.

The approaches for this section are those you have come to know: **0** Open, **3** Percutaneous, **4** Percutaneous Endoscopic, **7** Via Natural or Artificial Opening, **8** Via Natural or Artificial Opening Endoscopic, and **X** External.

Character Position 6: Substance

Character Position	Character Meaning
1	Section of the ICD-10-PCS book
2	Physiological system or anatomical region
3	Root operation term
4	Body system or region
5	Approach used by physician
6	**Substance**
7	Qualifier

In this character position, you will identify the substance being administered. Be careful! The Substance characters reported for Circulatory (second character 0) and those reported for Physiological Systems and Anatomical Regions (second character E) have different meanings for the same letters. This is a great example of why it is so important to read each table carefully and completely and to avoid assuming that the same letter means the same from table to table, even in the same section.

> **EXAMPLES**
>
> 30***G* Administration, Circulatory, ***, Bone marrow, *
>
> 3E***G* Administration, Physiological Systems, ***, Other Therapeutic Substance, *

> **CODING BITES**
>
> Check out the appendix ***Substance Key/Substance Definitions*** in your ICD-10-PCS code book as well as *Physicians' Desk Reference (PDR)* or another drug index.

Character Position 7: Qualifier

Character Position	Character Meaning
1	Section of the ICD-10-PCS book
2	Physiological system or anatomical region
3	Root operation term
4	Body system or region
5	Approach used by physician
6	Substance
7	**Qualifier**

This character will provide additional detail about the substance, if necessary.

EXAMPLES

Autologous . . . Character: **0**

Nonautologous . . . Character: **1**

Oxazolidinones . . . Character: **8**

No Qualifier . . . Character: **Z**

LET'S CODE IT! SCENARIO

Sean McRoyale, a 41-year-old male, was admitted into McGraw Hospital. Dr. Toller administered nonautologous pancreatic islet cells, intravenously.

Let's Code It!

Let's go through the steps of coding for ICD-10-PCS and determine the code or codes that should be reported for this encounter between Dr. Toller and Sean McRoyale.

From which section will you report this? The documentation actually tells you, where it states, "*administered.*"

First character: Section: Administration . . . 3

There are three choices, as you learned, for body system in this section. While it might make sense to think that Circulatory would be correct when the documentation states, "*intravenously*," as you read the Table, however, you can see that there is only one Root Operation Term under this body system, and this is Transfusion [Putting in blood or blood products], and this does not fit at all. Next is Indwelling Device, and that does not fit either. Therefore, the only realistic option is Physiological Systems and Anatomical Regions.

Second character: Physiological Systems and Anatomical Regions . . . E

You have only two options for a Root Operation Term for this body system in the ***Administration*** section: Introduction and Irrigation. You know Irrigation [Putting in or on a cleansing substance] does not fit. And the following details will help you confirm this decision.

Third character: Root Operation: Introduction . . . 0

The documentation states, "*intravenously.*" This means this substance was administered into a vein. This narrows down the options to Central Vein or Peripheral Vein. Venipuncture is typically done in the cubital fossa (inside the elbow), which includes three peripheral veins. Of course, in real life, when you are on the job, you must confirm this with additional documentation or the provider. For now, we will accept this was done via a peripheral vein.

Fourth character: Body Region: Peripheral Vein . . . 3

(continued)

Venipuncture is performed percutaneously, directly into the vein.

Fifth character: Approach: Percutaneous . . . 3

There are many, many choices in this sixth character column. The documentation states "*pancreatic islet cells*" as the substance. Find it, and make certain it is on the same row as Peripheral Vein.

Sixth character: Substance: Pancreatic Islet Cells . . . U

What type of cells? The documentation states, "*nonautologous*."

Seventh character: Qualifier: Nonautologous . . . 1

The ICD-10-PCS code you will report is

3E033U1 Introduction of nonautologous pancreatic islet cells, percutaneous, to peripheral vein

Good job!

36.3 Reporting Services from the Measurement and Monitoring Section

Character Definitions

The meanings for the ***Measurement and Monitoring*** section characters are shown in the following table:

Character Position	Character Meaning
1	Section of the ICD-10-PCS book
2	Physiological system
3	Root operation term
4	Body system
5	Approach used by physician
6	Function/device
7	Qualifier

For the most part, these character positions have different meanings than those in the other sections you have already learned about.

Character Position 1: Measurement and Monitoring Section 4

Character Position	Character Meaning
1	Section of the ICD-10-PCS book
2	Physiological system
3	Root operation term
4	Body system
5	Approach used by physician
6	Function/device
7	Qualifier

Procedures reported from the ***Measurement and Monitoring*** section will all begin with the number **4**.

Character Position 2: Physiological System

Character Position	Character Meaning
1	Section of the ICD-10-PCS book
2	**Physiological system**
3	Root operation term
4	Body system
5	Approach used by physician
6	Function/device
7	Qualifier

There are only two options for the second character:

Physiological Systems . . . Character: **A**

Physiological Devices . . . Character: **B**

Character Position 3: Root Operation

Character Position	Character Meaning
1	Section of the ICD-10-PCS book
2	Physiological system
3	**Root operation term**
4	Body system
5	Approach used by physician
6	Function/device
7	Qualifier

There are only two root operation terms used to report procedures in this section.

Measurement: Determining the level of a physiological or physical function at a point in time . . . Character: **0**

Monitoring: Determining the level of a physiological or physical function repetitively over a period of time . . . Character: **1**

EXAMPLE

An ECG measures the electrical activity of the heart at one point in time, whereas a Holter monitor continuously monitors the heart's rhythms over 24–48 hours.

1. ECG reported with **4A02X4Z Measurement of cardiac electrical activity, external**
2. Holter reported with **4A12XFZ Monitoring cardiac rhythms, externally**

Character Position 4: Body System

Character Position	Character Meaning
1	Section of the ICD-10-PCS book
2	Physiological system
3	Root operation term
4	**Body system**

(continued)

Character Position	Character Meaning
5	Approach used by physician
6	Function/device
7	Qualifier

The specific body system being measured or monitored is identified by the character in the fourth position. Note that this section includes **measurement** or monitoring of a patient's metabolism, temperature, or sleep. These are reported with a body system of **Z** None.

> **Measurement**
> To determine a level of a physiological or physical function.

EXAMPLES

Central Nervous System . . . Character: **0**

Cardiac System . . . Character: **2**

Respiratory System . . . Character: **9**

Character Position 5: Approach

Character Position	Character Meaning
1	Section of the ICD-10-PCS book
2	Physiological system
3	Root operation term
4	Body system
5	**Approach used by physician**
6	Function/device
7	Qualifier

The approaches for this section are those you have come to know: **0** Open, **3** Percutaneous, **4** Percutaneous Endoscopic, **7** Via Natural or Artificial Opening, **8** Via Natural or Artificial Opening Endoscopic, and **X** External.

Character Position 6: Function/Device

Character Position	Character Meaning
1	Section of the ICD-10-PCS book
2	Physiological system
3	Root operation term
4	Body system
5	Approach used by physician
6	**Function/device**
7	Qualifier

In this character position, you will identify the specific body function being measured or monitored, such as rhythm (**F**) of the heart or pressure (**B**) of the blood within the veins. This character may also report a device, such as a pacemaker (**S**), defibrillator (**T**) or cerebrospinal fluid shunt (W).

Characters are available for measuring and/or monitoring a patient's metabolism (**6**), temperature (**K**), or sleep (**Q**), such as a sleep study. These three functions use a body system character of **Z** None.

EXAMPLES

4A0HXCZ External measurement of fetal heart rate

4A1ZXQZ 48 hour sleep study, external monitoring

Character Position 7: Qualifier

Character Position	Character Meaning
1	Section of the ICD-10-PCS book
2	Physiological system
3	Root operation term
4	Body system
5	Approach used by physician
6	Function/device
7	**Qualifier**

This character will provide additional detail about either the body part or system or the procedure performed.

EXAMPLES

4A10X4G Monitoring of central nervous system activity, intraoperatively, external

4A143J1 Monitoring of peripheral pulse, venous, external

LET'S CODE IT! SCENARIO

Katrina Vales is a 17-year-old female with a history of asthma who was admitted with status asthmaticus. Once they were able to stop the current attack, Dr. Giffen measures her respiratory volume using a spirometer.

Let's Code It!

Let's go through the steps of coding for ICD-10-PCS and determine the code or codes that should be reported for this encounter between Dr. Giffen and Katrina Vales.

Which section? The documentation states, "*Dr. Giffen measures. . . .*"

First character: Section: Measurement and Monitoring . . . 4

Now, you have two choices for the body system: Physiological Systems or Physiological Devices. The measurement was of Katrina's respiratory function.

Second character: Body Region: Physiological Systems . . . A

You have two options for the root operation term: Measurement or Monitoring. The documentation states, "*Dr. Giffen measures. . . .*"

Third character: Root Operation: Measurement . . . 0

What body system is being measured? The documentation states, "*respiratory.*"

Fourth character: Body System: Respiratory . . . 9

(continued)

The documentation states, "*using a spirometer,*" meaning that you must know how a spirometer works to determine the next character. Use your medical dictionary or Google to find the facts about this method.

Fifth character: Approach: External . . . X

The documentation states, "*measures her respiratory volume. . . .*"

Sixth character: Function/Device: Volume . . . L

On this row, there is only one option for the seventh character.

Seventh character: Qualifier: No Qualifier . . . Z

The ICD-10-PCS code you will report is

4A09XLZ Measurement of respiratory volume

Good job!

36.4 Reporting Services from the Extracorporeal or Systemic Assistance and Performance Section

Character Definitions

The meanings for the ***Extracorporeal or Systemic Assistance and Performance*** section characters are shown in the following table:

Character Position	Character Meaning
1	Section of the ICD-10-PCS book
2	Physiological system
3	Root operation term
4	Body system
5	Duration
6	Function
7	Qualifier

For the most part, the character positions for the ***Extracorporeal or Systemic Assistance and Performance*** section have similar meanings as in the other sections about which you have already learned.

Character Position 1: Extracorporeal or Systemic Assistance and Performance Section 5

Character Position	Character Meaning
1	**Section of the ICD-10-PCS book**
2	Physiological system
3	Root operation term
4	Body system
5	Duration
6	Function
7	Qualifier

Procedures reported from the ***Extracorporeal or Systemic Assistance and Performance*** section will all begin with the number **5**.

Character Position 2: Physiological System

Character Position	Character Meaning
1	Section of the ICD-10-PCS book
2	**Physiological system**
3	Root operation term
4	Body system
5	Duration
6	Function
7	Qualifier

There is only one option for the second character:

Physiological Systems . . . Character: **A**

Character Position 3: Root Operation

Character Position	Character Meaning
1	Section of the ICD-10-PCS book
2	Physiological system
3	**Root operation term**
4	Body system
5	Duration
6	Function
7	Qualifier

There are only three root operation terms used to report procedures in this section:

Assistance: Taking over a portion of a physiological function by extracorporeal means . . . Character: **0**

Performance: Completely taking over a physiological function by extracorporeal means . . . Character: **1**

Restoration: Returning, or attempting to return, a physiological function to its original state by extracorporeal means . . . Character: **2**

EXAMPLE

5A05221 Hyperbaric oxygenation of a wound, continuous (an example of assistance because this is done to improve—or assist—the healing of the wound)

Character Position 4: Body System

Character Position	Character Meaning
1	Section of the ICD-10-PCS book
2	Physiological system
3	Root operation term
4	**Body system**
5	Duration
6	Function
7	Qualifier

The specific body systems being supported by these procedures are

Cardiac System . . . Character: **2**

Circulatory System . . . Character: **5**

Respiratory System . . . Character: **9**

Biliary System . . . Character: **C**

Urinary System . . . Character: **D**

EXAMPLE

5A1D00Z Filtration of a single period of duration, urinary system (hemodialysis takes over the physiological function of the urinary system by extracorporeal means)

Character Position 5: Duration

Character Position	Character Meaning
1	Section of the ICD-10-PCS book
2	Physiological system
3	Root operation term
4	Body system
5	**Duration**
6	Function
7	Qualifier

The fifth character position will report the length of time, or the number of times, the patient received this treatment:

Single . . . Character: **0** [*one time or one session*]

Intermittent . . . Character: **1** [*occasionally*]

Continuous . . . Character: **2** [*nonstop ongoing*]

Less than 24 Consecutive Hours . . . Character: **3** [*nonstop for a period of time*]

24–96 Consecutive Hours . . . Character: **4** [*nonstop for a period of time*]

Greater than 96 Consecutive Hours . . . Character: **5** [*nonstop for a period of time*]

Multiple . . . Character: **6** [*more than one time or one session*]

Intermittent, Less than 6 hours per day . . . Character: **7**

Prolonged Intermittent, 6–18 hours per day . . . Character: **8**

Continuous, Greater than 18 hours per day . . . Character: **9**

Intraoperative ... Character **A**

EXAMPLE

After the surgery, Brandon was kept on a ventilator for 31 hours.

5A1945Z Respiratory ventilator, 24–96 consecutive hours

Character Position 6: Function

Character Position	Character Meaning
1	Section of the ICD-10-PCS book
2	Physiological system
3	Root operation term
4	Body system
5	Duration
6	**Function**
7	Qualifier

In this character position, you will identify the specific physiological function occurring during this procedure:

Filtration . . . Character: **0**

Output . . . Character: **1**

Oxygenation . . . Character: **2**

Pacing . . . Character: **3**

Rhythm . . . Character: **4**

Ventilation . . . Character: **5**

EXAMPLE

5A2204Z Restoration of heart rhythm, single event (performing CPR)

Character Position 7: Qualifier

Character Position	Character Meaning
1	Section of the ICD-10-PCS book
2	Physiological system
3	Root operation term
4	Body system
5	Duration
6	Function
7	**Qualifier**

Extracorporeal
Outside of the body.

When a device or piece of equipment is used in the provision of the **extracorporeal** assistance or performance, the Qualifier will specify what was used:

	Character
Balloon Pump	**0**
Hyperbaric	**1**
Manual	**2**
Membrane	**3**
Nonmechanical	**4**
Pulsatile Compression	**5**
Other Pump	**6**
Continuous Positive Airway Pressure (CPAP)	**7**

Intermittent Positive Airway Pressure (IPAP)	**8**
Continuous Negative Airway Pressure (CNAP)	**9**
High Flow/Velocity Cannula	**A**
Intermittent Negative Airway Pressure (INAP)	**B**
Supersaturated	**C**
Impeller Pump	**D**
Membrane, Central	**F**
Membrane, Peripheral Veno-arterial	**G**
Membrane, Peripheral Veno-venous	**H**
Peripheral Veno-venous	**L**
No Qualifier	**Z**

ICD-10-PCS

LET'S CODE IT! SCENARIO

Linus Garza, a 63-year-old male, was in the hospital for surgery on his leg. During Linus's admission, Dr. Reagan ordered a CPAP machine to treat Linus's obstructive sleep apnea, only at night.

Let's Code It!

Let's go through the steps of coding for ICD-10-PCS and determine the code or codes that should be reported for this encounter between Dr. Reagan and Linus Garza for the CPAP treatment.

You already learned that *extracorporeal* means "outside of the body." You also need to know how a CPAP machine works.

First character: Section: Extracorporeal or Systemic Assistance and Performance . . . 5

There is only one body system option for this section.

Second character: Body System: Physiological Systems . . . A

A CPAP machine helps the body's breathing; it does not breathe for the patient. Therefore, assistance is the appropriate root operation term.

Third character: Root Operation: Assistance . . . 0

The CPAP assists the patient's breathing, so this is the Respiratory system.

Fourth character: Body System: Respiratory . . . 9

How long was Linus to be using the CPAP continuously? The documentation states, "*only at night*," therefore, less than 24 hours.

Fifth character: Duration: Less than 24 Consecutive Hours . . . 3

There is only one option for the sixth character, but it fits because *ventilation*, in health care, is breathing.

Sixth character: Function: Ventilation . . . 5

What does CPAP stand for?

Seventh character: Qualifier: Continuous Positive Airway Pressure . . . 7

The ICD-10-PCS code you will report is:

5A09357 **CPAP ventilation, less than 24 consecutive hours**

Good job!

36.5 Reporting Services from the Extracorporeal or Systemic Therapies Section

Character Definitions

The meanings for the ***Extracorporeal or Systemic Therapies*** section characters are shown in the following table:

Character Position	Character Meaning
1	Section of the ICD-10-PCS book
2	Physiological systems
3	Root operation
4	Body system
5	Duration
6	Qualifier
7	Qualifier

For the most part, the character positions for the ***Extracorporeal or Systemic Therapies*** section have similar meanings as in the other sections about which you have already learned. The difference between the procedures reported from this section and those from the ***Extracorporeal or Systemic Assistance and Performance*** section is that these therapies do not involve the process of assisting a physiological function or performing that function for the body.

Character Position 1: Extracorporeal or Systemic Therapies Section 6

Character Position	Character Meaning
1	**Section of the ICD-10-PCS book**
2	Physiological systems
3	Root operation
4	Body system
5	Duration
6	Qualifier
7	Qualifier

Procedures reported from the ***Extracorporeal or Systemic Therapies*** section will all begin with the number **6**.

Character Position 2: Physiological Systems

Character Position	Character Meaning
1	Section of the ICD-10-PCS book
2	**Physiological systems**
3	Root operation
4	Body system
5	Duration
6	Qualifier
7	Qualifier

There is only one option for the second character:

Physiological Systems . . .Character: **A**

Character Position 3: Root Operation

Character Position	Character Meaning
1	Section of the ICD-10-PCS book
2	Physiological systems
3	**Root operation**
4	Body system
5	Duration
6	Qualifier
7	Qualifier

There are 11 root operation terms used to report procedures in this section.

Atmospheric Control: Extracorporeal control of atmospheric pressure and composition . . . Character: **0**

Decompression: Extracorporeal elimination of undissolved gas from body fluids . . . Character: **1**

Electromagnetic Therapy: Extracorporeal treatment by electromagnetic rays . . . Character: **2**

Hyperthermia: Extracorporeal raising of body temperature . . . Character: **3**

Hypothermia: Extracorporeal lowering of body temperature . . . Character: **4**

Pheresis: Extracorporeal separation of blood products . . . Character: **5**

Phototherapy: Extracorporeal treatment by light rays . . . Character: **6**

Ultrasound Therapy: Extracorporeal treatment by ultrasound . . . Character: **7**

Ultraviolet Light Therapy: Extracorporeal treatment by ultraviolet light . . . Character: **8**

Shock Wave Therapy: Extracorporeal treatment by shock waves . . . Character: **9**

Perfusion: Extracorporeal treatment by diffusion of therapeutic fluid . . . Character: **B**

- The root operation term *decompression* is specific to a hyperbaric chamber used for treating decompression sickness, also known as the bends.
- When a *hyperthermic* procedure is used to treat a temperature imbalance, this is the section from which to report the code. However, if hyperthermia is used as an adjunct radiation treatment for a malignancy, this procedure is reported from the ***Radiation Therapy*** section (character **D**).
- The procedure *pheresis* is used primarily for two purposes:
  1. to treat a condition during which too much of a specific blood component is produced by the body (such as leukemia) and
  2. to remove a blood product from donor blood for purposes of transfusion to another patient, such as platelets.
- The *phototherapy* process removes blood from the patient into a machine that exposes that blood to light rays, recirculates it, and then returns this blood to the body.
- Note that *Shock Wave Therapy* is placed in the Tables section in numeric order (following table 8, Ultraviolet Light Therapy) and not in alphabetic order.

Character Position 4: Body System

Character Position	Character Meaning
1	Section of the ICD-10-PCS book
2	Physiological systems
3	Root operation
4	**Body system**

(continued)

Character Position	Character Meaning
5	Duration
6	Qualifier
7	Qualifier

The specific body systems being supported by these procedures are

Skin . . . Character: **0**

Urinary . . . Character: **1**

Central Nervous . . . Character: **2**

Musculoskeletal . . . Character: **3**

Circulatory . . . Character: **5**

Respiratory System . . . Character: **B**

Hepatobiliary System and Pancreas . . . Character: **F**

Urinary System . . . Character: **T**

None . . . Character: **Z**

Therapies such as atmospheric control, hyperthermia, and hypothermia are performed on the entire body and, therefore, have a body system of **Z** None.

Character Position 5: Duration

Character Position	Character Meaning
1	Section of the ICD-10-PCS book
2	Physiological systems
3	Root operation
4	Body system
5	**Duration**
6	Qualifier
7	Qualifier

The fifth character position will report the length of time, or the number of times, the patient received this treatment:

Single . . . Character: **0** [*one time or one session*]

Multiple . . . Character: **1** [*more than one time or one session*]

Character Position 6: Qualifier

Character Position	Character Meaning
1	Section of the ICD-10-PCS book
2	Physiological systems
3	Root operation
4	Body system
5	Duration
6	**Qualifier**
7	Qualifier

In this character position, there is one option for the 6AB Perfusion Table:

Donor Organ . . . Character: B

For all other Tables in this section, you have one option:

No Qualifier . . . Character: Z

Character Position 7: Qualifier

Character Position	Character Meaning
1	Section of the ICD-10-PCS book
2	Physiological systems
3	Root operation
4	Body system
5	Duration
6	Qualifier
7	**Qualifier**

When *pheresis* is performed, the Qualifier will specify what was used:

Erythrocytes . . . Character: **0**

Leukocytes . . . Character: **1**

Platelets . . . Character: **2**

Plasma . . . Character: **3**

Stem Cells, Cord Blood . . . Character: **T**

Stem Cells, Hematopoietic . . . Character: **V**

Ultrasound therapies performed on the circulatory system will utilize a Qualifier character to identify which specific vessels are being treated, when applicable:

Head and Neck Vessels . . . Character: **4**

Heart . . . Character: **5**

Peripheral Vessels . . . Character: **6**

Other Vessels . . . Character: **7**

No Qualifier . . . Character: **Z**

All other root operation terms (therapies) reported from this section have only one option:

No Qualifier . . . Character: **Z**

LET'S CODE IT! SCENARIO

Nathan Teeger, a 17-year-old male, was out walking near the ski resort where he was vacationing. He fell into a soft bed of snow and could not get out. The ski patrol took 5 hours to find him. At the hospital, Dr. Golden used hyperthermia to warm his body gently back to normal temperature. A single treatment was sufficient.

Let's Code It!

Let's go through the steps of coding for ICD-10-PCS and determine the code or codes that should be reported for this encounter between Dr. Golden and Nathan Teeger for this therapy.

Hyperthermia, from outside of Nathan's body, was used to help improve Nathan's health. You learned that this means it is a therapeutic procedure. Therefore, ***Extracorporeal or Systemic Therapies*** will be the section from which you will report the code for this procedure.

First character: Section: Extracorporeal or Systemic Therapies . . . 6

(continued)

There is only one option for body system in this section.

Second character: Body Region: Physiological Systems . . . A

The documentation states, "*used hyperthermia.*"

Third character: Root Operation: Hyperthermia . . . 3
Fourth character: Body System: None . . . Z

How many times did Dr. Golden use hyperthermia to treat Nathan? The documentation states, "*A single treatment. . .*"

Fifth character: Duration: Single . . . 0
Sixth character: Qualifier: None . . . Z
Seventh character: Qualifier: None . . . Z

The ICD-10-PCS code you will report is

6A3Z0ZZ **Hyperthermia for temperature imbalance**

Good job!

36.6 Reporting Osteopathic Services

Character Definitions

The meanings for the ***Osteopathic*** section characters are shown in the following table:

Character Position	Character Meaning
1	Section of the ICD-10-PCS book
2	Anatomical regions
3	Root operation term
4	Body region
5	Approach
6	Method
7	Qualifier

The ***Osteopathic*** section is very direct and straightforward.

Character Position 1: Osteopathic Section 7

Character Position	Character Meaning
1	Section of the ICD-10-PCS book
2	Anatomical regions
3	Root operation term
4	Body region
5	Approach
6	Method
7	Qualifier

Procedures reported from the ***Osteopathic*** section will all begin with the number 7.

Character Position 2: Anatomical Regions

Character Position	Character Meaning
1	Section of the ICD-10-PCS book
2	**Anatomical regions**
3	Root operation term
4	Body region
5	Approach
6	Method
7	Qualifier

There is only one option for the second character:

Anatomical Regions . . . Character: **W**

Character Position 3: Root Operation

Character Position	Character Meaning
1	Section of the ICD-10-PCS book
2	Anatomical regions
3	**Root operation term**
4	Body region
5	Approach
6	Method
7	Qualifier

There is only one root operation used when reporting osteopathic services:

Somatic
Related to the body, especially separate from the brain or mind.

Treatment: Manual treatment to eliminate or alleviate somatic dysfunction and related disorders . . . Character: **0**

EXAMPLE

7W03X2Z General mobilization of the lumbar region

Character Position 4: Body Region

Character Position	Character Meaning
1	Section of the ICD-10-PCS book
2	Anatomical regions
3	Root operation term
4	**Body region**
5	Approach
6	Method
7	Qualifier

The specific body regions supported by osteopathic services are

Head . . . Character: **0**

Cervical . . . Character: **1**

Thoracic . . . Character: **2**

Lumbar . . . Character: **3**

Sacrum . . . Character: **4**

Pelvis . . . Character: **5**

Lower Extremities . . . Character: **6**

Upper Extremities . . . Character: **7**

Rib Cage . . . Character: **8**

Abdomen . . . Character: **9**

EXAMPLE

7W06X8Z Isotonic muscle energy application to lower extremities

Character Position 5: Approach

Character Position	Character Meaning
1	Section of the ICD-10-PCS book
2	Anatomical regions
3	Root operation term
4	Body region
5	**Approach**
6	Method
7	Qualifier

All osteopathic services use an *external* approach, reported with character **X**.

Character Position 6: Method

Character Position	Character Meaning
1	Section of the ICD-10-PCS book
2	Anatomical regions
3	Root operation term
4	Body region
5	Approach
6	**Method**
7	Qualifier

In this character position, you will identify the specific method used by the doctor during this session:

Articulatory-Raising . . . Character: **0**

Facial Release . . . Character: **1**

General Mobilization . . . Character: **2**

High Velocity–Low Amplitude . . . Character: **3**

Indirect . . . Character: **4**

Low Velocity–High Amplitude . . . Character: **5**

Lymphatic Pump . . . Character: **6**

Muscle Energy—Isometric . . . Character: **7**

Muscle Energy—Isotonic . . . Character: **8**

Other Method . . . Character: **9**

EXAMPLE

7W05X4Z Indirect treatment of the pelvic region

Character Position 7: Qualifier

Character Position	Character Meaning
1	Section of the ICD-10-PCS book
2	Anatomical regions
3	Root operation term
4	Body region
5	Approach
6	Method
7	**Qualifier**

There is only one option for this character in the ***Osteopathic*** section:

No Qualifier . . . Character: **Z**

LET'S CODE IT! SCENARIO

Diane DeLucca, a 39-year-old female, was admitted due to a nerve condition in her face. After the results of the tests were analyzed, Dr. Slack diagnosed her with Bell's palsy. Dr. Slack, an osteopath, performed a facial release.

Let's Code It!

Let's go through the steps of coding for ICD-10-PCS and determine the code or codes that should be reported for this encounter between Dr. Slack and Diane DeLucca for this treatment.

There is nothing related to *facial release* in the Alphabetic Index. The best clue you have here is that Dr. Slack is an osteopath. For this section, you will find only one option presented for each of the first three characters.

First character: Section: Osteopathic . . . 7

Second character: Anatomical Regions . . . W

Third character: Root Operation: Treatment . . . 0

The treatment was applied to Diane's face; however, this is not one of the options provided for the fourth character. There is one option that is close.

Fourth character: Body System: Head . . . 0

There is only one option for the fifth character.

Fifth character: Approach: External . . . X

(continued)

What method did Dr. Slack use? The documentation states, "*a facial release*."

Sixth character: Method: Facial Release . . . 1

Seventh character: Qualifier: None . . . Z

The ICD-10-PCS code you will report is

7W00X1Z **Facial release**

Good job!

36.7 Reporting from the Other Procedures Section

Character Definitions

The meanings for the ***Other Procedures*** section characters are shown in the following table:

Character Position	Character Meaning
1	Section of the ICD-10-PCS book
2	Body system
3	Root operation term
4	Body region
5	Approach
6	Method
7	Qualifier

For the most part, the character positions for the ***Other Procedures*** section have similar meanings as in the other sections about which you have already learned.

Character Position 1: Other Procedures Section 8

Character Position	Character Meaning
1	**Section of the ICD-10-PCS book**
2	Body system
3	Root operation term
4	Body region
5	Approach
6	Method
7	Qualifier

Procedures reported from the ***Other Procedures*** section all begin with the number **8**.

Character Position 2: Body System

Character Position	Character Meaning
1	Section of the ICD-10-PCS book
2	**Body system**
3	Root operation term
4	Body region

(continued)

Character Position	Character Meaning
5	Approach
6	Method
7	Qualifier

There are only two options for the second character:

Indwelling Device . . . Character: **C**

Physiological Systems and Anatomical Regions . . . Character: **E**

Character Position 3: Root Operation

Character Position	Character Meaning
1	Section of the ICD-10-PCS book
2	Body system
3	**Root operation term**
4	Body region
5	Approach
6	Method
7	Qualifier

There is just one root operation term used to report procedures in this section.

Other Procedures: Methodologies that attempt to remediate or cure a disorder or disease . . . Character: **0**

EXAMPLE

8C01X6J Collection of cerebrospinal fluid

Character Position 4: Body Region

Character Position	Character Meaning
1	Section of the ICD-10-PCS book
2	Body system
3	Root operation term
4	**Body region**
5	Approach
6	Method
7	Qualifier

There are several body regions represented in this section.

EXAMPLE

Nervous System . . . Character: **1**

Circulatory System . . . Character: **2**

Head and Neck Region . . . Character: **9**

Integumentary System and Breast . . . Character: **H**

Lower Extremity . . . Character: **Y**

Character Position 5: Approach

Character Position	Character Meaning
1	Section of the ICD-10-PCS book
2	Body system
3	Root operation term
4	Body region
5	**Approach**
6	Method
7	Qualifier

The fifth character position, reporting the approach, will provide you with options with which you have become familiar: **0** Open, **3** Percutaneous, **4** Percutaneous Endoscopic, **7** Via Natural or Artificial Opening, **8** Via Natural or Artificial Opening Endoscopic, and **X** External.

EXAMPLE

8E0W8CZ Procedure on trunk region, via natural or artificial opening endoscopic, robotic-assisted

Character Position 6: Method

Character Position	Character Meaning
1	Section of the ICD-10-PCS book
2	Body system
3	Root operation term
4	Body region
5	Approach
6	**Method**
7	Qualifier

In this character position, you will identify the method employed during this procedure:

Acupuncture . . . Character: **0**

Therapeutic Massage . . . Character: **1**

Collection . . . Character: **6**

Computer Assisted Procedure . . . Character: **B**

Robotic Assisted Procedure . . . Character: **C**

Near Infrared Spectroscopy . . . Character: **D**

Other Method . . . Character: **Y**

Character Position 7: Qualifier

Character Position	Character Meaning
1	Section of the ICD-10-PCS book
2	Body system
3	Root operation term
4	Body region

(continued)

Character Position	Character Meaning
5	Approach
6	Method
7	**Qualifier**

The Qualifier will provide additional details as available or necessary.

You can see from this list, the Qualifier options range from anesthesia to in vitro fertilization to the use of imaging.

Anesthesia . . . Character: **0**

In Vitro Fertilization . . . Character: **1**

Breast Milk . . . Character: **2**

Sperm . . . Character: **3**

Yoga Therapy . . . Character: **4**

Meditation . . . Character: **5**

Isolation . . . Character: **6**

Examination . . . Character: **7**

Suture Removal . . . Character: **8**

Piercing . . . Character: **9**

Prostate . . . Character: **C**

Rectum . . . Character: **D**

With Fluoroscopy . . . Character: **F**

With Computerized Tomography . . . Character: **G**

With Magnetic Resonance Imaging . . . Character: **H**

No Qualifier . . . Character: **Z**

LET'S CODE IT! SCENARIO

Gillian Petrovic, a 31-year-old female, just gave birth via c-section. The nurse provided a pump so that Gillian could collect breast milk for the baby.

Let's Code It!

Let's go through the steps of coding for ICD-10-PCS and determine the code or codes that should be reported for this procedure.

This is not a typical type of hospital procedure, so that might give you a good hint to start with this section, ***Other Procedures***.

First character: Section: Other Procedures . . . 8

There are two options for the second character: Indwelling Device or Physiological Systems and Anatomical Regions. Gillian does not have an indwelling device related to this service, so this leaves one option.

Second character: Physiological Region: Physiological System and Anatomic Regions . . . E

There is only one option for the third character.

Third character: Root Operation: Other procedures . . . 0

(continued)

Don't decide too quickly for the body region. A woman's breast is considered part of the integumentary system, not the female reproductive system.

Fourth character: Body Region: Integumentary System and Breast . . . H

Pumping breast milk is done from outside of the body.

Fifth character: Approach: External . . . X

The pump "collects" the milk.

Sixth character: Method: Collection . . . 6

The qualifier explains what is being collected.

Seventh character: Qualifier: Breast Milk . . . 2

The ICD-10-PCS code you will report is

8E0HX62 Collection of breast milk

Good job!

36.8 Reporting Inpatient Chiropractic Services

Character Definitions

The meanings for the ***Chiropractic*** section characters are shown in the following table:

Character Position	Character Meaning
1	Section of the ICD-10-PCS book
2	Anatomical regions
3	Root operation term
4	Body region
5	Approach
6	Method
7	Qualifier

The ***Chiropractic*** section is very direct and straightforward.

Character Position 1: Chiropractic Section 9

Character Position	Character Meaning
1	**Section of the ICD-10-PCS book**
2	Anatomical regions
3	Root operation term
4	Body region
5	Approach
6	Method
7	Qualifier

Procedures reported from the ***Chiropractic*** section will all begin with the number **9**.

Character Position 2: Anatomical Regions

Character Position	Character Meaning
1	Section of the ICD-10-PCS book
2	**Anatomical regions**
3	Root operation term
4	Body region
5	Approach
6	Method
7	Qualifier

There is only one option for the second character:

Anatomical Regions . . . Character: **W**

Character Position 3: Root Operation

Character Position	Character Meaning
1	Section of the ICD-10-PCS book
2	Anatomical regions
3	**Root operation term**
4	Body region
5	Approach
6	Method
7	Qualifier

There is only one root operation used when reporting chiropractic services:

Manipulation: Manual procedure that involves a directed thrust to move a joint past the physiological range of motion, without exceeding the anatomical limit . . . Character: **B**

EXAMPLE

9WB1XBZ Non-manual manipulation of the cervical region

Character Position 4: Body Region

Character Position	Character Meaning
1	Section of the ICD-10-PCS book
2	Anatomical regions
3	Root operation term
4	**Body region**
5	Approach
6	Method
7	Qualifier

The specific body regions supported by chiropractic services are:

Head . . . Character: **0**

Cervical . . . Character: **1**

Thoracic . . . Character: **2**

Lumbar . . . Character: **3**

Sacrum . . . Character: **4**

Pelvis . . . Character: **5**

Lower Extremities . . . Character: **6**

Upper Extremities . . . Character: **7**

Rib cage . . . Character: **8**

Abdomen . . . Character: **9**

EXAMPLE

9WB7XKZ Manipulation of upper extremities, externally, with mechanical assistance

Character Position 5: Approach

Character Position	Character Meaning
1	Section of the ICD-10-PCS book
2	Anatomical regions
3	Root operation term
4	Body region
5	**Approach**
6	Method
7	Qualifier

All chiropractic services use an *external* approach, reported with character **X**.

Character Position 6: Method

Character Position	Character Meaning
1	Section of the ICD-10-PCS book
2	Anatomical regions
3	Root operation term
4	Body region
5	Approach
6	**Method**
7	Qualifier

Extra-articular
Located outside a joint.

In this character position, you will identify the specific method used by the doctor during this session:

Non-Manual . . . Character: **B**

Indirect Visceral . . . Character: **C**

Extra-articular . . . Character: **D**

Direct Visceral . . . Character: **F**

Long Lever Specific Contact . . . Character: **G**

Short Lever Specific Contact . . . Character: **H**

Long and Short Lever Specific Contact . . . Character: **J**

Mechanically Assisted . . . Character: **K**

Other Method . . . Character: **L**

EXAMPLE

9WB4XFZ Manipulation of sacrum, external direct visceral method

Character Position 7: Qualifier

Character Position	Character Meaning
1	Section of the ICD-10-PCS book
2	Anatomical regions
3	Root operation term
4	Body region
5	Approach
6	Method
7	**Qualifier**

There is only one option for this character in the ***Chiropractic*** section:

No Qualifier . . . Character: **Z**

LET'S CODE IT! SCENARIO

Ethan Logan, a 49-year-old male, works in a warehouse and hurt his back. He was admitted into the hospital for tests to determine the extent of the injury. While in the hospital, Dr. Maggun, a chiropractor, performed mechanically assisted manipulation on his lumbar region.

You Code It!

Let's go through the steps of coding for ICD-10-PCS and determine the code or codes that should be reported for this encounter between Dr. Maggun and Ethan Logan.

The documentation tells you that Dr. Maggun is a chiropractor, so this is a good reason to turn to the ***Chiropractic*** section of ICD-10-PCS.

You will find only one option for each of the first three characters in this section.

First character: Section: Chiropractic . . . 9

Second character: Body Region: Anatomical Regions . . . W

Third Character: Root Operation: Manipulation . . . B

What region of Ethan's body did Dr. Maggun treat?

Fourth character: Body Region: Lumbar . . . 3

There is only one option here for the fifth character, and it works because chiropractic treatments are done from outside the body.

Fifth character: Approach: External . . . X

(continued)

What method did Dr. Maggun use on Ethan? The documentation states, "*mechanically assisted. . . .*"

Sixth character: Method: Mechanically Assisted . . . K

Seventh character: Qualifier: None . . . Z

The ICD-10-PCS code you will report is

9WB3XKZ Chiropractic manipulation of the lumbar region using mechanical assistance

Good job!

36.9 Sections 2–9: Putting It All Together

Throughout this chapter, you have learned about each of the seven components of an ICD-10-PCS code used to report a procedure, service, or treatment from these sections. Now, let's put it all together and determine some codes all the way through.

LET'S CODE IT! SCENARIO

PATIENT: Alex Renetta

ADMITTING DIAGNOSIS: Crush fracture of left lower leg and foot

PAIN MANAGEMENT: The patient has stated that he is in severe pain. However, he is a recovering drug addict, clean 7 years, and will not accept any narcotics.

Dr. Donnatelli, an acupuncture physician, came in and used acupuncture methodologies to result in anesthesia effect for the left extremity. The patient was relieved by the treatment and the orthopedic surgeon was able to manipulate and cast the leg.

Code for Dr. Donnatelli.

Let's Code It!

Dr. Donnatelli used acupuncture to administer anesthesia so Alex could have his injury treated. As per the ICD-10-PCS Alphabetic Index, this is reported from the ***Other Procedures*** section.

First character: Section: Other Procedures . . . 8

Second character: Physiological Systems and Anatomical Regions . . . E

Third character: Root Operation: Other Procedures . . . 0

Remember that anesthesia is a process that uses needles in the skin to accomplish its goal . . .

Fourth character: Body Region: Integumentary System and Breast . . . H

Acupuncture is performed by inserting tiny needles gently into the epidermis.

Fifth character: Approach: Percutaneous . . . 3

Sixth character: Method: Acupuncture . . . 0

Seventh character: Qualifier: Anesthesia . . . 0

Put it all together and report code . . .

8E0H300 Anesthesia administered using acupuncture methodologies

Good job!

LET'S CODE IT! SCENARIO

PATIENT: Travis Clayton

PREOPERATIVE DIAGNOSES:
1. C5–6 facet fracture
2. Left C6 radiculitis

POSTOPERATIVE DIAGNOSES:
1. C5–6 facet fracture
2. Left C6 radiculitis

OPERATIONS PERFORMED:
Attempted closed reduction of vertebral fracture and subluxation with traction.

OPERATION: The patient was taken to the OR and placed in the supine position. Using 1% lidocaine and antibiotic ointment, Gardner-Wells tongs were placed in line with the external auditory meatus approximately a centimeter above the ear. The anesthesiologist, Dr. Mastrioni, administered conscious sedation. The patient tolerated the placement of tongs very well.

Ten pounds of traction were then added and a lateral C-arm image obtained, which showed persistent subluxation. Manual traction was then applied and maneuvers attempted with rotation as well as flexion and extension in an attempt to reduce the fracture. However, persistent subluxation was noted, and the decision was made to proceed with open reduction.

The patient was then administered general anesthetic with use of in-line traction. SSEP and EMG monitoring leads were placed. A Foley catheter was in place. Preoperative antibiotics were administered. SCDs were applied. The patient's arms were tucked to the side. The cervical spine and the left anterior iliac crests were prepped and draped in the standard sterile fashion.

Let's Code It!

Read the documentation of this procedure, and let's take it step by step, one character at a time, to build the correct code:

Traction is . . . placed onto the body, so . . .

First character: Section: Placement . . . 2

The neck is not an orifice, so you have one choice:

Second character: Anatomical Regions . . . W

Third character: Root Operation: Traction . . . 6

In this case, it may be easiest to look at the diagnosis to identify the specific body region being treated. The documentation states, "*C5–6 facet fracture*," which is in the neck.

Fourth character: Body Region: Neck . . . 2

Fifth character: Approach: External . . . X

Sixth character: Device: Traction Apparatus . . . 0

Seventh character: Qualifier: No Qualifier . . . Z

Now, put it all together and report this ICD-10-PCS code:

2W62X0Z Traction apparatus, neck

Good job!

LET'S CODE IT! SCENARIO

Bruce Diaz, a 73-year-old male, was in a car accident and was admitted into the hospital with a concussion and a fractured shoulder. His recent medical history reveals reduced renal function, so Dr. Wester ordered a session of 5 hours of dialysis daily, to be done bedside. Teena Strunk came up to his room with a mobile unit and performed the hemodialysis.

Let's Code It!

Bruce had one hemodialysis session provided to him, bedside. Hemodialysis is when a machine does the job of filtering the blood because the kidneys are not functioning properly. Turn to the ICD-10-PCS Alphabetic Index and find

Hemodialysis *see* Performance, Urinary, 5A1D

The Alphabetic Index has provided you with the first four characters; therefore, you need to check in the Tables section to determine the last three. Turn to the 5A1 Table:

First character: Section: Extracorporeal or Systemic Assistance and Performance . . . 5

Second character: Physiological Systems . . . A

The machine is taking over the function of the kidney, so this is the root operation term: Performance.

Third character: Root Operation: Performance . . . 1

Fourth character: Body System: Urinary . . . D

Fifth character: Duration: Intermittent, less than 6 hours per day . . . 7

Sixth character: Function: Filtration . . . 0

Seventh character: Qualifier: No Qualifier . . . Z

Now put it all together and report this code, with confidence:

5A1D70Z External filtration of the urinary system, single session

Good work!

Chapter Summary

This chapter has given you the opportunity to walk through the

(2) *Placement*,

(3) *Administration*,

(4) *Measurement and Monitoring*,

(5) *Extracorporeal or Systemic Assistance and Performance*,

(6) *Extracorporeal or Systemic Therapies*,

(7) *Osteopathic*,

(8) *Other Procedures*, and

(9) *Chiropractic* sections of ICD-10-PCS.

You have seen how each character position is important to reporting all of the pertinent details of a procedure, service, or treatment. You have learned that, in each section, the same character can have a different meaning. However, you always have the tables there to provide the options and their meanings to build the accurate code.

CODING BITES

Placement section codes report procedures that put a device in or on an anatomical site.

Administration section codes report procedures and services that introduce a therapeutic, prophylactic, protective, diagnostic, nutritional, or physiological substance.

Measurement and Monitoring section codes report those procedures that are done to determine a level of physiological or physical function.

Extracorporeal or Systemic Assistance and Performance section codes report the use of equipment to support or actually perform a physiological function from the outside of the body.

Extracorporeal or Systemic Therapies section codes report the use of equipment (machines) for a therapeutic purpose–other than assisting or performing a physiological function.

Osteopathic section codes report the provision of osteopathic manipulative treatments.

Other Procedures section codes report services including, but not limited to, acupuncture, in vitro fertilization, or simple suture removal.

Chiropractic section codes report the provision of chiropractic manipulative therapies.

CHAPTER 36 REVIEW
Placement through Chiropractic Sections

Let's Check It! Terminology

Match each key term to the appropriate definition.

1. **LO 36.4** Outside of the body.
2. **LO 36.1** To place a device in or on an anatomical site.
3. **LO 36.3** To determine a level of a physiological or physical function.
4. **LO 36.6** Related to the body, especially separate from the brain or mind.
5. **LO 36.8** Located outside a joint.
6. **LO 36.2** To introduce a therapeutic, prophylactic, protective, diagnostic, nutritional, or physiological substance.

A. Administration
B. Extra-articular
C. Extracorporeal
D. Measurement
E. Placement
F. Somatic

Let's Check It! Concepts

Part I: Placement (2), Administration (3), Measurement & Monitoring (4)

Choose the most appropriate answer for each of the following questions.

1. **LO 36.1** Within the Placement section, character position 2 Anatomical Region/Orifices, Anatomical Orifices is identified by which character?

   a. Y **b.** W **c.** X **d.** Z

2. **LO 36.1** Within the Placement section, character position 3 Root Operation, Putting pressure on a body region (identified with number 1), is which of the following?

   a. Dressing **b.** Immobilization **c.** Compression **d.** Traction

3. **LO 36.1** Within the Placement section, character position 4 Body Region/Orifice, the upper extremity, right, is identified by which character or number?

   a. A **b.** 8 **c.** C **d.** 9

4. **LO 36.1** Within the Placement section, character position 5 Approach, which is the correct approach?

   a. Open **b.** Percutaneous
   c. Via natural or artificial opening **d.** External

5. **LO 36.1** Johnny was playing at school and fractured his left arm. Dr. Keller applied a cast to Johnny's left arm. Within the Placement section, character position 6 Device, what number identifies the cast?

   a. 1 **b.** 2 **c.** 3 **d.** 4

6. **LO 36.2** All procedures reported from the Administration section will begin with which section number?

   a. 1 **b.** 2 **c.** 3 **d.** 4

7. **LO 36.2** Within the Administration section, character position 2 Physiological System/Anatomical Region, an indwelling device would be identified with which character or number?

   a. 0 **b.** C **c.** E **d.** X

8. **LO 36.2** A blood transfusion would be reported from which section?

   a. Obstetrics **b.** Placement
   c. Administration **d.** Measurement and Monitoring

9. **LO 36.2** Within the Administration section, character position 4 Body System/Region, when an irrigating substance (such as saline solution) is administered into an indwelling device (reported as body system Indwelling Device . . . C), the body system/region will be reported with which character?

   a. Z **b.** X **c.** C **d.** G

10. **LO 36.2** Within the Administration section, character position 7 Qualifier, Oxazolidinones is reported with which character or number?

    a. 1 **b.** Z **c.** 8 **d.** X

11. **LO 36.3** Within the Measurement and Monitoring section, character position 6 represents which of the following?

    a. Physiological system **b.** Body system **c.** Function/device **d.** Qualifier

12. **LO 36.3** Within the Measurement and Monitoring section, character position 2, a physiological device would be represented by which of the following characters or numbers?

    a. A **b.** 1 **c.** B **d.** 2

13. **LO 36.3** Within the Measurement and Monitoring section, character position 3 Root Operation, determining the level of a physiological or physical function repetitively over a period of time (identified by number 1) is known as

    a. An abortifacient **b.** Monitoring **c.** Measurement **d.** Laminaria

14. **LO 36.3** Within the Measurement and Monitoring section, character position 6, measuring a patient's temperature would be reported with which character?

    a. F **b.** S **c.** Q **d.** K

15. **LO 36.3** Within the Measurement and Monitoring section, character position 6, a sleep study would be reported with which character?

    a. B **b.** Q **c.** X **d.** Z

Part II: Extracorporeal or Systemic Assistance and Performance (5), Extracorporeal or Systemic Therapies (6), Osteopathic (7), Other Procedures (8), and Chiropractic (9) Sections

1. **LO 36.4** Within the Extracorporeal or Systemic Assistance and Performance section, character position 6 represents which of the following?

   a. Body system **b.** Root operation term **c.** Duration **d.** Function

2. **LO 36.4** Which of these is a term meaning "outside the body"?
   a. Phototherapy **b.** Extracorporeal **c.** Extra-articular **d.** Somatic
3. **LO 36.4** All of the Extracorporeal or Systemic Assistance and Performance procedures will begin with which section number?
   a. 5 **b.** 4 **c.** 2 **d.** 1
4. **LO 36.4** Within the Extracorporeal or Systemic Assistance and Performance section, character position 3 Root Operation, all of the following are root operation terms *except*
   a. Assistance **b.** Performance **c.** Manipulation **d.** Restoration
5. **LO 36.5** Within the Extracorporeal or Systemic Therapies section, character position 5 represents which of the following?
   a. Body system **b.** Root operation term **c.** Duration **d.** Function
6. **LO 36.5** Within the Extracorporeal or Systemic Therapies section, character position 3 Root Operation, which of the following is/are a root operation term(s)?
   a. Atmospheric control **b.** Hypothermia **c.** Pheresis **d.** All of these
7. **LO 36.5** Within the Extracorporeal or Systemic Therapies section, character position 4 Body System, number 3 represents which of the following?
   a. Urinary **b.** Central nervous **c.** Musculoskeletal **d.** Circulatory
8. **LO 36.5** Within the Extracorporeal or Systemic Therapies section, character position 7 Qualifier, ultrasound therapies performed on the circulatory system, peripheral vessels, would be reported with which character or number?
   a. 6 **b.** X **c.** 5 **d.** Z
9. **LO 36.6** Within the Osteopathic section, character position 6 represents which of the following?
   a. Anatomical region **b.** Method **c.** Body region **d.** Qualifier
10. **LO 36.6** All of the Osteopathic section procedures will begin with which section number?
    a. 5 **b.** 4 **c.** 7 **d.** 1
11. **LO 36.6** Within the Osteopathic section, which of the following is an option for character position 3 Root Operation?
    a. Treatment **b.** Manipulation **c.** Phototherapy **d.** Electromagnetic therapy
12. **LO 36.6** Within the Osteopathic section, character position 6, which number identifies low velocity-high amplitude?
    a. 0 **b.** 3 **c.** 5 **d.** 8
13. **LO 36.7** All of the Other Procedures section procedures will begin with which section number?
    a. 5 **b.** 8 **c.** 7 **d.** 9
14. **LO 36.7** Within the Other Procedures section, character position 2 Body System, an indwelling device is identified with which of the following characters?
    a. H **b.** E **c.** Y **d.** C
15. **LO 36.7** Within the Other Procedures section, character position 5 Approach, a procedure performed via natural or artificial opening is identified with which character or number?
    a. 7 **b.** 3 **c.** 8 **d.** X
16. **LO 36.7** Within the Other Procedures section, character position 6 Method, acupuncture would be identified with which character or number?
    a. B **b.** 6 **c.** 0 **d.** D
17. **LO 36.8** All of the Chiropractic section procedures will begin with which section number?
    a. 5 **b.** 8 **c.** 7 **d.** 9
18. **LO 36.8** Within the Chiropractic section, character position 2 Anatomical Regions, you have one option for the character. Which of the following represents the anatomical regions?
    a. B **b.** W **c.** X **d.** Z

19. LO 36.8 Within the Chiropractic section, character position 5 Approach, you have one option for the character. Which of the following represents the approach?

   a. Open
   b. Percutaneous
   c. Via natural or artificial opening
   d. External

20. LO 36.8 Within the Chiropractic section, character position 6 Method, a long and short lever specific contact will be reported with which character?

   a. G
   b. F
   c. J
   d. L

Let's Check It! Rules and Regulations

Please answer the following questions from the knowledge you have gained after reading this chapter.

1. **LO 36.1** List the seven root operation terms used in the Placement section, character position 3; explain each root operation term, and include the character that identifies each term.
2. **LO 36.2** Within the Administration section, character position 4, Body System/Region, there is an exception. What is that exception?
3. **LO 36.3** Within the Measurement and Monitoring section, character position 3, Root Operation, what are the root operation terms? Include the description and character identifier.
4. **LO 36.4** List the seven Extracorporeal or Systemic Assistance and Performance section character positions; include each character's meaning.
5. **LO 36.8** Within the Chiropractic section, character position 1 is identified by what section number?

ICD-10-PCS

YOU CODE IT! Practice

Using the techniques described in this chapter, carefully read through the case studies and determine the most accurate ICD-10-PCS code(s) for each case study.

1. Marvin Dunham, a 68-year-old male, is admitted to the hospital with a deep laceration to the forehead. Dr. Wallace applies a pressure dressing to his head to control the bleeding.
2. Tony Botnet, a 62-year-old male, has a nose bleed that will not stop bleeding. Tony's hemoglobin has dropped, so he is admitted to the hospital. Dr. Caulkins packed his nasal cavity, external approach, to control the bleeding.
3. Harry Watson, a 32-year-old male, is admitted to the hospital with a hemoglobin of 5.6 g/dL. Dr. Hanks performs a red blood cell transfusion, peripheral vein, percutaneous, nonautologous.
4. Angela Niles, a 58-year-old female, has been in the hospital for 3 days with a peritoneal cavity indwelling device. Dr. Adams performs an irrigation of the peritoneal cavity with irrigation substance, percutaneous approach.
5. Cynthia Yackey, a 9-year-old female, is admitted to Westward Hospital with an unexplained high fever. Dr. Hamilton measures Cynthia's temperature, external approach.
6. Steven Wallace, an 18-year-old male, wanted to join his college's football team. The team physical examination revealed a cardiac abnormality. Steven is admitted to Westward Hospital, where Dr. Jefferson monitors Steven's total cardiac activity under stress.
7. Meagan Garrison, a 43-year-old female, presents today with shortness of breath and a dry cough. Dr. Mansfield admits Meagan to the hospital and monitors her respiratory capacity, external approach.
8. Mason Dugan, a 57-year-old male, has been hospitalized for a week. Mason's lungs were not performing; he was placed on a respiratory ventilator 5 days ago.
9. Kwakita Sumwalt, a 39-year-old female, presents today in cardiac dysrhythmia. Dr. Tumbokon admits Kwakita to Westward Hospital and restores Kwakita's normal sinus rhythm.
10. Barbara Bell, a 33-year-old female, has been in the hospital for 4 days. Barbara has been complaining of right foot pain, so Dr. Harrison performs extracorporeal shockwave therapy, right heel, single treatment.

(continued)

11. Duncan Bowens, a 64-year-old male, has been hospitalized with diabetic polyneuropathy. He has also been diagnosed with urinary incontinence. Today Duncan receives a single treatment of electromagnetic therapy for his incontinence. Code today's treatment.
12. Kimberly Morgan, a 59-year-old female, was in a car accident and has been hospitalized for 2 days. She is currently having lower back pain. Today she receives an osteopathic treatment, lumbar region, low velocity-high amplitude, external approach, to relieve the pain. Code today's treatment.
13. Twanda Walters, a 34-year-old female diagnosed with trigeminal neuralgia, was admitted to Westward Hospital for stereotacic radiosurgery, which is scheduled for later in the week. Today Twanda is in pain and receives an acupuncture treatment, integumentary system, percutaneous approach, no qualifier. Code today's treatment.
14. Robert Thompson, a 16-year-old male, is admitted to the hospital with severe neck pain. Dr. Bell performs a chiropractic manipulation of the cervical region, mechanically assisted, external approach, to try and relieve the pain.
15. Susan Chapman, a 37-year-old female, is having chronic hip pain and has been admitted to Westward Hospital. Dr. Dugan performs a chiropractic manipulation of the pelvic region with long and short lever specific contact, external approach.

ICD-10-PCS YOU CODE IT! Application

The following exercises provide practice in abstracting physicians' notes and learning to work with documentation from our health care facility, Westward Hospital. These case studies are modeled on real patient encounters. Using the techniques described in this chapter, carefully read through the case studies and determine the most accurate ICD-10-PCS code(s) for each case study.

WESTWARD HOSPITAL

591 Chester Road

Masters, FL 33955

DISCHARGE SUMMARY

PATIENT: NATHANSON, MYRA

DATE OF ADMISSION: 08/30/26

DATE OF DISCHARGE: 09/01/26

ADMITTING DIAGNOSIS: Status asthmaticus

DISCHARGE DIAGNOSIS: 1. Status asthmaticus.

2. Bronchiolitis, empirically treated.

CONSULTANTS: None.

BRIEF HISTORY: The patient is a 17-year-old white female with known history of asthma since infancy, possible environmental allergies, who presented with progressive wheezing and respiratory distress for the past 2 days. The patient had been doing well on only p.r.n. medications per family's report. However, just previous to admission, the patient was exposed to dust and other particles after moving into a new house. After conservative treatment at home, the patient was brought into the emergency room, where she did not improve on albuterol, Atrovent treatments, or intravenous steroids immediately. Initial examination showed tachycardia of 128, rest tachypnea of about 35–40, and inspiratory and expiratory wheezes and rhonchi on lung examination. The patient was referred for admission for evaluation of worsening asthma and possible pneumonia.

STUDIES: The admission chest x-ray showed clear lungs. Clean catch urine culture showed only mixed skin flora.

HOSPITAL COURSE:

1. Status asthmaticus: The patient was admitted to the pediatric intensive care unit in moderate to severe respiratory distress with continuous albuterol treatments, Atrovent treatments q. 4 hours Decadron intravenously, and empiric treatment of respiratory infection with azithromycin intravenously. The patient responded to this aggressive treatment and within 1 day was transferred to the regular pediatric medical floor. The patient was afebrile with normal oxygen saturations and appearing much better. Before discharge, she received asthma education and social counseling along with the family and was connected with social work to help provide a home nebulizer for use.

(continued)

2. Empiric respiratory infection treatment: The patient did not show any specific indications of pneumonia or bronchitis by lab work; however, her initial physical examination showed possible pneumonia. She was started on intravenous antibiotics and was transferred to oral antibiotics before discharge.

DISCHARGE DISPOSITION: To home.

DISCHARGE INSTRUCTIONS

ACTIVITY: Ad lib.

DIET: Regular, as appropriate for age.

MEDICATIONS: Zithromax for 2 remaining days, albuterol one dose nebulizer treatment q.i.d. and p.r.n., and Flovent 110 mcg two puffs b.i.d.

FOLLOW-UP: Follow up with primary care physician in 1 week.

Benjamin Johnston, MD

Determine the most accurate ICD-10-PCS code(s) for the administration of the medications.

WESTWARD HOSPITAL

591 Chester Road

Masters, FL 33955

DISCHARGE SUMMARY

PATIENT: WARTTEL, JUDITH

DATE OF ADMISSION: 07/15/26

DATE OF SURGERY: 07/29/26

DATE OF DISCHARGE: 08/01/26

ADMITTING DIAGNOSIS: Peripheral vascular disease

DISCHARGE DIAGNOSIS: Peripheral vascular disease, status post right above-knee amputation

PROCEDURES:

1. Hyperbaric oxygen therapy.
2. Hemodialysis.
3. Lower extremity arterial Doppler.
4. A 2D echocardiogram with left ventricular hypertrophy, inferior septal hypokinesis and mildly impaired left ventricular function, sclerotic aortic valve, moderate mitral and severe tricuspid insufficiency.
5. Lower extremity Doppler negative for deep venous thrombosis. Initial lower extremity Doppler positive for calf deep venous thrombosis in the right lower extremity.

DISCHARGE DIAGNOSES:

1. Peripheral vascular disease, status post right above-knee amputation.
2. End-stage renal disease.
3. Non-insulin diabetes mellitus.
4. Hypertension.
5. Atrial fibrillation.
6. Mild congestive heart failure.
7. Protein depletion.
8. Anemia of chronic disease and postoperative anemia.
9. Hypothyroidism.

(continued)

HOSPITAL COURSE: The patient was initially admitted with right lower extremity calf thrombosis and cellulitis of the right calf. The patient was seen by renovascular surgery and infectious disease. At that time, she was started on IV antibiotics. She was continued with hyberbaric oxygen therapy (HBO), which had been performed as an outpatient. The patient had a repeat lower extremity Doppler, which did not reveal DVT; anticoagulation was discontinued at that time. The patient was seen by the pain management service. The patient was seen by cardiology for wide complex tachycardia that was self-limiting. No further workup was warranted by cardiology other than echo at this time. The patient's Coumadin was stopped and she was placed on Plavix due to bleeding. The patient continued on IV antibiotics and wound care. The patient's family requested a second opinion on above-knee amputation, as they were wishing for a below-knee amputation. Dr. Gerald saw the patient and advised the same. The patient underwent an AKA by Dr. Gerald without significant complications.

The patient was somewhat weak after surgery. She will continue with HBO and antibiotics. She was transferred to the floor from the PCU. She will continue with good pulmonary toilet. She was started back on Plavix and Coumadin was not restarted. She continued on hemodialysis, intermittent, 4 hours per day. Accu-Chek and sliding scale insulin were performed. The patient was arranged for skilled nursing facility (SNF) placement; however, prior to SNF placement, she slipped out of the bed and fell on her stump. Initial x-ray showed possible fracture. CT showed no fracture. The patient also had a full spinal x-ray and right shoulder x-ray performed without significant abnormalities. There was an area seen on the right shoulder x-ray, in the right parotid region, that appeared calcified; however, the patient does wear a bridge and had it on at the time of the x-ray, most likely representing these findings. I would recommend follow-up x-ray in 1 month of the right mandibular area to ensure this is unchanged.

The patient is discharged to skilled nursing facility at this time. She has finished HBO at this time. She will continue with hemodialysis as an outpatient. She is no longer on antibiotics. She will continue with blood sugar control. I still recommend a follow-up right mandibular x-ray in 3 to 4 weeks to ensure there are no changes and this definitely was the patient's bridge. She will follow with renovascular surgery, ID, cardiology, and skilled nursing facility MD once discharged.

Roxan Kernan, MD

Determine the most accurate ICD-10-PCS code(s) for the hyperbaric oxygen therapy and hemodialysis.

WESTWARD HOSPITAL

591 Chester Road

Masters, FL 33955

PATIENT: SHEPARD, JANIS

DATE OF ADMISSION: 09/14/26

ADMITTING DIAGNOSIS: Staghorn calculi

ATTENDING PHYSICIAN: Julio Yearlin, MD

Pt is a 69-year-old female who was admitted to the hospital with hematuria, nausea, and vomiting. A routine ECG is taken today in preparation for the surgical removal of the stones, which is scheduled for tomorrow.

Julio Yearlin, MD

Determine the most accurate ICD-10-PCS code(s) for the EKG.

WESTWARD HOSPITAL

591 Chester Road

Masters, FL 33955

DISCHARGE SUMMARY

PATIENT: KENSINGTON, CHARLES

DATE OF ADMISSION: 01/15/26

DATE OF DISCHARGE: 01/17/26

(continued)

ADMITTING DIAGNOSIS: Confusion, staring

DISCHARGE DIAGNOSIS: Possible TIA

This is an outpatient 58-year-old right-handed white male with a history of episodes of confusion and staring. He had an abnormal EEG in the past.

Routine 18-channel digital EEG was obtained to rule out any seizure activity or focal abnormalities.

FINDINGS: Background rhythm during awake stage shows well-organized, well-developed, average voltage 8 to 9 Hertz alpha activity in the posterior regions. It blocks with eye opening and it is bilaterally synchronous and symmetrical. No spike-and-wave discharges or any lateralizing abnormalities are seen. Photic stimulation did not produce any abnormalities. Hyperventilation was performed for 3 minutes. No abnormalities were found during the procedure. Intermittent EMG artifacts were seen. Stage II sleep was not achieved.

IMPRESSION: Normal awake study. No epileptiform discharges or any other paroxysmal activities or focal abnormalities seen. Clinical correlation is recommended.

Kenzi Bloomington, MD

Determine the most accurate ICD-10-PCS code(s) for the EEG.

WESTWARD HOSPITAL

591 Chester Road

Masters, FL 33955

DISCHARGE SUMMARY

PATIENT: HELMSLEY, GRAYSON

DATE OF ADMISSION: 10/07/26

DATE OF DISCHARGE: 10/09/26

ADMITTING DIAGNOSIS: Abnormal liver function, weight loss

DISCHARGE DIAGNOSIS: Metastatic pancreatobiliary carcinoma and metastatic disease to the peritoneal wall and the dome of the bladder

The patient is a 57-year-old male who was recently admitted to the hospital with significant weight loss associated with abnormal liver function tests. A CAT scan of the abdomen and pelvis noted a large mass in the tail of the pancreas and multiple hypodensities in the liver. He was seen in consultation and was subjected to a CAT scan–guided liver biopsy. He was also subjected to tumor markers that included a CEA and a CA19-9. He was noted to have markedly elevated CA19-9 at 2050. His CEA was 4.3 and his alfa-fetoprotein was less than 1.2.

The CAT-guided liver biopsy noted a high-grade infiltrating adenocarcinoma that was CK-7 and CAM 5.2 positive. The hepar antigen was negative. Based on this immunohistochemical staining, he was noted to have a metastatic pancreatobiliary carcinoma. His staging workup with CAT scan of the chest noted nonspecific mediastinal and axillary lymphadenopathy. The bone scan was essentially negative for metastatic disease. The CAT scan of the pelvis noted an enlarged prostate with questionable inflammatory changes on the dome of the bladder. Based on this evaluation, he was diagnosed with metastatic pancreatobiliary carcinoma and metastatic disease to the peritoneal wall and the dome of the bladder.

Following his diagnosis, he was referred to me and has been started on palliative chemotherapy with Gemzar. He has been tolerating Gemzar without much adverse effects. He was admitted to the hospital early this morning with uncontrolled blood sugars. The most likely etiology of his uncontrolled blood sugars is prednisone therapy.

Phillip Carlsson, MD

Determine the most accurate ICD-10-PCS code(s) for the administration of the chemotherapy.

37

Imaging, Nuclear Medicine, and Radiation Therapy Sections

Key Terms

Densitometry

High Osmolar

Intravascular Optical Coherence

Low Osmolar

Learning Outcomes

After completing this chapter, the student should be able to:

LO 37.1 Recognize the details reported from the Imaging section.

LO 37.2 Evaluate the details to determine the correct code reported from the Nuclear Medicine section.

LO 37.3 Determine the specifics required to build a code from the Radiation Therapy section.

LO 37.4 Analyze all of the details to build an accurate seven-character code for sections B, C, and D.

STOP! **Remember, you need to follow along in your ICD-10-PCS code book for an optimal learning experience.**

37.1 Reporting from the Imaging Section

Character Definitions

The meanings for the ***Imaging*** section characters are shown in the following table:

Character Position	Character Meaning
1	Section of the ICD-10-PCS book
2	Body system
3	Root type
4	Body part (specific anatomical site)
5	Contrast
6	Qualifier
7	Qualifier

You might have noticed that character positions here have many of the same meanings as for those in the ***Medical and Surgical*** section. You learned a lot about imaging services when you learned about coding from the ***Radiology*** section of CPT, so you have a bit of a head start for these procedures.

Character Position 1: Imaging Section B

Character Position	Character Meaning
1	**Section of the ICD-10-PCS book**
2	Body system
3	Root type
4	Body part (specific anatomical site)
5	Contrast
6	Qualifier
7	Qualifier

All of the codes from this section will begin with the letter **B**.

Character Position 2: Body System

Character Position	Character Meaning
1	Section of the ICD-10-PCS book
2	**Body system**
3	Root type
4	Body part (specific anatomical site)
5	Contrast
6	Qualifier
7	Qualifier

The body systems of the ***Imaging*** section are very similar to those you learned about for the ***Medical and Surgical*** section:

Central Nervous System . . . Character: **0**

Heart . . . Character: **2**

Upper Arteries . . . Character: **3**

Lower Arteries . . . Character: **4**

Veins . . . Character: **5**

Lymphatic system . . . Character: **7**

Eye . . . Character: **8**

Ears, Nose, Mouth and Throat . . . Character: **9**

Respiratory System . . . Character: **B**

Gastrointestinal System . . . Character: **D**

Hepatobiliary System . . . Character: **F**

Endocrine System . . . Character: **G**

Skin, Subcutaneous Tissue and Breast . . . Character: **H**

Connective Tissue . . . Character: **L**

Skull and Facial Bones . . . Character: **N**

Non-Axial Upper Bones . . . Character: **P**

Non-Axial Lower Bones . . . Character: **Q**

Axial Skeleton, Except Skull and Facial Bones . . . Character: **R**

Urinary System . . . Character: **T**

Female Reproductive System . . . Character: **U**

Male Reproductive System . . . Character: **V**

Anatomical Regions . . . Character: **W**

Fetus and Obstetrical . . . Character: **Y**

Two things to remember:

- The dividing line between *upper* and *lower* is the diaphragm.
- The *axial skeleton* is the torso (the body) and the *appendicular (non-axial) skeleton* is comprised of the extremities.

Character Position 3: Root Type

Character Position	Character Meaning
1	Section of the ICD-10-PCS book
2	Body system
3	**Root type**
4	Body part (specific anatomical site)
5	Contrast
6	Qualifier
7	Qualifier

The root type describes the type of imaging technology being used:

Plain Radiography (X-ray) . . . Character: **0**
Fluoroscopy . . . Character: **1**
Computerized Tomography (CT Scan) . . . Character: **2**
Magnetic Resonance Imaging (MRI) . . . Character: **3**
Ultrasonography . . . Character: **4**

- *Plain Radiography (X-ray):* Radiography is the use of electromagnetic radiation to visualize the visceral aspects (internal structures) of the human body.
- *Fluoroscopy:* Fluoroscopy is the emission of continuous x-ray beams to produce a real-time, dynamic image. High-density contrast agents, such as barium, might be administered to enable comparative data.
- *Computerized Tomography (CT Scan):* An x-ray beam is emitted, aimed through the anatomical site being studied, and then recorded by detectors. Then, the emissions are reconstructed to create a two- or three-dimensional image—a cross-sectional slice through the patient at a specific point. Each consecutive image is acquired at a slightly different angle, providing a more complete picture of the internal aspects.
- *Magnetic Resonance Imaging (MRI):* Three-dimensional views of internal body organs are created in real time, with greater visibility of variations within soft tissues. This technique makes visualization of brain, spine, muscles, joints, and other structures more detailed.
- *Ultrasonography:* Ultrasound, also known as ultrasonography, uses high-frequency sound waves to capture cross-sectional images of visceral organs, including the arteries, veins, and lymph nodes.

Character Position 4: Body Part

Character Position	Character Meaning
1	Section of the ICD-10-PCS book
2	Body system
3	Root type
4	**Body part (specific anatomical site)**
5	Contrast
6	Qualifier
7	Qualifier

From the brain to the toes, each body part is listed, specific to the body system in conjunction with the root type.

EXAMPLES

Brain . . . Character: **0**, under Central Nervous System, CT Scan

Coronary Artery, Single . . . Character: **0**, under Heart, Fluoroscopy

Thoracic Aorta . . . Character: **0**, under Upper Arteries, Plain Radiography

Abdominal Aorta . . . Character: **0**, under Lower Arteries, MRI

Epidural Veins . . . Character: **0**, under Veins, Plain Radiography

Character Position 5: Contrast

Character Position	Character Meaning
1	Section of the ICD-10-PCS book
2	Body system
3	Root type
4	Body part (specific anatomical site)
5	**Contrast**
6	Qualifier
7	Qualifier

As you learned earlier in this textbook, there are several types of imaging procedures performed with contrast materials. These materials may be barium or an iodine dye that is injected to highlight or make the visceral organs and body parts more clearly seen in the image.

High Osmolar
An ionic water-soluable iodinated contrast medium.

Low Osmolar
A non-ionic water-soluble iodinated contrast medium.

High Osmolar . . . Character: **0**

Low Osmolar . . . Character: **1**

Other Contrast . . . Character: **Y**

None . . . Character: **Z**

- *High Osmolar:* Also known as ionic contrast media. Examples include diatrizoate, metrizoate, and iothalamate.
- *Low Osmolar:* Also known as organic or non-ionic contrast media. Examples include iopamidol, ioxilan, and ioversol.

EXAMPLE

You might see something like this in the documentation about an MRI taken:

> *". . . Multiplanar sagittal, coronal and axial images were obtained through the left forearm prior to and following contrast administration using diatrizoate. Markers have been placed near the patient's indicated site of swelling, which includes the dorsum of the distal left forearm and also over the wrist. . . ."*

Multiplanar imaging typically refers to Magnetic Resonance Imaging (MRI). Never assume. Query the radiologist once and then you will know for certain going forward.

Character Position 6: Qualifier

Character Position	Character Meaning
1	Section of the ICD-10-PCS book
2	Body system
3	Root type
4	Body part (specific anatomical site)
5	Contrast
6	**Qualifier**
7	Qualifier

As you can see, a character placed in the sixth position will identify an additional detail specific to that table.

Intravascular Optical Coherence
A high-resolution, catheter-based imaging modality used for the optimized visualization of coronary artery lesions.

Unenhanced and Enhanced . . . Character: **0**

Laser . . . Character: **1**

Intravascular Optical Coherence . . . Character: **2**

None . . . Character: **Z**

Character Position 7: Qualifier

Character Position	Character Meaning
1	Section of the ICD-10-PCS book
2	Body system
3	Root type
4	Body part (specific anatomical site)
5	Contrast
6	Qualifier
7	**Qualifier**

The seventh character is required and may enable you to share additional details about this specific imaging procedure:

Densitometry
The process used to measure bone density, most often done to assess the patient's risk for osteopenia or osteoporosis.

Intraoperative . . . Character: **0**

Densitometry . . . Character: **1**

Intravascular . . . Character: **3**

Transesophageal . . . Character: **4**

Guidance . . . Character: **A**

None . . . Character: **Z**

EXAMPLE

You might see something like this in the operative report:

". . . The wire was then passed down to the superior vena cava without difficulty under direct fluoroscopy. . . ."

". . . With fluoroscopy, the catheter was then checked. It was noted to be in the superior vena cava just above the right atrium. . . ."

As you read the first snippet, you can see that the fluoroscopy is providing guidance so the wire could be placed accurately. So, this code's 7th character should be **A** Guidance.

In the second snippet, the fluoroscopy was used during a procedure on the patient's heart, directing you to report a 7th character of **0** Interoperative.

LET'S CODE IT! SCENARIO

Belinda Crandel, a 59-year-old female, has a family history of osteoporosis and was admitted into the hospital with a hairline fracture of the right hip. Dr. Franklin took a plain radiographic densitometry of her right hip to see if osteoporosis was an underlying cause of the fracture.

Let's Code It!

Let's go through the steps of coding for ICD-10-PCS and determine the code or codes that should be reported for the procedure that was performed.

First character: Section: Imaging . . . B

What body system was imaged? The documentation states, "*her right hip*," which is a non-axial (not the head or torso) lower bone.

Second character: Body System: Non-Axial Lower Bones . . . Q

What type of imaging was used? The documentation states, "*plain radiographic.*"

Third character: Root Operation: Plain Radiography . . . 0 (as in Zero)

Which specific body part was imaged? The documentation states, "*her right hip.*"

Fourth character: Body Part: Hip, Right . . . 0

There is no mention of any contrast being used, and there is only one option for the sixth character.

Fifth character: Contrast: None . . . Z

Sixth character: Qualifier: None . . . Z

The documentation does provide the detail for you to determine the accurate seventh character, where it states, "*densitometry.*"

Seventh character: Qualifier: Densitometry . . . 1

The ICD-10-PCS code you will report is

BQ00ZZ1 Plain radiography densitometry, right hip

Good job!

37.2 Reporting from the Nuclear Medicine Section

Character Definitions

The meanings for the ***Nuclear Medicine*** section characters are shown in the following table:

Character Position	Character Meaning
1	Section of the ICD-10-PCS book
2	Body system
3	Root type
4	Body part
5	Radionuclide
6	Qualifier
7	Qualifier

Character Position 1: Nuclear Medicine Section C

Character Position	Character Meaning
1	**Section of the ICD-10-PCS book**
2	Body system
3	Root type
4	Body part
5	Radionuclide
6	Qualifier
7	Qualifier

The procedures reported with codes from the ***Nuclear Medicine*** section describe the use of radioactive material administered into the patient's body to enable the creation of an image for further study. This modality is beneficial as a diagnostic tool for the assessment of metabolic functions and/or a therapeutic tool for the treatment of pathologic conditions.

NOTE: When radioactive materials are used to treat malignancies, the procedure is reported from the ***Radiation Therapy*** section, discussed later in this chapter.

Character Position 2: Body System

Character Position	Character Meaning
1	Section of the ICD-10-PCS book
2	**Body system**
3	Root type
4	Body part
5	Radionuclide
6	Qualifier
7	Qualifier

The character descriptors of body systems in this section are those with which you have become familiar in this code set.

EXAMPLES

Central nervous system . . . Character: **0**

Lymphatic and Hematologic System . . . Character: **7**

Respiratory System . . . Character: **B**

Urinary System . . . Character: **T**

Character Position 3: Root Type

Character Position	Character Meaning
1	Section of the ICD-10-PCS book
2	Body system
3	**Root type**
4	Body part
5	Radionuclide
6	Qualifier
7	Qualifier

The codes from the ***Nuclear Medicine*** section only report procedures that are noninvasive, meaning that the outer layer of the skin is not punctured and no incision is made.

Planar Nuclear Medicine Imaging: Introduction of radioactive materials into the body for single-plane display of images developed from the capture of radioactive emissions . . . Character: **1**

Tomographic (Tomo) Nuclear Medicine Imaging: Introduction of radioactive materials into the body for three-dimensional display of images developed from the capture of radioactive emissions . . . Character: **2**

Positron Emission Tomographic (PET) Imaging: Introduction of radioactive materials into the body for three-dimensional display of images developed from the simultaneous capture, 180 degrees apart, of radioactive emissions . . . Character: **3**

Nonimaging Nuclear Medicine Uptake: Introduction of radioactive materials into the body for measurements of organ function, from the detection of radioactive emissions . . . Character: **4**

Nonimaging Nuclear Medicine Probe: Introduction of radioactive materials into the body for the study of distribution and fate of certain substances by the detection of radioactive emissions; or alternatively, measurement of absorption of radioactive emissions from an external source . . . Character: **5**

Nonimaging Nuclear Medicine Assay: Introduction of radioactive materials into the body for the study of body fluids and blood elements, by the detection of radioactive emissions . . . Character: **6**

Systemic Nuclear Medicine Therapy: Introduction of unsealed radioactive materials into the body for treatment . . . Character: **7**

Character Position 4: Body Part

Character Position	Character Meaning
1	Section of the ICD-10-PCS book
2	Body system
3	Root type
4	**Body part**
5	Radionuclide
6	Qualifier
7	Qualifier

The list of body parts or systems for this section is similar to the list shown in the ***Imaging*** section. Combination descriptors–such as Ear, Nose, Mouth, and Throat–as well as regions–such as Lower Extremity Veins, Right–are included along with specific body parts, such as thyroid gland and spleen.

Character Position 5: Radionuclide

Character Position	Character Meaning
1	Section of the ICD-10-PCS book
2	Body system
3	Root type
4	Body part
5	**Radionuclide**
6	Qualifier
7	Qualifier

The options in this list include the descriptors of radioactive materials–the source of the radiation. Be careful–some of these are very similar.

Technetium 99m (Tc-99m) . . . Character: **1**

Cobalt 58 (Co-58) . . . Character: **7**

Samarium 153 (Sm-153) . . . Character: **8**

Krypton (Kr-81m) . . . Character: **9**
Carbon 11 (C-11) . . . Character: **B**
Cobalt 57 (Co-57) . . . Character: **C**
Indium 111 (In-111) . . . Character: **D**
Iodine 123 (I-123) . . . Character: **F**
Iodine 131 (I-131) . . . Character: **G**
Iodine 125 (I-125) . . . Character: **H**
Fluorine 18 (F-18) . . . Character: **K**
Gallium 67 (Ga-67) . . . Character: **L**
Oxygen 15 (O-15) . . . Character: **M**
Phosphorus 32 (P-32) . . . Character: **N**
Strontium 89 (Sr-89) . . . Character: **P**
Rubidium 82 (Rb-82) . . . Character: **Q**
Nitrogen 13 (N-13) . . . Character: **R**
Thallium 201 (Tl-201) . . . Character: **S**
Xenon 127 (Xe-127) . . . Character: **T**
Xenon 133 (Xe-133) . . . Character: **V**
Chromium (Cr-51) . . . Character: **W**
Other Radionuclide . . . Character: **Y**
None . . . Character: **Z**

CODING BITES

If the documentation shows that more than one radiopharmaceutical is used during one encounter, report a separate code for each identified substance.

The **Y** Other Radionuclide option is available to report any newly approved radionuclides. It is recommended to append documentation to the claim using this character to explain the specific radiation source utilized on the patient. And you may need to report a HCPCS Level II code, if available, to specify the radionuclide.

Character Position 6: Qualifier

Character Position	Character Meaning
1	Section of the ICD-10-PCS book
2	Body system
3	Root type
4	Body part
5	Radionuclide
6	**Qualifier**
7	Qualifier

This section has only one option for the character reported in the sixth position:

None . . . Character: **Z**

Character Position 7: Qualifier

Character Position	Character Meaning
1	Section of the ICD-10-PCS book
2	Body system
3	Root type
4	Body part
5	Radionuclide
6	Qualifier
7	**Qualifier**

There are no details reported by this Qualifier position, so the only option is . . .

None . . . Character: **Z**

LET'S CODE IT! SCENARIO

Oscar Farrell, an 83-year-old male, was admitted into the hospital with dyspnea and chest pain. Dr. Lowenthal did a PET imaging of his lungs and bronchi, using Fluorine 18.

Let's Code It!

Let's go through the steps of coding for ICD-10-PCS and determine the code or codes that should be reported for this encounter between Dr. Lowenthal and Oscar Farrell.

If you don't know, you can find PET imaging in the Alphabetic Index of ICD-10-PCS, which will direct you to the ***Nuclear Medicine*** section.

First character: Section: Nuclear Medicine . . . C

What body system was imaged? The documentation states, "*his lungs and bronchi,*" which are parts of the respiratory system.

Second character: Body System: Respiratory System . . . B

What type of imaging was performed? The documentation states, "*PET imaging.*"

Third character: Root Type: Positron Emission Tomographic (PET) Imaging . . . 3

What specific body parts were imaged? The documentation states, "*his lungs and bronchi.*"

Fourth character: Body Part: Lungs and Bronchi . . . 2

What radionuclide was used? The documentation states, "*Fluorine 18.*"

Fifth character: Radionuclide: Fluorine 18 . . . K

No additional details are required, and you only have one option for each of the last two characters.

Sixth character: Qualifier: None . . . Z
Seventh character: Qualifier: None . . . Z

The ICD-10-PCS code you will report is this:

CB32KZZ **PET imaging of lungs and bronchi, with Fluorine 18**

Good job!

37.3 Reporting from the Radiation Therapy Section

Character Definitions

The meanings for the ***Radiation Therapy*** section characters are shown in the following table:

Character Position	Character Meaning
1	Section of the ICD-10-PCS book
2	Body system
3	Root type (Modality)
4	Treatment site
5	Modality qualifier
6	Isotope
7	Qualifier

Character Position 1: Radiation Therapy Section D

Character Position	Character Meaning
1	**Section of the ICD-10-PCS book**
2	Body system
3	Root type (Modality)
4	Treatment site
5	Modality qualifier
6	Isotope
7	Qualifier

Procedures reported from the ***Radiation Therapy*** section will all begin with the letter **D**.

Character Position 2: Body System

Character Position	Character Meaning
1	Section of the ICD-10-PCS book
2	**Body system**
3	Root type (Modality)
4	Treatment site
5	Modality qualifier
6	Isotope
7	Qualifier

Again, the list for body system character descriptors in this section is very similar to other sections' lists for body systems.

Character Position 3: Root Type

Character Position	Character Meaning
1	Section of the ICD-10-PCS book
2	Body system
3	**Root type (Modality)**
4	Treatment site
5	Modality qualifier
6	Isotope
7	Qualifier

There are only four root types used to describe the modality of these procedures:

Beam Radiation . . . Character: **0**

Brachytherapy . . . Character: **1**

Stereotactic Radiosurgery . . . Character: **2**

Other Radiation . . . Character: **Y**

- *Beam Radiation:* Also known as external beam therapy (EBT), it uses one or more beams of high-energy x-rays directed at a patient's tumor.
- *Brachytherapy:* This method uses radioactive seeds that are placed in, or near, the tumor (internally). These seeds produce a high radiation dose in a limited manner, directly to the tumor. Use of this process controls the radiation exposure to surrounding, healthy tissues.
- *Stereotactic Radiosurgery:* This radiation methodology uses a focused high-power energy on a small area of the body, sometimes using a tool known as a CyberKnife. *NOTE:* Radiosurgery is not a surgical procedure; it is a treatment with no incisions made into the body.

Character Position 4: Treatment Site

Character Position	Character Meaning
1	Section of the ICD-10-PCS book
2	Body system
3	Root type (Modality)
4	**Treatment site**
5	Modality qualifier
6	Isotope
7	Qualifier

Consistent with other sections, these anatomical sites are very specific. *NOTE:* The same character is used to identify different body parts throughout this section. It changes from body system to body system.

EXAMPLES

Brain Stem . . . Character: **1**, under Central and Peripheral Nervous System

Thymus . . . Character: **1**, under Lymphatic and Hematologic System

Nose . . . Character: **1**, under Ear, Nose, Mouth, and Throat

Bronchus . . . Character: **1**, under Respiratory System

Character Position 5: Modality Qualifier

Character Position	Character Meaning
1	Section of the ICD-10-PCS book
2	Body system
3	Root type (Modality)
4	Treatment site
5	**Modality qualifier**
6	Isotope
7	Qualifier

This character will provide additional detail about the modality.

Photons <1 MeV . . . Character: **0**
Photons 1–10 MeV . . . Character: **1**
Photons >10 MeV . . . Character: **2**
Electrons . . . Character: **3**
Heavy Particles (Protons, Ions) . . . Character: **4**
Neutrons . . . Character: **5**
Neutron Capture . . . Character: **6**
Contact Radiation . . . Character: **7**
Hyperthermia . . . Character: **8**
High Dose Rate (HDR) . . . Character: **9**
Low Dose Rate (LDR) . . . Character: **B**
Intraoperative Radiation Therapy (IORT) . . . Character: **C**
Stereotactic Other Photon Radiosurgery . . . Character: **D**
Plaque Radiation . . . Character: **F**
Isotope Administration . . . Character: **G**

Stereotactic Particulate Radiosurgery . . . Character: **H**
Stereotactic Gamma Beam Radiosurgery . . . Character: **J**
Laser Interstitial Thermal Therapy . . . Character: **K**

Character Position 6: Isotope

Character Position	Character Meaning
1	Section of the ICD-10-PCS book
2	Body system
3	Root type (Modality)
4	Treatment site
5	Modality qualifier
6	**Isotope**
7	Qualifier

In this character position, you will identify the specific radioactive substance used during this procedure.

Cesium 137 (Cs-137) . . . Character: **7**
Iridium 192 (Ir-192) . . . Character: **8**
Iodine 125 (I-125) . . . Character: **9**
Palladium 103 (Pd-103) . . . Character: **B**
Californium 252 (Cf-252) . . . Character: **C**
Iodine 131 (I-131) . . . Character: **D**
Phosphorus 32 (P-32) . . . Character: **F**
Strontium 89 (Sr-89) . . . Character: **G**
Strontium 90 (Sr-90) . . . Character: **H**
Other Isotope . . . Character: **Y**
None . . . Character: **Z**

EXAMPLES

You may read something like these in the documentation:

". . . Palladium 103 radioactive seeds were implanted according to the preplanned computer calculation—a total of 56 seeds through 16 needles, each seed containing 1.04 mCi per seed. . . ."

". . . We implanted a total of 54 iodine-125 radioactive seeds through 12 needles with each seed containing 0.373 millicurie per seed. . . ."

Character Position 7: Qualifier

Character Position	Character Meaning
1	Section of the ICD-10-PCS book
2	Body system
3	Root type (Modality)
4	Treatment site
5	Modality qualifier
6	Isotope
7	**Qualifier**

This character will report that this radiation treatment was provided during a surgical procedure—or not.

Intraoperative . . . Character: **0**

No Qualifier . . . Character: **Z**

LET'S CODE IT! SCENARIO

Richard Raddison has been having severe pain in his stomach and was admitted into the hospital for tests. It was determined that Richard had malignant lesions in the fundus and pylorus areas of his stomach. Dr. Benjamin performed brachytherapy on Richard Raddison's stomach using Cesium 137, high dose rate.

Let's Code It!

Let's go through the steps of coding for ICD-10-PCS and determine the code or codes that should be reported for this encounter between Dr. Benjamin and Richard Raddison.

Brachytherapy was provided, and you already know this is a type of radiation therapy.

First character: Section: Radiation Therapy . . . D

What body system was being treated? The documentation states, "*his stomach*," which is a part of the gastrointestinal system.

Second character: Body System: Gastrointestinal System . . . D

What type of radiation therapy was used? The documentation states, "*brachytherapy*."

Third character: Root Type: Brachytherapy . . . 1

What specific body part was treated? The documentation states, "*his stomach*."

Fourth character: Treatment Site: Stomach . . . 1

What was the modality qualifier? The documentation states, "*high dose rate*."

Fifth character: Modality Qualifier: High Dose Rate . . . 9

What isotope was used? The documentation states, "*Cesium 137*."

Sixth character: Isotope: Cesium 137 (Cs-137) . . . 7

There is only one option to report for the seventh character.

Seventh character: Qualifier: None . . . Z

The ICD-10-PCS code you will report is this:

DD1197Z **Brachytherapy, stomach, high dose rate, Cs-137**

Good job!

NOTE: Isotopes Delivered by Implanted Device

When brachytherapy seeds are delivered via an implanted device, this is reported from the Medical and Surgical section, using the root term "Insertion" and the device character 6 used to describe that isotope.

Example: Palladium 103 brachytherapy seeds, embedded in a collagen matrix, were implanted into the patient's brain after a tumor was re-sectioned. This procedure would be reported with a code from the Medical and Surgical section of ICD-10-PCS: 00H005Z Insertion of a radioactive element Palladium 103 Collagen device into the brain, open approach.

37.4 Sections B, C, and D: Putting It All Together

LET'S CODE IT! SCENARIO

PATIENT: Carl Bergeron

ORDERING PHYSICIAN: Elias Madison, MD

HPI: Patient was admitted yesterday after falling in his office with no apparent reason. A 5 cm laceration on his scalp confirms that he hit his head on the desk as he fell.

IMAGING: *MRI OF THE HEAD*

The MRI of the head shows diffuse atrophy. There is no abnormality of the craniocervical junction. There is a small probable mucus retention cyst in the inferior right maxillary sinus. The brainstem is grossly intact. There is a slight increase in atrophy with regards to the left temporal lobe in comparison to the right. This is mild asymmetry, however. No large territorial defects are noted.

There is, however, noted on both the T2 and FLAIR images an area of very vague high signal along the left mid lateral ventricle region. This area of white matter suggests some probable demyelination. This is brought up in particular because, when contrast was given, there was a very vague sliver of enhancement directly in that area. This is seen on coronal imaging as well. This could be related to some collateral vessels and they are seen with contrast. Collateral vessels will be necessary due to the absence of good flow to the left MCA and ICA distribution on the left on the MRA, which will be described further following this report. Therefore, that is felt the most likely etiology. Other etiologies on this very vague and subtle enhancement would be tumor or luxury blood flow around a recent small ischemic insult. I would recommend that this simply be followed up over time in approximately 6 to 9 months or sooner if symptoms change.

There is no other area of enhancement of concern that is noted. We do see some asymmetry to the vascular venous drainage pattern with the gadolinium on the axial images in the posterior fossa and around the temporal lobe region on the left, which most likely again is related to the change in collateral flow to the left cerebral hemisphere.

The IAC and cerebellopontine angle regions do not show masses. No enhancing abnormality is noted to suggest an acoustic tumor. The inner ear and mastoid air cells are well aerated.

IMPRESSION:

1. *Diffuse atrophy.*
2. *FLAIR and T2 weighted images suggest some ischemic high signal changes in the white matter adjacent to the left lateral ventricle. In this area, with gadolinium, a small sliver of enhancement persists on both axial and coronal images. This sliver of enhancement may be related to collateral blood flow or luxury perfusion or recent ischemic insult. It could, though felt less likely, be related to mild enhancement of an underlying tumor. I feel this is less likely, and in light of no change in clinical symptoms, I would recommend simply a repeat MRI with gadolinium in approximately 6 to 9 months.*
3. *No other abnormal enhancement is noted.*
4. *There is a mild increase in atrophy with regards to the left temporal lobe when compared to the right; however, this is diffuse and subtle.*
5. *The internal auditory canal and cerebellopontine angle regions are normal in appearance.*

Lawrence Katenberg, MD, Radiology

Let's Code It!

According to the documentation, Dr. Katenberg is interpreting an MRI done of Carl's head. Let's determine the seven characters needed to build this code.

First character: Section: Imaging . . . B

Second character: Anatomical Regions . . . W

Third character: Root Operation: Magnetic Resonance Imaging (MRI) . . . 3

Fourth character: Body Part: Head . . . 8

(continued)

Was contrast used? The documentation states, "*when contrast was given.*" There is only one choice to report that contrast was used.

Fifth character: Contrast: Other Contrast . . . Y

Sixth character: Qualifier: Unenhanced and Enhanced . . . 0

Seventh character: Qualifier: None . . . Z

Now, put it all together and report, with confidence, this code:

BW38Y0Z MRI, head, unenhanced and enhanced

Good work!

ICD-10-PCS

LET'S CODE IT! SCENARIO

The patient is a 71-year-old female who was admitted last night due to subacute progressive spasticity over the last 7 months, increased difficulty walking, increased difficulty moving her right arm and hand, as well as increased rigidity. Her primary care physician has taken multiple MRIs, which included contrast, and there did not seem to be any abnormalities on his review.

She was given a provisional diagnosis of cerebral palsy, which does not fit with the natural course of this disease, as she was normal when she was a child. There seems to be an extrapyramidal as well as pyramidal component on examination today, but I do not appreciate spastic paraparesis as she was previously evaluated to have. The time course and progression of symptoms suggest a degenerative process with pyramidal and extrapyramidal component that could be part of secondary Parkinsonian spectrum disease. Perhaps there is a hereditary component to this.

I ordered lab work today to include ferritin, ceruloplasmin, copper, and liver function tests and Wilson disease screening. Also, as per my earlier order, she has just had a PET imaging with C-11 of her brain.

Let's Code It!

For this case, you are going to code for the PET imaging only. Remember, or use your medical dictionary, to confirm that PET stands for positron emission tomographic imaging, and find it in the ICD-10-PCS Alphabetic Index:

Positron Emission Tomographic (PET) Imaging

Brain C030

Terrific! Turn to the C03 Table in your ICD-10-PCS code book and let's determine the seven characters to build a correct code:

First character: Nuclear Medicine . . . C

What body system includes the brain? The *central nervous system* . . . that's right!

Second character: Central Nervous System . . . 0

Third character: Root Operation: Positron Emission Tomographic (PET) Imaging . . . 3

Fourth character: Body Part: Brain . . . 0

What radionuclide was used during this patient's imaging? The documentation states, "*with C-11.*"

Fifth character: Radionuclide: Carbon 11 (C-11) . . . B

Sixth character: Qualifier: None . . . Z

Seventh character: Qualifier: None . . . Z

Now, you can put it all together and report, with confidence, this ICD-10-PCS code:

C030BZZ PET imaging, brain, with Carbon 11 (C-11)

LET'S CODE IT! SCENARIO

PATIENT: Eric Periquinn

PREOPERATIVE DIAGNOSIS: Adenocarcinoma of the prostate

POSTOPERATIVE DIAGNOSIS: Adenocarcinoma of the prostate

PROCEDURE PERFORMED: Prostate brachytherapy

SURGEON: Gerald Crenshaw, MD

ANESTHESIA: General anesthesia via laryngeal mask airway (LMA)

DRAINS: One 18-French Foley catheter per urethra

INDICATIONS FOR PROCEDURE: This patient has a recent diagnosis of adenocarcinoma of the prostate diagnosed due to a very slowly rising PSA. His current PSA level is only 2.1, but prostate ultrasound biopsies were performed showing adenocarcinoma of the prostate at the left base of the prostate, and two biopsies were positive out of eight with a Gleason score of 6. Treatment options have been discussed, and he wishes to proceed with prostate brachytherapy. Informed consent has been obtained.

DESCRIPTION OF PROCEDURE: The patient was placed on the operating table in the supine position. General anesthesia was administered via laryngeal mask airway. He was then placed in the dorsal lithotomy position and sterilely prepped and draped in the usual fashion. The prostate ultrasound was inserted. The prostate was visualized using the preplanned study as a guide. Low dose prostate brachytherapy was performed. The patient tolerated the procedure well and had no immediate intraoperative or postoperative complications.

We implanted a total of 54 iodine-125 radioactive seeds through 12 needles with each seed containing 0.373 millicurie per seed. During the procedure, the patient received 4 mg of Decadron IV and 400 mg of Cipro IV. Subsequent fluoroscopy showed good distribution of the seeds throughout the prostate. The patient will have a CAT scan of the pelvis and simulation for his seed localization. Total target dose is 14,500 cGy.

The patient will be discharged with prescriptions for Cardura 1 mg a day for a month with two refills and Tylenol No. 3 one t.i.d. p.r.n. for pain, a total of 20, Pyridium Plus one b.i.d. for 10 days, Cipro 500 mg b.i.d. for 5 days, and prednisone 10 mg t.i.d. for a week.

Discharge instructions were explained to the patient and his wife. He will return to see me in my office in 3 weeks for a follow-up.

Let's Code It!

Dr. Crenshaw performed brachytherapy, which is radiation therapy, on Eric. Turn in the ICD-10-PCS Alphabetic Index to:

Brachytherapy [*read down the long list until you get to . . .*] Prostate DV10

Turn to the DV1 Table to complete this code:

First character: Section: Radiation Therapy . . . D

Second character: Male Reproductive System . . . V

Third character: Root Operation: Brachytherapy . . . 1

Fourth character: Treatment Site: Prostate . . . 0

Was this high dose or low dose rate? The documentation states, "*Low dose prostate brachytherapy.*"

Fifth character: Modality Qualifier: Low Dose Rate . . . B

What isotope was used? The documentation states, "*iodine-125 radioactive seeds.*"

Sixth character: Isotope: Iodine 125 . . . 9

Seventh character: Qualifier: None . . . Z

Now, put it all together and, with confidence, report this code:

DV10B9Z **Low dose brachytherapy, prostate, with iodine 125**

Really good work!

Chapter Summary

Imaging is a wonderful way for a physician to see inside the body to help determine a diagnosis. Nuclear medicine techniques enable the assessment of metabolic functions and can be used for either diagnostic or therapeutic purposes. And radiation therapies provide an efficacious way to treat malignancy. When provided to a patient who has been admitted into the hospital, these services and treatments are reported with a code from one of these sections.

CODING BITES

For those ***Imaging, Nuclear Medicine***, and ***Radiation Therapy*** services that use pharmaceuticals, you will need an additional code to report more details about the specific contrast material. You can find these drug codes in your HCPCS Level II code book.

Examples

(Contrast) High Osmolar contrast material, up to 149 mg/ml iodine concentration, per ml . . . code **Q9958**

(Contrast) Low Osmolar contrast material, 400 or greater mg/ml iodine concentration, per ml . . . code **Q9951**

(Radionuclide) Technetium 99m arcitumomab, diagnostic, per study dose, up to 45 millicuries . . . code **A9568**

(Isotope) Iodine I-125 serumalbumin, diagnostic, per 5 microcuries . . . code **A9532**

CHAPTER 37 REVIEW
Imaging, Nuclear Medicine, and Radiation Therapy Sections

Let's Check It! Terminology

Match each key term to the appropriate definition.

1. **LO 37.1** A non-ionic water-soluble iodinated contrast medium.
2. **LO 37.1** A high-resolution, catheter-based imaging modality used for the optimized visualization of coronary artery lesions.
3. **LO 37.1** The process used to measure bone density, most often done to assess the patient's risk for osteopenia or osteoporosis.
4. **LO 37.1** An ionic water-soluble iodinated contrast medium.

A. Densitometry
B. High Osmolar
C. Intravascular Optical Coherence
D. Low Osmolar

Let's Check It! Concepts

Choose the most appropriate answer for each of the following questions.

1. **LO 37.1** Within the Imaging section, character position 5 represents which of the following?
   a. Body system **b.** Contrast **c.** Device **d.** Qualifier
2. **LO 37.1** All of the codes reporting an Imaging section procedure will begin with what section letter?
   a. A **b.** B **c.** D **d.** F
3. **LO 37.1** All of the following would be found within the Imaging section, character position 3, Root Type, *except*
   a. x-ray **b.** CT scan **c.** PET **d.** MRI
4. **LO 37.1** Within the Imaging section, character position 6 Qualifier, which of the following are available options?
   a. Unenhanced and enhanced **b.** Laser
   c. Intravascular optical coherence **d.** All of these

5. **LO 37.2** Within the Nuclear Medicine section, character position 1 is identified by which of the following section letters?
   a. E **b.** B **c.** D **d.** C

6. **LO 37.2** Within the Nuclear Medicine section, which character position represents the radioactive materials–the source of the radiation being used?
   a. 5 **b.** 4 **c.** 3 **d.** 2

7. **LO 37.2** Introduction of radioactive materials into the body for three-dimensional display of images developed from the capture of radioactive emissions, identified by the character 2, is known as
   a. positron emission tomographic (PET) imaging
   b. planar nuclear medicine imaging
   c. nonimaging nuclear medicine uptake
   d. tomographic (tomo) nuclear medicine imaging

8. **LO 37.3** Within the Radiation Therapy section, which character position describes the modality of the procedure?
   a. 5 **b.** 4 **c.** 3 **d.** 2

9. **LO 37.3** Californium would be classified as
   a. a treatment site **b.** an isotope **c.** a modality **d.** a qualifier

10. **LO 37.3** Within the Radiation Therapy section, character position 7 Qualifier, which of the following characters represents the radiation treatment provided during a surgical procedure?
   a. Z **b.** 0 **c.** X **d.** 1

Let's Check It! Rules and Regulations

Please answer the following questions from the knowledge you have gained after reading this chapter.

1. **LO 37.1** List the five root types found within the Imaging section, character position 3, including the character that identifies each.
2. **LO 37.1** List the types of qualifiers found in the Imaging section, character position 7, Qualifier; include the character that identifies each.
3. **LO 37.3** When radioactive materials are used to treat malignancies, the procedure is reported from which ICD-10-PCS section?
4. **LO 37.2** List five types of radionuclides found within the Nuclear Medicine section, character position 5; include the character that identifies each.
5. **LO 37.3** There are only four root types used to describe the modality in the Radiation Therapy section, character position 3. What are they? Include the character that identifies each.

ICD-10-PCS

YOU CODE IT! Practice

Using the techniques described in this chapter, carefully read through the case studies and determine the most accurate ICD-10-PCS code(s) for each case study.

1. Edward Baker, a 26-year-old male, was riding his dirt bike and fell off, hurting his left ankle. Ed presents to Wynguard Hospital, where Dr. Dyson takes an x-ray, without contrast, of the ankle. Dr. Dyson also notes hemarthrosis and admits Ed to Wynguard Hospital. Code the x-ray.
2. Phoebe Eaddy, a 16-year-old female, complains of urinary dribbling and feels like her bladder is still full after voiding. Phoebe was diagnosed with type 1 diabetes 3 years ago. Dr. Barbato admits Phoebe to Weston Hospital and performs an ultrasound of Phoebe's urethra, which reveals nerve damage caused by her diabetes. Code the ultrasound.
3. Hugo Abbott, a 49-year-old male, has been diagnosed with osteosarcoma of his right knee. Hugo has been having difficulty, so Dr. Simmons admits Hugo to Westward Hospital, where an MRI, without contrast, of his right knee is performed.
4. Gregg Huggins, a 25-year-old male diagnosed with Graves' disease, is admitted to the hospital for a planar nuclear medicine imaging procedure of his thyroid gland, iodine 123 (I-123).

(continued)

5. Hazel Baker, a 51-year-old female, is admitted to the hospital for a tomographic nuclear medicine imaging procedure of her parathyroid glands, radionuclide–technetium 99m (Tc-99m).
6. Susan Gibbons, a 43-year-old female, is admitted to Westward Hospital for a positron emission tomographic (PET) imaging procedure of the lungs and bronchi, radionuclide–fluorine 18 (F-18).
7. Glenda McMahon, a 41-year-old female, is admitted to the hospital due to severe abdominal pain. Dr. Harmon performed a liver and spleen tomography using radionuclide Technetium 99m.
8. Joe Jefferson, a 72-year-old male, is admitted to the hospital with heart palpitations and edema of his legs and feet. Dr. Moss performs a heart positron emission tomographic (PET) scan.
9. Frank Ogburn, a 48-year-old male, has unexplained skeletal pain and is admitted to Westward Hospital so Dr. Cannon can perform a systemic nuclear medicine therapy whole body scan, strontium 89 (Sr-89).
10. Ozie Lewis, a 73-year-male, has been diagnosed with esophageal cancer. Ozie was admitted to Westward Hospital for beam radiation therapy to the esophagus, photons 1-10 MeV.
11. Jeff McCord, a 37-year-old male, was admitted to Westward Hospital 3 days ago and has been diagnosed with lymphatic cancer. Today Jeff receives his first treatment of brachytherapy of the inguinal lymphatic nodes, low dose rate, iridium 192 (Ir-192).
12. Harry Glover, a 38-year-old male, was admitted to Westward Hospital for stereotactic gamma beam radiosurgery on his eye.
13. Alna Lindsay, a 68-year-old female, was admitted to Westward Hospital today for brachytherapy of the hypopharynx, low dose rate, iodine 125 (I-125) treatment.
14. Charles Medlin, a 31-year-old male, has been diagnosed with a lung tumor and was admitted to Westward Hospital for stereotactic particulate radiosurgery.
15. Brandon Russell, a 37-year-old female, was admitted to Westward Hospital 2 days ago and has been diagnosed with osteosarcoma. Today she receives beam radiation therapy to the femur, photons >10 MeV.

YOU CODE IT! Application

The following exercises provide practice in abstracting physicians' notes and learning to work with documentation from our health care facility, Westward Hospital. These case studies are modeled on real patient encounters. Using the techniques described in this chapter, carefully read through the case studies and determine the most accurate ICD-10-PCS code(s) for each case study.

WESTWARD HOSPITAL
591 Chester Road
Masters, FL 33955

PATIENT: ALTERMANN, AMANDA

DIAGNOSIS: Concussion

REFERRING PHYSICIAN: Jacob Huffman, MD

Pt is a 52-year-old female who presented to the emergency room accompanied by her husband, Ron. Pt is complaining of a severe headache and seeing stars. Her husband said she was standing on a ladder when she fell off, striking her head; she lost consciousness for approximately 3 minutes. Dr. Huffman notes some disorientation, slurred speech, and a delay in response to his questions. Amanda is admitted to the hospital with a concussion. A skull x-ray without contrast and brain MRI without contrast are both performed.

Benjamin Johnston, MD

Determine the most accurate ICD-10-PCS code(s) for the imaging procedure(s).

(continued)

WESTWARD HOSPITAL

591 Chester Road

Masters, FL 33955

RADIOLOGIST REPORT

PATIENT: GRIFFTH, KERRAN

DATE OF ADMISSION: 08/19/26

DATE OF DISCHARGE: 08/23/26

PREOP DIAGNOSIS: Right ureteral obstruction secondary to colon cancer

POSTOP DIAGNOSIS: Right ureteral obstruction secondary to colon cancer

SURGEON: Roger Abernathy, MD

ANESTHESIA: Moderate sedation

Operation:

1. Cystoscopy
2. Right retrograde pyelogram with low Osmolar contrast material
3. Removal and replacement of double-J stent

HISTORY/INDICATIONS: This is a 32-year-old female with a history of colon cancer of the cecum and secondary right ureteral obstruction who had a stent inserted a number of months ago. At this time, she is in the hospital and it is time for a stent change. Consequently, the patient presents for the procedure.

PROCEDURE: The patient was taken to the operating room and there she was given midazolam, 0.5 mg, positioned in the dorsal lithotomy position, and the genitalia scrubbed and prepped with Betadine. Sterile towels and sheets were utilized to drape the patient in the usual fashion. A cystoscope was introduced into the bladder. The ureteral catheter was identified. It was grabbed and removed without any difficulty. Subsequently, the cystoscope was reinserted into the bladder and the right ureteral orifice was identified over a Pollack catheter. A glide wire was inserted into the right collecting system. Some contrast was injected and a hydronephrotic right side was noted. Then, the wire was placed through the Pollack catheter. With the wire in position, over the wire a 7 French 26-cm double-J stent was inserted. Excellent coiling was noted fluoroscopically in the kidney and distally with a cystoscope. The bladder was then drained and again it was inspected prior to removal. There was no evidence of any tumors or lesions in the bladder. The stent was in good position. The cystoscope was removed and the patient was taken to the recovery room awake and in stable condition.

Roger Abernathy, MD

Determine the most accurate ICD-10-PCS code(s) for the pyelogram.

WESTWARD HOSPITAL

591 Chester Road

Masters, FL 33955

RADIOLOGY SUMMARY

PATIENT: LACTANA, LAVINIA

DATE OF ADMISSION: 10/05/26

DATE OF DISCHARGE: 10/17/26

ADMITTING DIAGNOSIS: Bilateral breast asymmetry and ptosis, status post left lumpectomy and radiation therapy for cancer.

(continued)

DISCHARGE DIAGNOSIS: Bilateral breast asymmetry and ptosis, status post left lumpectomy and radiation therapy for cancer.

This 41-year-old single female is status post surgery cleared for bilateral high dose brachytherapy with palladium 103.

Patient tolerated her first treatment and was returned to her room.

Jennell Goren, MD

Determine the most accurate ICD-10-PCS code(s) for brachytherapy.

WESTWARD HOSPITAL

591 Chester Road

Masters, FL 33955

PATIENT: HARRINGTON, ROSA

DATE OF ADMISSION: 11/15/26

DATE OF DISCHARGE: 11/17/26

DIAGNOSIS: Appendicitis

ATTENDING PHYSICIAN: Dennis Beckham, MD

HISTORY OF PRESENT ILLNESS: This is a 39-year-old previously healthy female. She awoke this morning with pain in her abdomen. Her pain continued, periumbilical, and apparently now has traversed to the right lower quadrant. On a 1 to 10 pain scale she states a 7 for pain. She has had some nausea and vomiting. No history of inflammatory bowel disease, colon cancer, abdominal operations, or bleeding. No urinary tract symptomatology.

PAST MEDICAL HISTORY: Noncontributory.

MEDICATIONS: None.

ALLERGIES: None.

SOCIAL HISTORY: No smoking.

FAMILY HISTORY: Unremarkable.

REVIEW OF SYSTEMS: As per ER intake chart.

PHYSICAL EXAMINATION:

HEENT: No scleral icterus.
NECK: Unremarkable.
HEART: No findings.
LUNGS: No findings.
ABDOMEN: Exquisite right lower quadrant tenderness. Positive focal rebound. No masses.
RECTAL: Unremarkable.
EXTREMITIES: Unremarkable.

LABORATORY AND DIAGNOSTIC STUDIES: White blood count is 25, otherwise unremarkable. An ultrasound of the appendix was performed. The patient has clear-cut possible retrocecal appendicitis.

RECOMMENDATIONS/PLAN: The patient has received antibiotics. The patient has consented to a laparoscopic, possible open, appendectomy. She was counseled concerning the benefits and risks of the surgery, including but not limited to bleeding, infection, death, and injury. All questions were answered and she agreed to the procedure. We will place bilateral sequential compression devices and call the operating room to have her scheduled as soon as possible.

Dennis Beckham, MD

Determine the most accurate ICD-10-PCS code(s) for the ultrasonography.

(continued)

WESTWARD HOSPITAL

591 Chester Road

Masters, FL 33955

HISTORY OF PRESENT ILLNESS ADMISSION

PATIENT: WAYFIELD, PORTER

DATE OF ADMISSION: 10/07/26

DATE OF DISCHARGE: 10/09/26

ADMITTING DIAGNOSIS: Cervical sprain C1–C7; lumbar strain L4–L5; multiple subluxation of cervical spine.

ATTENDING PHYSICIAN: Joanne Stafford, MD

This 31-year-old male was admitted after being involved in a two-car MVA 2 weeks ago. He saw his family physician, Dr. Ashley Proctor, after experiencing constant neck pain radiating into the shoulders. Pain medication and rest (no movement) provided temporary relief. Dr. Proctor suggested admission for further evaluation.

In addition to neck pain, Pt states pain radiating across the lower back area beginning approximately 2 hours after the MVA. He states it hurts to move, bend, and walk. Pt denies similar pain in back or neck before.

BP 122/85, P60. After review of patient history questionnaire, PE indicates general appearance is age appropriate with average build and a protective gait. Normal lymph nodes: cervical; axillae; groin. Upper and lower extremities appear normal with the exception of muscle strength in both arms and left leg. Toe-walk exam rates 3 of 5. Limited-to-no ROM with pain C1–C7 and L4–L5. Pt exhibits spinal tenderness: cervical, dorsal, and lumbar. Evidence of edema: cervical and lumbar regions. Muscle spasms evident: scalenes, traps, lat, and paraspinal.

Patient sent to Radiology for x-rays: cervical and lumbar. Radiologic results show multiple subluxations of the cervical vertebrae with pain on movement. Dens and spinous process are intact. No breaks or fractures. Lumbar spine is intact with no breaks or fractures.

JOANNE STAFFORD, MD

Determine the most accurate ICD-10-PCS code(s) for the imaging procedure(s).

38

Physical Rehabilitation and Diagnostic Audiology through New Technology Sections

Key Terms

Audiology
Biofeedback
Detoxification
Psychotherapy
Rehabilitation
Substance Abuse

Learning Outcomes

After completing this chapter, the student should be able to:

LO 38.1 Recognize the details reported from the Physical Rehabilitation and Diagnostic Audiology section.
LO 38.2 Evaluate the details to determine services reported from the Mental Health section.
LO 38.3 Determine the specifics required to accurately report services from the Substance Abuse Treatment section.
LO 38.4 Interpret the documentation to report services from the New Technology section.
LO 38.5 Analyze documentation to report ICD-10-PCS codes from sections F–X.

STOP! Remember, you need to follow along in your ICD-10-PCS code book for an optimal learning experience.

38.1 Reporting Services from the Physical Rehabilitation and Diagnostic Audiology Section

Character Definitions

The meanings for the ***Physical Rehabilitation and Diagnostic Audiology*** section characters are shown in the following table:

Character Position	Character Meaning
1	Section of the ICD-10-PCS book
2	Section qualifier
3	Root type
4	Body system & region
5	Type qualifier
6	Equipment
7	Qualifier

For the most part, these character positions have different meanings than in the other sections you have already learned about.

Character Position 1: Physical Rehabilitation and Diagnostic Audiology Section F

Character Position	Character Meaning
1	Section of the ICD-10-PCS book
2	Section qualifier
3	Root type
4	Body system & region
5	Type qualifier
6	Equipment
7	Qualifier

Procedures reported from the ***Physical Rehabilitation and Diagnostic Audiology*** section begin with the letter **F**.

Character Position 2: Section Qualifier

Character Position	Character Meaning
1	Section of the ICD-10-PCS book
2	Section qualifier
3	Root type
4	Body system & region
5	Type qualifier
6	Equipment
7	Qualifier

There are only two options for the second character:

Rehabilitation . . . Character: **0**

Diagnostic Audiology . . . Character: **1**

Rehabilitation
Health care that is committed to improving, maintaining, or returning physical strength, cognition, and mobility.

Audiology
The study of hearing, balance, and related disorders.

Character Position 3: Root Type

Character Position	Character Meaning
1	Section of the ICD-10-PCS book
2	Section qualifier
3	Root type
4	Body system & region
5	Type qualifier
6	Equipment
7	Qualifier

The root type terms are unique to report procedures in this section.

Under *Rehabilitation*, you will find these third character options:

Speech Assessment . . . Character: **0**

Motor and/or Nerve Function Assessment . . . Character: **1**

Activities of Daily Living Assessment . . . Character: **2**

Speech Treatment . . . Character: **6**

Motor Treatment . . . Character: **7**

Activities of Daily Living Treatment . . . Character: **8**

Hearing Treatment . . . Character: **9**

Cochlear Implant Treatment . . . Character: **B**

Vestibular Treatment . . . Character: **C**

Device Fitting . . . Character: **D**

Caregiver Training . . . Character: **F**

Under *Diagnostic Audiology*, you will find these third character options:

Hearing Assessment . . . Character: **3**

Hearing Aid Assessment . . . Character: **4**

Vestibular Assessment . . . Character: **5**

Character Position 4: Body System & Region

Character Position	Character Meaning
1	Section of the ICD-10-PCS book
2	Section qualifier
3	Root type
4	**Body system & region**
5	Type qualifier
6	Equipment
7	Qualifier

The specific body system being assessed or rehabilitated will be identified in this character position. In some cases, these may not be specified, such as with some speech assessment procedures or caregiver training. These are reported with a body system of **Z** None.

EXAMPLES

Neurological System—Whole Body . . . Character: **3**
Circulatory System—Upper Back/Upper Extremity . . . Character: **5**
Genitourinary System . . . Character: **N**

Character Position 5: Type Qualifier

Character Position	Character Meaning
1	Section of the ICD-10-PCS book
2	Section qualifier
3	Root type
4	Body system & region
5	**Type qualifier**
6	Equipment
7	Qualifier

The character placed in this position will provide additional detail about the root type.

EXAMPLES

Under Root Type **Speech Assessment**, the fifth character may identify

Motor Speech (**B**) or Fluency (**D**)

while under Root Type **Activities of Daily Living**, the fifth character may report

Feeding/Eating (**2**) or Home Management (**4**)

Character Position 6: Equipment

Character Position	Character Meaning
1	Section of the ICD-10-PCS book
2	Section qualifier
3	Root type
4	Body system & region
5	Type qualifier
6	**Equipment**
7	Qualifier

In this character position, you will report any equipment that was used during the assessment or treatment.

EXAMPLES

F06Z9PZ Orofacial myofunctional speech treatment using a computer

F13ZC1Z Hearing assessment pure tone Stenger, with audiometer

Character Position 7: Qualifier

Character Position	Character Meaning
1	Section of the ICD-10-PCS book
2	Section qualifier
3	Root type
4	Body system & region
5	Type qualifier
6	Equipment
7	**Qualifier**

The only option in this position is

None . . . Character: **Z**

LET'S CODE IT! SCENARIO

Elias Garmine, a 67-year-old male, was admitted after having a stroke (CVA). Anita Cohen, a certified physical therapist, is working with him on functional ambulation due to right-side hemiplegia.

Let's Code It!

Let's go through the steps of coding for ICD-10-PCS and determine the code or codes that should be reported for this encounter between Anita Cohen and Elias Garmine.

The documentation states that a certified physical therapist is performing the treatment, so this will lead you to the ***Physical Rehabilitation*** section.

First character: Section: Physical Rehabilitation & Diagnostic Audiology . . . F

Second character: Section Qualifier: Rehabilitation . . . 0

What is the type of treatment, or for what purpose is this being done? The documentation states, "*functional ambulation*," which addresses motor function. Read carefully. This is *motor treatment*, not *assessment*.

Third character: Root Type: Motor Treatment . . . 7

Read the long list of body system/region options. You will note that none of them actually fits this circumstance.

Fourth character: Body Region: None . . . Z

What type of treatment is Anita providing to Elias? The documentation states, "*functional ambulation*."

Fifth character: Type Qualifier: Gait Training/Functional Ambulation . . . 9

Did Anita use any equipment in her work with Elias? None is documented.

Sixth character: Equipment: None . . . Z

There is only one option for the seventh character.

Seventh character: Qualifier: None . . . Z

The ICD-10-PCS code you will report is this:

F07Z9ZZ Gait training/functional ambulation

Good job!

38.2 Reporting Services from the Mental Health Section

Character Definitions

The meanings for the ***Mental Health*** section characters are shown in the following table:

Character Position	Character Meaning
1	Section of the ICD-10-PCS book
2	Body system
3	Root type
4	Type qualifier
5	Qualifier
6	Qualifier
7	Qualifier

Character Position 1: Mental Health Section G

Character Position	Character Meaning
1	**Section of the ICD-10-PCS book**
2	Body system
3	Root type
4	Type qualifier
5	Qualifier
6	Qualifier
7	Qualifier

Procedures reported from the ***Mental Health*** section will begin with the letter **G**.

Character Position 2: Body System

Character Position	Character Meaning
1	Section of the ICD-10-PCS book
2	**Body system**
3	Root type
4	Type qualifier
5	Qualifier
6	Qualifier
7	Qualifier

There is only one option for the second character:

None . . . Character: **Z**

Character Position 3: Root Type

Character Position	Character Meaning
1	Section of the ICD-10-PCS book
2	Body system
3	**Root type**
4	Type qualifier
5	Qualifier
6	Qualifier
7	Qualifier

There are 12 root types used in this section.

Psychotherapy
The treatment of mental and emotional disorder through communication or psychologically rather than medical means.

Psychological Tests: Include developmental, intellectual, psychoeducational, neurobehavioral, cognitive, neuropsychological, personality, and/or behavioral testing . . . Character: **1**

Crisis Intervention: Includes defusing, debriefing, counseling, psychotherapy, and/or coordination of care with other providers or agencies . . . Character: **2**

Medication Management: Analyzing and varying the dosage of medication to find the most efficacious balance, especially when the patient is taking several different pharmaceuticals . . . Character: **3**

Biofeedback
Training to gain voluntary control of automatic bodily functions.

Individual Psychotherapy: Includes behavior, cognitive, interactive, interpersonal, psychoanalysis, psychodynamic, psychophysiological, and/or supportive . . . Character: **5**

Counseling: Exploration of vocational interest, aptitudes, and required adaptive behavior skills to develop and carry out a plan for achieving a successful vocational placement, enhancing work-related adjustment, and/or pursuing viable options in training education or preparation . . . Character: **6**

Family Psychotherapy: Remediation of emotional or behavioral problems presented by one or more family members when psychotherapy with more than one family member is indicated . . . Character: **7**

Electroconvulsive Therapy: Includes appropriate sedation and other preparation of the individual . . . Character: **B**

Biofeedback: Includes electroencephalogram (EEG), blood pressure, skin temperature, or peripheral blood flow, electrocardiogram (ECG), electrooculogram, electromyogram (EMG), respirometry or capnometry, galvanic skin response (GSR) or electrodermal response (EDR), perineometry to monitor and regulate bowel or bladder activity and electrogastrogram to monitor and regulate gastric motility . . . Character: **C**

Hypnosis: Induction of a state of heightened suggestibility by auditory, visual, and tactile techniques to elicit an emotional or behavioral response . . . Character: **F**

Narcosynthesis: Administration of intravenous barbiturates in order to release suppressed or repressed thoughts . . . Character: **G**

Group Psychotherapy: Treatment of two or more individuals with a mental health disorder by behavioral, cognitive, psychoanalytic, psychodynamic, or psychophysiological means to improve functioning or well-being . . . Character: **H**

Light Therapy: Application of specialized light treatments to improve functioning or well-being . . . Character: **J**

Character Position 4: Type Qualifier

Character Position	Character Meaning
1	Section of the ICD-10-PCS book
2	Body system
3	Root type
4	**Type qualifier**
5	Qualifier
6	Qualifier
7	Qualifier

This character will explain whether the procedure was educational or vocational, providing more detail about the encounter. The descriptors presenting these additional details will be represented by the same characters, but they change by the root type.

EXAMPLES

Developmental . . . Character: **0**, under Psychological Tests
Interactive . . . Character: **0**, under Individual Psychotherapy
Educational . . . Character: **0**, under Counseling
Unilateral-Single Seizure . . . Character: **0**, under Electroconvulsive Therapy

Character Position 5: Qualifier

Character Position	Character Meaning
1	Section of the ICD-10-PCS book
2	Body system
3	Root type
4	Type qualifier
5	**Qualifier**
6	Qualifier
7	Qualifier

The only option in this position is

None . . . Character: **Z**

Character Position 6: Qualifier

Character Position	Character Meaning
1	Section of the ICD-10-PCS book
2	Body system
3	Root type
4	Type qualifier
5	Qualifier
6	**Qualifier**
7	Qualifier

The only option in this position is

None . . . Character: **Z**

Character Position 7: Qualifier

Character Position	Character Meaning
1	Section of the ICD-10-PCS book
2	Body system
3	Root type
4	Type qualifier
5	Qualifier
6	Qualifier
7	**Qualifier**

The only option in this position is

None . . . Character: **Z**

ICD-10-PCS

LET'S CODE IT! SCENARIO

While in the hospital for repair of a stomach ulcer, Carlos Weiner, a 53-year-old male, was behaving oddly. Dr. Albessi performed some neuropsychological testing.

(continued)

Let's Code It!

Let's go through the steps of coding for ICD-10-PCS and determine the code or codes that should be reported for this encounter between Dr. Albessi and Carlos Weiner.

Psychological testing brings us to the ***Mental Health*** section.

First character: Section: Mental Health . . . G

There is only one option for the body region in this section.

Second character: Body Region: None . . . Z

What was done? The documentation states, "*neuropsychological testing*."

Third character: Root Type: Psychological Tests . . . 1

Specifically . . .

Fourth character: Type Qualifier: Neuropsychological . . . 3

There are no more details to be reported with the last three characters.

Fifth character: Qualifier: None . . . Z

Sixth character: Qualifier: None . . . Z

Seventh character: Qualifier: None . . . Z

The ICD-10-PCS code you will report is

GZ13ZZZ Neuropsychological testing

Good job!

38.3 Reporting from the Substance Abuse Treatment Section

Character Definitions

The meanings for the ***Substance Abuse*** section characters are shown in the following table:

Character Position	Character Meaning
1	Section of the ICD-10-PCS book
2	Body systems
3	Root type
4	Type qualifier
5	Qualifier
6	Qualifier
7	Qualifier

Character Position 1: Substance Abuse Section H

Character Position	Character Meaning
1	**Section of the ICD-10-PCS book**
2	Body systems
3	Root type
4	Type qualifier

(continued)

Character Position	Character Meaning
5	Qualifier
6	Qualifier
7	Qualifier

Procedures reported from the **Substance Abuse** *Treatment* section will all begin with the letter **H**.

> **Substance Abuse**
> Regular consumption of a substance with manifestations.

Character Position 2: Body Systems

Character Position	Character Meaning
1	Section of the ICD-10-PCS book
2	**Body systems**
3	Root type
4	Type qualifier
5	Qualifier
6	Qualifier
7	Qualifier

There is only one option for the second character:

None . . . Character: **Z**

Character Position 3: Root Type

Character Position	Character Meaning
1	Section of the ICD-10-PCS book
2	Body systems
3	**Root type**
4	Type qualifier
5	Qualifier
6	Qualifier
7	Qualifier

There are seven root operation terms used to report procedures in this section:

> **Detoxification**
> The process of removing toxic substances or qualities.

Detoxification Services: Not a treatment modality but helps the patient stabilize physically and psychologically until the body becomes free of drugs and the effects of alcohol . . . Character: **2**

Individual Counseling: Comprising several techniques, which apply various strategies to address drug addiction . . . Character: **3**

Group Counseling: Provides structured group counseling sessions and healing power through the connection with others . . . Character: **4**

Individual Psychotherapy: Treatment of an individual with addictive behavior by behavioral, cognitive, psychoanalytic, psychodynamic, or psychophysiological means . . . Character: **5**

Family Counseling: Provides support and education for family members of addicted individuals. Family member participation seen as critical to substance abuse treatment . . . Character: **6**

Medication Management: Monitoring or adjusting the use of replacement medications for the treatment of addiction . . . Character: **8**

Pharmacotherapy: The use of replacement medications for the treatment of addiction . . . Character: **9**

Character Position 4: Type Qualifier

Character Position	Character Meaning
1	Section of the ICD-10-PCS book
2	Body systems
3	Root type
4	**Type qualifier**
5	Qualifier
6	Qualifier
7	Qualifier

This character will add detail to the description of the root type.

EXAMPLES

12-Step . . . Character: **3**, under Individual Counseling
Interactive . . . Character: **5**, under Individual Psychotherapy
Nicotine Replacement . . . Character: **0**, under Pharmacotherapy

Character Position 5: Qualifier

Character Position	Character Meaning
1	Section of the ICD-10-PCS book
2	Body systems
3	Root type
4	Type qualifier
5	**Qualifier**
6	Qualifier
7	Qualifier

In this character position, the only option is

None . . . Character: **Z**

Character Position 6: Qualifier

Character Position	Character Meaning
1	Section of the ICD-10-PCS book
2	Body systems
3	Root type
4	Type qualifier
5	Qualifier
6	**Qualifier**
7	Qualifier

In this character position, the only option is

None . . . Character: **Z**

Character Position 7: Qualifier

Character Position	Character Meaning
1	Section of the ICD-10-PCS book
2	Body systems
3	Root type
4	Type qualifier
5	Qualifier
6	Qualifier
7	**Qualifier**

In this character position, the only option is

None . . . Character: **Z**

LET'S CODE IT! SCENARIO

Harrison Argan has been in the New Horizons Substance Abuse Rehabilitation Hospital for 2 weeks now. Today, Dr. Lerner meets with Harrison for medication management with his methadone maintenance treatment plan.

Let's Code It!

Let's go through the steps of coding for ICD-10-PCS and determine the code or codes that should be reported for this encounter between Dr. Lerner and Harrison Argan.

For a patient that has been admitted to a Substance Abuse Rehabilitation Hospital, the section choice is clear.

First character: Section: Substance Abuse . . . H

There is only one option for the second character.

Second character: Body System: None . . . Z

What was Dr. Lerner doing for Harrison at this session? The documentation states, "*for medication management.*"

Third character: Root Type: Medication Management . . . 8

What specifics were focused on? The documentation states, "*methadone maintenance.*"

Fourth character: Type Qualifier: Methadone Maintenance . . . 1

There are no additional details to be reported with the last three characters.

Fifth character: Qualifier: None . . . Z

Sixth character: Qualifier: None . . . Z

Seventh character: Qualifier: None . . . Z

The ICD-10-PCS code you will report is

HZ81ZZZ **Medication management for methadone maintenance**

Good job!

38.4 Reporting from the New Technology Section

Character Definitions

As you learned earlier, every ICD-10-PCS code has seven characters, and each character position has a meaning. While all of these codes have the same number of characters, each section uses each character position differently. So, let's review the meanings for the ***New Technology*** section characters:

Character Position	Character Meaning
1	Section of the ICD-10-PCS book
2	Body system being treated
3	Root operation term
4	Body part (specific anatomical site)
5	Approach used by physician
6	Device/Substance/Technology
7	Qualifier, if applicable

You might have noticed that these are different meanings from those used in the ***Medical and Surgical*** and other sections.

GUIDANCE CONNECTION

Read the ICD-10-PCS Official Guidelines for Coding and Reporting, **New Technology Section Guidelines (Section X)**, subsection **D. New Technology Section**, subhead **General guidelines**, paragraph **D1**.

Character Position 1: New Technology Section X

Character Position	Character Meaning
1	**Section of the ICD-10-PCS book**
2	Body system being treated
3	Root operation term
4	Body part (specific anatomical site)
5	Approach used by physician
6	Device/Substance/Technology
7	Qualifier

The codes reported from the ***New Technology*** section (beginning with the character **X**) are used to identify a specific procedure. They are not to be used to add detail or information about a procedure reported from another section, nor do they require any additional codes to supplement their meaning. They are complete in and of themselves to explain what was provided to the patient.

Character Position 2: Body System Being Treated

Character Position	Character Meaning
1	Section of the ICD-10-PCS book
2	**Body system being treated**
3	Root operation term
4	Body part (specific anatomical site)

(continued)

Character Position	Character Meaning
5	Approach used by physician
6	Device/Substance/Technology
7	Qualifier

Currently, in this section, the body systems from which to choose are:

Nervous System . . . Character: **0**

Cardiovascular System . . . Character: **2**

Gastrointestinal System . . . Character: **D**

Hepatobiliary System and Pancreas . . . Character: **F**

Skin, Subcutaneous Tissue, Fascia, and Breast . . . Character: **H**

Muscles, Tendons, Bursae, and Ligaments . . . Character: **K**

Bones . . . Character: **N**

Joints . . . Character: **R**

Urinary System . . . Character: **T**

Anatomical Regions . . . Character: **W**

Physiological Systems . . . Character: **X**

Extracorporeal . . . Character: **Y**

Character Position 3: Root Operation

Character Position	Character Meaning
1	Section of the ICD-10-PCS book
2	Body system being treated
3	**Root operation term**
4	Body part (specific anatomical site)
5	Approach used by physician
6	Device/Substance/Technology
7	Qualifier

The options are limited for the choice of this character, as well:

Assistance: Taking over a portion of a physiological function by extracorporeal means . . . character: **A**

Bypass: Altering the route of passage of the contents of a tubular body part . . . Character **K**

Destruction: Physical eradication of all or a portion of a body part by the direct use of energy, force, or a destructive agent . . . Character: **5**

Dilation: Expanding an orifice or the lumen of a tubular body part . . . Character: **7**

Division: Cutting into a body part, without draining fluids and/or gases from the body part, in order to separate or transect a body part ... Character 8

Extirpation: A procedure where the physician is cutting out or taking out solid matter from a body part . . . character: **C**

Fusion: Joining together portions of an articular body part rendering the articular body part immobile . . . character: **G**

Irrigation: Putting in or on a cleaning substance . . . Character **P**

Insertion: Putting in a nonbiological appliance that monitors, assists, performs, or prevents a physiological function but does not physically take the place of a body part...Character **H**

Inspection: Visually and/or manually exploring a body part . . . Character **J**

Introduction: The process of putting in, or on, a substance for therapeutic, diagnostic, nutritional, physiological, or prophylactic purposes. Blood and blood products are excluded . . . character: **0**

Measurement: Determining the level of a physiological or physical function at a point in time . . . Character: **E**

Monitoring: Monitoring is described in ICD-10-PCS as the determination, repeatedly over a period of time, of the level(s) of a physiological or a physical function . . . character: **2**

Other Procedures: Methodologies which attempt to remediate or cure a disorder or disease... Character **Z**

Replacement: Putting in or on biological or synthetic material that physically takes the place and/or function of all or a portion of a body part . . . character: **R**

Reposition: Moving to its normal location, or other suitable location, all or a portion of a body part . . . character: **S**

Supplement: Putting in or on biological or synthetic material that physically reinforces and/or augments the function of a portion of a body part ...Character **U**

Transfusion: Putting in blood or blood products... Character **1**

Restriction: Partially closing an orifice or the lumen of a tubular body part . . . Character **V**

Character Position 4: Body Part

Character Position	Character Meaning
1	Section of the ICD-10-PCS book
2	Body system being treated
3	Root operation term
4	**Body part (specific anatomical site)**
5	Approach used by physician
6	Device/Substance/Technology
7	Qualifier

The options for the body part that is the objective of this procedure are also limited in number:

Cardiovascular System

Coronary Artery, One Artery . . . Character: **0**

Coronary Artery, Two Arteries . . . Character: **1**

Coronary Artery, Three Arteries . . . Character: **2**

Coronary Artery, Four or More Arteries . . . Character: **3**

Innominate Artery and Left Common Carotid Artery . . . Character: **5**

Aortic Valve . . . Character: **F**

Skin, Subcutaneous Tissue, Fascia, and Breast

Skin . . . Character: **P**

Muscles, Tendons, Bursae, and Ligaments

Muscle . . . Character: **2**

Bones

Lumbar Vertebra . . . Character: **0**

Cervical Vertebra . . . Character: **3**

Thoracic Vertebra . . . Character: **4**

Joints

Knee Joint, Right . . . Character: **G**

Knee Joint, Left . . . Character: **H**

Occipital-Cervical Joint . . . Character: **0**

Cervical Vertebral Joint . . . Character: **1**

Cervical Vertebral Joints, 2 or more . . . Character: **2**

Cervicothoracic Vertebral Joint . . . Character: **4**

Thoracic Vertebral Joint . . . Character: **6**

Thoracic Vertebral Joints, 2 to 7 . . . Character: **7**

Thoracic Vertebral Joints, 8 or more . . . Character: **8**

Thoracolumbar Vertebral Joint . . . Character: **A**

Lumbar Vertebral Joint . . . Character: **B**

Lumbar Vertebral Joints, 2 or more . . . Character: **C**

Lumbosacral Joint . . . Character: **D**

Male Reproductive System

Prostate . . . Character: **0**

Anatomical Regions

Peripheral Vein . . . Character: **3**

Central Vein . . . Character: **4**

Mouth and Pharynx . . . Character: **D**

Extracorporeal

Vein Graft . . . Character: **4**

Character Position 5: Approach

Character Position	Character Meaning
1	Section of the ICD-10-PCS book
2	Body system being treated
3	Root operation term
4	Body part (specific anatomical site)
5	Approach used by physician
6	Device/Substance/Technology
7	Qualifier

This position's character options should be familiar to you, at this point.

Open: An open approach is one that uses cutting through the skin or mucous membrane and any other body layers necessary to expose the site of the procedure . . . Character: **0**

Percutaneous: A percutaneous approach is described by ICD-10-PCS as entry, by puncture or minor incision, of instrumentation through the skin or mucous membrane and any other body layers necessary to reach the site of the procedure . . . Character: **3**

Percutaneous Endoscopic: Entry, by puncture or minor incision, of instrumentation through the skin or mucous membrane and any other body layers necessary to reach and visualize the site of the procedure . . . Character: **4**

Via Natural or Artificial Opening: Entry of instrumentation through a natural or artificial external opening to reach the site of the procedure . . . Character: **7**

Via Natural or Artificial Opening Endoscopic: Entry of instrumentation through a natural or artificial external opening to reach the site of the procedure . . . Character: **8**

External: Procedures performed directly on the skin or mucous membrane and procedures performed indirectly by the application of external force through the skin or mucous membrane . . . Character: **X**

Character Position 6: Device/Substance/Technology

Character Position	Character Meaning
1	Section of the ICD-10-PCS book
2	Body system being treated
3	Root operation term
4	Body part (specific anatomical site)
5	Approach used by physician
6	Device/Substance/Technology
7	Qualifier

The devices described in this column's options are new and different from those most of us have encountered. They are listed by the body system being treated.

Cardiovascular System

Cerebral Embolic Filtration, Dual Filter: Cerebral embolic dual-filtration units are designed to protect the brain from injury caused by embolic debris, specifically in patients diagnosed with aortic stenosis having a transcatheter aortic valve replacement (TAVR) procedure . . . Character: **1**

Orbital Atherectomy Technology: Orbital atherectomy is used to treat patients with severely calcified coronary lesions as well as symptomatic peripheral arterial disease (PAD) within the major and branch arteries of the leg. The FDA also cleared the orbital atherectomy system (OAS) to treat stenosis in synthetic arteriovenous shunts that are often used to provide vascular access for dialysis patients . . . Character: **6**

Zooplastic Tissue, Rapid Deployment Technique: The use of zooplastic tissue with rapid deployment technique on an aortic valve can now be reported . . . Character: **3**

Skin, Subcutaneous Tissue, Fascia, and Breast

Skin Substitute, Porcine Liver Derived: The use of porcine liver skin substitute can now be reported accurately . . . Character: **L**

Muscles, Tendons, Bursae, and Ligaments

Concentrated Bone Marrow Aspirate: . . . Character: **0**

Bones

Magnetically Controlled Growth Rod(s): Magnetically controlled growth rods are new innovations, especially for children requiring spinal surgery for scoliosis. Instead of sequential surgical procedures to adjust the rods as children grow, the surgeon can use a magnetic device, in the office, to lengthen the rods, in just minutes . . . Character: **3**

Joints

Intraoperative Knee Replacement Sensor: Intraoperative sensors are a disposable tibial insert used to aid orthopedic surgeons in placing prosthetic joint components during knee replacement surgery . . . Character: **2**

Interbody Fusion Device, Nanotextured Surface: The fusion of vertebral joints is not new, but the use of the nanotextured surface is now reported with a code built from this new table . . . Character: **9**

Interbody Fusion Device, Radiolucent Porous: . . . Character: **F**

Male Reproductive System

Robotic Waterjet Ablation: This is a new method, used as an alternative to TURP (transurethral resection of the prostate) as a treatment for BPH (benign prostate hyperplasia) . . . Character: **A**

Anatomical Regions

Ceftazidime-Avibactam Anti-infective: This is provided for the treatment of adult patients with complicated intra-abdominal infections and complicated urinary tract infections including pyelonephritis caused by designated susceptible bacteria, including certain *Enterobacteriaceae* and *Pseudomonas aeruginosa* . . . Character: **2**

Idarucizumab, Dabigatran Reversal Agent: Idarucizumab is an antibody fragment that was developed to reverse the anticoagulant effects of dabigatran (Pradaxa) . . . Character: **3**

Isavuconazole Anti-infective: This is used for the treatment of invasive aspergillosis and treatment of invasive mucormycosis in patients 18 years and older . . . Character: **4**

Blinatumomab Antineoplastic Immunotherapy: This is used for the treatment of patients with Philadelphia chromosome-negative relapsed or refractory B-cell precursor acute lymphoblastic leukemia . . . Character: **5**

Andexanet Alfa, Factor Xa Inhibitor Reversal Agent: Andexanet Alfa is a new drug that reverses the blood-thinning reactions caused by Factor Xa inhibitors (an anticoagulant that directly works on Factor X of the coagulation cascade in the blood), when a Factor Xa has been administered in the wrong dosage or in error . . . Character: **7**

Uridine Triacetate: Uridine triacetate is a new drug that, when taken orally, combats the adverse effects of chemotherapy overdoses, as well as helps those who manifest life-threatening toxicities within four days of having chemotherapy administered. Currently, this treatment is effective when fluorouracil or capecitabine is the drug causing this adverse effect . . . Character: **8**

Defibrotide Sodium Anticoagulant: Defibrotide Sodium anticoagulant is administered as a therapeutic treatment for patients diagnosed with hepatic veno-occlusive disease (VOD) after having a hematopoietic stem cell transplantation (HSCT) [also known as a bone marrow transplant] . . . Character: **9**

Bezlotoxumab Monoclonal Antibody: Bezlotoxumab is a version of human monoclonal antibody designed to neutralize the toxin produced by the *C. diff* bacteria that is known to possibly damage the patient's intestinal walls . . . Character: **A**

Cytarabine and Daunorubicin Liposome Antineoplastic: Liposomal daunorubicin may be helpful in overcoming multidrug resistance in high-risk acute leukemia . . . Character: **B**

Engineered Autologous Chimeric Antigen Receptor T-cell Immunotherapy: Chimeric antigen receptor (CAR) therapy can be compared to autologous bone marrow transplantation. T cells are collected by apheresis, and then expanded and genetically modified . . . Character: **C**

Other New Technology Therapeutic Substance: . . . Character: **F**

Plazomicin Anti-infective: This is an aminoglycoside antibacterial for the treatment of complicated urinary tract infections (UTI) . . . Character: **G**

Synthetic Human Angiotensin II: A solution administered to patients with sepsis or distributive shock to support increase of blood pressure . . . Character: **H**

Extracorporeal

Endothelial Damage Inhibitor: Endothelial dysfunction describes manifestations of cardiovascular risk including diminished production and reduced availability of nitric oxide as well as the possible imbalance in the relative contribution of endothelium-derived relaxing and contracting factors . . . Character: **8**

Character Position 7: Qualifier

Character Position	Character Meaning
1	Section of the ICD-10-PCS book
2	Body system being treated
3	Root operation term
4	Body part (specific anatomical site)
5	Approach used by physician
6	Device/Substance/Technology
7	**Qualifier**

Each year, this character changes for the new codes added to this specific section. So, for 2025, the seventh character options are

New Technology Group 1 . . . Character: **1**

New Technology Group 2 . . . Character: **2**

New Technology Group 3 . . . Character: **3**

New Technology Group 4 . . . Character: **4**

New Technology Group 5 . . . Character: **5**

New Technology Group 6 . . . Character: **6**

New Technology Group 7 . . . Character: **7**

New Technology Group 8 . . . Character: **8**

New Technology Group 9 . . . Character: **9**

New Technology Group 10 . . . Character: **A**

New Technology Group 11 . . . Character: **B**

This will continue each year, as new details are placed into the code set.

LET'S CODE IT! SCENARIO

Darla Wellington, 61-year-old female, was diagnosed with malignant hypertension, resistant to pharmaceutical control with seven different antihypertensive drugs. Dr. Malvern performed a renal sympathetic nerve ablation, which was done percutaneously, reducing risk and Darla's length of stay in the hospital.

(continued)

Let's Code It!

Let's go through the steps of coding for ICD-10-PCS and determine the code or codes that should be reported for the procedure that was performed.

In the Alphabetic Index, look up

Destruction > sympathetic nerve(s), ultrasound > ablation X051329

Turn to the ICD-10-PCS Table beginning X05

First character: Section: New Technology . . . X

The notes state the patient is having synpathetic nerves treated, which are part of the nervous system.

Second character: Body System: Nervous System . . . 0

The ablation of the renal nerves fits the root operational term of destruction

Third character: Root Operation: Destruction . . . 5

The body part being ablated is stated as the renal sympathetic nerve(s).

Fourth character: Body Part: Renal sympathetic nerve(s) . . . 1

The notes state the procedure was performed percutaneously.

Fifth character: Approach: Percutaneous . . . 3

The notes state that ultrasound ablation was used.

Sixth character: Device: ultrasound ablation . . . 2
Seventh character: Qualifier: New Technology Group 9 . . . 9

The ICD-10-PCS code you will report is this:

X051329 **Ultrasound ablation of renal sympathetic nerve(s), percutaneously**

New Technology Codes for COVID-19

Since 2024, ICD-10-PCS procedure codes describe the introduction or infusion of both COVID-19 treatments and vaccinations, including monoclonal antibodies, provided to inpatients.

Details on submitting claims to Medicare for the administration of COVID-19 vaccine to an inpatient, current information can be found at: https://www.cms.gov/medicare/payment/covid-19/medicare-billing-covid-19-vaccine-shot-administration. It is important to check with each individual third-party payer for their own directions.

As you read the individual code descriptions, you can the anatomical location of introduction, as well as the specific substance.

38.5 Sections F–X: Putting It All Together

LET'S CODE IT! SCENARIO

PATIENT NAME: Alfredo Sugerman

DATE OF EVALUATION: 11/16/2026

ATTENDING PHYSICIAN: Oscar Clarice, MD

HISTORY OF PRESENT ILLNESS: This is a 71-year-old male with a history of end-stage COPD, previous CVA, seizure disorder, chronic headaches, and chronic pain syndrome who was admitted to the hospital yesterday for increasing pain all over the body. He has also expressed feelings of severe depression, and a psychiatric consultation was requested for evaluation of

(continued)

the same. The patient reports that he had been going through a lot for the past few months. He was referring to his medical problems, chronic obstructive pulmonary disease, especially the pain all over the body for which no clear organic reason has been found so far. He says that he is in pain all the time, constantly. He is tired of it. He cannot take care of himself, and he was recently in a nursing home but had a bad experience over there. He does not want to go back to the nursing home. He was living with a woman for 15 years, but she is not able to take care of him. He was very helpless and hopeless, and he voices passive death wishes but denies any active intentions. He says that he will never do that to himself. Patient admits to having insomnia and extremely depressed crying episodes and reports very poor energy level, motivation, loss of interest, and feeling sad and unhappy all the time. He had some depression symptoms in the past, related to the medical problems, and was placed on Lexapro and Seroquel for sleep for the past few weeks, but it is not helping. Seroquel helped for his sleep, but he does not want this medication as he knows this is an antipsychotic. He denies any delusions or hallucinations.

PAST PSYCHIATRIC HISTORY: No history of any psychiatric illness or psychiatric hospitalization or any suicidal attempts in the past.

CURRENT MEDICATIONS: On admission, Protonix, Synthroid, Nitro-Dur patches, Tenormin 25 mg once a day, Ditropan, Atrovent, Nasonex, multivitamins, Os-Cal, Bumex, Imdur, Micro-K, Lexapro 10 mg daily, magnesium oxide, Klonopin 0.25 mg every 12 hours, Seroquel 100 mg nightly, Phenergan p.r.n., and Pulmicort inhaler.

ALLERGIES: Nonsteroidal anti-inflammatory drugs and sulfa drugs.

PSYCHIATRIC MENTAL STATUS EXAMINATION: The patient is a thinly built male who appears to be in moderate distress from pain. He is generally cooperative and pleasant; he shows significant psychomotor retardation but no agitation. He speaks in a very low volume voice. He is alert and oriented in all three spheres. Memory grossly intact in all modalities. Speech is coherent. Mood is depressed, tearful, constricted affect. No evidence of any overt psychosis or hypomania. He does have passive death wishes; however, he denies any active suicidal intentions or thoughts. Insight and judgment questionable. Intellectual abilities in average normal range.

IMPRESSIONS: Neurobehavioral and cognitive status tests along with my observations lead to these impressions:

Axis I: Major depression, single episode, moderate to severe with anxiety component.

Axis II: Deferred.

Axis III: Chronic pain syndrome, narcotic dependence, chronic obstructive pulmonary disease, status post cerebrovascular accident, and seizure disorder.

RECOMMENDATIONS: The patient does not appear to be responding to his current psychotropic medications, so we will discontinue the Lexapro and Seroquel. Instead, we will use Effexor XR 37.5 mg once a.m. and also Desyrel 50 mg nightly. We will continue to monitor the patient closely.

Let's Code It!

Dr. Clarice performed neurobehavioral and cognitive status psychological tests as a part of his evaluation of Mr. Sugerman. Let's work our way through the ***Mental Health*** section . . . because this was a psychological evaluation.

First character: Section: Mental Health . . . G
Second character: System: None . . . Z

What did Dr. Clarice actually do? The documentation states, "*Psychiatric mental status examination.*"

Third character: Root Operation: Psychological Tests . . . 1

Review the options for the fourth character in Table GZ1. The documentation states, "*Neurobehavioral and cognitive status tests.*"

Fourth character: Type Qualifier: Neurobehavioral and Cognitive Status . . . 4
Fifth character: Qualifier: None . . . Z
Sixth character: Qualifier: None . . . Z
Seventh character: Qualifier: None . . . Z

Now, you can report this ICD-10-PCS code with confidence:

GZ14ZZZ Neurobehavioral and cognitive status psychological tests

LET'S CODE IT! SCENARIO

PATIENT: Francis Fredericks

The patient had been seen by this department for a clinical swallowing evaluation. At that time, he had reported 3 to 4 months of coughing with liquids, approximately one time per week. He had a barium swallow, which showed one episode of aspiration with appropriate cough response. Given the patient's complaints of coughing with thin liquids and possible reflux-related symptoms, an objective swallowing evaluation was recommended. However, the patient chose not to follow up for further objective testing at that time.

Admitted today for left side weakness, he is reporting that dysphagia has persisted, and now he feels as though he can cough or choke several times a day with either liquids or solids. He is on a regular diet. He takes his pills with water without difficulty. He has a reported 5- to 10-pound weight loss over the past several months that has been unexplained. His physician has asked him to gain some weight to improve his nutritional status. He has no recent history of pneumonia. The patient does complain of feeling as though he has sluggish passage of his meals and sometimes this will cause him to stop eating early. He has a feeling of increased mucus with frequent throat clearing throughout the day, and he complains of frequent heartburn. He is not on any proton pump inhibitor regimen at this time.

PAST MEDICAL HISTORY: Coronary artery disease requiring LAD stent placement, hypertension, hyperlipidemia, asymptomatic right carotid stenosis, chronic anemia due to renal disease, chronic renal insufficiency that is stable.

CLINICAL OBSERVATIONS: I am performing this swallow dysfunction study at the request of Dr. King. He uses a walker due to knee trouble and the weakness, but he is brought to our office by an orderly in a wheelchair. He is fully alert and oriented, slightly hard of hearing. He is able to provide a comprehensive history. Good speech intelligibility. Vocal quality is slightly raspy, although otherwise within normal limits for age and gender.

ORAL PERIPHERAL EXAM: The patient has naturally present dentition, in poor condition. There is bilateral palatal elevation, good lingual and labial strength and range of motion, and good ability to maintain intraoral pressure. Cough is strong and unproductive. There is good hyolaryngeal elevation and excursion to palpation.

SWALLOWING EVALUATION: Administered p.o. trials of ice chips, thin puree, and particulate solid.

ORAL PHASE: The patient is able to self-feed appropriately. He has good bolus containment and timely anterior to posterior transit with mildly delayed trigger of pharyngeal swallow overall. Question premature spillage with multiple sips of thin liquids.

PHARYNGEAL PHASE: Audible and question slightly discoordinated swallowing pattern for multiple sips of thin liquids. One swallow required for single sips of thin, puree, and particulate solids. No overt clinical signs or symptoms of aspiration after any p.o. trial, although the patient reports that he had slight difficulty with the initial sip of water, feeling like it might head down the wrong pipe.

SUMMARY AND IMPRESSION: The patient is an 87-year-old male with a several-year history of reported dysphagia to solids and liquids. This can happen several times per day. Clinically, he does not show significant overt clinical signs of aspiration, although question discoordinated swallowing pattern for thin liquids, especially when given larger quantities. This is likely consistent with the one incidence of symptomatic aspiration on a barium swallow in the past. The patient also complains of multiple symptoms that appear consistent with laryngopharyngeal reflux, and these include increased mucus, throat clearing, and globus sensation. He reports frequent heartburn and sensation of slow esophageal passage. At this time, would recommend objective testing to further evaluate oropharyngeal swallowing mechanism to determine if coordination of swallowing pattern has been affected over time. Further differential diagnosis would be considerable reflux in current complaints. The patient may benefit from a proton pump inhibitor regimen if deemed appropriate by his physicians. At today's session, discussed aspiration precautions, especially given that the patient self-reported drinks multiple sips at a time. In addition, reflux precautions were recommended, including sitting upright 90 degrees with all p.o. and for 1 hour after meals. The patient was also counseled to monitor his nutritional intake. If he is indeed shortening meals due to sensation of sluggish passage, would recommend multiple smaller meals a day rather than three large ones to allow for adequate nutritional intake. The patient understands all given recommendations and is in agreement for a follow-up with an objective swallowing test.

RECOMMENDATIONS:

1. Regular diet with thin liquids.
2. Medications one at a time with water.
3. Further objective testing via modified barium swallow.
4. Upright 90 degrees with all p.o. and for 1 hour after meals.
5. Decrease bolus size and rate of presentation.
6. Single bites and single sips.

(continued)

7. Consideration of proton pump inhibitor regimen if reflux is deemed by the patient's physicians to be playing a role in the patient's current symptoms.
8. Further recommendations will be made pending outcome of objective study.

Gail Robbins

Speech-Language Pathologist

Let's Code It!

This assessment contains a speech evaluation and a swallow study. Look in the ICD-10-PCS Alphabetic Index; there is no listing for *swallow* or *swallow study*. Let's try this:

Speech Assessment F00

At least it is a place to start, so turn to the F00 Table:

First character: Section: Physical Rehabilitation and Diagnostic Audiology . . . F

This makes sense. The category of speech and swallow studies is considered part of *physical rehabilitation*.

Second character: System: Rehabilitation . . . 0
Third character: Root Operation: Speech Assessment . . . 0

You may be thinking that this cannot be correct because this was really a swallow study. That's good thinking, but let's continue to review the options in this Table before we go looking elsewhere.

Fourth character: Body System/Region: None . . . Z

Read carefully all of the options for the fifth character. Bedside Swallowing and Oral Function sounds close, except the documentation states, "*he is brought to our office by an orderly in a wheelchair.*" This tells us this was not done bedside. The next row has a good possibility that works:

Fifth character: Type Qualifier: Instrumental Swallowing and Oral Function . . . J

Review the options for the sixth character. This is straightforward.

Sixth character: Equipment: Swallowing . . . W
Seventh character: Qualifier: None . . . Z

When we take this coding process one step at a time, it is not as confusing as one might perceive. You can now put this all together and, with confidence, report this code:

F00ZJWZ Instrumental swallowing and oral function assessment

LET'S CODE IT! SCENARIO

George is a 19-year-old male, self-referred for inpatient treatment due to drug and alcohol abuse. He is currently unemployed and homeless, and has charges pending due to a number of "bounced" checks written over the past several months. George reports that both of his parents were drug addicts, and he experienced physical, sexual, and emotional abuse throughout childhood at their hands. His father died of liver disease at the age of 37.

George also reports that, at the age of 12, he was kicked out of his family's home because his father suspected that he was gay. Although they live in the same town, he has not had any contact with either parent for 7 years. George describes his relationship with his younger sister as "fair." He is not presently involved in a steady relationship but does have a network of friends in the local gay community with whom he has been staying off and on. At the time that he left home, George survived by becoming involved in sexual relationships with older men, many of whom were also abusive. He has had numerous sexual partners (both male and female) over the past 7 years, has traded sex for drugs and money, has had sex under the influence of drugs and alcohol, and has been made to have sex against his will. George identifies himself as bisexual, not gay.

George first used alcohol at age 11, when he had his first sexual encounter with a man. He began using other drugs, including inhalants and marijuana, by age 16 and amphetamines and cocaine by age 17. At 18, 3 months prior to entering treatment, he began using crack.

(continued)

This first individual counseling session was focused on this basic, interpersonal foundation to enable us to establish an efficacious treatment plan. George is strong in his desire to get clean, and I have assured him that we can help him here.

Let's Code It!

George has admitted himself into a substance abuse inpatient treatment program, and this is documentation of his first individual counseling session. Turn to the ***Substance Abuse Treatment*** section and let's build an ICD-10-PCS code:

First character: Section: Substance Abuse Treatment . . . H

Second character: System: None . . . Z

Third character: Root Operation: Individual Counseling . . . 3

Fourth character: Type Qualifier: Interpersonal . . . 4

Fifth character: Qualifier: None . . . Z

Sixth character: Qualifier: None . . . Z

Seventh character: Qualifier: None . . . Z

Now, put it all together and, with confidence, report this code:

HZ34ZZZ **Interpersonal-based individual counseling for substance abuse treatment**

Chapter Summary

This chapter has given you the opportunity to walk through the ***Physical Rehabilitation and Diagnostic Audiology*** (F), ***Mental Health*** (G), ***Substance Abuse Treatment*** (H), and ***New Technology*** (X) sections of ICD-10-PCS. You have seen how each character position is important to reporting all of the pertinent details of a procedure, service, or treatment. You have learned that, in each section, the same character can have a different meaning. However, you always have the Tables there to provide the options and their meanings to build the accurate code.

CODING BITES

More Information:

Physical Medicine and Rehabilitiation

https://medlineplus.gov/ency/article/007448.htm

National Alliance on Mental Illness (NAMI)

https://www.nami.org/Learn-More/Treatment

Substance Abuse and Mental Health Services Administration

http://www.samhsa.gov/treatment

CHAPTER 38 REVIEW
Physical Rehabilitation and Diagnostic Audiology through New Technology Sections

Let's Check It! Terminology

Match each key term to the appropriate definition.

1. **LO 38.2** Training to gain voluntary control of automatic bodily functions.
2. **LO 38.2** The treatment of mental and emotional disorder through communication or psychologically rather than medical means.
3. **LO 38.3** Regular consumption of a substance with manifestations.
4. **LO 38.1** Health care that is committed to improving, maintaining, or returning physical strength, cognition, and mobility.
5. **LO 38.1** The study of hearing, balance, and related disorders.
6. **LO 38.3** The process of removing toxic substances or qualities.

A. Abuse
B. Audiology
C. Biofeedback
D. Detoxification
E. Psychotherapy
F. Rehabilitation

Let's Check It! Concepts

Choose the most appropriate answer for each of the following questions.

1. **LO 38.1** Within the Physical Rehabilitation and Diagnostic Audiology section, character position 6 represents which of the following?

   a. Section qualifier **b.** Type qualifier **c.** Equipment **d.** Qualifier

2. **LO 38.1** Within the Physical Rehabilitation and Diagnostic Audiology section, character position 2 Section Qualifier, which of the following characters represents diagnostic audiology?

   a. 0 **b.** 1 **c.** 2 **d.** 3

3. **LO 38.1** Within the Physical Rehabilitation and Diagnostic Audiology section, character position 3 Root Type, which of the following characters represents a hearing aid assessment?

   a. B **b.** 2 **c.** D **d.** 4

4. **LO 38.2** All of the codes reporting a Mental Health section procedure will begin with which section letter?

   a. G **b.** H **c.** I **d.** J

5. **LO 38.2** Within the Mental Health section, character position 3 Root Type, the encounter documents *Includes behavior, cognitive, interactive, interpersonal, psychoanalysis, psychodynamic, psychophysiological, and/or supportive*, identified by the character 5. This encounter is known as

   a. psychological tests. **b.** individual psychotherapy.
   c. counseling. **d.** crisis intervention.

6. **LO 38.2** Within the Mental Health section, which character position identifies whether the procedure was educational or vocational?

   a. 2 **b.** 3 **c.** 4 **d.** 5

7. **LO 38.3** All of the codes reporting a Substance Abuse Treatment section procedure will begin with which section letter?

   a. F **b.** H **c.** J **d.** K

8. **LO 38.3** Within the Substance Abuse Treatment section, the encounter documents *Not a treatment modality but helps the patient stabilize physically and psychologically until the body becomes free of drugs and the effects of alcohol,* represented by the character 2. This is known as

   a. individual psychotherapy. **b.** medication management.
   c. pharmacotherapy. **d.** detoxification services.

9. **LO 38.3** Within the Substance Abuse Treatment section, what character position adds detail to the description of the Root Type?

   a. 4 **b.** 5 **c.** 6 **d.** 7

10. **LO 38.4** All of the codes reporting a New Technology procedure will begin with the section letter

    a. Z **b.** X **c.** Y **d.** W

Let's Check It! Rules and Regulations

Please answer the following questions from the knowledge you have gained after reading this chapter.

1. **LO 38.1** List the Physical Rehabilitation and Diagnostic Audiology section, character position 2, Section Qualifier, options, including the character that identifies each.
2. **LO 38.1** Within the Physical Rehabilitation and Diagnostic Audiology section, character position 4, Body System and Region, if the encounter is for caregiver training, what would be the character assignment to represent the encounter?
3. **LO 38.2** List six Mental Health section, character position 3, Root Type, options; include the description and the character that identify each.
4. **LO 38.3** Within the Mental Health section, what does the character position 4, Type Qualifier, explain?
5. **LO 38.4** List six options from the New Technology section, character position 6, Device/Substance/Technology; include the description and the character that identify each.

YOU CODE IT! Practice

Using the techniques described in this chapter, carefully read through the case studies and determine the most accurate ICD-10-PCS code(s) for each case study.

1. Bennie Hallmon, a 67-year-old male, has been in Westward Hospital for a week and is showing signs of deteriorating speech. Dr. Lindler performs a bedside swallowing and oral function speech assessment, no equipment.
2. Merry Gilbert, a 22-year-old female, was hospitalized 7 days ago due to an automobile accident resulting in left hemiplegia. Dr. Tarrant performs an ADL home management assessment using assistive, adaptive, supportive, and protective equipment.
3. Fred Copeland, a 14-month-old male, was admitted to Westward Hospital because he does not react to sudden loud noises and has not begun to use simple words. Fred is diagnosed with severe sensorineural hearing loss and has a multiple channel cochlear implant. Today, Dr. Cantey performs a cochlear implant rehabilitation treatment. Code today's session.
4. Patricia Swartzenturber, a 23-year-old female, has been experiencing recurring episodes of vertigo and some hearing loss. Dr. Wooton admits Patricia to Westward Hospital, where she is diagnosed with Ménière's disease. Pat complains of ringing in her ears. Dr. Wooton fits a tinnitus masker, no equipment used.
5. Vickie Fulmer, a 61-year-old female, presents to Dr. Derry with trembling and twitchy motions she states are involuntary. Dr. Derry also notes diaphoresis and admits Vickie to the hospital, where she is later diagnosed with generalized anxiety disorder. Today, while in the hospital, Vickie participates in an individual interpersonal psychotherapy session. Code today's session.

(continued)

6. Ralph Canopus, a 37-year-old male, was very agitated and restless and threatened suicide. Dr. Patterson admitted Ralph to Westward Hospital, where he was diagnosed with major depression. Today, while in the hospital, Ralph and his family participate in a family psychotherapy session led by Dr. Patterson. Code today's session.
7. AKA: Grover Humphrey, age unknown, male, was found wondering the streets with no memory or ability to reason. A card with a name was found in one of his pockets. He was admitted to Westward Hospital, where Dr. Hatfield performed a cognitive status psychological test.
8. Hugo Parsons, a 15-year-old male, is brought to Westward Hospital by his parents. Hugo's parents have noticed a dramatic personality change recently as well as unexplained anger. Dr. Smyth completes a physical examination and finds Hugo has a substance abuse issue. Dr. Smyth admits Hugo to Westward Hospital and begins detoxification treatment.
9. Jessica Abbott, a 41-year-old female, has been admitted to Westward Hospital for esophageal cancer. Jessica has been smoking cigarettes since she was 16 years old. Dr. Barbato manages her nicotine replacement medication.
10. Eloise Baker, a 56-year-old female, had been diagnosed as an alcoholic and is having severe delirium tremens and seizures. Dr. Hewitt admits Eloise to Westward Hospital. Today, while in the hospital, Eloise participated in a 12-step individual psychotherapy session.
11. Edward Skipper, a 24-year-old male, has been diagnosed with human immunodeficiency virus (HIV). Ed attends a post-test group counseling session held by Dr. Dyson at Westward Hospital.
12. Rinika Simms, a 72-year-old female, was admitted to Westward Hospital for a percutaneous cerebral embolic filtration, single integrated distal filter, left common carotid artery, new technology group 11.
13. Thomas Balakrishnan, a 59-year-old male, presents with leg cramping, numbness, and weakness following physical activity. On examination, Dr. Oliver finds a diminished pulse in his right leg and foot. Thomas is diagnosed with peripheral artery disease and admitted to Westward Hospital. Dr. Oliver dilates the right anterior tibial artery using a resorbable, everolimus-eluting intraluminal scaffold(s), percutaneous approach. The procedure involves multiple dilation sites and employs New Technology Group 10.
14. Margie Lewis, a 49-year-old female, was admitted to Westward Hospital and was diagnosed with Spondylolisthesis. Dr. Marten inserts a Titanium stand-alone ALIF System, open, interbody fusion device, custom-made anatomically designed, new technology group 7.
15. John Hook, a 9-month-old male, was diagnosed with early onset scoliosis. John is admitted to Westward Hospital for reposition of a thoracic, magnetically controlled growth rod, open approach, new technology group 2.

ICD-10-PCS YOU CODE IT! Application

The following exercises provide practice in abstracting physicians' notes and learning to work with documentation from our health care facility, Westward Hospital. These case studies are modeled on real patient encounters. Using the techniques described in this chapter, carefully read through the case studies and determine the most accurate ICD-10-PCS code(s) for each case study.

WESTWARD HOSPITAL
591 Chester Road
Masters, FL 33955
PROGRESS NOTES

PATIENT: HOUGH, BETH

DATE OF ADMISSION: 05/30/26

DATE OF DISCHARGE: 06/01/26

ADMITTING DIAGNOSIS: Acute pyelonephritis caused by *E. coli*

DISCHARGE DIAGNOSIS: Acute pyelonephritis caused by *E. coli*

(continued)

The patient is a 29-year-old female suffering with burning on urination. She stated she also noticed a fishy odor after urination. The urinalysis and culture lab results showed positive for acute pyelonephritis caused by *E. coli.* She was referred to me. I then admitted her to the hospital for treatment with Cefiderocol Anti-infective, peripheral vein introduction.

Benjamin Johnston, MD

Determine the most accurate ICD-10-PCS code(s) for the Ceftazidime-Avibactam Anti-infective.

WESTWARD HOSPITAL

591 Chester Road

Masters, FL 33955

DISCHARGE SUMMARY

PATIENT: GILLINS, MARTIN

DATE OF ADMISSION: 07/15/26

DATE OF SURGERY: 07/29/26

DATE OF DISCHARGE: 08/01/26

DIAGNOSIS: Left below-knee amputation

DISCHARGE DIAGNOSIS: Pt is a 67-year-old male with a history of peripheral arterial disease and lower extremity bypass surgeries who was admitted with gangrene of left foot. The patient underwent left below-knee amputation.

PAST MEDICAL HISTORY: Hyperlipidemia and hypertension.

SOCIAL HISTORY: Lives with wife.

FAMILY HISTORY: Noncontributory.

PHYSICAL EXAMINATION: At the time of admission, the patient was afebrile. Vital signs are stable. Temperature 97.7. Blood pressure 131/71. Oral mucosa was moist. Sclerae anicteric. Lungs: Bilaterally clear to auscultation. Heart: Regular. Abdomen: Scaphoid. Right foot intact. Minimal erythema. Minimal edema.

HOSPITAL COURSE: Dr. Norcross notes patient is medically stable. Compression was not used due to the significant ischemia. The patient was placed on Avelox. Bowels moved on a regular basis. The patient responded to rehabilitation well. Appetite is improving. Albumin was 2.7. Hemoglobin was 11.4. The patient was able to perform all ADLs with supervision. Good range of motion was noted to the left knee. No dehiscence was found. Wife will act as caregiver and was trained in wound care management. The patient was discharged to wife.

MEDICATIONS: Avelox 400 mg daily, aspirin one tablet daily, Roxicodone 5–10 mg every 6 hours as needed for pain, Cardizem 60 mg three times a day, Nitro-Dur patch daily, and Lanoxin 0.25 mg daily.

The patient will follow up with Dr. Norcross on Wednesday. A dry dressing, wrapping with Kling and stockinette, no compression is to be maintained. The patient was prescribed front-wheel walker, 3-in-1 commode, shower chair, and ADL kit. The patient was prescribed home health nursing, physical therapy, occupational therapy, and aide. The patient was also given a wheelchair. All instructions were given.

Karen Norcross, MD

Determine the most accurate ICD-10-PCS code(s) for the caregiver training.

(continued)

WESTWARD HOSPITAL

591 Chester Road

Masters, FL 33955

PATIENT: WRIGHT, ROBBIN

DATE OF ADMISSION: 06/05/26

DATE OF DISCHARGE: 06/17/26

ADMITTING DIAGNOSIS: Marijuana abuse

ATTENDING PHYSICIAN: Jennell Goren, MD

Robbin Wright, a 16-year-old female, presented to Dr. Goren complaining of a cough and a sore throat, lasting about 1 week. She and her mother deny fever, nasal congestion, or runny nose. She says she feels more tired than usual and her mom states that she hasn't been getting out of bed to go to camp or any other activities. Mom seems most worried that she is much less active than she usually is and that she has been hanging out with her friends until late at night. Patient states that her "mom won't get off my back." She admits that her grades had been dropping before summer break, and she quit the baseball team. Mom leaves the room, and patient admits to smoking pot every day, usually several times a day, for the past 8 or 9 months or so. She denies any other drug use and states smoking pot is "no big deal."

After discussion with the patient and her parents, Robbin is admitted into a substance abuse hospital to treat her high level of irritability and anxiety and for daily individual and group behavioral counseling.

Upon admission:

PE: Physical examination is remarkable only for a mildly erythematous throat without petechiae. Lungs are slightly congested, and the rest of her exam is normal. Vital signs are also unremarkable. A rapid strep screen is negative.

FIRST DAY—INDIVIDUAL COUNSELING: Discussion with patient about side effects and risks of abusing pot. She states she has tried to quit but can't make it through an entire day without smoking. It is pointed out to her that her pot use is already having a negative impact on her life (absence and lack of interest in school). We discussed options and methodologies for her quitting with reduced effects. Blood is taken to record the levels of THC, and she agrees to regular surveillance.

PLAN: Marijuana abuse behavioral counseling; daily individual counseling; daily group counseling. Reevaluation after six (6) full days of residential treatment.

Jennell Goren, MD

Determine the most accurate ICD-10-PCS code(s) for the counseling.

WESTWARD HOSPITAL

591 Chester Road

Masters, FL 33955

PHYSICAL REHABILITATION ASSESSMENT

PATIENT: LEWTER, GENE

DATE OF ADMISSION: 11/15/26

DATE OF DISCHARGE: 11/17/26

DIAGNOSIS: 1. Acute myofascial strain.
2. Acute exacerbation of chronic low back pain.

SUBJECTIVE: The patient is a 47-year-old male. The patient came in for back pain. He was initially evaluated by Dr. Bruce Allen for back pain for the last 2 days. He said it was in the mid back, going down to the left knee, with some paresthesias in the feet and numbness in the feet. Movement, remaining still, and laying on a side seem to relieve pain. Lying directly on his back increases the pain. No problems with urination. No fever or chills. No nausea, vomiting, or diarrhea. No abdominal pain.

(continued)

PAST MEDICAL HISTORY: Significant for back injury. He had anterior fusion of L3–L4 in the past. He has had multiple episodes, about one a month, since the surgery of exacerbation of his chronic back pain. This typical pain pattern with numbness and radiation down the leg, he states, is nothing unusual for the last multiple episodes. He has had no bladder or bowel dysfunction.

SOCIAL HISTORY: He is a smoker.

OBJECTIVE: The patient is alert, in no acute distress, obviously uncomfortable however. C-spine is negative. He is tender over the mid back, L2 through L4, with paravertebral muscle spasm that is palpable, also quite tender. Decreased range of motion. The patient is alert and orientated x3. No motor deficits. Strength 5/5. He does have diminished left patellar reflex. Decreased sensory on the left great and little toes, medial aspect of the foot, and lateral aspect on the plantar surface of the foot. Sensory is intact.

INTERVENTION: Motor and nerve function assessment, range of motion, and joint integrity of lower back and lower extremity were performed.

ASSESSMENT:

1. Acute myofascial strain.

2. Acute exacerbation of chronic low back pain.

PLAN: Percocet 5 mg 1–2 q. 4–6 hours as needed for pain, Soma one, three times a day, Indocin SR 75 mg b.i.d. with food. Follow up with the specialist who did his back surgery for reevaluation of his increasing back pain over the last several years. Any acute problems, recheck sooner. Any problems with bladder or bowel, recheck immediately.

Roberta Opell, PT

Determine the most accurate ICD-10-PCS code(s) for the motor function assessment.

WESTWARD HOSPITAL

591 Chester Road

Masters, FL 33955

HISTORY OF PRESENT ILLNESS ADMISSION

PATIENT: JETT, JAMES

DATE OF ADMISSION: 10/07/26

DATE OF DISCHARGE: 10/09/26

ADMITTING DIAGNOSIS: Schizophrenia and polysubstance abuse

HISTORY OF PRESENT ILLNESS: This is a 27-year-old male with a history of schizophrenia and polysubstance abuse referred by his case manager due to increased hallucinations, including auditory, and new onset of olfactory, gustatory, and tactile hallucinations. Since the onset of the hallucinations, the patient has become acutely suicidal with multiple plans. He has a history of polysubstance abuse with alcohol and crack but has been sober for greater than 3 months and has been in rehab. He also complains of headaches recently. The patient presented frightened and tearful and continued to endorse suicidal thoughts.

PAST PSYCHIATRIC HISTORY: Paranoid schizophrenia, substance abuse.

PAST MEDICAL HISTORY: Left shoulder injury with chronic pain and a seizure one time in the past.

FAMILY HISTORY: The patient does have a brother with schizophrenia and a mother who died from complications of diabetes.

SOCIAL HISTORY: The patient currently is in rehab. Divorced. Did finish high school and went to junior college for a little while but did not get a degree. He has been unable to hold a steady job for most of his life.

REVIEW OF SYSTEMS: Included headache and some blurry vision. He denies constitutional symptoms. He denied chest pain, difficulty breathing, GI symptoms, dysuria. He does endorse left shoulder pain. He denied any skin conditions and he does endorse numbness of his distal feet.

(continued)

MENTAL STATUS EXAMINATION: Neurobehavioral and Cognitive Status Exam: Appearance and Behavior: He had good eye contact, well groomed, fair hygiene. Speech and Language: Normal volume, tone, and rate, nonpressured. Mood and Affect: Mood was depressed and affect was congruent and restricted. Thought processes linear and goal directed. Thought Content: He does have some paranoia, believing that people, including the doctors, are experimenting on him. HI/SI: He denies currently having suicidal ideations. Perceptual Abnormalities: He reports visual, auditory, gustatory, and tactile hallucinations. Orientation: He is alert and oriented x3. Memory and abstractions are fair. Fund of knowledge and IQ are average and insight and judgment are limited and poor. His initial physical exam was significant for pain and decreased range of motion in the left shoulder on passive abduction and extension and a mild paresthesia of the plantar surface of his right second toe; otherwise, neurologic exam was normal.

JOANNE STAFFORD, MD

Determine the most accurate ICD-10-PCS code(s) for the cognitive status test.

39

Inpatient Coding Capstone

Learning Outcomes

After completing this chapter, the student should be able to:

LO 39.1 Correctly abstract patient records to determine accurate coding using ICD-10-CM and ICD-10-PCS code sets.

Reporting the procedures provided to a patient who has been admitted into an inpatient facility can cover a broad spectrum. The cases in this chapter will support your learning using ICD-10-PCS procedure codes.

Remember, read carefully and completely.

CASE STUDY #1: NESTOR GONZALEZ

ICD-10-CM ICD-10-PCS

H&P

Nestor Gonzalez, a 69-year-old previously healthy male, was seen in my office with a cough productive of thick purulent sputum of 3-days duration. Fever was present and he reported dyspnea on exertion.

Vital signs—BP 96/60 mmHg, P 116 beats/min, RR 24 breaths/min, T 103.5°F rectal.

On examination, he appeared acutely ill.

Lung examination revealed scattered ronchi, which were greater on the right than the left.

I determined that the patient needed to be admitted into the hospital right away.

Upon admission: Bronchoscopic aspiration specimen culture, C&S, and gram stain. Blood tests and sputum culture were ordered and a chest x-ray taken.

RESULTS: Chest x-ray showed increased opacity in the lung field indicating pneumonia, as suspected; culture confirmed *E. coli* with Shiga toxin.

Dx: Community-acquired pneumonia due to *Escherichia coli* 0157 (E. coli) with Shiga toxin

Treatment: IV ciprofloxacin 300 mg q 12h, infused over 60 minutes

Dr. Ryan MacDoule

CASE STUDY #2: TINA LEBROCK

H&P

Patient is Tina LeBrock, a 71-year-old female with known unstable angina due to coronary artery disease. During the week prior to admission, she underwent an outpatient procedure of diagnostic heart catheterization. At the time of this heart catheterization procedure, the patient was found to have occlusion of the left anterior descending coronary artery in two separate locations.

Due to the findings from this diagnostic procedure, the patient is now admitted for a scheduled percutaneous transluminal coronary angioplasty (PTCA) with a plan for stent insertions. The patient also has known secondary diagnoses of hypertension, hyperlipidemia, and current tobacco use. The hypertension, hyperlipidemia, and unstable angina are currently being treated with medications.

The patient was taken to the procedure room and underwent a PTCA of the left anterior descending coronary artery with insertion of two Taxus drug-eluting stents, one at each occlusion site.

Dr. Lawrence Marcheon

CASE STUDY #3: GRAYSON CARLYLE

Patient: Grayson Carlyle

15 May 2026

MRN: C18-54662517

Surgeon: Annalissa Brubaker, MD

PREOPERATIVE: gonarthrosis deformans; four ipsilateral periprosthetic fractures

HPI: A 43-year-old otherwise healthy male patient with a diagnosis of osteoarthrosis was admitted in 2025 for elective left-knee arthroplasty. He had a history of three nonsignificant knee traumas, and an arthrotomy with synovectomy had been performed on the left knee due to synovitis in 2024. His physical examination at admission showed severe insufficiency of the medial collateral ligament and rotational instability of the left knee joint. Other joints showed no abnormal findings.

X-ray revealed gonarthrosis deformans stage II with 5° varus angulation. The patient underwent total arthroplasty (Allopro *NPK*, Switzerland) of the left knee on March 4, 2024. Postoperative x-ray revealed good alignment of the prosthesis; both components were centered in the midline of the joint, and overall knee alignment was 8° in valgus.

Two 1-g prophylactic doses of the antibiotic cefuroxime were administered perioperatively. The patient developed a fever on the third postoperative day, and the same antibiotic was administered intravenously (750 mg three times a day, postoperative days 3–10).

The patient was discharged in good general condition on March 18, 2024, and he had no medical problems during the outpatient follow-up period.

A year later, on May 26, 2025, the patient fell at home and was admitted to the hospital with a supracondylar fracture of the left distal femoral metaphysis (displacement in flexion and varus). Skeletal traction with 7 kg was applied primarily, and the patient underwent surgery. The tibial component of the endoprosthesis was loose and was removed; the femoral shaft was fixed with a dynamic condylar screw device, and a revision arthroplasty using a long-stem endoprosthesis was done.

The patient had no postoperative complications. The outpatient follow-up period was uneventful, and after 3 months, he returned to work.

The patient started experiencing pain and swelling in his left knee joint approximately 1 year after the second surgery. An x-ray performed in August 27, 2025, showed radiolucency around the tibial component, which had also migrated anteroinferiorly. Based on these findings and also on clinical and laboratory data, infection of the endoprosthesis was diagnosed, and the patient was admitted for 1-stage revision arthroplasty. Microbiological culture from joint aspirations showed the presence of *Pseudomonas aeruginosa* sensitive to Tazocin (piperacillin sodium and tazobactam sodium), ceftazidime, imipenem, amikacin, gentamicin, and ciprofloxacin.

The patient had surgery on September 1, 2025. Because the previous femoral supracondylar fracture was consolidated, the DCS fixator and endoprosthesis were removed and revision arthroplasty with long-stem rotational endoprosthesis (*Link Endo-Model Total Hinge Knee*) was performed. The tibial defect was additionally filled with 15-mm spacer.

Microbiological cultures taken during surgery confirmed the diagnosis of *P. aeruginosa* infection. During the hospital stay, antibiotics were administered intravenously according to microbe sensitivity (antibiogram) and our infection protocol: gentamicin 240 mg once a day and ciprofloxacin 200 mg twice a day for the first 5 postoperative days. Starting on the sixth postoperative day, gentamicin combined with ceftazidime 500 mg twice a day was administered, and was continued for 9 days.

The patient was discharged home with no complaints. He was prescribed oral rifampicin 300 mg twice a day for the next 2 months. Full weight-bearing was allowed after 6 weeks.

Three months later, the patient fell on a slippery street and sustained an axially displaced fracture of proximal metaphysis of tibia and fibula. This time treatment was conservative: closed reduction was achieved and maintained in a long-leg cast. Follow-up x-ray on December 14, 2025, showed that bone fragments were still in satisfactory alignment and there was evidence of callus formation. The patient returned to work and his usual activities in January 2026.

On March 9, 2026, the patient was admitted to the hospital again because of a spiral dislocated fracture in left femoral distal diaphysis. The femur was shortened and displaced axially in varus position. Skeletal traction (5 kg) was applied primarily, and surgery was performed later. Offstripping of femoral periosteum in both fragments was seen during surgery. Internal fixation of the left femoral bone was achieved with an AO plate and screw. The patient recovered and was discharged on March 17, 2026. He was told to limit weight-bearing for the next 2.5 months and to walk with crutches.

Unfortunately the patient didn't follow these instructions, and the plate broke off the bone in its distal part due to walking. An open reosteosynthesis (exchange of screws and repositioning of the plate) was performed this morning (May 15, 2026).

CASE STUDY #4: DAMARIS ALBAQSHI

Patient: Damaris Albaqshi

MRN: D9513597135

Attending Physician: Markesha Cacciola, MD

A 42-year-old female patient was admitted to the hospital with a swelling on the right tibia. Past history revealed that the patient was operated upon 24 years ago for a pathological fracture of the right tibia and the diagnosis at that time had been adamantinoma. The preoperative radiograph of the right leg showed osteolysis of the bone, and the chest radiograph revealed lung metastases. Regional computed tomography (CT) of the right leg showed that the tumor was invading the surrounding soft tissues. The cortex appeared moderately expanded and attenuated. Bone scanning showed intensive positivity in the middle of the right tibia. The CT scan of the thorax demonstrated two lung metastases. One of these was in close contact with the right anterior pulmonary artery and the other was located in the left posterior lobe. Fine needle aspiration (FNA) biopsy confirmed the diagnosis of adamantinoma of right tibia suggesting local recurrence.

The patient underwent surgery wherein the tumor was widely resected and the tibia reconstructed with specific recombined osteosynthesis (salvage surgery). The pathological examination of the excised tumor confirmed the diagnosis of adamantinoma set by FNA biopsy. The histological examination revealed a multiforming adamantinoma with basaloid, spindle cellular, and tubular characteristics. Examination of the adamantinoma that had been excised earlier revealed the same characteristics. The postoperative period was without complications and the patient walked in 15 days.

CASE STUDY #5: MICHAELA DEMARCO

Patient: Michaela DeMarco

MRN: K3357151

14 July 2026

Attending Physician: Cecilia Rowens, MD

HISTORY: This patient is a 5-year-old female with normal birth history and development with the exception of an episode of maternal hemiplegia during pregnancy. Family history is not significant of any neurologic issues. Her medical history is unremarkable except for celiac disease. Due to this, she is sustained with a gluten-free diet.

Five months ago, she was found to have scarlet fever. Resulting therefrom, she experienced episodes of left hand tremor lasting about 5–7 seconds with no alteration of consciousness. Four weeks later, she had additional events and was taken to the nearby emergency department, where an EEG was performed.

The results of the EEG evidenced a normal background with right centrotemporal spikes. A second EEG, performed the next day, showed similar findings yet recorded sleep and sleep activation of the discharges.

With these results, she was placed on ethosuximide. An MRI of the brain was completed and showed unremarkable results with the exception of "*slight signal alteration involving the posterior periventricular white substance of both sides of a nonspecific nature.*" Opacification of the sinuses and otomastoiditis was also observed.

The patient exhibited some "restlessness of her limbs" during sleep, but has had no additional seizures. However, this past month, she then had two larger events. She was then placed on divalproex sodium at 750 mg divided per day for 14 days.

<u>Family history:</u>

Mother experienced a transitory left hemiplegia during pregnancy. Both the father and 18-month-old sister are reported to be in good health. No family history is known related to epilepsy or mental retardation.

<u>Medical background:</u>

Delivered during normal spontaneous delivery at 39th week + 2.

No pre-, peri-, and postnatal anguish reported. Neonate exhibited good suction. Mother breastfed the infant up until 6 months, then weaned.

(continued)

During physical examination, it was noted that the neonate's psychomotor development was within normal limits. Seated posture at 4.5 months, standing unassisted at 11 months, first words when 8 months. Alvus and diuresis WNL, feeding non-gluten diet due to celiac disease. Her sleep-wake rhythm is also reported within normal limits. NKA. Patient diagnosed previously with celiac disease.

Five months ago, she was placed on a regime of antibiotic therapy due to an episode of scarlet fever. Four weeks later, while under antibiotic therapy, she developed a fever and then started to show brief episodes evidenced by right hand tremors, with a duration of approximately 5–7 seconds each, without any concomitant consciousness alterations.

The parents report that these episodes began approximately 7 months ago, and both described these episodes as occasional. Currently, similar episodes of tremors were observed prompting her parents to take her to urgent care.

The child was transferred and admitted to the hospital's pediatric neurology floor. This is when a diagnosis of "*Focal epilepsy of myoclonic nature in patient with normal psychomotor development*" was determined. During this admission, tests were ordered and completed:

- Blood tests: within normal limits with the exception of Hb (Hemoglobin) 11.03 g/dl (v.n. 12–14), MCV 64.9 fl (v.n. 75–85), Platelets 607 (v.n. 130–400), iron in the blood 39 mcg/dl (v.n. 50–80).
- EEG: Right centrotemporal paroxysmal abnormalities with tendency to omo and contralateral spreading in tracing with normal background rhythm.
- EEG during sleeping: 2 right centrotemporal paroxysmal abnormalities with tendency to spreading and with activation when sleeping.

The patient was discharged with prescriptions for:

Ethosuximide 80 mg × 2 a day at 8 a.m. and 8 p.m. for 1 week

Ethosuximide 80 mg + 160 mg at 8 a.m. and 8 p.m. for 1 week

Ethosuximide 160 mg × 2 a day at 8 a.m. and 8 p.m. continuing

Brain MRN was performed under sedation with results within normal limits, except for the "*slight signal alteration involving the posterior peri-ventricular white substance of both sides, of nonspecific nature, and bilateral otomastoiditis, opacification of maxillary sinuses, of ethmoid cells and of sphenoidal sinuses bilaterally. Asymmetry of temporal-basal superficial vessels, due to ectasia of a vessel on the right side, is observed.*"

The child's parents observed some type of restless limbs (both arms and legs) when she was sleeping occasionally, after about 3 hours as well as early in the morning. Additionally, and perhaps more of a concern, these restless limbs in the evenings (about 7 p.m.), as well as when the child goes to bed (approximately 10:00 p.m.). They reported that she often complains about being cold, repeating this multiple times.

This month, she experienced two epileptic seizures. The first one occurred during an afternoon nap — waking up catatonic, staring, with hardly any response to questions. There were times that right-sided rigidity was also noted. These events typically lasted about 10 minutes and she would then fall asleep. Once awaking, the child took about 90 minutes to recover her mood. At times, she also complained stomach pain.

The second epileptic seizure was noted when the child was being seen in the clinic to check her medication dosage and a follow-up visit. Once awake, she experienced a 25-seconds-long crisis, with remarkable tremors to arms, legs, eyes, and twisted and munching mouth.

Following these events, her attending physician changed her medication regime with:

Valproic acid oral suspension 80 mg at 8 a.m. and 80 mg at 8 p.m. for 7 days

Valproic acid oral suspension 120 mg at 8 a.m. and 120 mg at 8 p.m. for 7 days

Valproic acid oral suspension 160 mg at 8 a.m. and 160 mg at 8 p.m. on-going

No substantial crisis occurred after the first 7 days of treatment with the minimum dosage. During sleep, the child moves constantly, wriggling her limbs at about 3 a.m. (intensely for 30 minutes at a time until she falls back to sleep) or at about 5:00 a.m. In addition, when she wakes up, she moves uncontrollably for approximately 5 minutes.

Evaluation and consultations have determined two possible diagnoses:

1) Focal-Onset Epilepsy. The patient's seizures began on the right side of her brain (causing the effect to the left side of the body including shaking and rigidity). Should these spread to the entire brain, this could result in the entire body shaking, This was evidenced with her second seizure. The MRI was unremarkable as to a cause for the seizure (such as a tumor, stroke, or malformation). This is an encouraging indication with an improved opportunity for the child to outgrow seizures. Observations of the sinuses and mastoid showed nothing that would cause the seizures. We recommend that an ENT specialist should evaluate these incidental findings.

(continued)

2) Benign Rolandic Epilepsy. This is the most common epilepsy syndrome in childhood (not counting febrile seizures) and onset can occur anywhere from age 1–15 (however, typically by age 7). These seizures are typically similar to the partial seizures described by her parents. It should be noted that these seizures can occur on either side of the brain and commonly occur just after falling asleep or just upon waking. The diagnostic EEG reveals centrotemporal spikes that are more frequent during sleep (similar to this patient's). On an EEG, these spikes can be identified only on one side or they might alternate between the right and left sides, showing from one test to the next. When the spikes are only seen consistently on one side, then subsequent EEGs would reveal discharges on the opposite side. Virtually all children outgrow this type of epilepsy, around puberty if not earlier. The restlessness of the limbs during sleep is not epileptic; however, it is common in epileptic children. They often exhibit restless sleep or jerking motions of the limbs (sleep myoclonus). These are benign.

TREATMENT: A 24-hour EEG is ordered during this current admission.

DISCHARGE: The 24-hour EEG evidenced abnormalities consistently on only the left side, confirming a diagnosis of idiopathic focal-onset epilepsy. Her normal development is very reassuring and can be seen with this type of epilepsy. Some children with this type of seizure can experience problems with attention/focus/memory as they get older, but this is usually mild and gets better as the condition normalizes.

CASE STUDY #6: POPPY BROWNING

Patient: Poppy Browning

MRN: A399523147

Physician: Carla Firmann, MD

Second hospitalization, 1 month later, following appearance of arising colics, difficult to treat with pain medications, high body temperature, and increase in inflammation ratings, symptoms consistent with picture of infective cholangitis. Therefore, the picture was resolved with antibiotic therapy and with carrying out a papillotomy by means of ERCP. Discharged under antibiotic therapy with Ciprofloxacin, Cortisone, and Azathioprine.

Third hospitalization, 3 days after discharge from previous hospitalization, following arising colics with progressive ultrasound scan dilatation of bile ducts and evidence of dropsy of the gallbladder. Moreover, 48 hours following hospitalization, amylase increase (600 UI/l) was detected. The IgG4 dosage (18 mg/dl) was within normal limits, excluding a possible autoimmune hepatitis/pancreatitis syndrome.

ERCP performed with dilatation and cleaning of the common bile duct that involved the spillage of corpuscular material and bile with purulent appearance bringing about a fast improvement of symptomatology and a rapid reduction in the amylase values. Later on, laparoscopic cholecystectomy was carried out. During postsurgery, after a short period of wellness, the patient suffered from an abdominal pain. Reappearance interpreted, at the beginning, as a light pancreatitis (treated with antibiotic therapy). Subsequently, persisting painful crises were observed despite blood tests showing substantial stability.

Therefore, an MR cholangiography was carried out (images enclosed on CD) that has revealed an appearance of intra- and extrahepatic bile duct dilatation, evident also at common bile duct level where the picture seems to reveal a relevant stenosis: "Intrahepatic bile ducts with clear wall irregularity and with minimal stenosis followed by dilatations in a picture to be related to the base pathology. Irregularity at the extrahepatic bile ducts and at the common bile duct level too, the common bile duct distal region appears moderately reduced in diameter, also in papillary region, also as a result of papillotomy."

In light of the aforesaid, a biliary stent was placed during ERCP in order to guarantee bile ducts patency. The clinical picture, after surgery, was stable with occasional presence of pains involving mainly the right hypochondrium without any characteristics of biliary colics. At discharge, blood tests showed evidence of improvement of the hepatic cytolisys index (AST 28, ALT 38) with still elevated values of gammaGt (197) and APC 2.02 mg/dl probably linked to the inflammatory pathology rather than to an infective event. Discharge with indication to follow a therapy with Deltacortene to scale down the Azathioprine and antibiotic therapy with Augmentin.

Fourth hospitalization, 1 month later, in gastroenterology department for clinical test: The patient reported slight painful crisis in epigastric region; at examinations APC negativization (0.59) and a further reduction in GGTs with transaminase substantially stable. Therefore, the therapy with Amoxicillin + Clavulanic Acid was suspended and Metronidazole 250 mg was prescribed three times a day every other week.

(continued)

Fifth hospitalization during the same month, following an episode of infective cholangitis with blood tests that showed transaminase on the increase (ALT 248, AST 114, GGT 281) with leukocytosis (WBCs 13,000, neutrophils 88%, lymphocytes 7.9%) and elevated APC (4.48). Therapy started with Augmentin (1 g three times a day) for 7 days and then end. At the end of the 7 days, preventive treatment prescribed with Cotrimoxazole (tablet 160 + 800) one tablet twice a day.

Sixth hospitalization, 2 weeks after the previous one, following epigastric pain and nausea, occurred after 1 day from Augmentin interruption and 1 day after the beginning of therapy with Cotrimoxazole.

The most significant lab examinations at admission: CRP = 1.92 mg/dl; GGT 129 U/L; AST = 29 U/L; ALT = 97 U/L.

Abdomen ultrasound scan with evidence of common bile duct dilatation. "Dilatation of the proximal and medial segment of the common bile duct, with diameter up to 10 mm, in whose context binary images are appreciated referable to the well-known stent. A moderate ectasia of intrahepatic bile ducts is connected, in particular in the left parts."

To treat the severe painful symptomatology, a therapy with Ketorolac Tromethamine 90 mg in 250 cc in continuous infusion was started.

Because of the increase in the inflammation ratings and in the dilatation of the common bile duct at the abdominal ultrasound scan, supposing an occlusion of the biliary stent with overlapped cholangitis, an antibiotic therapy has been started with Meropenem 1 g × 3, IV, and a high osmolar ERCP was carried out.

ERCP didn't show any materials obstructing the stent. Biliary washing was within normal limits.

Therapy prescribed at home: Augmentin (1 g × 3); Ciproxin (500 mg × 2); Folina 5 mg (one tablet every other day); Deltacortene (25 mg daily); Azathioprine (100 mg daily); Lansoprazole (30 mg daily); Ursodesossicolic Acid (300 mg three times a day).

CASE STUDY #7: DAVID CHANG

Patient: David Chang

MRN: C55359541

Attending Physician: Evangeline DeRupo, MD

HPI: A 13-year-old boy had been well until 4 weeks before admission, when he developed a cough, periorbital edema, ankle swelling, headaches, and upper abdominal discomfort. On admission, he was febrile with facial and ankle edema; there were generalized, superficial lymphadenopathy; numerous adventitial sounds in the lungs; and mild hypertension (BP 140/110). His hemoglobin was 72 g/l with a normal white-cell count and an erythrocyte sedimentation rate (ESR) of 137 mm/h. His blood urea was high (27.5 mmol/l) with a low serum bicarbonate (13.6 mmol/l) and serum albumin (19 g/l). His creatinine clearance was 45 ml/min/m^2 with urinary protein loss of 6.7 g/day. His serum CH_{50} was low (14 U/ml; NR 25–45), as was his C3 level (0.20 g/l; NR 0.8–1.4); his C4 level was normal (0.30 g/l; NR 0.2–0.4). A chest x-ray showed several rounded opacities in both lungs. These were presumed to be infective and treated with amoxycillin and flucloxacillin with resolution of the radiological findings.

The association of a low C3 with acute glomerulonephritis suggested acute poststreptococcal disease as the most likely diagnosis, although no streptococci were isolated and streptococcal antibodies were not raised. Over the following 3 weeks, his blood urea fell but the proteinuria and hypertension persisted.

CURRENT ADMISSION: Although he feels better, he still has heavy proteinuria with a low serum albumin (22 g/l; NR 35–50). Surprisingly, the serum CH_{50} and C3 levels are still low at 18 U/ml and 0.4 g/l, respectively. This pattern was not consistent with the working diagnosis. It suggested continued complement activation via the alternate pathway, either due to some circulating activating factor or because of a regulatory defect caused by absence of the inhibitors I or H. However, his serum levels of I and H are normal. Electrophoresis of fresh serum and plasma showed the presence of C3 breakdown products and his serum was able to break down C3 in normal serum due to the presence of C3 nephritic factor.

C3 nephritic factor shows a strong association with membranoproliferative glomerulonephritis, but not with acute poststreptococcal glomerulonephritis. Because these conditions have different prognoses, a bilateral renal biopsy was performed yesterday. The results show 11 glomeruli, all of which were swollen with proliferation of mesangial, endothelial, and epithelial cells. On electron microscopy, the capillary loops showed basement membrane thickening with electron-dense deposits within the GBM. On immunofluorescence, intense C3 deposition is present in the GBM without immunoglobulin staining. These appearances, together with the finding of circulating C3 nephritic factor, are characteristic of *membranoproliferative glomerulonephritis* with *dense intramembranous deposits* (type II MPGN). Alternate-day prednisolone 10 mg PO per day was started, with prescription for 5 mg PO every other day for 30 days, although this disease nearly always shows a slow progression to chronic renal failure.

CASE STUDY #8: MARYBELLE OSENKOWSKY

Patient: Marybelle Osenkowsky

Physician: Fiona McNally, MD

History

This 87-year-old female has been a patient of the McGraw Health Center and Clinic since 2024. Chronic conditions: pernicious anemia, osteoarthritis, and urinary incontinency. She is fully functional and fully independent. She provides care for her homebound husband, who has severe COPD. They live in a home chosen because it was "close to the hospital" to ensure access to house calls for her husband.

In September 2024, the husband died as a result of respiratory arrest. Her only relative is a niece who talks with her about once a month. In October 2025, her home was broken into and our patient was raped and robbed. She was taken to a local hospital specializing in rape. Here, she is distressed, delusional, and reported to be very emotionally distraught.

Examination

I saw the patient about 3 weeks after the rape in a community nursing home, where she was moved after a 4-day stay at the hospital. She was very distressed, delusional, and confused. She slowly improved over 2 months and was discharged to a senior living center.

In March of 2026, the patient was seen in the office. She is still very emotionally unstable. She is crying, depressed (not suicidal), and stressed about her new home. She wants to move to a different senior housing unit because it would be on the bus route, making it easier to get around. She has also hired a middle-aged woman as a caregiver.

Today, 9 months after moving to the new facility, she becomes acutely ill with psychotic symptoms and severe paranoia. She hallucinates that men and women are in her bed and calls others all hours of the day. I admitted her into a hospitalized psychiatric unit and she shows improvement over about 14 days without antipsychotic medication. IV Haloperidol 2.5 mg q30 min x3 h.

Diagnosis: Delusional disorder, Acute Post Traumatic Stress Disorder

CASE STUDY #9: ROGER WESTERMAN

Patient: Roger Westerman

Physician: LaTisha Rodriquez, MD

H&P

History:

05/13/26: trouble w balance × 1 year, fatigue, fall × 4 (retropulse × 3)

Walking slowly for few years—getting worse

Trouble going to standing from sitting position

No tremor, handwriting OK, no shuffling gait

Urinary incontinence without urgency—just leaks, not at night

Inattentive per wife

Cooks, but wife must redirect at times

Gave up driving 1 yr ago because he was nervous about his skills

Decline in function—no aerobics × 2–3 yrs

Depressive symptoms—had seen a psychiatrist for years. Had been on Prozac but it "made him feel too great" and he gave it up

Overall, there had been a significant deterioration in function

(continued)

Past Medical History

2017: Serial TIAs—anterior circulation symptoms—Carotid ultrasound (–), treated with aspirin 81 mg qd

2019: Another TIA—ASA 325 mg. Repeat carotid ultrasound (–)

2020: Right hemisensory symptoms—Left thalamic infarct on MRI

2023: Neurology evaluation—problems with balance, coordination, reduced exercise tolerance

February 1, 2026: MRI—mild prominence 3rd and lateral vents, periventricular white matter changes, old left thalamic lacune. Low normal B12. Normal: TSH, folate, ESR, CBC, HbA1C

Examination

SH: retired kindergarten teacher

Recently moved to an apartment house in the city

Requires help with instrumental activities of daily living

Physical Examination

Cranial nerves normal

Motor: normal x LUE extensor, LE flex 4/5

Normal tone, no cogwheeling, no shuffle, normal facies

3+ patellar DTR, 1+ ankles DTR, toes downgoing

- Retropulses with challenge
- Normal cerebellar exam
- Gait—ataxia present

Data and Scans

Review of head MRI/CTs from '07, '09, '14, '16:

Enlarging ventricles over time

Substantial white matter changes

Thalamic infarct

MRI, 11/01/2026 shows differential diagnosis of:

Sequelae of stroke (ataxia) vs. Normal pressure hydrocephalus

Surgery: Open procedure to insert monitoring device into cerebrum. Successful.

Code for monitoring device surgery.

CASE STUDY #10: KARL ATTENDA

PREOPERATIVE DIAGNOSIS: Bilateral inguinal hernia

POSTOPERATIVE DIAGNOSIS: Bilateral inguinal hernia, direct

OPERATION PERFORMED: Laparoscopic bilateral inguinal hernia repair

SURGEON: Lawrence Podentale, MD

ANESTHESIA: General endotracheal

ESTIMATED BLOOD LOSS: Minimal

DESCRIPTION OF OPERATION: With the patient under general endotracheal anesthesia, the abdomen was prepped with ChloraPrep solution and draped in the usual manner. A transverse skin incision was made below and to the right of the umbilicus to a length of approximately 4 cm. The incision was carried through the subcutaneous tissue. Bleeders were cauterized. The right rectus sheath was identified and incised lateral to the midline. The preperitoneal space was then developed following insertion of a Spacemaker balloon, which was inflated under direct vision.

(continued)

Following removal of the Spacemaker balloon, a #10 trocar was placed in the preperitoneal space and the preperitoneal space was insufflated with CO_2. Two #5 trocars were placed in the lower midline. Video laparoscope was inserted in the preperitoneal space. Landmarks including symphysis pubis, right Cooper ligament, and right inferior epigastric vessels were identified. Dissection was then continued lateral to the transverse abdominis muscle. The internal ring was then explored for the presence of an indirect hernia sac. No indirect hernia sac was identified. The patient had a cord lipoma, which was reduced under direct vision. Exploration of the medial space showed a medial defect suggesting a direct hernia. A large-size Bard 3D mesh was placed in the preperitoneal space and anchored to the symphysis pubis and anterior abdominal wall along the upper edge of the mesh with a stapler. The lower edge of the mesh was affixed to the abdominal wall with Tisseel fibrin glue.

Following this, the left preperitoneal space was explored in the same fashion. Landmarks including symphysis pubis, Cooper ligament, and inferior epigastric vessels were identified. The dissection was continued laterally to the transverse abdominis muscle. The internal ring was then explored for the presence of an indirect hernia sac. No indirect hernia sac was identified. A cord lipoma was reduced. The patient was found to have a medial defect suggesting a direct hernia. A large-size left 3D Prolene mesh was then placed in the preperitoneal space and placed over the floor of the inguinal canal and stapled to the symphysis pubis and anterior abdominal wall along the upper edge of the mesh with a stapler.

The lower edge was anchored to the abdominal wall with Tisseel fibrin glue. The preperitoneal space was then deflated. All trocars were withdrawn. The defect in the rectus sheath was closed with figure-of-eight 0 Vicryl suture. The skin incisions were closed with subcuticular 5-0 Monocryl suture. Sterile dressings were then applied. The patient tolerated the procedure well and was brought to the recovery room in stable condition. Needle and sponge counts were correct.

PROCEDURE: Laparoscopic repair of bilateral inguinal hernias

Lawrence Podentale, MD

CASE STUDY #11: KEASHA FROENMAN

PREOPERATIVE DIAGNOSIS: Degenerative joint disease, left shoulder

POSTOPERATIVE DIAGNOSIS: Degenerative joint disease, left shoulder, with degenerative labral tear and chondral flap tear of glenoid

OPERATION PERFORMED: Arthroscopic exam of glenohumeral joint with arthroscopic debridement of labral tears, chondroplasty, and microfracture of glenoid

SURGEON: Cassandra LeRoy, MD

ASSISTANT SURGEON: Rose Carter, MD

ANESTHESIA: General

DESCRIPTION OF OPERATION: The patient was brought to the operating room and placed in a supine position on the operating room table. General anesthetic was administered. The left shoulder was prepped and draped in a sterile orthopedic fashion after she was placed in a beach-chair position. A time-out was performed confirming left shoulder pathology, and she also had 1 gram of Ancef administered intravenously. After the sterile orthopedic prep and drape, a posterior stab wound was created and the arthroscope was introduced into the glenohumeral joint. The joint was inspected. There were degenerative changes of the labrum circumferentially. Through an anterior portal, a full-radius resector was inserted and these areas debrided back to stable tissue, and this was supplemented with use of the ArthroCare wand on a setting of one. There was a flap tear of the anterior portion of the mid glenoid region. This was easily displaceable. Using a 4.2 full-radius resector, this was debrided back to stable tissue and then an awl was used to microfracture the bone. The inflow pump was then stopped and bloody fluid could be seen coming from the microfracture area. The undersurface of the rotator cuff was inspected and found to be without pathology. The arthroscope was then placed into the anterior portal, and through the posterior portal, the ArthroCare wand and a full-radius resector were inserted and the most inferior aspect and posterior aspect of the glenoid and labrum debrided. There were no frank tears of the posterior labrum. The arthroscope was then placed in the subacromial space, which did appear to be pristine. There was no evidence of impingement. All instruments were then removed and the stab wounds were closed with a single Monocryl suture and Steri-Strips. Dry sterile dressings were placed over the wound. The patient was placed in a shoulder sling and then sent to the recovery room in stable condition.

CASE STUDY #12: REISHICA DECLERQUE

DATE OF ADMISSION: 09/09/2026

DATE OF DISCHARGE: 09/11/2026

DISCHARGE DIAGNOSES:

1. Intrauterine gestation at term
2. History of two previous cesarean sections
3. Delivered viable male infant
4. Multiparity, fertility, desired sterilization

PROCEDURES PERFORMED:

1. Repeat low transverse cesarean section
2. Bilateral tubal ligation

COMPLICATIONS: None

PERTINENT FINDINGS/HISTORY AND PHYSICAL: Refer to the detailed admission dictation.

The patient is a 35-year-old gravida 6, now para 3-0-3-3 female, who was admitted at term for repeat cesarean section and sterilization. The patient had previous cesarean sections for labor arrest, for an infant weighing 9 pounds 12 ounces, and elective repeat. The patient strongly desired repeat cesarean section. She also wanted to have a tubal ligation and signed the appropriate consent forms. Patient is well aware of the risks, options, failure rates, and permanency of sterilization procedures. Her antenatal course was significant for development of A1 diabetes with blood sugars in excellent control, on diet only. The patient declined genetic screening because of advanced maternal age.

LABORATORY INVESTIGATIONS: The patient's admission hemoglobin was 11.1 with hematocrit of 33.4 and platelet count 196,000. Her postoperative hematocrit was 32.2.

HOSPITAL COURSE: The patient was admitted on the morning of her scheduled surgery. Detailed informed consent was again obtained. Under spinal anesthesia, uncomplicated repeat low transverse cesarean section and bilateral tubal ligation were performed. A viable male infant with Apgars of 9 and 9 with birth weight of 8 pounds 6 ounces was delivered. The patient's postoperative course was uneventful. She remained afebrile with stable vital signs. She returned quickly to good ambulation and regular diet. She had normal GI function return. Her incision healed nicely. Her lochia was light.

Discharge examination revealed negative HEENT, neck, heart, lung, extremities, and abdominal examinations.

CONDITION ON DISCHARGE: Stable.

DISPOSITION: Discharged to home.

DISCHARGE INSTRUCTIONS:

ACTIVITY: Slow increase as tolerated. No heavy lifting. Strict pelvic rest.

DIET: Regular.

MEDICATIONS: Colace p.r.n., Tylenol p.r.n., and prenatal vitamins. The patient is breastfeeding. Prescriptions for Percocet 325/5 tablets, #30, no refills, 1 to 2 p.o. q.4–6 h. p.r.n. pain and ibuprofen 800 mg, #20, no refills, 1 p.o. q.8 h. p.r.n. pain.

Follow up as an outpatient in the office in 1 week.

The patient has received routine verbal instructions and agrees to comply. She knows to contact us immediately should she develop any signs or symptoms of complications such as fevers, chills, drainage from the incision, abdominal distention, nausea, vomiting, heavy vaginal bleeding, leg redness or swelling, chest pain, chest pressure, or shortness of breath.

CASE STUDY #13: WARREN ELLIS

REFERRING PHYSICIAN: Charles Craigen, MD

REASON FOR CONSULTATION: Evaluation and management of painful lymphadenitis.

Thank you for this infectious disease consultation.

(continued)

HISTORY OF PRESENT ILLNESS: The patient is a 41-year-old male who about 3 days prior to admission noticed what appeared to be a painful inguinal lymph node on the left that seemed to progressively increase in size. This started while on a business trip, but after he returned to work, he noticed it became a lot more tender and swollen. He finally presented to the emergency department after having a couple of days of onset of fever and was admitted for further evaluation. The patient on arrival did have a low-grade temperature of 100. He was started initially on Flagyl and Cipro, that was changed to doxycycline and Rocephin, and now he is on Zithromax, PO and vancomycin, IV.

The patient does not have any known infection as far as he knows. The patient has not had any exposure to tuberculosis, although he said that he has had weight loss and some night sweats, but this has only started since the onset of his symptoms about a week ago. He has not had any long-term weight loss or long-term night sweats or cough. The patient had traveled for that weekend prior to getting his onset of symptoms, but he did not do any camping. He does have two cats at home but no obvious cat bite or scratches as far as he knows. The patient has also been involved in a new sexual relationship about several months ago and has not had an HIV test recently. He had one 2 years ago that he reports was negative. No other history of sexually transmitted diseases to his knowledge.

REVIEW OF SYSTEMS: Unremarkable other than mentioned above. The patient had diarrhea 1 day prior to admission and currently still has diarrhea.

PAST MEDICAL HISTORY: Hypertension, history of kidney stones, depression, migraines.

PAST SURGICAL HISTORY: Cyst removed from the right leg.

ALLERGIES: No known allergies.

MEDICATIONS: List is currently reviewed and the antibiotics are listed above in the HPI.

SOCIAL HISTORY: The patient does not use tobacco, alcohol, or drugs. He is divorced from his first wife but is living with a new girlfriend. He has four children, all of whom live at home with him.

FAMILY HISTORY: Negative for immune dysfunction.

PHYSICAL EXAMINATION: General: The patient is alert and oriented and in no acute distress. He is afebrile. Temperature 96.5, pulse 70, respirations 19, and blood pressure 115/73. HEENT: Pupils are equal and reactive. Head is normocephalic and atraumatic. Sinuses are nontender. Oropharynx is clear without lesions. Neck: Supple without lymphadenopathy. Heart: Regular rate and rhythm. Lungs: Clear to auscultation bilaterally. Abdomen: Soft, nontender, and nondistended with no rebound or guarding. Good bowel sounds are heard. Genitourinary: The left groin reveals tender adenopathy. There is definite swelling and a mass felt in the left inguinal area. There is no obvious cut or scratches seen. The rest of the inguinal area appears fairly unremarkable without lesions or blisters seen. Lower extremities are without edema, clubbing, or cyanosis, and appeared normal. Skin: Reveals no rashes. Neurologic: Grossly nonfocal.

LABORATORY DATA: Laboratory data have been reviewed and showed an elevated white count of 16. There is a band neutrophilia of 27%. Liver function tests are unremarkable. Creatinine is normal. UA is unremarkable. Chlamydia and gonorrhea DNA probe are negative.

DIAGNOSTIC STUDIES: CT of the abdomen was done that was unremarkable. There is a nonspecific enlargement of a lymph node within the left inguinal region as seen on the CT of the pelvis.

IMPRESSION:

1. Painful lymph node lymphadenitis with a broad differential.

2. Diarrhea, which is new onset, right before admission.

DISCUSSION: The differential is broad. This could be suppurative bacterial process, which is usually due to staph and strep. It is less likely to be tularemia or Yersinia. We also need to consider fungal, TB, and sexually transmitted diseases including HIV. We also need to consider cat scratch disease.

RECOMMENDATIONS:

1. I will do a percutaneous biopsy of the inguinal mass.

2. We will order HIV antibody and quantitative viral load.

3. We will check Bartonella antibodies as well as *Chlamydia trachomatis* titers.

4. We will check PPD.

5. Check *Clostridium difficile* toxin.

6. Daptomycin antibiotic to replace the vancomycin.

We will continue to follow. Thank you for asking us to participate in this patient's care.

Code for the biopsy of the inguinal mass.

CASE STUDY #14: HILLARY ROMINEY

ORDERING PHYSICIAN: Harrison Brady, MD

DATE OF INTERPRETATION OF STUDY:

Echocardiogram was obtained for assessment of left ventricular function. The patient has been admitted with diagnosis of syncope. Overall, the study was suboptimal due to poor sonic window.

FINDINGS:

1. Aortic root appears normal.
2. Left atrium is mildly dilated. No gross intraluminal pathology is recognized, although subtle abnormalities could not be excluded. Right atrium is of normal dimension.
3. There is echo dropout of the interatrial septum. Atrial septal defects could not be excluded.
4. Right and left ventricles are normal in internal dimension. Overall left ventricular systolic function appears to be normal. Eyeball ejection fraction is around 55%. Again, due to poor sonic window, wall motion abnormalities in the distribution of lateral and apical wall could not be excluded.
5. Aortic valve is sclerotic with normal excursion. Color flow imaging and Doppler study demonstrate trace aortic regurgitation.
6. Mitral valve leaflets are also sclerotic with normal excursion. Color flow imaging and Doppler study demonstrate trace to mild degree of mitral regurgitation.
7. Tricuspid valve is delicate and opens normally. Pulmonic valve is not clearly seen. No evidence of pericardial effusion.

CONCLUSIONS:

1. Poor quality study.
2. Eyeball ejection fraction is 55%.
3. Trace to mild degree of mitral regurgitation.
4. Trace aortic regurgitation.

CASE STUDY #15: ELENA BEVERLY

DATE OF ADMISSION: 03/01/2026

DATE OF DISCHARGE: 03/09/2026

DISCHARGE DIAGNOSES:

AXIS I:

1. Bipolar disorder, depressed, with psychotic features, symptoms in remission.
2. Attention deficit hyperactivity disorder, symptoms in remission.

AXIS II: Deferred.

AXIS III: None.

AXIS IV: Moderate.

AXIS V: Global assessment of functioning 65 on discharge.

REASON FOR ADMISSION: The patient was admitted with a chief complaint of suicidal ideation. The patient was brought to the hospital after her guidance counselor found a note the patient wrote, which detailed to whom she was giving away her possessions when she dies. The patient told the counselor that she hears voices telling her to hurt herself and others. The patient reports over the last month these symptoms have exacerbated. The patient had a fight in school recently, which the patient blames on the voices. Three weeks ago, she got pushed into a corner at school and threatened to cut herself and others with a knife. The patient was suspended for that remark.

(continued)

PROCEDURES AND TREATMENT:

1. Individual cognitive and group psychotherapy.
2. Psychopharmacologic management.
3. Family therapy conducted by social work department with the patient and the patient's family for the purpose of education and discharge planning.

HOSPITAL COURSE: The patient responded well to individual and group psychotherapy, milieu therapy, and medication management. As stated, family therapy was conducted.

DISCHARGE ASSESSMENT: At the time of discharge, the patient is alert and fully oriented. Mood euthymic. Affect broad range. She denies any suicidal or homicidal ideation. IQ is at baseline. Memory intact. Insight and judgment good.

PLAN: The patient may be discharged as she no longer poses a risk of harm toward herself or others. The patient will continue on the following medications: Ritalin LA 60 mg q.a.m., Depakote 500 mg q.a.m. and 750 mg q.h.s., Abilify 20 mg q.h.s. Depakote level on date of discharge was 110. Liver enzymes drawn were within normal limits. The patient will follow up with Dr. Petrikas for medication management and Dr. Sanders for psychotherapy. All other discharge orders per the psychiatrist, as arranged by social work.

PART VI

REIMBURSEMENT, LEGAL, AND ETHICAL ISSUES

INTRODUCTION

A professional coding specialist's responsibilities may not stop when the last code is determined. Remember, the codes you determine are used on requests for payment, known as reimbursement claims. *Whenever money is involved, there are always legal and ethical issues attached, and you must familiarize yourself with all of the aspects for doing a complete and professional job for your facility, whether it is a small physician's office or a huge hospital. Understanding these components ensures that you will have a career draped in honesty, integrity, and success.*

40

Reimbursement

Key Terms

Automobile Insurance
Capitation Plans
Centers for Medicare & Medicaid Services (CMS)
Dependents
Diagnosis-Related Group (DRG)
Disability Compensation
Discounted FFS
Electronic Media Claim (EMC)
Electronic Remittance Advice (ERA)
Eligibility Verification
Episodic Care
Explanation of Benefits (EOB)
Fee-for-Service (FFS) Plans
Gatekeeper
Health Care
Health Maintenance Organization (HMO)
Insurance Premium
Liability Insurance
Managed Care
Point-of-Service (POS)
Preferred Provider Organization (PPO)
Remittance Advice (RA)
Third-Party Payer
Tracer
TriCare
Usual, Customary, and Reasonable (UCR)
Workers' Compensation

Learning Outcomes

After completing this chapter, the student should be able to:

LO 40.1 Define the role of health insurance and managed care plans in the delivery of health care services.
LO 40.2 Identify and define the types of health insurance plans.
LO 40.3 Explain the types of compensation used in health care reimbursement.
LO 40.4 Describe the information available for proper coding from NCCI edits and NCD and LCD.
LO 40.5 Utilize Place-of-Service and Type-of-Service codes as required.
LO 40.6 Create a system for organizing claims, understanding denials, and filing appeals.

40.1 The Role of Insurance in Health Care

A health insurance policy is a contractual agreement between an insurance carrier (company) and an individual related to health care issues. And the basis of this contract is risk. Insurance is just like gambling in Las Vegas. Basically, the insurance company is betting that a certain event will *not* happen to you, such as you getting sick. If that happens, it would have to pay your medical bills. On the other side of the table, you are betting (by paying an **insurance premium**) that you *will* have a major illness or health catastrophe. Think about it—if you knew for a fact that you would never get ill or have any injury, and would only have to go to the doctor for your annual checkups, would you pay all that money every month for insurance premiums? Of course not. You are betting that you will, at some point, get all that money back, when you need it to pay for some type of treatment.

When **managed care** was developed, the health insurance industry realized that it could lower its risk (and save money) if it could keep people healthy by encouraging them to go to the doctor for regular checkups, tests, and so forth. This thinking created a major change in the health insurance industry and in the medical care industry, increasing the focus of health care delivery to include preventive care, rather than only therapeutic (medical) care.

Medical care is the identification and treatment of illnesses and injuries—in other words, whatever a health care provider does to help you with a health problem or concern that you have (**Figure 40-1**).

Preventive care is provision of services designed to prevent the problem from manifesting (developing) or to discover it in early stages when it is more easily corrected. Preventive care includes well-baby visits (**Figure 40-2**), screenings, diagnostics, and routine checkups.

The term **health care** refers to a combination of these two types of services.

Insurance Premium
The amount of money, often paid monthly, by a policyholder or insured, to an insurance company to obtain coverage.

Managed Care
A type of health insurance coverage that controls the care of each subscriber (or insured person) by using a primary care provider as a central health care supervisor.

Health Care
The total management of an individual's well-being by a health care professional.

CODING BITES

Medical Care + Preventive Care = Health Care

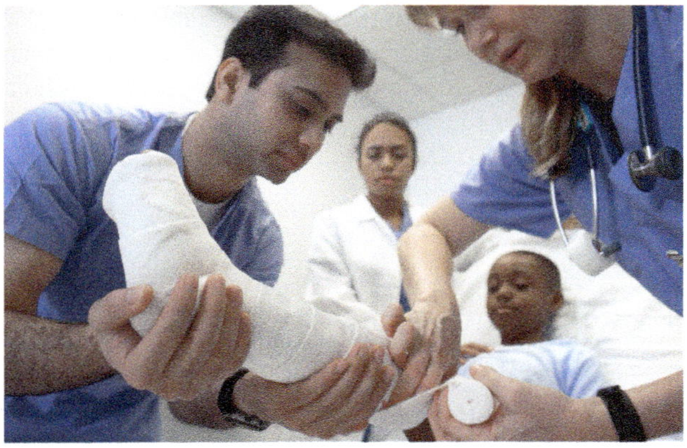

FIGURE 40-1 Treatment of a broken leg is an example of medical care

ERproductions Ltd/Blend Images LLC

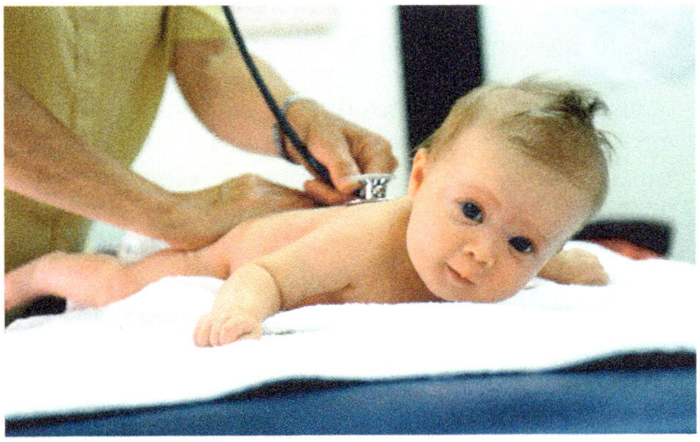

FIGURE 40-2 Well-baby visits are an example of preventive care

Pixtal/AGE Fotostock

EXAMPLES

Dr. Michaelson examines Paul and gives him a shot of antibiotics to help Paul get rid of an infection. The doctor has identified Paul's illness and is treating that illness. This is medical care.

Dr. Calavari knows Katrina works at a day care center and gives her a flu shot to help her avoid getting the flu. The doctor is preventing Katrina from becoming ill. This is preventive care.

We all know that every organization needs to have money coming in so that it can stay in business. The physician provides a service to his or her patients and expects to be paid for those services. That money is what keeps a practice open and allows it to pay your salary. If enough people don't pay their bills, then an office must lay off people (and that could mean you!). Or you might not be able to get that next raise, even if you deserve it.

By now, you understand how important all of this information is and how you have a personal stake in completing claim forms correctly. As you transfer information from patient registration forms and other documents, be certain to

- Double-check your work to make sure it is accurate.
- Confirm that the form is completely filled out, with no necessary information missing.
- Verify the spelling of every name and the accuracy of every number.

It all must be absolutely correct.

> **CODING BITES**
>
> The process of getting information and submitting claims to the third-party payer is key to the survival of your health care facility and all the people it employs.

Most third-party payers, including Medicare, prefer claim forms to be submitted electronically. An **electronic media claim (EMC)**, also called an electronic claim, is evaluated more quickly than a print claim form. Accepted claims are paid faster. Years ago, it was not unusual for health care facilities to wait 4 to 6 months to receive payment from an insurance company. With electronic claims, this time has been reduced to 2 to 3 weeks.

Electronic Media Claim (EMC)
A health care claim form that is transmitted electronically.

Increased use of technology in this process also means that there is an excellent chance a computer will be reviewing your claim form. During the initial processing of a claim you have sent, the computer will only compare letter to letter and number to number, looking for an exact match to the letters and numbers in its files. Then, claims with errors, such as invalid policy numbers or missing information, will be rejected and returned to you.

EXAMPLE

The computer cannot scan your claim form and say, "Oh, I can see this is a typo. They really meant to put a *W* instead of a *U*." No, all the computer knows is that the letter is supposed to be a *U* and it is not. And the claim will be rejected.

Third-Party Payer
An individual or organization that is not directly involved in an encounter but has a connection because of its obligation to pay, in full or part, for that encounter.

CODING BITES

Party #1: The health care provider

Party #2: The patient

Party #3: The insurance carrier

The Participants

Essentially, there are three participants in each health care encounter, or visit:

1. The physician or health care provider.
2. The patient–the person seeking services.
3. The insurance carrier covering the costs of health care activities for the patient.

Some people get their health insurance policies through a program at their place of employment, some through the government, and others directly with the insurance carriers as individual policyholders. It doesn't matter very much to the health care facility. In any case, a **third-party payer** will pay, in part, the patient's bills for services that your facility will provide. Health insurance carriers are often referred to as third-party payers. This means that someone not directly involved in the health care relationship is paying for the service. The health care provider is party #1, the patient is party #2, and the insurance carrier is party #3–the third party. Therefore, the insurance company is the third-party payer.

The Role of AI in Health Insurance

The implementation of artificial intelligence (AI) is growing in many different industries, including health care and health insurance. According to two surveys conducted within the health insurance industry, approximately 79% of these third-party payers are either currently using AI, planning to use AI, or plan to investigate the use of AI and ML (machine learning) in their day-to-day operations.

Health Maintenance Organization (HMO)
A type of health insurance that uses a primary care physician, also known as a gatekeeper, to manage all health care services for an individual.

Gatekeeper
A physician, typically a family practitioner or an internist, who serves as the primary care physician for an individual. This physician is responsible for evaluating and determining the course of treatment or services, as well as for deciding whether or not a specialist should be involved in care.

CODING BITES

HMOs use a "home base" concept, with a primary care physician (PCP), also known as the gatekeeper, serving as the central base to supervise each individual's health care.

Many third-party payers are already using AI as they automate claims processing, having these computer programs review each claim as it is submitted. It is natural to understand that these companies also use AI to prevent and detect fraudulent claims as well as early identification of those who attempt to abuse the system. Plus, providers get the benefit as requests for prior authorizations are made easier using the third-party payer website which activates AI. This software will evaluate the information submitted and the policy coverage details to determine which procedures for which beneficiaries are approved. This has been shown to smooth this process and issue approvals quicker.

The future of healthcare is woven with computer software programs, such as AI and ML, to support more efficient and effective delivery of healthcare.

40.2 Types of Insurance Plans

There are many types of health plans that people may purchase, or contract for, with companies that specialize in insurance.

Health Maintenance Organization (HMO)

In a **health maintenance organization (HMO)**, members, also called enrollees, prepay for health care services. The members are encouraged to get preventive treatment to promote wellness (and keep medical costs down). In addition, each member has a primary care physician (PCP), also known as a **gatekeeper**. The PCP is responsible for monitoring the individual's well-being and making all decisions regarding care. It is the PCP who determines if a specialist is required for a certain evaluation or procedure. When this occurs, it is the PCP who is responsible for completing the patient referral form and getting approval from the HMO for the patient to visit the specialist. Generally, HMOs do not require a patient to satisfy a deductible before benefits begin. (See the section ***Patient/Beneficiary Out-of-Pocket Contributions*** later in this chapter.)

Preferred Provider Organization (PPO)

In a **preferred provider organization (PPO)**, physicians, hospitals, and other health care providers join together and agree to offer services to members of a group (often called subscribers) at a lower cost or discount. These plans usually permit the individual subscriber (the patient) to choose the physician or specialist to see, with a discount for staying in the network by using a physician who is a member of the plan. If the individual chooses a physician who does not belong to the network, or is not participating with that PPO, the individual will pay a penalty or receive less of a discount in the cost of those services. This can give the individual more control over his or her health care. It can save time and money, as well.

Preferred Provider Organization (PPO)
A type of health insurance coverage in which physicians provide health care services to members of the plan at a discount.

Some PPO plans require the patient to satisfy a deductible first before benefits begin. (See the section ***Patient/Beneficiary Out-of-Pocket Contributions*** later in this chapter.) Typically, a higher deductible will translate into a lower monthly premium for this type of insurance coverage.

EXAMPLE

If a person covered under a PPO plan is having problems sneezing and knows the problem is his or her allergies, the individual can choose an allergist—a provider who specializes in the treatment of allergies—from the PPO network without having to go to his or her primary care physician for a referral. If the plan were an HMO, the person would have to make an appointment with the PCP first in order to get the referral to the allergist. Then, the person could make an appointment to see the allergist.

CODING BITES

PPOs typically **P**ermit the **P**atient to **O**pt (or choose) his or her physician or specialist.

Point-of-Service (POS) Plan

Giving individuals a little more flexibility, a **point-of-service (POS)** plan is almost a combination of an HMO and a PPO. Each insured person has a primary care physician (PCP) and a list of providers that participate in the HMO. When health care providers within the HMO network are used, the insured pays only a regular copayment amount or a small charge. There is no deductible or co-insurance payment involved. However, this plan may also include a self-referral option, in which the individual insured can choose to go to an out-of-network provider. In that case, the individual may be responsible for paying both a deductible and a co-insurance payment.

Point-of-Service (POS)
A type of insurance plan that will allow an HMO enrollee to choose his or her own nonmember physician at a lower benefit rate, costing the patient more money out-of-pocket.

CODING BITES

POS plans combine features of an HMO and a PPO.

Federal Government Plans

Centers for Medicare & Medicaid Services (CMS)

In 1977, the Health Care Financing Administration (HCFA, pronounced hic-fah) was created to coordinate federal health services programs. On July 1, 2001, HCFA became the **Centers for Medicare & Medicaid Services (CMS)**. Many health care professionals still refer to this agency as "HicFah" and to the CMS-1500 claim form as the "HicFah 1500." Old habits take a while to change. At least you now understand that these two acronyms refer to the same federal organization.

Centers for Medicare & Medicaid Services (CMS)
The agency under the Department of Health and Human Services (DHHS) in charge of regulation and control over services for those covered by Medicare and Medicaid.

Medicare is a national health insurance program that pays, or reimburses, for health care services provided to those over the age of 65 (see **Figure 40-3**). In addition, this plan may cover individuals who are under the age of 65 and are permanently disabled (such as the blind), as well as those with end-stage renal disease (ESRD) who are suffering from permanent kidney failure and require either dialysis or a kidney transplant.

Medicaid is a plan that pays for, or reimburses, medical assistance and health care services for people who are indigent (low-income) (see **Figure 40-4**). The program is jointly funded

CODING BITES

Medica**RE** = **RE**tired people (who are over the age of 65)

Medica**ID** = **I**n**D**igent, or low-income, individuals

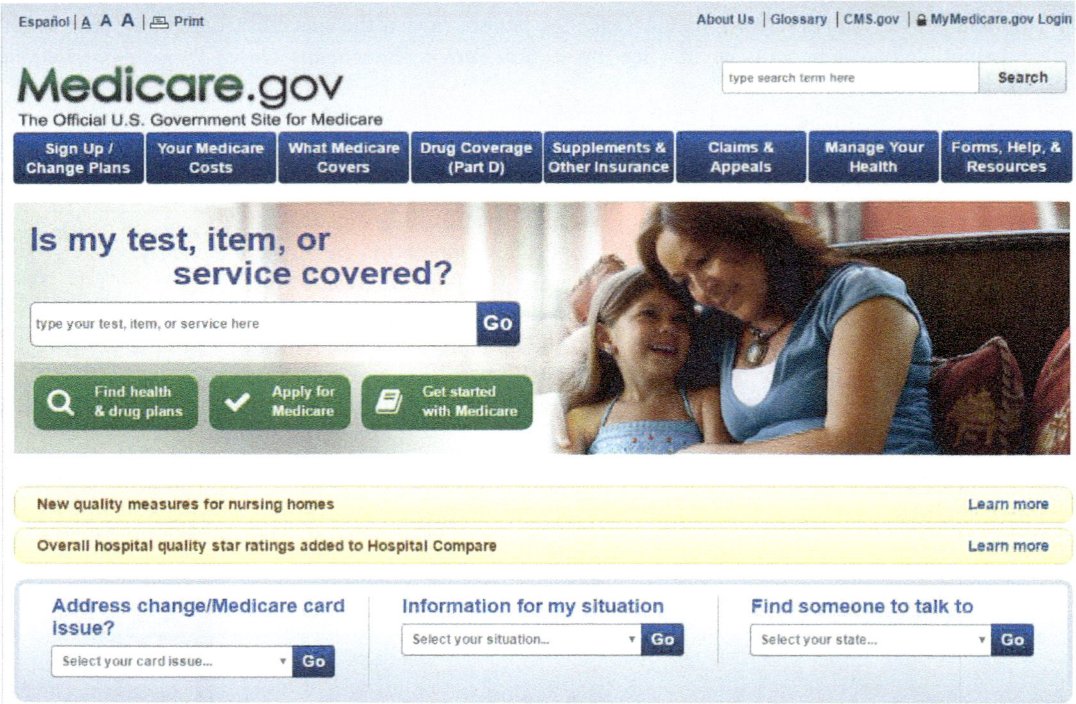

FIGURE 40-3 Medicare.gov, the official U.S. government site for Medicare

Source: Medicare.gov

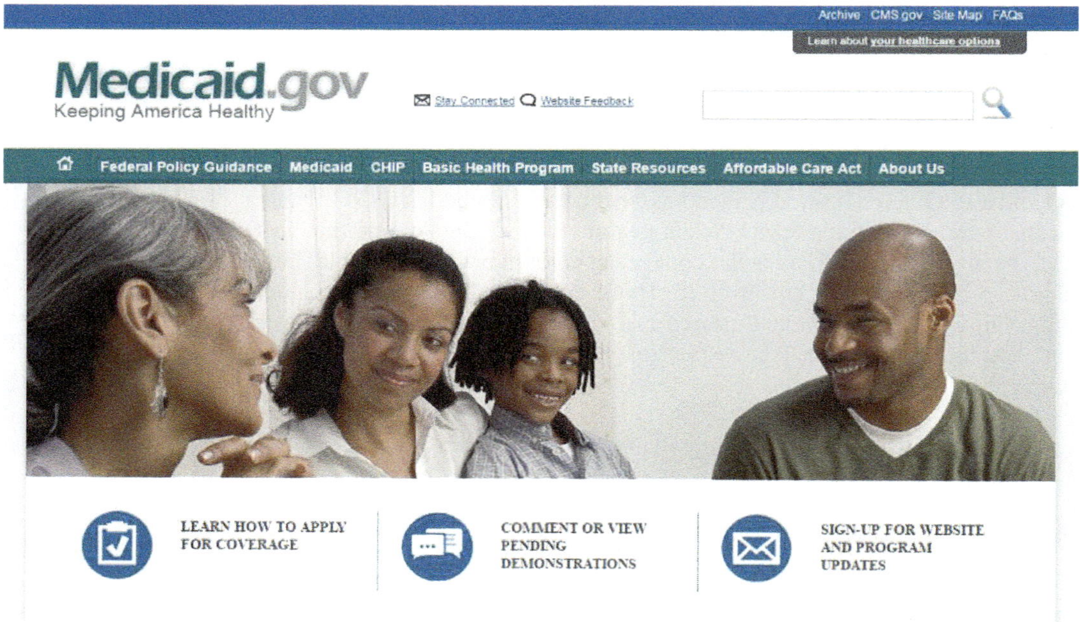

FIGURE 40-4 Medicaid.gov, the official U.S. government website of Medicaid

Source: Medicaid.gov

by the federal and state governments. Each state government then administers its own plan. This means that each state determines who is eligible and what services are covered. It is important to know that each state has its own requirements, in case you have a patient that has just moved to your state. Each state may even have a unique name or term for its program. For example, in California the program is called Medi-Cal.

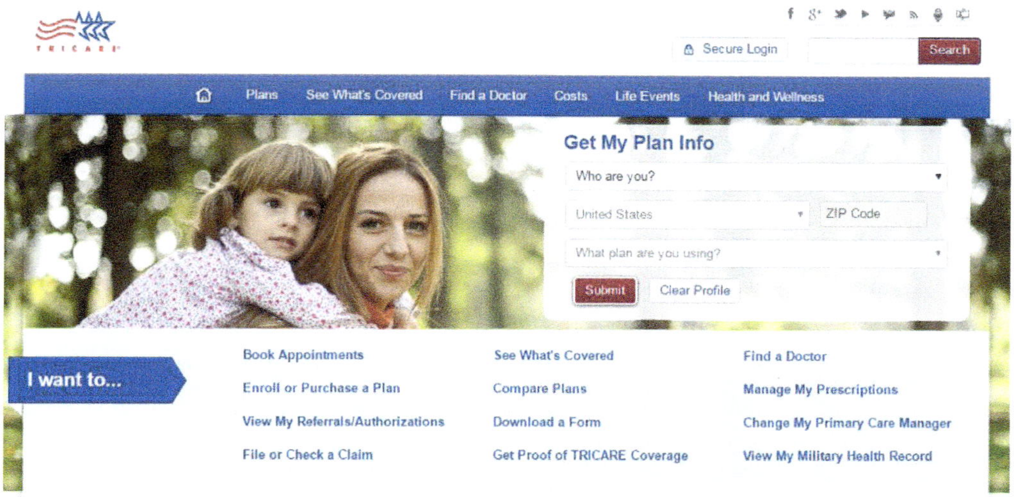

FIGURE 40-5 TriCare.mil, the official U.S. government website of TRICARE

Source: Tricare.mil

TriCare

TriCare offers the most common health care plans you will encounter when caring for individuals in the military and their families (see **Figure 40-5**). This program was formerly known as CHAMPUS.

TriCare
A government health plan that covers medical expenses for the dependents of active-duty service members, CHAMPUS-eligible retirees and their families, and the dependents of deceased active-duty members.

TriCare was created to help the following individuals receive better access to improved health care services:

- Active-duty service members (ADSM), also known as sponsors.
- The **dependents** (spouses and children) of ADSMs.
- Surviving spouses and surviving children of deceased ADSMs.
- Retired service members, their spouses, and their children.
- Surviving spouses and children of deceased retired members.

Dependents
Individuals who are supported, either financially or with regard to insurance coverage, by others.

TriCare was created to provide health care benefits for the dependents of those serving in the uniformed services and retirees. ADSMs are those from any of the seven uniformed services, including the U.S. military (the Army, Navy, Air Force, Marine Corps, and Coast Guard), as well as those serving in the Public Health Service, National Guard and Reserve, and the National Oceanic and Atmospheric Administration (NOAA). Eligibility for TriCare is determined by the services, and information is maintained in the Defense Enrollment Eligibility Reporting System (DEERS).

Other Insurance Plans

Workers' compensation is an insurance program designed to pay the medical costs for treating those injured, or made ill, at their place of work or by their job. This includes injuries resulting from a fall off a ladder while performing a job-related task, getting hurt in an accident while driving a company car on a business trip, or developing a lung disorder caused by toxic fumes in the office. Generally, a workers' compensation plan covers only specific medical bills, such as laboratory bills, physicians' fees, and other medical services. Most often, lost income is not covered by this policy. Each state oversees the workers' compensation contracts with particular insurance carriers.

Workers' Compensation
An insurance program that covers medical care for those injured or for those who become ill as a consequence of their employment.

Disability compensation is an insurance plan that reimburses disabled individuals for a percentage of what they used to earn each month. This plan does not pay physicians' bills or for therapy treatments. A disability plan only provides insureds with money to replace a portion of their lost paycheck because they are unable to work. Disability payments might come through a federal government agency such as the Social Security Administration, or patients may have a private insurance plan (such as AFLAC).

Disability Compensation
A plan that reimburses a covered individual a portion of his or her income that is lost as a result of being unable to work due to illness or injury.

YOU INTERPRET IT!

Joe Hines works as an electrician for a small company. One day, he falls off a ladder at work and injures his back severely. He is taken to the emergency room by ambulance, and the attending physician orders x-rays and a CT scan. The tests confirm that Joe's spine is broken in two places and a cast is applied around Joe's entire torso. After a week in the hospital, Joe is discharged. The physician's discharge orders state that Joe is to stay in bed for 7 months, in traction, while the fracture heals. A home health agency is contracted to provide a trained health care professional to go to Joe's house to care for him and attend to his needs around the clock.

1. In this scenario, what type of insurance will be responsible for the payment of each of Joe's expenses due to this accident?

Liability Insurance
A policy that covers loss or injury to a third party caused by the insured or something belonging to the insured.

Automobile Insurance
Auto accident liability coverage will pay for medical bills, lost wages, and compensation for pain and suffering for any person injured by the insured in an auto accident.

Liability insurance is commonly part of a person's homeowners or business owners insurance. This type of policy covers losses to a third party caused by the insured or something owned by the insured. In other words, the insurance company will pay for, or reimburse for, any harm or damage done to someone else (not a member of the household or the business).

Automobile insurance might become an issue for your office if you treat someone for an injury that was caused by the individual's involvement in an automobile accident. Full-coverage automobile policies usually include liability insurance that covers these expenses.

YOU INTERPRET IT!

Sarah goes over to Margaret's house for dinner. After a delicious meal, Sarah walks toward the door to leave and go home. As she turns to say goodnight to Margaret, Sarah trips and falls. Margaret calls the paramedics, and, at the hospital, the x-rays ordered by the attending physician confirm that Sarah has indeed broken her wrist. A cast is applied, and Sarah is sent home with a prescription for pain medication. The attending physician advises Sarah to see her primary care physician in 1 week for a follow-up.

2. What type of insurance will cover Sarah's medical expenses?

YOU INTERPRET IT!

Kyle, a fifth-grade student, slipped down the stairs at school. Typically, the school's liability policy would cover the damage, or medical expenses. The school is the insured, and the student is the third party.

3. If a faculty member and a student are walking through the cafeteria of the school and both slip and fall, what types of policies will cover any injuries that might be caused by the fall?

CODING BITES

And you need these details for determining the external cause codes, too!

Details Are Required

As you can see from all this information, different types of insurance policies might be responsible for an individual's medical treatment. Therefore, in your job as medical insurance coder/biller, you must make certain that if an individual comes to the provider for treatment for an *injury* (rather than an *illness*), you must find out the *details* of how and where the injury occurred. This will help determine which carrier will cover the charges.

40.3 Methods of Compensation

There are several payment plans that insurance carriers (third-party payers) use to pay physicians and other health care providers for their services.

Fee-for-Service (FFS) Plans

In **fee-for-service (FFS) plans**, the insurance company pays the health care provider for each individual service supplied to the patient, as reported by the procedure codes listed on the claim, according to an agreed-upon price list (also known as a fee schedule). When the physician's office agrees to participate in the plan, it is also agreeing to provide services and accept the amount of money indicated on that schedule for each of those services. This is like going to a restaurant with an à la carte menu. The menu lists a price for each item: the salad, the roast beef, the apple pie. The restaurant accepts the amount of money the guest pays for each item received. Different plans may pay different amounts of money for one particular service, just as different restaurants may charge different amounts for a similar dish.

Fee-for-Service (FFS) Plans
Payment agreements that outline, in a written fee schedule, exactly how much money the insurance carrier will pay the physician for each treatment and/or service provided.

Sometimes, when one insurance carrier pays a provider at a lower rate than other carriers, it is referred to as a **discounted FFS**. In a typical discounted FFS, the payments are reduced from the physician's regular rate. This is similar to the discount you might get at a store when showing your student ID card–you get a discount because you are a member of the school.

Discounted FFS
An extra reduction in the rate charged to an insurer for services provided by the physician to the plan's members.

EXAMPLE

Three people, each with a different insurance carrier, go to the same physician for a flu shot (injection). Insurance carrier #1 has agreed to pay the physician $20 for giving the injection. Insurance carrier #2 has agreed to pay the physician $22.50, and insurance carrier #3 has agreed to pay the physician $18 for the same injection. Your office should charge all patients the same amount. This is known as the *charged amount*. However, insurance carriers working with your office on a fee-for-service contract will pay only the amount stated on their fee schedule. That's all they will pay and no more. This is called the *allowed amount*.

Capitation Plans
Agreements between a physician and a managed care organization that pay the physician a predetermined amount of money each month for each member of the plan who identifies that provider as his or her primary care physician.

CODING BITES

CAPitation plans pay by the *cap*. One cap goes on one head, and the insurance carrier is going to pay the physician for each cap, or head–that is, per person.

Capitation Plans

With **capitation plans**, the insurance company pays the physician a fixed amount of money for every individual covered by that plan (often called members or subscribers) being seen by that physician. Physicians get this amount of money every month, as long as they are listed as the physician of record (primary care physician (PCP)) for that individual. Whether the insured person goes to see that physician once, three times, or not at all during a particular month, the physician's office will be paid the same amount. This plan is like the dinner special at your local restaurant. You pay one price, which includes soup, salad, all-you-can-eat entrée, and dessert. If you don't eat your soup, you do not pay any less; if you get seconds on the entrée, you do not pay any more.

Episodic Care

An **episodic care** agreement between insurer and physician means the provider is paid one flat fee for the expected course of treatment for a particular injury or illness. This is like the meal deal of health care. One package price includes all of the services and treatments necessary for the proper care of the patient's condition in accordance with the accepted standards of care.

Episodic Care
An insurance company pays a provider one flat fee to cover the entire course of treatment for an individual's condition.

EXAMPLE

Audrey Callahan fell off her bicycle and broke her arm. The x-ray shows that it is a simple, clean fracture, and the physician applies a cast. The doctor schedules a follow-up appointment for her and expects that she will not need much other attention until the cast comes off in 6 weeks. At that time, an x-ray will confirm that the fracture has healed properly and the cast will be removed. This entire sequence of events, and treatment, is very predictable for a routine simple fracture. Therefore, the insurance company has agreed to pay the physician one flat fee for this event, rather than having the physician's office file a claim for each procedure and service individually: the first encounter; the first x-ray; the application of the cast; the follow-up encounter; the last encounter; the last x-ray; and removal of the cast.

Audrey Callahan's physician is being reimbursed under an episodic care agreement with the insurance carrier.

Diagnosis-Related Group (DRG)
An episodic care payment system basing reimbursement to hospitals for inpatient services upon standards of care for specific diagnoses grouped by their similar usage of resources for procedures, services, and treatments.

Diagnosis-related groups (DRGs) are a type of episodic care payment plan used by Medicare to pay for treatments and services provided to beneficiaries who have been admitted into an acute care hospital (inpatients). DRGs are categorized by the principal (first-listed) diagnosis code and take into consideration elements such as the patient's age and gender and the presence of any complications or manifestations (additional diagnoses or conditions). You read more about DRGs in the chapter titled ***Inpatient (Hospital) Diagnosis Coding***.

The CMS Transforming Episode Accountability Model (TEAM)

Beginning on January 1, 2026, there is a new mandatory episodic (bundled) payment model, titled CMS Transforming Episode Accountability Model (TEAM), that will directly focus on hospitals (acute care facilities) ensuring their responsibility for follow-up when caring for patients covered by Original Medicare. The intent of this program looks at the 30-day period after discharge, starting with post-care coordination and transition of care for those patients having one of these five procedures:

- Coronary Artery Bypass Graft (CABG) surgery
- Major Bowel Surgery
- Lower Extremity Joint Replacement (LEJR) surgery
- Surgical Hip and Femur Fracture Treatment (SHFFT)
- Spinal fusion surgery

Included is the requirement for a referral to a primary care provider confirming continuity of care and thereby encompassing Medicare Parts A and B services as they relate to the complete post-operative care of this patient. This TEAM model has been structured based on evidence leading to improved healthcare outcomes.

You, as the medical coding professional, will confirm participation using MS-DRG and CPT (HCPCS) code assignments:

All participants are accountable for all episode categories unsess an exclusion applies.

Episode Category	MS-DRG and/or HCPCS codes
CABG (inpatient)	MS-DRG: 231, 232, 233, 234, 235, 236
Major Bowel Procedure (inpatient)	MS-DRG: 329, 330, 331
LEJR (inpatient/outpatient)	MS-DRG: 469, 470, 521, 522 HCPCS: 27447, 27130, 27702
SHFFT (inpatient)	MS-DRG: 480, 481, 482
Spinal Fusion (inpatient/outpatient)	MS-DRG: 402, 426, 427, 428, 429, 430, 447, 448, 450, 451, 471, 472, 473 HCPCS: 22551, 22554, 22612, 22630, 22633

Source: https://www.cms.gov/priorities/innovation/innovation-models/team-model

Patient/Beneficiary Out-of-Pocket Contributions

Patients with insurance policies often contribute to reimbursing providers for their health care services, in addition to paying monthly premiums. The following are the most common methods used for the individual's payments:

Usual, Customary, and Reasonable (UCR)
The process of determining a fee for a service by evaluating the *usual* fee charged by the provider, the *customary* fee charged by most physicians in the same community or geographical area, and what is considered *reasonable* by most health care professionals under the specific circumstances of the situation.

1. *Copayment (also known as the copay).* The copayment is usually a fixed amount of money that the individual will pay each time he or she goes to a health care provider. It may be $10, $15, $20, or more. Each policy is different. As a matter of fact, the copay on the same policy for the same patient may be different, depending on whether this is a visit to a family physician, a specialist, or the hospital.
2. *Co-insurance.* Co-insurance is different from the copayment because it is based on a percentage of the total charge rather than a fixed amount. The percentage that the patient pays is most often calculated on the **usual, customary, and reasonable (UCR)** charge that has been determined for this type of visit or procedure. Frequently, the individual is required to pay 20% of the total allowed amount by the physician or facility, but that might differ for various types of policies and carriers.
3. *Deductible.* This is the amount of money that patients must pay, out of their own pockets, before the insurance benefits begin. The deductible might be as little as $250 or as much as $1,000 or more. Patients have to pay the total amount until they have paid the whole deductible for that calendar year. After that, they will usually pay just the copayment and/or the co-insurance amount.

CODING BITES

The various amounts for the copay, the co-insurance, and the deductible are good examples of why it is so essential that you contact the insurance carrier for every patient to verify the patient's coverage and eligibility for certain procedures and treatments and to see if the deductible has been met for the year.

MACRA

Medicare Access and CHIP Reauthorization Act (MACRA) was designed to reward health care providers for quality patient care and to ultimately reduce costs. As a part of this, the Quality Payment Program also was implemented. This program incorporates important advances to ensure that electronic health information will be available when and where clinicians need it so optimal care can be provided.

The Quality Payment Program includes two paths:

- Advanced Alternative Payment Models (APMs)
- Merit-Based Incentive Payment System (MIPS)

Both of these paths require use of certified EHR technology to exchange information across providers and with patients to support improved care delivery, including patient engagement and care coordination. In addition, this program requires EHR manufacturers to publish application programming interfaces (API), which increase interoperability (making it easier for software programs such as smartphone apps to access information from other programs) for certified health IT.

Physicians have options and began participating in this program back in 2017.

40.4 NCCI Edits and NCD/LCD

National Correct Coding Initiative (NCCI)

The CMS developed the National Correct Coding Initiative (NCCI) to reinforce accurate and proper coding in addition to preventing reimbursement of inaccurate amounts as the result of noncompliance coding methods in Part B claims (physician and outpatient services). This system was founded with coding policies based on

- The official coding guidelines, as published in the American Medical Association's CPT code book.
- National (NCD) and local (LCD) policies and edits.
- Coding guidelines developed by national societies.
- Analysis of standard medical and surgical practices.
- Review of current coding practices.

There are two types of edits within the NCCI focus: PTP and MUE.

Procedure-to-Procedure (PTP) Edits

Within the long lists of procedures, services, and treatments performed by health care providers, there are those that cannot, or should not, be provided to the same patient on the same date of service. CMS computers evaluate submitted claims to look for pairs of codes being reported that are known to be mutually exclusive procedures, also known as procedure-to-procedure (PTP) edits.

EXAMPLE

23680 Open treatment of shoulder dislocation, with surgical or anatomical neck fracture, with manipulation

20690 Application of a uniplane (pins or wires in 1 plane), unilateral, external fixation system

These codes report two procedures that would not be performed at the same time for the same patient, according to the standards of care. This is an example of a PTP edit.

Medically Unlikely Edits (MUE)

The purpose of the NCCI medically unlikely edits (MUE) is to prevent improper payments when services are reported with incorrect units of service. An MUE for an HCPCS/CPT code is the maximum units of service that a provider would report under most circumstances for a single beneficiary on a single date of service.

EXAMPLE

72270 Myelography, 2 or more regions, radiological supervision and interpretation

The MUE edit for this code is a maximum of one for a patient per date of service because the code description states "two or more." Therefore, reporting this code more than once for the same patient on the same date would not be accurate.

National Coverage Determinations (NCD) and Local Coverage Determinations (LCD)

CODING BITES

Submitting a claim for a service or item not covered by the patient's policy is considered fraud . . . even if it gets paid. It is your responsibility to know! Not the patient. Not the doctor. You, the professional coding specialist.

In some circumstances, a National Coverage Determination (NCD) is created to clearly establish the criteria for coverage of an item or service applicable to all Medicare beneficiaries nationwide. When there is no NCD, there may be a Local Coverage Determination (LCD) in effect. An LCD is a decision by a fiscal intermediary (FI) or carrier as to when and for what reasons a particular service or item is covered in that area (a state or region). The Medicare Coverage Database (MCD), available at https://www.cms.gov (see **Figure 40-6**), contains all NCDs and LCDs in a searchable database.

Virtually all third-party payers issue coverage determinations valid nationally or in a particular state or locale. Therefore, you should have the ability to verify coverage for an item or service *prior* to providing it, and certainly before creating and submitting the claim.

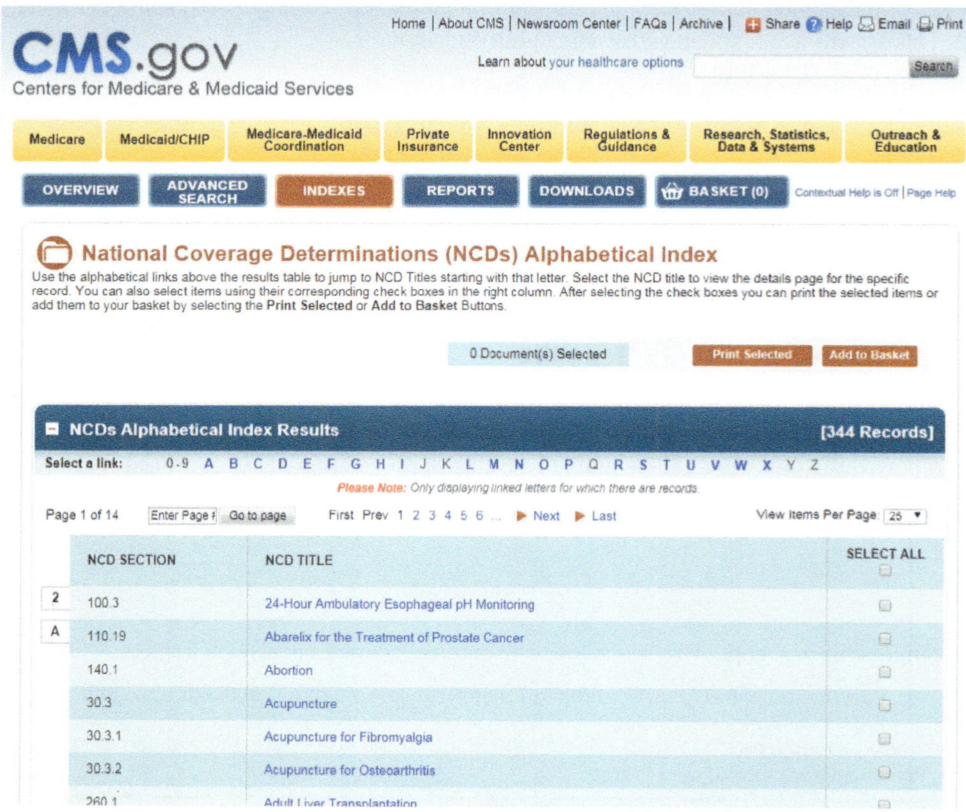

FIGURE 40-6 National Coverage Determinations (NCDs) Alphabetic Index

Source: CMS.gov

Once you find a coverage determination on the service or item the physician wants to provide to the patient, you can obtain the details about the criteria for coverage. In this Medicare NCD on Adult Liver Transplantation (**Figure 40-7**), the procedure would be categorized (**Benefit Category**) as an Inpatient Hospital Service. Next, the section **Item/Service Description** is provided to ensure that everyone understands precisely what procedure, service, or item is being discussed. Read further down the page to the section **Indications and Limitations of Coverage: B. Nationally Covered Indications** and you can see the diagnoses considered as medically necessary for this procedure. Earlier in this text, you learned about medical necessity in the chapter ***Introduction to the Languages of Coding***. The next section clarifies what types of **Follow-Up Care** will be covered, as well.

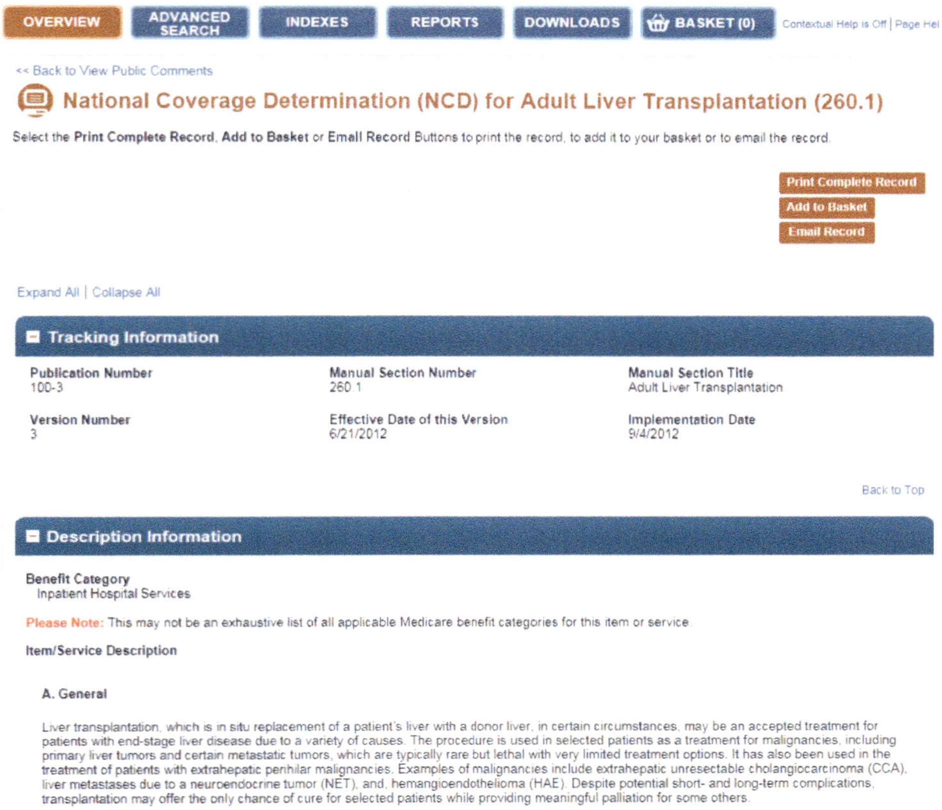
OVERVIEW | ADVANCED SEARCH | INDEXES | REPORTS | DOWNLOADS | BASKET (0) | Contextual Help is Off | Page Hel

<< Back to View Public Comments

National Coverage Determination (NCD) for Adult Liver Transplantation (260.1)

Select the **Print Complete Record**, **Add to Basket** or **Email Record** Buttons to print the record, to add it to your basket or to email the record.

Print Complete Record
Add to Basket
Email Record

Expand All | Collapse All

Tracking Information

Publication Number	Manual Section Number	Manual Section Title
100-3	260.1	Adult Liver Transplantation
Version Number	**Effective Date of this Version**	**Implementation Date**
3	6/21/2012	9/4/2012

Back to Top

Description Information

Benefit Category
Inpatient Hospital Services

Please Note: This may not be an exhaustive list of all applicable Medicare benefit categories for this item or service.

Item/Service Description

A. General

Liver transplantation, which is in situ replacement of a patient's liver with a donor liver, in certain circumstances, may be an accepted treatment for patients with end-stage liver disease due to a variety of causes. The procedure is used in selected patients as a treatment for malignancies, including primary liver tumors and certain metastatic tumors, which are typically rare but lethal with very limited treatment options. It has also been used in the treatment of patients with extrahepatic perihilar malignancies. Examples of malignancies include extrahepatic unresectable cholangiocarcinoma (CCA), liver metastases due to a neuroendocrine tumor (NET), and, hemangioendothelioma (HAE). Despite potential short- and long-term complications, transplantation may offer the only chance of cure for selected patients while providing meaningful palliation for some others.

FIGURE 40-7 NCD for Adult Liver Transplantation (in part)

Source: CMS.gov

GUIDANCE CONNECTION

Go to the **Medicare Coverage Database**:

https://www.cms.gov/medicare-coverage-database/search.aspx

On the right side is the Quick Search bar to sort through all National Coverage Determinations (NCDs) and Local Coverage Determinations (LCDs).

40.5 Place-of-Service and Type-of-Service Codes

Place-of-Service Codes

Place-of-Service (POS) codes are used on professional claims to identify the specific location where procedures, services, and treatments were provided to the patient.

Place of Service Code(s)	Place of Service Name	Place of Service Description
01	Pharmacy	A facility or location where drugs and other medically related items and services are sold, dispensed, or otherwise provided directly to patients.
02	Telehealth	The location where health services and health-related services are provided or received, through a telecommunication system.
03	School	A facility whose primary purpose is education.
04	Homeless Shelter	A facility or location whose primary purpose is to provide temporary housing to homeless individuals (e.g., emergency shelters, individual or family shelters).
05	Indian Health Service Free-Standing Facility	A facility or location, owned and operated by the Indian Health Service, that provides diagnostic, therapeutic (surgical and nonsurgical), and rehabilitation services to American Indians and Alaska Natives who do not require hospitalization.
06	Indian Health Service Provider-Based Facility	A facility or location, owned and operated by the Indian Health Service, that provides diagnostic, therapeutic (surgical and nonsurgical), and rehabilitation services rendered by, or under the supervision of, physicians to American Indians and Alaska Natives admitted as inpatients or outpatients.
07	Tribal 638 Free-Standing Facility	A facility or location, owned and operated by a federally recognized American Indian or Alaska Native tribe or tribal organization under a 638 agreement, that provides diagnostic, therapeutic (surgical and nonsurgical), and rehabilitation services to tribal members who do not require hospitalization.
08	Tribal 638 Provider-Based Facility	A facility or location, owned and operated by a federally recognized American Indian or Alaska Native tribe or tribal organization under a 638 agreement, that provides diagnostic, therapeutic (surgical and nonsurgical), and rehabilitation services to tribal members admitted as inpatients or outpatients.
09	Prison/ Correctional Facility	A prison, jail, reformatory, work farm, detention center, or any other similar facility maintained by federal, state, or local authorities for the purpose of confinement or rehabilitation of adult or juvenile criminal offenders.
10	Unassigned	N/A
11	Office	Location, other than a hospital, skilled nursing facility (SNF), military treatment facility, community health center, state or local public health clinic, or intermediate care facility (ICF), where the health professional routinely provides health examinations, diagnosis, and treatment of illness or injury on an ambulatory basis.
12	Home	Location, other than a hospital or other facility, where the patient receives care in a private residence.
13	Assisted Living Facility	Congregate residential facility with self-contained living units providing assessment of each resident's needs and on-site support 24 hours a day, 7 days a week, with the capacity to deliver or arrange for services including some health care and other services.
14	Group Home	A residence, with shared living areas, where clients receive supervision and other services such as social and/or behavioral services, custodial service, and minimal services (e.g., medication administration).
15	Mobile Unit	A facility/unit that moves from place-to-place equipped to provide preventive, screening, diagnostic, and/or treatment services.
16	Temporary Lodging	A short-term accommodation such as a hotel, camp ground, hostel, cruise ship, or resort where the patient receives care, and that is not identified by any other POS code.
17	Walk-in Retail Health Clinic	A walk-in health clinic, other than an office, urgent care facility, pharmacy, or independent clinic and not described by any other Place-of-Service code, that is located within a retail operation and provides, on an ambulatory basis, preventive and primary care services.
18	Place of Employment-Worksite	A location, not described by any other POS code, owned or operated by a public or private entity where the patient is employed, and where a health professional provides ongoing or episodic occupational medical, therapeutic, or rehabilitative services to the individual.

(continued)

Place of Service Code(s)	Place of Service Name	Place of Service Description
19	Off-Campus Outpatient Hospital	A portion of an off-campus hospital provider-based department that provides diagnostic, therapeutic (both surgical and nonsurgical), and rehabilitation services to sick or injured persons who do not require hospitalization or institutionalization.
20	Urgent Care Facility	Location, distinct from a hospital emergency room, an office, or a clinic, whose purpose is to diagnose and treat illness or injury for unscheduled, ambulatory patients seeking immediate medical attention.
21	Inpatient Hospital	A facility, other than psychiatric, that primarily provides diagnostic, therapeutic (both surgical and nonsurgical), and rehabilitation services by, or under, the supervision of physicians to patients admitted for a variety of medical conditions.
22	On-Campus Outpatient Hospital	A portion of a hospital's main campus that provides diagnostic, therapeutic (both surgical and nonsurgical), and rehabilitation services to sick or injured persons who do not require hospitalization or institutionalization.
23	Emergency Room—Hospital	A portion of a hospital where emergency diagnosis and treatment of illness or injury is provided.
24	Ambulatory Surgical Center	A free-standing facility, other than a physician's office, where surgical and diagnostic services are provided on an ambulatory basis.
25	Birthing Center	A facility, other than a hospital's maternity facilities or a physician's office, that provides a setting for labor, delivery, and immediate post-partum care as well as immediate care of newborn infants.
26	Military Treatment Facility	A medical facility operated by one or more of the Uniformed Services. Military Treatment Facility (MTF) also refers to certain former U.S. Public Health Service (USPHS) facilities now designated as Uniformed Service Treatment Facilities (USTF).
27–30	Unassigned	N/A
31	Skilled Nursing Facility	A facility that primarily provides inpatient skilled nursing care and related services to patients who require medical, nursing, or rehabilitative services but does not provide the level of care or treatment available in a hospital.
32	Nursing Facility	A facility that primarily provides to residents skilled nursing care and related services for the rehabilitation of injured, disabled, or sick persons, or, on a regular basis, health-related care services above the level of custodial care to other than individuals with intellectual disabilities.
33	Custodial Care Facility	A facility that provides room, board, and other personal assistance services, generally on a long-term basis, and that does not include a medical component.
34	Hospice	A facility, other than a patient's home, in which palliative and supportive care for terminally ill patients and their families are provided.
35–40	Unassigned	N/A
41	Ambulance—Land	A land vehicle specifically designed, equipped, and staffed for lifesaving and transporting the sick or injured.
42	Ambulance—Air or Water	An air or water vehicle specifically designed, equipped, and staffed for lifesaving and transporting the sick or injured.
43–48	Unassigned	N/A
49	Independent Clinic	A location, not part of a hospital and not described by any other Place-of-Service code, that is organized and operated to provide preventive, diagnostic, therapeutic, rehabilitative, or palliative services to outpatients only.
50	Federally Qualified Health Center	A facility located in a medically underserved area that provides Medicare beneficiaries preventive primary medical care under the general direction of a physician.
51	Inpatient Psychiatric Facility	A facility that provides inpatient psychiatric services for the diagnosis and treatment of mental illness on a 24-hour basis, by or under the supervision of a physician.

(continued)

Place of Service Code(s)	Place of Service Name	Place of Service Description
52	Psychiatric Facility—Partial Hospitalization	A facility for the diagnosis and treatment of mental illness that provides a planned therapeutic program for patients who do not require full-time hospitalization, but who need broader programs than are possible from outpatient visits to a hospital-based or hospital-affiliated facility.
53	Community Mental Health Center	A facility that provides the following services: outpatient services, including specialized outpatient services for children, the elderly, individuals who are chronically ill, and residents of the CMHC's mental health services area who have been discharged from inpatient treatment at a mental health facility; 24-hour-a-day emergency care services; day treatment, other partial hospitalization services, or psychosocial rehabilitation services; screening for patients being considered for admission to state mental health facilities to determine the appropriateness of such admission; and consultation and education services.
54	Intermediate Care Facility/ Individuals with Intellectual Disabilities	A facility that primarily provides health-related care and services above the level of custodial care to individuals but does not provide the level of care or treatment available in a hospital or SNF.
55	Residential Substance Abuse Treatment Facility	A facility that provides treatment for substance (alcohol and drug) abuse to live-in residents who do not require acute medical care. Services include individual and group therapy and counseling, family counseling, laboratory tests, drugs and supplies, psychological testing, and room and board.
56	Psychiatric Residential Treatment Center	A facility or distinct part of a facility for psychiatric care that provides a total 24-hour therapeutically planned and professionally staffed group living and learning environment.
57	Nonresidential Substance Abuse Treatment Facility	A location that provides treatment for substance (alcohol and drug) abuse on an ambulatory basis. Services include individual and group therapy and counseling, family counseling, laboratory tests, drugs and supplies, and psychological testing.
58–59	Unassigned	N/A
60	Mass Immunization Center	A location where providers administer pneumococcal pneumonia and influenza virus vaccinations and submit these services as electronic media claims, paper claims, or using the roster billing method. This generally takes place in a mass immunization setting, such as a public health center, pharmacy, or mall but may include a physician office setting.
61	Comprehensive Inpatient Rehabilitation Facility	A facility that provides comprehensive rehabilitation services under the supervision of a physician to inpatients with physical disabilities. Services include physical therapy, occupational therapy, speech pathology, social or psychological services, and orthotics and prosthetics services.
62	Comprehensive Outpatient Rehabilitation Facility	A facility that provides comprehensive rehabilitation services under the supervision of a physician to outpatients with physical disabilities. Services include physical therapy, occupational therapy, and speech pathology services.
63–64	Unassigned	N/A
65	End-Stage Renal Disease Treatment Facility	A facility, other than a hospital, that provides dialysis treatment, maintenance, and/or training to patients or caregivers on an ambulatory or home-care basis.
66–70	Unassigned	N/A
71	Public Health Clinic	A facility maintained by either state or local health departments that provides ambulatory primary medical care under the general direction of a physician.
72	Rural Health Clinic	A certified facility that is located in a rural medically underserved area that provides ambulatory primary medical care under the general direction of a physician.
73–80	Unassigned	N/A

(continued)

Place of Service Code(s)	Place of Service Name	Place of Service Description
81	Independent Laboratory	A laboratory certified to perform diagnostic and/or clinical tests independent of an institution or a physician's office.
82–98	Unassigned	N/A
99	Other Place of Service	Other place of service not identified above.

Type-of-Service Codes

In addition to providing pre-categorization of procedures, Type-of-Service (TOS) codes are also used to ensure that procedures, services, and treatments, along with the Place-of-Service codes, are used to determine appropriateness of location and service.

Type of Service Indicators

0 Whole Blood

1 Medical Care

2 Surgery

3 Consultation

4 Diagnostic Radiology

5 Diagnostic Laboratory

6 Therapeutic Radiology

7 Anesthesia

8 Assistant at Surgery

9 Other Medical Items or Services

A Used DME

B High-Risk Screening Mammography

C Low-Risk Screening Mammography

D Ambulance

E Enteral/Parenteral Nutrients/Supplies

F Ambulatory Surgical Center (Facility Usage for Surgical Services)

G Immunosuppressive Drugs

H Hospice

J Diabetic Shoes

K Hearing Items and Services

L ESRD Supplies

M Monthly Capitation Payment for Dialysis

N Kidney Donor

P Lump Sum Purchase of DME, Prosthetics, Orthotics

Q Vision Items or Services

R Rental of DME

S Surgical Dressings or Other Medical Supplies

T Outpatient Mental Health Treatment Limitation

U Occupational Therapy

V Pneumococcal/Flu Vaccine

W Physical Therapy

40.6 Organizing Claims: Resubmission, Denials, and Appeals

> **CODING BITES**
>
> You are responsible for following up on every claim you send.

One thing that is very important for a professional insurance biller to do is to keep track of all the claims sent out on behalf of his or her medical facility, whether it is a physician's office or a hospital. Even with the help of computers and clearinghouses, a claim can get lost. It happens on occasion with letters sent through the post office, and it can happen electronically as well. One little power surge or a computer with a virus can make your claim disappear. The only way you may know about this happening is the absence of a response, such as a payment, a statement of rejection, or a denial. Therefore, you have to keep track of every claim form you submit.

The following are two simple steps for staying organized.

1. Keep a log of every claim as you send it. If you are using a clearinghouse, you will receive a report, listing all the claims sent (complete with date and time sent) and to which payer they were forwarded. Place these notices in a file folder on your computer's desktop or print out these reports and place them in a three-ring binder or another type of file. If you are sending claims directly from your office, you should create a separate master index for logging in this information. If you prefer, you can keep a master index in a notebook on your desk and handwrite a notation for each claim you send, indicating the following:
    - Carrier name (the third-party payer to whom you sent the claim)
    - Patient name
    - Date of service
    - Date and time you sent the claim
2. Build into your schedule a specific day and time each week for following up claims. When you set an appointment with yourself, such as every Friday at 9 a.m., or Mondays after the morning staff meeting, you will reduce the number of times that your workday will prevent you from doing this. It is so easy to say, "Once a week I am going to follow up on the claims" and just never have the time for this very important task. Each week, or as often as required by the number of claims you send out, go over the list and separate the claims into three "piles":
    - Pile 1: Claims that have been paid by the insurers
    - Pile 2: Claims for which you have received rejection or denial notices
    - Pile 3: Claims for which you have received no notices or payment

Pile 1: Claims That Have Been Paid by the Insurers

> **Remittance Advice (RA)**
> Notification identifying details about a payment from the third-party payer.

> **Electronic Remittance Advice (ERA)**
> Remittance advice that is sent to the provider electronically.

> **Explanation of Benefits (EOB)**
> Another type of paper remittance advice, more typically sent to the policyholder. However, some in the industry use the term *EOB* interchangeably with *RA*.

The HIPAA Health Care Payment and Remittance Advice is the electronic transmission of this payment, using HIPAA-approved secure data sets. The transmission has two parts: the transaction and the document.

- The document is a **remittance advice (RA)** or an **electronic remittance advice (ERA)**. Some health care professionals also refer to this document as an **explanation of benefits** or **EOB**. However, an EOB is sent to the patient or beneficiary, not the provider.
- The transaction is an electronic funds transfer (EFT) that sends the payment directly into your facility's bank account, like a direct deposit.

The RA will provide all the details of this payment, including

- The exact amount of monies your office is receiving
- For which patient
- For which procedures performed
- On which service dates

Once you are certain that a claim has been approved and your office has received payment from the third-party payer, the first thing you should do is mark this claim as paid in your master index. Be very careful when doing this.

When you enter the deposits into the computer (and into the bank, if the funds were not electronically transferred), you must be very diligent. You might have two claims for the same patient for different dates or two patients with the same name or similar names. You do not want to mark the wrong claim paid and leave the wrong claim marked unpaid. This will cause a lot of confusion and aggravation in dealing with the insurance carrier.

Pile 2: Claims for Which You Have Received Denial Notices

You have learned how to avoid many denied claims by checking, double-checking, and triple-checking your work. Make certain that

1. Insurance coverage is confirmed (eligibility verification).
2. All the information (such as policyholder and policy number) is entered correctly.
3. The best, most appropriate codes are used.
4. Medical necessity has been established by those codes.
5. All the information has been correctly placed on the correct claim form.

Despite doing everything correctly, some claims are denied and come back unpaid. However, this does not mean that you either have to go after the guarantor for the money or have your office go without the money it deserves. There are many reasons an insurance carrier, or payer, may deny a claim. Let's review some of the most common reasons for a claim to be denied and what you can do about it.

Denied Due to Office Personnel Error

If you discover that the claim has been denied by the insurance carrier due to an error made by you or someone in your office, this can be fixed. Simply find out what the error was and correct it.

Compare the policy number on the claim to the copy of the insurance card that you made when the patient was seen in your office for this encounter. It is important that you specifically check it against the copy taken at the encounter for which this claim form is billing the insurance company. The patient may have been in your office more recently with a new policy because his or her insurance changed between the most recent visit and the visit for which this claim was submitted.

CODING BITES

Get into the habit of dating the copy you make of the insurance card each time the patient comes in to see the physician.

You might find that, when you keyed the number into the computer, you inadvertently switched two numbers. It can happen when you are in a busy, hectic, noisy office with many people talking to you at the same time.

If you find that the policy number matches the ID card, you will have to continue looking for the typo, going over the claim form one box at a time to check every piece of information that was entered. Once you find the error, all you have to do is correct it and resubmit a corrected claim form.

You should have caught the error when you double-checked your work, but . . . OK. It happens. You have wasted time (and if you are using a clearinghouse, you have wasted money as well), and you have delayed payment to your office, but follow the third-party payer's procedure for resubmitting corrected claims and the money will arrive.

CODING BITES

Make certain that you mark a resubmission with the words "Corrected Claim" so there is no mistake that you are not double billing (which is against the law).

EXAMPLES

The policy number or a CPT code is invalid (nonexistent) because it was entered improperly.

Anyone could look at the number 546998823 and accidentally key in 546999823.

Denied Due to Lack of Coverage

You look at the denial notice and it doesn't make sense. You have documentation in the file that, when you called for **eligibility verification**, the insurance carrier representative confirmed that the patient's coverage was valid and the policy carried no exclusions. The copayment, co-insurance, and deductible were also confirmed. However, the claim was returned as denied, with the reason that the patient was not covered.

Eligibility Verification
The process of confirming with the insurance carrier that an individual is qualified for benefits that would pay for services provided by your health care professional on a particular day.

What may have happened is that, between your verification of the patient's coverage and the arrival of the claim at the insurance carrier's office, the policy was canceled or changed. When your claim arrived, the computer, or the person, simply looked at the file, saw that the policy was no longer in effect, and therefore denied the claim. If this is the case:

1. You will need to send a letter, not make a phone call, to the insurance carrier. In the letter, carefully state the date and time of the eligibility verification and the name of the insurance representative who told you the patient was covered for services by your office. (Make certain your office's procedure for eligibility verification includes the documentation of all of these details for just this reason.) Emphasize the date of the phone call or print out the electronic verification, as well as the date(s) of treatment or service, and attach a fresh printout of the claim form.
2. Before you submit this letter, call the company and confirm the name, title, and address of the employee responsible for receiving your appeal request. If you send this information to the wrong person, it may get lost within the company or, at the very least, it will delay your satisfaction of this issue.
3. Make certain you keep copies of everything, and follow up in a week or two if you have not heard from the insurer.

In other cases, claims have been denied because the individual's policy was canceled prior to your treatment and the insurance representative did not have (or did not tell you) up-to-date information. Therefore, your office provided treatment based on misinformation. As a matter of policy, typically the insurance carrier will claim that its staff member's confirmation of coverage does not represent a guarantee that your office will be paid. Again, you do not want to take no for an answer.

Both federal and state courts have ordered insurance carriers to pay claims based on their statements of eligibility at the time treatment and services were provided. These courts have established that the insurance representative's, or the electronic, confirmation of benefits serves as encouragement to the physician, or other provider, to offer that treatment or service.

When you think about it, if the insurance carrier had stated that the patient did not have coverage at the time you called for verification, your office may have chosen to not see the patient, to not take an x-ray, or to ask the patient to pay cash at that time. The fact that the insurance carrier told you, or a member of your office, that it would pay the claim encouraged your physician to treat the individual and reasonably expect to be paid for his or her work. Again, you must do the following:

1. Write a letter of appeal to the appropriate person at the insurance company, stating all the details of the verification conversation.
2. If your office does eligibility verification electronically, you should copy the printout of the electronic confirmation and attach it to the letter.
3. Always keep hard copy (paper) documentation or notes indicating to whom you spoke, what was said, and the date and time of the conversation.

If your appeal is denied again, your office may need to enlist the services of an attorney. The bottom line is that your office is entitled to this payment, but there are times you may need to fight for it.

Denied Due to Lack of Medical Necessity

Should your office receive a denial based on lack of medical necessity, there are some things you must do:

1. Go back and confirm the diagnosis (ICD-10-CM) and procedure (CPT or ICD-10-PCS) codes that appear on the claim form are the best, most accurate codes.
   a. There is a possibility that there was a simple error in keying in the code (such as transposing two of the numbers or leaving off a digit). More than once, a health care office and a patient have gone through months of arguing with the insurance carrier for the coverage of a procedure, only to find that the entire problem was a simple typographical error.
   b. Perhaps there was an error in coding. Go back and look at the physician's notes. Start from the beginning and recode the encounter. If there is another coder in your office, you might ask him or her to look at the notes and code the diagnosis and procedure(s). Then compare the other coder's determination of the best, most appropriate codes with yours. If you come up with different and/or additional codes this time, you might go ahead and resubmit the claim with the new codes. Or this review might confirm that the codes were correct on the original claim.
   c. Review the linking of the procedure codes to diagnosis codes (paper claim form CMS-1500 Box 24E or eClaim 837P Loop ID 2400). Confirm the links are correct.
2. Contact the insurance carrier and get a written copy of its definition of medical necessity, or check its website and print it out. Often the list of criteria for medical necessity consists of any treatment or service that
   a. Is commonly performed by health care practitioners (considered accepted standard of care) for the treatment of the condition, illness, or injury as indicated by the diagnosis code(s) provided.
   b. Is provided at the most efficient level of care that ensures the patient's safety.

c. Is not experimental.
d. Is not elective.

Using the criteria for medical necessity from the insurance carrier that denied the claim (different carriers may have different criteria), review the patient's health record to confirm that this individual and this particular encounter meet all of the requirements. Again,

- Double-check the diagnosis and procedure codes to make certain they all accurately represent what occurred during that visit.
- Call and speak with the claims examiner to identify exactly what he or she thought the problem was with the claim. This conversation may give you some insight into what you should be looking for as you review the patient's chart.
- Get support materials from your health care professionals, particularly the attending physician on this case. Copies of articles or pages from credible sources, such as *The Merck Manual*, the *New England Journal of Medicine*, or other qualified sources of research, will help support your claim.
- If this patient encounter was the result of another provider referring the individual to your physician for additional treatment, the referring physician might agree to write a letter supporting your office.

3. Write a letter to the third-party payer's appeals board, or to whomever the claims representative instructs you to send the documentation, outlining all of the information you have gathered to corroborate specifically why the denial should be overturned.
   a. Include copies of supporting documentation, such as pages from the National Library of Medicine's website or a letter from the referring provider.
   b. In addition, request that a qualified health care professional licensed in the area of treatment or service under discussion be the one to review your appeal. This may provide a more agreeable opinion as to the medical necessity of your claim and get it approved.

EXAMPLE

Christopher Novack, a 67-year-old male, is seen by his family physician after stating that he was driving to his office earlier and felt so dizzy he had to pull over. While waiting for the dizziness to pass, he felt his heart beating rapidly, and he began to sweat. He was worried that he was having a heart attack and came right over to see Dr. Bennetti.

Dr. Bennetti, knowing that Chris had been diagnosed with type 2 diabetes mellitus, checked his glucose levels and found them to be grossly abnormal, causing the dizziness and sweating. He administered an injection of insulin. Then, Dr. Bennetti checked Chris's heart with a 12-lead EKG. The results were negative.

When you perform your medical necessity review, you can see that the code for type 2 diabetes mellitus will justify the glucose test and the injection of the insulin.

However, if you do not have a second diagnosis code for his rapid heartbeat, the claim would be rejected. Without the code for rapid heartbeat, there is no medical justification provided on the claim form for performing an EKG.

Denied Due to Preexisting Condition

Note: ACA requires all health insurance policies to cover preexisting conditions. However, some issues may still arise from this issue. Pay close attention.

A denial on the grounds that the patient was treated for a preexisting excluded condition or illness reinforces the need for accurate confirmation of eligibility before the patient is seen and treated by the physician. If, in fact, your physician is about to treat a patient for a specific diagnosis, you must determine if the insurance carrier has excluded that condition, illness, or injury from coverage. This should be done during the eligibility verification. However, if you get to the point at which a submitted claim has been denied due to a preexisting condition that has been excluded, you still have several options to try to get your claim paid:

1. Start by reviewing the diagnosis code. There may be a difference in the diagnosis codes, now and for past treatment, making your claim valid.
2. Request a copy of the insurance carrier's definition of a preexisting condition. Once you clearly understand the requirements, you will be able to better analyze the details of this claim and its validity.
3. A review of the patient's past medical records also may assist you in appealing this denial. Examining specific diagnosis codes and physician's notes' diagnostic statements may find an opportunity to justify the insurance carrier's coverage of this claim.

When you have the information to support your claim, write an appeal letter outlining why the denial should be reversed.

Denied Due to Benefit Limitation on Treatment by an Assistant

Some medical offices have physician's assistants (PA) and nurse practitioners (NP) treat patients for routine examinations, vaccinations, and other medical services. However, some insurance carriers limit the types of treatments and services for which they will pay when provided by a health care worker who is not a licensed physician. There are a couple of approaches to appeal this type of denial.

1. Begin by authenticating the qualifications of the person who provided the service or treatment. You will also want to reinforce, in your appeal, that having this health care professional perform this procedure, under the supervision of the licensed physician, was the most cost-efficient way to provide the service to the patient.
2. Obtain a copy of the carrier's written policy regarding treatment to patients by assistants and search for language that specifically denies payment for services provided by a professional with the credentials of your staff member. If you do not find any such language, your appeal letter should include that the insurance carrier's policy does not specifically exclude services provided by this level of professional.

Subsequent Denials

There are additional steps that can be taken to appeal a second or third denial. Sometimes an insurance carrier will deny a claim, hoping that you will give up and it will not have to pay. However, most of the time, subsequent denials are just a matter of poor communication between the insurance carrier and the health care facility. Remember, although it is an insurance carrier's responsibility and obligation to pay claims, it is also its responsibility and obligation to protect its assets from fraud. Primarily, it is this intention that creates the circumstance of a falsely denied claim. However, after you have exhausted all efforts within the insurance carrier's organization to get the carrier to see your side and pay the claim, you have additional options:

1. Many states have state boards and/or review panels for this type of situation. Experienced health care providers, with varying areas of specialization, sit on these review boards. Their duty is to go over all the details of the case; examine the patient's health record, the claim form, and all other documentation; and evaluate the insurance carrier's basis for denying the claim. They have the right, empowered by the state government, to override the insurance carrier's decision and force the carrier to pay the claim. Bringing an appeal to this type of review board is an option to both health care professionals and individuals alike.
2. If the patient is covered under an employer's self-insured health plan, the state board is usually not an option for appeal. However, the federal government oversees and regulates self-insured plans and can provide you with an appeals process. At the very least, these insurers are required to have an in-house appeal board that will hear your case.

Surprisingly, you have an excellent chance of winning an appeal when you handle it properly. Researchers have found very high success rates for providers who file appeals. Therefore, if a claim is denied, it is worth the time to look into the reasons for denial and possibly exercise the right to appeal.

Writing Letters of Appeal

When a claim has been denied and you have gathered all the documentation to support your position that the denial is incorrect, you need to write a formal letter of appeal. This letter should contain the following:

Recipient: Check the website or call the third-party payer and get the name, title, and address of the person to whom you should address this letter. Make certain you double-check the spelling of the person's name–don't assume. Even a name as straightforward as John can also be spelled Jon or Jahn. Just ask!

RE: In the space between the recipient's name and address, and the salutation, you need to include identification regarding the person to whom this letter refers. This should be indented to your one-inch tab position. The details that should be shown in this area of the letter are

Patient Name:

Policyholder Name:

Policy Number:

Date(s) of Service:

Claim Number:

Total Amount of Claim: $

Salutation: Always begin the letter with a proper business salutation to the recipient by name. For example, Dear Mr. Smith: or Dear Ms. Jones (followed by a colon). Avoid generic salutations such as To Whom It May Concern unless the insurance carrier will not release the name of the person designated to receive appeal letters and has instructed you to address this letter to a department or title.

Paragraph 1: State briefly and directly why you are writing this letter. This is a summary or condensed version of the rest of the letter. Be factual, not emotional. Be specific about when and/or how you were informed that the claim was denied and the reasons stated by the insurance carrier for the denial. This paragraph is to make certain that you and the reader of this letter are on the same page (pardon the pun!). It is difficult to capture and retain someone's attention to what you are saying if he or she doesn't know to what or whom you are referring.

EXAMPLES

Our claims service representative, Raul Vega, told us that the above claim was denied due to a lack of medical necessity. This letter is an official notice that we wish to appeal this decision.

On November 3, 2024, our office received a notice stating that the above-mentioned claim was denied because of lack of coverage. This letter is to appeal this decision.

Paragraph 2: Itemize all the facts/evidence you have to support your position that you should be paid. Explain what documentation you have to encourage them to change their minds and approve/pay your claim. This list may contain highlights from the physician's notes outlining why the procedure was medically necessary. You might include statistics proving that this procedure is no longer considered experimental but is now widely accepted as the new standard of care. Attach copies (never originals) of documents that contain the information and refer to those attachments in this portion of the letter. In reality, this section of the letter may need to be longer than one paragraph. Write what you need to establish your rationale, but remember that this is not creative writing. Do not use flowery language or get long in your explanation. Be direct and to the point and include just the facts.

EXAMPLES

As you can see in the attached documentation, the x-rays confirmed that the patient had a compound fracture requiring immediate surgery.

On Thursday, September 4, 2024, at 1:35 p.m. Eastern, I spoke with Emma Longwood in your Eligibility Verification department, who confirmed that Mr. Smith was fully covered by your HMO plan for the following procedures. . . .

Paragraph 3: Use paragraph 3 (the last paragraph) to clearly define where this discussion should go next. Of course, you want them to just reconsider and pay the claim; however, you will need to keep this a bit more open-ended. Offer to provide any additional documentation the insurance carrier may feel necessary. Supply your contact information (office phone number, e-mail address, fax number) even if it is right there on the letterhead. Set an appointment generally (i.e., "I will call you next week") to follow up with this person. The purpose of this statement is to keep this appeal moving in a direction toward acceptance and payment. You do not want this letter to get buried on a busy desk. In addition, mark your calendar and call when you said you would. It is your responsibility to keep this issue on the top of the insurance carrier's priority list. You know that old saying, "The squeaky wheel gets the grease." This means that those that speak up get the attention.

EXAMPLES

If you need any more information, to bring this to a quick resolution, please contact me at. . . .

I will call you at the end of the week to discuss this matter further. In the meantime, if you need to contact me, please do so at. . . .

Closing and Signature: All business letters should contain a closing, as well as the signature and title of the person sending the correspondence. *Sincerely* or *Sincerely yours* (followed by a comma) are the most common closings. After leaving four lines blank to make room for your signature, key in your full name. Directly underneath your name, key in your title (e.g., Insurance Specialist). If you are going to attach copies of important documentation to this letter, you need to note this under your signature. Leave one empty line under your title, and key in Enclosure or Enclosures or Enc. This notation points the recipient to the additional pages included in the envelope.

Pile 3: Claims for Which You Have Received No Notices or Payment

If a reasonable time has passed after sending a claim and you have received no notices or payment, you will need to follow up with the insurance carrier. (The term *reasonable time* is specifically defined by each third-party payer.)

1. Go to the third-party payer's website and check the status of the claim, or call and speak with someone in customer service to determine which examiner or representative will be handling your claim. Try to confirm that he or she has received your claim by getting a date and time of receipt and ask which staff member received it. If you cannot get this information, or you get a vague statement, such as "Oh, I'm sure we have it somewhere. We are very busy. We'll get to it soon," you will need to take the next step.
2. Go back over all the paperwork that accompanied claims paid by this carrier in the same time frame, such as an electronic remittance advice (ERA), or a remittance advice (RA). There may have been a mistake and the wrong claim was marked paid in your file (meaning that this claim has really already been paid) and it is another claim that is still outstanding.
3. Once you are certain the insurance company has not responded to this claim in any way, you may need to send a **tracer**, also known as a duplicate billing or second submission. A tracer is an official request for a third-party payer to search its system to find a missing health claim form. It is also a term used for a replacement health claim form resubmitted to replace one that was lost.

Tracer
An official request for a third-party payer to search its system to find a missing health claim form. It is also a term used for a replacement health claim form resubmitted to replace one that was lost.

Most insurance carriers require you to wait a specific number of days or weeks after the original date of submission before you are permitted to send a tracer claim. Check with the carrier, as each may have a different waiting period. This second version of the same claim must be marked "Tracer." This is to make sure that the insurance carrier knows you are not attempting to bill a second time for the same services. Double billing is against the law; however, sending a bill a second time because you believe that the first claim has been lost is good business.

Make a note in your master index of the date and time that you refiled the claim. That way, you can follow up again if you need to.

AUDITING CLAIMS

The Job of a Claims Auditor

An important part of the reimbursement process is a sub-sector known as claims auditing. It can be included in the job description for a medical coding professional or a medical reimbursement specialist or it may be a separate job description. Those responsible for auditing claims are, essentially, checking for accuracy throughout the claim, along with other details involved in the process, such as:

- Confirm that all details entered onto a claim are accurate; demographic information as well as medical codes supported by documentation in adherence with official guidelines and policies
- Resolve concerns regarding rejected or denied claims, as well as overpayments
- Analyze the response status of all claims, including paid in full, paid in part, and those placed in determination
- Prepare reports identifying trends including response times and other issues in the claims process
- Alert needs for re-training or additional education necessary to ensure compliance with the False Claims Act and other applicable laws and regulations

In addition to healthcare facilities, such as hospitals and physician groups, claims auditors are hired by third-party payers, including virtually all private payers such as Humana and United Healthcare, as well as Medicare and the Veteran's Administration.

Different Types of Audits

As you review these responsibilities of a claims auditor, the next aspect to understand is the scope of an audit you are about to complete. Briefly, the key parameters are:

- *Retrospective Audits*: In these cases, the auditor would review healthcare claims created and submitted over a past period of time, such as the last six months. The review can cover, not only the specific content of the claim as submitted but include the response from the third-party payer. This additional insight can be very informative with regard to the individual processes of your department's reimbursement methodologies.
- *External Audits* are conducted by authorities outside of this facility, such as a MAC (Medicare Administration Contractor) or possibly the Office of the Inspector General. Most often, these audits are triggered by a suspicion garnered from computerized reviews of every claim submitted by this facility to a specific third-party payer. The typical external audit will

review the previous three (3) years of claims submitted. If the audit reveals any improper actions, this can be extended back an additional seven (7) years.

- *Concurrent (Prospective) Audits*: This auditing process is inserted between the reimbursement specialist's completion of a claim and the actual submission of the claim to the third-party payer. Performing concurrent audits allows the facility to ensure that every claim submitted is completely accurate and is requesting optimal reimbursement. Conducting a concurrent audit supports the compliance with the False Claims Act and other applicable laws and regulations, reducing the facility's potential liability.
- *Internal Audits* are initiated by the facility itself with the intention of ensuring their reimbursement process is legally compliant and functioning efficiently to obtain optimal compensation.

Chapter Summary

A fundamental part of an insurance coding and medical billing specialist's job is to work with the insurance companies that will reimburse your health care facility for the services and procedures you provide to your patients. You need to understand how your facility will be paid (such as fee-for-service, capitation, or episodic care); be able to distinguish among the types of policies (such as HMOs, PPOs, and managed care policies, as well as Medicare, Medicaid, and TriCare plans); and quickly identify which is responsible for sending payment to you. This will help your billing efforts be more efficient and you get paid more quickly.

The procedures you develop and abide by for tracking the health insurance claim forms you submit is almost as important as the coding process itself. Some health care offices do not have a routine for handling situations, such as lost claims or denied claims. However, you must realize how important this is to the overall financial well-being of your facility.

When you are organized, and keep a tracking log of all the claims you submit, your work is easier and your success rate is higher. Appealing denied claims is a part of your career, and it is an important part of the entire medical billing and insurance claims process.

CODING BITES

The basic reimbursement methods are applicable across all types of health care, and include capitation, fee for service, episodic (global) payment, and cost reimbursement.

It is the provider's responsibility to confirm the method of reimbursement prior to providing services.

For more information on the MACRA program, go to

https://www.cms.gov/medicare/quality/value-based-programs/chip-reauthorization-act

You Interpret It! Answers

1. Workers' compensation and disability compensation, **2.** Margaret's liability insurance, **3.** Facility member = workers' compensation; student = school's liability insurance

CHAPTER 40 REVIEW Reimbursement

Let's Check It! Terminology

Match each term to the appropriate definition.

Part I

1. **LO 40.2** A physician, typically a family practitioner or an internist, who serves as the primary care physician for an individual. This physician is responsible for evaluating and determining the course of treatment or services, as well as for deciding whether or not a specialist should be involved in care.

A. Automobile Insurance

B. Capitation Plans

2. **LO 40.1** A type of health insurance coverage that controls the care of each subscriber (or insured person) by using a primary care provider as a central health care supervisor.
3. **LO 40.2** A type of health insurance that uses a primary care physician, also known as a gatekeeper, to manage all health care services for an individual.
4. **LO 40.2** A policy that covers loss or injury to a third party caused by the insured or something belonging to the insured.
5. **LO 40.1** The total management of an individual's well-being by a health care professional.
6. **LO 40.3** An insurance company pays a provider one flat fee to cover the entire course of treatment for an individual's condition.
7. **LO 40.2** The agency under the Department of Health and Human Services (DHHS) in charge of regulation and control over services for those covered by Medicare and Medicaid.
8. **LO 40.3** Payment agreements that outline, in a written fee schedule, exactly how much money the insurance carrier will pay the physician for each treatment and/or service provided.
9. **LO 40.3** An extra reduction in the rate charged to an insurer for services provided by the physician to the plan's members.
10. **LO 40.1** The amount of money, often paid monthly, by a policyholder or insured, to an insurance company to obtain coverage.
11. **LO 40.2** Auto accident liability coverage will pay for medical bills, lost wages, and compensation for pain and suffering for any person injured by the insured in an auto accident.
12. **LO 40.3** Agreements between a physician and a managed care organization that pay the physician a predetermined amount of money each month for each member of the plan who identifies that provider as his or her primary care physician.
13. **LO 40.2** A plan that reimburses a covered individual a portion of his or her income that is lost as a result of being unable to work due to illness or injury.
14. **LO 40.2** Individuals who are supported, either financially or with regard to insurance coverage, by others.

C. Centers for Medicare & Medicaid Services (CMS)
D. Dependents
E. Disability Compensation
F. Discounted FFS
G. Episodic Care
H. Fee-for-Service (FFS) Plans
I. Gatekeeper
J. Health Care
K. Health Maintenance Organization (HMO)
L. Insurance Premium
M. Liability Insurance
N. Managed Care

Part II

1. **LO 40.6** An official request for a third-party payer to search its system to find a missing health claim form. It is also a term used for a replacement health claim form resubmitted to replace one that was lost.
2. **LO 40.3** The process of determining a fee for a service by evaluating the *usual* fee charged by the provider, the *customary* fee charged by most physicians in the same community or geographical area, and what is considered *reasonable* by most health care professionals under the specific circumstances of the situation.
3. **LO 40.6** Remittance advice that is sent to the provider electronically.
4. **LO 40.2** A type of insurance plan that will allow an HMO enrollee to choose his or her own nonmember physician at a lower benefit rate, costing the patient more money out-of-pocket.
5. **LO 40.1** An individual or organization that is not directly involved in an encounter but has a connection because of its obligation to pay, in full or part, for that encounter.
6. **LO 40.6** Another type of paper remittance advice, more typically sent to the policyholder. However, some in the industry use the term *EOB* interchangeably with *RA*.
7. **LO 40.2** A type of health insurance coverage in which physicians provide health care services to members of the plan at a discount.
8. **LO 40.2** A government health plan that covers medical expenses for the dependents of active-duty service members, CHAMPUS-eligible retirees and their families, and the dependents of deceased active-duty members.
9. **LO 40.2** An insurance program that covers medical care for those injured or for those who become ill as a consequence of their employment.
10. **LO 40.1** A health care claim form that is transmitted electronically.

A. Electronic Media Claim (EMC)
B. Electronic Remittance Advice (ERA)
C. Eligibility Verification
D. Explanation of Benefits (EOB)
E. Point-of-Service (POS)
F. Preferred Provider Organization (PPO)
G. Remittance Advice (RA)
H. Third-Party Payer
I. Tracer
J. TriCare

11. **LO 40.6** The process of confirming with the insurance carrier that an individual is qualified for benefits that would pay for services provided by your health care professional on a particular day.
12. **LO 40.6** Notification identifying details about a payment from the third-party payer.

K. Usual, Customary, and Reasonable (UCR)
L. Workers' Compensation

Part III

1. **LO 40.2** May cover medical expenses caused by a car accident.
2. **LO 40.2** Preferred provider organization.
3. **LO 40.3** A fixed amount paid each visit by the individual.
4. **LO 40.3** Payment, per service provided, from the insurance company.
5. **LO 40.2** A government program for indigent and needy people.
6. **LO 40.3** An episodic-care payment system basing reimbursement to hospitals for inpatient services upon standards of care for specific diagnoses grouped by their similar usage of resources for procedures, services, and treatments.

A. Copayment
B. DRG
C. Fee-for-Service
D. PPO
E. Medicaid
F. Auto Insurance Policy

Let's Check It! Concepts

Choose the most appropriate answer for each of the following questions.

1. **LO 40.1** Medical care is defined as
   - **a.** identification and treatment of illness and/or injury.
   - **b.** services to prevent illness such as a routine checkup or wellness visit.
   - **c.** laboratory services.
   - **d.** only those services performed by a medical doctor.
2. **LO 40.2** An organization that depends on the services of a gatekeeper is
   - **a.** a preferred provider organization.
   - **b.** Medicare.
   - **c.** a health maintenance organization.
   - **d.** a not-for-profit hospital.
3. **LO 40.3** A capitation plan pays the provider
   - **a.** per specific service.
   - **b.** per member every month.
   - **c.** for treatments in a hospital only.
   - **d.** one flat fee per illness or condition.
4. **LO 40.2** Medicare is a government plan that covers primarily
   - **a.** military personnel.
   - **b.** poor and needy.
   - **c.** those over the age of 65.
   - **d.** government employees.
5. **LO 40.4** When CMS computers evaluate submitted claims to look for pairs of codes being reported that are known to be mutually exclusive procedures, this is also known as ________ edits.
   - **a.** LCD
   - **b.** NCD
   - **c.** PTP
   - **d.** MUE
6. **LO 40.2** TriCare provides health care benefits for the dependents of
   - **a.** state workers.
   - **b.** those serving in the uniformed services.
   - **c.** athletes.
   - **d.** health care workers.
7. **LO 40.5** What specific location does POS code 23 identify?
   - **a.** Urgent Care Facility
   - **b.** Assisted Living Facility
   - **c.** Telehealth
   - **d.** Emergency Room–Hospital

8. **LO 40.6** The HIPAA Health Care Payment and Remittance Advice is the electronic transmission of payment, using HIPAA-approved secure data sets. The transmission has two parts: the ________ and the ________.
   - **a.** claim, transaction
   - **b.** transaction, document
   - **c.** document, claim
   - **d.** date, carrier name
9. **LO 40.3** When an individual pays a percentage of the total charge, it is called the
   - **a.** deductible.
   - **b.** copayment.
   - **c.** coinsurance.
   - **d.** premium.
10. **LO 40.2** CMS stands for
    - **a.** Centers for Medical Services.
    - **b.** Corporation of Medical Systems.
    - **c.** Centers for Medicare & Medicaid Services.
    - **d.** Cycle of Medical Selections.

Let's Check It! Which Type of Insurance?

Match the situation with the type of insurance that would cover the expenses. Answers may be used more than once.

1. **LO 40.2** Mrs. Matthews, a teacher at Medical Coder Academy, slipped in her office, fell, and hurt her back.
2. **LO 40.2** Ralph broke his leg and must be in traction for 9 months. What plan will help him pay his rent and electric bill?
3. **LO 40.2** Mary Lou was at the mall, shopping for a birthday present, when she slipped on a wet floor and broke her hip.
4. **LO 40.1** Keith was walking down the stairs in his house, fell over his son's toy, and twisted his ankle.
5. **LO 40.2** Marlene was driving to work when another car hit her from behind. The EMTs took her to the hospital with a sprained ankle and sore neck.
6. **LO 40.2** Harvey caught a cold when he went fishing last weekend.
7. **LO 40.2** Jared enrolled in the insurance coding program at the local college. While leaving after his first class, another student bumped into him, he banged his head on a shelf, and he got a scalp laceration.
8. **LO 40.2** At home after his 85th birthday party, Jack tripped on the rug, fell, and broke his hip.
9. **LO 40.2** Suzette's husband is in the Marines. She is pregnant with their first child.
10. **LO 40.2** James is out of work and has no prospects. He is broke and has a really bad sore throat.

- **A.** Health Insurance
- **B.** Workers' Compensation
- **C.** Medicaid
- **D.** Disability Compensation
- **E.** Liability Insurance
- **F.** TriCare
- **G.** Automobile Insurance
- **H.** Medicare

Let's Check It! Rules and Regulations

Please answer the following questions from the knowledge you have gained after reading this chapter.

1. **LO 40.4** What does NCCI stand for, and what is its purpose?
2. **LO 40.4** What is a procedure-to-procedure edit, who performs it, and when is it performed?
3. **LO 40.4** What is the purpose of medically unlikely edits?
4. **LO 40.6** What does it mean when a claim is denied due to an office personnel error, and can it be corrected?
5. **LO 40.6** What should you do if your office receives a claim denial due to lack of medical necessity?

Let's Check It! Auditing

Choose the most appropriate answer for each of the following questions.

1. LO 40.6 Joaquin Trenton, a 33-year-old male, was working in a warehouse when a large crate containing lawn mower engines fell on his left foot. He was taken to the ED, x-rays were taken confirming a fracture, and a cast was applied before his discharge home. The medical reimbursement specialist created the claim and readied it to be submitted it to Mr. Trenton's health insurance company. The auditor, conducting a concurrent audit, flagged the claim. The impending error was ____

A: That the hospital should have admitted him

B: This claim should be submitted to Workers' Compensation, not health insurance.

C: There are no errors. This is correct.

D: That prior authorization was not obtained

2. LO 40.6 Yasmine Katzman, a 27-year-old female, went last week to have her annual mammogram. She knew this was provided at no charge under the Affordable Care Act, so she was surprised to receive an invoice from the provider for $150. She contacted the provider to question the charge. When reviewing the claim, the internal auditor discovered that the medical coder failed to append modifier ___ to the code for the mammogram.

A: Modifier 32 Mandated Services

B: Modifier 59 Distinct Procedural Service

C: Modifier 50 Bilateral Procedure

D: Modifier 33 Preventive Services

3. LO 40.6 During a retrospective internal audit, it was found that the same code for a procedure provided frequently in this practice was repeatedly reported even when the documentation included additional details which would have required a different procedure code to be accurate. The more accurate procedure code would have reimbursed at $500 higher in each instance, denying the facility a substantial amount of money. Three of these claims were submitted and paid over the last six months. Based on these facts, the auditor recommends ___.

A: Writing off these three claims

B: Requiring all medical coders to enroll in a degree program

C: Re-coding the claims and submitting them as "Corrected"

D: Charging the difference to the patient

4. LO 40.6 During a concurrent review, the auditor discovered a claim for patient, Leslie Garner. The problem was that this claim identified Leslie as a female, when in fact this patient is a male. Thanks to this auditor, the claim was corrected prior to submission and having the claim ____ was avoided.

A: Rejected

B: Denied

C: Placed in determination

D: Marked fraudulent

5. LO 40.6 This family practice has been supporting this community for the last 75 years when Dr. Joe's father opened its doors. They care for multiple generations. During a retrospective review, the auditor discovered a claim reporting services provided to Jason Channing, III was denied. In reality, these services were actually provided to Jason Channing Sr. The elder Channing is covered by Medicare while his grandson is covered by Humana, via his job. What should be done next?

A: Create a new claim for Channing Sr and submit to Humana

B: Write it off

C: Send an invoice to the patient to be paid out-of-pocket

D: Create a new claim for Channing Sr and submit to Medicare

41

Introduction to Health Care Law and Ethics

Key Terms

- Administrative Laws
- Civil Law
- Coding for Coverage
- Common Law
- Covered Entities
- Criminal Law
- Disclosure
- Double Billing
- Executive Orders
- HIPAA's Privacy Rule
- Mutually Exclusive Codes
- Protected Health Information (PHI)
- Release of Information (ROI)
- Statutory Laws
- Supporting Documentation
- Unbundling
- Upcoding
- Use

Learning Outcomes

After completing this chapter, the student should be able to:

LO 41.1 Identify the sources for directives governing behavior.
LO 41.2 Understand the rules for ethical and legal coding.
LO 41.3 Apply the requirements of the False Claims Act.
LO 41.4 Translate the components of the Health Insurance Portability and Accountability Act's Privacy Rule.
LO 41.5 Elaborate the responsibilities of the Health Care Fraud and Abuse Control Program.
LO 41.6 Adhere to the codes of ethics of our industry.
LO 41.7 Analyze the reasons for creating a compliance plan.

41.1 Sources for Legal Guidance

The health care industry is responsible for providing services to maintain and repair the human body. For all of those providing health care services, the federal and state governments have crafted and enacted laws and regulations designed to ensure honest, safe, and appropriate behaviors from all involved. In addition, these laws and regulations provide a remedy—compensation or restitution—when individuals step outside of these approved boundaries. As a health care professional, you must be familiar with the government's directives so you can conduct yourself and your facility accordingly. This text is written to provide you with the necessary foundation of legal and ethical knowledge and understanding to support a successful career in health care. This chapter will introduce you to the basic concepts.

The *Federal Register*

The *Federal Register* is the daily journal of the U.S. federal government. The Office of the Federal Register (OFR), in conjunction with the U.S. Government Printing Office (GPO), created and maintains the website version of this publication.

Created in 1935, the *Federal Register*'s purpose is to inform "*citizens of their rights and obligations, documents the actions of Federal agencies, and provides a forum for public participation, in the democratic process.*" Included in its contents are executive orders, presidential proclamations, policy statements, proposed rules, notices of scheduled hearings, and other government actions.

Take a look at a small section of the *Federal Register* in **Figure 41-1** and access the full *Federal Register* at https://www.federalregister.gov/.

Sources of Directives

Many different types of laws and regulations exist to direct certain behaviors of those individuals working in health care, on both the clinical side and the administrative side. Federal and state governments and their agencies initiate these directives.

There is a hierarchy established that sets the level of authority, which begins at the top with the U.S. Constitution as the first and foremost directive. In 1787, at the Constitutional Convention in Philadelphia, Pennsylvania, the Constitution of the United States was determined to be the highest and foremost of enacted law. Article VI of the Constitution states:

> *"This Constitution, and the Laws of the United States which shall be made in Pursuance thereof; and all Treaties made, or which shall be made, under the Authority of the United States, shall be the supreme Law of the Land; and the Judges in every State shall be bound thereby, any Thing in the Constitution or Laws of any State to the Contrary notwithstanding."*

39186 Federal Register / Vol. 78, No. 126 / Monday, July 1, 2013 / Rules and Regulations

List of Subjects

21 CFR Part 21

Privacy.

45 CFR Part 5b

Privacy.

Therefore, the Department of Health and Human Services is amending 21 CFR part 21 and 45 CFR part 5b to read as follows:

Title 21

PART 21—PROTECTION OF PRIVACY

■ 1. The authority citation for 21 CFR part 21 continues to read as follows:

Authority: 21 U.S.C. 371; 5 U.S.C. 552, 552a.

■ 2. Section 21.61 is amended by adding paragraph (d) to read as follows:

§ 21.61 Exempt systems.

* * * * *

DEPARTMENT OF HEALTH AND HUMAN SERVICES

Office of the Secretary

45 CFR Part 5b

[Docket No. NIH–2011–0001]

Privacy Act; Implementation

ACTION: Final rule.

SUMMARY: The Department of Health and Human Services (HHS or Department), through the National Institutes of Health (NIH), is exempting a system of records from certain requirements of the Privacy Act to protect the integrity of NIH research misconduct proceedings and to protect the identity of confidential sources in such proceedings.

DATES: *Effective Date:* This rule is effective July 31, 2013.

FOR FURTHER INFORMATION CONTACT: Jerry Moore, NIH Regulations Officer, Office of Management Assessment, Division of Management Support, 6011 Executive

support is contrary to the interests of the PHS and the Federal government and to the health and safety of the public, to the integrity of research, and to the conservation of public funds" 42 CFR 93.100(a).

Under the Privacy Act, individuals have a right of access to information pertaining to them that is contained in a system of records. At the same time, the Privacy Act permits certain types of systems to be exempt from some of the Privacy Act requirements. For example, section (k)(2) of the Privacy Act allows Agency heads to exempt from certain Privacy Act provisions a system of records containing investigatory material compiled for law enforcement purposes. This exemption's effect on the record access provision is qualified in that if the maintenance of the material results in the denial of any right, privilege, or benefit that the individual would otherwise be entitled to by federal law, the individual must be granted access to the material except to the extent that the access would reveal

FIGURE 41-1 U.S. Congress's *Federal Register* showing official details relating to the Privacy Act (in part)

Source: gpo.gov

Following the U.S. Constitution is federal law–those laws established by the U.S. Congress. State constitutions, state statutory laws, and then local laws complete the bottom tiers.

Statutory Laws
Laws that are enacted by federal and state legislature.

Statutory laws, most often referred to as *statutes*, are created and enacted by the federal and state legislatures (Congress). Members of Congress are responsible for writing the law. Then, once passed by votes in the House and the Senate, it is said to be "enacted." Because federal statutes take precedence over state statutory laws, state and local legislatures are not permitted to enact a law that contradicts any current federal law. This way, no one has to worry about which law takes dominance because this order of priority is already established.

There are circumstances, however, where the federal law provides some flexibility in behavior and the state law is more exact about the required behavior. In these cases, the state law would take precedence. For example, the federal law commonly called HIPAA's Privacy Rule (Health Insurance Portability and Accountability Act) empowers a health care provider to use his or her judgment whether or not to reveal protected health information to authorities when a patient is diagnosed with a contagious disease. However, virtually every state has a law that makes the reporting to authorities of a patient diagnosed with a contagious disease mandatory. The state law does not conflict with the federal law; it is actually more specific in its directive about behavior, so it overrules the federal law. This example is one that illustrates how important it is for all health care professionals to be familiar with both federal and state laws that govern their job responsibilities.

EXAMPLES

The Emergency Medical Treatment and Active Labor Act (EMTALA)
The Affordable Care Act (ACA)
Equal Employment Opportunity Act (EEO)

Executive Orders
Official policies issued by the president of the United States.

Executive orders are official documents issued by the president of the United States to set policy. They do not require approval from the legislature (Congress); however, they are issued, typically, under statutory authority and, therefore, have the full effect and force of a federal statute. The federal courts have upheld this.

Common Law
Also known as case law, this is created by judicial decisions made during court trials.

Common law, also referred to as case law, is created by a judicial decision made during a court trial. These decisions, documented in law books for local, state, and federal court cases, create precedents–they establish a position. If you have ever watched a television show or movie with a court scene, you might remember the attorneys stating something like, "In *Brown v. The Board of Education*. . . ." This statement refers to a specific court case (*Brown v. The Board of Education*) and the decision made by that presiding judge. Those decisions are already accepted by the court, and therefore provide the current presiding judge with an established opinion.

You can see an example of the use of case law in the small portion of the Supreme Court opinion shown in **Figure 41-2**, the last three lines. A previous case–*PLIVA, Inc. v. Mensing*, 564 U.S. ___–is cited and this document goes on to explain the decision determined in that case and how it is related to this current case.

Private Practice Implements Safeguards for Waiting Rooms

Covered Entity: Private Practice

Issue: Safeguards; Impermissible Uses and Disclosures

A staff member of a medical practice discussed HIV testing procedures with a patient in the waiting room, thereby disclosing PHI to several other individuals. Also, computer screens displaying patient information were easily visible to patients. Among other corrective actions to resolve the specific issues in the case, OCR required the provider to develop and implement policies and procedures regarding appropriate administrative and physical safeguards related to the communication of PHI. The practice trained all staff on the newly developed policies and procedures. In addition, OCR required the practice to reposition its computer monitors to prevent patients from viewing information on the screens, and the practice installed computer monitor privacy screens to prevent impermissible disclosures.

FIGURE 41-2 The use of case law

Source: Department of Health and Human Services

EXAMPLES

United States v. Windsor

Mutual Pharmaceutical Co. v. Bartlett

Adoptive Couple v. Baby Girl

Administrative Laws
Also known as rules and regulations, these are created and adjudicated by administrative agencies given authority by Congress.

Administrative laws are those created and monitored by administrative agencies that have been given the responsibility to oversee specific areas, such as health care. The creation and implementation of specific rules and regulations have been delegated to those agencies created by Congress, under the Administrative Procedures Act, so each agency can ensure its assigned tasks can be accomplished. For example, Congress created the Centers for Disease Control and Prevention (CDC) as an administrative agency of the federal government to oversee issues related to contagious diseases. The CDC, therefore, has the authority to establish rules and regulations and to enforce those regulations (as long as they are consistent with the statute under which the agency was created). One of these rules is the mandated reporting of infectious diseases. Several surveillance information systems are used to enable the required reporting of these diagnoses; some are direct to the CDC while others are channeled through state departments of health first. However, if a particular diagnosis of an infectious disease is not reported, as required, the CDC has the authority to take action for noncompliance.

In **Figure 41-3**, you can see a screen shot of the website Regulations.gov. This website provides you with a searchable database of all federal agency regulations.

EXAMPLE

Centers for Medicare & Medicaid Services (CMS) has established its "rules of participation" for health care participating providers.

Criminal Law
Laws governing the behavior of the actions of the population related to health and well-being.

Criminal law seeks to control the behavior of people and companies when their actions are related to the health, welfare, and safety of an individual or property with the intention of protecting public order. Criminal activity is divided into two types, determined by the severity of the infraction: misdemeanors and felonies.

- A *misdemeanor* is a lesser offense, such as driving under the influence, public nuisances, and certain traffic violations. These infractions are adjudicated in local courts and are punishable with fines, penalties, and possible sentences of incarceration to county jail for up to 364 days.
- A *felony* is much more serious. This is a crime in violation of state or federal law and often carries a sentence of anywhere from 1 year to life in prison. Health care claims that are fraudulent and abusive of the reimbursement system constitute criminal activity and are an example of a felony. The Department of Justice, in conjunction with states' attorneys general, investigates accusations of these improper actions.

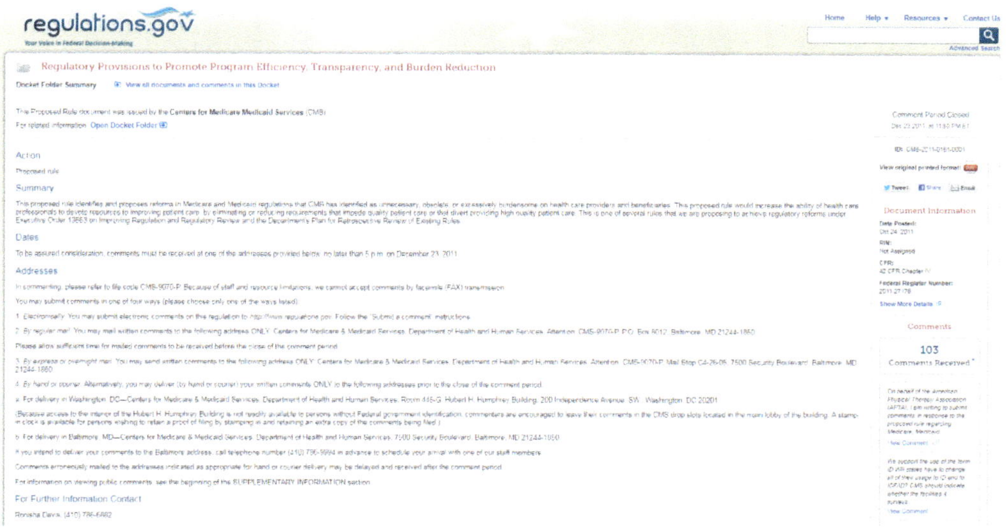

FIGURE 41-3 A snapshot of the website Regulations.gov, which offers a searchable database of federal agency rules and regulations

Source: Regulations.gov

In **Figure 41-4**, you can see a release from the FBI reporting a guilty plea from a company who was investigated and found guilty of criminal activity–involving violations of the False Claims Act as a result of a qui tam lawsuit.

FOR IMMEDIATE RELEASE

Friday, July 21, 2023

Booz Allen Agrees to Pay $377.45 million to Settle False Claims Act Allegations

The settlement resolved a lawsuit filed under the qui tam provision of the False Claims Act.

The qui tam lawsuit was filed by Sarah Feinberg, a former employee, and is captioned United States ex rel. Feinberg v. Booz Allen Hamilton, Inc.

Ms. Feinberg will receive $69,828,832 in connection with the settlement

FIGURE 41-4 A brief summary of a case resulting from a qui tam health care fraud lawsuit

Source: https://www.justice.gov/opa/pr/booz-allen-agrees-pay-37745-million-settle-false-claims-act-allegations

Civil Law
Laws that govern the relationships between people, and between businesses.

Civil law governs the conduct of those involved in a relationship: between private companies, individuals, and sometimes the government. Most often, a civil complaint or lawsuit will result from one party accusing the other of failure to comply with the terms of a contract. There are many instances of contractual relationships throughout the health care industry. Physicians and health care facilities may contract with a managed care organization; some facilities use contract workers to fill in for staff members on vacation; a family may contract with a home health care agency for services to a homebound patient; and the federal government may contract for health care services from a professional that does not include direct patient care. **Figure 41-5** shows specific language that may be included in one of these contracts. The violation of a patient's confidentiality falls into this category because, in the United States, privacy is considered a civil right. This is why an alleged violation of privacy laws is handled through the Office of Civil Rights (OCR) within the Department of Health and Human Services (DHHS) of the federal government.

41.2 Rules for Ethical and Legal Coding

As a coder, you have a very important responsibility–to yourself, your patients, and your facility. The work you do results in the creation of health claim forms and other reports that are legal documents. What you do can contribute to your facility staying healthy (businesswise) or being fined and possibly shut down by the Office of the Inspector General and your state's attorney general. You might make an error that could cause a patient to be unfairly denied health insurance coverage. It is important that you clearly understand the ethical and legal aspects of your position. Following are some issues, with regard to the ethics and legalities of coding, with which you should become very familiar.

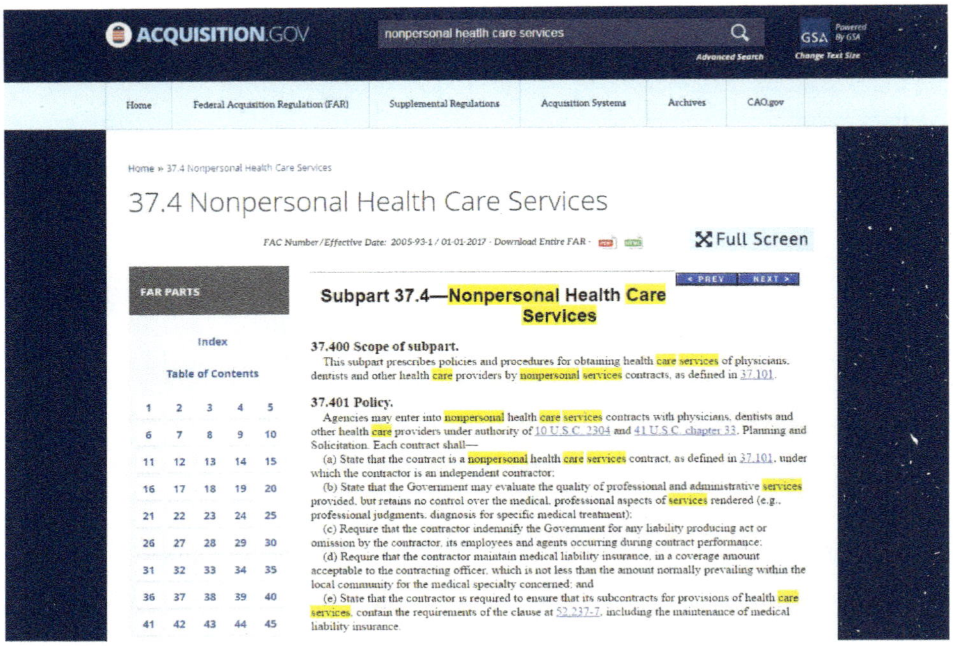

ACQUISITION.GOV

Home | Federal Acquisition Regulation (FAR) | Supplemental Regulations | Acquisition Systems | Archives | CAO.gov

Home » 37.4 Nonpersonal Health Care Services

37.4 Nonpersonal Health Care Services

FAC Number/Effective Date: 2005-93-1 / 01-01-2017 · Download Entire FAR ·

Subpart 37.4—Nonpersonal Health Care Services

37.400 Scope of subpart.

This subpart prescribes policies and procedures for obtaining health care services of physicians, dentists and other health care providers by nonpersonal services contracts, as defined in 37.101.

37.401 Policy.

Agencies may enter into nonpersonal health care services contracts with physicians, dentists and other health care providers under authority of 10 U.S.C. 2304 and 41 U.S.C. chapter 33. Planning and Solicitation. Each contract shall—

(a) State that the contract is a nonpersonal health care services contract, as defined in 37.101, under which the contractor is an independent contractor;

(b) State that the Government may evaluate the quality of professional and administrative services provided, but retains no control over the medical, professional aspects of services rendered (e.g., professional judgments, diagnosis for specific medical treatment);

(c) Require that the contractor indemnify the Government for any liability producing act or omission by the contractor, its employees and agents occurring during contract performance;

(d) Require that the contractor maintain medical liability insurance, in a coverage amount acceptable to the contracting officer, which is not less than the amount normally prevailing within the local community for the medical specialty concerned; and

(e) State that the contractor is required to ensure that its subcontracts for provisions of health care services, contain the requirements of the clause at 52.237-7, including the maintenance of medical liability insurance.

FIGURE 41-5 A partial example of language used in a contract for health care services that does not always include direct patient contact

Source: Acquisition.gov

> **Supporting Documentation**
> The paperwork in the patient's file that corroborates the codes presented on the claim form for a particular encounter.

1. It is very important that the codes indicated on the health claim form represent the services actually performed and the reasons why they are provided as supported by the documentation in the patient's health record. Don't use a code on a claim form without ensuring the **supporting documentation** is there in the file.

EXAMPLE

Coral Robinson's file indicates that Dr. Longmire ordered a blood test to determine whether or not she is pregnant. There is no report showing the results of the test. You see Dr. Longmire, and he tells you that Coral is pregnant and you should go ahead and code that diagnosis so the claim can be sent in. He promises to place the lab report and update the notes in her file later. Until the physician documents in the patient's chart that the patient is pregnant, you are not permitted to code the pregnancy.

> **Coding for Coverage**
> Choosing a code on the basis of what the insurance company will cover (pay for) rather than accurately reflecting the truth.

2. Some health care providers may improperly encourage **coding for coverage**. This term refers to the process of determining diagnostic and procedural codes not by the accuracy of the code but with regard to what the insurance company will pay for or "cover." That is dishonest and is considered fraud. If you find yourself in an office or facility that insists you "code for coverage" rather than code to accurately reflect the documentation and the services actually performed, you should immediately discuss your situation with someone you trust. Some providers will rationalize the process by saying they are doing it so the patients can get the treatment they really need paid for by the insurance company. Altruism aside, it is still illegal and, once discovered, financial penalties and possible jail time can be assessed.

EXAMPLE

Corbin Bloom wants a nose job (rhinoplasty); however, he cannot afford it. The insurance carrier will not pay for cosmetic surgery, so the coder changes the code to indicate that Corbin has a deviated septum requiring surgical correction so that the insurance carrier will pay for the procedure. That is *coding for coverage* and is fraud.

3. If you find yourself in an office or facility that insists that you include codes for procedures that you know, or believe, were never performed at a level of intensity or complexity as described by the code, this might be fraudulent behavior known as **upcoding**—the process of using a code that claims a higher level of service, or a more severe illness, than is true. Upcoding is considered falsifying records. Even if all you do is fill out the claim form, you are participating in something unethical and illegal.

Upcoding
Using a code on a claim form that indicates a higher level of service than that which was actually performed.

EXAMPLE

Erica Forney, a 69-year-old female, in the hospital for a broken hip, had her glucose level checked by the nurse, and it was at an abnormal level. Dr. Magnus ordered additional tests to rule out diabetes mellitus. Coding that Erica has diabetes is *upcoding* her condition and will fraudulently increase reimbursement from Medicare by changing the diagnosis-related group (DRG). In addition, placing a chronic disease on her health chart when she doesn't have it will cause her problems later on.

4. It is not permissible to code and bill for individual (also known as *component*) elements when a comprehensive or combination (bundle) code is available. This is referred to as **unbundling** and is illegal.
   For Medicare billing, refer to the Medicare National Correct Coding Initiative (CCI), which lists standardized bundled codes. The CCI is used to find coding conflicts, such as unbundling, the use of **mutually exclusive codes**, and other unacceptable reporting of CPT codes. When these errors are discovered, those claims are pulled for review and may be subject to possible suspension or rejection.

Unbundling
Coding individual parts of a specific procedure rather than one combination, or bundle, that includes all the components.

Mutually Exclusive Codes
Codes that are identified as those that are not permitted to be used on the same claim form with other codes.

EXAMPLE

Dr. Hayden's notes indicate that Rico was experiencing nausea and vomiting. Instead of coding **R11.2 Nausea with vomiting**, the coder unbundles, coding **R11.0 Nausea** alone and **R11.11 Vomiting** alone.

Double Billing
Sending a claim for the second time to the same insurance company for the same procedure or service, provided to the same patient on the same date of service.

5. If you resubmit a claim that has been lost, identify it as a "tracer" or "second submission." If you don't, you might be found guilty of **double billing**, billing the insurance company twice for a service provided only once. This also constitutes fraud.
6. You must code all conditions or complications that are relevant to the current encounter. Separating the codes relating to one specific encounter and placing them on several different claim forms over the course of several different days is neither legal nor ethical. It not only indicates a lack of organization of the office but also can cause suspicion of duplicating service claims, known as double billing. Even if you are reporting procedures that were actually done for diagnoses that actually exist, remember that the claim form is a legal document. All data on that claim form, including dates of service, must be accurate. Do not submit the claim form until you are certain it is complete, with all diagnoses and procedures listed. If it happens that, after you submit a claim, an additional service provided comes to light (such as a lab report with an extra charge that didn't come across your desk until after you filed the claim), then you must file an amended claim. While not illegal because you are identifying that the claim contains an adjustment, most third-party payers really dislike amended claims. You can expect an amended claim to be scrutinized.

CODING BITES

Always read the complete description in the provider's notes in addition to referencing the encounter form or superbill, and then carefully find the best available code that supports medical necessity according to the documentation.

All the activities mentioned here are considered fraud and are against the law. It is not worth breaking the law and being charged with any of these penalties just to hang on to a job.

CODING BITES

Office of the Inspector General (OIG)

https://oig.hhs.gov/reports-and-publications/workplan/index.asp

Office of the Inspector General (OIG) Workplan

The Office of the Inspector General (OIG), in the Department of Health and Human Services, is the agency that investigates and prosecutes failure to comply with the legal requirements for coding. The OIG plans in advance, for the upcoming year, what specific violations will be reviewed and investigated. This is valuable information to support the development of internal policies and procedures as well as foci for internal audits. When you can uncover and correct coding and billing errors *BEFORE* the federal or state auditors show up, this lessens fines and penalties considerably.

The workplan is released each year by October 1 for the upcoming calendar year. It is subsectioned by the type of facility affected, so you don't have to read through everything to find that which applies to your organization. Sometimes the issue is directly related to billing and coding; others may be more administrative.

EXAMPLES

HOSPITALS

Hospital Reporting of Patient Harm Events per CMS and State Requirements

Hospitals collect information about patient harm events to meet Medicare requirements to measure, analyze, and track adverse patient harm events. Hospitals are also required to report certain types of harm events to meet CMS program and State legal requirements. Prior OIG work found that hospitals reported few harm events to State reporting systems (Few Adverse Events in Hospitals Were Reported to State Adverse Event Reporting Systems (OEI-06-09-00092)). We will determine the extent to which hospitals reported harm events as required per CMS program and State requirements. We will use harm events OIG identified through medical review for the study Adverse Events in Hospitals: A Quarter of Medicare Patients Experienced Harm in October 2018 (OEI-06-18-00400) as the basis for this review. This is a supplemental product to our ongoing study that is examining hospital identification of patient harm events (OEI-06-18-00401).

Medicare Inpatient Hospital Billing for Sepsis

Sepsis is the body's extreme response to an infection. It is a life-threatening, emergency medical issue that often progresses quickly and responds best to early intervention. The definition of and guidance for sepsis have changed over the years in attempts to identify it more accurately. The definition of sepsis was updated in 2016 by an international task force to better differentiate sepsis from a general infection. This narrower definition is widely recognized by groups such as the World Health Organization. However, CMS and CDC currently recognize an older, broader definition. Sepsis is a frequently billed diagnosis in Medicare. There are concerns that hospitals may be taking advantage of this broader definition, as they have a financial incentive to do so. This study will analyze Medicare claims to assess patterns in the inpatient hospital billing of sepsis in 2023 and describe how the billing of sepsis varied among hospitals. We will also estimate the costs to Medicare associated with using the broader, rather than the narrower, definition of sepsis.

EXAMPLE

HOME HEALTH SERVICES

Medicare Payments for Home Dialysis Services

Medicare Part B covers outpatient dialysis services for enrollees diagnosed with end-stage renal disease (ESRD). Treatments can be provided in an outpatient or home setting and must be monitored by certified ESRD facilities. Prior OIG work identified inappropriate Medicare payments for dialysis services. Specifically, OIG identified claims for which there were neither dialysis treatment notes for home dialysis sessions nor documentation of the dispensing or administration of medication billed. Additionally, OIG found claims with medication billed exceeding a physician-prescribed amount, as well as other issues with comprehensive assessments, plans of care, and physicians' monthly progress notes. We will review claims for Medicare Part B home dialysis services provided to ESRD patients to determine whether such services complied with Medicare requirements. Also, we will review the impact of home dialysis services on enrollees and whether enrollees' quality of care could be affected.

41.3 False Claims Act

The federal False Claims Act (FCA) was enacted by Congress to make the submission of a claim to a federal agency containing false information an illegal act. After this law was put into place, virtually every individual state passed its own version. This means that an individual may be charged with violation of both the federal law *AND* the state law, magnifying the fines, penalties, and consequences of this fraudulent behavior.

Who Is Liable?

Which staff members are responsible for ensuring that a facility or provider complies with FCA? All individuals and facilities that are involved in the creation and submission of claims–requests for reimbursement–based on coverage provided by governmental programs, such as Medicare or Medicaid, are responsible for complying with this law. Legally, these entities are referred to as federal contractors. Some people read the word *contractor* and immediately think of construction projects. However, in these cases, this phrase refers to one signing a contract to do business with a government program, that is, a participating provider. The Department of Justice takes enforcement of the FCA seriously (see **Figure 41-6** for just one example).

APRN and Medical Practice to Pay Over $600k and Cease Connecticut Medicaid Participation to Settle False Claims Act Allegations

Wednesday, August 6, 2025

David X. Sullivan, United States Attorney for the District of Connecticut, today announced that ARMAND NTCHANA and his various entities have entered into a civil settlement agreement with the federal and state governments and agreed to pay more than $600,000 to resolve allegations that they violated the federal and state False Claims Acts by causing false claims to be submitted to Medicare and Connecticut Medicaid. Ntchana currently resides in Alexandria, Louisiana.

The federal and state governments allege that from January 2016 through October 2020, Ntchana and IPS violated the federal and state False Claims Acts by improperly billing Medicare and Connecticut Medicaid for services not rendered, the services of an unlicensed provider, and for upcoded or duplicative claims.

FIGURE 41-6 An extract from a press release from the Department of Justice concerning a case enforcing the False Claims Act

Source: "APRN and Medical Practice to pay Over $600k ..." August 6, 2025.

What Is a Claim?

Needless to say, this law requires the proper behavior of individuals filing claims for reimbursement. So, let's begin with the FCA's specific definition of what a claim is: "*a demand for money or property made directly to the Federal Government or to a contractor, grantee, or other recipient.*"*

Under the requirements of the individual state governments, this would be a demand for reimbursement from the state government or other entity within.

The Knowledge Requirement

In addition, this law includes a "knowledge requirement." This portion of the law states that the simple action of submitting a claim with false information is not a violation. The individual must *know* that the information on the claim is false. What does "*know*" mean?

- *Actual knowledge* . . . knowing for a fact that the information is false.
- *Willful ignorance*, also known as deliberate ignorance . . . those who should know due to their job position, training, or responsibilities within the organization with regard to filing the claim but purposely don't ask about the validity of the information, or ignore the falsity of the information.
- *Disregard* of the truth or falsity . . . behavior that exhibits an indifference to confirming that the information is true.

*Source: Federal False Claims Act, Department of Justice.

> **EXAMPLES**
>
> *Actual knowledge:*
>
> *"I know that the procedures documented in the patient's record were not actually performed."*
>
> *Willful ignorance:*
>
> *"I don't know for a fact, and I don't want to know."*
>
> *Disregard of the truth:*
>
> *"It's not my concern. I just do what I am told."*

Essentially, this means that an individual is required to comply with this law if, as part of his or her job, the individual *knows* the accuracy of the information on the claim, or *should know* the accuracy of the information. If your job involves anything to do with the creation and submission of a claim to any third party, it is your responsibility to know for a fact that the information is true. And no court will accept your excuse that you "didn't know."

The Qui Tam Provision

The *qui tam provision* within the FCA, commonly known as the *Whistleblower Statute*, empowers private citizens (typically those who work within organizations that do not comply) to file a lawsuit on behalf of the federal or state government against the facility for noncompliance. Sadly, there are health care professionals who will not listen to a staff member explaining that a particular behavior or sequence of actions is not legal. The intent of this statute is to recruit those honest individuals who witness an organization that is committing, or encouraging, fraudulent activities to step up and help to stop the illegal actions by reporting the fraud or filing a qui tam suit.

The government knows how scary and difficult it can be to come forward. Therefore, they reward the person or persons reporting the fraud with a percentage of the total amount recovered by the federal or state government as a result of the qui tam lawsuit. This reward can be anywhere from 15% to 30%.

> **CODING BITES**
>
> Want more details about qui tam lawsuits? Here is an interesting article: "***Qui Tam Whistleblower Guide,***" from the *National Law Review* (June 27, 2024):
>
> https://natlawreview.com/article/qui-tam-whistleblower-guide

> **EXAMPLE**
>
> Settlements and judgments under the False Claims Act exceeded $2.9 billion in the fiscal year ending Sept. 30, 2024,... The government and whistleblowers were party to 558 settlements and judgments, the second highest total after last year's record of 566 recoveries, and whistleblowers filed 979 qui tam lawsuits, the highest number in a single year. Settlements and judgments since 1986, when Congress substantially strengthened the civil False Claims Act, now total more than $78 billion.

> **CODING BITES**
>
> Be very careful when writing or typing this acronym. It is HIPAA . . . one P and two As.

41.4 Health Insurance Portability and Accountability Act (HIPAA)

The Health Insurance Portability and Accountability Act of 1996, known as HIPAA (pronounced *hip-aah*), was enacted by the federal government and directly applies to you as a coding professional. Like most federal laws, HIPAA covers many different issues and concerns. The Privacy Rule is one part of this law that you are obligated to know and understand.

> **HIPAA's Privacy Rule**
> A portion of HIPAA that ensures the availability of patient information for those who should see it while protecting that information from those who should not.

HIPAA's Privacy Rule

HIPAA's Privacy Rule was written to protect an individual's privacy with regard to personal health information, without getting in the way of the flow of data that is necessary to provide appropriate care for that patient. Essentially, the lawmakers tried to make certain that *a patient's information is easily accessible to those who should have access to it* [such as the physician, insurance coder and biller, and therapist] *and, at the same time, keep it secured against unauthorized people* [such as potential employers, coworkers, or neighborhood gossips] so that they do not see things they have no business seeing.

Who Is Responsible for Obeying This Law

HIPAA's Privacy Rule went into effect on April 14, 2003, and concerns every physician's office, clinic, hospital, and health insurance carrier—every type of business that is directly involved in the delivery of and/or payment for health care services, no matter how big or small. The largest of corporations owning hundreds of hospitals around the country and an office with one physician working alone are all included. HIPAA calls these businesses **covered entities**, and they all must comply with the terms of the law.

Covered Entities
Health care providers, health plans, and health care clearinghouses—businesses that have access to the personal health information of patients.

Covered entities are divided into three categories:

- Health care providers
- Health plans
- Health care clearinghouses

You probably already know the definition of a *health care provider*: any person or organization that gives health care services as the primary business purpose.

EXAMPLE

Health care providers as defined by HIPAA: physicians, dentists, hospitals, clinics, pharmacies, laboratories, and so on.

CODING BITES

Respecting a patient's privacy is also a sign of respect for the person. When you are the patient, you want to be treated with respect. So following HIPAA's Privacy Rule is not just the law of the United States; it is the law of treating people fairly.

Health plans are described as organizations that provide and/or pay for health care services as their main reason for being in business. They include health insurance carriers, HMOs, employee welfare benefit plans, government health plans (such as TriCare, Medicare, and Medicaid), and group health plans provided through employers and associations. It doesn't matter whether the plan is offered to an individual or a group—all companies offering this coverage are included.

EXAMPLE

Health care plans as defined by HIPAA: Medicare, Medicaid, TriCare, BlueCross BlueShield, Prudential, and so on.

In addition, technology has created another type of organization involved in this process, called a *health care clearinghouse*. These companies help process electronic health insurance claims. Medical billing services, medical review services, and health information management system companies are included in this definition.

EXAMPLE

Health care clearinghouses as defined by HIPAA: National Clearinghouse, NDC Electronic Claims, WebMD Network Services, and others.

The workforces of covered entities are also included under HIPAA. A covered entity's workforce consists of every person who is involved with the company—full time, part time, volunteer, intern, extern, physician, nurse, assistant—and this has nothing to do with whether they are paid. Everyone must comply with the terms of this law.

EXAMPLE

A covered entity's workforce as defined by HIPAA: full-time staff members, part-time staff members, volunteers, interns, externs, janitorial staff members, and so on.

CODING BITES

HIPAA's Privacy Rule is mostly about protecting your patient's privacy.

What This Law Covers

You are certainly familiar with the topic of doctor–patient confidentiality. It means that anything a patient tells his or her doctor must be kept private. The doctor is not allowed, under most circumstances, to reveal to anyone what was said. This includes family members, parents (in many cases), and friends. This is important so that an individual will feel comfortable being open and honest and tell the physician things that are very, very personal, possibly even embarrassing or private facts that this person has never told anyone else. However, in order for the physician to properly treat this individual, the physician must know everything.

In order for you to do your job properly, you have access to all this confidential information. You need to know very personal and private facts about every one of your patients in order to accurately report the data.

> **Protected Health Information (PHI)**
> Any patient-identifiable health information regardless of the form in which it is stored (paper, computer file, etc.).

You know what is wrong with them (their diagnoses) now and in the past; you know why they came to see this health care provider and why they saw others before they came to your facility; and you know what the health care provider thinks (observations and impressions) about these patients, as well as what has been done, is being done, and will be done to treat them. You know all these things because you have access to patients' health care records, including all the physician's notes. HIPAA calls this personal health care information (past, present, and future conditions) individually identifiable health information. In other words, it is information that anyone could look at and know exactly which individual is being discussed–one specific person. Specific pieces of data, called **protected health information (PHI)**, are pieces of information related to an individual that must be kept confidential, the grouping of facts that might have someone say, "Oh, I know him! Oh, and he has that!"

EXAMPLE

Nicholas is a patient of Dr. Molinaro, and the information inside his chart (paper or electronic) consists of his records, charts, lab reports, and physician's notes documenting everything Nicholas has ever discussed with his physician. Karyn needs all this information to do her job as the office's coding specialist. At this moment, Karyn has stepped away from her desk. Nicholas's file is sitting on Karyn's desk, lying open.

From the color of the folder, even from a distance, it is obvious that this is a patient of Dr. Molinaro's. The top piece of paper indicates that his patient has been diagnosed with a sexually transmitted disease. *At this point, any unauthorized person couldn't really know whose chart this is because Dr. Molinaro has hundreds of patients.*

Right above the diagnosis anyone can see that this patient is a male. Although this will eliminate some of Dr. Molinaro's patients, there are still too many to know for certain.

Upon closer examination of the paperwork in the folder, anyone could see that this male patient with the sexually transmitted disease lives on Main Street in Our Town, Florida. *The list of Dr. Molinaro's patients that is being referred to is getting very short now.*

In the upper right corner, anyone can see Dr. Molinaro's male patient, who lives on Main Street, Our Town, Florida, who has a sexually transmitted disease, was born on June 13, 1985. *Oh my, did you know Nicholas lives on Main Street in Our Town, and his birthday is June 13th? It must be Nicholas who has that terrible disease!*

Did Karyn fulfill her responsibility to protect Nicholas's privacy? What could she have done differently to ensure that this patient's PHI was protected?

Nicholas's private health record is no longer private. His diagnosis of a sexually transmitted disease is health information. After discovering his gender, address, and birth date, someone can connect this diagnosis directly to one particular person. All these details, and any other pieces of information like these, are protected to be private under the law. This means that all this information is confidential, and it is against the law for you to reveal any of it, with only a few exceptions:

1. You can tell other health care professionals who are directly involved in the course of doing your job.
2. You can tell someone when given written permission from the patient to do so.
3. You can tell in situations, as outlined in the law, based on "best professional judgment."

> **Use**
> (1) The sharing of information between people working in the same health care facility for purposes of caring for the patient. (2) Occasional consumption of a substance without clinical manifestations.

The Use and Disclosure of PHI

HIPAA's Privacy Rule is very specific as to how you can handle the PHI that you work with every day. The guidelines offer two terms to describe how you might deal with these data.

The term **use** (with regard to HIPAA) means that the information is being shared between people who work together in the same office and need to exchange PHI in order to better serve the patient.

EXAMPLE

You are getting ready to code the diagnosis for Herman Farber's recent visit and need additional information. You speak with the attending physician, Dr. Yaw, to discuss Herman's PHI so that you can make certain you find the best, most appropriate diagnosis code. You are using that patient's PHI because the information is being shared between you and the physician in the same office for the benefit of the patient.

Disclosure
The sharing of information between health care professionals working in separate entities, or facilities, in the course of caring for the patient.

The second term is **disclosure**. HIPAA defines the term *disclosure* to mean that PHI is being revealed to someone outside the health care office or facility. For example, you prepare a health insurance claim form to send to the patient's insurance company so it will pay your office for the procedures provided. On that claim form, you must put the patient's full name and address, birth date, diagnosis codes, and procedure codes. As you learned earlier in this chapter, each piece of data is not necessarily confidential. When you put all this information together in one place, it becomes PHI because this health information (diagnosis and procedure codes) is now connected to a specific person (identified by the name, address, birth date, etc.) on one piece of paper. However, you must disclose this information to the insurance carrier in order to get paid. You are disclosing the information because the insurance company personnel who will read this claim form do not work for your health care facility—they are an outside company.

EXAMPLE

Dr. Royan indicates that his patient, Caleb Carter, needs some lab work. Dr. Royan will use Mr. Carter's PHI in his orders for which tests should be performed. Then you need to call the laboratory and disclose Mr. Carter's PHI (his name and diagnosis) along with what specific tests should be performed by the lab.

Remember that everyone in your office and everyone at the insurance carrier and the lab is a member of a covered entity's workforce. You are all bound by the same terms of the HIPAA law and cannot reveal any patient's PHI, except under particular circumstances (such as use and disclosure), unless you have the patient's written permission (**Figure 41-7**).

"To date [October 31, 2024], OCR settled or imposed a civil money penalty in 152 cases resulting in a total dollar amount of $144,878,972.00. OCR has investigated complaints against many different types of entities including: national pharmacy chains, major medical centers, group health plans, hospital chains, and small provider offices."

FIGURE 41-7 Enforcement Results, as of October 31, 2024

Source: https://www.hhs.gov/hipaa/for-professionals/compliance-enforcement/data/enforcement-highlights/index.html

Getting Written Approval

Release of Information (ROI)
The form (either on paper or electronic) that a patient must sign to give legal permission to a covered entity to disclose that patient's PHI.

In most situations, other than those already mentioned, the health care provider must get a patient's written permission to disclose the PHI. Although there are many preprinted **Release of Information (ROI)** forms that your office or facility may purchase, the Privacy Rule of HIPAA insists that all these documents have the following characteristics:

1. Are written in plain language (not legalese) so that the average person can understand what he or she is signing.
2. Are very specific as to exactly what information will be disclosed or used.
3. Specifically identify the person or organization that will be disclosing the information.
4. Specifically identify the person(s) who will be receiving the information.
5. Have a definite expiration date.
6. Clearly explain that the person signing this release may retract this authorization in writing at any time.

Figure 41-8 is an example of a form that your facility might use for this purpose.

Permitted Uses and Disclosures

The Privacy Rule outlines six circumstances in which health care professionals are permitted, with or without written patient permission, to use their best professional judgment as to whether or not they should use and/or disclose a patient's PHI.

FORM APPROVED: OMB NO. 0917-0030
Expiration Date: 09/30/2023
See OMB Statement on Reverse.

DEPARTMENT OF HEALTH AND HUMAN SERVICES
Indian Health Service

AUTHORIZATION FOR USE OR DISCLOSURE OF PROTECTED HEALTH INFORMATION

COMPLETE ALL SECTIONS, DATE, AND SIGN

I. I, ______________________________ *(Name of Patient)*, hereby voluntarily authorize the disclosure of information from my health record.

II. The information is to be disclosed by:	**And is to be provided to:**
NAME OF FACILITY	NAME OF PERSON/ORGANIZATION/FACILITY
ADDRESS	ADDRESS
CITY/STATE	CITY/STATE

III. The purpose or need for this disclosure is:

☐ Further Medical Care ☐ Attorney ☐ School ☐ Research
☐ Personal Use ☐ Insurance ☐ Disability ☐ Other *(Specify)* ____________

IV. The information to be disclosed from my health record: *(check appropriate box(es))*

☐ Only information related to *(specify)* ____________

☐ Only the period of events from ____________ to ____________
☐ Other *(specify) (CHS, Billing, etc.)* ____________
☐ Entire Record

If you would like any of the following sensitive information disclosed, check the applicable box(es) below:

☐ Alcohol/Drug Abuse Treatment/Referral ☐ HIV/AIDS-related Treatment
☐ Sexually Transmitted Diseases ☐ Mental Health *(Other than Psychotherapy Notes)*
☐ Psychotherapy Notes ONLY (by checking this box, I am waiving any psychotherapist-patient privilege)

V. I understand that I may revoke this authorization in writing submitted at any time to the Health Information Management Department, except to the extent that action has been taken in reliance on this authorization. If this authorization was obtained as a condition of obtaining insurance coverage or a policy of insurance, other law may provide the insurer with the right to contest a claim under the policy. If this authorization has not been revoked, it will terminate one year from the date of my signature unless a different expiration date or *expiration event* is stated.

____________ *(Specify new date)*

I understand that IHS will not condition treatment or eligibility for care on my providing this authorization except if such care is: (1) research related or (2) provided solely for the purpose of creating Protected Health Information for disclosure to a third party.

I understand that information disclosed by this authorization, except for Alcohol and Drug Abuse as defined in 42 CFR Part 2, may be subject to redisclosure by the recipient and may no longer be protected by the Health Insurance Portability and Accountability Act Privacy Rule [45 CFR Part 164] and the Privacy Act of 1974 [5 USC 552a].

SIGNATURE OF PATIENT OR PERSONAL REPRESENTATIVE *(State relationship to patient)*	DATE
SIGNATURE OF WITNESS *(If signature of patient is a thumbprint or mark)*	DATE

This information is to be released for the purpose stated above and may not be used by the recipient for any other purpose. Any person who knowingly and willfully requests or obtains any record concerning an individual from a federal agency under false pretenses shall be guilty of a misdemeanor (5 USC 552a(i)(3)).

PATIENT IDENTIFICATION

NAME *(Last, First, MI)*	RECORD NUMBER
ADDRESS	
CITY/STATE	DATE OF BIRTH

PSC Graphics (301) 443-1090 EF

FIGURE 41-8 Example of authorization form to release health information

Source: Department of Health and Human Services, Form OMB 0817-0030

1. *To the individual.* Health care professionals can *use their best professional judgment to decide whether or not a patient should be told* certain things contained in his or her health care record. Questions come up especially when mental health issues and terminal conditions (when a patient is almost certain to die in the near future) are concerned and there is doubt if the patient can deal with the medical facts. In almost all cases, providing patients with their own PHI is allowed.
2. *Treatment, payment, and/or operations (TPO).* This means that health care professionals are free to use and/or disclose PHI when it comes to making decisions, coordinating, and managing the *treatment* of a patient's condition.
   In addition, PHI can be disclosed for *payment* activities, such as billing and claims processing, as mentioned earlier in this chapter. In this description, the term *operations* refers to the health care facility's own management of case coordination and quality evaluations.

EXAMPLE

A physician needs to be able to discuss PHI details with a therapist so that, together, they can establish a proper course of treatment for the patient.

3. *Opportunity to agree or object.* This relates to a more informal situation where the patient is present and alert and has the ability to give verbal permission or not with regard to a specific disclosure.

   One important point to remember: Although it is much easier to simply ask someone for his or her oral approval than to go get a form and make the patient sign first, it is in your best interest to get written approval whenever possible. People's memories may fail, or they may change their mind later about what they really did tell you. If there is nothing on paper, you cannot prove what was said. For your own protection, get it in writing whenever possible!

EXAMPLE

Asher Grimm is about to hear Dr. Brant explain his test results. Asher's wife is in the waiting room. Dr. Brant may ask Asher if it is okay to invite his wife in and permit her to hear this information, too. Asher can then say, "Yes, that is fine" or "No, I don't want her to know about this." Dr. Brant then must abide by what the patient requests.

4. *Incidental use and disclosure.* As long as reasonable safeguards are in place, this portion of the rule addresses the fact that information might accidentally be used or disclosed during the regular course of business.

EXAMPLE

Dr. Holloway comes out of an examining room and approaches Nurse Miller standing at the desk. This is a back area, and patients are not generally in this hallway, so Dr. Holloway speaks to the nurse in a normal tone of voice to instruct her on preparing Mrs. Hunter for a procedure. All of a sudden, another patient comes around the corner, lost on her way back to the waiting room, and overhears the conversation.

CODING BITES

Incidental is close to the word *accidental*—if someone accidentally overhears what you say.

This is called incidental use and is understandable in a working environment; therefore, it is not considered a violation of the law.

However, it is important for conversations like this to include only the minimum necessary PHI to accomplish the goal. *Minimum necessary* refers to the caution that should be used to release only the smallest amount of information required to accomplish the task and no more. Not only is it unnecessary to release more, it is unprofessional.

EXAMPLE

In the hallway outside the exam room, the physician would only need to say, "Serita, please prepare Mrs. Hunter for her examination." She would not need to include other details about Mrs. Hunter, such as, "Serita, please prepare Mrs. Hunter for her examination. You know she has a terrible rash on her thighs. I suspect that it's poison ivy. However, it could be a sexually transmitted disease. We'll have to find out how many sexual partners she has had in the last 6 months." All that extra information is unnecessary to the proper care of Mrs. Hunter at this moment.

> **CODING BITES**
>
> Remember that, when there is a state or federal mandate to report (that means you have no choice; you must report to the proper authorities), this does not apply *only* to the physician of your practice but also applies to you.

5. *Public interest.* There are times when the public's best interest may prompt disclosing what you know about a patient. Very often, this is mandated by state laws, which would then take priority over the federal HIPAA law. In other words, if the federal law says you are allowed to tell, and your state's law says you must tell–then, you must! These situations include the reporting of suspected abuse (child abuse, elder abuse, neglect, domestic violence) and the reporting of sexually transmitted and other contagious diseases. You are included in the health care team and must think about the community, which must be warned if someone is walking around with a contagious (communicable) disease. Most states require notification to the police in cases where the patient has been shot or stabbed. It is your responsibility to find out what the laws are in your state and how to correctly file a report.

   If the physician does not report suspected child abuse of one of your patients, it is your obligation to pick up the phone and call.
6. *Limited data set.* For research, public health statistics, or other health care operations, PHI can be revealed, but only after it has been depersonalized. In other words, if the data that connect this information to a specific individual are removed or blacked out, the information is no longer individually identifiable health information, so it does not need to be protected any longer.

> **EXAMPLE**
>
> You can release a health record that has no name, address, telephone number, e-mail address, Social Security number, or photographs attached to it. Even certain physician's notes can be released after they have been stripped of personal data. Following is a sample portion of a record that can be shown without fear of violating anyone's privacy:
>
> "XXX ________ is 33 years old. Back in April, ________ was in a motor vehicle accident while he was on the job. ________ is complaining about some neck pain. ________ has tingling into the left hand."
>
> The example above is a direct quote from the medical record of an actual patient after the specified direct identifiers have been removed. You cannot connect this health information to any one particular person. Therefore, the information is no longer protected and can be used for research and in other ways that may help the community.

> **CODING BITES**
>
> This law simply assures every person coming to your health care facility that his or her personal and private information will be protected and treated with respect.

Privacy Notices

HIPAA instructs all its covered entities to create policies and procedures with regard to the use and disclosure of PHI. In addition, the law actually states that, once policies and procedures are developed, the facilities must follow these policies. Copies of the written policy must be given to every patient and posted in a general area where it can be seen by all patients.

Notices of Privacy written in compliance with HIPAA's Privacy Rule must contain the following points:

1. A full description of how the covered entity may use and/or disclose a patient's PHI.
2. A statement about the covered entity's responsibility to protect a patient's privacy.
3. Complete information about the patient's rights, including contact information for the Department of Health and Human Services (DHHS), should the patient wish to lodge a complaint that his or her privacy was violated.
4. The name of a specific employee of the covered entity, who must be named as *privacy officer*. This person's name, as well as contact information, must be included in the written notice to handle patients' questions and complaints.

The covered entity must receive written acknowledgment from each patient stating that he or she received the written privacy practices notice. This is usually one of the papers that a patient has to sign when going to a health care facility for the first time.

One of the most important aspects of this portion of the Privacy Rule is that the law specifically says that the covered entity not only has to create these policies and procedures but also has to abide by them. If it doesn't, it is considered to be in violation of federal law and punishable by fines and/or imprisonment.

Although some health care staff members feel that HIPAA and its Privacy Rule are a pain in the neck, think about what this law actually means: respecting your patients' privacy and dignity. Isn't that what you expect from your health care professionals when you go for help? It is not enough that only the doctor be bound to protect the patient's information as confidential because the doctor is no longer the only person who has access. Your health care facility is no place for gossip. You might find this person's hemorrhoids funny or that person's rash gross. As a professional, you should not be concerned with entertaining your friends with your patients' private circumstances. How would you feel if it were *your* personal problem that your health care team members were giggling about with their friends? Or you might consider telling your brother that his girlfriend came in with a sexually transmitted disease. You cannot! Everyone is entitled to privacy. As difficult as it may be, you must remain a professional.

CODING BITES

Just because you *can* take a look at any patient's chart doesn't mean you should. In your facility, you will probably be granted permission to access patients' charts so you can do your work. Under certain circumstances you may be tempted to look, not for your job but because the patient is your friend or neighbor or a celebrity. You may think no harm is being done, just caring or curiosity. But there is harm, and you are prohibited, by law, to do this.

In June 2023, Yakima Valley Memorial Hospital agreed to pay $240,000 and implement a plan to update policies and procedures after hospital security guards were found to illegally access 419 patient medical records.

You could be the president of the hospital and have your best friend come into the ED of your hospital. Without specific permission from that patient, you would be forbidden from looking at the record. Every individual has the right to make his or her own decision about who should know what about his or her own health information.

Violating HIPAA's Privacy Rule

Any individual who discovers that his or her privacy has been misused or disclosed without permission can file a complaint with the Department of Health and Human Services (DHHS) that the health care provider, health plan, or clearinghouse has not followed HIPAA's regulations. When writing this law, Congress included specifications for both civil and criminal penalties to be applied against any covered entity that fails to protect its patients' PHI. These penalties include fines–up to $250,000–and up to 10 years in prison (**Figure 41-9**).

Enforcement Results as of October 31, 2024
Since the compliance date of the Privacy Rule in April 2003, OCR has received over 374,321 HIPAA complaints and has initiated over 1,193 compliance reviews. We have resolved ninety-nine percent of these cases (370,578).
OCR has investigated and resolved over 31,191 cases by requiring changes in privacy practices and corrective actions by, or providing technical assistance to, HIPAA covered entities and their business associates. Corrective actions obtained by OCR from these entities have resulted in change that is systemic and that affects all the individuals they serve. OCR has successfully enforced the HIPAA Rules by applying corrective measures in all cases where an investigation indicates noncompliance by the covered entity or their business associate. To date, OCR settled or imposed a civil money penalty in 152 cases resulting in a total dollar amount of $144,878,972.00. OCR has investigated complaints against many different types of entities including: national pharmacy chains, major medical centers, group health plans, hospital chains, and small provider offices.
https://www.hhs.gov/hipaa/for-professionals/compliance-enforcement/data/enforcement-highlights/index.html

FIGURE 41-9 Information summary of OCR investigations into HIPAA violations

Source: https://www.hhs.gov/hipaa/for-professionals/compliance-enforcement/data/enforcement-highlights/index.html

A covered entity is responsible for any violation of HIPAA requirements by any of its employees, business associates, or other members of its workforce, such as interns and volunteers. Generally, the senior officials of the covered entity may be punished for the lack of compliance; however, middle managers and staff members are not exempt.

Civil Penalties

1. $100 with no prison for each single violation of a HIPAA regulation with a maximum of $25,000 for multiple violations of the same portion of the regulation during the same calendar year.

EXAMPLE

You tell your best friend that Oliver Tesca, whom you both went to school with, came into your physician's office and tested positive for a sexually transmitted disease. You, of course, swear her to secrecy. Later that day, she bumps into Oliver's fiancée and feels obligated to tell her about Oliver's condition. Oliver puts two and two together, after his fiancée breaks up with him, and he files a complaint that you disclosed his PHI without permission. You and/or your physician is fined $100.

Criminal Penalties

2. Up to $50,000 *and* up to 1 year in jail for the unauthorized or inappropriate disclosure of individually identifiable health information.

> **EXAMPLE**
>
> After you are fined the $100 civil penalty for the inappropriate disclosure of Oliver Tesca's PHI, you and/or your physician is charged with criminal penalties for the same disclosure, including a fine of $50,000 and a year in jail.

3. Up to $100,000 *and* up to 5 years in prison for the unauthorized or inappropriate disclosure of individually identifiable health information through deception.

> **EXAMPLE**
>
> Your best friend since high school, Sally-Anne Hoskins, just got a great job as a pharmaceutical representative. To help her, you give her a list of 250 patients from your facility who have been diagnosed with diabetes so she can advertise her company's new drug to them. You and she both know this is illegal, so you tell Sally-Anne that you got permission from each of the patients to release the information (and that is a lie). After a patient complains to DHHS, the investigation discovers your relationship with Sally-Anne. You and your physician are fined $100,000 per occurrence (that's for each person on the list), as well as sentenced to 5 years in prison. FYI: 250 × $100,000 = $25 million!

4. Up to $250,000 *and* up to 10 years in prison for the unauthorized or inappropriate disclosure of individually identifiable health information through deception with intent to sell or use for business-related benefit, personal gain, or hateful detriment.

> **EXAMPLE**
>
> A famous television star is a patient of the physician's office down the hall from yours. You get a call from a tabloid newspaper offering you $50,000 for any information on the celebrity's health. So you call the manager of the pathology lab and tell him you are filling in at the other physician's office and need test results for Mr. TV. Then you call the tabloid reporter and tell him what you found out. You used deception (you lied about working in the other physician's office) to gain PHI, which you then sold for personal financial gain. You (and possibly your physician) are fined a quarter of a million dollars and sentenced to 10 years in prison—definitely not worth it!

Refusing to Release Patient Information

Sometimes, it seems that everyone agrees with the importance of protecting a patient's privacy until he or she asks for someone's details and is refused. It happens with parents and spouses all too often, and you must be prepared for how to say "no" and deal with the impact that may ensue.

When asked *why* you will not release details about a man's wife or mother's teenage daughter, educate the individual with the facts. Frequently, simply replying, "That is our policy" accomplishes little more than infuriating them, so instead, explain why you cannot share the information. Explain that health care staff are all required, by federal law, to protect our patients' privacy with no exceptions. Say that, as soon as possible, he or she should speak with the patient and enable the patient to tell the story about his or her health care encounter. Ask nicely for the individual's understanding.

41.5 Health Care Fraud and Abuse Control Program

The Health Insurance Portability and Accountability Act (HIPAA) created the Health Care Fraud and Abuse Control Program (HCFACP). This program, under the direction of the attorney general and the secretary of the DHHS, acts in accordance with the Office of the Inspector General (OIG) and coordinates with federal, state, and local law enforcement agencies to discover those who attempt to defraud or abuse the health care system, including Medicare and Medicaid patients and programs.

The Health Care Fraud and Abuse Control Program FY 2023 reports more than $3.4 billion total recovered to the Federal Government or paid to private persons in FY 2023. This program has proven to be a valuable effort with more than $3 returned to the Medicare Trust Funds and the Federal Medicaid budget (CMS) for every $1 spent to conduct these inquiries. Investigations resulted in $1.4 billion in recoveries which included:

- 1,151 convictions (including 817 for fraud and 334 for patient abuse or neglect)
- $961 million in criminal recoveries
- $407 million in civil recoveries
- 493 civil settlements and judgments
- 1,042 exclusions of individuals and entities from federally funded programs

Source: **https://oig.hhs.gov/reports/all/2024/health-care-fraud-and-abuse-control-program-report-fiscal-year-2023/**

The report reviews the many different methods used to get money illegally, including: kickbacks for ordering and conducting tests that were not medically necessary; claims for reimbursement for unnecessary durable medical equipment (DME); ordering and performing genetic testing scams; and illicit claims for home health services and hospice practices that were not in line with valid or quality of care.

When you look at these 2023 numbers, you can see that people are being caught trying to get money for health care services to which they are not entitled. This is an important reminder that if individuals try to get you to participate in illegal or unethical behaviors, the question is not "Will you be caught?" but "When will you be caught?"

CODING BITES

In FY 2023, civil health care fraud settlements and judgments under the False Claims Act exceeded $1.8 billion, in addition to other health care administrative impositions won or negotiated by the Federal Government.

Source: https://oig.hhs.gov/reports/all/2024/health-care-fraud-and-abuse-control-program-report-fiscal-year-2023/

41.6 Codes of Ethics

There are two premier trade organizations for professional coding specialists. Each has published a code of ethics to guide members of our industry on the best professional way to conduct themselves.

American Health Information Management Association Code of Ethics

The American Health Information Management Association (AHIMA) is the preeminent professional organization for health information workers, including insurance coding specialists. The AHIMA House of Delegates designated the elements as being critical to the highest level of honorable behavior for its members.

In this era of reimbursements based on diagnostic and procedural coding, the professional ethics of health information coding professionals continue to be challenged. Standards of ethical coding practices for coding professionals were developed by AHIMA's Coding Policy and Strategy Committee and approved by AHIMA's board of directors.

GUIDANCE CONNECTION

AHIMA Code of Ethics

You can find the AHIMA Code of Ethics at:

http://bok.ahima.org/doc?oid=105098#.XFM6hlxKg3U

AHIMA Standards of Ethical Coding

Coding is one of the foundational functions of the health information management department. As complex as is the process of coding accurately, there are multipart, intricate regulations that impact that process. In addition, professional coding specialists must make ethical decisions that would benefit from an appropriate and knowledgeable source. The AHIMA Standards of Ethical Coding are presented to all members of the industry to support their ethical and legal decisions and behaviors, as well as to reinforce and evidence the commitment of coding professionals to integrity. These Standards are offered for use to all AHIMA members or nonmembers, in all types of health care facilities and organizations.

GUIDANCE CONNECTION

AHIMA Standards of Ethical Coding

The Standards of Ethical Coding can be found at:

http://bok.ahima.org/CodingStandards#.XFTCCs9Kg8Y

AAPC Code of Ethical Standards

American Academy of Professional Coders (AAPC) is an influential organization in the health information management industry. Its members, and their certifications, are well respected throughout the United States and the world. Its Code of Ethical Standards also illuminates the importance of an insurance coding and billing specialist's exhibiting the most ethical and moral conduct.

GUIDANCE CONNECTION

AAPC Code of Ethical Standards

Members of the American Academy of Professional Coders shall be dedicated to providing the highest standard of professional coding and billing services to employers, clients and patients. Professional and personal behavior of AAPC members must be exemplary.

AAPC members shall maintain the highest standard of personal and professional conduct. Members shall respect the rights of patients, clients, employers and all other colleagues.

Members shall use only legal and ethical means in all professional dealings and shall refuse to cooperate with, or condone by silence, the actions of those who engage in fraudulent, deceptive or illegal acts.

Members shall respect and adhere to the laws and regulations of the land and uphold the mission statement of the AAPC.

Members shall pursue excellence through continuing education in all areas applicable to their profession.

Members shall strive to maintain and enhance the dignity, status, competence and standards of coding for professional services.

Members shall not exploit professional relationships with patients, employees, clients or employers for personal gain.

Above all else we will commit to recognizing the intrinsic worth of each member.

This code of ethical standards for members of the AAPC strives to promote and maintain the highest standard of professional service and conduct among its members. Adherence to these standards assures public confidence in the integrity and service of professional coders who are members of the AAPC.

Failure to adhere to these standards, as determined by AAPC, will result in the loss of credentials and membership with the American Academy of Professional Coders.

Source: American Academy of Professional Coders.

41.7 Compliance Programs

A formal compliance program has been strongly recommended by the OIG (Office of Inspector General) of the DHHS (Department of Health and Human Services) to help all health care facilities establish their organizations' respect for the laws and their agreement to follow the direction from those laws. However, there are certain health care providers for whom this is not only suggested but mandated by law.

The Deficit Reduction Act of 2005, which went into effect January 1, 2007, mandates a compliance program for all health care organizations that receive $5 million or more a year from Medicaid. This law is very specific that the facility's compliance program include written guidance and policies about employees' responsibilities under the False Claims Act.

On March 23, 2010, the Patient Protection and Affordable Care Act was signed into law. Among the many other elements of health care covered by this law, there is a provision in Section 6401 that providers participating in Medicare and Medicaid create compliance programs. This includes physicians' offices and suppliers.

A compliance program will officially create policies and procedures, establish the structure to adhere to those policies, set up a monitoring system to ensure that it works, and correct conduct that does not comply. The foundation of the compliance program is the creation of an organizational culture of honesty and compliance with the laws; the discouragement of fraud, waste, and abuse; the discovery of any fraudulent activities as soon as possible using internal policies and audits; and immediate corrective action when fraud and abuse do occur.

The federal sentencing guidelines manual provides a seven-step list of the components of an effective compliance program.

GUIDANCE CONNECTION

Federal Sentencing Guidelines Manual: The Seven Steps to Due Diligence

1. Establish compliance standards and procedures
2. Assign overall responsibility to specific high-level individual(s)
3. Use due care to avoid delegation of authority to individuals with an inclination to get involved in illegal actions
4. Effectively communicate standards and procedures to all staff
5. Utilize monitoring and auditing system to detect non-compliant conduct
6. Enforce adequate disciplinary sanctions when appropriate
7. Respond to episodes of non-compliance by modifying program, if necessary

Source: United States Sentencing Commission, *2014 USSC Guidelines Manual* (November 1, 2014), ussc.gov.

Chapter Summary

Knowing your legal and ethical responsibilities as a health care professional will give you a strong foundation for a healthy career. HIPAA's Privacy Rule, along with the codes of ethics from both AHIMA and AAPC, should help guide you through any challenges.

For all of those providing health care services, the federal and state governments have crafted and enacted laws and regulations designed to ensure honest, safe, and appropriate behaviors from all involved. The *Federal Register* is the daily journal of the U.S. federal government, used to inform citizens of the actions of the federal government. The hierarchy established for the levels of authority begin with the U.S. Constitution, followed by federal statutory law, state constitutions, state statutory laws, and local laws. Executive orders, issued by the president of the United States, have the same authority as federal statutes. Common law, also known as case law, is created by judicial decisions made during court trials, establishing precedents. Administrative laws are the rules and regulations established by administrative agencies in their efforts to encourage compliance so they can complete their assigned tasks. The violation of criminal law may be a misdemeanor (lessor offense) or a felony (more serious offense). Civil laws govern the conduct of two individuals or entities in a contractual agreement or a civil wrongdoing, known as a tort.

Confidentiality, honesty, and accuracy are the watchwords that all health information management professionals should live by.

CODING BITES

Medical records, also known as patient charts, whether in paper or electronic form, are legal documents. As business records, they can be used as evidence in a court of law, and can be required by issuance of a *subpoena duces tecum*.

As per the HIPAA Privacy Rule, a "designated record set" must be specified by each health care organization. Essentially, this is a collection of files (paper or electronic) that include:

- the medical records and billing records about individuals maintained by, or for, a covered health care provider;
- the enrollment, payment, claims adjudication, case study, or medical management record systems maintained by or for a health plan; or
- documentation used for the provider or plan to make decisions about individuals.

CHAPTER 41 REVIEW
Introduction to Health Care Law and Ethics

Let's Check It! Terminology

Match each term to the appropriate definition.

1. **LO 41.2** Choosing a code on the basis of what the insurance company will cover (pay for) rather than accurately reflecting the truth.
2. **LO 41.1** Laws governing the behavior of the actions of the population related to health and well-being.
3. **LO 41.2** Coding the individual parts of a specific diagnosis or procedure rather than one combination or bundle that includes all of those components.
4. **LO 41.1** Official policies issued by the president of the United States.
5. **LO 41.1** Also known as rules and regulations, these are created and adjudicated by administrative agencies, given authority by Congress.
6. **LO 41.4** Health care providers, health plans, and health care clearinghouses–businesses that have access to the personal health information of patients.
7. **LO 41.4** Any patient-identifiable health information regardless of the form in which it is stored (paper, computer file, etc.).
8. **LO 41.1** Laws that are enacted by federal and state legislature.
9. **LO 41.2** Using a code on a claim form that indicates a higher level of service or a more severe aspect of disease or injury than that which was actual and true.
10. **LO 41.4** A portion of HIPAA that ensures the availability of patient information for those who should see it while protecting that information from those who should not.
11. **LO 41.4** The sharing of information between people working in the same health care facility for purposes of caring for the patient.
12. **LO 41.4** The sharing of information between health care professionals working in separate entities, or facilities, in the course of caring for the patient.
13. **LO 41.1** Also known as case law, this is created by judicial decisions made during court trials.
14. **LO 41.2** The paperwork in the patient's file that corroborates the codes presented on the claim form for a particular encounter.
15. **LO 41.2** Sending a claim for the second time to the same insurance company for the same procedure or service, provided to the same patient on the same date of service.

A. Administrative Law
B. Coding for Coverage
C. Common Law
D. Covered Entities
E. Criminal Law
F. Disclosure
G. Double Billing
H. Executive Orders
I. HIPAA's Privacy Rule
J. Protected Health Information (PHI)
K. Statutory Laws
L. Supporting Documentation
M. Unbundling
N. Upcoding
O. Use

Let's Check It! Concepts

Choose the most appropriate answer for each of the following questions.

1. **LO 41.4** The intent of HIPAA's Privacy Rule is to
   a. protect an individual's privacy.
   b. not interfere with the flow of information necessary for care.
   c. restrict health care professionals from doing their jobs.
   d. protect an individual's privacy and not interfere with the flow of information necessary for care.
2. **LO 41.4** Protected health information (PHI) is
   a. any health information that can be connected to a specific individual.
   b. a listing of diagnosis codes.
   c. current procedural terminology.
   d. covered entity employee files.

3. **LO 41.4** According to HIPAA, covered entities include all *except*
   - **a.** health care providers.
   - **b.** health plans.
   - **c.** health care computer software manufacturers.
   - **d.** health care clearinghouses.

4. **LO 41.4** The term *use* per HIPAA's Privacy Rule refers to the exchange of information between health care personnel
   - **a.** and health care personnel in other health care facilities.
   - **b.** and family members.
   - **c.** in the same office.
   - **d.** and the pharmacist.

5. **LO 41.4** The term *disclosure* per HIPAA's Privacy Rule refers to the exchange of information between health care personnel
   - **a.** and health care personnel in other covered entities.
   - **b.** and family members.
   - **c.** in the same office.
   - **d.** and the patient.

6. **LO 41.4** Which of the following is *not* a covered entity under HIPAA?
   - **a.** County hospital
   - **b.** BlueCross BlueShield Association
   - **c.** Physician Associates medical practice
   - **d.** Computer technical support

7. **LO 41.6** There are two premier trade organizations for professional coding specialists. Each organization has a code of ethics to guide members on the best professional way to conduct themselves. These two organizations are
   - **a.** AHIMA and OFR.
   - **b.** GPO and AAPC.
   - **c.** AHIMA and AAPC.
   - **d.** HIPAA and EEO.

8. **LO 41.4** According to HIPAA's rules and regulations, a covered entity's workforce includes
   - **a.** only paid, full-time employees.
   - **b.** only licensed personnel working in the office.
   - **c.** volunteers, trainees, and employees, part time and full time.
   - **d.** business associates' employees.

9. **LO 41.4** HIPAA's Privacy Rule has been carefully crafted to
   - **a.** protect a patient's health care history.
   - **b.** protect a patient's current medical issues.
   - **c.** protect a patient's future health considerations.
   - **d.** all of these.

10. **LO 41.4** A written form to release PHI should include all *except*
    - **a.** specific identification of the person who will be receiving the information.
    - **b.** the specific information to be released.
    - **c.** legal terminology so it will stand up in court.
    - **d.** an expiration date.

11. **LO 41.4** Those who are permitted to file an official complaint with DHHS are
    - **a.** health care providers.
    - **b.** any individual.
    - **c.** health plans.
    - **d.** clearinghouses.

12. **LO 41.4** Penalties for violating any portion of HIPAA apply to
    - **a.** patients.
    - **b.** patients' families.
    - **c.** all covered entities.
    - **d.** health care office managers.

13. **LO 41.3** An individual who files a false claim can be charged for violations by
    - **a.** federal law.
    - **b.** state law.
    - **c.** both federal and state law.
    - **d.** Filing a false claim is not a violation of law.

14. **LO 41.1** DHHS stands for
    - **a.** Department of Home and Health Services.
    - **b.** Division of Health and Health Care Sciences.
    - **c.** Department of Health and Human Services.
    - **d.** District of Health and HIPAA Systems.

15. **LO 41.2** Changing a code from one that is most accurate to one you know the insurance company will pay for is called
    - **a.** coding for coverage.
    - **b.** coding for packaging.
    - **c.** unbundling.
    - **d.** double billing.

16. **LO 41.2** Unbundling is an illegal practice in which coders
    - **a.** bill for services never provided.
    - **b.** bill for services with no documentation.
    - **c.** bill using several individual codes instead of one combination code.
    - **d.** bill using a code for a higher level of service than what was actually provided.

17. **LO 41.2** Upcoding is an illegal practice in which coders
    - **a.** bill for services never provided.
    - **b.** bill for services with no documentation.
    - **c.** bill using several individual codes instead of one combination code.
    - **d.** bill using a code for a higher level of service than what was actually provided.

18. **LO 41.2** Medicare's CCI investigates claims that include
    - **a.** unbundling.
    - **b.** the improper use of mutually exclusive codes.
    - **c.** unacceptable reporting of CPT codes.
    - **d.** all of these.

19. **LO 41.5** The Health Care Fraud and Abuse Control Program FY 2023 reports more than _______ billion total recovered to the Federal Government or paid to private persons in FY 2023.
    - **a.** $3.4
    - **b.** $1.75
    - **c.** $3.6
    - **d.** $2.5

20. **LO 41.7** According to the federal sentencing guidelines manual, all of the following are components of the seven steps to due diligence for an effective compliance program *except*
    - **a.** establish compliance standards and procedures.
    - **b.** assign overall responsibility to specific high-level individual(s).
    - **c.** utilize monitoring and auditing systems to detect noncompliant conduct.
    - **d.** cease disciplinary sanctions.

Let's Check It! Rules and Regulations

Please answer the following questions from the knowledge you have gained after reading this chapter.

1. **LO 41.4** Why was HIPAA's Privacy Rule written?
2. **LO 41.2** Explain double billing. Is it permissible practice for a professional coding specialist?
3. **LO 41.1** Explain civil law in relation to the health care industry.
4. **LO 41.3** What is the False Claims Act's definition of a claim and what is the knowledge requirement?
5. **LO 41.7** What are the federal sentencing guidelines manual's seven steps to due diligence for an effective compliance program?

ICD-10-PCS

YOU CODE IT! Application

Following are some health care scenarios. Determine the best course of action that you, as the health information management professional for the facility, should take. Identify any legal and/or ethical issues that may need to be considered and explain how you would deal with the situation.

(continued)

PRADER, BRACKER, & ASSOCIATES

A Complete Health Care Facility

159 Healthcare Way • SOMEWHERE, FL 32811 • 407-555-6789

PATIENT: HOLLAND, FELECIA

ACCOUNT/EHR #: HOLLFE001

Attending Physician: Oscar R. Prader, MD

This 31-year-old female is 32-weeks pregnant. She presents today in tears. She is suffering from hemorrhoids and cannot stand it anymore. The pain and itching are making life difficult for her, as it hurts to sit for any length of time, and she cannot sleep. As it is difficult for her to lie on her stomach, due to the pregnancy, she can only find some comfort by either walking around or lying on her side. She is asking (more like begging) for a hemorrhoidectomy—a simple surgical procedure that can be done in the office and will almost immediately provide her with complete relief.

The correct CPT code for the treatment of Felecia's condition is

46260 Hemorrhoidectomy, internal and external, 2 or more columns/groups

However, Felecia's insurance carrier will not pay for a hemorrhoidectomy with a diagnosis that indicates there are no complications. According to the insurance customer service representative, it will only pay in full for the procedure

46250 Hemorrhoidectomy, external, 2 or more columns/groups

Felecia's husband, Ben, is a civilian who works for a defense contractor and is currently in Iraq supporting the troops. Money is tight for the family because Ben's paycheck has been delayed due to a mix-up in paperwork when he was transferred to the Middle East. There is no way they can afford to pay cash for the hemorrhoidectomy.

All you need to do is change the one number of the code and Felecia can have the relief she so desperately needs. As the professional coding specialist in this office, what should you do?

PRADER, BRACKER, & ASSOCIATES

A Complete Health Care Facility

159 Healthcare Way • SOMEWHERE, FL 32811 • 407-555-6789

PATIENT: OKONEK, MARC

ACCOUNT/EHR #: OKONMA001

Attending Physician: Andrew Bracker, MD

As the coding specialist for this facility, you are given the chart for this patient after his recent encounter with Dr. Bracker. On the face sheet you notice that Dr. Bracker has indicated the procedure provided to this patient to be Excision dermoid cyst, nose; simple, skin, subcutaneous. However, there is nothing at all in the rest of the documentation, including the encounter notes and lab reports, to support medical necessity for this procedure.

As a professional coding specialist in this office, what should you do?

(continued)

PRADER, BRACKER, & ASSOCIATES

A Complete Health Care Facility

159 Healthcare Way • SOMEWHERE, FL 32811 • 407-555-6789

PATIENT: RIALS, ELIZABETH

ACCOUNT/EHR #: RIALEL001

Attending Physician: Oscar R. Prader, MD

Today, Tonya Baliga comes into your office. She states that she is Elizabeth Rials's sister and that she has been asked by her sister to collect a copy of her complete medical record. Ms. Baliga tells you that her sister has moved to another town and needs the records for an upcoming medical appointment with her new doctor. She hands you a printout of an e-mail, supposedly from Ms. Rials, to serve as documentation that she should have the records.

As a professional coding specialist in this office, what should you do?

PRADER, BRACKER, & ASSOCIATES

A Complete Health Care Facility

159 Healthcare Way • SOMEWHERE, FL 32811 • 407-555-6789

PATIENT: SINGELTON, SANDRA

ACCOUNT/EHR #: SINGSA001

Attending Physician: Andrew Bracker, MD

The patient is a 17-year-old female who came in for counseling on birth control.

Today, Angela Thurman came into the office. She stated that she is Sandra's mother and found an appointment card for this facility in her daughter's jeans. She demands to know why her daughter came to see the physician. She is angry and frustrated and states that she will not leave until she is told why her daughter saw the doctor.

As a professional coding specialist in this office, what should you do?

PRADER, BRACKER, & ASSOCIATES

A Complete Health Care Facility

159 Healthcare Way • SOMEWHERE, FL 32811 • 407-555-6789

PATIENT: EVERFIELD, CARL

ACCOUNT/EHR #: EVERCA001

Attending Physician: Oscar R. Prader, MD

The patient came to see the physician because he hates his nose. His self-esteem is very low, and, as a teenage boy, he has developed severe social anxiety. His family does not have the money to pay for a rhinoplasty (nose job), and the only way that the insurance company will pay for this cosmetic surgery is for medical necessity, such as a deviated septum.

You have been told to code the diagnosis of deviated septum to support medical necessity for the rhinoplasty. The doctor and office manager both tell you that this is the "right" thing to do.

As a professional coding specialist in this office, what should you do?

APPENDIX

E/M Coding Rubric Worksheet

Begin by narrowing down the entire E/M chapter to the appropriate subsection:

Step 1. Location	New Patient/Initial	Established/Subsequent
Office/Outpatient	99347–99350	99211–99215
Hospital—Observation	99218–99220	99224–99226
Hospital—Inpatient	99221–99223	99231–99233
Emergency Department	99281–99285	
Nursing Facility	99304–99306	99307–99310
Domiciliary (Assisted Living)	99324–99328	99334–99337
Home Services	99341–99345	99347–99350

Step 2. Key Components	New Patient/Initial	Established/Subsequent
History		
Problem-Focused: Chief complaint; brief history of present illness or problem.		
Expanded Problem-Focused: Chief complaint; brief history of present illness; problem-pertinent system review		
Detailed: Chief complaint; extended history of present illness; problem-pertinent system review extended to include a review of a limited number of additional systems; pertinent past, family, and/or social history directly related to patient's problem(s).		
Comprehensive: Chief complaint; extended history of present illness; review of systems that are directly related to the problem(s) identified in the history of the present illness plus a review of all additional body systems; complete past, family, and social history.		

CodePath: For more information on determining level of history, see *Let's Code It!* **Chapter 23**, **Section 23.4** ***Types of E/M Services - Level of Patient History*** (beginning on page 648).

Step 3. Key Components	New Patient/Initial	Established/Subsequent
Physical Examination		
Problem-Focused: A limited exam of the affected body area or organ system		
Expanded Problem-Focused: A limited exam of the affected body area or organ system and other symptomatic or related organ system(s)		
Detailed: An extended exam of the affected body area(s) and other symptomatic or related organ system(s)		
Comprehensive: A general multisystem exam -or- a complete exam of a single organ system		

CodePath: For more information on determining level of Physical Examination, see *Let's Code It!* **Chapter 23**, **Section 23.4** ***Types of E/M Services - Level of Physical Examination***.

Step 4. Key Components	New Patient/Initial	Established/Subsequent
Medical Decision Making		
Straightforward: Minimal number of possible diagnoses and/or treatment options; minimal quantity of information to be obtained, reviewed, and analyzed; and minimal risk of significant complications, morbidity, and/or mortality		
Low Complexity: Limited number of possible diagnoses and/or treatment options; limited quantity of information to be obtained, reviewed, and analyzed; and limited risk of significant complications, morbidity, and/or mortality		
Moderate Complexity: Multiple number of possible diagnoses and/or treatment options; moderate quantity of information to be obtained, reviewed, and analyzed; and moderate risk of significant complications, morbidity, and/or mortality		
High Complexity: Extensive number of possible diagnoses and/or treatment options; extensive quantity of information to be obtained, reviewed, and analyzed; and high risk of significant complications, morbidity, and/or mortality		

CodePath: For more information on determining level of Medical Decision Making, see *Let's Code It!* **Chapter 23**, **Section 23.4** ***Types of E/M Services - Level of Medical Decision Making.***

Combining Multiple Levels in One Code

Once you have determined what level of history was taken, what level of physician exam was performed, and what level of MDM was provided by the physician as documented in the case notes, this all needs to be put together into one code. When all three key components point to the same code, this is a piece of cake. But what about when the three levels point toward different E/M codes? How do you mesh them all into one code? The CPT guidelines state, "*. . . must meet or exceed the stated requirements to qualify for a particular level of E/M service.*"

You must find the one level that is satisfied by ALL THREE levels of care when you are reporting for a NEW patient, or TWO out of THREE for established patients. Find the only code that has ALL THREE levels equal to or greater than the code's key component descriptors, as identified on your above worksheets, to determine which one E/M code should be reported.

CodePath: For new Patients . . . You can only code as high as your lowest key component.

GLOSSARY

A

Ablation The destruction or eradication of tissue.

Abnormal Findings Test results that indicate a disease or condition may be present.

Abortifacient A drug used to induce an abortion.

Abortion The end of a pregnancy prior to or subsequent to the death of a fetus.

Abstracting The process of identifying the relevant words or phrases in health care documentation in order to determine the best, most appropriate code(s).

Abuse Regular consumption of a substance with manifestations.

Accessory Organs Organs that assist the digestive process and are adjacent to the alimentary canal: the gallbladder, liver, and pancreas.

Accommodation Adaptation of the eye's lens to adjust for varying focal distances.

Acute Severe; serious.

Administration To introduce a therapeutic, prophylactic, protective, diagnostic, nutritional, or physiological substance.

Administrative Laws Also known as rules and regulations, these are created and adjudicated by administrative agencies given authority by Congress.

Advanced Life Support (ALS) Life-sustaining, emergency care provided, such as airway management, defibrillation, and/or the administration of drugs.

Adverse Effect An unexpected bad reaction to a drug or other treatment.

Agglutination The process of red blood cells combining together in a mass or lump.

Allogeneic The donor and recipient are of the same species, e.g., human → human, dog → dog (also known as an *allograft*).

Allotransplantation The relocation of tissue from one individual to another (both of the same species) without an identical genetic match.

Alphabetic Index The section of a code book showing all codes, from A to Z, by the short code descriptions.

Alphanumeric Section The section of the HCPCS Level II code book listing all of the codes in alphanumeric order.

Alphanumeric Containing both letters and numbers.

Ambulatory Surgery Center (ASC) A facility specially designed to provide surgical treatments without an overnight stay; also known as a *same-day surgery center.*

AMCC Automated Multi-Channel Chemistry—Automated organ disease panel tests performed on the same patient, by the same provider, on the same day.

Anatomical Site A specific location within the anatomy (body).

Anemic Any of various conditions marked by deficiency in red blood cells or hemoglobin.

Anesthesia The loss of sensation, with or without consciousness, generally induced by the administration of a particular drug.

Anesthesiologists Physicians specializing in the administration of anesthesia.

Angina Pectoris Chest pain.

Angiography The imaging of blood vessels after the injection of contrast material.

Anomaly An abnormal, or unexpected, condition.

Antibodies Immune responses to antigens.

Anticipatory Guidance Recommendations for behavior modification and/or other preventive measures.

Antigen A substance that promotes the production of antibodies.

Anus The portion of the large intestine that leads outside the body.

Anxiety The feelings of apprehension and fear, sometimes manifested with physical manifestations such as sweating and palpitations.

Anxiolytic A drug used to reduce anxiety.

Approach The path the physician took to access the body part upon which the treatment or procedure was targeted.

Approach The specific technique used for the procedure.

Arthrodesis The immobilization of a joint using a surgical technique.

Arthrography The recording of a picture of an anatomical joint after the administration of contrast material into the joint capsule.

Arthropathy Disease or dysfunction of a joint [plural: arthropathies].

Articulation A joint.

Ascending Colon The portion of the large intestine that connects the cecum to the hepatic flexure.

Assume Suppose to be the case, without proof; guess the intended details.

Asymptomatic No symptoms or manifestations.

Atherosclerosis A condition resulting from plaque buildup on the interior walls of the arteries, causing reduced blood flow; also known as *arteriosclerosis.*

Atrium A chamber that is located in the top half of the heart and receives blood.

Audiology The study of hearing, balance, and related disorders.

Autologous The donor tissue is taken from a different site on the same individual's body (also known as an *autograft*).

Automobile Insurance Auto accident liability coverage will pay for medical bills, lost wages, and compensation for pain and suffering for any person injured by the insured in an auto accident.

Avulsion Injury in which layers of skin are traumatically torn away from the body.

Axis of Classification A single meaning within the code set; providing a detail.

B

Bacteria Single-celled microorganisms that cause disease.

Basic Life Support (BLS) The provision of emergency CPR, stabilization of the patient, first aid, control of bleeding, and/or treatment of shock.

Basic Personal Services Services that include washing/bathing, dressing and undressing, assistance in taking medications, and assistance getting in and out of bed.

Behavioral Disturbance A type of common behavior that includes mood disorders (such as depression, apathy, and euphoria), sleep disorders (such as insomnia and hypersomnia), psychotic symptoms (such as delusions and hallucinations), and agitation (such as pacing, wandering, and aggression).

Benign Nonmalignant characteristic of a neoplasm; not infectious or spreading.

Benign Prostatic Hyperplasia (BPH) Enlarged prostate that results in depressing the urethra.

Biofeedback Training to gain voluntary control of automatic bodily functions.

Bladder Cancer Malignancy of the urinary bladder.

Blepharitis Inflammation of the eyelid.

Blister A bubble or sac formed on the surface of the skin, typically filled with a watery fluid or serum.

Blood Fluid pumped throughout the body, carrying oxygen and nutrients to the cells and wastes away from the cells.

Blood Type A system of classifying blood based on the antigens present on the surface of the individual's red blood cells; also known as *blood group*.

Body Part The anatomical site upon which the procedure was performed.

Body System The physiological system, or anatomical region, upon which the procedure was performed.

Bulbar Conjunctiva A mucous membrane on the surface of the eyeball.

Bulla A large vesicle that is filled with fluid.

Burn Injury by heat or fire.

C

Capitation Plans Agreements between a physician and a managed care organization that pay the physician a predetermined amount of money each month for each member of the plan who identifies that provider as his or her primary care physician.

Carbuncle A painful, pus-filled boil due to infection of the epidermis and underlying tissues, often caused by staphylococcus.

Carcinoma A malignant neoplasm or cancerous tumor.

Care Plan Oversight Services E/M of a patient, reported in 30-day periods, including infrequent supervision along with preencounter and postencounter work, such as reading test results and assessment of notes.

Carrier An individual infected with a disease who is not ill but can still pass it to another person; an individual with an abnormal gene that can be passed to a child, making the child susceptible to disease.

Cataract Clouding of the lens or lens capsule of the eye.

Category I Codes The codes listed in the main text of the CPT book, also known as CPT codes.

Category II Codes Codes for performance measurement and tracking.

Category II Modifiers Modifiers provided for use with Category II CPT codes to indicate a valid reason for a portion of a performance measure to be deleted from qualification.

Category III Codes Codes for emerging technology.

Catheter A thin, flexible tube, inserted into a body part, used to inject fluid, to extract fluid, or to keep a passage open.

Cecum A pouchlike organ that connects the ileum with the large intestine; the point of connection for the vermiform appendix.

Centers for Medicare & Medicaid Services (CMS) The agency under the Department of Health and Human Services (DHHS) in charge of regulation and control over services for those covered by Medicare and Medicaid.

Cerebral Infarction An area of dead tissue (necrosis) in the brain caused by a blocked or ruptured blood vessel.

Cerebrovascular Accident (CVA) Rupture of a blood vessel causing hemorrhaging in the brain or an embolus in a blood vessel in the brain causing a loss of blood flow; also known as *stroke*.

Certified Registered Nurse Anesthetist (CRNA) A registered nurse (RN) who has taken additional, specialized training in the administration of anesthesia.

Character A letter or number component of an ICD-10-PCS code.

Chelation Therapy The use of a chemical compound that binds with metal in the body so that the metal will lose its toxic effect. It might be done when a metal disc or prosthetic is implanted in a patient, eliminating adverse reactions to the metal itself as a foreign body.

Cholelithiasis Gallstones.

Chondropathy Disease affecting the cartilage [plural: chondropathies].

Choroid The vascular layer of the eye that lies between the retina and the sclera.

Chronic Long duration; continuing over an extended period of time.

Chronic Kidney Disease (CKD) Ongoing malfunction of one or both kidneys.

Chronic Obstructive Pulmonary Disease (COPD) An ongoing obstruction of the airway.

Ciliary Body The vascular layer of the eye that lies between the sclera and the crystalline lens.

Civil Law Laws that govern the relationships between people, and between businesses.

Class A Finding Nontraumatic amputation of a foot or an integral skeletal portion.

Class B Finding Absence of a posterior tibial pulse; absence or decrease of hair growth; thickening of the nail, discoloration of the skin, and/or thinning of the skin texture; and/or absence of a posterior pedal pulse.

Class C Finding Edema, burning sensation, temperature change (cold feet), abnormal spontaneous sensations in the feet, and/or limping.

Classification Systems The term used in health care to identify ICD-10-CM, CPT, ICD-10-PCS, and HCPCS Level II code sets.

Clinical Laboratory Improvement Amendment (CLIA) Federal legislation created for the monitoring and regulation of clinical laboratory procedures.

Clinically Significant Signs, symptoms, and/or conditions present at birth that may impact the child's future health status.

Closed Treatment The treatment of a fracture without surgically opening the affected area.

Co-morbidity A separate diagnosis existing in the same patient at the same time as an unrelated diagnosis.

Coagulation Clotting; the change from a liquid into a thickened substance.

Coding for Coverage Choosing a code on the basis of what the insurance company will cover (pay for) rather than accurately reflecting the truth.

Coding Process The sequence of actions required to interpret physician documentation into the codes that accurately report what occurred during a specific encounter between health care professional and patient.

Common Bile Duct The juncture of the cystic duct of the gallbladder and the hepatic duct from the liver.

Common Law Also known as case law, this is created by judicial decisions made during court trials.

Complex Closure A method of sealing an opening in the skin involving a multilayered closure and a reconstructive procedure such as scar revision, debridement, or retention sutures.

Complication An unexpected illness or other condition that develops as a result of a procedure, service, or treatment provided during the patient's hospital stay.

Computed Tomography (CT) A specialized computer scanner with very fine detail that records imaging of internal anatomical sites; also known as computerized axial tomography (CAT).

Computed Tomography Angiography (CTA) A CT scan using contrast materials to visualize arteries and veins all over the body.

Concurrent Coding System in which coding processes are performed while a patient is still in the hospital receiving care.

Condition The state of abnormality or dysfunction.

Cone A receptor in the retina that is responsible for light and color.

Confirmed Found to be true or definite.

Congenital A condition existing at the time of birth.

Conjunctivitis Inflammation of the conjunctiva.

Conscious Sedation The use of a drug to reduce stress and/or anxiety.

Consultation An encounter for purposes of a second physician's opinion or advice, requested by another physician, regarding the management of a patient's specific health concern. A consultation is planned to be a short-term relationship between a health care professional and a patient.

Cornea Transparent tissue covering the eyeball; responsible for focusing light into the eye and transmitting light.

Corneal Dystrophy Growth of abnormal tissue on the cornea, often related to a nutritional deficiency.

Corrosion A burn caused by a chemical; chemical destruction of the skin.

Covered Entities Health care providers, health plans, and health care clearinghouses—businesses that have access to the personal health information of patients.

CPT Code Modifier A two-character code that may be appended to a code from the main portion of the CPT book to provide additional information.

Criminal Law Laws governing the behavior of the actions of the population related to health and well-being.

Critical Care Services Care services for an acutely ill or injured patient with a high risk for life-threatening developments.

Cushing's Syndrome A condition resulting from the hyperproduction of corticosteroids, most often caused by an adrenal cortex tumor or a tumor of the pituitary gland.

Cyst A fluid-filled or gas-filled bubble in the skin.

Cytology The investigation and identification of cells.

D

Dacryocystitis Lacrimal gland inflammation.

Decubitus Ulcer A bedsore or wound created by lying in the same position, on the same irritant without relief.

Deformity A size or shape (structural design) that deviates from that which is considered normal.

Demographic Demographic details include the patient's name, address, date of birth, and other personal details, not specifically related to health.

Densitometry The process used to measure bone density, most often done to assess the patient's risk for osteopenia or osteoporosis.

Dependence Ongoing, regular consumption of a substance with resulting significant clinical manifestations, and a dramatic decrease in the effect of the substance with continued use, therefore requiring an increased quantity of the substance to achieve intoxication.

Dependents Individuals who are supported, either financially or with regard to insurance coverage, by others.

Depressive An emotional state that includes sadness, hopelessness, and gloom.

Dermis The internal layer of the skin; the location of blood vessels, lymph vessels, hair follicles, sweat glands, and sebum.

Descending Colon The segment of the large intestine that connects the splenic flexure to the sigmoid colon.

Detoxification The process of removing toxic substances or qualities.

Device The identification of any materials or appliances that may remain in or on the body after the procedure is completed.

Diabetes Mellitus (DM) A chronic systemic disease that results from insulin deficiency or resistance and causes the body to improperly metabolize carbohydrates, proteins, and fats.

Diagnosis A physician's determination of a patient's condition, illness, or injury.

Diagnosis-Related Group (DRG) An episodic care payment system basing reimbursement to hospitals for inpatient services upon standards of care for specific diagnoses grouped by their similar usage of resources for procedures, services, and treatments.

Differential Diagnosis When the physician indicates that the patient's signs and symptoms may closely lead to two different diagnoses; usually written as "diagnosis A versus diagnosis B."

Disability Compensation A plan that reimburses a covered individual a portion of his or her income that is lost as a result of being unable to work due to illness or injury.

Disclosure The sharing of information between health care professionals working in separate entities, or facilities, in the course of caring for the patient.

Discounted FFS An extra reduction in the rate charged to an insurer for services provided by the physician to the plan's members.

Dislocation The movement of a muscle away from its normal position.

DMEPOS Durable medical equipment, prosthetic, and orthotic supplies.

Donor Area (Site) The area or part of the body from which skin or tissue is removed with the intention of placing that skin or tissue in another area or body.

Dorsopathy Disease affecting the back of the torso [plural: dorsopathies].

Double Billing Sending a claim for the second time to the same insurance company for the same procedure or service, provided to the same patient on the same date of service.

Duodenum The first segment of the small intestine, connecting the stomach to the jejunum.

Duplex Scan An ultrasonic scanning procedure to determine blood flow and pattern.

Durable Medical Equipment (DME) Apparatus and tools that help individuals accommodate physical frailties, deliver pharmaceuticals, and provide other assistance that will last for a long time and/or be used to assist multiple patients over time.

Durable Medical Equipment Regional Carrier (DMERC) A company designated by the state or region to act as the fiscal intermediary for all DME claims.

Dyslipidemia Abnormal lipoprotein metabolism.

E

Early and Periodic Screening, Diagnostic, and Treatment (EPSDT) A Medicaid preventive health program for children under 21.

Ectopic Out of place, such as an organ or body part.

Edema An overaccumulation of fluid in the cells of the tissues.

Edentulism Absence of teeth.

Electronic Media Claim (EMC) A health care claim form that is transmitted electronically.

Electronic Remittance Advice (ERA) Remittance advice that is sent to the provider electronically.

Elevated Blood Pressure An occurrence of high blood pressure; an isolated or infrequent reading of a systolic blood pressure above 120 mmHg and/or a diastolic blood pressure above 80 mmHg.

Eligibility Verification The process of confirming with the insurance carrier that an individual is qualified for benefits that would pay for services provided by your health care professional on a particular day.

Embolus A thrombus that has broken free from the vessel wall and is traveling freely within the vascular system.

End-Stage Renal Disease (ESRD) Chronic, irreversible kidney disease requiring regular treatments.

Enteral Within, or by way of, the gastrointestinal tract.

Epidermis The external layer of the skin, the majority of which is squamous cells.

Episodic Care An insurance company pays a provider one flat fee to cover the entire course of treatment for an individual's condition.

Eponym A disease or condition named for a person.

Esophagus The tubular organ that connects the pharynx to the stomach for the passage of nourishment.

Established Patient A person who has received professional services from the physician/qualified health care professional or another physician/qualified health care professional of the exact same specialty and subspecialty who belongs to the same group practice, within the past three years.

Etiology The original source or cause for the development of a disease; also, the study of the causes of disease.

Evaluation and Management (E/M) The codes that describe the specific components of a meeting between a health care professional and a patient.

Exacerbation An increase in the severity of a disease or its symptoms.

Excision The full-thickness removal of a lesion, including margins; includes (for coding purposes) a simple closure.

Executive Orders Official policies issued by the president of the United States.

Experimental A procedure or treatment that has not yet been accepted by the health care industry as the standard of care.

Explanation of Benefits (EOB) Another type of paper remittance advice, more typically sent to the policyholder. However, some in the industry use the term *EOB* interchangeably with *RA*.

Extent The percentage of the body that has been affected by the burn or corrosion.

External Cause An event, outside the body, that causes injury, poisoning, or an adverse reaction.

Extra-articular Located outside a joint.

Extracorporeal Outside of the body.

Extraocular Muscles The muscles that control the eye.

F

Fee-for-Service (FFS) Plans Payment agreements that outline, in a written fee schedule, exactly how much money the insurance carrier will pay the physician for each treatment and/or service provided.

First-Degree Burn Redness of the epidermis (skin).

First-Listed "First-listed diagnosis" is used, when reporting outpatient encounters, instead of the term "principal diagnosis."

Fluoroscope A piece of equipment that emits x-rays through a part of the patient's body onto a fluorescent screen, causing the image to identify various aspects of the anatomy by density.

Fornix The conjunctival fornix is the area between the eyelid and the eyeball. The superior fornix is between the upper lid and eyeball; the inferior fornix is between the lower lid and the eyeball [plural: fornices].

Fracture Broken cartilage or bone.

Full-Thickness A measure that extends from the epidermis to the connective tissue layer of the skin.

Functional Activity Glandular secretion in abnormal quantity.

Fundus The domed section of an organ farthest from its opening.

Fungi Group of organisms, including mold, yeast, and mildew, that cause infection [singular: fungus].

Furuncle A staphylococcal infection in the subcutaneous tissue; commonly known as a *boil.*

G

Gallbladder A pear-shaped organ that stores bile until it is required to aid the digestive process.

Gangrene Necrotic tissue resulting from a loss of blood supply.

Gatekeeper A physician, typically a family practitioner or an internist, who serves as the primary care physician for an individual. This physician is responsible for evaluating and determining the course of treatment or services, as well as for deciding whether or not a specialist should be involved in care.

General Anesthesia The administration of a drug in order to induce a loss of consciousness in the patient, who is unable to be aroused even by painful stimulation.

Genetic Abnormality An error in a gene (chromosome) that affects development during gestation; also known as a *chromosomal abnormality.*

Gestation The length of time for the complete development of a baby from conception to birth; on average, 40 weeks.

Gestational Diabetes Mellitus (GDM) Usually a temporary diabetes mellitus occurring during pregnancy; however, such patients have an increased risk of later developing type 2 diabetes.

Gestational Hypertension Hypertension that develops during pregnancy and typically goes away once the pregnancy has ended.

Glands of Zeis Altered sebaceous glands that are connected to the eyelash follicles.

Glaucoma The condition that results when poor draining of fluid causes an abnormal increase in pressure within the eye, damaging the optic nerve.

Global Period The length of time allotted for postoperative care included in the surgical package, which is generally accepted to be 90 days for major surgical procedures and up to 10 days for minor procedures.

Global Surgical Package A group of services already included in the code for the operation and not reported separately.

Glomerular Filtration Rate (GFR) The measurement of kidney function; used to determine the stage of kidney disease. GFR is calculated by the physician using the results of a creatinine test in a formula with the patient's gender, age, race, and other factors; normal GFR is 90 and above.

Gross Examination The visual study of a specimen (with the naked eye).

Gynecologist (GYN) A physician specializing in the care of the female genital tract.

H

Hair A pigmented, cylindrical filament that grows out from the hair follicle within the epidermis.

Hair Follicle A saclike bulb containing the hair root.

Harvesting The process of taking skin or tissue (on the same body or another).

HCPCS Level II Modifier A two-character alphabetic or alphanumeric code that may be appended to a code from the main portion of the CPT book or a code from the HCPCS Level II book.

Health Care The total management of an individual's well-being by a health care professional.

Health Maintenance Organization (HMO) A type of health insurance that uses a primary care physician, also known as a gatekeeper, to manage all health care services for an individual.

Hematopoiesis The formation of blood cells.

Hemoglobin (hgb or Hgb) The part of the red blood cell that carries oxygen.

Hemolysis The destruction of red blood cells, resulting in the release of hemoglobin into the bloodstream.

Hemorrhage Excessive or severe bleeding.

Hemostasis The interruption of bleeding.

Hernia A condition in which one anatomical structure pushes through a perforation in the wall of the anatomical site that normally contains that structure.

High Osmolar An ionic water-soluable iodinated contrast medium.

HIPAA's Privacy Rule A portion of HIPAA that ensures the availability of patient information for those who should see it while protecting that information from those who should not.

Hospice Care that is provided to all patients with a terminal illness with a prognosis of 6 months or less to live.

Hospital-Acquired Condition (HAC) A condition, illness, or injury contracted by the patient during his or her stay in an acute care facility; also known as *nosocomial condition.*

Human Immunodeficiency Virus (HIV) A condition affecting the immune system.

Hyperglycemia Abnormally high levels of glucose.

Hypertension High blood pressure, usually a chronic condition; often identified by a systolic blood pressure above 140 mmHg and/or a diastolic blood pressure above 90 mmHg.

Hypnotic A drug that induces sleep.

Hypoglycemia Abnormally low glucose levels.

Hypoglycemics Prescription, non-insulin medications designed to lower a patient's glycemic level.

Hypotension Low blood pressure; systolic blood pressure below 90 mmHg and/or diastolic measurements of lower than 60 mmHg.

Hypothyroidism A condition in which the thyroid converts energy more slowly than normal, resulting in an otherwise unexplained weight gain and fatigue.

I

Ileum The last segment of the small intestine.

Immunization To make someone resistant to a particular disease by vaccination.

Index to External Causes The alphabetic listing of the external causes that might cause a patient's injury, poisoning, or adverse reaction.

Infarction Tissue or muscle that has deteriorated or died (necrotic).

Infection The invasion of pathogens into tissue cells.

Infectious A condition that can be transmitted from one person to another.

Inflammation The reaction of tissues to infection or injury; characterized by pain, swelling, and erythema.

Influenza An acute infection of the respiratory tract caused by the influenza virus.

Infusion The introduction of a fluid into a blood vessel.

Injection Compelling a fluid into tissue or cavity.

Inpatient An individual admitted for an overnight or longer stay in a hospital.

Inpatient Facility An establishment that provides health care services to individuals who stay overnight on the premises.

Insurance Premium The amount of money, often paid monthly, by a policyholder or insured, to an insurance company to obtain coverage.

Intermediate Closure A multilevel method of sealing an opening in the skin involving one or more of the deeper layers of the skin. Single-layer closure of heavily contaminated wounds that required extensive cleaning or removal of particulate matter also constitutes intermediate closure.

Interpret Explain the meaning of; convert a meaning from one language to another.

Interval The time measured between one point and another, such as between physician visits.

Intervertebral Disc A fibrocartilage segment that lies between vertebrae of the spinal column and provides cushioning and support.

Intravascular Optical Coherence A high-resolution, catheter-based imaging modality used for the optimized visualization of coronary artery lesions.

Iris The round, pigmented muscular curtain in the eye.

Isogeneic The donor and recipient individuals are genetically identical (i.e., monozygotic twins).

J

Jejunum The segment of the small intestine that connects the duodenum to the ileum.

K

Keratitis An inflammation of the cornea, typically accompanied by an ulceration.

L

Laboratory A location with scientific equipment designed to perform experiments and tests.

Laceration Damage to the epidermal and dermal layers of the skin made by a sharp object.

Lacrimal Apparatus A system in the eye that consists of the lacrimal glands, the upper canaliculi, the lower canaliculi, the lacrimal sac, and the nasolacrimal duct.

Laminaria Thin sticks of kelp-related seaweed, used to dilate the cervix, that can induce abortive circumstance during the first 3 months of pregnancy.

Laminectomy The surgical removal of a vertebral posterior arch.

Laterality The right or left side of anatomical sites that have locations on both sides of the body; e.g., right arm or left arm; *unilateral* means one side and *bilateral* means both sides.

Lens A transparent, crystalline segment of the eye, situated directly behind the pupil, that is responsible for focusing light rays as they enter the eye and travel back to the retina.

Level of Patient History The amount of detail involved in the documentation of patient history.

Level of Physical Examination The extent of a physician's clinical assessment and inspection of a patient.

Liability Insurance A policy that covers loss or injury to a third party caused by the insured or something belonging to the insured.

Linking Confirming medical necessity by pairing at least one diagnosis code to at least one procedure code.

Liters per Minute (LPM) The measurement of how many liters of a drug or chemical are provided to the patient in 60 seconds.

Liver The organ, located in the upper right area of the abdominal cavity, that is responsible for regulating blood sugar levels; secreting bile for the gallbladder; metabolizing fats, proteins, and carbohydrates; manufacturing some blood proteins; and removing toxins from the blood.

Local Anesthesia The injection of a drug to prevent sensation in a specific portion of the body; includes local infiltration anesthesia, digital blocks, and pudendal blocks.

Locum Tenens Physician A physician who fills in, temporarily, for another physician.

Low Birth Weight (LBW) A baby born weighing less than 5 pounds 8 ounces, or 2,500 grams.

Low Osmolar A non-ionic water-soluble iodinated contrast medium.

M

Macule A flat lesion with a different pigmentation (color) when compared with the surrounding skin.

Magnetic Resonance Arthrography (MRA) MR imaging of an anatomical joint after the administration of contrast material into the joint capsule.

Magnetic Resonance Imaging (MRI) A three-dimensional radiologic technique that uses nuclear technology to record pictures of internal anatomical sites.

Main Section The section of the CPT code book listing all of the codes in numeric order.

Major Complication and Co-morbidity (MCC) A complication or co-morbidity that has an impact on the treatment of the patient and makes care for that patient more complex.

Malformation An irregular structural development.

Malignant Invasive and destructive characteristic of a neoplasm; possibly causing damage or death.

Malunion A fractured bone that did not heal correctly; healing of bone that was not in proper position or alignment.

Managed Care A type of health insurance coverage that controls the care of each subscriber (or insured person) by using a primary care provider as a central health care supervisor.

Manic An emotional state that includes elation, excitement, and exuberance.

Manifestation A condition that develops as the result of another, underlying condition.

Manipulation The attempted return of a fracture or dislocation to its normal alignment manually by the physician.

Mass Abnormal collection of tissue.

Measurement To determine a level of a physiological or physical function.

Medical Decision Making (MDM) The level of knowledge and experience needed by the provider to determine the diagnosis and/or what to do next.

Medical Necessity The assessment that the provider was acting according to standard practices in providing a procedure or service for an individual with a specific diagnosis.

Meibomian Glands Sebaceous glands that secrete a tear film component that prevents tears from evaporating so that the area stays moist.

Mesentery A fold of a membrane that carries blood to the small intestine and connects it to the posterior wall of the abdominal cavity.

Metastasize To proliferate, reproduce, or spread.

Microscopic Examination The study of a specimen using a microscope (under magnification).

Modifier A two-character code that affects the meaning of another code; a code addendum that provides more meaning to the original code.

Moll's Glands Ordinary sweat glands.

Monitored Anesthesia Care (MAC) The administration of sedatives, anesthetic agents, or other medications to relax but not render the patient unconscious while under the constant observation of a trained anesthesiologist; also known as "twilight" sedation.

Morbidity Unhealthy.

Morphology The study of the configuration or structure of living organisms.

Mortality Death.

Mutually Exclusive Codes Codes that are identified as those that are not permitted to be used on the same claim form with other codes.

Myalgia Pain in a muscle.

Myocardial Infarction (MI) Malfunction of the heart due to necrosis or deterioration of a portion of the heart muscle; also known as a *heart attack*.

Myopathy Disease of a muscle [plural: myopathies].

N

Neoplasm Abnormal tissue growth; tumor.

Neoplasm Table The Neoplasm Table lists all possible codes for benign and malignant neoplasms, in alphabetic order by anatomical location of the tumor.

Nevus An abnormally pigmented area of skin. A birthmark is an example.

New Patient A person who has not received any professional services within the past 3 years from either the provider or another provider of the same specialty and the same subspecialty who belongs to the same group practice.

Nodule A tissue mass or papule larger than 5 mm.

Nonessential Modifiers Descriptors whose inclusion in the physician's notes are not absolutely necessary and that are provided simply to further clarify a code description; optional terms.

Nonphysician A nonphysician can be a nurse practitioner, certified registered nurse anesthetist, certified registered nurse, clinical nurse specialist, or physician assistant.

Nonunion A fractured bone that did not heal back together; no mending or joining together of the broken segments.

Nosocomial A hospital-acquired condition; a condition that develops as a result of being in a health care facility.

Not Elsewhere Classifiable (NEC) Specifics that are not described in any other code in the ICD-10-CM book; also known as *not elsewhere classified.*

Not Otherwise Specified (NOS) The absence of additional details documented in the notes.

Notations Alerts and warnings that support more accurate use of codes in a specific code set.

NSTEMI A nontransmural elevation myocardial infarction—a heart event during which the coronary artery is partially occluded (blocked).

Nuclear Medicine Treatment that includes the injection or digestion of isotopes.

Nursing Facility A facility that provides skilled nursing treatment and attention along with limited medical care for its (usually long-term) residents, who do not require acute care services (hospitalization).

O

Obstetrics (OB) A health care specialty focusing on the care of women during pregnancy and the puerperium.

Obstruction A blockage or closing.

Official Guidelines A listing of rules and regulations instructing how to use a specific code set accurately.

Open Treatment Surgically opening the fracture site, or another site in the body nearby, in order to treat the fractured bone.

Ophthalmologist A physician qualified to diagnose and treat eye disease and conditions with drugs, surgery, and corrective measures.

Optometrist A professional qualified to carry out eye examinations and to prescribe and supply eyeglasses and contact lenses.

Oral Cavity The opening in the face that begins the alimentary canal and is used for the input of nutrition; also known as the *mouth.*

Orbit The bony cavity in the skull that houses the eye and its ancillary parts (muscles, nerves, blood vessels).

Orthotic A device used to correct or improve an orthopedic concern.

Other Specified Additional information the physician specified that isn't included in any other code description.

Otorhinolaryngology The study of the human ears, nose, and throat (ENT) systems.

Outpatient A patient who receives services for a short amount of time (less than 24 hours) in a physician's office or clinic, without being kept overnight.

Outpatient facility An **outpatient facility** includes a hospital emergency room, ambulatory care center, same-day surgery center, or walk-in clinic.

Outpatient Services Health care services provided to individuals without an overnight stay in the facility.

Overlapping Boundaries Multiple sites of carcinoma without identifiable borders.

P

Palpebrae The eyelids [singular: palpebra].

Palpebral Conjunctiva A mucous membrane that lines the palpebrae.

Pancreas A gland that secretes insulin and other hormones from the islet cells into the bloodstream and manufactures digestive enzymes that are secreted into the duodenum.

Pancreatic Islets Cells within the pancreas that secrete insulin and other hormones into the bloodstream.

Papule A raised lesion with a diameter of less than 5 mm.

Parasites Tiny living things that can invade and feed off other living things.

Parathyroid Glands Four small glands situated on the back of the thyroid gland that secrete parathyroid hormone.

Parenteral By way of anything other than the gastrointestinal tract, such as intravenous, intramuscular, intramedullary, or subcutaneous.

Parenteral Enteral Nutrition (PEN) Nourishment delivered using a combination of means other than the gastrointestinal tract (such as IV) in addition to via the gastrointestinal tract.

Past, Family, and Social History (PFSH) Collection of details, related to the chief complaint, regarding possible signs, symptoms, behaviors, genetic connection, etc.

Patch A flat, small area of differently colored or textured skin; a large macule.

Pathogen Any agent that causes disease; a microorganism such as a bacterium or virus.

Pathology The study of the nature, etiology, development, and outcomes of disease.

Percutaneous Skeletal Fixation The insertion of fixation instruments (such as pins) placed across the fracture site. It may be done under x-ray imaging for guidance purposes.

Perforation An atypical hole in the wall of an organ or anatomical site.

Perinatal The time period from before birth to the 28th day after birth.

Personnel Modifier A modifier adding information about the professional(s) attending to the provision of this procedure or treatment to the patient during this encounter.

Phalanges Fingers and toes [singular: phalange or phalanx].

Phobia Irrational and excessive fear of an object, activity, or situation.

Physical Status Modifier A two-character alphanumeric code used to describe the condition of the patient at the time anesthesia services are administered.

***Physicians' Desk Reference* (PDR)** A series of reference books identifying all aspects of prescription and over-the-counter medications, as well as herbal remedies.

Placement To put a device in or on an anatomical site.

Plasma The fluid part of the blood.

Platelets (PLTs) Large cell fragments in the bone marrow that function in clotting; also known as *thrombocytes.*

Pneumonia An inflammation of the lungs.

Pneumothorax A condition in which air or gas is present within the chest cavity but outside the lungs.

Point-of-Service (POS) A type of insurance plan that will allow an HMO enrollee to choose his or her own nonmember physician at a lower benefit rate, costing the patient more money out-of-pocket.

Polydipsia Excessive thirst.

Polyuria Excessive urination.

Preferred Provider Organization (PPO) A type of health insurance coverage in which physicians provide health care services to members of the plan at a discount.

Prematurity Birth occurring prior to the completion of 37 weeks gestation.

Prenatal Prior to birth; also referred to as *antenatal.*

Present-On-Admission (POA) A one-character indicator reporting the status of the diagnosis at the time the patient was admitted to the acute care facility.

Pressure Ulcer An open wound or sore caused by pressure, infection, or inflammation.

Preventive A type of action or service that stops something from happening or from getting worse.

Preventive Care Health-related services designed to stop the development of a disease or injury.

Principal Diagnosis The condition, after study, that is the primary, or main, reason for the admission of a patient to the hospital for care; the condition that requires the largest amount of hospital resources for care.

Problem-Pertinent System Review The physician's collection of details of signs and symptoms, as per the patient, affecting only those body systems connected to the chief complaint.

Procedure Action taken, in accordance with the standards of care, by the physician to accomplish a predetermined objective (result); a surgical operation.

Products of Conception The zygote, embryo, or fetus, as well as the amnion, umbilical cord, and placenta.

Proptosis Bulging out of the eye; also known as *exophthalmos*.

Prostatitis Inflammation of the prostate.

Prosthetic Fabricated artificial replacement for a damaged or missing part of the body.

Protected Health Information (PHI) Any patient-identifiable health information regardless of the form in which it is stored (paper, computer file, etc.).

Psychotherapy The treatment of mental and emotional disorder through communication or psychologically rather than medical means.

Puerperium The time period from the end of labor until the uterus returns to normal size, typically 3 to 6 weeks.

Pupil The opening in the center of the iris that permits light to enter and continue on to the lens and retina.

Push The delivery of an additional drug via an intravenous line over a short period of time.

Pustule A swollen area of skin; a vesicle filled with pus.

Q

Qualifier Any additional feature of the procedure, if applicable.

Qualitative The determination of character or essential element(s).

Quantitative The counting or measurement of something.

Query To ask.

R

Radiation The high-speed discharge and projection of energy waves or particles.

Recipient Area The area, or site, of the body receiving a graft of skin or tissue.

Rectum The last segment of the large intestine, connecting the sigmoid colon to the anus.

Red Blood Cells (RBCs) Cells within the blood that contain hemoglobin responsible for carrying oxygen to tissues; also known as *erythrocytes*.

Regional Anesthesia The administration of a drug in order to interrupt the nerve impulses without loss of consciousness.

Rehabilitation Health care that is committed to improving, maintaining, or returning physical strength, cognition, and mobility.

Reimbursement The process of paying for health care services after they have been provided.

Relationship The level of familiarity between provider and patient.

Release of Information (ROI) The form (either on paper or electronic) that a patient must sign to give legal permission to a covered entity to disclose that patient's PHI.

Remittance Advice (RA) Notification identifying details about a payment from the third-party payer.

Respiratory Disorder A malfunction of the organ system relating to respiration.

Retina A membrane in the back of the eye that is sensitive to light and functions as the sensory end of the optic nerve.

Retinal Detachment A break in the connection between the retinal pigment epithelium layer and the neural retina.

Retinopathy Degenerative condition of the retina.

Rh (Rhesus) Factor An antigen located on the red blood cell that produces immunogenic responses in those individuals without it.

Risk Factor Reduction Intervention Action taken by the attending physician to stop or reduce a behavior or lifestyle that is predicted to have a negative effect on the individual's health.

Rod An elongated, cylindrical cell within the retina that is photosensitive in low light.

Root Operation Term The category or classification of a particular procedure, service, or treatment.

Rule of Nines A general division of the whole body into sections that each represents 9%; used for estimating the extent of a burn.

S

Salivary Glands Three sets of bilateral exocrine glands that secrete saliva: parotid glands, submaxillary glands, and sublingual glands.

Saphenous Vein Either of the two major veins in the leg that run from the foot to the thigh near the surface of the skin.

Scale Flaky exfoliated epidermis; a flake of skin.

Schizophrenia A psychotic disorder with no known cause.

Sclera The membranous tissue that covers all of the eyeball (except the cornea); also known as *the white of the eye*.

Screening An examination or test of a patient who has no signs or symptoms that is conducted with the intention of finding any evidence of disease as soon as possible, thus enabling better patient outcomes.

Second-Degree Burn Blisters on the skin; involvement of the epidermis and the dermis layers.

Secondary Diabetes Mellitus Diabetes caused by medication or another condition or disease.

Secondary Hypertension The condition of hypertension caused by another condition or illness.

Sedative A tranquilizer; a drug used to calm or soothe.

Self-Administer To give medication to oneself, such as a diabetic giving herself an insulin injection.

Sepsis Condition typified by two or more systemic responses to infection; a specified pathogen.

Septic Shock Severe sepsis with hypotension; unresponsive to fluid resuscitation.

Septicemia Generalized infection spread through the body via the bloodstream; blood infection.

Sequela A cause-and-effect relationship between an original condition that has been resolved with a current condition; also known as a late effect.

Sequela (Late Effects) A condition directly caused by another condition which may not appear until after the initial condition has cleared; (2) cause-and-effect relationship between an original condition, illness, or injury and an additional problem caused by the existence of that original condition. Time is not a requirement for a diagnosis as a late effect because the additional concern may be present at any time.

Services Spending time with a patient and/or family about health care situations.

Service-Related Modifier A modifier relating to a change or adjustment of a procedure or service provided.

Severe Sepsis Sepsis with signs of acute organ dysfunction.

Severity The level of seriousness.

Sigmoid Colon The dual-curved segment of the colon that connects the descending colon to the rectum; also referred to as the *sigmoid flexure.*

Signs Measurable indicators of a patient's health status.

Simple Closure A method of sealing an opening in the skin (epidermis or dermis), involving only one layer. It includes the administration of local anesthesia and/or chemical or electrocauterization of a wound not closed.

Site The specific anatomical location of the disease or injury.

Skin The external membranous covering of the body.

Somatic Related to the body, especially separate from the brain or mind.

Somatoform Disorder The sincere belief that one is suffering an illness that is not present.

Sonogram The use of sound waves to record images of internal organs and tissues; also called an *ultrasound.*

Specialty Care Transport (SCT) Continuous care provided by one or more health professionals in an appropriate specialty area, such as respiratory care or cardiovascular care, or by a paramedic with additional training.

Specimen A small part or sample of any substance obtained for analysis and diagnosis.

Sphincter A circular muscle that contracts to prevent passage of liquids or solids.

Spondylopathy Disease affecting the vertebrae [plural: spondylopathies].

Standard of Care The accepted principles of conduct, services, or treatments that are established as the expected behavior.

Status Asthmaticus The condition of asthma that is life-threatening and does not respond to therapeutic treatments.

Statutory Laws Laws that are enacted by federal and state legislature.

STEMI An ST elevation myocardial infarction—a heart event during which the coronary artery is completely blocked by a thrombus or embolus.

Stomach A saclike organ within the alimentary canal designed to contain nourishment during the initial phase of the digestive process.

Subcutaneous The layer beneath the dermis; also known as the *hypodermis.*

Substance Abuse Regular consumption of a substance with manifestations.

Supplemental Report A letter or report written by the attending physician or other health care professional to provide additional clarification or explanation.

Supporting Documentation The paperwork in the patient's file that corroborates the codes presented on the claim form for a particular encounter.

Surgical Approach The methodology or technique used by the physician to perform the procedure, service, or treatment.

Surgical Pathology The study of tissues removed from a living patient during a surgical procedure.

Symbols Marks, similar to emojis, that provide additional direction to use codes correctly and accurately.

Symptom A subjective sensation or departure from the norm as related by the patient.

Systemic Spread throughout the entire body.

Systemic Condition A condition that affects the entire body and virtually all body systems, therefore requiring the physician to consider this in his or her medical decision-making for any other condition.

Systemic Inflammatory Response Syndrome (SIRS) A definite physical reaction, such as fever, chills, etc., to an unspecified pathogen.

T

Table of Drugs and Chemicals The section of the ICD-10-CM code book listing drugs, chemicals, and other biologicals that may poison a patient or result in an adverse reaction.

Tables The section of the ICD-10-PCS code book listing all of the codes in alphanumeric order, based on the first three characters of the code.

Tabular List The section of the ICD-10-CM code book listing all of the codes in alphanumeric order.

Teeth Small, calcified protrusions with roots in the jaw [singular: tooth].

Third-Degree Burn Destruction of all layers of the skin, with possible involvement of the subcutaneous fat, muscle, and bone.

Third-Party Payer An individual or organization that is not directly involved in an encounter but has a connection because of its obligation to pay, in full or part, for that encounter.

Thrombus A blood clot in a blood vessel [plural: thrombi].

Thyroid Gland A two-lobed gland located in the neck that reaches around the trachea laterally and connects anteriorly by an isthmus. The thyroid gland produces hormones used for metabolic function.

Topical Anesthesia The application of a drug to the skin to reduce or prevent sensation in a specific area temporarily.

Topography The classification of neoplasms primarily by anatomical site.

Tracer An official request for a third-party payer to search its system to find a missing health claim form. It is also a term used for a replacement health claim form resubmitted to replace one that was lost.

Transfer of Care When a physician gives up responsibility for caring for a patient, in whole or with regard to one specific condition, and another physician accepts responsibility for the care of that patient.

Transfusion The provision of one person's blood or plasma to another individual.

Transplantation The transfer of tissue from one site to another.

Transverse Colon The portion of the large intestine that connects the hepatic flexure to the splenic flexure.

Treatment The provision of medical care for a disorder or disease.

TriCare A government health plan that covers medical expenses for the dependents of active-duty service members, CHAMPUS-eligible retirees and their families, and the dependents of deceased active-duty members.

Tuberculosis An infectious condition that causes small rounded swellings on mucous membranes throughout the body.

Type 1 Diabetes Mellitus A sudden onset of insulin deficiency that may occur at any age but most often arises in childhood and adolescence; also known as *insulin-dependent diabetes mellitus (IDDM), juvenile diabetes*, or *type I.*

Type 2 Diabetes Mellitus A form of diabetes mellitus with a gradual onset that may develop at any age but most often occurs in adults over the age of 40; also known as *non-insulin-dependent diabetes mellitus (NIDDM)* or *type II.*

U

Ulcer An erosion or loss of the full thickness of the epidermis.

Unbundling Coding individual parts of a specific procedure rather than one combination, or bundle, that includes all the components.

Underlying Condition One disease that affects or encourages another condition.

Uniform Hospital Discharge Data Set (UHDDS) A compilation of data collected by acute care facilities and other designated health care facilities.

Unlisted Codes Codes shown at the end of each subsection of the CPT used as a catch-all for any procedure not represented by an existing code.

Unspecified The absence of additional specifics in the physician's documentation.

Upcoding Using a code on a claim form that indicates a higher level of service than that which was actually performed.

Urea A compound that is excreted in urine.

Urea Reduction Ratio (URR) A formula to determine the effectiveness of hemodialysis treatment.

Urinary System The organ system responsible for removing waste products that are left behind in the blood and the body.

Urinary Tract Infection (UTI) Inflammation of any part of the urinary tract: kidney, ureter, bladder, or urethra.

Use (1) The sharing of information between people working in the same health care facility for purposes of caring for the patient. (2) Occasional consumption of a substance without clinical manifestations.

Usual, Customary, and Reasonable (UCR) The process of determining a fee for a service by evaluating the *usual* fee charged by the provider, the *customary* fee charged by most physicians in the same community or geographical area, and what is considered *reasonable* by most health care professionals under the specific circumstances of the situation.

Uveal Tract The middle layer of the eye, consisting of the iris, ciliary body, and choroid.

V

Vascular Referring to the vessels (arteries and veins).

Venography The imaging of a vein after the injection of contrast material.

Ventricle A chamber that is located in the bottom half of the heart and receives blood from the atrium.

Vermiform Appendix A long, narrow mass of tissue attached to the cecum; also called *appendix.*

Vertebra A bone that is a part of the construction of the spinal column [plural: vertebrae].

Viruses Microscopic particles that initiate disease, mimicking the characteristics of a particular cell; viruses can reproduce only within the body of the cell that they have invaded.

Vitreous Chamber The interior segment of the eye that contains the vitreous body.

W

White Blood Cells (WBCs) Cells within the blood that help to protect the body from pathogens; also known as *leukocytes.*

Withdrawal Abruptly stopping the use of a drug that has been used continuously prior to the cessation, which can result in both physical and psychological conditions.

Workers' Compensation An insurance program that covers medical care for those injured or for those who become ill as a consequence of their employment.

X

Xenogeneic The donor and recipient are of different species, e.g., bovine cartilage → human (also known as a *xenograft* or *heterograft*).

INDEX

Note: Page numbers followed by *f* and *t* indicate figures and tables, respectively. Page numbers in boldface indicate definitions of terms.

A

B

C

F

G

H

J

K

L

M

P

S